HEALTHCARE–ASSOCIATED INFECTIONS IN AUSTRALIA

Principles and Practice of Infection Prevention and Control

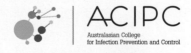

ACIPC
Australasian College
for Infection Prevention and Control

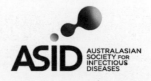

ASID
AUSTRALASIAN
SOCIETY FOR
INFECTIOUS
DISEASES

HEALTHCARE-ASSOCIATED INFECTIONS IN AUSTRALIA

Principles and Practice of Infection Prevention and Control

Editor-in-Chief

Professor Ramon Z. Shaban

Editors

Professor Brett G. Mitchell

Dr Deborough Macbeth

Professor Philip L. Russo

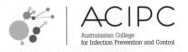

ACIPC
Australasian College
for Infection Prevention and Control

ELSEVIER

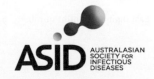

ASID
AUSTRALASIAN
SOCIETY FOR
INFECTIOUS
DISEASES

ELSEVIER

Elsevier Australia. ACN 001 002 357
(a division of Reed International Books Australia Pty Ltd)
Tower 1, 475 Victoria Avenue, Chatswood, NSW 2067

ISBN: 978-0-7295-4364-4

Notice

National Library of Australia Cataloguing-in-Publication Data

---

 A catalogue record for this book is available from the National Library of Australia

---

Cover photos courtesy of Stefanie Zingsheim, Western Sydney Local Health District, the University of Sydney, and the Australian Dental Association (NSW Branch) Ltd.

Content Strategist: Libby Houston and Natalie Hunt
Content Project Manager: Shubham Dixit
Edited by Claire Linsdell
Proofread by Annabel Adair
Permissions Editing and Photo Research: Regina Lavanya Remigius
Cover design by Georgette Hall
Internal Design by Natalie Bowra
Index by Innodata

Typeset by GW India

Printer in India by Multivista Global Pvt. Ltd.

Last digit is the print number: 9   8   7   6   5   4   3   2   1

Contents

Foreword Australasian College for Infection Prevention and Control (ACIPC)

This comprehensive work offers invaluable insights and practical guidance for infection prevention and control within the Australian healthcare system. By promoting knowledge, expertise and best practices, *Healthcare-Associated Infections in Australia: Principles and Practice of Infection Prevention and Control* will contribute to reducing the burden of healthcare-associated infections and enhance patient safety in Australia.

We congratulate and commend the authors of the chapters within this textbook, the first to be edited and authored by infection prevention and control experts and address the unique challenges faced within the Australian context.

We are confident the text will be an invaluable tool for infection control professionals, administrators, educators, academics and students.

We extend our congratulations to the editors of the text, Ramon Shaban, Brett Mitchell, Deborough Macbeth and Philip Russo, and all the contributors to this pivotal text.

Kristie Popkiss
President
Australasian College for Infection Prevention and Control Ltd

Foreword Australasian Society for Infectious Diseases (ASID)

The Australasian Society for Infectious Diseases is delighted to endorse this comprehensive and informative book *Healthcare-associated Infections in Australia: Principles and Practice of Infection Prevention and Control*. It provides a contemporary update on all matters relating to infection prevention and control in the Australian context, a topic of extreme importance as highlighted during the recent COVID-19 pandemic. Topics span from the guiding principles to contemporary practice across multiple healthcare settings including veterinary practice.

Optimal infection prevention and control practices are of utmost importance as we face the impact of global warming on global infectious disease spread and outbreak threats, increased outbreaks of vaccine-preventable diseases such as measles due to declining vaccine uptake and global travel and rising antimicrobial resistance, including pan-resistant organisms.

This book provides a cutting-edge practical toolkit for optimal Infection Prevention and Control in Australia and is highly recommended by society.

Katie Flanagan
President
Australasian Society for Infectious Diseases (ASID)

Preface

It is with great pleasure that we present the first edition of *Healthcare-Associated Infections in Australia: Principles and Practice of Infection Prevention and Control*. The release of this book heralds the introduction of the first comprehensive, contemporary, practical and evidence-based Australian text for infection control practitioners, healthcare workers and students to guide their everyday work, practice and study. It is an invaluable resource for the everyday clinician and healthcare professional, containing information that is specifically tailored to a wide range of local practice environments and informed by best-available global evidence.

This text addresses a critical gap in the context-specific academic literature with respect to healthcare-associated infection and the science and practice of IPC in Australia. Whereas our peer professions of infectious diseases, medical microbiology, nursing and others have comprehensive Australian textbooks on their subjects, up until now there has been no such resource on IPC. This notable void has been amplified by the COVID-19 pandemic, which resulted in unparalleled disruption to the health and wellbeing of individuals globally. As new issues related to communicable diseases and IPC continue to emerge and evolve—such as increasing antimicrobial resistance and the dawning of a global 'post antibiotic era'—the need for such a resource became paramount. Here, we thoroughly address this gap in the literature but also prepare professionals and clinicians to respond effectively to the ever-changing landscape of disease and infection control.

Each of the 45 chapters contains information derived from the most recent published research as well as benefitting from the author team's extensive wealth of experience in the practice of IPC in Australia. Our 72 contributing authors are recognised professionals of standing in Australia or New Zealand and all were chosen for their expertise.

The text is organised into two sections. Section 1 comprehensively documents the core principles that underpin contemporary IPC practice in Australia. These chapters include the origins and history of IPC; manifestations of its contemporary construct; IPC programs and plans; the role of the infection control professional; governance and standards; risk assessment and management; and One Health. In addition, their underpinning sciences are discussed, including microbiology and sciences of infection and disease, clinical infectious diseases, epidemiology and surveillance, outbreak management, public health and research for evidence-based practice.

Building on this, Section 2 covers the contemporary practice of IPC in Australia, beginning with comprehensive overviews of core practices, such as Standard and Transmission-based Precautions, followed by an examination of the most relevant contemporary healthcare-associated infections. The final 20 chapters examine contemporary practices and systems in 20 different healthcare contexts in Australia. The context-specific environments and unique risks associated with these are described, and guidance is provided on the specific practices that should feature in their associated infection control management plans.

The chapters are indexed and cross-referenced so that readers can readily integrate relevant sections in ways that mirror what happens in practice, and case studies enable consolidation of knowledge for practice. As with all textbooks and all forms of infection, it is critical that readers continue to search for the most recent sources of appropriate information to guide their practice. To assist with this, useful websites are provided throughout the text.

We commend *Healthcare-Associated Infections in Australia: Principles and Practice of Infection Prevention and Control* to you in support of our shared efforts to prevent and control healthcare-associated infections—the leading complication and challenge to the provision of high-quality, safe and effective care for patients, their families and the community.

Ramon Z. Shaban
Brett G. Mitchell
Deborough Macbeth
Philip L. Russo

Editorial Board

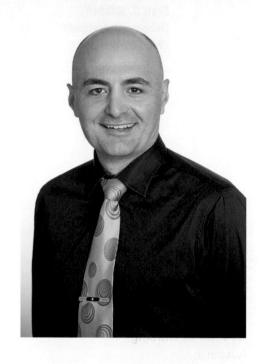
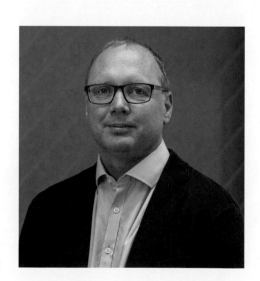

Dr Deborough Macbeth

BN MAAppEthics PhD RN CICP-E PSM

Assistant Director of Nursing (Infection Control), Gold Coast Hospital and Health Service, Southport, Queensland, Australia

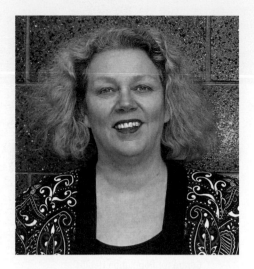

Professor Philip L. Russo

BN MClinEpid PhD RN CICP-E MACN FACICPC

Professor of Nursing and Director of Research, School of Nursing and Midwifery, Monash University, Melbourne, Victoria, Australia;
Director of Nursing Research, Cabrini Health, Melbourne, Victoria, Australia;
Adjunct Associate Professor of Nursing, School of Nursing and Health, Avondale University, Lake Macquarie, New South Wales, Australia

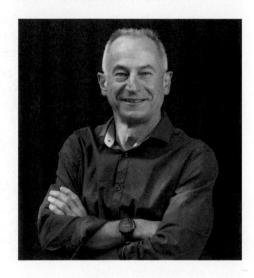

Contributors

Prof Eugene Athan MBBS(Hon) MD PhD FRACP MPH
Professor
Infectious Disease
School of Medicine, Deakin University and Barwon Health
Geelong, VIC
Australia
ORCiD 0000-0001-9838-6471

Dr Shopna Kumari Bag MBBS BSc(Med) MIPH FAFPHM
Director
Centre for Population Health
Western Sydney Local Health District
North Parramatta, NSW
Australia
ORCiD 0000-0001-9838-6471

Dr Jocelyne Marie Basseal BSc(Hons) PhD GradCertInfCon
Associate Director
Sydney Infectious Diseases Institute, Faculty of Medicine and Health
The University of Sydney
Sydney, NSW
Australia
ORCiD 0000-0002-4434-7079

Assoc Prof Justin Beardsley MBChB PhD FRACP
Associate Professor
Department of Infectious Diseases
Westmead Hospital
Western Sydney Local Health District
Sydney, NSW
Australia

Assoc Prof Noleen Bennett RN MPH PhD
Infection Control Consultant
Victorian Healthcare Associated Infection Surveillance System (VICNISS)
The Peter Doherty Institute for Infection and Immunity
Parkville, VIC
Australia

Karen Therese Booth RN DipAppSc(Nursing) BHScN GAICD
President
Australian Primary Health Care Nurses Association (APNA)
Melbourne, VIC
Australia

Dr Lynette Bowen RN PhD
Lecturer, Head of Undergraduate
School of Nursing
Avondale University
Lake Macquarie, NSW
Australia
ORCiD 0000-0002-8136-1398

Dr Emma Charters BSc(SpPath) PhD
Speech Pathologist
Head and Neck, Allied Health
Chris O'Brien Lifehouse
Sydney, NSW
Australia
ORCiD 0000-0001-8246-210X

Prof Sharon C-A. Chen PhD MBBS FRACP FRCPA
Professor
Infectious Diseases and Microbiology
Westmead Hospital
Westmead, NSW
Australia

Penelope Clarke
Program Lead, Communicable Diseases Team
Centre for Population Health
Western Sydney Local Health District
North Parramatta, NSW
Australia

Assoc Prof Valery Combes BSc(Hons) MSc PhD
Associate Professor
School of Life Sciences, Faculty of Science
University of Technology Sydney
Ultimo, NSW
Australia
ORCiD 0000-0003-2178-3596

Assoc Prof Louise Anne Cooley MBBS FRACP FRCPA
Department of Microbiology and Infectious Diseases
Royal Hobart Hospital
Hobart, TAS
Australia

Assoc Prof Stephen J Corbett MBBS MPH FAFPHM
Associate Professor
Western Sydney Clinical School
The University of Sydney
Sydney, NSW
Australia
ORCiD 0000-0003-0009-5532

Dr Susan E. Coulson BAppSc(Physio) GradCertEdStudies(Higher Ed) MAppSc(Exercise&SportSc) PhD
Physiotherapist
Discipline of Physiotherapy
Sydney School of Health Sciences, Faculty of Medicine and Health
The University of Sydney
Sydney, NSW
Australia
ORCiD 0000-0002-3586-2562

Kathy Dempsey RN DipAppSc BSc(Nursing)
MNSc(InfCon&HospEpidemiol) SHEA/CDC CertInfCon CertMedMicro,
DipLdrshp&Mgt CICP-E
NSW Chief ICP / HAI advisor
Healthcare-associated Infection/ Infection Prevention and
Control Program
Clinical Excellence Commission
Sydney, NSW
Australia

Prof Dale Dominey-Howes BSc(Hons) PhD FGS FRGS
Professor
School of Geosciences
The University of Sydney
Sydney, NSW
Australia
ORCiD 0000-0003-2677-2837

Assoc Prof Mark Douglas BSc(Med)(Hons) MBBS(Hons) PhD
FRACP
Associate Professor
Storr Liver Centre and Sydney Infectious Diseases Institute
Faculty of Medicine and Health
The University of Sydney and Westmead Hospital
Sydney, NSW
Australia

Dr Tiffany Jane Dwyer BAppSc(Phty)(Hons1) PhD
Physiotherapist
Discipline of Physiotherapy
Sydney School of Health Sciences, Faculty of Medicine and
Health
The University of Sydney
Sydney, NSW
Australia
ORCiD 0000-0001-6403-2894

Dr Oyebola Fasugba MBBS MPHTM PhD
Senior Research Officer
Nursing Research Institute
St Vincent's Health Network Sydney
St Vincent's Hospital
Melbourne, VIC
School of Nursing
Midwifery and Paramedicine
Australian Catholic University
Sydney, NSW
Australia

Dr Patricia Ellen Ferguson BMed(Hons) MMed(Clin Epi)
PhD FRACP
Infectious Diseases Physician
Centre for Infectious Diseases and Microbiology
Westmead Hospital
Westmead, NSW
Australia

Dr Roslyn Lee Franklin BDSc GCert Inf Prev & Cnt
Dentist and Director
Amalgamate2020 Pty Ltd
Bunbury, WA
Australia
ORCiD 0000-0002-5904-8215

Christine Fuller DipAppSc(Nursing) BAppSc(NursingAdmin)
MHealthAdmin GAICD
Deputy CEO / Chief Nursing Officer
Head Office
Correct Care Australasia
Melbourne, VIC
Australia

Sylvia Gandossi BN
Infection Control Consultant
Microbiology
Western Diagnostic Pathology
Jandakot, WA
Australia

Dr Priya Garg BSc MBBS DTM&H FRACP
Doctor (Specialist)
Infectious Diseases
Westmead Hospital
Westmead, NSW
Australia
ORCiD 0000-0002-7724-3428

Dr Katherine Garnham MBBS FRACP(Infectious Diseases)
FRCPA(Microbiology)
Infectious Diseases Physician and Microbiologist
Gold Coast Hospital and Health Service
Gold Coast, QLD
Australia

Dr John Gerrard BSc(Med) MBBS MSc DTM&H FRACP
Queensland Chief Health Officer
Gold Coast University Hospital
Brisbane, QLD
Australia

Prof Gwendolyn L. Gilbert AO MBBS MD MBioethics FRACP
FRCPA
Honorary Professor
Sydney Infectious Diseases Institute, Faculty of Medicine and
Health
The University of Sydney
Sydney, NSW
Australia
ORCiD 0000-0001-7490-6727

Dr Nicole Gilroy MBBS MAppEpid MPH FRACP
Specialist Infectious Diseases
Centre for Infectious Diseases and Microbiology
Westmead Hospital
Westmead, NSW
Australia

Assoc Prof Gary Dean Grant BPharm GradCertHigherEd PhD
Associate Professor
School of Pharmacy and Medical Sciences
Griffith University
Gold Coast, QLD
Australia

Dr Fiona Ellen Hawke BAppSc(Podiatry)(Hons)
GradCertTertiaryTeaching PhD
Podiatrist
College of Health, Medicine and Wellbeing
University of Newcastle
Newcastle, NSW
Australia
ORCiD 0000-0002-1511-8701

Assoc Prof Jane Heller BSc BVSc DipVetClinStud
DiplECVPH PhD MANZCVS
Associate Professor in Veterinary Epidemiology and Public
Health
School of Agricultural, Environmental and Veterinary Sciences
Charles Sturt University
Wagga Wagga, NSW
Australia

Belinda C. Henderson BN MAdvancedPrac FACIPC CICP-E
Infection Prevention and Control Advisor
Queensland Department of Health
Brisbane, QLD
Australia

Gareth Hockey RN BN MPH
Clinical Nurse Consultant
Infection Prevention and Control
Prince of Wales Hospital
Randwick, NSW
Australia

Tejaswini Ashish Kalkundri BPharm MPharm
School of Pharmacy and Medical Sciences
Griffith University
Gold Coast, QLD
Australia
ORCiD 0000-0002-5021-1987

Prof Martin Kiernan RN DipN MPH MClinRes
Richard Wells Research Centre
University of West London
Brentford, West London
UK

Dr Myong Gyu Kim MD FRACP
Specialist Infectious Diseases
Centre for Infectious Diseases and Microbiology
Westmead Hospital
Westmead, NSW
Australia
ORCiD 0000-0003-4282-414X

Assoc Prof Maurizio Labbate BSc(Hons) PhD
Associate Professor
School of Life Sciences, Faculty of Science
University of Technology Sydney
Ultimo, NSW
Australia

Debra Gay Lee RN Master of Infection Prevention and Control
GradCert Public Health
Principal Advisor Occupational Health
Office of Industrial Relations Queensland
Redcliffe, QLD
Australia

Dr Cecilia Z. Li PhD
Research Fellow
Infection Prevention and Control
Susan Wakil School of Nursing and Midwifery, Faculty of
Medicine and Health
The University of Sydney
Sydney, NSW
Australia

Dr Lyn-li Lim MBBS GradDipClinEpi MPH FRACP
Infectious Diseases Physician
Victorian Healthcare Associated Infection Surveillance System
(VICNISS)
The Peter Doherty Institute for Infection and Immunity
Parkville, VIC
Australia
ORCiD 0000-0003-1782-7875

Dr Deborough Macbeth BN MA(AppEthics) PhD
Assistant Director of Nursing
Infection Control
Gold Coast Hospital and Health Service
Southport, QLD
Australia
ORCiD 0000-0001-5615-6889

Dr Susan Maddocks MBBS PhD DTM&H FRACP FRCPA
Doctor
Centre for Infectious Diseases and Microbiology
Westmead Hospital
Westmead, NSW
Australia
ORCiD 0000-0002-7843-551X

Terry McAuley RN MSc Medical Device Decontamination Grad Dip
Education and Training Cert Mgt Decontamination Reusable Medical
Devices Cert Sterilization and Infection Control Cert Perioperative
Nursing Cert Operating Suite Management MACORN MACIPC MCNA
Director
STEAM Consulting Pty Ltd
Greenvale, VIC
Australia

Dr Gerald McDonnell BSc PhD
Vice President
Microbiological Quality and Sterility Assurance
Johnson & Johnson
Raritan, NJ
USA

Prof Brett Gerard Mitchell DipTN BN MAdvPrac
GradCertTeach&Assess PhD
Professor
School of Nursing
Avondale University
Wahroonga, NSW
Australia

Dr David Mitchell MBBS MMedSci(Epi) FRACP FRCPA
Senior Staff Specialist
Centre for Infectious Diseases and Microbiology
Westmead Hospital
Westmead, NSW
Australia

Dr Lyndall J. Mollart RM RN PhD
Lecturer
School of Nursing and Midwifery
University of Newcastle
Gosford, NSW
Australia
ORCiD 0000-0002-8390-0658

Cathi Montague RN ENB998 MClinNursing FCENA
Nurse Consultant, Infection Prevention and Control
Drug and Alcohol Services South Australia
SA Health
Adelaide, SA
Australia
ORCiD 0000-0002-7652-5140

Dr Shizar Nahidi MD PhD
Senior Lecturer (Adjunct)
Faculty of Medicine, Nursing and Health Sciences
Monash University
Melbourne, VIC
Hospital Medical Officer (HMO)
Latrobe Regional Hospital
Traralgon, VIC
Australia
ORCiD 0000-0003-0443-4626

Rachel Newell BAppSci(Nursing) MN(Neonatal) GradDip(Midwifery)
School of Nursing and Midwifery
University of Newcastle
Gosford, NSW
Australia
ORCiD 0000-0002-3522-0682

Prof Jacqueline Maree Norris BVSc MVSt PhD FASM RCVS
(Vet micro)
Professor in Veterinary Microbiology and Infectious Diseases,
Head of School and Dean
Sydney School of Veterinary Science
The University of Sydney
Sydney, NSW
Australia
ORCiD 0000-0002-0003-6930

Dr Chong Wei Ong MBBS(Hons) FRACP FRCPA
Deputy Director
Department of Clinical Microbiology
Canberra Health Services
Canberra, ACT
Australia

Dr Matthew Vincent Neil O'Sullivan MBBS(Hons) MMed(ClinEpi)
DTM&H PhD FRACP FRCPA
Senior Staff Specialist in Clinical Microbiology and Infectious
Diseases
Centre for Infectious Diseases and Microbiology
New South Wales Health Pathology, ICPMR
Westmead, NSW
Australia
ORCiD 0000-0001-8783-5323

Prof Sue Randall RGN SFHEA PhD
Professor of Rural and Remote/Primary Health Care Nursing
The University of Sydney's Department of Rural Health
(Broken Hill) and the Susan Wakil School of Nursing
and Midwifery
Faculty of Medicine and Health
Broken Hill, NSW
Australia
ORCiD 0000 0003 2068

Dr Roselle Robosa MBBS
Institute of Clinical Pathology and Medical Research
Westmead Hospital
Westmead, NSW
Australia

Dr Christine Roder BSc(Hons) MBiotechnology PhD
Infectious Disease Researcher
Barwon South West Public Health Unit
Barwon Health
Geelong, VIC
Australia

Prof Philip L. Russo BN MClin(Epi) PhD
Professor
School of Nursing and Midwifery
Monash University
Melbourne, VIC
Australia

Prof Ramon Zenel Shaban BSc(Med) BN GradCertInfCon
PGDipPH&TM MEd MCommHealthPrac(Hons1) PhD RN FCENA FACN
FACIPC CICP-E
Professor and Clinical Chair, Communicable Disease Control
and Infection Prevention
Sydney Infectious Diseases Institute and Sydney Nursing
School, Faculty of Medicine and Health
The University of Sydney
Sydney, NSW
Australia
ORCiD 0000-0002-5203-0557

Dr Benjamin Silberberg MBBS MRes MPH DFPH
Advanced Trainee in Public Health Medicine
Centre for Population Health
Western Sydney Local Health District
North Parramatta, NSW
Australia
ORCiD 000-0001-8394-7774

Paul Simpson BA(Nursing)(Hons) MSc(InfCon)
Clinical Nurse Consultant
Infection Prevention and Control Service
Redcliffe Hospital, Metro North Health
Brisbane, QLD
Australia

Clinical Prof Tony Skapetis BDS MEd(AdultEd) PhD FIADT
The University of Sydney School of Dentistry
Clinical Director Education, Oral Health
Education Unit Westmead Centre for Oral Health
Westmead, NSW
Australia
ORCiD 0000-0003-0401-9908

Dr Cristina Sotomayor-Castillo DVM MSc PhD
Affiliate Research Fellow
Susan Wakil School of Nursing and Midwifery, Faculty of
Medicine and Health
The University of Sydney
Sydney, NSW
Australia

Dr Vanessa Sparke RN BN GradCertCriticalCareNursing
GradCertResearchMethods GradDipEducation&Training MPH&TM PhD
Senior Lecturer
Nursing and Midwifery
James Cook University
Smithfield, QLD
Australia

Assoc Prof Andrew James Stewardson MBBS MS(Epi) PhD FRACP
Associate Professor
Department of Infectious Diseases
The Alfred Hospital and Central Clinical School
Monash University
Melbourne, VIC
Australia
ORCiD 0000-0001-6805-1224

Prof Thea F. van de Mortel BSc(Hons) MHlthSc PhD Intensive
Care Certificate FACIPC FACN SFHEA
Professor
School of Nursing and Midwifery
Griffith University
Southport, QLD
Australia

Dr Herdeza Verzosa DMD CertDent(ADC) DipMgt
Senior Dental Officer
Education Unit
Westmead Centre for Oral Health
Westmead, NSW
Australia

Dr Catherine Viengkham BPsych(Hons) PhD
Research Fellow
Susan Wakil School of Nursing and Midwifery
The University of Sydney
Sydney, NSW
Australia
ORCiD 0000-0002-7802-4219

Dr Sanchia Warren MBBS(Hons) FRACP FRCPA
Infectious Diseases Physician and Clinical Microbiologist
Department of Microbiology and Infectious Diseases
Royal Hobart Hospital
Hobart, TAS
Australia

Prof Donna Louise Waters RN BA MPH PhD
Professor
Faculty of Medicine and Health
The University of Sydney
Sydney, NSW
Australia

Dr James Erle Wolfe BSc(Adv)(Hons) MD FRACP
Infectious Diseases Physician
Department of Microbiology and Infectious Diseases
Royal Hobart Hospital
Hobart, TAS
Australia

Margaret Wymarra BNSc
Academic Tutor (Bachelor of Nursing Science)
Indigenous Education and Research Centre
James Cook University
Ngulaigau Mudh Campus
Thursday Island, QLD
Australia

Dr Peta-Anne Patricia Zimmerman RN BN MHSc GradCert
HigherEd DPH CICP-E FACIPC SFHEA
Senior Lecturer/Program Advisor
School of Nursing and Midwifery
Griffith University
Gold Coast, QLD
Australia
ORCiD 0000-0003-3764-1277

Reviewers

Ruth Barratt RN BSc MAdvPrac(Hons) CICP-E
Infection Prevention and Control Consultant
Health Quality and Safety Commission New Zealand
Christchurch
New Zealand

Silvana Bettiol BSc(Hons) MPH PhD
Senior Lecturer, Public Health and Communicable Disease
Tasmanian School of Medicine
Hobart, TAS
Australia

Claire Boardman PSM BAppSci(Nursing) GradCertInfCon MPH
Lecturer
School of Nursing and Midwifery
Monash University
Clayton, VIC
Australia

Stéphane Bouchoucha RN BSc(Hons) MSc GradCertIPC PhD
Associate Head of School
School of Nursing and Midwifery
Deakin University
Melbourne, VIC
Australia

Lynette Bowen RN PhD
Lecturer, Head of Undergraduate
College of Health, Medicine and Wellbeing
School of Nursing and Midwifery
University of Newcastle
Callaghan, NSW
Australia

Lynne Brown RN BN(Distinction) MN(Hons)
Lecturer
School of Nursing and Midwifery – Nursing
Griffith University
Brisbane, QLD
Australia

Penelope Burns BMed MPH&TM
Clinical Associate Professor
ANU School of Medicine and Psychology
General Practitioner
Sydney, NSW
Australia

Evonne T. Curran NursD
Honorary Senior Research Fellow
School of Health and Life Sciences
Glasgow Caledonian University
Glasgow
Scotland

Julie Dally RN BN GCUT GCACN MN
Lecturer
School of Nursing and Midwifery
The University of Notre Dame
Fremantle, WA
Australia

Mandy Davidson RN GradCertInfCon MPHTM CertIIISterilisation CertIVTAE
Clinical Nurse Consultant
Townsville Hospital and Health Service
Douglas, QLD
Australia

Katherine Garnham MBBS FRACP(Infectious Diseases) FRCPA(Microbiology)
Department of Infectious Diseases
Gold Coast University Hospital
Department of Microbiology
Griffith University
Gold Coast, QLD
Australia

Lyn Grattidge GradCertInfPrev&Mgt
Clinical Nurse Specialist
Infection Prevention and Management
Royal Perth Bentley Group
Bentley, WA
Australia

Susan Jain MIPH PhD
Principal Advisor, Infection Prevention and Control
Clinical Excellence Commission
University of New South Wales
St Leonards, NSW
Australia

Natasha Nunes BSc(Nursing) MNursing(Ldrshp&Mgt)
Coordinator of Nursing
Infection Prevention and Control
South Metropolitan Health Service
Fiona Stanley Hospital
Murdoch, WA
Australia

Suzanne Rogers RN ENB329(IPC) CertEd&ClinSupervision GradCertOHS GradCertPublicHealth GradDipMentalHealth MN(Clinical)
Nurse Coordinator
Canterbury Hauora Coordination Hub
Te Whatu Ora – Health New Zealand
Canterbury
New Zealand

Sharron Smyth-Demmon MACN RN MCN BEd(ProfHons)
MACORN MNSWOTA MACPAN
Nurse Educator, Higher Education
Australian College of Nursing
Parramatta, NSW
Australia

Vanessa Sparke BA(Nursing) GradCertCriticalCareNursing
GradDipEd&Training GradCertResearchMethods MPH&TM PhD
Senior Lecturer/Site Coordinator, Nursing and Midwifery, Cairns
Campus
Course Coordinator, Graduate Certificate of Infection Control
College of Healthcare Sciences
Division of Tropical Health and Medicine
James Cook University
Douglas, QLD
Australia

Sinu Thomas RN BN CertIVTA GradCertEmergencyNursing
GradDipCriticalCare MNCriticalCare
Course Coordinator for Acute Care Nursing
Australian College of Nursing
Parramatta, NSW
Australia

Catherine Viengkham BPsych(Hons) PhD
Research Fellow
Susan Wakil School of Nursing and Midwifery
The University of Sydney
Sydney, NSW
Australia

Annie Wells RN BN MAdvPrac(ICP)
Nursing Director
Communicable Disease Prevention Unit
Department of Health
Public Health Services Tasmania
Hobart, TAS
Australia

Pre-Proposal Reviewers

Lynette Bowen
Lecturer, Head of Undergraduate
College of Health, Medicine and Wellbeing
School of Nursing and Midwifery
University of Newcastle
Callaghan, NSW
Australia

Rebecca McCann
Program Manager
Healthcare Associated Infection Unit, Department of Health
Perth, WA
Australia

Thea van de Mortel
Professor
School of Nursing and Midwifery
Griffith University
Brisbane, QLD
Australia

Kristie Popkiss
Quality and Risk Manager
St John of God Midland Public and Private Hospitals
Midland, WA
Australia

Annie Wells
Nursing Director, Communicable Disease Prevention Unit
Department of Health
Public Health Services Tasmania
Hobart, TAS
Australia

Acknowledgements

There are many people to whom we owe an enormous vote of thanks. Sincerest thanks to the many contributing authors and peer reviewers—our colleagues—for their time and generosity in sharing their knowledge and experience to make our aim a reality, particularly during the most difficult of times, the public health emergency phase of the COVID-19 pandemic. We thank the boards of directors and members of the Australasian College for Infection Prevention and Control (ACIPC) and the Australasian Society for Infectious Diseases (ASID) for their support and endorsement of this title. Lastly, we extend special thanks to Dr Catherine Viengkham for her tremendous support with managing the development process.

Ramon Z. Shaban
Brett G. Mitchell
Deborough Macbeth
Philip L. Russo

SECTION 1

PRINCIPLES

CHAPTER 1

The history of healthcare-associated infections and infection prevention and control in Australia

PROFESSOR GWENDOLYN L. GILBERT[i-ii]

Chapter highlights

- Precedents and global trends—19th and early 20th century microbiologists and medical practitioners rediscovered commonsense infection prevention and control (IPC) principles and began to publish solid evidence to support them
- Pathogens—of the numerous microorganisms that contribute to hospital-acquired infections, a few, such as *Staphylococcus aureus* and the blood-borne viruses, stand out because of their profound influence on hospital IPC practices
- People and programs—the recollections and observations of some of the microbiologists and nurses who participated in the development of hospital IPC programs and establishment of IPC as a clinical specialty complement the limited published information on the history of hospital IPC in Australia
- Policies and practices—hospital IPC policies and practices were formalised in IPC programs during the latter part of the 20th century, and modified in response to changing microbial epidemiology, antibiotic resistance, emerging pathogens and healthcare priorities, but were inconsistently implemented

i   Sydney Infectious Diseases Institute, Faculty of Medicine and Health, University of Sydney, Sydney, NSW
ii Westmead Hospital, Westmead, NSW

Introduction

This chapter presents a history of post-World War II healthcare-associated infections (HAIs)[i] and hospital infection prevention and control (IPC) in Australia in—mainly—the 20th century. Like all history, it is selective. Some topics have been omitted or skimmed over, while others are explored in detail or embellished with anecdotes that aim to illuminate the relationships between the story's *dramatis personae* (hospital patients and healthcare workers [HCWs][ii]) and the *stages*—or hospitals—on which they act.

Throughout the chapter, the reflections of 23 doctors and nurses[iii] who were involved in the early history of IPC in Australia, and who were interviewed in 2019, are interspersed. Their insights add light and colour to the story. They are quoted here with their consent but without naming them, unless similar information had been published elsewhere. Otherwise, the chapter relies on published literature by Australian authors where possible. Inevitably, the story and the literature cited are influenced by the author's many years of experience as an infectious disease physician and medical microbiologist.

Infectious disease threats are influenced by past and current global events and knowledge. Part A, Precedents and global trends, outlines the status of HAIs and early hospital IPC programs in other industrialised countries in the 19th and early 20th centuries, as background to their evolution in 20th century Australia.

Part B, Pathogens, aims to show how a few key microbes have been most influential in determining the trajectory of IPC. In Part C, People and programs, the origins and early years of hospital IPC programs and the establishment of IPC as a specialty in Australia are portrayed, mainly from the perspective of people who participated in or observed them close up. Part D, Policies and practices, describes a few illustrative IPC practices that have been incorporated into national policies, then often challenged or forgotten, only to be 'rediscovered' during infectious disease outbreaks.

Healthcare-associated infections bridge the hypothetical barrier between the community and hospitals. Whether pathogens are introduced by a patient, visitor or staff member, or bred in situ by excessive antimicrobial use, they can be amplified among vulnerable hospital patients and peripatetic staff and reintroduced into the community. This means that IPC is not only essential for patient safety, but also for public health. The impact of infectious diseases, including HAIs, has diminished dramatically since the 19th century, at least in wealthy countries, but preventable HAIs persist, and hospitals and healthcare systems are often poorly prepared for outbreaks. This partly reflects their failure either to remember or apply lessons from the past. Recently, the SARS-CoV-2/COVID-19 pandemic has contributed to increased awareness and, perhaps, compliance with old IPC practices, some of which have been 'discovered', *de novo*, since the pandemic began. It remains to be seen which memories will outlive this latest crisis.

PART A
PRECEDENTS AND GLOBAL TRENDS

1.1 19th century

In the early–mid 19th century in industrialised countries, urban crowding, squalor and poverty contributed to escalating mortality rates from infectious disease in the community and from hospital sepsis in dirty overcrowded hospitals.[1,2] By the turn of the century, sanitation, improved living conditions and hospital reforms had contributed to a major decline in premature death rates.[3-5] Still, when sepsis occurred, outcomes were poor and 'remedies', such as purging, bleeding or toxic infusions, were largely ineffective.[6]

1.1.1 Disease transmission debates

Two ancient theories of disease transmission remained contentious in the 19th century.[7] Whether disease was spread by contact (contagion) or by noxious vapours from decaying organic matter (miasmas)[8,9] had social, economic and political implications. Contagion could

---

[i]Infections acquired during, but not present or incubating before, a hospital admission were referred to as 'nosocomial' or 'hospital-acquired' throughout much of the period covered in this chapter. Currently, the preferred term is 'healthcare-associated' to reflect the fact that a) many procedures or episodes of care that once occurred in hospitals are now performed in outpatient or day surgery clinics, b) invasive devices remain in situ after discharge and c) hospital-acquired infections are often not apparent until after discharge.

[ii]In this chapter the term healthcare workers (HCWs) is used broadly to include all hospital employees, including managers and visiting staff or consultants, unless otherwise specified.

[iii]They were former or current nurses (mainly infection control professionals [ICP]; n=11), medical microbiologists (MM; n=10), of whom 4 were also infectious disease physicians, and hospital scientists who had worked, formally or informally, as ICPs (HS; n=2). They have been identified only by codes: ICP, MM, or HS and an arbitrarily assigned number.

be controlled by quarantine, but only at the expense of free trade and personal liberty; on the other hand, control of miasmas required government-funded public health bureaucracies to oversee sanitation and urban renewal to banish miasmas.[10] Both theories had passionate supporters and opponents.

The controversy was particularly salient in the context of rising puerperal fever and maternal mortality rates.[11] Alexander Gordon's observation, in 1795, that doctors and midwives spread puerperal fever from patient to patient,[12] was largely ignored until the 1840s when James Young Simpson and Oliver Wendell Holmes, among others, publicly supported this view and, controversially, implicated physicians in particular.[13-15] A strident opponent of this contention, Charles Meigs, asserted that puerperal fever was due to 'accident or providence' and, to hold doctors responsible 'would mark, ... with a black and ineffaceable spot, the hard-won reputation of every physician ...'.[iv 16,17]

Simpson, who regarded puerperal and surgical infections as 'intercommunicable', coined the term 'hospitalism' to describe sepsis. He claimed that the risk of death, in the 'vitiated atmosphere of hospitals', was greater than for soldiers 'entering ... the bloodiest and more fatal battlefields'.[13,18]

1.1.2 Effective interventions

In 1847, Ignaz Semmelweis was perplexed by the high maternal mortality in the 1st Division of Vienna Lying-in Hospital, where deliveries were performed by medical students. By comparison, the mortality rate in the 2nd Division, where midwives presided, was much lower.[19] When a colleague died from wound sepsis from an autopsy-related injury, Semmelweis was struck by similarities between the findings of his colleague's autopsy and those of women dying from puerperal sepsis. He hypothesised that medical students who, unlike midwives, performed autopsies, carried 'cadaveric poison' on their hands to women in labour. In May 1847, he ordered students to wash their hands in 'chlorina liquida', before entering the labour ward. The results were dramatic. Maternal death rates, in the 1st and 2nd Divisions, which had been 11.4% and 2.7%, in 1846, fell to 1.27% and 1.3%, respectively, in 1848.[20] When Semmelweis belatedly published these results in 1861, they were largely ignored or ridiculed until years later.[21] This was partly because of his difficult personality and poor communication skills, but also because his thesis,

that puerperal fever was caused by 'cadaverous particles', was inconsistent with prevailing theories.[22]

Meanwhile, in England, the sanitarian movement had gained momentum. Sanitarians produced statistical evidence that sanitation, waste disposal and slum clearance not only controlled noxious smells (miasmas) but also saved lives.[4] In 1854, a London Times correspondent's report of appalling conditions and a high mortality among soldiers at the British Military hospital, in the Crimea, caused public outrage. Florence Nightingale was sent to investigate. She found filthy, overcrowded, vermin-infested wards and deployed her formidable nursing and administrative skills to introduce strict hygiene and other measures, based on sanitarian principles.[23,24] In her report to the British parliament she presented data, using sophisticated statistical methods, showing that infectious diseases had been a far more common cause of death than war wounds and that, following her reforms, the soldiers' death rate fell from 33% in the first, to 2%, in the third quarter of 1855.[23] Nightingale's Crimean experience influenced her later hospital and nursing reforms on which the 'nursing model of care' is based.[25,26]

1.1.3 Germ theory and antisepsis

Louis Pasteur's germ theory—that microscopic organisms in the air were responsible for fermentation and putrefaction—was published in the 1860s.[27] Joseph Lister recognised its relevance to wound sepsis:[28,29] '[W]hen it had been shown ... that the septic property of the atmosphere depended on minute organisms, which owe their energy to their vitality, it occurred to me that decomposition in the injured part might be avoided by ... destroying the floating particles'.[30] With this insight, Lister applied carbolic acid, liberally, to operative sites and kept wounds covered with carbolic acid-soaked dressings for several weeks. After this regimen was introduced, in 1867, deaths from compound fractures fell from 46% to 15%.[30-32] Although these results were initially greeted with scepticism, antisepsis was soon widely accepted. In Australia, it was introduced by a Melbourne Hospital surgeon, William Gilbee, soon after publication of Lister's results, and was well established by the 1880s.[33]

By the end of the century, asepsis was beginning to replace antisepsis. Sterile gowns and caps were first used in the 1880s, and sterile rubber gloves in 1899. Although gloves were not used consistently until the

---

[iv]Throughout the chapter, quotations not in italics are from published material; those in italics are from participants in the qualitative study described above.

1920s,[34] surgical hand scrubs and no-touch technique were adopted earlier.[35] During the 1930–40s, there was extensive research into the best types, and number of layers, of gauze for use in masks,[35-37] and ongoing controversy about when they should be used.[11]

By the end of the 19th century, the main principles of hospital IPC and epidemiology, including the importance of environmental and personal hygiene, surveillance and statistical analysis, and asepsis had been established. However, the principles continued to be disputed and related IPC practices were highly variable.

1.1.4 19th century health professions and the health revolution

In the mid-19th century, longstanding physicians', apothecaries' and barber-surgeons' craft guilds were transformed into professional organisations. Colleges and medical associations were established to regulate standards, provide licences-to-practice to those deemed to have appropriate (university) qualifications, and protect doctors' 'ownership' of rapidly expanding medical knowledge. The 'medical model' based on Pasteur's germ theory and Koch's postulates, included the concept that diseases have specific causes and characteristic anatomical and/or physiological lesions that can be treated by specific remedies.[38-40] At last, medical research was generating effective therapies, and doctors (upper-class men) were acquiring increasing social, economic and political capital.[41]

By contrast, most nurses were poorly paid, uneducated women who were little more than domestic servants, apart from a few middle-class women for whom nursing was a religious vocation or philanthropic interest.[42] In England, Nightingale campaigned for nursing to be accepted as a respectable profession for educated women. Many doctors saw this as a challenge to their authority, but they needed trained nurses to implement increasingly complex treatments. To gain doctors' support, Nightingale decreed that nurses must obey doctors' orders relating to medical treatment, but would be accountable to the nursing hierarchy for training, practice standards and discipline.[43]

1.2 20th century

In the early 20th century, life expectancy was further extended by antimicrobial therapies that cured many previously fatal diseases and made it possible to introduce lifesaving therapies that required iatrogenic immunosuppression.[1,2] After World War II, doctors eagerly embraced the use of antibiotics for life-threatening infections. Because they seemed so safe, antibiotics were also used to treat minor (often viral) infections and for prophylaxis. Hospital hygiene seemed less imperative. '[T]he belief that infectious diseases had been successfully overcome was pervasive in biomedical circles from as early as 1948 ...'.[44] The belief was encouraged by an expanding repertoire of vaccines[45] and a plethora of antibiotics, aggressively promoted by the manufacturers. Although resistance was already emerging by the 1950s,[46] it was assumed that, if bacteria developed resistance to one antibiotic, others would be available to replace it.

This optimism was naïve.[47] In hospitals, surgical site infection (SSI) rates were increasing. The main culprit was the versatile *Staphylococcus aureus*,[v] which had replaced group A streptococcus (GAS) as the major hospital pathogen. Initially, *S. aureus* was susceptible to most antibiotics, but it soon showed its capacity to become resistant to almost any agent to which it was exposed.[48] In 1955, Edward Lowbury observed: 'the dilemma of hospital infection has been complicated rather than solved by chemotherapy'.[49] By the late 20th century, any hope of 'closing the book on infectious diseases'[44] was dashed by a succession of emerging pathogens (e.g. human immunodeficiency virus [HIV] and hepatitis B and C viruses) and the re-emergence of others that, ostensibly, had been controlled.[50]

1.2.1 Antimicrobial resistance (AMR[vi]) and transmission of multidrug-resistant organisms (MROs)

Naturally-occurring penicillinase was identified in 1928, before penicillin was used therapeutically in the 1940s.[51] Penicillin-resistant *S. aureus* (PRSA) and multidrug (streptomycin and tetracycline) resistant *S. aureus* (mPRSA) were already appearing in hospitals in the 1950s.[46,52,53] Meanwhile, recognition that nosocomial *S. aureus* infections were associated with both environmental contamination and nasal colonisation had reactivated longstanding controversies about transmission routes and the preventive roles of personal protective equipment (PPE) and hand hygiene.[11,54] Bacteriologists

---

[v]In the 19th century, pyogenic micrococci were divided into 'streptococci' and 'staphylococci' based on microscopic appearance (chains or grape-like clusters, respectively). The 'golden' staphylococcus was originally called *Staphylococcus pyogenes* but changed to *S. aureus* to distinguish it from *Streptococcus pyogenes*, which is now more commonly called group A (haemolytic) streptococcus (GAS).

[vi]The original antimicrobial agents, which were mainly antibacterial, were referred to collectively, but not always accurately, as antibiotics. Later, antifungal, antiviral and antiparasitic agents were included in the term 'antimicrobial agents' and resistance referred to as AMR.

in the UK and Australia were among the first to use bacteriophage typing to investigate *S. aureus* transmission.[11] They showed that 66–80% of PRSA isolates belonged to phage group III, whereas susceptible strains were more diverse.[55-57] The increasing prevalence of PRSA/mPRSA prompted the development of methicillin and other penicillinase-resistant beta-lactam antibiotics,[vii] which were expected to solve the problem. Spraying methicillin into ward air was proposed, to break the cycle of colonisation and hospital cross-infection;[58] unsurprisingly, promising early results were transient. Clinical isolates of methicillin-resistant *S. aureus* (MRSA) were first identified in 1961, and hospital outbreaks[viii] reported soon afterwards.[59-61] MRSA was to dominate the next chapter in the ongoing 'hospital staph' saga.[62,63]

As antibiotics were used with increasing frequency in hospitals during the 1960s, environmental Gram-negative bacteria (GNB), such as *Pseudomonas aeruginosa*, which were intrinsically resistant to most early antibiotics, became established as opportunistic hospital pathogens. Soon they began to acquire resistance to newer broad-spectrum (anti-pseudomonal) agents developed to combat them. Endogenous GNB (e.g. Enterobacteriaceae), that were initially susceptible to early broad-spectrum beta-lactams (e.g. ampicillin, first generation cephalosporins) and aminoglycosides (e.g. gentamicin), also began to develop resistance, spread by R-factors (plasmids) that carried resistance to several antibiotics.[64,65] Evidence-based antibiotic prescribing to reduce the *emergence* of MROs, and enhanced administrative, environmental and behavioural IPC measures to limit their *transmission* were urgently needed.[66-68]

1.2.2 HAI surveillance, IPC programs and hospital epidemiology

In the 1950s, it was recognised that the burden of HAIs was generally underestimated.[67] An epidemiological approach was required, including bacterial strain typing and systematic surveillance with timely feedback of results to clinicians.[48] Some countries established HAI surveillance and IPC programs during the 1960s. The UK and Australia[55] were among the first to establish infection control committees (ICCs) and appoint infection control officers (ICOs).[68] The role of ICO was envisaged, in 1955, as '... one individual whose responsibility it is to direct and coordinate all the activities which make for safety from infection, [including] ... whether the blankets were being sterilised, ... sterilisers were functioning properly, [or] there were carriers of streptococci working in the ward [etc.] ...'.[67]

Initially, most ICOs were doctors, who soon found that the role demanded more time than they had available. The first infection control sister/professional (ICS/ICP)[ix] was appointed in England in 1959[69] and in many other countries, including Australia,[70] during the 1960s. A nurse with similar duties had been appointed in the USA, in 1956.[48] At the first International Conference on Nosocomial Infections, in 1970, Sir Robert E. O. Williams challenged delegates to provide concrete evidence that appropriate IPC practices could improve patient outcomes, so as to encourage clinicians to comply with them more consistently.[64]

CASE STUDY 1

Study on the Efficacy of Nosocomial Infection Control (SENIC)

SENIC responded to Williams' challenge. Its objectives were, briefly to determine whether, and by how much: a) infection surveillance and control programs (ISCPs) reduced HAI rates; and b) hospital/patient characteristics and individual ISCP components contributed to the

---

viiIncluding isoxazolyl penicillins, such as flucloxacillin, and first generation cephalosporins, such as cephalothin, which have excellent activity against methicillin-susceptible *S. aureus*. Until recently, MRSA was resistant to all beta-lactam antibiotics.

viiiHAI 'outbreak' of an MRO usually implies transmission of the organism between patients who become colonised. Outbreaks are recognised either when a small minority of colonised patients develops overt infection or by active screening of patients because of a recognised risk of transmission. Staff are often vectors of transmission and sometimes become colonised, but are rarely overtly infected.

ixHCWs responsible for IPC have varied over time. Initially, most ICOs were bacteriologists, whose familiarity with laboratory results from all over the hospital, and access to strain typing results, provided insight into cross-infection. Sometimes they, or a clinician (often a surgeon), initiated the appointment of an experienced senior nursing sister (ICS) or relatively junior infection control nurse (ICN). Recently ICSs and ICNs (and others in similar roles) have been referred to, variously, as IC practitioner or professional (ICP) or (in the USA), infection preventionist.

outcomes.[71] Over six years (1974-9), the SENIC included: a survey of USA acute hospitals; Interviews with key personnel from a sample of hospitals with different types of ISCP; and two rounds of medical record reviews of selected patients in each of the hospitals sampled, to determine changes in rates of four well-defined HAIs.[72]

By 1976, 64% of >6500 US hospitals surveyed had an ISCP, supervised by a physician or microbiologist, and 42% employed an ICP.[73] The most effective ISCP components varied for different types of HAI. For example, timely feedback of data to surgeons was associated with reduced SSI rates; and active control measures, such as staff training in catheter care, with reduced urinary tract and bloodstream infection (BSI) rates. Overall, the most effective ISCP component was the employment of one full-time equivalent (FTE) ICP per 250 beds. The average HAI rate among the >330 hospitals sampled was ~6%. Between 1970 and 1975-6, HAI rates *increased* by 18%, in hospitals *without* effective ISCPs; but they *fell* by 32%, in hospitals *with* effective programs.[72] Another critical finding was that 'an infection control nurse working with a physician ... and practicing epidemiologic surveillance and control techniques, can prevent up to one third of the nosocomial infections ...'.[72] SENIC also confirmed that reliable, well-presented data could motivate preventive action by clinicians and administrators.

PART B
PATHOGENS

This section is an overview of some of the microbes that have influenced the trajectory of IPC history in Australia. The selection of what to include was influenced by interviews with IPC pioneers and the author's own experience. Perhaps the most prominent microbial influence on hospital IPC in the 20th century was *S. aureus*, a persistent, ubiquitous and adaptable hospital pathogen. Environmental and enteric bacteria are generally less prevalent but can cause serious hospital outbreaks; they are discussed more briefly. Blood-borne viruses (BBVs) are, arguably, the most influential group of viral pathogens. Among many community viruses, seasonal influenza is an important but often underestimated cause of hospital outbreaks. It is discussed briefly, along with some other epidemic viruses.

1.3 The dominant role of *Staphylococcus aureus*

1.3.1 Healthcare-associated staphylococcal infection in (mainly) adults—1940s–80s

By the mid–late 1940s, GAS had almost disappeared as a major hospital pathogen, in the wake of widespread penicillin use.[74,75] It re-emerged briefly in the 1950s, usually as a co-pathogen with PRSA, in SSIs that occurred despite penicillin prophylaxis. '[W]hen streptococcus is implanted into a surgical wound along with a staphylococcus that is a potent penicillinase-producer, parenteral penicillin cannot be relied upon to prevent streptococcal colonisation of the wound'.[76] GAS retreated again when penicillin prophylaxis was discontinued.[77] PRSA increased steadily during the 1950s–60s[52,78,79] and some phage types[x] spread within hospitals.[55] *S. aureus* contaminated the environment, blankets and anterior nares of staff and patients. Oiling of blankets reduced environmental contamination but did not affect the nasal carriage or SSI rates.[75,77,80,81] Patients colonised after admission often infected their own wounds with the same strain.[82] During the 1960s, widespread use of a new topical antibiotic, neomycin, in an attempt to reduce SSI rates, rapidly led to resistance[53,56] (Table 1.1, Q1;1).

1.3.2 *Staphylococcus aureus* phage type 80/81—from neonatal units to global pandemic

In 1949–50, the increasing prevalence of neonatal *S. aureus* colonisation was causing concern in Sydney nurseries. Although infections were uncommon, the fact that most isolates were penicillin resistant caused concern.[83-85] In 1952, Sydney paediatrician Dr Clair Isbister reported clusters of more severe *S. aureus* infections in neonates and their mothers. They were caused by a new PRSA phage type which was later identified as 80/81, and shown to have caused 70 of 86 neonatal nursery outbreaks in Australia during the 1950s. It spread to neonates' families, hospital staff and patients, and the general community, causing skin and soft tissue infections (Table 1.1, Q1;2), osteomyelitis in children and, less commonly, life-threatening pneumonia, particularly in

---

[x]Bacteriophage (phage) typing of *S. aureus* was introduced, in 1948, by [xi]Dr Phyllis Rountree, the senior bacteriologist at Royal Prince Alfred Hospital (RPAH), who led a National Health and Medical Research Council (NHMRC)-funded national staphylococcal reference laboratory. It was critical for epidemiological studies of *S. aureus*.

TABLE 1.1 Pathogens

Q1;1	*'Neomycin-resistant* Staph aureus *was causing havoc. Every second surgeon had a little puffer of neomycin powder in his pocket ... whenever he looked at a wound, he sprinkled* [some] *on it. We persuaded the staff to ban all topical antibiotics ...* [despite] *tremendous resistance. It had great results ... gradually neomycin-resistant staph disappeared'* [MM1].
Q1;2	*'When I started at the hospital, in the 1950s, ... there'd be 10 to 12 doctors or nurses, off with boils and carbuncles'* [HS1].
Q1;3	[At a Sydney hospital] *'... in 1958, we were losing one neonate a week from staph. infection, phage type 80/81. Phisohex was like magic. When we started bathing the babies it disappeared'* [MM1].
Q1;4	*'I started to use* [prophylactic] *vancomycin to reduce the MRSA infection in the vascular unit ...* [but] *I produced an epidemic of Klebsiella ...'* [MM2].
Q1;5	*'*[In 1971–72] *in the neonatal ICU, three babies had pseudomonas meningitis. My registrar grabbed some of the feeds and found that every one of them had pseudomonas in them. We had a pyocin typing scheme* [and] *initially we went around to all the sinks and found* P. aeruginosa, *but always the wrong pyocin type. We went to the milk kitchen, which was using chlorine disinfectants, and found it wasn't properly disinfecting the jugs used for making up the mixture—that was the problem'* [MM3].
Q1;6	*'*[Also in 1971–2, there was] *... a terrible epidemic of disease in patients having open heart surgery due to one contaminated bottle of cardioplegia solution with Enterobacter aerogenes in it.* [Another outbreak] *was ... of sternal split infections with a lathering brush that some surgical dresser had brought in to use before shaving the patients'* [MM3].
Q1;7	*MRSA was the big focus, but there were also aminoglycoside resistant Gram negatives—Klebsiellas and Pseudomonas. They didn't spread as readily as MRSA. They affected particular patients who were immunosuppressed and on antibiotics. They were in the background but trying to get people to use narrow spectrum antibiotics, where they could, was not just directed at MRSA'* [MM4].
Q1;8	*'We had an anaesthetist who picked it* [hepatitis B] *up. He was the stimulus to get the anaesthetists to wear gloves ... We had huge issues with medical staff getting hep B vaccinated. They said it was their business and they weren't going to do it, including the head of the Infection Control Committee ...'* [ICP1].
Q1;9	*'It became apparent that there were a couple of hep B colonised foreign-born doctors spreading it in NSW hospitals ... It was not until the '80s we realised what a problem we had with hep B ... by then medical staff were hammering to make sure that needlesticks were monitored'* [MM3].
Q1;10	*'The episode of HIV transmission in that operating session was very important for HIV and infection control.* [W]*hen we got to investigate it, a lot of fundamental things in infection control were missing, including not to use multidose vials. That was what brought in universal precautions as a sort of new genre of infection control in Australia ... CDC and everyone was doing exactly the same thing, at the same time, for the same reasons'* [MM5].
Q1;11	*'AIDS was terrible, but it wasn't going to be transmitted in the wards. The surgeons were reluctant, but common sense eventually prevailed. The head of surgery said, "It's our job to look after these people"'* [MM3].

HS: hospital scientist; MM: medical microbiologist; ICP: infection control professional.
Note: These quotes are from participants in a qualitative study conducted by the author, in 2019, on the history of IPC in Australia (see Introduction and footnote iii for further information). The quotes have been edited for clarity and flow, but care has been taken not change the meaning. Individual participants are not named but gave permission for their comments to be used in any publication arising from the interviews.

infants.[56,86-88] *S. aureus* 80/81 probably arose in either Australia or Canada, but soon spread to many other countries.[56]

In some neonatal nurseries, 'overcrowding, under-staffing and a poor general level of nursery hygiene'[89] contributed to cross-infection. Infants in communal nurseries were handled four times more frequently, on average, by more nurses and had more infections than those rooming-in with their mothers.[89] After the

introduction of rooming-in at a Geelong nursery, the *S. aureus* infection rate fell from 34% to 12%.[90] In a Melbourne neonatal unit, *S. aureus* infections remained a problem despite rooming-in, but routine bathing of infants with hexachlorophene (Phisohex) reduced staphylococcal colonisation from 70% to 31%, and sepsis from 17% to 1.3%.[91] Hexachlorophene almost certainly prevented many neonatal deaths (Table 1.1, Q1;3). However, despite its efficacy and lack of adverse effects in thousands of infants in whom it was used, it was withdrawn in the late 1960s, because of fear of neurotoxicity.[92]

1.3.3 The MRSA era in Australian hospitals—1980s

In Australia, methicillin was first used in 1961 and MRSA was first isolated in Sydney, in 1966. MRSA was often resistant to other antibiotics but remained relatively uncommon,[63,93] until a new clone appeared in the late 1970s and spread to many hospitals in the eastern states.[56,68,94] In Melbourne, gentamicin-resistant MRSA was first identified in 1978, and by 1979 it had increased from 6% to 70% of MRSA isolates.[95,96] In 1979, 40% of Melbourne hospitals reported having MRSA-colonised inpatients, many of whom developed serious infections.[93] At the Royal Melbourne Hospital (RMH), 53% of HA *S. aureus* BSIs (SABSIs) were due to MRSA.[97] Outbreaks occurred in all four Melbourne neonatal intensive care units (ICUs), in 1980–81. Of >300 infants who were colonised, ~10% developed serious, sometimes fatal, infections.[98] Hospital MRSA outbreaks occurred in Sydney hospitals in 1981–3.[99] At a Brisbane hospital, between 1979–89, the average annual SABSI count increased from 40 to 138 and the proportion due to MRSA from 4% to 37%.[100] To control outbreaks, some hospitals opened isolation wards, screened patients and staff in high-risk wards or temporarily reintroduced hexachlorophene washing of neonates.[93,98-100] An attempt to prevent MRSA SSIs with routine vancomycin prophylaxis was associated with an unanticipated outcome (Table 1.1, Q1;4).

In Western Australia (WA), MRSA was rare until 1982, when the admission of an MRSA-colonised interstate patient to Royal Perth Hospital (RPH) initiated a prolonged outbreak.[101] Thereafter, a 'search and destroy' policy was adopted in WA. New patients and staff from outside WA were screened for MRSA and carriers were isolated or excluded until cleared. Over two years, 4% of patients screened were colonised but, although ~40% of them had clinical infections, cross-infection occurred only once. In the 1980s, only 0.4% of *S. aureus* isolates in WA were MRSA, compared with 10–30% elsewhere in Australia.[102] The prevalence increased over the next decade due to the emergence of community-associated non-multiresistant MRSA in northern WA. The proportion of HA SABSIs due to MRSA, in five Perth teaching hospitals, increased from zero in 1990 to 14% in 1997–9[103]—but still far less than the 40% reported in 17 non-WA hospitals in 1999–2002.[104]

1.4 Environmental and enteric bacteria

1.4.1 Multidrug-resistant Gram-negative bacilli (MDR GNB)

Although overshadowed by *S. aureus*, GNB were increasingly responsible for HAI outbreaks during the 1960s–70s, as the antibiotics to which they were naturally resistant (streptomycin, tetracycline, chloramphenicol) were used more often. Outbreaks of *P. aeruginosa* and other GNB infections, among burns, ICU, neonatal and immunosuppressed patients, were often linked to moist ward environments or contaminated equipment or solutions. Epidemiological studies often identified a point source, but cross-infection was also implicated[105-110] (Table 1.1, Q1;5–6).

Despite the production of new antibiotics with potent Gram-negative activity, resistance continued to emerge, including among the Enterobacteriaceae. In 1975, a gentamicin-resistant *Klebsiella pneumoniae* outbreak at a Melbourne hospital involved 42 patients, more than half of whom had significant infections.[111] Later gentamicin- and tobramycin-resistant *P. aeruginosa* were isolated from patients in two Sydney hospitals.[112] The first 'Antibiotic Guidelines' was published in 1978,[113] but changing doctors' prescribing habits proved to be difficult (Table 1.1, Q1;7). During the next 20 years, multiresistant Enterobacteriaceae and *Acinetobacter baumanii* caused troublesome hospital outbreaks.[114-117] GNB became progressively resistant to aminoglycosides and extended-spectrum penicillins, cephalosporins and carbapenems. An increasing variety of mobile genetic elements carrying multiple resistance genes was identified. Extended-spectrum beta-lactamase (ESBL) producing Enterobacteriaceae and other MDR GNB were introduced, sporadically, from high prevalence countries, but they were still uncommon in Australian hospitals before 2000.[118-120]

1.4.2 Vancomycin-resistant enterococci (VRE)—*Enterococcus faecalis* and *Enterococcus faecium*

The Gram-positive enterococci are also opportunists. In the 1970s, use of third generation cephalosporins (3GCs), to which enterococci are resistant, led to an increase in enterococcal infections, most commonly due to *E. faecalis*. Enterococci had been reliably susceptible to vancomycin (a glycopeptide), but resistance emerged in Europe and the USA in the 1980s, due to acquisition of a mobile gene cluster, usually *vanA* or *vanB*, typically by *E. faecium*.[121] In Europe, VRE in humans was often linked to foodborne transmission from animals treated with another glycopeptide, avoparcin. In the USA, predominantly nosocomial transmission was attributed to extensive vancomycin and 3GC use.[122]

VRE were first isolated in Australia in 1994, and their numbers increased slowly.[123] The most prevalent genotype in New South Wales (NSW), *vanB E. faecium*, was also responsible for most enterococcal BSIs nationally; *vanA* was more prevalent in other states.[122] During the 1990s, glycopeptide use was increasing in Australia, in both humans and animals. Their relative contributions to the emergence of VRE was debated, but it was generally agreed that human consumption of vancomycin and 3GCs were the main drivers.[124,125]

The first reported VRE hospital outbreak in Australia (due to *vanA E. faecium*) was in Brisbane, in 1999.[126] In two VRE outbreaks, in Melbourne and Perth in 2001 (due to *vanB E. faecium*), transmission was associated with 3GC and vancomycin use, diarrhoea in colonised patients, inter-ward transfers and inadequate isolation facilities.[127,128] When reinforcement of routine IPC measures failed to control these outbreaks, additional measures were introduced including: screening of all hospital patients; isolation or cohorting of carriers and contacts; enhanced cleaning and hand hygiene campaigns; and restriction of 3GCs.[127,128] A minority of patients were clinically infected, but the cost of eradication was justified by the difficulty of treating VRE BSI.[127] These outbreaks showed that eradication of a new nosocomial pathogen may be feasible when it is first introduced. However, it is much more difficult once the pathogen is established. By the early 2000s, VRE was endemic in many Australian hospitals; new, more transmissible strains of the globally disseminated, hospital-adapted clonal complex 17 had emerged, and the incidence of VRE BSIs was increasing.[129]

1.5 Blood-borne viruses (BBVs)

During the 1960s, 700–800 patients with acute hepatitis were admitted to Fairfield Infectious Diseases Hospital (FIDH) in Melbourne, annually. Most cases were probably due to 'infectious' hepatitis A and the rest to serum or post-transfusion hepatitis B but, without diagnostic tests, the cause could only be inferred by the clinical features. In the 1950s–60s, Saul Krugman's controversial experiments in institutionalised children confirmed that infectious and serum hepatitis were distinct, and each was followed by homologous immunity. Krugman also showed that serum hepatitis could be spread by close contact or ingestion and was followed, in a minority of cases, by chronic infection.[130]

1.5.1 Hepatitis B virus (HBV)

When the 'Australia antigen' was discovered in the 1960s, and shown to be the HBV surface antigen (HBsAg), it provided a tool for epidemiological investigations.[131] In early Australian serosurveys, HBsAg was detected in stored sera from 50% of transfusion-acquired, 3% of non-transfusion-acquired, 7–20% of undifferentiated acute, and 12% of chronic, hepatitis cases.[132-134]

Admissions to FIDH due to acute hepatitis B increased during the 1970s; many cases were HAIs, affecting patients and HCWs. Others were linked to intravenous drug use (IVDU) or tattooing.[135] HBsAg screening of blood donors began in 1970. In a 1982 survey, 18 (2%) of 842 cardiac surgical patients most of whom had non-A, non-B hepatitis (NANBH), developed post-transfusion hepatitis. However, three had HBV infection, despite donor screening,[136] which indicated that screening for HBV core antibody (anti-HBc), in addition to HBsAg, was required to identify all HBV-infected donors. HBV outbreaks were a recognised, but preventable, hazard in haemodialysis units. In a special dialysis unit for HBV carriers at FIDH, strict IPC precautions were observed, including post-exposure HB immunoglobulin prophylaxis. Only one transmission event occurred over 10 years (1970–79), among 48 patients and 43 staff.[137] HBeAg—a protein detected in HBV carriers with active infection—was shown to correlate with increased risks of chronic liver disease, mother-to-baby transmission, and HBV transmission following contaminated needlestick injury.[138-141]

The immediate effect of HBV in hospitals was mainly confined to high-risk units, but additional precautions to protect all HCWs were recommended, in Australia, in the 1970s.[135] An inactivated, plasma-derived HBV vaccine was licensed in Australia in 1982, and recommended for high-risk adults (including HCWs) and infants of HBsAg-positive mothers, in 1986. It was replaced by recombinant vaccine in 1987.[142] Uptake by HCWs was slow, initially, because of an (unfounded) fear of vaccine-induced infection (Table 1.1, Q1;8). Unvaccinated HCWs were at considerable risk of HBV infection, from sharps injury, contamination while handling laboratory specimens, or eating/drinking in contaminated areas. Serological surveys in the USA showed that up to 20% of HCWs had markers of HBV infection. Patients were also at risk from HBV-infected staff performing exposure-prone procedures[135,143.] (Table 1.1, Q1;9)

Meanwhile, after prolonged searching, HAV had been identified in 1973.[144,145] With tests for both HBV and HAV[xi] available, most hepatitis cases could be identified, but there was circumstantial evidence of several NANBH viruses, including at least one BBV (HCV).

1.5.2 Human immunodeficiency virus (HIV)

In June 1981, clusters of previously rare *Pneumocystis carinii* pneumonia, Kaposi's sarcoma, and other opportunistic infections were reported among young gay men, in the USA. By early 1983, ~1200 cases of acquired immune deficiency syndrome (AIDS) had been diagnosed in the USA, with 450 deaths. Most were in gay men, but blood product recipients (e.g. haemophiliacs), IVDUs, female partners of men with AIDS and their infants were also affected.[146] Human immunodeficiency virus (HIV) was identified as the cause in 1983–4 and diagnostic tests (for HIV antibody) became available in 1985.[147,148] In the USA, the Centers for Disease Control and Prevention (CDC) issued guidance for protection of HCWs and prevention of vertical transmission in 1982–5.[149-151]

In Australia, AIDS was first reported in 1982.[152] In November 1984, in Queensland, the deaths of several babies after receiving HIV-contaminated transfusions provoked a backlash against the unwittingly HIV-infected blood donors.[153] Blood donor screening for HIV antibody began in 1985 and prospective surveillance in 1986. By 1994, AIDS case numbers had begun to decline. Back-projection of dates of HIV-acquisition indicated that it had been first introduced into Australia around 1980.[xii] New infections reached a peak in 1984, before declining until 1999–2000,[154] when they began to increase gradually.[155]

HIV HAIs were rare and HIV seroprevalence in HCWs was no higher than in the general population.[141,156] Globally, there were three reported clusters of HCW-to-patient transmission, presumably during exposure-prone-procedures.[157] In NSW, in 1989, five cases of patient-to-patient transmission occurred during minor procedures in a surgeon's consulting room. Four women, with no HIV risk factors, and one man,

who reported having had sex with men, were affected. The surgeon was HIV-negative and no breach of IPC was identified,[158] but the incident prompted review of IPC practices (Table 1.1, Q1;10).

In 1987, the first antiretroviral drug became available in Australia.[159] Zidovudine (azidothymidine [AZT]), and other individual antiretroviral drugs, suppressed HIV infection temporarily, but resistance soon developed. Combination therapy (highly active antiretroviral therapy [HAART]) was introduced in 1996. HAART effectively reduced viral load and delayed disease progression in most people with HIV infection.[160,161] By the early 2000s, AIDS-related hospital admissions and premature deaths had declined markedly.[162]

Australia's response to AIDS was acknowledged as among the most effective worldwide. It included leadership by, and collaboration between, the gay community and health authorities; the adoption of evidence-based policies, including needle-syringe exchange and methadone replacement programs, free anonymous HIV testing and subsidised therapy; and a supportive political environment.[153,163] Despite a relatively enlightened official response, people living with AIDS encountered stigmatisation and discriminatory treatment.[164] Children with AIDS were described as 'innocent victims', implying that unwittingly infected blood donors were 'guilty'. Some surgeons demanded universal presurgical HIV screening and special management of HIV-positive patients, including postponement or cancellation of surgery. Both strategies were promptly rejected as impractical, uneconomic and unethical (Table 1.1, Q1;11). Despite a low HAI risk, many ICPs believed that HIV influenced hospital IPC more than other BBVs.

1.5.3 Hepatitis C virus (HCV)

HCV was eventually identified in 1988, when its genome was cloned and HCV antigen became available for serological tests.[165,166] Australian seroprevalence studies, using stored sera from the 1970s showed a high prevalence (~60%) of HCV antibody in haemophiliacs and IVDUs, but a much lower prevalence in haemodialysis patients and gay men (<10%).[167] Blood donor screening for HCV antibody (anti-HCV) began in 1990. A review of HCV epidemiology, in the period 1970-90, estimated that the incidence of HCV

[xi]Hepatitis A, until recently, was diagnosed by detection of HAV-IgM in acute serum or by IgG seroconversion, in patients with acute hepatitis. HAV does not cause chronic infection. Past infection is diagnosed by detection of HAV IgG.
[xii]Newly-acquired HIV infection is commonly followed, after 10-14 days, by an acute, nonspecific (and often undiagnosed), self-limiting febrile illness, sometimes associated with rash and lymphadenopathy ('seroconversion illness'). There is a variable window period before HIV-antibody is detectable and an incubation period of months to years (median 12) before clinical evidence of immune deficiency and/or an 'AIDS-defining illness' occur.

infection among IVDUs was 15–40 per 100 person-years of drug use.[168] In South Australia, in 1995, HCV seroprevalence in pregnant women was 1.1% and IVDU the only independent positive predictor. It was therefore decided that routine antenatal screening was not warranted.[169]

Retrospective testing of ~170,000 Australian blood donor sera, collected before routine anti-HCV screening began, showed that 0.26% were HCV-RNA-positive[xiii] and, therefore, potentially infectious.[170] In Sydney, 1% of >700 cardiac surgical patients, who had received unscreened blood, developed post-transfusion HCV hepatitis (one per 1000 donations).[171] Retrospective screening of their ~3500 donors found that 0.75% were anti-HCV-positive and 0.2% HCV-RNA-positive.

Sexual and vertical transmission of HCV were much less common than of either HBV or HIV, and nosocomial infection with HCV much less common than with HBV.[172] However, a cluster of nosocomial infections occurred in Sydney, in 1993. Two women developed acute hepatitis several weeks after minor surgery at a private hospital. Subsequent investigation showed that they, and three others (two women, one man) who had had procedures in the same operating session, were anti-HCV-positive and infected with the same HCV genotype. None of the women had risk factors, but the man had a history of IVDU. He was the first on the operating list to be infected and the most likely index case. No route of transmission was identified. It was hypothesised that contamination of a reusable piece of the anaesthetic circuit, by the index patient's respiratory secretions, had been transferred to the other patients via laryngeal masks, which are known to cause minor mucosal trauma.[173]

There is no HCV vaccine. Early therapies in the 1980s and 90s were relatively ineffective, but since the early 2000s, increasingly effective combination antiviral therapy means that most cases of chronic HCV infection are now curable. Nevertheless, HCV remains a significant public health challenge globally, because of unidentified chronic infection and associated cirrhosis and cancer.

1.6 Epidemic/community viruses

Before the introduction of vaccines, epidemic infectious diseases were often introduced into hospitals by patients or staff. Most major cities had infectious diseases hospitals or wards within major hospitals (see Part D), which reduced the risk. But infections, introduced into a general hospital by patients with mild or atypical symptoms, often spread before control measures could be implemented, especially if routine IPC practices were suboptimal. Even after the introduction of vaccines, outbreaks of measles, pertussis and varicella, among others, occurred sporadically, despite widespread (sometimes mandatory) HCW immunisation against 'childhood' infections. Modified pertussis and varicella can occur, even in fully immunised adults, and measles can be introduced by unimmunised patients or staff. Even small outbreaks can cause serious disease, especially among vulnerable (e.g. newborn, elderly or immunocompromised) patients, and require costly control measures.[174-176] Annual influenza vaccination is recommended and is usually free but not mandatory for most HCWs in Australia; however, uptake has been variable and often poor.[177] Nosocomial outbreaks of seasonal influenza and other respiratory and gastrointestinal (e.g. norovirus) viral infections, for which there are no vaccines, regularly cause staff absenteeism and potentially serious disease in vulnerable patients.[178-181]

PART C
PEOPLE AND PROGRAMS

The most important influences on hospital IPC are, of course, people, including the patients and the diverse groups of actors on whom their care depends: frontline HCWs (nursing, medical and allied health professionals and support staff); IPC and infectious disease specialists (ICPs, microbiologists, infectious disease physicians, epidemiologists); and hospital and health service administrators who determine priorities and allocate resources. This section explores how their roles, attitudes and interactions have evolved and influenced IPC programs, policies and practices since the 1960s.

1.7 1960s—Surgeons, bacteriologists and early ICP appointments

IPC was relatively neglected during the early 20th century, but reinvigorated intermittently, particularly during

---

[xiii]HCV ribonucleic acid (RNA) in serum is a marker of active/chronic HCV infection in a minority of people who have been infected with HCV (as shown by the presence of anti-HCV). HCV-RNA is detected by reverse-transcriptase polymerase chain reaction (RT-PCR).

HAI outbreaks. Until the 1970s, surgical asepsis, operating theatre rituals and hygienic ward practices were largely enforced by senior surgeons or charge sisters. Bacteriologists in clinical pathology departments were able to identify HAI outbreaks and trends. Some took the initiative to investigate causes and suggest remedies, by observation and discussion with staff in wards and departments. Others undertook HAI-related research, often in collaboration with clinicians. There were few hospital medical microbiologists at the time, but some scientist-bacteriologists made major contributions to HAI epidemiology. They were, effectively, the first ICPs.[182-184]

One hospital scientist-bacteriologist, who took on an informal role as 'hospital detective', was a participant in the qualitative study. As a new science graduate, in 1956, he was appointed to the Alfred Hospital's Department of Bacteriology, where the senior bacteriologist, Glen Buckle, had a longstanding interest in hospital cross-infection.[185] Buckle encouraged him to *spend time in the wards because that's where all the action was* (see Table 1.2, Q2;1). He visited the wards, where the charge sisters were *usually ex-army and very frightening* but tolerated his presence if he obeyed their rules. By checking laboratory results, he identified infection clusters and investigated causes[182,183] (Table 1.2, Q2;2).

Dr Phyllis Rountree was a prominent, post-war, hospital research scientist at Royal Prince Alfred Hospital (RPAH) in Sydney. She documented many aspects of the bacteriology, antibiotic resistance and epidemiology of *S. aureus* infections.[185] Her numerous publications had a profound influence on hospital IPC in Australia and internationally during the 1940s–70s. She described *S. aureus* colonisation, SSI and neonatal infection rates and transmission routes, the emergence of new strains and the effects of widespread antibiotic use on resistance.[53,74,75,81,186]

During the 1960s, the few medical microbiologists in Australian hospitals included Drs Ahalya (Babi) Rao (Princess Alexandra Hospital [PAH], Brisbane), Sydney Bell (Prince of Wales Hospital [POWH], Sydney), Robin Pavillard (Royal Perth Hospital [RPH]) and Bryan Stratford (St Vincent's Hospital, Melbourne)[185] among others. They were concerned about increasing HAI rates, and were often instrumental in the formation of ICCs and appointment of ICPs. As ICC members they largely determined what the ICPs' roles would be and often closely supervised their work (Table 1.2, Q2;3-5).

At PAH, in Brisbane, a senior surgeon initiated the formation of an ICC, the members of which were himself, the medical microbiologist and the surgical supervisor. They appointed Nancy Wernigk in 1962, as the first Australian ICP.[70,187] Wernigk was influential among the nursing and other hospital staff, but her activities were directed and closely supervised by the medical microbiologist (Table 1.2, Q2;4–6). She and members of the ICC, separately, published detailed descriptions of her duties.[70,187] Her primary roles were to monitor surgical wounds and report SSI rates to the ICC, but she also instructed ward nurses in aseptic wound dressing technique, checked sterilisation methods throughout the hospital and undertook special projects, such as screening of operating theatre staff for *S. aureus* colonisation and decolonising carriers.[187] According to the consultants who initiated her appointment, '...her very presence in the wards and in the theatres is a reminder of the problems of hospital infection'.[70] Moreover, the surgeons acknowledged her essential contribution to their research. 'It would be difficult to conduct a trial such as this unless there was a special person—for example, an infection control sister—available to record the results without the distraction of other major duties'.[188]

The spread of neomycin-resistant *S. aureus* at POWH in Sydney (Table 1.2, Q2;7) prompted the formation of an ICC and appointment of an ICP, in 1965. Alva Sparks was the first ICP in NSW.[189,190] She developed rapport with the ward sisters, implemented a strict wound dressing protocol, established a comprehensive IPC program, and trained a team of ICPs (Table 1.2, Q2;8). Her appointment to the microbiology department was controversial, because the Director of Nursing believed all nurses should be part of the nursing division (Table 1.2, Q2;9–10).

In Perth, Dr Robin Pavillard, a UK-trained medical microbiologist, was appointed to the RPH in 1966. He was particularly interested in IPC and familiar with developments in the USA and UK. He appointed a senior ICS not long after he arrived in Perth[185] (Table 1.2, Q2;11). Several other ICPs were appointed during the 1960s, including at Royal Alexandra Hospital for Children in Sydney, Royal Adelaide Hospital and Adelaide Children's Hospital.[190]

According to participants in the qualitative study, these early ICPs were experienced nurses who had worked as charge sisters in other wards or departments. They were knowledgeable and confident enough to take on and define a hospital-wide ICP role and implement practice improvements to prevent or manage HAI risks, often with limited support or even opposition from the nursing hierarchy. Because some of their self-appointed roles impinged on ward sisters' domains and were not sanctioned

TABLE 1.2 People and programs: medical microbiologists

Q2;1	'That's where I started my infection control, though it wasn't called that. I classed myself as the hospital detective, like Mr Buckle. He knew every engineer, every cleaner, everybody in the hospital and they knew him.' '[I] inveigled my way into every department in the hospital, so I knew about the kitchens, I knew how they cooked the food, [and] how it was delivered, I knew the air-conditioning, the water systems, I knew every system in the hospital' [HS1].
Q2;2	'A lot of outbreaks were [due to] poor sterilisation, poor disinfection, lack of cleaning of instruments, design of pan flushers, urinals' [HS1].
Q2;3	'The Infection Control Committee was dominated by medical staff, I don't recall anyone from nursing being there—medical administrator, the microbiologist, I think someone from the medical side, and a surgical person' [ICP2].
Q2;4	'She was stationed in the microbiology department. I taught her about bacteria. She had access to all the figures, and every morning [would ask] 'Have we got any new staphylococcal infections?' She would look at the wounds [and] collect any material that was not being sent' [MM6].
Q2;5	'The infection control sister gave advice from the angle of nursing, but we kept medical advice under medical control. We didn't let nursing become the head. [ICC members] took a daily interest—you have to really hold the reins' [MM6].
Q2;6	[A senior surgeon] 'wanted to know the rate of infection [but] there were surgeons in the hospital who did not want us to look at their wounds. One very senior surgeon was antagonistic; he was a powerful man, so we had to be very careful. We did it with diplomacy, but he wouldn't allow us to follow his cases' [MM6].
Q2;7	'We'd been gathering the information for a year ... and we had a problem with neomycin-resistant Staph aureus. Every second surgeon had a little puffer of neomycin powder in his pocket ... whenever he looked at a wound, he sprinkled [some] on it. We formed an infection control committee and persuaded the staff to ban the use of all topical antibiotics. At first there was tremendous resistance, but we persuaded them. In fact, the surgical staff became the greatest converts and would report anybody they saw using topical neomycin. It had great results, gradually neomycin-resistant staph disappeared' [MM1].
Q2;8	'Alva Sparks was a nurse of the old school—starched uniform, starched white veil. She kept her own meticulous records, by hand. She became interested in cross-infection with pseudomonas in neonatal humidicribs and started the practice of drying them in the sunlight ... to eliminate surface carriage. She kept control by strict hygiene, Listerian principles, and antibiotic restrictions' [MM1].
Q2;9	'One of the biggest problems I had with the appointment of the infection control sister was the matron. [She] was really up in arms. The board appointed [the ICS] responsible to me and no way could you have a nurse responsible to anybody but the matron. These arguments went on for years. [The] compromise, was that the [ICS] was professionally responsible to the microbiologist and administratively to the matron' [MM1].
Q2;10	"Sparksy" stayed on for years and worked with microbiology. The nursing administration had to tolerate it, because Sparksy was a formidable person. I think they saw the value [but] the position never survived in micro after she retired in the '80s' [MM8].
Q2;11	'[At RPH] Robin was very interested in infection control. He appointed infection control nurses and set up a small infection control laboratory. He was widely read [and aware of] what the Americans were doing but also of what Graham Ayliffe and others in the UK were doing. The first infection control nurse was recording post-operative infections [and] it was pretty obvious which ward had the highest rates. Robin was quite diplomatic. He'd make sure the information was accurate and talk to the surgeons first and usually got them onside. He would work with the nursing staff too, usually starting with the Director of Nursing' [MM7].
Q2;12	'[The first ICP at RMH] was appointed not long after Robin—he wanted an infection control nurse; he saw them as the frontline troops. She was based in microbiology, [which] wasn't an issue. Robin had good liaison with the senior medical staff and heads of nursing and medical administration. He was the first clinical microbiologist at RMH. Before then the clinical pathologists sat in the lab and never got out. Robin was a new phenomenon, who didn't restrict himself to the lab' [MM4].
Q2;13	'[He] was particularly interested in hospital hygiene and cleanliness. [He would do] ward rounds with the cleaners [and] tell them how important it was to have a clean hospital... "to suck up the skin squames and pus, and the staph, in vacuum cleaners with filters ... You guys are terribly important for keeping infection at bay". He had good rapport and they did a damn good job' [MM4].
Q2;14	'He had an interesting vision of the importance of minutiae in the hospital and the operating theatres. We used to monitor them with settle plates. At 6 am there's nothing on the settle plates, but when you get the bustling of the nurses setting up, the surgeons coming in, germs start appearing. It's people germs come from, the more people you have rushing in and out, the more problems' [MM4].
Q2;15	'She would periodically find that there was so much staphylococcal colonisation on the ward that she would have it closed. She was powerful enough to do that—a scientist in charge of microbiology who would say to the Professor of Surgery, "This ward's going to be closed until we've cleaned it and the patients who are colonised are sent somewhere else." In my time at the hospital, I never managed to have a ward closed for any reason—surgeons wouldn't allow it, so it didn't happen' [MM3].

TABLE 1.2 People and programs: medical microbiologists—cont'd

Q2;16	'The matron had a simple philosophy that every nurse is her own infection control officer. She said that's our job, and there's no need to have anyone particular doing it because we all do it' [MM3].
Q2;17	'The medical administration became totally involved when hospital accreditation became important ... Unless we had a properly operating infection control committee, regular meetings and minutes, we weren't going to get accredited. This was in the late '70s ... we did this because we had to' [MM3].
Q2;18	'I had pretty much carte blanche to do what I thought was sensible. I took away from the US quite a lot of information about hospital epidemiology. I made a ploy to have infection control one of the senior nursing initiatives and so a post for infection control and epidemiology was established. [I appointed] a senior nurse who'd been in a variety of semi-administrative nursing roles and a very canny manager' [MM5].
Q2;19	'It was an academic initiative that arose out of the wound infections scenario. It had a high profile in the hospital and seemed to be a good thing. That's how infection control was seen to be an essential way to go. We didn't have to prove anything' [MM5].

by nursing directors, they needed tact and diplomacy to win the support and respect of their colleagues.

1.8 1970s–90s—Hesitant beginnings and evolution of hospital IPC programs

1.8.1 Medical microbiologists and IPC

The implementation of early IPC programs was the responsibility of individual hospitals, and often dependent on the initiative of individual microbiologists or clinicians, with variable support from hospital administrators. Most Australian hospitals did not establish IPC programs or appoint ICPs until the 1970–80s, and then it was often in response to accreditation requirements. The Australian Council on Healthcare Standards (ACHS) was formed in 1974 to establish practice standards and implement (voluntary) hospital accreditation.[191] Its requirements for infection surveillance and control programs included the need for hospitals to establish a multidisciplinary ICC, appoint a full- or part-time ICN, review reports of HAIs, identify patients requiring isolation, and monitor disinfection, sterilisation and environmental cleaning practices. How these requirements were to be fulfilled was undefined and there was little specific guidance, except from overseas literature.[189] In 1980 the New South Wales Health Commission defined the ICP's primary role, vaguely, as coordinating IPC policies set by the ICC.[192]

Medical microbiologists were appointed to many major teaching hospitals during the 1970s, often when multidisciplinary clinical pathology services were split into specialty departments. In 1975, Pavillard moved to Melbourne, where he was appointed as the first medical microbiologist at the RMH. MRSA was already causing concern and 'he and his deputy ... were fearless in their campaigns to educate surgeons'.[185] Pavillard appointed an ICP soon after he arrived (Table 1.2, Q2;12)

and rapidly established collaborative relationships with medical, surgical, nursing and administrative hierarchies. He had a particular interest in environmental cleanliness. He established a rapport with the cleaners and monitored their work, by personal observation and extensive bacteriological sampling. Pavillard was a visible and influential presence in the hospital (Table 1.2; Q2;12-14).

Another medical microbiologist, appointed in the early 1970s, reflected ruefully that, as a newly qualified consultant, he had far less influence than his senior-scientist predecessor, who had been a formidable presence at RPAH for many years (Table 1.2, Q2;15). Faced with major HAI outbreaks, including 'rampant MRSA' and serious Gram-negative infections, he was convinced the hospital needed to appoint an ICP. Despite his lobbying, the matron refused, since she believed that IPC was the role of every nurse (Table 1.2, Q2;16). So, the task fell to the infectious diseases registrar, who investigated several serious HAI outbreaks during the 1970s. Cases of *P. aeruginosa* meningitis in the neonatal ICU were traced to inadequate disinfection of jugs used to mix infant formula, and a cluster of *Enterobacter aerogenes* SSIs in cardiac surgical patients, to contaminated cardioplegia solution. It was not until several years later, with accreditation imminent, that an ICP was appointed (Table 1.2, Q2;17).

A newly appointed Professor/Director of Microbiology at Flinders Medical Centre in Adelaide had a very different experience (Table 1.2, Q2;18). He appointed an ICP, who 'came in to help' with 'an intensive postoperative monitoring system' which he had initiated, with the Professor of Surgery. Having documented an unacceptably high rate of SSIs, following colorectal surgery, they appointed a full-time wound manager and secured pharmaceutical company funds for a trial of perioperative antibiotic prophylaxis. They demonstrated the value of SSI surveillance with a successful intervention, by demonstrating a significant reduction in SSI rates[193] (see Part D). This established the value of IPC, and the role of the ICP was readily accepted by hospital staff and administration (Table 1.2, Q2;19).

1.8.2 A new wave of administration-initiated ICP appointments

Many more hospital IPC programs were established during the 1970s. By 1980, at least 14 major Sydney hospitals[189] and many large hospitals in other states had appointed ICPs. However, most smaller hospitals only did so when 'voluntary' accreditation became unavoidable, and then they often appointed relatively junior, part-time ICNs, without relevant training, experience or a position description (Table 1.3, Q3;1–2). Even senior nurses with experience as operating theatre or ward sisters rarely had IPC training. They were expected to get on with it and, fortunately, most of them did (Table 1.3, Q3;3). Nursing

TABLE 1.3 People and programs: infection control professionals

Q3;1	'I knew nothing. I didn't even know where to go for help. It wasn't like just ringing around and saying, what do you do with your infection control? In those two days, I had to find a few hours to find out about infection control' [ICP3].
Q3;2	'I was just "a nurse". I didn't get any acknowledgement. The Director of Nursing appointed someone because it would look good at accreditation ... I never felt I was responsible to anyone. I had to develop an infection control program from scratch. It was early days and you had to be very careful because people didn't like somebody walking into the wards to see what was going on' [ICP1].
Q3;3	'When I started, nobody knew about IPC, and nobody wanted to know about it. In my pushy way I changed all that. I just told them to do it' [ICP4].
Q3;4	'The Director of Nursing wanted an infection control program that was only education. She didn't want you to look into anything and say, "Well, perhaps there are things we could do better". She just wanted a program for accreditation' [ICP1].
Q3;5	'In 1985 I had a part-time job in [a small private hospital which] had just embarked upon accreditation, and they'd booked an accreditation survey. I was working there as a ward nurse and the director of nursing said "We need someone to be responsible for infection control, staff health, quality management and environmental services— you're the perfect person!". I learnt on the job. I had very few people that I could go to for information. The public sector had a few ICPs that you could contact if you really needed assistance but generally, they weren't offering a lot of support to the private sector. They didn't have a lot of support themselves either' [ICP5].
Q3;6	'I went to [a nearby teaching] hospital, where [two people] were working in infection control and I started talking to them and getting some ideas about what I should do and working with the microbiologists, because I thought that might be where I could start to see what organisms look like. I'd read the plates every day ... I'd look to see if it was an MRSA or a staph, I'd go and have a look at the wound, so that I was well known on the wards' [ICP3].
Q3;7	[In Adelaide] 'We started getting together because none of us knew what we were supposed to be doing really. We'd meet, we'd chat, we'd support each other, because we all had different structures in our hospitals. We formed the Infection Control Group, probably 1978, and started meeting regularly. We functioned quite well as a group, but we were predominantly led by the microbiology people' [ICP2].
Q3;8	[In Sydney] 'We had an association, but because we were so thinly spread, we broke it up into [local groups] so we could get together. We had a monthly meeting and people like Yvonne Cossart, from the University of Sydney who was very supportive of infection control, organised guest speakers ...' [ICP1].
Q3;9	'The private sector was isolated and education was lacking, so we set up an educator's forum amongst the independent private hospitals in New South Wales with good representation, monthly teleconferences, sharing information, policies and procedures—if you're having a problem somebody else must be too' [ICP5].
Q3;10	'I got into infection control when someone took maternity leave in 1989. I didn't have any experience ... The infection control team was one of the first who had historically worked as a team of nurses, microbiologists and infectious diseases physicians. It was well-supported and collaborative. You weren't working in isolation. We had support from the surgeons, because we'd all worked at that hospital for so long ...' [ICP6].
Q3;11	'... people didn't like somebody walking into the wards to see what was going on. The other problem then was "I'm a doctor, I don't want you to look at what I'm doing, I know what I'm doing and it's correct" [ICP1]
Q3;12	'In the early days, we were pushing against it. After an infection control meeting, when I'd said, "We need to do this, if we're going to get accreditation ..." [a senior doctor] whispered to me as I walked out, "Listen, girly, we don't do it that way here"' [ICP1].
Q3;13	'A new CEO said, "There's no point having [an ICP] if they're not listening to what you're saying and doing something". He said, "If you're going down to the wards to see a patient you need to document it in the notes". I got hauled before the Medical Director for daring to write in a patient's notes, but the CEO intervened and said, "Well, why did you call her down there?"' [ICP1].
Q3;14	'We are now expected to do so much documentation and reporting and the work involved in so many different committees ... it's pandemonium. I had to make the effort to go up to the ward just to get out and talk to people and find out what's happening. The amount of documentation for the new accreditation guidelines drives ICPs mad' [ICP1].

Directors' expectations of these new ICPs varied from minimal to unrealistic (Table 1.3, Q3;4–5). The ICPs' main sources of support were either the hospital microbiologist or colleagues at other hospitals, with whom they shared knowledge, experiences and encouragement in informal groups, which developed into state-based infection control associations (Table 1.3, Q3;6–9).

In October 1985, representatives of the state-based associations met in Sydney and agreed to form a national group, the Australian Infection Control Association (AICA). Its first annual meeting was in Fremantle, in 1986, and the first national conference in Canberra, in 1987. The first 10 years of AICA's history were documented in detail by Elaine Graham, the first ICP at Canberra Hospital and a member and vice-president of the first AICA executive.[190]

By the late 1980s, most major hospitals had well-established IPC units, with one or more ICPs. A nurse appointed to one of these units, even with no IPC experience, could learn on the job, with guidance from experienced colleagues (Table 1.3, Q3;10). By then, there were also more opportunities for IPC training and education. Courses of varying structure, content and duration were offered by the College of Nursing and at Fremantle and Sydney Hospitals in the 1980s, and later at the Albion Street Centre in Sydney and Mayfield Centre in Melbourne, among others. Many larger hospitals ran in-house courses that others could attend. Griffith University was the first to offer graduate IPC courses (certificate and masters) in the 1990s. The cost and availability of financial support and approved leave for ICPs to attend these courses varied.

The ICP's role was, and still is, contested in some hospitals. This was largely due to a lack of clarity or consistency about the qualifications required, if any, or the ICP's authority and status within the hospital. Consequently, the experience, training and competence of nurses appointed to these positions varied. Some faced hostility or indifference from senior nursing and medical staff because they were perceived to be interfering with or policing clinical care; or because their role was perceived to be one of data collector, without clinical responsibility (Table 1.3, Q3;11–12). Active support from the hospital administration was essential for them to be effective, but also highly variable (Table 1.3, Q3;13).

PART D
POLICIES AND PRACTICES

Many IPC practices were well established during the 20th century, but variably implemented in Australian hospitals. The effectiveness of IPC practice was (and is) highly dependent on administrative leadership and governance, the physical environment, properly implemented evidence-based policies, the capacity (time available, training and experience) of ICPs and the co-operation of HCWs, patients and visitors. This section briefly summarises the development of several illustrative IPC practices that are particularly important in protecting hospital patients and staff, and the general community, from HAIs.

1.9 Segregating people who are (or may be) infectious

1.9.1 Isolation and quarantine

Sick people with contagious diseases have been isolated, to protect others, since antiquity. The concept of confining healthy but potentially infectious people for 40 days after a known or likely exposure to a contagious disease probably originated with Hippocrates. The term 'quarantine' dates from the 14th century, when ships arriving in Venice and other coastal cities, from plague-infected ports, were required to anchor off-shore for 40 days.[194] A similar practice, in 19th century Sydney, protected the settlement from the introduction of diseases that had broken out during the long voyage from England, such as typhus, smallpox or measles.[195,196]

In the late 19th century, several specialist infectious diseases hospitals were established in Australia, including the Coast (later Prince Henry) Hospital, at Little Bay in Sydney (1881); Victoria (later Metropolitan) Infectious Diseases Hospital, at Shenton Park in Perth (1893); and the Queens Memorial (later Fairfield) Infectious Diseases Hospital, in Melbourne (1904). These hospitals, and infectious disease wards in general hospitals, cared for sick people with diseases such as smallpox, diphtheria, typhoid, scarlet fever and measles. In 1919, when pandemic influenza reached Australia, hospital facilities were rapidly overwhelmed and makeshift hospitals were set up in tents and public buildings.[197] Once many of the common epidemic diseases had been all but eliminated by sanitation, immunisation and/or antibiotic therapy, most infectious disease hospitals were closed or repurposed.

In the 1970s, patients colonised with MROs were often segregated to prevent transmission to other patients. Sometimes wards were closed as a short-term solution, but in the 1980s, as the prevalence of MROs increased, the supply of new antibiotics began to dwindle, and BBVs emerged, different solutions were needed. Some hospitals opened or reopened isolation wards or referred patients to former isolation hospitals; some made do with limited numbers of single rooms (Table 1.4, Q4;1–4).Vulnerable patients were sometimes protected from exposure to MRSA by segregating them instead (Table 1.4, Q4;5).

1.9.2 Universal and standard precautions

In 1988, the CDC published recommendations for the protection of HCWs against BBV infections, including blood and body fluid precautions when caring for all patients, irrespective of their infection status.[198] Universal precautions specified the use of PPE, including gloves, gowns and face protection, to protect skin

TABLE 1.4 Policies and practices

Isolation of (potentially) infectious patients	
Q4;1	'Shenton Park Rehabilitation Hospital had six high security isolation rooms, with access to the outside. Each room had a garden and an anteroom at negative pressure to the corridor, and the room was at negative pressure to the ante room. They were high quality in terms of infection control' [MM7].
Q4;2	'We had a mixture of people, who were there [at Shenton Park] because of their TB or whatever. The spinal unit took patients from all over the world for rehabilitation. A man from India had a multi-resistant Pseudomonas in a wound that had broken down, that was really difficult to contain' [ICP7].
Q4;3	'We had a staph isolation ward in the old Marks Pavilion, at Prince Henry Hospital, when it ceased to be full of infectious diseases patients. [Later] they converted Marks to an AIDS ward' [MM8].
Q4;4	'They tried putting some of the infections in Marks. It was a bit of a disaster because "out of sight, out of mind"— they were neglected, but they had strict isolation. In the old wards at Prince of Wales, they had four side rooms and they were isolated—[the ICP] made sure they had their own staff' [MM1].
Q4;5	'In the '80s MRSA came back with a vengeance. It was a real concern. One of our orthopaedic surgeons solved the problem. The Department of Health wanted to close [an old hospital] that had a couple of operating theatres. He said "We'd like to have that for clean orthopaedic surgery. We'll make sure no-one who is MRSA colonised is allowed in this hospital". We had a strict apartheid system for clean orthopaedic surgery which worked unbelievably well. We never had problems with MRSA' [MM3].
Q4;6	[At a Children's Hospital]: 'Because of the AIDS epidemic and scare we had a huge issue if people didn't do universal/ standard precautions. They'd say "children are innocent, they couldn't possibly have anything, you don't need to wear gloves". But I was concerned because we had cardiac patients from overseas who had hep B. A lot of infection control practitioners used HIV/AIDS to get people to wear gloves working near body fluids' [ICP1].
Q4;7	'HIV/AIDS changed IPC ... excessive glove use came in, that has made [a] nightmare for us. It led the foray into proper personal protective equipment, better sharps management. Prior to 1985 nurses really never wore gloves. Now they wear them all the time, to the point that it's obsessive-compulsive behaviour, some wear gloves everywhere. The minute they get to work they put a pair of gloves on, and they wash them. Trying to change that behaviour is hopeless' [ICP9].
Q4;8	'In the 80s, we had a couple of haemophiliac children with HIV and the dentists refused to do dental work on them. We implemented universal precautions, which was seen as the panacea. Then we realised, when you still had respiratory patients, and patients with gastro, that didn't resolve all the problems. We were starting to get MROs, and resistant Haemophilus influenzae patients. That's when standard precautions came back, with transmission-based precautions' [ICP2].
HAI surveillance	
Q4;9	'... the Professor of Surgery reckoned we should be able to do better than 30–40% post-colectomy wound infection ... so we put in a very intensive postoperative monitoring system. We appointed a full-time nurse as a wound manager/research person to document postoperative symptoms and established it was time to go to short-course perioperative medication' [MM5].
Q4;10	'The national survey wasn't useful because it was in the middle of a surgeons' strike [in NSW]' [ICP1].
Q4;11	'CHRISP had three streams of research: hand hygiene, the economics of infection costs in hospitals, and surveillance. Central coordination of antibiotic policy started in Queensland, as part of CHRISP's remit. Eventually there was an acceptance that [CHRISP] would write the infection control policies that were implemented throughout the state [for] hospitals that were to be accredited by ACHS' [MM2].

TABLE 1.4 Policies and practices—cont'd

	Hand hygiene
Q4;12	[1950s]: *'There wasn't the same carry on like they do now, but before they attended a patient, they were required to wash their hands. And they did'* [MM1].
Q4;13	[1960s]: *'Some did, some didn't, but the big thing was diplomacy, because people didn't like to be told what to do... you* [had to] *approach them diplomatically ...'* [MM6].
Q4;14	[1970s]: *'Surgeons were conscientious about the routine pre-operative "scrub". In the theatres there were rituals that were pretty much adhered to; in the wards, they were god-like of course, but I don't think they washed their hands'* [MM3].
Q4;15	*'In the '70s, there were escalating attempts to encourage handwashing and endless correspondence about what's safe for nurses to use. Any company that had a product ... was entitled to come along and lobby the administrators and accountants to have the products introduced. The hospital was full of all sorts of products, but by the end of the '70s we were rationalising'* [MM3].
Q4;16	*'We didn't have Gram-negative infections. I guess it was to do with hand hygiene. In 1991 we had a handwashing campaign. There was a jingle about handwashing on hold on the switchboard that drove everyone mad but created awareness. I became known as the handwashing king. They'd see me in the corridor and say, "Oh, I washed my hands today"* [MM8].
Q4;17	*'The hand hygiene program has been a good model—to raise awareness of infection prevention and control and provide opportunities to do some measurement, even if it's not particularly robust, to see whether hand hygiene impacts upon other areas of risk, e.g. SABS. But we need to evolve because it is a very labour-intensive program, and the hand hygiene compliance data does not reflect what is truly happening at the bedside'* [ICP5].
Q4;18	*'I think the NHHI is hopeless. I mean it's a Hawthorne effect. If people are watching, they know what they're supposed to be doing and so people go and do it. I think it's actually not a very useful use of money'* [MM2].
Q4;19	*'I've always thought that Hand Hygiene Australia was too onerous, and I've had problems with direct observation. The data are not accurate. The auditors watch the teams come on their rounds and they insist that every time they come out of every room, everyone uses the product. And that just doesn't make sense—they're being treated like kindergarten children'* [ICP6].
Q4;20	*'Doctors' hand hygiene is really poor in comparison to nurses, between 62–72% compliant.* [However] *doctors in our ICU do really well. We've had a big improvement, but they had a very low baseline to start. That was on the direction of their director. He sent a letter to all visiting consultants that basically said, "if you fail to comply with 'bare below the elbows' and our hand hygiene and PPE practices, you'll be asked not to come back". He only had to send one of the vascular surgeons on their way, for everyone to start to do the right thing'* [ICP8]

and mucous membranes, when exposure to blood or body fluid was anticipated; safe handling and disposal of needles and other sharps; and handwashing before and after patient contact, whether or not gloves were used. In Australia, the Australian National Council on AIDS (ANCA) and NHMRC, jointly, published 'Universal body substance precautions', in 1990. An updated version, 'Management guidelines for the control of infectious disease hazards in healthcare', was published in 1993, following investigation of the patient-to-patient HIV transmission event.[158] This was Australia's first national IPC guidelines and (one of) the first, globally, to include respiratory precautions[199] (Table 1.1, Q1;10).

The principle of universal precautions was that all patients should be managed as if they had a BBV infection.[198] This avoided stigmatisation of patients with known HIV infection and protected HCWs caring for an unrecognised BBV carrier. Some HCWs questioned the practicability and effectiveness of universal precautions and compliance was often poor, especially among doctors (Table 1.4, Q4;6), who often lobbied for stronger measures for patients known to be infected.[200,201] A survey of Australian anaesthetists found that two-thirds of them wanted universal preoperative screening for HBV, HIV and HCV. However, many of them admitted to not observing basic precautions; most did not ask patients about risk factors for BBV infections, two-thirds said that they routinely resheathed needles and many had suffered needlestick injuries, and most did not wear gloves while giving anaesthetics.[202,203] By contrast, many ICPs believed that HCWs, overall, frequently used gloves in excess of recommended indications (Table 1.4, Q4;7).

In 1996, CDC replaced universal precautions with standard precautions which, like the earlier Australian guidelines, included routine contact and respiratory precautions (Table 1.4, Q4;8). Additional/transmission-based precautions were recommended for patients with suspected or known infection.[199] In 2007, CDC recommended contact precautions and single room isolation (CPI) or cohorting of patients who were colonised with MRSA, VRE or other target MROs.[204]

1.9.3 Contact precautions and single room isolation (CPI)

A version of CPI for MRO-colonised patients had been widely practised in Australia since the 1980s, when the prevalence of MRSA and some MDR GNBs increased rapidly. However, the goals of CPI were poorly defined. Was it intended to eradicate the target pathogen or reduce its prevalence? What were the measures of success or failure? Were there adverse effects? In the absence of answers, this practice continued as established practice in many hospitals, without evaluation of its effectiveness.

CPI, plus hospital-wide patient screening and enhanced routine IPC measures, undoubtedly contributed to the control or even eradication of MRSA[98,101,205] or VRE[126,127,206] in non-endemic settings, but such stringent measures could not be sustained indefinitely. Compliance with contact precautions is variable and universal patient screening impractical.[207] Two recent reviews[206,208] identified methodological flaws, including simultaneous introduction of other measures and/or a lack of control groups, in most studies designed to assess the effectiveness of CPI. These reviews and recent Australian commentaries[209,210] concluded that the evidence for a significant benefit of CPI over standard precautions, to prevent MRO transmission, was weak at best.

Moreover, there was strong circumstantial evidence that CPI could be harmful. It could interfere with patient care and was associated with increased risks of preventable injury, medication errors and adverse psychological effects, and led to excess use of resources.[206,208,211-213] Genomic evidence has shown that de novo/endogenous generation of VR E. faecium, during broad spectrum antibiotic therapy, is as important as cross-transmission.[214] 'Horizontal' IPC measures, applied irrespective of MRO colonisation, can reduce transmission as effectively as CPI. These include full compliance with recommended IPC practices, including standard precautions, HAI surveillance with feedback to clinicians, and antibiotic stewardship. Disinfectant skin washing of patients in

high-risk settings is an effective additional measure.[215-217] A practice such as CPI that is minimally effective (if at all) and compromises patient safety, and for which there are suitable alternatives, must be regarded as unethical.[209] The limited indications for CPI should be clearly defined and the practice implemented appropriately, to prevent patient harm and optimise benefit, only when required.[210,218]

1.10 HAI surveillance— 19th and early 20th century

Since the 19th century, many clinicians and researchers have recognised the important role of monitoring of HAI rates, identifying risk factors and causes, and evaluating the effectiveness of preventive measures. In Australia, HAI surveillance has been sporadic. Many different approaches, of variable reliability, have been used: in-hospital monitoring or project-based surveys by microbiologists or clinicians; mandatory or voluntary laboratory or clinician reporting to public health authorities or specialist agencies; and automated collection of medical record-based administrative data.

Rountree's studies and published reports of the prevalence, strain types, antibiotic resistance and clinical effects of S. aureus, over many years, often prompted timely local interventions. They provided invaluable insights into the epidemiology of S. aureus infection with ongoing relevance to IPC practices generally. Recognition of rising SSI rates and rapid emergence of antibiotic resistance associated with topical use based on in-hospital surveillance prompted the appointments of Australia's first ICPs (see Parts B and C). However, the full potential of HAI surveillance to improve patient outcomes requires long-term commitment, clearly defined goals, timely interventions and periodic review. Without them, surveillance can be little more than costly and ineffectual data collection.

In 1973, a group of Brisbane surgeons published the results of the (until then) largest-ever prospective study of SSI rates, spanning nine years.[219] A single ICP classified 20,822 operative procedures, inspected and graded surgical wounds, collected swabs for culture as required and documented SSI rates. The paper provides detailed and interesting data on a wide range of different types of operation, but there is no mention of feedback of results to surgeons or interventions resulting from them. SSI rates fluctuated, over time, but there were no consistent reductions. For some types of operation, the rates were described as 'unacceptable'. Based on this, it is not clear whether the prolonged surveillance and co-pious data collected, contributed (or was intended to contribute) to better patient outcomes.

By contrast, a shorter prospective survey of SSI rates and an effective intervention clearly demonstrated benefit. It was a well-planned (and funded) double-blind, controlled trial of short-course perioperative IV cefoxitin, in colorectal surgery, which resulted in a significantly lower SSI rate in recipients of prophylactic cefoxitin (3%) than in controls (27%).[193] The study provided benefit to almost half of the study participants and, by providing robust evidence of the effectiveness of short-course perioperative prophylaxis, to many future patients (Table 1.4, Q4;9). According to one of the investigators, it established the value of IPC and hospital epidemiology in the hospital where it was done (Table 1.2, Q2;19).

1.10.1 Further development of HAI surveillance

Australia's first and, until recently, only national HAI prevalence survey was conducted in 1984. Data were collected using standardised methodology, in July 1984, on 28,643 patients in 269 metropolitan, rural, public and private hospitals with >50 acute beds. The overall HAI prevalence was 6.3%, of which surgical wound (34%), urinary tract (22%), respiratory (19%), skin (4.4%), gastrointestinal (3.4%) and bloodstream (1.6%) infections accounted for the majority.[220] The HAI prevalence, in hospitals with >500 beds (8.6%), was similar to that (9%) in a comparable 1980 survey of large hospitals in England and Wales.[221] Prevalence surveys can provide valuable data on large patient samples and identify high-risk targets for prospective surveillance and remedial action needed to reduce HAI morbidity and costs; but they have limitations.[222] They are biased towards longer stay patients, at increased risk of HAI; data are collected by numerous surveyors, which can introduce inconsistencies; and they represent a snapshot in time, so are subject to unpredictable factors (Table 1.4, Q4;10).

In 1993, the ACHS introduced clinical indicators for hospitals seeking accreditation. HAI indicators were surgical wound infections (SWIs) and healthcare-associated bacteraemias.[223] These indicators were unreliable; neither standardised definitions nor risk stratification were used, and a minority of hospitals contributed data.[224] In a critique of the ACHS clinical indicator program McLaws et al argued that its cost–effectiveness would be improved by a focus on high-risk procedures and the use of standardised definitions, such as those used by USA's National Nosocomial Infection Surveillance System (NNIS).[224] Critics who were opposed to clinical indicators argued that HAI surveillance was too complex and costly, and potentially misleading.[225] This was undoubtedly true for the clinical indicator program as it was, with ill-defined methodology and inadequate resources. A survey of ICPs in 1999 found that most hospitals employed fewer than the recommended ICP FTEs. Surveillance occupied much of their time, but many lacked adequate training, clerical support or access to computers.[192]

Meanwhile, in the absence of reliable national surveillance, several states initiated their own. In NSW, the Hospital Infection Standardised Surveillance (HISS) program was piloted in 1998-9,[226] but not fully implemented. The Victorian Nosocomial Infection Surveillance System (VICNISS) coordinating centre was established in 2002[227] and is still operational. The Centre for Healthcare Related Infection Surveillance and Prevention (CHRISP) was established in Queensland in 2000.[228] CHRISP introduced sophisticated statistical methods to assess incidence trends for low prevalence HAIs[229] and incorporated state-wide IPC and antimicrobial prescribing support for smaller hospitals, in addition to HAI surveillance (Table 1.4, Q4;11). Its funding was withdrawn after a change in government.

International evidence has shown that well-structured *national* HAI surveillance programs are associated with lower HAI rates, reduced healthcare costs, more efficient data management and benchmarking, targeted IPC programs and standardised training. In 2000, ACHS finally adopted standardised SWI and BSI case definitions, developed by AICA.[230] A few years later, all states had surveillance programs using AICA or NNIS definitions, but there were still many differences between them, for example, in procedures surveyed, risk stratification methods and resources available.[231] There has been further progress in Australia since 2008, including national surveillance of SABSIs and hand hygiene compliance, with significant improvements in both. However, a comprehensive national HAI surveillance program, in Australia, remains elusive.[232]

1.11 Hand hygiene

Common sense and the observations of 19th century pioneers showed that frequent handwashing by HCWs, while caring for patients, could reduce pathogen transmission. Throughout the 20th century, hand hygiene was recognised as one of the most important IPC measures but, in practice, it was often neglected. Compliance improved during outbreaks but was otherwise variable and rarely monitored (Table 1.4, Q4;12–14). Nurses were generally more observant than doctors, but acceptable overall compliance rates were hard to achieve. There were practical problems, such as too few handbasins, often in corridors distant from the bedside; however, improved accessibility did not necessarily increase compliance.[233] The time required and frequency of recommended handwashing regimes were regarded as impractical, likely to interfere with patient care,[234] and cause skin damage.[235] The choice of handwashing product was complicated by determined marketing by manufacturers (Table 1.4, Q4;15).

Hand hygiene campaigns during the 1990s showed low baseline compliance rates and variable, perceived (Table 1.4, Q4;16) or documented, improvements. A study of doctors' handwashing practices, in 1996, was conducted in a newly opened paediatric ICU, where handbasins were located within 2–3 metres of each bed, with a choice of four handwash solutions, including alcoholic chlorhexidine. Handwashing rates were similar before and after patient contact and, at baseline, were only 11–12%. After several periods of overt observation and performance feedback, they rose to >65%, before falling to 55% a few weeks later when the study ended.[236]

A recurring barrier to hand hygiene compliance has been a perceived lack of evidence of patient benefit.[237] A review of studies from the 1970s–90s concluded that evidence for a causal relationship between improved hand hygiene compliance and lower HAI rates was convincing but limited.[235] In the late 1990s in Geneva, a hospital-wide campaign to promote the use of bedside alcohol-based hand rub (ABHR) led to overall improvement in hand hygiene compliance from 48% to 66% over three years, mainly among nurses. This was associated with decreases in MRSA transmission and HAIs.[238] ABHR with emollient was as effective as water-based products, less damaging to skin and, if supplied at the bedside, far less time consuming to use.[234,237] In Australia, this study stimulated hand hygiene campaigns in several states and a National Hand Hygiene Initiative (NHHI).

At a Melbourne teaching hospital, implementation of a suite of interventions, including the introduction of ABHR, improved cleaning procedures and a comprehensive culture-change program led to an increase in hand hygiene compliance from 21% at baseline to 49% a year later. Over the next three years, MRSA clinical isolate and BSI rates fell significantly.[216] Subsequently, a coordinated pilot study in six Victorian hospitals, followed by a rollout of a state-wide program

using the same methodology, showed similar improvements in hand hygiene compliance and reductions in MRSA infections.[239] In NSW, in 2006, the 'Clean Hands Save Lives' campaign in all public hospitals promoted the use of ABHR. Average compliance increased from 47% at baseline to 61% across three post-implementation surveys, 5–12 months later. There was sustained improvement among all professional groups, except doctors, whose compliance reverted to pre-implementation levels.[240] Although there were significant reductions in two ACHS MRSA indicators in NSW hospitals after the campaign, they could not be accepted as evidence of its effectiveness, since there were similar reductions in other states.[241] Different outcomes between the NSW and Victorian programs may reflect differences in baseline compliance and MRSA indicators used; additional measures, in the Victorian program, probably contributed.

Following these studies[216,238-241] the Australian NHHI, based on the World Health Organization's 'My 5 Moments of Hand Hygiene' program,[242] was launched in 2009. Over eight years, 2009–17, the number of participating hospitals increased from 105 to 937 and the average audited hand hygiene compliance rate, from 64% to 84% (albeit with wide variation between 'moments' and HCW groups). Across 132 major public hospitals, improved compliance was associated with significant reductions in HA-SABSI rates.[243] There were mixed reactions to the NHHI among participants in the qualitative study, many of whom were sceptical about whether the reported 84% compliance was an accurate reflection of day-to-day ward practice, and many believed that audit requirements were too onerous (Table 1.4, Q4;17–19). Local leadership was an important determinant of doctors' compliance (Table 1.4, Q4;20).

PART E
CONCLUSIONS—WHAT HAS HISTORY TAUGHT US ABOUT IPC IN AUSTRALIA?

This review of IPC history in Australia has confirmed what ICPs have known since the 1960s and 70s—that the basic principles of IPC, established during the 19th and early 20th centuries, are still valid. Moreover, proponents of both major transmission theories—contagion and miasma—were at least partly correct; infectious disease pathogens can spread by contact and/or via the air (and several other routes). Some pathogens favour one route over others, but few are exclusive. Some clinical effects of infectious diseases, such as cough or diarrhoea, promote transmission and influence the primary route, but some pathogens can also spread from people who are colonised or infected but asymptomatic. Transmission also depends on the pathogen's infectious dose, the infected person's behaviour, the susceptibility of the person exposed, the type of exposure and the environment in which it occurs.

Our modern understanding of transmission routes confirms the validity of basic IPC principles that have been recognised for centuries but forgotten and rediscovered periodically, particularly in the mid-19th century, when certain factors were shown, convincingly, to reduce HAIs, including:

- *A physical environment* that is spacious enough to allow adequate separation of patients and has suitable facilities for the isolation of infectious patients; is sufficiently well ventilated to ensure dispersal of airborne pathogens; and where surfaces, equipment and other fomites are cleaned (and, when appropriate, disinfected or sterilised) to minimise (or eliminate) contamination.
- *Administrative and governance systems* that ensure there are enough appropriately trained staff to care for all patients, safely, in a safe working environment, and senior administrators and clinical leaders who consult with, support and respect the experience and expertise of frontline staff, including IPC and infectious disease specialists.
- *IPC policies and practices* that protect patients and staff from unwitting exposure to infection and ensure that staff are consulted and informed about context-specific implementation of policies and practices, and adequately trained, equipped and supported to comply with them.
- *HAI/MRO surveillance and auditing of IPC practices* to ensure that they are effective in minimising preventable HAI rates and compliance is not unnecessarily burdensome; that timely feedback of results to clinicians, administrators and consumers leads to effective intervention, if indicated; and that policies and practices are reviewed or reinforced, in consultation with stakeholders.

Some additional principles recognised during the 20th century include that:

- Antimicrobial agents and vaccines, while enormously beneficial, are not panaceas but tools that must be used judiciously to preserve their efficacy. They complement, but cannot replace, other IPC measures; pathogenic microbes have an almost infinite capacity to outwit our most innovative efforts to eliminate them.
- ICPs and infectious disease physicians, working together and employing epidemiological surveillance and control techniques, can prevent a significant proportion of HAIs.

The spread of pathogens and MROs in healthcare (and similar) settings can usually be attributed to failure to maintain one or more of these principles. The COVID-19 pandemic has provided ample opportunity to reflect on the degree to which such failures may have contributed to SARS-CoV-2 transmission in healthcare or residential facilities that provide physical care to sick or incapacitated people. An immunologically naïve population and the high transmissibility and low infectious dose of SARS-CoV-2—especially its later variants—may have overwhelmed even the most stringently applied IPC measures. However, the pandemic has highlighted failures to apply even basic IPC measures during 'business-as-usual' or to implement learnings from past outbreaks.

1.12 Physical environment

During the COVID-19 pandemic, old arguments about transmission of respiratory pathogens (contact/droplet vs airborne) resurfaced. Early epidemiological evidence indicated that close personal contact and respiratory droplets were the predominant modes of transmission; but it was known that aerosol-generating procedures presented an increased risk of airborne transmission. It soon became apparent that aerosol-generating *behaviours*, such as coughing, shouting or singing by people infected with SARS-CoV-2, also increased the risk of airborne transmission, particularly in poorly ventilated indoor environments. It was shown that the heating, ventilation and air-conditioning (HVAC) systems in many facilities were not maintained or adjusted properly, to ensure sufficient air exchanges or flow, to disperse a highly transmissible pathogen such as SARS-CoV-2. This was highlighted when older people with dementia were admitted to hospital with COVID-19 and became distressed in the unfamiliar environment; their aerosol-generating behaviours increased the risk of transmission to HCWs.[244] When the limitations of existing HVAC systems were recognised, some could be adjusted to increase air exchange frequency; others needed to be replaced. Meanwhile other solutions, such as the use of portable 'air scrubbers', were successfully deployed.[245-247]

1.13 Administration and governance

Administrative support for IPC programs is sometimes not adequate to ensure that policies are appropriately implemented. There may be too few ICP FTEs for the number and types of beds, or the ICPs' status and authority in the hospital are not recognised, even though many have years of experience, specialist professional credentials and postgraduate qualifications. Regrettably, there is a tendency for some senior managers and doctors—who may have had little interest in IPC under 'normal' circumstances—to assume control during a crisis and override the authority of ICPs.

Before the pandemic, increasing demands for data collection and documentation required for accreditation had eroded ICPs' available time for ward-based staff support, surveillance or outbreak investigation (Table 1.3, Q3;14). Chronic staff shortages in many hospitals meant that regular IPC education and training were often neglected because staff were not allowed time to participate. Training of emergency department and ICU staff in the use of high-level PPE had often lapsed after a flurry of activity during the 2015–16 West African Ebola outbreak. Many staff had not been fit-tested or trained in the safe use of P2/N95 respirators[248,249] and so, when the pandemic began, they were ill prepared.

Hospital administrators, managers and senior clinicians were also ill prepared. HCWs' perceptions of centralised control, indecisive leadership, and inadequate communication with frontline staff, led to mistrust.[250] HCWs' fear for their own, their families' and their patients' safety may have been ameliorated by better preparation and support.[251] Their anxiety was intensified by uncertainty about transmission routes, disease severity and the likely trajectory of the pandemic, by public disagreement among 'experts'—whose expertise was variable and often in fields other than IPC or infectious diseases—and frequent changes of, or conflicting, IPC/PPE guidelines. Some HCWs believed they were being denied access to best-quality equipment and reported bullying in response to their safety concerns, which engendered a sense of inequity and loss of confidence in leadership.[251,252]

Their concerns were confirmed when they or their colleagues were infected with COVID-19 at work. Early in the pandemic, most HCWs who developed COVID-19 were infected overseas or in the community, at rates comparable to those in the general population but during the second wave, particularly in Victoria, their infection rates were significantly higher than in the community. Transmission often occurred in nonclinical areas of the hospital (meeting rooms, offices, cafeterias), almost as often as in the wards.[253] High rates of absenteeism, due to illness or exposure to COVID-19 (requiring quarantine), greatly exacerbated preexisting staff shortages.

Coda

The basic IPC principles and lessons from past infectious disease crises have been forgotten and rediscovered numerous times over at least the past 200 years. There have been significant recent improvements in IPC programs nationally, but inconsistencies between states and territories limit their effectiveness and waste resources. More improvement is needed for Australian healthcare services to be better prepared for the next (inevitable) infectious disease outbreak or pandemic. The overarching lesson is that a culture of IPC safety must be supported and maintained during business-as-usual, not merely during crises. This will require enhancements of physical infrastructure, administrative and clinical leadership and governance, and adequate numbers of appropriately trained staff, including ICPs with enough time, support and authority to implement and maintain effective IPC programs.

References

1. Aiello AE, Larson EL, Sedlak R. The health revolution: medical and socioeconomic advances. Am J Infect Control. 2008;36(10 Suppl):S116-127.
2. Armstrong GL, Conn LA, Pinner RW. Trends in infectious disease mortality in the United States during the 20th century. JAMA. 1999;281(1):61-66.
3. Larson E. Innovations in health care: antisepsis as a case study. Am J Public Health. 1989;79(1):92-99.
4. Aiello AE, Larson EL, Sedlak R. Hidden heroes of the health revolution: sanitation and personal hygiene. Am J Infect Control. 2008;36(10 Suppl):S128-151.
5. Gawande A. Two hundred years of surgery. N Engl J Med. 2012;366(18):1716-1723.
6. Funk DJ, Parrillo JE, Kumar A. Sepsis and septic shock: a history. Crit Care Clin. 2009;25(1):83-101, viii.
7. Karamanou M, Panayiotakopoulos G, Tsoucalas G, Kousoulis AA, Androutsos G. From miasmas to germs: a historical

approach to theories of infectious disease transmission. Infez Med. 2012;20(1):58–62.

8. Condrau F, Worboys, M. Second opinions: epidemics and infections in nineteenth-century Britain. Soc Hist Med. 2007;20(1):147–158.

9. Noymer A, Jarosz, C. Causes of death in nineteenth century New England: the dominance of infectious disease. Soc Hist Med. 2008;21(3):573–578.

10. Ackerknecht EH. Anticontagionism between 1821 and 1867: the Fielding H. Garrison Lecture. 1948. Int J Epidemiol. 2009;38(1):7–21.

11. Ayliffe GAJ, English, MP. Hospital infection. From miasmas to MRSA. Cambridge, UK: Cambridge University Press, 2003.

12. Gordon A. Treatise on the epidemic puerperal fever of Aberdeen. Internet Archive Open Knowledge Commons and Harvard Medical School ed. London: G.G. & J. Robinson, 1795, 2010.

13. Selwyn S. Sir James Simpson and hospital cross infection. Med Hist. 1965;9:241–248.

14. Holmes OW. The contagiousness of puerperal fever. The Harvard Classics. 38. New York: PF Collier & Son Company 1909–14. New York Bartleby.com, 2001; 1843 (reprinted 2001 from N. Engl, Quart J Med, Surg).

15. Parsons GP. The British medical profession and contagion theory: puerperal fever as a case study, 1830–1860. Med Hist. 1978;22(2):138–150.

16. Parsons GP. Puerperal fever, anticontagionists, and miasmatic infection, 1840–1860: toward a new history of puerperal fever in antebellum America. J Hist Med Allied Sci. 1997;52(4):424–452.

17. Meigs CD. On the nature, signs, and treatment of childbed fevers: in a series of letters addressed to the students of his class. Letter VI Philadelphia: Blanchard and Lea, 1854.

18. Simpson JY. Clinical lectures. Med Times & Gaz. 1859;39.

19. Nuland SB. The enigma of Semmelweis—an interpretation. J Hist Med Allied Sci. 1979;34(3):255–272.

20. Semmelweis IP. Die Aetioloies, der Begriff und die Prophylaxis des Kinderbettfiebers. (The etiology, concept and prophylaxis of childbed fever). Wisconsin: University of Wisconsin Press, 1861 (1983).

21. Stewardson A, Pittet D. Ignac Semmelweis—celebrating a flawed pioneer of patient safety. Lancet. 2011;378(9785):22–23.

22. Gillies D. Hempelian and Kuhnian approaches in the philosophy of medicine: the Semmelweis case. Stud Hist Philos Biol Biomed Sci. 2005;36(1):159–181.

23. Gill CJ, Gill GC. Nightingale in Scutari: her legacy reexamined. Clin Infect Dis. 2005;40(12):1799–1805.

24. Davies R. 'Notes on nursing: what it is and what it is not'. (1860): by Florence Nightingale. Nurse Educ Today. 2012;32(6):624–626.

25. Aravind M, Chung KC. Evidence-based medicine and hospital reform: tracing origins back to Florence Nightingale. Plast Reconstr Surg. 2010;125(1):403–409.

26. Artioli G, Foa C, Taffurelli C. An integrated narrative nursing model: towards a new healthcare paradigm. Acta Biomed. 2016;87(4–S):13–22.

27. Toledo-Pereyra LH. Louis Pasteur surgical revolution. J Invest Surg. 2009;22(2):82–7.

28. Toledo-Pereyra LH. Joseph Lister's surgical revolution. J Invest Surg. 2010;23:241–3.

29. Nakayama DK. Antisepsis and asepsis and how they shaped modern surgery. Am Surg. 2018;84(6):766–771.

30. Lister J. On the antiseptic principle in the practice of surgery. Br Med J. 1867;2(351):246–248.

31. Lister J. An address on the effect of the antiseptic treatment upon the general salubrity of surgical hospitals. Br Med J. 1875;2(782):769–771.

32. Newsom SW. Pioneers in infection control—Joseph Lister. J Hosp Infect, 2003;55(4):246–253.

33. Lewis MJ. Medicine in colonial Australia, 1788 1900 Med J Aust. 2014;201(1 Suppl):S5–S10.

34. Adams LW, Aschenbrenner CA, Houle TT, Roy RC. Uncovering the history of operating room attire through photographs. Anesthesiology. 2016;124(1):19–24.

35. Spooner JL. History of surgical face masks. AORN J. 1967;5(1):x–80.

36. Rockwood CA, Jr., O'Donoghue DH. The surgical mask: its development, usage, and efficiency. A review of the literature, and new experimental studies. Arch Surg. 1960;80:963–71.

37. Matuschek C, Moll F, Fangerau H, Fischer JC, Zanker K, van Griensven M, et al. The history and value of face masks. Eur J Med Res. 2020;25(1):23.

38. Mendelsohn JA. 'Like all that lives': biology, medicine and bacteria in the age of Pasteur and Koch. Hist Philos Life Sci. 2002;24(1):3–36.

39. Bury M. Medical Model. In: Gabe JM, L.E., editor. Key concepts in medical sociology. 2nd ed. Los Angeles: Sage Publications Ltd, 2013, p. 111–115.

40. Wade DT, Halligan PW. Do biomedical models of illness make for good healthcare systems? BMJ. 2004;329(7479):1398–1401.

41. Porter R. The greatest benefit to mankind. A medical history of humanity. London: W. W. Norton & Company Inc, 1997.

42. Helmstadter C. Shifting boundaries: religion, medicine, nursing and domestic service in mid-nineteenth-century Britain. Nurs Inq. 2009;16(2):133–143.

43. MacMillan KM. The challenge of achieving interprofessional collaboration: should we blame Nightingale? J Interprof Care. 2012;26(5):410–415.

44. Spellberg B, Taylor-Blake B. On the exoneration of Dr William H. Stewart: debunking an urban legend. Infect Dis Poverty. 2013;2(1):3.

45. Plotkin S. History of vaccination. Proc Natl Acad Sci U S A. 2014;111(34):12283–12287.

46. Barber M, Rozwadowska-Dowzenko M. Infection by penicillin-resistant staphylococci. Lancet. 1948;2(6530): 641–644.

47. Gilbert GL, Kerridge, I. Hospital infection prevention and control and antimicrobial stewardship: dual strategies to reduce antibiotic resistance in hospitals. In: Jamrozik E, Selgelid M, ed. Ethics and drug resistance: collective responsibility for global public health. Public Health Ethics Analysis: Springer, 2020.

48. Wise RI, Ossman EA, Littlefield DR. Personal reflections on nosocomial staphylococcal infections and the development of hospital surveillance. Rev Infect Dis. 1989;11(6):1005–1019.

49. Lowbury EJ. Cross-infection of wounds with antibiotic-resistant organisms. Br Med J. 1955;1(4920):985–990.

50. Snowden FM. Emerging and reemerging diseases: a historical perspective. Immunol Rev. 2008;225:9–26.

51. Davies J, Davies D. Origins and evolution of antibiotic resistance. Microbiol Mol Biol Rev. 2010;74(3):417–433.

52. Rountree PM, Thomson EF. Incidence of antibiotic-resistant staphylococci in a hospital. Lancet. 1952;2(6728):262–265.

53. Rountree PM, Beard MA. The spread of neomycin-resistant staphylococci in a hospital. Med J Aust. 1965;1(14):498–502.

54. Jackson MM, Lynch P. Infection control: in search of a rational approach. Am J Nurs. 1990;90(10):65–68, 71–47.

55. Rountree PM. Bacteriophage typing of strains of staphylococci isolated in Australia. Lancet. 1953;1(6759):514–516.

56. Rountree PM. History of staphylococcal infection in Australia. Med J Aust. 1978;2(12):543–546.

57. Isbister C, Durie EB, Rountree PM, Freeman BM. Further study of staphylococcal infection of the new-born. Med J Aust. 1954;2(23):897-900.
58. Elek SD, Fleming PC. A new technique for the control of hospital cross-infection. Experience with BRL. 1241 in a maternity unit. Lancet. 1960;2(7150):569-572.
59. Barber M. Methicillin-resistant staphylococci. J Clin Pathol. 1961;14:385-393.
60. Jevons MP, Coe AW, Parker MT. Methicillin resistance in staphylococci. Lancet. 1963;1(7287):904-907.
61. Stewart GT, Holt RJ. Evolution of natural resistance to the newer penicillins. Br Med J. 1963;1(5326):308-311.
62. Benner EJ, Kayser FH. Growing clinical significance of methicillin-resistant *Staphylococcus aureus*. Lancet. 1968;2(7571):741-744.
63. Rountree PM, Beard MA. Hospital strains of *Staphylococcus aureus*, with particular reference to methicillin-resistant strains. Med J Aust. 1968;2(26):1163-1168.
64. Forder AA. A brief history of infection control—past and present. S Afr Med J. 2007;97(11 Pt 3):1161-1164.
65. Davies J. Vicious circles: looking back on resistance plasmids. Genetics. 1995;139(4):1465-1468.
66. Williams REO, Blowers R, Garrod LP, Shooter RA. Hospital infection: causes and prevention. 2nd ed. London: Lloyd-Luke (Medical Books) Ltd, 1966.
67. Colebrook L. Infection acquired in hospital. Lancet. 1955;269(6896):885-891.
68. Hillier K. Babies and bacteria: phage typing, bacteriologists, and the birth of infection control. Bull Hist Med. 2006;80(4):733-761.
69. Gardner AM, Stamp M, Bowgen JA, Moore B. The infection control sister. A new member of the control of infection team in general hospitals. Lancet. 1962;2(7258):710-711.
70. Davis NC, Garlick F, Fielding G, Rao A. The infection control sister: her role in a large hospital. Lancet. 1963;2(7321):1321-1322.
71. Haley RW, Quade D, Freeman HE, Bennett JV. The SENIC Project: study on the efficacy of nosocomial infection control (SENIC Project). Summary of study design. Am J Epidemiol. 1980;111(5):472-485.
72. Haley RW, Culver DH, White JW, Morgan WM, Emori TG, Munn VP, Hooton TM. The efficacy of infection surveillance and control programs in preventing nosocomial infections in US hospitals. Am J Epidemiol. 1985;121(2):182-205.
73. Haley RW, Shachtman RH. The emergence of infection surveillance and control programs in US hospitals: an assessment, 1976. Am J Epidemiol. 1980;111(5):574-591.
74. Rountree PM. Cross-infection of surgical wounds. Med J Aust. 1951;2(23):766-769.
75. Rountree PM. Cross-infection of wounds in a surgical ward during a trial of the use of oiled blankets. Med J Aust. 1947;1(14):427-430.
76. Rountree PM. *Streptococcus pyogenes* infections in a hospital. Lancet. 1955;269(6882):172-173.
77. Rountree PM. The treatment of hospital blankets with oil emulsions and the bactericidal action of fixanol C (cetyl pyridinium bromide). Med J Aust. 1946;1:539-544.
78. Rountree PM, Thomson EF. Incidence of penicillin-resistant and streptomycin-resistant staphylococci in a hospital. Lancet. 1949;2(6577):501-504.
79. Rountree PM, Barbour RG. Incidence of penicillin-resistant and streptomycin-resistant staphylococci in a hospital. Lancet. 1951;1(6652):435-436.
80. Rountree PM, Armytage JE. Hospital blankets as a source of infection. Med J Aust. 1946;1:503-506.
81. Rountree PM, Barbour RG. Nasal carrier rates of *Staphylococcus pyogenes* in hospital nurses. J Pathol Bacteriol. 1951;63(2):313-324.
82. Rountree PM, Harrington M, Loewenthal J, Gye R. Staphylococcal wound infection in a surgical unit. Lancet. 1960;2(7140):1-6.
83. Coventry KJ, Isbister C. A bacteriological and clinical study of infection in newborn babies in a maternity hospital nursery. Med J Aust. 1951;2(12):394-396.
84. Isbister C. A clinical study of infections of the newborn occurring in a maternity hospital over a six-month period. Med J Aust. 1951;2(12):386-394.
85. Rountree PM, Barbour RG. *Staphylococcus pyogenes* in new-born babies in a maternity hospital. Med J Aust. 1950;1(16):525-528.
86. Rountree PM, Freeman BM. Infections caused by a particular phage type of *Staphylococcus aureus*. Med J Aust. 1955;42(5):157-161.
87. Rountree PM, Beard MA. Further observations on infection with phage type 80 staphylococci in Australia. Med J Aust. 1958;45(24):789-795.
88. Taft LI. Recent experiences with staphylococcal infection in childhood. Med J Aust. 1955;42(24):970-976.
89. Campbell K. Cross infection in the neo-natal nursery. Med J Aust. 1954;2(9):329-331.
90. Plueckhahn VD. The staphylococcus and the newborn child. Br Med J. 1961;2(5255):779-785.
91. Hill AM, Butler HM, Laver JC. Reduction of staphylococcal infection in the newly born. Med J Aust. 1959;46(2):633-634.
92. Plueckhahn VD. Hexachlorophene toxicity, the new-born child and the Staphylococcus. Med J Aust. 1972;1(18):897-903.
93. Pavillard R, Harvey K, Douglas D, Hewstone A, Andrew J, Collopy B, et al. Epidemic of hospital-acquired infection due to methicillin-resistant *Staphylococcus aureus* in major Victorian hospitals. Med J Aust. 1982;1(11):451-454.
94. Stratford BC. Practical problems in antibiotic therapy. Med J Aust. 1965;1(12):434-436.
95. Perceval A, McLean AJ, Wellington CV. Emergence of gentamicin resistance in *Staphylococcus aureus*. Med J Aust. 1976;2(2):74.
96. McDonald M, Ward P, Harvey K. Antibiotic-associated diarrhoea and methicillin-resistant *Staphylococcus aureus*. Med J Aust. 1982;1(11):462-464.
97. McDonald M, Hurse A, Sim KN. Methicillin-resistant *Staphylococcus aureus* bacteraemia. Med J Aust. 1981;2(4):191-194.
98. Gilbert GL, Asche V, Hewstone AS, Mathiesen JL. Methicillin-resistant *Staphylococcus aureus* in neonatal nurseries. Two years' experience in special-care nurseries in Melbourne. Med J Aust. 1982;1(11):455-459.
99. King K, Brady L, Thomson M, Harkness JL. Antibiotic-resistant staphylococci in a teaching hospital. Med J Aust. 1982;2(10):461-465.
100. Faoagali JL, Thong ML, Grant D. Ten years' experience with methicillin-resistant *Staphylococcus aureus* in a large Australian hospital. J Hosp Infect. 1992;20(2):113-119.
101. Pearman JW, Christiansen KJ, Annear DI, Goodwin CS, Metcalf C, Donovan FP, et al. Control of methicillin-resistant *Staphylococcus aureus* (MRSA) in an Australian metropolitan teaching hospital complex. Med J Aust. 1985;142(2):103-108.
102. Dailey L, Coombs GW, O'Brien FG, Pearman JW, Christiansen K, Grubb WB, et al. Methicillin-resistant *Staphylococcus aureus*, Western Australia. Emerg Infect Dis. 2005;11(10):1584-1590.

103. Cordova SP, Heath CH, McGechie DB, Keil AD, Beers MY, Riley TV. Methicillin-resistant *Staphylococcus aureus* bacteraemia in Western Australian teaching hospitals, 1997-1999: risk factors, outcomes and implications for management. J Hosp Infect. 2004;56(1):22-28.

104. Collignon P, Nimmo GR, Gottlieb T, Gosbell IB, Australian Group on Antimicrobial R. *Staphylococcus aureus* bacteremia, Australia. Emerg Infect Dis. 2005;11(4):554-561.

105. Shallard MA, Williams AL. A study of the carriage of gram-negative bacilli by new-born babies in hospital. Med J Aust. 1965;1:540-542.

106. Deighton MA, Tagg JR, Mushin R. Epidemiology of *Pseudomonas aeruginosa* infection in hospitals. 2. 'Fingerprinting' of Ps. aeruginosa strains in a study of cross-infection in a children's hospital. Med J Aust. 1971;1(17):892-896.

107. Rubbo SD, Gardner JF, Franklin JC. Source of *Pseudomonas aeruginosa* infection in premature infants. J Hyg (Lond). 1966;64(1):121-128.

108. Garland SM, Mackay S, Tabrizi S, Jacobs S. *Pseudomonas aeruginosa* outbreak associated with a contaminated blood-gas analyser in a neonatal intensive care unit. J Hosp Infect. 1996;33(2):145-151.

109. Buttery JP, Alabaster SJ, Heine RG, Scott SM, Crutchfield RA, Bigham A, et al. Multiresistant *Pseudomonas aeruginosa* outbreak in a pediatric oncology ward related to bath toys. Pediatr Infect Dis J. 1998;17(6):509-513.

110. Tagg JR, Mushin R. Epidemiology of *Pseudomonas aeruginosa* infection in hospitals. 1. Pyocine typing of Ps. aeruginosa. Med J Aust. 1971;1(16):847-852.

111. Forbes I, Gray A, Hurse A, Pavillard R. The emergence of gentamicin-resistant klebsiellae in a large general hospital. Med J Aust. 1977;1(1-2):14-16.

112. Sinclair MI, Asche V, Morgan AF, Holloway BW. Plasmid-determined tobramycin and gentamicin resistance in strains of *Pseudomonas aeruginosa* from two Sydney hospitals. Med J Aust. 1981;2(6):283-286, 287.

113. Harvey K, Dartnell J, Hemming M. Improving antibiotic use: 25 years of antibiotic guidelines and related initiatives. Commun Dis Intell Q Rep. 2003;27 Suppl:S9-12.

114. Clarke BG. Infection in the intensive care unit. Med J Aust. 1977;2(3 Pt 2 Suppl):27-29.

115. Mutton KJ, Brady LM, Harkness JL. Serratia cross-infection in an intensive therapy unit. J Hosp Infect. 1981;2(1):85-91.

116. Riley TV, Webb SA, Cadwallader H, Briggs BD, Christiansen L, Bowman RA. Outbreak of gentamicin-resistant *Acinetobacter baumanii* in an intensive care unit: clinical, epidemiological and microbiological features. Pathology. 1996;28(4):359-363.

117. Peleg AY, Seifert H, Paterson DL. *Acinetobacter baumannii*: emergence of a successful pathogen. Clin Microbiol Rev. 2008;21(3):538-582.

118. Bell JM, Turnidge JD, Gales AC, Pfaller MA, Jones RN, Sentry ASG. Prevalence of extended spectrum beta-lactamase (ESBL)-producing clinical isolates in the Asia-Pacific region and South Africa: regional results from SENTRY Antimicrobial Surveillance Program (1998-99). Diagn Microbiol Infect Dis. 2002;42(3):193-198.

119. Looke DF, Gottlieb T, Jones CA, Paterson DL. Gram-negative resistance: can we combat the coming of a new 'Red Plague'? Med J Aust. 2013;198(5):243-244.

120. Harris P, Paterson D, Rogers B. Facing the challenge of multidrug-resistant gram-negative bacilli in Australia. Med J Aust. 2015;202(5):243-247.

121. Murray BE. The life and times of the enterococcus. Clin Microbiol Rev. 1990;3(1):46-65.

122. Bell JM, Paton JC, Turnidge J. Emergence of vancomycin-resistant enterococci in Australia: phenotypic and genotypic characteristics of isolates. J Clin Microbiol. 1998;36(8):2187-2190.

123. Kamarulzaman A, Tosolini FA, Boquest AL, Geddes JE, Richards MJ. Vancomycin-resistant *Enterococcus faecium* in a liver transplant recipient (abstract). Aust, N Z J Med. 1995;25:560.

124. Ferguson JK. Vancomycin-resistant enterococci: causes and control. Med J Aust. 1999;171(3):117-118.

125. Collignon PJ. Vancomycin-resistant enterococci and use of avoparcin in animal feed: is there a link? Med J Aust. 1999;171(3):144-146.

126. Bartley PB, Schooneveldt JM, Looke DF, Morton A, Johnson DW, Nimmo GR. The relationship of a clonal outbreak of *Enterococcus faecium vanA* to methicillin-resistant *Staphylococcus aureus* incidence in an Australian hospital. J Hosp Infect. 2001;48(1):43-54.

127. Christiansen KJ, Tibbett PA, Beresford W, Pearman JW, Lee RC, Coombs GW, et al. Eradication of a large outbreak of a single strain of vanB vancomycin-resistant *Enterococcus faecium* at a major Australian teaching hospital. Infect Control Hosp Epidemiol. 2004;25(5):384-390.

128. Cooper E, Paull A, O'Reilly M. Characteristics of a large cluster of vancomycin-resistant enterococci in an Australian hospital. Infect Control Hosp Epidemiol. 2002;23(3):151-153.

129. Coombs GW, Pearson JC, Daly DA, Le TT, Robinson JO, Gottlieb T, et al. Australian enterococcal sepsis outcome programme annual report, 2013. Commun Dis Intell Q Rep. 2014;38(4):E320-6.

130. Krugman S. Viral hepatitis: overview and historical perspectives. Yale J Biol Med. 1976;49(3):199-203.

131. Blumberg BS, Sutnick AI, London WT, Millman I. Australia antigen and hepatitis. N Engl J Med. 1970;283(7):349-354.

132. Ferris AA, Kaldor J, Lucas CR. Australia antigen and viral hepatitis: a brief review and a preliminary Australian report. Pathology. 1970;2(1):1-8.

133. Hawkes RA. Australia antigen and viral hepatitis in Sydney. A hospital series. Med J Aust. 1970;2(12):519-525.

134. Gust ID, Lucas CR. Australia antigen in acute hepatitis in Melbourne. Med J Aust. 1971;1(5):260-262.

135. Forbes JA, Bennett NM, Lucas CR. Practical aspects of the hepatitis B problem. Med J Aust. 1974;2(6):216-219.

136. Cossart YE, Kirsch S, Ismay SL. Post-transfusion hepatitis in Australia. Report of the Australian Red Cross study. Lancet. 1982;1(8265):208-213.

137. Lucas CR, Williamson HG, Dimitrakakis M, Gust ID. Maintenance dialysis of patients infected with hepatitis B virus. Med J Aust. 1981;1(7):343-345.

138. Beasley RP, Hwang LY, Lin CC, Chien CS. Hepatocellular carcinoma and hepatitis B virus. A prospective study of 22 707 men in Taiwan. Lancet. 1981;2(8256):1129-1133.

139. Beasley RP, Hwang LY, Lin CC, Stevens CE, Wang KY, Sun TS, et al. Hepatitis B immune globulin (HBIG) efficacy in the interruption of perinatal transmission of hepatitis B virus carrier state. Initial report of a randomised double-blind placebo-controlled trial. Lancet. 1981;2(8243):388-393.

140. Gilbert GL. Prevention of vertical transmission of hepatitis B. The place of routine screening in antenatal care, and the case for immunization of infants at risk. Med J Aust. 1984;141(4):213-216.

141. Lanphear BP. Trends and patterns in the transmission of blood-borne pathogens to health care workers. Epidemiol Rev. 1994;16(2):437-450.

142. National Centre for Immunisation Research and Surveillance NCIRS. Significant events in hepatitis B

vaccination practice in Australia. 2018. Available from: https://www.ncirs.org.au/sites/default/files/2018-11/Hepatitis-B-history-July-2018.pdf.

143. Bell DM, Shapiro CN, Ciesielski CA, Chamberland ME. Preventing blood-borne pathogen transmission from health-care workers to patients. The CDC perspective. Surg Clin North Am. 1995;75(6):1189-1203.

144. Feinstone SM, Kapikian AZ, Purceli RH. Hepatitis A: detection by immune electron microscopy of a viruslike antigen associated with acute illness. Science. 1973;182(4116):1026-1028.

145. Locarnini SA, Ferris AA, Stott AC, Gust ID. The relationship between a 27-nm virus-like particle and hepatitis A as demonstrated by immune electron microscopy. Intervirology. 1974;4(2):110-118.

146. Centers for Disease Control and Prevention (CDC). Current trends prevention of acquired immune deficiency syndrome (AIDS): report of inter-agency recommendations. MMWR. 1983;32(8):101-103.

147. Barre-Sinoussi F, Chermann JC, Rey F, Nugeyre MT, Chamaret S, Gruest J, et al. Isolation of a T-lymphotropic retrovirus from a patient at risk for acquired immune deficiency syndrome (AIDS). Science. 1983;220(4599):868-871.

148. Gallo RC, Salahuddin SZ, Popovic M, Shearer GM, Kaplan M, Haynes BF, et al. Frequent detection and isolation of cytopathic retroviruses (HTLV-III) from patients with AIDS and at risk for AIDS. Science. 1984;224(4648):500-503.

149. CDC. Current trends acquired immunodeficiency syndrome (AIDS); precautions of clinical and laboratory staffs. MMWR. 1982;31(43):577-580.

150. CDC. AIDS Precautions for health-care workers and allied health professionals. MMWR. 1983;32(34):450-451.

151. CDC. Current trends recommendations for assisting in the prevention of perinatal transmission of human T-lymphotropic virus type III/lymphadenopathy-associated virus and acquired immunodeficiency syndrome. MMWR. 1985;34(48):721-726; 731-732.

152. Penny R, Marks R, Berger J, Marriott D, Bryant D. Acquired immune deficiency syndrome. Med J Aust. 1983;1(12):554-557.

153. Plummer D, Irwin L. Grassroots activities, national initiatives and HIV prevention: clues to explain Australia's dramatic early success in controlling the HIV epidemic. Int J STD AIDS. 2006;17(12):787-793.

154. Kaldor J, McDonald A. HIV/AIDS surveillance systems in Australia. J Acquir Immune Defic Syndr. 2003;32 Suppl 1:S18-23.

155. Guy RJ, McDonald AM, Bartlett MJ, Murray JC, Giele CM, Davey TM, et al. HIV diagnoses in Australia: diverging epidemics within a low-prevalence country. Med J Aust. 2007;187(8):437-440.

156. Chamberland ME, Ciesielski CA, Howard RJ, Fry DE, Bell DM. Occupational risk of infection with human immunodeficiency virus. Surg Clin North Am. 1995;75(6):1057-1070.

157. National Health Service (NHS). HIV infected health care workers: guidance on management and patient notification. London: Department of Health (UK), 2005 July, 2005. Available from: https://www.ilo.org/wcmsp5/groups/public/—-ed_protect/—-protrav/—-ilo_aids/documents/legaldocument/wcms_127515.pdf.

158. Chant K, Lowe D, Rubin G, Manning W, O'Donoughue R, Lyle D, et al. Patient-to-patient transmission of HIV in private surgical consulting rooms. Lancet. 1993;342(8886-8887):1548-1549.

159. Solomon PJ, Wilson SR, Swanson CE, Cooper DA. Effect of zidovudine on survival of patients with AIDS in Australia. Med J Aust. 1990;153(5):254-257.

160. Gulick RM, Mellors JW, Havlir D, Eron JJ, Gonzalez C, McMahon D, et al. Treatment with indinavir, zidovudine, and lamivudine in adults with human immunodeficiency virus infection and prior antiretroviral therapy. N Engl J Med. 1997;337(11):734-739.

161. Hammer SM, Squires KE, Hughes MD, Grimes JM, Demeter LM, Currier JS, et al. A controlled trial of two nucleoside analogues plus indinavir in persons with human immunodeficiency virus infection and CD4 cell counts of 200 per cubic millimeter or less. AIDS Clinical Trials Group 320 Study Team. N Engl J Med. 1997;337(11):725-733.

162. Porter K, Babiker A, Bhaskaran K, Darbyshire J, Pezzotti P, Porter K, et al. Determinants of survival following HIV-1 seroconversion after the introduction of HAART. Lancet. 2003;362(9392):1267-1274.

163. Bowtell W. Australia's response to HIV/AIDS 1982-2005. Sydney, Australia: Lowy Institute for International Policy, 2005. Available from: https://archive.lowyinstitute.org/sites/default/files/pubfiles/Bowtell%2C_Australia%27s_Response_to_HIV_AIDS_logo_1.pdf.

164. Bermingham S, Kippax S. HIV-related discrimination: a survey of New South Wales general practitioners. Aust N Z J Public Health. 1998;22(1):92-97.

165. Choo QL, Kuo G, Weiner AJ, Overby LR, Bradley DW, Houghton M. Isolation of a cDNA clone derived from a blood-borne non-A, non-B viral hepatitis genome. Science. 1989;244(4902):359-362.

166. Zuckerman AJ. The elusive hepatitis C virus. BMJ. 1989;299(6704):871-873.

167. Gust I, Nicholson S, Dimitrakis M, Hoy J, Lucas R. Prevalence of infection with hepatitis C virus in Australia. Med J Aust. 1989;151:719.

168. Crofts N, Jolley D, Kaldor J, van Beek I, Wodak A. Epidemiology of hepatitis C virus infection among injecting drug users in Australia. J Epidemiol Community Health. 1997;51(6):692-697.

169. Garner JJ, Gaughwin M, Dodding J, Wilson K. Prevalence of hepatitis C infection in pregnant women in South Australia. Med J Aust. 1997;167(9):470-472.

170. Allain JP, Coghlan PJ, Kenrick KG, Whitson K, Keller A, Cooper GJ, et al. Prediction of hepatitis C virus infectivity in seropositive Australian blood donors by supplemental immunoassays and detection of viral RNA. Blood. 1991;78(9):2462-2468.

171. Ismay SL, Thomas S, Fellows A, Keller A, Kenrick KG, Archer GT, et al. Post-transfusion hepatitis revisited. Med J Aust. 1995;163(2):74-77.

172. Liddle C. Hepatitis C. Anaesth Intensive Care. 1996;24(2):180-183.

173. Chant K, Kociuba K, Munro R, Crone S, Kerridge R, Quin J, et al. Investigation of possible patient-to-patient transmission of hepatitis C in a hospital. NSW Public Health Bulletin. 1994;5(5):47-51.

174. Faoagali JL, Darcy D. Chickenpox outbreak among the staff of a large, urban adult hospital: costs of monitoring and control. Am J Infect Control. 1995;23(4):247-250.

175. Flego KL, Belshaw DA, Sheppeard V, Weston KM. Impacts of a measles outbreak in Western Sydney on public health resources. Commun Dis Intell Q Rep. 2013;37(3):E240-245.

176. Paterson JM, Sheppeard V. Nosocomial pertussis infection of infants: still a risk in 2009. Commun Dis Intell Q Rep. 2010;34(4):440-443.

177. Seale H, Kaur R, MacIntyre CR. Understanding Australian healthcare workers' uptake of influenza vaccination:

examination of public hospital policies and procedures. BMC Health Serv Res. 2012;12:325.

178. Goldwater PN, Martin AJ, Ryan B, Morris S, Thompson J, Kok TW, et al. A survey of nosocomial respiratory viral infections in a children's hospital: occult respiratory infection in patients admitted during an epidemic season. Infect Control Hosp Epidemiol. 1991;12(4):231-238.

179. Russo PL, Spelman DW, Harrington GA, Jenney AW, Gunesekere IC, Wright PJ, et al. Hospital outbreak of Norwalk-like virus. Infect Control Hosp Epidemiol. 1997;18(8):576-579.

180. Ferguson PE, Sorrell TC, Bradstock K, Carr P, Gilroy NM. Parainfluenza virus type 3 pneumonia in bone marrow transplant recipients: multiple small nodules in high-resolution lung computed tomography scans provide a radiological clue to diagnosis. Clin Infect Dis. 2009;48(7):905-909.

181. Ferguson PE, Gilroy NM, Faux CE, Mackay IM, Sloots TP, Nissen MD, et al. Human rhinovirus C in adult haematopoietic stem cell transplant recipients with respiratory illness. J Clin Virol. 2013;56(3):255-259.

182. Coventry C, Harrington G, Johnston P, Strother, R. The story of the development of infection control at the Alfred. Part 1. Beginnings. Alfred Hospital faces and places. III Melbourne, Victoria: Alfred Hospital, 1996, p. 309-316.

183. Perceval A. Infection control at the Alfred—a bacteriologist's account. Alfred Hospital faces and places. III Melbourne, Victoria: Alfred Hospital, 1996, p. 319-326.

184. Butler HM. Infection control. Australian Nurses' Journal. 1972;2(2):24-25,32.

185. Fenner F. History of microbiology in Australia. Canberra: Brolga Press, 1990.

186. Rountree PM, Vickery AM. Further observations on methicillin-resistant staphylococci. 1973;1(21):1030-1034.

187. Wernigk N. The duties of an infection control sister. Source unknown, 1963.

188. Fielding G, Rao A, Davis NC, Wernigk N. Prophylactic topical use of antibiotics in surgical wounds: a controlled clinical trial using 'Polybactrin'. Med J Aust. 1965;2(4): 159-161.

189. Albera G, Murphy C, Gold J. Reflections on the beginnings of infection control in NSW. NSW Public Health Bull. 1996;5(7):75-76.

190. Graham-Robertson E. History of the Australian infection control association (AICA): the first ten years 1985 to 1995. 2006.

191. McIntosh A, McManus I, Party C. 40 years of ACHS history—a timeline through the ages. Australian Council on Health Standards, 2014. Available from: https://www1.achs.org.au/media/100550/achs_historic_timeline_final.pdf.

192. Murphy CL, McLaws ML. Who coordinates infection control programs in Australia? Am J Infect Control. 1999;27(3): 291-295.

193. Hoffmann CE, McDonald PJ, Watts JM. Use of peroperative cefoxitin to prevent infection after colonic and rectal surgery. Ann Surg. 1981;193(3):353-356.

194. Gensini GF, Yacoub MH, Conti AA. The concept of quarantine in history: from plague to SARS. J Infect. 2004;49(4):257-261.

195. Longhurst P. Quarantine matters: colonial quarantine at North Head, Sydney and its material and ideological ruins. Int J Hist Archaeol. 2016;20:589-600.

196. Hobbins P. Union Jack or Yellow Jack? Smallpox, sailors, settlers and sovereignty. J Imp Commonw Hist. 2017; 45(3):391-415.

197. Curson P, McCracken K. An Australian perspective of the 1918–1919 influenza pandemic. NSW Public Health Bull. 2006;17(7-8):103-107.

198. CDC. Perspectives in disease prevention and health promotion update: universal precautions for prevention of transmission of human immunodeficiency virus, hepatitis B virus and other blood-borne pathogens in health-care settings. MMWR. 1988;37(24):377-388.

199. Leaver M. Universal precautions to become standard: infection control news brief. Collegian. 1996;3(1):14.

200. Davidson G, Gillies P. Safe working practices and HIV infection: knowledge, attitudes, perception of risk, and policy in hospital. Qual Health Care. 1993;2(1):21-26.

201. Gerberding JL, Lewis FR, Jr., Schecter WP. Are universal precautions realistic? Surg Clin North Am. 1995;75(6): 1091-1104.

202. Richards MJ, Jenkin GA, Johnson PD. Universal precautions: attitudes of Australian and New Zealand anaesthetists. Med J Aust. 1997;166(3):138-140.

203. Kerridge RK. Universal precautions and anaesthetists: time for a rethink? Med J Aust. 1997;166(3):142.

204. Siegel JD, Rhinehart E, Jackson M, Chiarello L, Healthcare Infection Control Practices Advisory C. Management of multidrug-resistant organisms in health care settings, 2006. Am J Infect Control. 2007;35(10 Suppl 2):S165-193.

205. Jernigan JA, Titus MG, Groschel DH, Getchell-White S, Farr BM. Effectiveness of contact isolation during a hospital outbreak of methicillin-resistant Staphylococcus aureus. Am J Epidemiol. 1996;143(5):496-504.

206. Morgan DJ, Murthy R, Munoz-Price LS, Barnden M, Camins BC, Johnston BL, et al. Reconsidering contact precautions for endemic methicillin-resistant Staphylococcus aureus and vancomycin-resistant enterococcus. Infect Control Hosp Epidemiol. 2015;36(10):1163-1172.

207. Karki S, Houston L, Land G, Bass P, Kehoe R, Borrell S, et al. Prevalence and risk factors for VRE colonisation in a tertiary hospital in Melbourne, Australia: a cross sectional study. Antimicrob Resist Infect Control. 2012; 1(1):31.

208. Kullar R, Vassallo A, Turkel S, Chopra T, Kaye KS, Dhar S. Degowning the controversies of contact precautions for methicillin-resistant Staphylococcus aureus: a review. Am J Infect Control. 2016;44(1):97-103.

209. Harris J, Walsh K, Dodds S. Are contact precautions ethically justifiable in contemporary hospital care? Nurs Ethics. 2019;26(2):611-624.

210. Karki S, Leder K, Cheng AC. Should we continue to isolate patients with vancomycin-resistant enterococci in hospitals? Med J Aust. 2015;202(5):234-236.

211. Wyer M, Iedema R, Jorm C, Armstrong, G, Hor S-Y, Hooker C, et al. Should I stay or should I go? Patient understandings of and responses to source-isolation practices. Patient Experience Journal. 2015;2(2):60-68.

212. Stelfox HT, Bates DW, Redelmeier DA. Safety of patients isolated for infection control. JAMA. 2003;290(14):1899-1905.

213. Karki S, Leder K, Cheng AC. Patients under contact precautions have an increased risk of injuries and medication errors: a retrospective cohort study. Infect Control Hosp Epidemiol. 2013;34(10):1118-1120.

214. Howden BP, Holt KE, Lam MM, Seemann T, Ballard S, Coombs GW, et al. Genomic insights to control the emergence of vancomycin-resistant enterococci. mBio. 2013;4(4).

215. Karki S, Cheng AC. Impact of non-rinse skin cleansing with chlorhexidine gluconate on prevention of healthcare-associated infections and colonization with multi-resistant organisms: a systematic review. J Hosp Infect. 2012;82(2):71-84.

216. Johnson PD, Martin R, Burrell LJ, Grabsch EA, Kirsa SW, O'Keeffe J, et al. Efficacy of an alcohol/chlorhexidine hand hygiene program in a hospital with high rates of

nosocomial methicillin-resistant *Staphylococcus aureus* (MRSA) infection. Med J Aust. 2005;183(10):509-514.

217. Harrington G, Watson K, Bailey M, Land G, Borrell S, Houston L, et al. Reduction in hospitalwide incidence of infection or colonization with methicillin-resistant *Staphylococcus aureus* with use of antimicrobial hand-hygiene gel and statistical process control charts. Infect Control Hosp Epidemiol. 2007;28(7):837-844.

218. Morgan DJ, Kaye KS, Diekema DJ. Reconsidering isolation precautions for endemic methicillin-resistant *Staphylococcus aureus* and vancomycin-resistant enterococcus. JAMA. 2014;312(14):1395-1396.

219. Davis NC, Cohen J, Rao A. The incidence of surgical wound infection: a prospective study of 20,822 operations. Aust N Z J Surg. 1973;43(1):75-80.

220. McLaws ML, Gold J, King K, Irwig LM, Berry G. The prevalence of nosocomial and community-acquired infections in Australian hospitals. Med J Aust. 1988; 149(11-12):582-590.

221. Meers PD. Infection in hospitals. Br Med J (Clin Res Ed). 1981;282(6271):1246.

222. McLaws ML, Irwig LM, Mock P, Berry G, Gold J. Predictors of surgical wound infection in Australia: a national study. Med J Aust. 1988;149(11-12):591-595.

223. Collopy BT, Balding C. The Australian development of national quality indicators in health care. JT Comm J Qual Improv. 1993;19(11):510-518.

224. McLaws ML, Murphy C, Keogh G. The validity of surgical wound infection as a clinical indicator in Australia. Aust N Z J Surg. 1997;67(10):675-678.

225. Collopy BT. Measuring surgical wound infection. Aust N Z J Surg. 1997;67(10):673-674.

226. McLaws ML, Taylor PC. The Hospital Infection Standardised Surveillance (HISS) programme: analysis of a two-year pilot. J Hosp Infect. 2003;53(4):259-267.

227. Russo PL, Bull A, Bennett N, Boardman C, Burrell S, Motley J, et al. The establishment of a statewide surveillance program for hospital-acquired infections in large Victorian public hospitals: a report from the VICNISS Coordinating Centre. Am J Infect Control. 2006;34(7):430-436.

228. Morton AP, Clements AC, Doidge SR, Stackelroth J, Curtis M, Whitby M. Surveillance of healthcare-acquired infections in Queensland, Australia: data and lessons from the first 5 years. Infect Control Hosp Epidemiol. 2008; 29(8):695-701.

229. Morton AP, Whitby M, McLaws ML, Dobson A, McElwain S, Looke D, et al. The application of statistical process control charts to the detection and monitoring of hospital-acquired infections. J Qual Clin Pract. 2001;21(4):112-117.

230. Allricht E, Borgert J, Butler M, Cadwallader H, Collignon P, Cooper C, et al. Uniform national denominator definitions of infection control clinical indicators: surgical site and health care associated blood stream infection. Australian Infection Control 2001;6(2):47-59.

231. Richards MJ, Russo PL. Surveillance of hospital-acquired infections in Australia—one nation, many states. J Hosp Infect. 2007;65 Suppl 2:174-181.

232. Russo PL, Cheng AC, Richards M, Graves N, Hall L. Healthcare-associated infections in Australia: time for national surveillance. Aust Health Rev. 2015;39(1):37-43.

233. Whitby M, McLaws ML. Handwashing in healthcare workers: accessibility of sink location does not improve compliance. J Hosp Infect. 2004;58(4):247-253.

234. Voss A, Widmer AF. No time for handwashing!? Handwashing versus alcoholic rub: can we afford 100%

compliance? Infect Control Hosp Epidemiol. 1997;18(3): 205-208.

235. Larson E. Skin hygiene and infection prevention: more of the same or different approaches? Clin Infect Dis. 1999; 29(5):1287-1294.

236. Tibballs J. Teaching hospital medical staff to handwash. Med J Aust. 1996;164(7):395-398.

237. Vandenbroucke-Grauls CM. Clean hands closer to the bedside. Lancet. 2000;356(9238):1290-1291.

238. Pittet D, Hugonnet S, Harbarth S, Mourouga P, Sauvan V, Touveneau S, et al. Effectiveness of a hospital-wide programme to improve compliance with hand hygiene. Infection Control Programme. Lancet. 2000;356(9238):1307-1312.

239. Grayson ML, Jarvie LJ, Martin R, Johnson PD, Jodoin ME, McMullan C, et al. Significant reductions in methicillin-resistant *Staphylococcus aureus* bacteraemia and clinical isolates associated with a multisite, hand hygiene culture-change program and subsequent successful statewide roll-out. Med J Aust. 2008;188(11):633-640.

240. McLaws ML, Pantle AC, Fitzpatrick KR, Hughes CF. Improvements in hand hygiene across New South Wales public hospitals: clean hands save lives, part III. Med J Aust. 2009;191(S8):S18-24.

241. McLaws ML, Pantle AC, Fitzpatrick KR, Hughes CF. More than hand hygiene is needed to affect methicillin-resistant *Staphylococcus aureus* clinical indicator rates: clean hands save lives, part IV. Med J Aust. 2009;191(S8):S26-31.

242. World Health Organization. WHO guidelines on hand hygiene in health care: 2009. Geneva: WHO, 2009. Available from: http://whqlibdoc.who.int/publications/2009/9789241597906_eng.pdf.

243. Grayson ML, Stewardson AJ, Russo PL, Ryan KE, Olsen KL, Havers SM, et al. Effects of the Australian National Hand Hygiene Initiative after 8 years on infection control practices, health-care worker education, and clinical outcomes: a longitudinal study. Lancet Infect Dis. 2018;18(11):1269-1277.

244. Buising KL, Williamson D, Cowie BC, MacLachlan J, Orr E, MacIsaac C, et al. A hospital-wide response to multiple outbreaks of COVID-19 in health care workers: lessons learned from the field. Med J Aust. 2021;214(3): 101-104 e1.

245. Morawska L, Milton DK. It is time to address airborne transmission of coronavirus disease 2019 (COVID-19). Clin Infect Dis. 2020;71(9):2311-2313.

246. Morawska L, Tang JW, Bahnfleth W, Bluyssen PM, Boerstra A, Buonanno G, et al. How can airborne transmission of COVID-19 indoors be minimised? Environ Int. 2020; 142:105832.

247. Buising KL, Schofield R, Irving L, Keywood M, Stevens A, Keogh N, et al. Use of portable air cleaners to reduce aerosol transmission on a hospital coronavirus disease 2019 (COVID-19) ward. Infect Control Hosp Epidemiol. 2022; 43(8):987-992.

248. Barratt R, Gilbert GL, Shaban RZ, Wyer M, Hor SY. Enablers of, and barriers to, optimal glove and mask use for routine care in the emergency department: an ethnographic study of Australian clinicians. Australas Emerg Care. 2020;23(2):105-113.

249. Barratt R, Shaban RZ, Gilbert GL. Characteristics of personal protective equipment training programs in Australian and New Zealand hospitals: a survey. Infect Dis Health. 2020;25(4):253-261.

250. Broom J, Williams Veazey L, Broom A, Hor S, Degeling C, Burns P, et al. Experiences of the SARS-CoV-2 pandemic

amongst Australian healthcare workers: from stressors to protective factors. J Hosp Infect. 2022,121.75 81.

251. Ayton D, et al. Experiences of personal protective equipment by Australian healthcare workers during the COVID-19 pandemic, 2020: a cross-sectional study. PLoS One. 2022 Jun 7;17(6):e0269484. doi: 10.1371/journal.pone.0269484. eCollection 2022. Available from: https://www.ncbi.nlm.nih.gov/pubmed/35671287.

252. Broom J, Broom A, Williams Veazey L, Burns P, Degeling C, Hor S, et al. 'One minute it's an airborne virus, then it's a droplet virus, and then it's like nobody really knows...': experiences of pandemic PPE amongst Australian healthcare workers. Infect Dis Health. 2022;27(2):71-80.

253. Rafferty AC, Hewitt MC, Wright R, Hogarth F, Coatsworth N, Ampt F, et al. COVID-19 in health care workers, Australia 2020. Commun Dis Intell (2018). 2021;45.

CHAPTER 2

Contemporary infection prevention and control, and clinical infectious diseases in Australia

PROFESSOR RAMON Z. SHABAN[i-iv]

Dr CATHERINE VIENGKHAM[i-ii]

Dr JUSTIN BEARDSLEY[v]

Dr KATHERINE GARNHAM[vi]

Chapter highlights

- An overview of healthcare-associated infections (HAIs) and of the contemporary systems and structures for infection prevention and control (IPC) in Australia
- The types, categories and prevalence of HAIs
- The contemporary challenges associated with HAIs in Australia and the burden they place on populations and the Australian healthcare system
- The clinical assessment and management of the common and significant infectious diseases and HAIs most frequently encountered in Australian hospitals

i   Susan Wakil School of Nursing and Midwifery, Faculty of Medicine and Health, University of Sydney, Sydney, NSW
ii Sydney Infectious Diseases Institute, Faculty of Medicine and Health, University of Sydney, Sydney, NSW
iii Public Health Unit, Centre for Population Health, Western Sydney Local Health District, Westmead, NSW
iv New South Wales Biocontainment Centre, Western Sydney Local Health District, Westmead, NSW
v   Department of Infectious Diseases, Westmead Hospital, Western Sydney Local Health District, Sydney, NSW
vi Infectious Diseases and Microbiology, Gold Coast University Hospital and Health Service, Gold Coast, QLD

Introduction

Infectious diseases and healthcare-associated infections (HAIs) constitute a significant part of the work of all healthcare workers and pose major risks to patient safety. Healthcare-associated infections are those that are acquired in healthcare facilities ('nosocomial' infections) or because of healthcare interventions ('iatrogenic' infections), which may become evident after people leave the healthcare facility. They are a major patient safety problem, and a leading cause of significant morbidity, mortality and excess healthcare expenditure.[1-3] While research into infection prevention and control has led to improvements in our understanding of effective HAI prevention strategies, between 5–15% of all hospital inpatients will develop an HAI, with as many as 1 in 17 of these ultimately dying.[4] The excess length of stay attributable to HAIs in Australia can be as high as 8 days, consuming millions of dollars of health resources in additional diagnostic and management interventions.[5] Increasing rates of antimicrobial resistance (AMR) are compounding this already serious problem, as infections become both more difficult and more expensive to treat.[6]

There are both environmental and patient level risks to consider for infectious diseases and HAIs, and their attributable burden can be mitigated by interventions at the institutional as well as individual healthcare worker levels. Some of the environmental risk mitigations include ventilation, space cleaning, hand hygiene, and the regulation of how antimicrobials are used within the hospital. A hospital that is well designed, appropriately and regularly cleaned, where staff adhere to gold-standard hand hygiene practices, and where antimicrobial stewardship is implemented will expose its patients to the minimum risk. Healthcare workers must be aware of the risks of infectious diseases and HAIs and how to reduce them. This chapter will broadly introduce the clinical assessment, management and strategies for the control of the common and significant infectious diseases and HAIs most frequently encountered in Australian hospitals.

2.1 Healthcare in Australia

Australia is a federation of six states and two territories. The delivery of health and healthcare in Australia is the shared responsibility of the Australian Government and the state and territory governments. The states and territories have constitutional and sovereign responsibility and authority for providing care; and the responsibility for funding, policy development, regulation and service delivery is shared.[3]

The states and territories are responsible for the delivery of health services, each with their own health service organisations, systems and structures. State and territory governments administer public hospitals and associated health services through the local, area or district health jurisdictions, and each is responsible for the delivery of care and associated business activities. There are approximately 140 of these networks across Australia, of which approximately 120 are geographically based, and 20 are state- or territory-wide networks.[7] In addition, state and territory governments license and regulate private hospitals.[3]

2.2 The types, categories and prevalence of HAIs in Australia

Surveillance of HAIs and their epidemiology, as examined in Chapter 10, is the cornerstone of efforts to control and prevent them. As each Australian state and territory is responsible for, and administers, its own healthcare system, this includes the manner in which HAIs are defined, categorised and reported. Currently, there are multiple systems for the surveillance of HAIs in Australia and no single unified national system. At a macro level, we distinguish three broad types of HAI epidemiological data being collected and reported in different ways across Australian jurisdictions.

2.2.1 State and territory jurisdiction HAI data

First, all jurisdictions have systems for the surveillance and reporting of HAIs, but the extent of the reported data is incomplete and there are no jurisdiction reports on all of the listed HAIs. The HAIs currently reported by each jurisdiction are shown in Table 2.1. Victoria (VIC) and Western Australia (WA) report on all but two HAIs—urinary tract infections and pneumonia. Tasmania (TAS) reports on four types, South Australia (SA) on three and New South Wales (NSW), Queensland (QLD), the Northern Territory (NT) and the Australian Capital Territory (ACT) all report on only one. The only HAI that is reported across all jurisdictions is bloodstream infection caused by *Staphylococcus aureus*. This is because the rates of *Staphylococcus aureus* bacteraemia infection (SABSI) are a safety and quality indicator within the safety dimension of the Australia Health Performance Framework (AHPF).[3]

2.2.2 HAI peer-reviewed literature data

Second, some data are published in the peer-reviewed and grey literature. These publications may draw information from available state and territory surveillance systems, conduct independent surveys of specific infections or focus on particular Australian populations and groups,

TABLE 2.1 Publicly available HAI HAC data for each Australian state and territory

HAI HAC	NSW	VIC	QLD	SA	WA	TAS	NT	ACT
Urinary tract infection	–	–	–	–	–	–	–	–
Surgical site infection	–	✓	–	–	✓	–	–	–
Pneumonia	–	–	–	–	–	–	–	–
Bloodstream infection	✓	✓	✓	✓	✓	✓	✓	✓
Central line and peripheral line-associated bloodstream infection	–	✓	–	✓	✓	✓	–	–
Multidrug-resistant organisms (MROs)	–	✓	–	✓	✓	✓	–	–
Infection associated with prosthetics/implantable devices	–	✓	–	–	✓	–	–	–
Gastrointestinal infection	–	✓	–	–	✓	✓	–	–

or they may provide a systematic review of all available data. However, given the variability between studies in how HAIs are defined, how data is collected, and the characteristics of the population being examined, the estimations made for national rates of HAIs based on these data may be inaccurate.[3]

2.2.3 Healthcare-associated infection Hospital-acquired complications (HAI HACs)

Third, and most recently, there are HAI hospital-acquired complication (HAC) data. HACs are defined as a complication for which clinical risk mitigation strategies may reduce (but not necessarily eliminate) the risk of that complication occurring. There are 16 HAC categories and the Independent Hospital Pricing Authority (IHPA) collects data on each of the 16 categories of HACs identified by the Australian Commission on Safety and Quality in Health Care (ACSQHC). One of the HAC categories is HAIs, and specifically defines nine HAI HAC types. These are:

1. urinary tract infection
2. surgical site infection
3. pneumonia
4. bloodstream infection
5. central line and peripheral line-associated bloodstream infection
6. multidrug-resistant organism
7. infection associated with prosthetics/implantable devices
8. gastrointestinal infections
9. other high-impact infections.

These data are not publicly available, but can be accessed and reported at a limited capacity upon request.[3] Table 2.2 shows the distribution of eight listed HAIs

TABLE 2.2 Nationwide distribution for all eight HAI HACs by jurisdiction (%), 1 Jul 2018 to 30 Jun 2019[3]

HAI HAC	NSW	VIC	QLD	SA	WA	TAS	NT	ACT
Urinary tract infection	27.3	33.7	21.8	6.0	6.0	2.9	0.7	1.7
Surgical site infection	35.2	26.6	18.4	5.0	9.0	3.6	1.3	1.8
Pneumonia	28.2	32.7	16.0	10.2	6.4	3.1	1.3	2.1
Bloodstream infection	22.8	44.4	18.4	3.8	5.9	2.0	0.9	1.9
Central line and peripheral line-associated bloodstream infection	38.4	18.6	22.7	5.0	9.6	3.0	0.7	2.1
Multidrug-resistant organism	28.3	33.2	20.3	4.2	7.6	2.4	1.4	1.6
Infection associated with prosthetics/implantable devices	33.6	23.2	22.3	7.9	7.6	2.4	1.4	1.6
Gastrointestinal infection	31.8	30.2	15.2	8.1	7.5	3.3	0.8	3.2

Source: Shaban RZ, Mitchell BG, Macbeth D, Russo PL. Epidemiology of healthcare-associated infections in Australia. 1 ed. Sydney, Australia: Elsevier; 2021.

across each state and territory. As expected, NSW, VIC and QLD, being the most populous states, account for over 70% of the country's HAIs.

2.3 Contemporary challenges and the burden of HAIs on populations and the Australian healthcare system

2.3.1 Estimated prevalence of HAIs

Our ability to estimate the prevalence of HAIs is severely limited by the lack of a national aggregated dataset. As previously mentioned, the incidence of HAIs in acute healthcare facilities is not only incomplete but varies according to the data source. Early national reports released by the ACSQHC in 2009 estimated approximately 200,000 cases of HAIs occurred each year.[8,9] A later ACSQHC guideline, published in 2018, reported an incidence of 60,037 HAIs for the 2015–16 period, which were pulled directly from IHPA data sets.[10] A systematic review of published peer-reviewed literature that reported the incidence of HAIs in Australian hospitals from 2010–16 similarly estimated an incidence of 83,096 HAIs per year.[1] However, the researchers urged caution when interpreting these results due to the lack of complete data for several common infections, including pneumonia, gastroenterological and bloodstream infections. The study concluded that the true incidence of HAIs was likely double their estimated value, at around 165,000 cases per year. A 2018 point prevalence study conducted on 2767 patients across 19 Australian hospitals found that HAI prevalence rates ranged from 5.7% to 17% in acute adult inpatients.[11] It has been estimated that over 170,000 cases of HAIs and 7500 deaths resulting from HAIs occurred annually.[12]

To increase the robustness and reliability of these data, researchers have called for a national consensus on definitions and reporting of surveillance methodology. System-wide efforts to achieve the national mandate of eliminating preventable infections initially focused on financial penalties for specific events, such as bloodstream infections. This led to the Australian Government introducing system-wide financial penalties for hospital-associated complications from 2017. Fundamentally, HAIs, cross-contamination and the spread of infection and infectious disease are risks in all healthcare settings.

The following sections provide a brief overview of the epidemiology of each type of healthcare-associated infection.

2.3.2 Urinary tract infection (UTI)

Urinary tract infection refers to an infection affecting the bladder, urethra, ureters or kidneys. UTIs are one of the most commonly reported HAIs, accounting for approximately 20 to 30% of total HAIs in Australia and internationally.[10,11,13,14] Symptoms of a UTI include dysuria, suprapubic pain, increased need and urgency to urinate, incontinence and abnormal urine colour. Further effects of the infection may result in fever, fatigue, nausea, rigors and delirium.[15]

In the healthcare setting, catheter-associated UTIs (CAUTIs) account for up to 80% of total UTIs.[16] The high rates of UTIs are likely exacerbated by the frequent, and at times unnecessary, insertion of indwelling urinary catheters, with an estimated 15% to 25% of patients in general hospitals having a catheter placed during their stay.[17-19] The length of hospital stay for patients who experience a healthcare-associated UTI is 20.6 days longer compared to a patient without this complication.[10] No jurisdictions report data on UTIs. In peer-reviewed literature, several estimates for the rates of healthcare-associated UTIs and CAUTIs have been provided, however, there is high variability in how the infection is defined and the populations that are investigated. Two longitudinal studies have estimate the incidence of UTIs per patient admission in VIC and NSW at 1.4% and 1.7% respectively.[20,21] A subsequent multi-site study conducted across multiple states observed a point prevalence of 2.4%.[11]

2.3.3 Surgical site infection (SSI)

Surgical site infection refers to an infection that occurs in the region of the body where prior surgery has been performed. The characteristic of an SSI varies depending on the classification of the wound (e.g. clean, clean-contaminated, contaminated, dirty) and the locus of infection (superficial, deep or organ/space). Symptoms of SSIs are typically localised to the area of surgery and usually include heat, swelling, redness, pain and the production of pus and unpleasant smelling fluids.

It is a common complication that occurs following approximately 3% of surgical procedures.[10] Like UTIs, they are one of the most common types of HAIs.[11] SSIs are estimated to result in a total 206,527 excess bed days annually, and affected patients remain in hospitals for 20.3 days longer on average compared to those without the complication.[10] Jurisdictional data on SSIs are available from VIC and WA, which reported SSI incidence rates of 0.6% and 1.6% respectively, averaged across all categories of patient risk and surgical procedures.[22,23] It is notable, however, that VIC reports a wider range of surgical procedures compared to WA, including infection rates for cardiac bypass, colorectal and femoro-popliteal and femoro-tibial bypass grafts, which have the highest rates of SSIs (over 4%). This is broadly consistent with the rate of 3.6% reported in the multi-site, multi-state point prevalence study.[11]

2.3.4 Pneumonia

Pneumonia describes the infection and inflammation of the lungs. Bacteria and viruses are the most common causes of pneumonia; however, the specific causal agents differ between pneumonia acquired in the community and that acquired in healthcare settings. Approximately 35% of healthcare-associated pneumonia is classified as ventilator-associated pneumonia (VAP). The infection is characterised by a productive cough, chest pain, shortness of breath, fatigue, fever and nausea.

Globally, pneumonia is the second most common HAI, and is associated with the greatest patient morbidity and mortality.[24] Nineteen percent of patients with non-ventilator-associated pneumonia are transferred into the intensive care unit during their stay, and affected patients stay in hospital 19 days longer compared to those with no complication.[10] No jurisdictions currently report cases of healthcare-associated pneumonia. The prevalence of healthcare-associated pneumonia based on peer-reviewed literature reported a range between 2.4% to 12.4%, depending on the population of patients examined.[11,25]

2.3.5 Bloodstream infection (BSI)

Bloodstream infections describe the presence of viable bacterial or fungal microorganisms in the bloodstream. BSIs are identified by a positive blood culture and may occur in the healthcare setting following the presence of an indwelling medical device (e.g. intravascular line, urinary catheter), a surgical procedure or any other invasive procedure, therapy or incision. Symptoms of BSIs include increased heart rate, palpitations, fever, chills, lethargy, fatigue, altered mental state and low blood pressure.

On an international level, the ECDC identified that 3.5% of ICU patients acquired a BSI with an estimated attributable mortality of 5.0%.[26] In general, the length of hospital stay for those who acquire a BSI is greater by up to 20.6 days.[10,26] Rates of *Staphylococcus aureus* bacteraemia are a key safety and quality indicator for hospitals under the Australian Health Performance Framework (AHPF). As a result, it is the only HAI that is reported nationally and by all jurisdictions. This data is published by the Australian Institute of Health and Welfare

(AIHW).[27] The initial national benchmark was 2.0 cases per 10,000 patient days, which all jurisdictions met for 2016–17 with a national rate of 0.76 cases. Since then, the benchmark has been reduced from 2.0 cases to 1.0 cases per 10,000 patient days. The national rate of SABSI for 2019–20 was 0.71 cases per 10,000 patient days, ranging between 0.47 to 0.86 per 10,000 patient days across different jurisdictions.[28] BSIs are estimated to account for around 10% of total HAIs in Australian hospitals.[11]

2.3.6 Central line and peripheral line-associated bloodstream infection

As previously discussed, bloodstream infections may arise from several causes. Central line-associated bloodstream infections (CLABSIs) refer to bloodstream infections caused by the introduction of pathogens into the bloodstream via a central or peripheral line. Intravascular devices are commonly used in hospital patients for medical treatment and they increase the risk of acquiring a BSI.[29] Symptoms of CLABSIs are consistent with those of general BSIs.[10]

Patients with a hospital-acquired CLABSI increase their length of hospital stay by an average of 16.8 days compared to patients without the complication.[10] Approximately 15% of adults in acute wards have a central vascular device and 55% have a peripheral vascular device.[11] Point prevalence study data from the ECDC report that 33% of bloodstream infections identified were central vascular device-related, while 6% were peripheral vascular device-related.[30] Four out of eight jurisdictions report CLABSI data, though not all release these reports annually. Reports of CLABSI infection rate are typically presented as a proportion of total healthcare-associated BSI infection or as a proportion per 1000 line days. In SA, device-associated cases accounted for approximately 31% of total BSI cases, with central lines specifically accounting for 69% of device-associated episodes in 2020.[31] Similarly, 52% of BSI cases were IV device-related in TAS.[32] In VIC and WA, the rate of CLABSI in ICUs was 1 and 0.33 cases per 1000 central line days, respectively.[22,23]

2.3.7 Multidrug-resistant organisms (MROs)

The term multidrug-resistant organisms refers to bacteria that are resistant to one or more classes of antimicrobial agents.[10] This resistance results from the inappropriate administration of antimicrobials, which have been frequently prescribed since their discovery in the early 20th century. Multidrug-resistant organisms are becoming increasingly problematic due to their increasing resistance to many commercially available antimicrobial agents. This notably includes methicillin resistant *Staphylococcus aureus* (MRSA), a resistant form of *Staphylococcus aureus* bacteria responsible for many of the HAIs listed in this section. Patients with MROs generally fail to respond to antibiotics, leading to prolonged infection, higher risk of complications and the need for additional or alternative therapies with problematic side effects.

The complications associated with MROs are particularly difficult and lead to hospital stays that are approximately 29.6 days longer than patients without MRO infection.[10] Four out of eight jurisdictions currently publish independent data on MROs: VIC, WA, SA and TAS. Additionally, the ACSQHC administers the Antimicrobial Use and Resistance in Australia (AURA) Surveillance System, which collects data on hospital antimicrobial usage as well as antimicrobial resistance via CARAlert, Australian Passive AMR surveillance (APAS) and the Australian Group on Antimicrobial Resistance (AGAR). According to CARAlert, the MROs that are more commonly identified in hospitals compared to in the community include: *Enterobacter cloacae* complex; *Enterococcus faecalis*; *Enterococcus faecium*; *Escherichia coli*; *Pseudomonas aeruginosa*; *Staphylococcus aureus*; and methicillin-resistant *Staphylococcus aureus*.[33]

2.3.8 Infection associated with prosthetics/implantable devices

Infections associated with prosthetics and implantable devices are those caused by the insertion and care of medical devices that typically remain in the body permanently, such as shunts, cochlear implants, pacemakers and insulin pumps.[10] Symptoms of infection are usually localised and include pain, swelling and tenderness, as well as fever, chills, palpitations, hypotension, fatigue and impaired mental state. Although these infections are rarer compared to the others listed, their occurrence can inflict significant morbidity and mortality, with adverse outcomes ranging from impaired function to sepsis and amputation.[34,35]

Infections associated with prosthetics and implantable devices may prolong the length of hospital stay by an average of 19.9 days.[10] Jurisdictional data is reported by VIC and WA, and shares significant overlap with data on SSIs and is generally limited to data regarding knee and hip replacement surgery. When averaging across both types of surgery, as well as categories of patient risk, VIC reports 1.1 infections per 100 procedures and WA reports 0.7 infections per 100 procedures.[22,23] Estimated rates

from peer-reviewed literature are limited, with only one retrospective cohort study in QLD that found a 2.7% deep prosthetic joint infection rate following total knee arthroplasty.[36] This study specifically identified high humidity and temperature as important risk factors for infection.

2.3.9 Gastrointestinal infection

Gastrointestinal infections describe infections of the gastrointestinal tract, which typically lead to acute episodes of diarrhoea, abdominal cramps, nausea, vomiting, lethargy and dehydration. Common causes of healthcare-associated gastrointestinal infection include *Clostridium difficile*, rotavirus and norovirus.[37] *C. difficile* has been responsible for outbreaks of severe disease, and specific hypervirulent strains of *C. difficile* have been associated with significant morbidity and mortality.[38,39] *Clostridiodes difficile* infection (CDI) is linked to prolonged and unnecessary use of antimicrobials. Additionally, the infection can be transmitted between humans and survive on surfaces for long periods, making it a key marker for infection control programs in healthcare facilities.

Gastrointestinal infections may prolong hospital stays by an average of 25.3 days.[10] As of 2022, three jurisdictions report *C. difficile* infections. Victoria reported 1.6 *C. difficile* infections per 10,000 bed days in 2019–20.[22] Both TAS and WA reported high rates, at 6.1 and 5.1 CDIs per 10,000 bed days respectively in their most recently released HAI reports.[23,32] These rates were consistent with those observed in peer-reviewed studies conducted in hospitals in VIC[40,41] and WA.[42]

2.4 Clinical infectious diseases

2.4.1 Infections of the respiratory system

Respiratory infections are one of the most common causes of disease globally and in Australia. The respiratory system encompasses the lungs, air passages, pulmonary vessels and breathing muscles and is responsible for the uptake of oxygen into, and expulsion of carbon dioxide from, the body. The system is anatomically divided into two sections: the upper respiratory tract, which includes the nasal cavity, sinuses, pharynx and larynx; and the lower respiratory tract, which is composed of the trachea, lungs, bronchi and diaphragm. Infections that affect the lower respiratory tract are generally more serious compared to the upper. The following section provides a brief overview of common clinical respiratory infections.

See Chapter 20 for a more comprehensive description of respiratory infections in the context of healthcare and infection control.

Influenza: Influenza is a highly transmissible, viral respiratory infection. Influenza viruses have evolved over centuries and they continue to mutate rapidly to cause seasonal epidemics worldwide. In Australia, these epidemics occur mid-year, starting from April and ending in September. Occasionally, novel highly virulent influenza strains emerge and may cause pandemics, leading to significantly greater morbidity and mortality compared to seasonal epidemics. Several influenza pandemics have occurred since the beginning of the 20th century, including the 1918–19 pandemic which was estimated to have killed 40–50 million people worldwide.[43] Influenza remains one of the most notified infectious diseases in Australia and is a common reason for consultation with a general practitioner.

Four types of influenza virus have been identified and are currently in circulation globally: A, B, C and D (Table 2.3). Influenza A is the most commonly detected virus in notified cases, generally accounting for over 90% of influenza cases in Australia.[44] Human-to-human transmission of influenza occurs when an individual encounters the respiratory droplets or secretions of an infected person. This may be through inhaling the infected particles or by touching contaminated surfaces, which then transfer to the eyes, nose and mouth. From there, the influenza virus enters the respiratory tract and replicates within respiratory epithelial cells. Symptoms usually present 1–3 days after infection and include fever, chills, malaise and muscle pain, which is shortly thereafter followed by sore throat, cough and runny nose. Most symptoms resolve within a week of infection, although some respiratory symptoms, like the cough, may last for longer. Infection prevention for influenza is best aimed at reducing risk and household transmission.[45]

Pneumonia: Pneumonia is an infection of the lungs, which can be caused by a wide range of microorganisms, including bacteria, viruses and fungi. The infection is particularly threatening in children, the elderly and the immunocompromised. Patients with pneumonia typically present with a fever, cough and chest pain, although in some infections organs outside of the lungs may also be affected, leading to additional symptoms and complications such as diarrhoea and liver dysfunction. Eventual respiratory failure is observed with cases of severe pneumonia, which may end in death.

This distinction between community-acquired and hospital-acquired pneumonia is important, as the causes and subsequent severity of the disease commonly differ depending on where the disease was acquired. Hospital-acquired pneumonia (HAP) accounts for 7.6% of all hospital-acquired complications.[46] It increases the likelihood of death, causes significant morbidity, and prolongs the length of hospital stay by an average of almost 20 days.[5] Although many of the risk factors for HAP are non-modifiable host factors, there are some important strategies available to HCWs to reduce incidence of infection. For example, ventilator-associated pneumonia can be reduced by minimising the duration of mechanical ventilation, careful positioning of the patient and meticulous attention to oral hygiene.[47] Input from physiotherapists and swallow assessments can help reduce the incidence of other HAPs,[48] along with ensuring patients are appropriately vaccinated.

As for all infectious diseases, early diagnosis and therapy improves outcomes, so patients should be carefully monitored for signs and symptoms of HAP, which may include cough, breathlessness, chest pain, hypoxia, fevers and rising inflammatory markers. There is a higher risk for MROs causing HAP than community-acquired infection. If possible, microbiological diagnosis via culture of sputum or other lower respiratory tract specimen will help to guide therapy. Empiric

TABLE 2.3 Characteristics of healthcare-associated pneumonia infections

At-risk patients	Prevention	Signs (S) and investigations (I)	Usual organism(s)
Ventilated patients (20%) Elderly Aspiration	Swallow assessment Physiotherapy Mobilising/sitting out of bed or upright Positioning of ventilated patients	S: Hypoxia, elevated respiratory rate, cough, fever I: Chest x-ray Culture of lower respiratory tract sample, e.g. sputum	*Staphylococcus aureus** Gram-negative bacilli or cocci *Haemophilus influenza* *Klebsiella* spp.

*20–30% of healthcare-associated Staphylococcus aureus *infections will be methicillin-resistant* S. aureus.

therapy per the eTG is stratified by disease severity—severe cases need broad spectrum antimicrobials, including anti-pseudomonal cover. Empiric therapy for mild to moderate disease does not need to cover *Pseudomonas*, since it only accounts for a small proportion of infections, and it is reasonable to await microbiological confirmation.

SARS-CoV-2 and COVID-19: The emergence of novel infectious respiratory diseases continues to pose an unpredictable and serious challenge to the healthcare system. Since the beginning of the 21st century, there have been three global pandemics caused by new coronaviruses. The first was the 2002–04 severe acute respiratory syndrome (SARS) pandemic caused by SARS-CoV-1, which spread to over 30 countries and infected approximately 8000 people. This was followed a decade later by Middle East respiratory syndrome (MERS), caused by MERS-CoV, which continues to circulate in specific regions to this day with approximately 2500 cases reported. In late 2019, the first cases of the new respiratory disease COVID-19, caused by the coronavirus SARS-CoV-2, were observed. This disease was highly transmissible and spread rapidly between countries, and was officially declared a pandemic by the World Health Organization in March 2020.[49] Unlike SARS and MERS, COVID-19 had a considerably lower case fatality rate, but had far greater human-to-human transmission, leading to over one million confirmed cases within the first five months of the outbreak.

SARS-CoV-2 targets and replicates within the lungs. Mild presentations of illness account for approximately 80% of COVID-19 cases, with some individuals also remaining asymptomatic over the course of the disease. For those who are symptomatic, fever and cough are the most commonly reported symptoms, followed by shortness of breath, fatigue, myalgia, rhinorrhoea and chills. As mentioned above, human-to-human transmission occurs easily and most prominently via inhalation or direct contact with infected respiratory droplets. However, transmission via the handling of contaminated objects and airborne particles have also been implicated. To date, there have been over 500 million cases reported globally, with a crude fatality rate of approximately 1.1%. In general, children experience milder clinical symptoms compared to adults, and severe or fatal outcomes occur considerably more frequently in the elderly and those with comorbid conditions.

Similar to previous novel coronavirus outbreaks, COVID-19 poses a significant risk to healthcare workers.

The situation was particularly dire during the beginning of the pandemic when PPE was in short supply and may have been improperly donned or reused.[50-52] Outbreaks of novel diseases cause considerable issues with significant carry-on effects in the healthcare sector. Staff are responsible for the provision of care, while simultaneously burdened with the anxiety of becoming infected and passing the disease on to others, including members of their household. Protocols for isolating infected workers and suspected contacts provided the most effective interventions of infection control, but inevitably places a substantial strain on the remaining workforce.[53] At time of writing, vaccines for the disease have been introduced. Regardless, COVID-19 still circulates widely, and cases continue to accumulate with the relaxation of infection control regulations worldwide. Careful attention is being exercised to the epidemiology of the virus and its emerging variants, as well as changes in the protection offered by existing vaccinations over time.[54]

Tuberculosis: Tuberculosis (TB) is a disease caused by bacteria belonging to the *Mycobacterium tuberculosis* complex, which include *M. tuberculosis*, *M. bovis*, *M. africanum*, *M. microti* and *M. canettii*.[55] Of these, the most frequent and important agent of disease in humans is *M. tuberculosis*, a rod-shaped, non-spore-forming, aerobic bacterium which grows very slowly compared with other bacteria.[56] Rates of TB vary widely across the world, although it has declined significantly in most industrialised countries since the early 1900s (Fig 2.1). Rates of TB are low in Australia, with an approximate incident rate of 5.8 cases per 100,000 population since the mid-1980s.[57] However, specific sub-populations, such as Aboriginal and Torres Strait Islanders and people born overseas, exhibit four to five times as many cases compared to non-Indigenous Australian-born people.[55,57]

The initial signs and symptoms of active TB are often non-specific and insidious, and include fever and night sweats, weight loss, anorexia, general malaise and weakness. As the disease progresses a cough develops, accompanied by the production of purulent sputum that often becomes blood-streaked. Tuberculosis is usually diagnosed by clinical symptoms, chest x-ray findings and results of tuberculin skin testing, also known as a Mantoux Test.[56] The disease typically affects, and is localised to, the lungs (pulmonary tuberculosis) but has the potential to spread to other organs or tissues in the body and cause more severe disease (extrapulmonary tuberculosis). In such cases, the infection can spread to

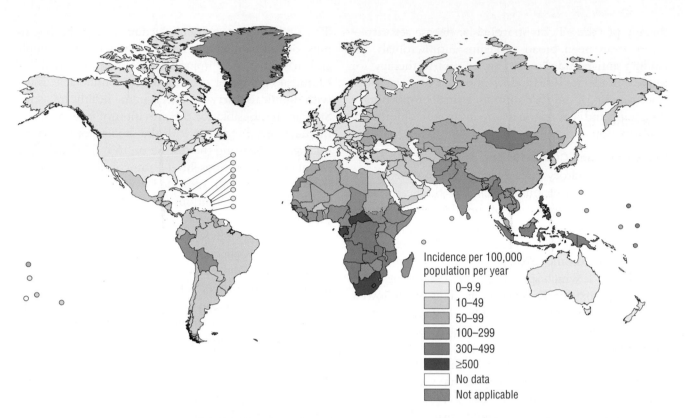

FIGURE 2.1 Estimated TB incidence rates by country, 2020
Source: World Health Organization. Global tuberculosis report 2021. Geneva, Switzerland: WHO; 2021

areas like the meninges, pleura, pericardium, kidneys, bones and joints, larynx, skin, intestines, peritoneum and eyes.[59,60] Immunocompromised people are most at risk of developing extrapulmonary TB, particularly those with human immunodeficiency virus (HIV), in which TB can be particularly lethal.

Tuberculosis can be categorised as either primary or secondary tuberculosis to distinguish between the two stages of infection. Primary tuberculosis defines the events following the initial infection with tubercle bacilli. Primary tuberculosis is asymptomatic in approximately 90% of immunocompetent people. The lesion formed in the lung at this time may not be detectable on chest x-ray and will heal spontaneously in the majority of cases.[55] Secondary tuberculosis describes the occurrence of the disease in the period following primary tuberculosis infection where dormant bacteria re-emerge and the latent infection is reactivated. This infection is usually localised to the lungs.[55] Secondary tuberculosis may occur many years after the initial infection, though the risks for reactivation increase with factors like age and impaired immune function. In general, persons infected with tuberculosis have, approximately, a 10% risk for developing active TB during their lifetime.[61]

The primary form of transmission is via the inhalation of infectious aerosol droplets, which may be expelled in enormous quantities when a person with active TB coughs, sneezes or/and talks. Viable bacteria can survive suspended in the air and in dust for long periods. The incubation period from infection to demonstrable primary lesion or significant tuberculin reaction is around 4–12 weeks.[61] Patients with active TB require transmission-based precautions for airborne transmission and should be placed in an enclosed, negative-pressure room. Healthcare workers and visitors should wear particulate filter masks when they are in the room of an infected patient and the patient should wear a surgical mask during transport. Diagnosis of TB is notifiable by law, and must be notified to the TB prevention and control service and health department.[9,62] In instances of latent TB infection, the individual does not develop symptoms, is not contagious, and there is no risk of transmission of the disease to others unless reactivation occurs.

TABLE 2.4 Types of viral hepatitis and their characteristics

Hepatitis	A	B	C	D	E
Virus	*Picornaviridae, Hepatovirus*	*Hepadnaviridae, Orthohepadnavirus*	*Flaviviridae, Hepacivirus*	Unassigned, *Deltavirus*	*Hepeviridae, Orthohepevirus*
Transmission	Faecal–oral	Blood, body fluid, sexual, perinatal	Blood, body fluid, sexual, perinatal	Blood, body fluid, sexual, perinatal	Faecal–oral
Incubation period	15–45 days	40–180 days	20–120 days	30–180 days	40 days
Hepatitis severity	Mild to moderate Increases with age	Moderate to severe 1% fulminant hepatic failure	Mild	Severe	Mild to moderate
Mortality	<0.2%, >1% for over 40 yrs old	0.2–2%	<1%	2–20%	0.2–1%; up to 20% in pregnancy
Chronicity	No	Yes; 2–7% in adults, >90% in newborns	Yes; up to 80%	Yes; 1–3% of co-infections; 70–80% of superinfection (with HBV)	No
Vaccination	Yes	Yes	No	Via HBV immunisation	No

2.4.2 Hepatic infections and viral hepatitis

Broadly speaking, hepatitis is the injury and inflammation of the liver. Viruses are a major cause of hepatitis, but other microorganisms and non-infectious causes may also be responsible.[63,64] Non-viral causes include drugs and chemicals such as carbon tetrachloride, ethylene glycol, rifampicin, methotrexate, monoamine oxide inhibitors, chlorpromazine and paracetamol.[65,66]

Viral hepatitis: Currently, there are five known strains of hepatitis virus: A, B, C, D and E (Table 2.4). While all five viruses cause disease of the liver and produce common signs and symptoms—such as fatigue, malaise, reduced appetite, abdominal pain, nausea and jaundice—the epidemiology, modes of transmission, severity of the illness and prevention methods differ considerably between viruses. For example, HAV and HEV are both transmitted via the faecal–oral route, facilitated by close personal contact, poor hygiene, unsanitary conditions or the consumption of contaminated food or water. On the other hand, HBV, HCV and HDV are all transmitted by some combination of exposure to infected blood or bodily fluids, sexual contact or from mother to child. In comparison to HAV and HEV, the blood-borne hepatitis viruses are more likely to lead to the development of chronic disease. As the clinical symptoms of acute hepatitis are similarly observed across all viruses, definitive diagnosis of the causative virus can only be made by laboratory testing. Figure 2.2 shows the notification rate of all hepatitis viruses in Australia over the past decade.

Treatment of viral hepatitis also differs heavily depending on the virus type and the severity of infection. In general, supportive care, such as rest, fluid intake and nutrition are provided for all presentations of acute viral hepatitis, and remain the only necessary treatment option for HAV and HEV, which are both self-limiting and generally resolve on their own.[68-70] Targeted pharmacological treatments and antivirals are administered in instances where the disease becomes chronic and are most commonly used to combat liver disease in patients with chronic HBV and HCV.[69,70] Severe presentations of hepatitis can manifest in cirrhosis, liver cancer and liver failure, at which point liver transplantation may be considered.[64]

Healthcare workers are at risk of acquiring hepatitis virus infections through exposure to patients' blood, bodily fluids or faeces. The risk is increased for those performing exposure-prone procedures, where there is exposure of the patient's open tissues to the blood of the healthcare worker. These procedures will commonly include the use of sharp instruments and needle tips and may involve situations where visibility of the healthcare

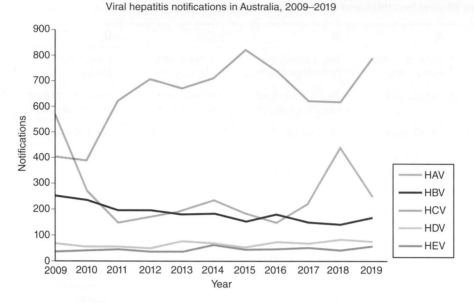

FIGURE 2.2 Viral hepatitis notifications in Australia, 2009–19

Source: Australian Institute of Health and Welfare. Infectious and communicable diseases Canberra, Australia: AIHW; 2020 [cited 2022 17 June]. Available from: https://www.aihw.gov.au/reports/australias-health/infectious-and-communicable-diseases.

worker's hands is obstructed. In general, adoption of prophylactic measures is the optimal strategy for preventing viral hepatitis infection. Vaccinations are widely available for HAV and HBV, the latter of which also offers indirect protection against HDV. Currently, neither HCV nor HEV have widely accessible vaccines.[68,69] For the blood-borne HCV, the best infection prevention measures include the safe use of needles, appropriate disposal of sharps and waste, and the active screening of blood donors. For HEV, prevention measures include maintaining a good standard of hygiene and sanitation at both facility and individual HCW levels.

2.4.3 Urinary tract infections

Catheter-associated urinary tract infections (CAUTI): Urinary tract infections are an important hospital-acquired infection, comprising 11% of all in-hospital complications according to the Australian Institute of Health and Welfare, and over 25% of all HAIs.[46] They are commonly related to catheters, and therefore removal as early as practicable is a key pillar of controlling these infections. It is important to monitor catheterised patients for signs of infection, which may include fevers, malaise, delirium and rising inflammatory markers (Table 2.5). Microbiologic culture of a clean midstream urine specimen is the most useful diagnostic test in non-catheterised patients but as discussed below, urine samples from catheterised patients can be difficult to interpret. The

International Society for Infectious Diseases estimates that the daily risk for developing bacteriuria with an indwelling catheter is 3–10%.[71] Approximately 10–25% of these patients will develop symptoms of urinary tract infection, and 5% of them will develop bacteraemia. This final link in the chain of events carries a mortality of 30%.

These figures highlight the risks of prolonged catheterisation, but also highlight another important matter: not all cases of bacteriuria turn into infections. The first stage in the development of CAUTIs is the development of bacterial biofilms in the lumen of the catheter. This is probably almost universal and does not indicate infection, and routine microbiology of catheter urine is not helpful. If the catheter is changed, a fresh urine specimen collected from the catheter insertion should be sent for microbiologic culture. The leading organisms for CAUTIs are *Escherichia coli, Pseudomonas aeruginosa, Klebsiella* and *Enterococcus faecalis.*[11] *Candida* is often isolated and requires investigation, although it is rarely a cause of infection and may not require therapy. The patients at particular risk for CAUTIs are females, older patients, diabetics and those who are immunocompromised. Management should begin with removal of the catheter wherever possible, which is often enough to resolve the infection. Where necessary, antibiotics directed against cultured organisms are administered. See Chapter 17 for more information on urinary tract infections.

TABLE 2.5 Characteristics of healthcare-associated urinary tract infections

At-risk patients	Prevention	Signs (S) and Investigations (I)	Usual organism(s)
Patients with current or recent indwelling urinary catheter Patients with preexisting renal tract abnormalities Post-urological intervention	Removal of unnecessary urinary catheters Care of perineum in bed-bound patients	S: Dysuria (uncatheterised), suprapubic or flank tenderness, fever I: Clean midstream urine for microbiologic culture. If IDC: change urinary catheter and send urine specimen collected during fresh insertion.	*Escherichia coli* *Enterococcus faecalis/ faecium* *Klebsiella* spp.

2.4.4 Bloodstream infections (BSIs)

Bloodstream infections pose a serious health risk to patients and are leading causes of morbidity and mortality within the Australian healthcare system. Bloodstream infections may occur from an uncontrolled infection at any site or through the direct introduction of organisms into the bloodstream. Patients with BSIs become acutely unwell and can deteriorate rapidly. Diagnosis is by blood culture and all positive blood cultures demand investigation.

Fever is frequently the first sign, which is why it is important to send blood cultures urgently as part of the initial investigation of fever. Patients quickly develop other signs of sepsis, including tachycardia, hypotension, delirium and respiratory decompensation. The attributable mortality odds ratio for BSIs ranges from 2.47–5.01%, depending on the organism.[5] Early initiation of empiric antibiotics improves outcomes with choice guided by suspected site of infection in accordance with evidence-based guidelines such as the eTG. Empiric antibiotics should be administered after blood cultures have been sent, but within the first hour of developing signs of sepsis. Once an organism is identified, antimicrobial therapy should be modified accordingly.

Any organism can cause a BSI. A large survey of over 8000 episodes of BSI in QLD showed that 47% were Gram-positive bacteria, 44% were Gram-negative bacteria, 5% were fungi, and 4% were other organisms.[72] There were over 15,000 cases of BSIs across Australia in 2015–16.[46] These occurred in a very heterogenous group of patients, ranging from otherwise healthy patients who had surgery within the preceding 30 days to profoundly immunosuppressed patients on chemotherapy.

Reducing the incidence of BSIs is an important focus of the Australian Safety and Quality Goals for Health Care. To standardise markers of quality and to enable the introduction of quality targets across different locations and different times, two specific bloodstream infections are closely monitored: hospital-acquired *Staphylococcus aureus* bloodstream infections (SABSI) and central line-associated bloodstream infections (CLABSI). There were 1573 episodes of hospital-acquired SABSI in 2018–19.[28] The rate of infection has reduced from 1.1 per 10,000 patient days in 2010–11 (when records began) to 0.71 per patient days most recently.[28,73] The national benchmark is 1.0 case per 10,000 patient days and is currently exceeded in all states and territories. These impressive results can be at least partially attributed to campaigns focusing on the key intervention available to reduce incidence: meticulous attention to hand hygiene.

Central line and peripheral line-associated bloodstream infections comprise 1.4% of all HAI and make up around 20% of all healthcare-acquired BSIs.[74] By definition, they require the presence of central or peripheral intravascular catheter. Ensuring that such lines are only inserted when absolutely necessary and removing them as soon as possible is the most important intervention we have to reduce incidence of CLABSIs. When placing a central line, good skin preparation and aseptic technique, including full barrier personal protective equipment (PPE), can reduce risk. Whenever staff are manipulating the line, careful attention to sterile technique and hand hygiene is vital. Furthermore, the insertion site should be closely monitored for any signs of infection, which may include redness, tenderness or swelling (Table 2.6). It is important that the date of insertion is clearly documented for all intravenous devices, and that the ongoing need for their presence is reviewed regularly. See Chapter 20 for more information on BSIs.

Human immunodeficiency virus (HIV)/Acquired immune deficiency syndrome (AIDS): Human immunodeficiency virus is a retrovirus that binds to cells with CD4 receptors, including T-cells, monocytes, macrophages and dendritic cells, which facilitate the coordination of the body's immune

TABLE 2.6 Characteristics of healthcare-associated bloodstream infections

At-risk patients	Prevention	Signs (S) and investigations (I)	Usual organism(s)
Post-operative patients Chronic disease Prolonged or recurrent exposure to antibiotics Patients with indwelling medical devices including PIVC Immunosuppression Preexisting skin conditions	Daily monitoring and documentation of IVC/PICC sites Removal of IVC in line with local guidelines	S: Fever, inflamed or tender venous catheter site, with or without exudate I: Collect 2 sets of peripheral blood cultures Collect culture from indwelling central or long lines May require ultrasound to assess for thrombophlebitis or clot at insertion site	*Staphylococcus aureus** *Escherichia coli* *Enterococcus* spp.

20–30% of healthcare-associated Staphylococcus aureus infections will be methicillin-resistant S. aureus.

response. As the infection progresses, the CD4 cell count declines, resulting in a substantially weakened immune system that is no longer able to effectively ward off subsequent infections. The incubation period for HIV can range from two weeks to several months. For most infected individuals, the first clinical symptom of disease is the development of an acute, self-limited mononucleosis-like illness lasting for 1–2 weeks. Following this, there is a period of asymptomatic infection, which may last from a few months to several years. During this stage, CD4 cells are in a gradual but constant state of decline. Onset of symptomatic HIV infection is usually insidious, with non-specific symptoms such as lymphadenopathy, appetite loss, chronic diarrhoea, weight loss, fever and fatigue.

Acquired immune deficiency syndrome is a severe, life-threatening consequence of HIV infection, and is generally defined when CD4 cell count is <200 cells/mm[3]. This syndrome represents the late clinical stage of infection with HIV and is most often the result of progressive damage to the immune and other organ systems. At this stage, HIV-infected people become highly susceptible to illnesses and opportunistic infections. These include several cancers, pulmonary and extrapulmonary tuberculosis, recurrent pneumonia, wasting syndrome, neurological disease (HIV dementia or sensory neuropathy) and invasive cervical cancer.[61]

HIV is transmitted by direct contact with blood or specific infected body fluids, through mucous membranes, broken skin or through percutaneous injury. Certain body fluids, such as saliva, urine and sweat, do not carry a risk of transmission unless blood is also present. The most common routes of transmission are through infected blood, sexual fluids and from infected mother to baby during pregnancy and delivery.[8] All persons in the acute or chronic stage of infection who are HIV-antibody-positive are potentially infectious, with the severity of disease also increasing with greater viral load. The period of infectivity is believed to begin shortly after primary infection and to continue throughout life.[75] Furthermore, infectivity may also increase with increasing immune deficiency, clinical symptoms and presence of other sexually transmitted infections.[61] The most commonly used diagnostic test for HIV infection is serologic detection of antibodies, as most individuals infected with HIV develop detectable antibodies within 1–3 months. This consists of an enzyme-linked immunoassay, which is then followed for confirmation by an additional test such as the Western blot or indirect immunofluorescence assay (IFA).

The risk to healthcare workers of acquiring HIV from an occupational exposure is very small, with the average risk for HIV infection estimated to be 0.3% after percutaneous exposure (needlestick injury) and 0.09% following mucous membrane exposure.[75] Nevertheless, exposure to HIV must be managed in accordance with established protocols including timely access to expert counselling and post-exposure prophylactic (PEP) treatments as required. Stringent practice of standard precautions is recommended, particularly the use of appropriate PPE when performing non-invasive and/or invasive procedures where the HCW may encounter blood or bodily fluids, and the safe and appropriate use and subsequent disposal of sharps and clinical waste.

2.4.5 Gastrointestinal infections

Gastrointestinal infections may be caused by viruses, bacteria or parasites, leading to an inflammation of the gastrointestinal tract, which encompasses all major organs of the digestive system. Many microorganisms can

TABLE 2.7 Examples of common organisms responsible for gastrointestinal infections and acute diarrhoea

Organism	Examples	Common causes	Length of illness
Bacteria	*Campylobacter*	Contaminated or improperly prepared animal-based food products	3–6 days
	Clostridium difficile	Poor hygiene and sanitation, hospital and healthcare settings	2–3 days
	Salmonella	Raw or undercooked meat, seafood and eggs, unpasteurised dairy products	2–7 days
	Yersinia	Contaminated food, raw or undercooked meat (esp. pork), unpasteurised milk	1–3 weeks
Viruses	Adenovirus	Faecally polluted water, human-to-human via respiratory droplets	1–2 weeks
	Rotavirus	Human-to-human via contact and faecal–oral routes	4–6 days
	Norovirus	Human-to-human via contact and faecal–oral routes	1–2 days
Parasites	*Cryptosporidium*	Contaminated food and water, travelling, poor sanitation, faecal–oral	1–2 weeks
	Giardia lamblia	Contaminated food and water, travelling, poor sanitation, faecal–oral	2–6 weeks

enter the human body, simply through the ingestion of food and drink. However, the digestive system has developed a series of natural defences, such as stomach acid and digestive enzymes, which effectively eliminate most of these microorganisms before they can reach the intestine. Several organisms have evolved to survive the body's defence mechanisms and subsequently cause infection and disease. These include, but are not limited to, adenovirus, rotavirus, norovirus, *Campylobacter* spp., *Clostridium difficile*, *Salmonella* spp., *Yersinia*, *Cryptosporidium* and *Giardia lamblia* (Table 2.7). Most pathogens will enter the gastrointestinal tract via the faecal–oral route, from contaminated hands, food or fluids.

Acute diarrhoeal disease: The most common outcome of gastrointestinal infection is acute diarrhoeal disease, which is characterised by a sudden onset of acute diarrhoea and the excretion of loose and watery stools that lasts one to several days. In prolonged cases, acute diarrhoeal disease will cause excessive fluid loss and dehydration, which may be serious. Infectious diarrhoea is usually distinguished into two categories: non-inflammatory diarrhoea, characterised by an acute and self-limiting presentation of watery stool without blood; and inflammatory diarrhoea (or dysentery), characterised by diarrhoea with presence of blood, mucus and pus.[76]

Non-inflammatory diarrhoeas are caused by organisms such as viruses, *Vibrio cholerae* and enterotoxigenic *Escherichia coli*, which adhere to the mucosa of the small intestine and disrupt the absorptive and/or secretory processes without causing significant tissue damage. The resulting diarrhoea is caused by an excessive secretion of fluids from the lining cells. Inflammatory diarrhoea is caused by organisms such as *Salmonella*, *Shigella*, *Campylobacter*, enteroaggregative and enterohemorrhagic *E. coli* and *Clostridium difficile*. The infection produces an inflammatory response which typically damages the mucosal lining of the colon and leads to the appearance of blood and mucus when passing stools. Inflammatory diarrhoea commonly presents with additional symptoms, such as fever and tenesmus. Both inflammatory and non-inflammatory cases may have associated abdominal cramps, while nausea and vomiting are typically limited to those with non-inflammatory, viral infections.

There are approximately 6.42 gastrointestinal infections per 10,000 hospitalisations in Australian hospitals.[46] In Australia, the most common causes of gastrointestinal disease are *C. difficile*, norovirus and rotavirus. The most recently estimated national incidence rate of *C. difficile* infection in Australia is 4.0 per 10,000.[77] Infection generally results from upsets to the microbiome, as a result of prolonged broad spectrum antibiotic use. Its incidence, therefore, will be reduced by improvements in antimicrobial stewardship (AMS)—ensuring that the narrowest spectrum antibiotic is used for the minimum duration required to treat underlying infections.[78] Norovirus is a common cause of non-bacterial gastroenteritis. Similarly, outbreaks of norovirus have also been frequently reported in the emergency department (ED), hospital wards and aged care facilities. Norovirus commonly occurs in winter months, and is a syndrome of acute nausea, vomiting and diarrhoea. Vomiting, in particular, causes widespread aerosol dissemination of viral particles, resulting in environmental contamination and subsequent spread.

Outbreaks of infectious gastrointestinal diseases can occur sporadically and there are organisms that cause infections seasonally. Infections in healthcare may arise from staff, clients, visitors, air, food, water, sterile products, the environment and vermin (see Table 2.8). They cause significant distress for patients and frequently prolong hospital stays. Whenever diarrhoea develops in a patient, especially those at risk of *C. difficile* infection (e.g. those with immunosuppression, exposure to antibiotics, prolonged hospital admission, shared space or bathroom facilities with a known case) it is important that a stool sample is sent for diagnostic testing. Once a diagnosis is suspected, and especially once confirmed, patients must be nursed under barrier precautions. It is important to note that alcohol-based hand rubs are not effective against *C. difficile* or norovirus, and that hands should be washed with soap and water. If locally available, infection prevention and control teams should become involved with any potential outbreak, to ensure that contact tracing is carried out and any patients potentially exposed receive appropriate follow-up. From a therapeutic perspective, often cessation of the causative antimicrobial is sufficient to improve symptoms. In more severe cases, however, treatment can range from a course of oral vancomycin to, in unremitting cases, faecal microbiota transplant. Further details on gastrointestinal HAIs, their diagnosis and management can be found in Chapter 21.

2.4.6 Wounds and skin infections

Wounds, particularly chronic ones, are challenging to manage. Infection occurs when replicating microorganisms, like *Staphylococcus aureus*, enter through the open wound and subsequently overcome the body's defence mechanisms. Local signs of infection include oedema, erythema and purulent exudate. If the infection becomes vascular, patients may deteriorate into sepsis or septic shock, a form of distributive shock with a higher risk of mortality.[79] Septic shock ultimately results in a cellular hypoxia, anaerobic metabolism and respiration and irreversible cell injury. Treating the infection is critical for resuscitation to be successful. Identifying, treating and preventing wound infection, and sepsis, is a major challenge in emergency trauma and care, and there are well-established screening tools that should be deployed, such as qSOFA. In instances of sepsis and septic shock, patients require aggressive resuscitation and rapid, broad-spectrum antibiotic therapy until microbiological culture and sensitivities, and antibiograms, can be performed.[80,81]

Skin and soft tissue infections (SSTIs): Healthcare-associated skin and soft tissue infections range from local cellulitis to fulminant, necrotising infections. They generally arise from breaches in the integument, such as haematomas, small wounds or skin tears, pressure areas and ulcers. Healthcare-associated SSTIs are well recognised but incompletely defined and studied. These infections are most commonly caused by *S. aureus*, which is more likely to be resistant to first-line antibiotics if acquired in a healthcare setting.[82] Signs of cellulitis include tender, warm, erythematous areas, sometimes with purulent discharge if involving a wound, skin tear or ulcer. Purulent discharge should be sampled with a bacterial swab and sent for microbiologic culture. Infections of chronic or pressure ulcers sometimes require assessment with imaging to exclude progression of the infection to underlying bone (osteomyelitis). General principles of therapy include appropriate analgesia, accurate antimicrobial choice (which may change based on the culture result), optimising nutrition and glycaemic control in the malnourished or diabetic patient, meticulous pressure care, and consultation with an experienced wound practitioner

TABLE 2.8 Characteristics of healthcare-associated gastrointestinal infections

At-risk patients	Prevention	Signs (S) and investigations (I)	Usual organism(s)
Protracted antimicrobial use Immunosuppression Elderly	Avoid unnecessary antibiotic use Hand hygiene Contact precautions for patients with diarrhoea	S: Diarrhoea, abdominal tenderness I: Stool specimen for MCS, *C. difficile* testing, viral testing (PCR or antigen)	*Clostridium difficile* Viral

TABLE 2.9 Characteristics of healthcare-associated skin and soft tissue infections

At-risk patients	Prevention	Signs (S) and investigations (I)	Usual organism(s)
Pressure area Skin tear Diabetes Immunosuppression Elderly Underweight or overweight	Pressure area risk assessment, prevention and care Nutrition Glycaemic control	S: Cellulitis, erythema, tenderness, exudate I: Swab ulcer or wound if present, send for bacterial culture	*Staphylococcus aureus** *Streptococcus pyogenes*

*20–30% of healthcare-associated Staphylococcus aureus *infections will be methicillin-resistant* S. aureus.

for advice on frequency and type of dressing if the SSTI is wound- or ulcer-related (Table 2.9).

Surgical site infections (SSIs): Surgical site infections complicate approximately 3% of all surgical procedures, with incidence rates varying according to the site of surgery.[11] The highest rates are reported in patients who have undergone vascular surgical interventions, making them a particular focus for close observation. There is good evidence that routine perioperative antibiotic prophylaxis reduces the incidence of SSIs.[83] The current eTG details which procedures require prophylaxis, and the appropriate choice of antibiotic. In general, prophylaxis is given at the time of surgery, and does not need to be continued after the patient returns to the ward. Patients undergoing longer procedures, or who are colonised with MROs, may require individualised antibiotic prophylaxis.

Surgical site infections present with inflammation, tenderness and exudate at the surgical wound site. Very severe necrotising infections, which are rare, may have associated gas gangrene (subcutaneous crepitus), and require prompt review. If exudate is present, a bacterial swab should be collected and sent for microbiologic culture. Management may include surgical debridement and antibiotic therapy directed against identified pathogens (Table 2.10). See Chapter 18 for more information on SSIs.

Wound care is made more complex with multiple resistant organisms such as MRSA. The emergence and re-emergence of rapid-spread MROs is an ongoing international health priority.[84] Historically, *Staphylococcus aureus* has been a major cause of wound infections, septic shock and hospital-associated infection. It is the leading cause of healthcare-associated SSIs, and the second leading cause of healthcare-associated BSIs. It is responsible for infections such as osteomyelitis, septic arthritis, skin infections, endocarditis and meningitis.[85] MRSA continues to challenge the safety and quality of modern healthcare, and in some settings MRSA can constitute as many as 20% of all HAIs. Endemic in most hospitals and epidemic in others, approximately 30% of all *S. aureus* infections present with some form of drug resistance.[86]

The main route of MRSA transfer is from one client to another. Individuals transmit infection by failing to decontaminate their hands effectively before and after contact with individuals colonised or infected with MRSA. Attempts to eliminate endemic MRSA in hospitals have proven difficult, costly and have been largely unsuccessful. In some settings, identification of known carriers, prospective surveillance of clients and hospital workers and use of nasal mupirocin have helped control drug-resistant *S. aureus* infection rates.[86,87] Reported costs of an HAI vary because of the wide range of study populations, sites of infection and methods used.[86]

TABLE 2.10 Characteristics of healthcare-associated surgical site infections

At-risk patients	Prevention	Signs (S) and investigations (I)	Usual organism(s)
Long surgery Diabetic	Appropriate perioperative antimicrobial prophylaxis Postoperative wound care Glycaemic control Hand hygiene	S: Erythema, exudate or tenderness at wound site I: Superficial swab of exudate for Gram stain bacterial culture	*Staphylococcus aureus**

*20–30% of healthcare-associated Staphylococcus aureus *infections will be methicillin-resistant* S. aureus.

2.4.7 High-risk patient populations

The primary risk factors for infectious disease and HAIs include advanced age, longer duration of hospitalisation, prolonged courses of antimicrobials and the presence of indwelling medical devices.[88] Other risk factors include any form of immunosuppression, including that related to chronic disease, especially diabetes and HIV infection.

Older populations: It should be noted that throughout this chapter, elderly individuals are frequently highlighted as populations who are at higher risk of acquiring specific infections and/or infectious diseases. The ageing process introduces several, usually unavoidable, physiological changes that predispose elderly individuals to greater morbidity and mortality from infectious disease. These include, but are not limited to, decreased mobility, impaired sight and hearing, weakened immune responses, multiple interacting pharmacological treatments, and most importantly, preexisting physical conditions like diabetes and hypertension. Additionally, cognitive impairment, resulting from conditions like dementia or Alzheimer's disease, may also act to impede diagnosis or inhibit the efficacy of certain infection control practice procedures. Moreover, infection may be difficult to diagnose "as many" older individuals have a pulse/temperature dissociation that masks the signs of infection.[89] Often, a change in behaviour or cognitive functioning, loss of appetite, or tachypnoea is the only symptom that indicates an infection is present in older individuals.[62]

The COVID-19 pandemic has had a disproportionately adverse impact on older people, particularly those in healthcare and residential-care settings who were more likely to have additional comorbidities and experience greater severity of COVID-19 symptoms and mortality.[90] In Australia, those over 60 years of age comprise less than 10% of cases, yet account for more than 90% of deaths.[91] See Chapter 29 for more information on infection prevention and control in aged care services and residential aged care facilities.

Paediatric populations: Children are also at increased risk of acquiring and experiencing more severe clinical outcomes from infections and infectious disease. Similar to older people, the immune system of young children is vulnerable as they have not had as much time to develop, relative to adults. This puts children at more risk from vaccine-preventable diseases because they often have not yet developed full immunity to these agents. Moreover, young children are still in the process of learning appropriate hygiene practices. Many young children will naturally exhibit a certain degree of oral fixation, which involves placing foreign and potentially contaminated objects into their mouths. As a result, bacteria and viruses, particularly those highlighted under gastrointestinal infections, are very frequent causes of infection in children due to their common faecal–oral and contact transmission pathways.

The respiratory rate is also higher in children compared to adults. When in combination with a disproportionate ratio of body-surface-area-to-weight, this puts them at a greater risk from inhaling aerosolised infectious agents. Respiratory infectious diseases are one of the most common health issues in paediatric patients encountered by emergency clinicians. Like adults, children are at risk from hospital-acquired infections, multidrug-resistant organisms and respiratory illnesses. Newborns and children with immunodeficiencies are at an increased risk from infection, especially during an infectious disease outbreak. See Chapter 43 for more information on infection control practices in paediatric and neonatal health.

Conclusion

While it is not possible to completely eliminate infectious diseases and HAIs, their incidence can be greatly reduced. Optimising environmental cleaning, hand hygiene and antimicrobial stewardship as well as patient nutrition, glycaemic control, wound and device care will all substantially reduce the burden. Knowledge of how to recognise and commence investigation of these infections improves outcomes for affected patients and is thus an important skill for all healthcare workers.

Useful websites/resources

- Communicable Diseases, Department of Health and Ageing, Australian Government. https://www.health.gov.au/health-topics/communicable-diseases
- Australian National Notifiable Diseases and Case Definitions, Communicable Diseases Network Australia. https://www1.health.gov.au/internet/main/publishing.nsf/Content/cdna-casedefinitions.htm

- Infectious Diseases, Health Direct. https://www.healthdirect.gov.au/infectious-diseases
- Infectious Diseases, New South Wales Ministry of Health. https://www.health.nsw.gov.au/Infectious/Pages/default.aspx
- Communicable Diseases Network Australia (CDNA). https://www1.health.gov.au/internet/main/publishing.nsf/Content/cda-cdna-index.htm
- The Blue Book Guidelines for the control of infectious diseases, first edition. Communicable Diseases Section, Public Health Group, Department of Health, Victoria. https://www.health.vic.gov.au/infectious-diseases/disease-information-and-advice
- Series of National Guidelines, Communicable Diseases Network Australia. https://www1.health.gov.au/internet/main/publishing.nsf/Content/cdnasongs.htm

References

1. Mitchell BG, Shaban RZ, Macbeth D, Wood C-J, Russo PL. The burden of healthcare-associated infection in Australian hospitals: a systematic review of the literature. Infect Dis Health. 2017;22(3):117-128.
2. Network NHS. Surveillance for Surgical Site Infection (SSI) Events. Atlanta: Centers for Disease Control, 2020.
3. Shaban RZ, Mitchell BG, Macbeth D, Russo PL. Epidemiology of healthcare-associated infections in Australia. Sydney: Elsevier, 2021.
4. Haque M, Sartelli M, McKimm J, Bakar MA. Health care-associated infections–an overview. Infect Drug Resist. 2018;11:2321-2333.
5. Lee X, Stewardson A, Worth L, Graves N, Wozniak T. Attributable length of stay, mortality risk, and costs of bacterial health care-associated infections in Australia: a retrospective case-cohort study. Clin Infect Dis. 2021;72(10):e506-e14.
6. Murray CJ, Ikuta KS, Sharara F, Swetschinski L, Aguilar GR, Gray A, et al. Global burden of bacterial antimicrobial resistance in 2019: a systematic analysis. Lancet. 2022. Feb 12;399(10325):629-655.
7. Australian Commission on Safety and Quality in Health Care. AURA 2019: third Australian report on antimicrobial use and resistance in human health. Sydney: ACSQHC, 2019.
8. Australian Commission on Safety and Quality in Health Care. Cruickshank M, Murphy C, eds. Reducing harm to patients from healthcare associated infections: an Australian infection prevention and control model for acute hospitals. Sydney: ACSQHC, 2009.
9. National Health and Medical Research Council. Australian guidelines for the prevention and control of infection in healthcare. Canberra: NHMRC, 2010.
10. Australian Commission on Safety and Quality in Health Care. Hospital-acquired complication - 3. Healthcare-associated infection fact sheet. Sydney: ACSQHC, 2018.
11. Russo PL, Stewardson AJ, Cheng AC, Bucknall T, Mitchell BG. The prevalence of healthcare associated infections among adult inpatients at nineteen large Australian acute-care public hospitals: a point prevalence survey. Antimicrob Resist Infect Control. 2019;8(1):1-8.
12. Lydeamore MJ, Mitchell BG, Bucknall T, Cheng AC, Russo PL, Stewardson AJ. Burden of five healthcare associated infections in Australia. Antimicrob Resist Infect Control. 2022;11(1):69.
13. Zarb P, Coignard B, Griskeviciene J, Muller A, Vankerckhoven V, Weist K, et al. The European Centre for Disease Prevention and Control (ECDC) pilot point prevalence survey of healthcare-associated infections and antimicrobial use. Eurosurveillance. 2012;17(46):20316.
14. Magill SS, Edwards JR, Bamberg W, Beldavs ZG, Dumyati G, Kainer MA, et al. Multistate point-prevalence survey of health care–associated infections. NEJM. 2014;370(13):1198-1208.
15. Elvy J, Colville A. Catheter associated urinary tract infection: what is it, what causes it and how can we prevent it? J Infect Prev. 2009;10(2):36-41.
16. Weber DJ, Sickbert-Bennett EE, Gould CV, Brown VM, Huslage K, Rutala WA. Incidence of catheter-associated and non-catheter-associated urinary tract infections in a healthcare system. Infect Control Hosp Epidemiol. 2011;32(8):822-823.
17. Jain P, Parada JP, David A, Smith LG. Overuse of the indwelling urinary tract catheter in hospitalized medical patients. Arch Intern Med. 1995;155(13):1425-1429.
18. Munasinghe RL, Yazdani H, Siddique M, Hafeez W. Appropriateness of use of indwelling urinary catheters in patients admitted to the medical service. Infect Control Hosp Epidemiol. 2001;22(10):647-649.
19. Warren JW. Catheter-associated urinary tract infections. Int J Antimicrob Agents. 2001;17(4):299-303.
20. Mitchell BG, Ferguson J, Anderson M, Sear J, Barnett A. Length of stay and mortality associated with healthcare-associated urinary tract infections: a multi-state model. J Hosp Infect. 2016;93(1):92-99.
21. Aubron C, Flint AW, Bailey M, Pilcher D, Cheng AC, Hegarty C, et al. Is platelet transfusion associated with hospital-acquired infections in critically ill patients? Critical Care. 2017;21(1):1-8.
22. Doherty Institute. Healthcare-associated infection in Victoria: surveillance report 2019-20. Melbourne: Doherty Institute, 2021.
23. Communicable Disease Control Directorate. Healthcare infection surveillance Western Australia: Annual Report 2017-18. Perth: Communicable Disease Control Directorate, 2018.
24. Rotstein C, Evans G, Born A, Grossman R, Light RB, Magder S, et al. Clinical practice guidelines for hospital-acquired pneumonia and ventilator-associated pneumonia in adults. Can J Infect Dis Med Microbiol. 2008;19(1):19-53.
25. Sanagou M, Leder K, Cheng A, Pilcher D, Reid C, Wolfe R. Associations of hospital characteristics with nosocomial pneumonia after cardiac surgery can impact on standardized infection rates. Epidemiol Infect. 2016;144(5):1065-1074.
26. European Centre for Disease Prevention and Control. Incidence and attributable mortality of healthcare-associated

infections in intensive care units in Europe, 2008–2012. Stockholm: ECDC, 2018.

27. Australian Institute of Health and Welfare. Staphylococcus aureus bacteraemia in Australian hospitals 2016–17. Canberra: AIHW, 2017.

28. Australian Institute of Health and Welfare. Bloodstream infections associated with hospital care 2019–20. Canberra: AIHW, 2021.

29. Maki DG, Kluger DM, Crnich CJ, eds. The risk of bloodstream infection in adults with different intravascular devices: a systematic review of 200 published prospective studies. Mayo Clin Proc; 2006;81(9):1159-1171.

30. European Centre for Disease Prevention and Control. Point prevalence survey of healthcare-associated infections and antimicrobial use in European acute care hospitals. Stockholm: ECDC, 2013.

31. Program SAH-aIS. Bloodstream infection. Annual report 2020. Adelaide: SA Health, 2021.

32. Department of Health, Tasmania. Tasmanian acute public hospitals healthcare associated infection surveillance annual report 2020. Hobart: Department of Health, Tasmania, 2021.

33. Australian Commission on Safety and Quality in Health Care. AURA 2021: fourth Australian report on antimicrobial use and resistance in human health. Sydney: ACSQHC, 2021.

34. Romero-Palacios A, Petruccelli D, Main C, Winemaker M, de Beer J, Mertz D. Screening for and decolonization of Staphylococcus aureus carriers before total joint replacement is associated with lower S aureus prosthetic joint infection rates. Am J Infect Control. 2020;48(5):534-537.

35. Hamilton WG, Balkam CB, Purcell RL, Parks NL, Holdsworth JE. Operating room traffic in total joint arthroplasty: identifying patterns and training the team to keep the door shut. Am J Infect Control. 2018;46(6):633-636.

36. Armit D, Vickers M, Parr A, Van Rosendal S, Trott N, Gunasena R, et al. Humidity a potential risk factor for prosthetic joint infection in a tropical Australian hospital. ANZ J Surg. 2018;88(12):1298-12301.

37. Crews JD. Healthcare-associated gastrointestinal infections. In: McNeil JC, Campbell JR, Crews JD, eds. Healthcare-associated infections in children: a guide to prevention and management. Cham: Springer International Publishing, 2019, p. 197-213.

38. Herbert R, Hatcher J, Jauneikaite E, Gharbi M, d'Arc S, Obaray N, et al. Two-year analysis of Clostridium difficile ribotypes associated with increased severity. J Hosp Infect. 2019;103(4):388-394.

39. Slimings C, Riley TV. Antibiotics and hospital-acquired Clostridium difficile infection: update of systematic review and meta-analysis. J Antimicrob Chemother. 2014;69(4): 881-891.

40. Worth L, Spelman T, Bull A, Brett J, Richards M. Epidemiology of Clostridium difficile infections in Australia: enhanced surveillance to evaluate time trends and severity of illness in Victoria, 2010–2014. J Hosp Infect. 2016;93(3):280-285.

41. Hebbard AI, Slavin MA, Reed C, Trubiano JA, Teh BW, Haeusler GM, et al. Risk factors and outcomes of Clostridium difficile infection in patients with cancer: a matched case-control study. Support Care Cancer. 2017;25(6):1923-1930.

42. Foster N, Collins D, Ditchburn S, Duncan C, Van Schalkwyk J, Golledge C, et al. Epidemiology of Clostridium difficile infection in two tertiary-care hospitals in Perth, Western Australia: a cross-sectional study. NMNI. 2014;2(3):64-71.

43. Australian Government: Department of Parliamentary Services. Australia's capacity to respond to an infectious disease outbreak. Canberra: Department of Parliamentary Services, 2004.

44. Australian Government: Department of Health and Aged Care. Australian influenza surveillance Report No. 05, 2022. Canberra: Department of Health and Aged Care, 2022.

45. Weber JT, Hughes JM. Beyond Semmelweis: moving infection control into the community. Ann Intern Med. 2004;140(5):397-398.

46. Australian Institute of Health and Welfare. Admitted patient care 2017-2018: Australian hospital statistics. Canberra: AIHW, 2019.

47. Boltey E, Yakusheva O, Costa DK. 5 Nursing strategies to prevent ventilator-associated pneumonia. Am Nurse Today. 2017;12(6):42-43.

48. Yang S, Choo YJ, Chang MC, eds. The preventive effect of dysphagia screening on pneumonia in acute stroke patients: a systematic review and meta-analysis. Healthcare (Basel). 2021;20;9(12):1764.

49. Australian Government: Department of Health and Aged Care. Coronavirus (COVID-19) at a glance – 20 December 2020. Canberra: Department of Health and Aged Care, 2020.

50. Li C, Sotomayor-Castillo C, Nahidi S, Kuznetsov S, Considine J, Curtis K, et al. Emergency clinicians' knowledge, preparedness and experiences of managing COVID-19 during the 2020 global pandemic in Australian healthcare settings. Australas Emerg Care. 2021;24(3):186-196.

51. Nguyen LH, Drew DA, Graham MS, Joshi AD, Guo C-G, Ma W, et al. Risk of COVID-19 among front-line health-care workers and the general community: a prospective cohort study. Lancet Public Health. 2020;5(9):e475-e83.

52. Chou R, Dana T, Buckley DI, Selph S, Fu R, Totten AM. Epidemiology of and risk factors for coronavirus infection in health care workers: a living rapid review. Ann Intern Med. 2020;173(2):120-136.

53. Australian Institute of Health and Welfare (AIHW). The first year of COVID-19 in Australia: direct and indirect health effects. Canberra: AIHW, 2021.

54. Tenforde MW, Self WH, Naioti EA, Ginde AA, Douin DJ, Olson SM, et al. Sustained effectiveness of Pfizer-BioNTech and Moderna vaccines against COVID-19 associated hospitalizations among adults—United States, March–July 2021. MMWR Morb Mortal Wkly Rep. 2021;70(34):1156.

55. Communicable Diseases Network Australia. National strategic plan for TB control in Australia beyond 2000. Canberra: Department of Health and Ageing, 2002.

56. Lee G. Respiratory tract infections. In: Lee G, Bishop P, eds. Microbiology and infection control for health professionals. 4th ed. Sydney: Pearson Education Australia, 2010, p. 397-423.

57. Bright A, Denholm JT, Coulter C, Waring J, Stapledon R. Tuberculosis notifications in Australia, 2015-2018. Canberra: National Tuberculosis Advisory Committee, Australian Government Department of Health, 2020.

58. World Health Organization. Global tuberculosis report 2021. Geneva: WHO, 2021.

59. Tally NJ, J. MC. Clinical gastroenterology: a practical problem based approach. Sydney: MacLennan & Petty, 1996.

60. Kasper DL, Braunwald E, Fauci AS, et al. Section 7: Infectious diseases. Harrison's manual of medicine. New York: McGraw-Hill, 2006.

61. Newberry L. Sheehy's emergency nursing: principles and practice. 5th ed. St Louis: Mosby, 2003.

62. National Health and Medical Research Council. Australian Guidelines for the Prevention and Control of Infection in Healthcare. Canberra, Australia: NHMRC, 2019.

63. Wasley A, Miller JT, Finelli L, Centers for Disease Control and Prevention (CDC). Surveillance for acute viral hepatitis—United States 2005. MMWR Surveillance Summary. 2007;56(3):24.

64. Lee G, Bishop P. Gastrointestinal tract infections. In: Lee G, ed. Microbiology and infection control for health professionals 4th ed. Sydney: Pearson Education Australia, 2010.

65. van der Poel CL, Cuypers HT, Reesink HV. Hepatitis C virus six years on. Lancet. 1994;334(8935):1475-1479.

66. Moseley RH. Evaluation of abnormal liver function tests. Med Clin North Am. 1996;80(5):10.

67. Australian Institute of Health and Welfare. Infectious and communicable diseases Canberra: AIHW, 2020 [cited 17 Jun 2022]. Available from: https://www.aihw.gov.au/reports/australias-health/infectious-and-communicable-diseases.

68. World Health Organization. Hepatitis A, Geneva: WHO, 2021 [cited 23 Mar 2022]. Available from: https://www.who.int/news-room/fact-sheets/detail/hepatitis-a.

69. World Health Organization. Hepatitis B, Geneva: WHO, 2021 [cited 23 Mar 2022]. Available from: https://www.who.int/news-room/fact-sheets/detail/hepatitis-b.

70. World Health Organization. Hepatitis C, Geneva: WHO; 2021 [cited 23 Mar 2022]. Available from: https://www.who.int/news-room/fact-sheets/detail/hepatitis-c.

71. Hooton TM, Bradley SF, Cardenas DD, Colgan R, Geerlings SE, Rice JC, et al. Diagnosis, prevention, and treatment of catheter-associated urinary tract infection in adults: 2009 International Clinical Practice Guidelines from the Infectious Diseases Society of America. Clin Infect Dis. 2010;50(5):625-663.

72. Si D, Runnegar N, Marquess J, Rajmokan M, Playford EG. Characterising health care-associated bloodstream infections in public hospitals in Queensland, 2008–2012. Med J Aust. 2016;204(7):276.

73. Australian Institute of Health and Welfare. Australian hospital statistics 2010–2011: Staphylococcus aureus bacteraemia in Australian public hospitals. Canberra, Australia: AIHW, 2011.

74. Australian Institute of Health and Welfare. Bloodstream infections associated with hospital care 2019–20 Canberra: AIHW, 2021.

75. Communicable Diseases Network Australia. Infection control guidelines for the prevention of transmission of infectious diseases in the health care setting. Canberra: Australian Government Department of Health and Ageing, 2004.

76. Navaneethan U, Giannella RA. Mechanisms of infectious diarrhea. Nat Clin Pract Gastroenterol Hepatol. 2008;5(11):637-647.

77. Australian Commission on Safety and Quality in Health Care. Clostridioides difficile infection—2019 data snapshot. Sydney: ACSQHC, 2021.

78. Australian Commission on Safety and Quality in Health Care. Antimicrobial stewardship in Australian health care. Sydney: ACSQHC, 2022.

79. Rhodes A, Evans LE, Alhazzani W, Levy MM, Antonelli M, Ferrer R, et al. Surviving Sepsis Campaign: international guidelines for management of sepsis and septic shock: 2016. Intensive Care Med. 2017; 43(3):304-377.

80. Burrell AR, McLaws ML, Fullick M, Sullivan RB, Sindhusake D. Sepsis kills: early intervention saves lives. Med J Aust. 2016;204(2):73 e1-7.

81. Lelubre C, Vincent JL. Mechanisms and treatment of organ failure in sepsis. Nat Rev Nephrol. 2018;14(7):417-427.

82. Zervos MJ, Freeman K, Vo L, Haque N, Pokharna H, Raut M, et al. Epidemiology and outcomes of complicated skin and soft tissue infections in hospitalized patients. J Clin Microbiol. 2012;50(2):238-245.

83. Allen J, David M, Veerman J. Systematic review of the cost-effectiveness of preoperative antibiotic prophylaxis in reducing surgical-site infection. BJS Open. 2018;2(3):81-98.

84. Australian Commission on Safety and Quality in Health Care. AURA 2021: Fourth Australian report on antimicrobial use and resistance in human health. Sydney: ACSQHC, 2021.

85. Lee G. Cardiovascular and multisystem infections. In: Lee G, Bishop P, eds. Microbiology and infection control for health professionals. 4th ed. Sydney: Pearson Education Australia, 2010.

86. Rubin RJ, Harrington CA, Poon A, Dietrick K, Greene JA, Moiduddin A. The economic impact of Staphylococcus aureus infection in New York City hospitals. Emerg Infect Dis. 1999;5(1):18.

87. Casewell MW. New threats to the control of methicillin-resistant Staphylococcus aureus. J Hosp Infect. 1995;30, Supplement (0):465-471.

88. Australian Commission on Safety and Quality in Health Care. National Safety and Quality Health Service Standards. Sydney: ACSQHC, 2021.

89. Johnson A, Roush RE, Howe JL, Sanders M, McBride MR, Sherman A, et al. Bioterrorism and Emergency Preparedness in Aging (BTEPA). Gerontol Geriatr Educ. 2008;26(4):23.

90. Shahid Z, Kalayanamitra R, McClafferty B, Kepko D, Ramgobin D, Patel R, et al. COVID-19 and older adults: what we know. J Am Geriatr Soc. 2020;68(5):926-929.

91. Australian Government Department of Health and Aged Care. Coronavirus (COVID-19) case numbers and statistics. Canberra: Department of Health and Aged Care, 2022 [cited 5 March 2022]. Available from: https://www.health.gov.au/health-alerts/covid-19/case-numbers-and-statistics.

CHAPTER 3

Sciences of infection and disease

ASSOCIATE PROFESSOR MAURIZIO LABBATE[i]

Dr VALERY COMBES[i]

Chapter highlights

- An overview of pathogens important in Australian healthcare, including their structure, taxonomy and methods of transmission
- General strategies of specific groups of pathogens, showing how they cause disease in human and animal hosts
- Details of how the host immune system works against pathogens and therapies that assist in the treatment and prevention of infectious disease
- A summary of common assays used in the diagnosis of pathogens, and the therapies associated with their identification and management

i   School of Life Sciences, Faculty of Science, University of Technology Sydney, Ultimo, NSW

Introduction

COVID-19 has reminded us that pathogens are devastating and have significant individual, societal and population implications for human health and wellbeing. Pathogens that affect humans are diverse and can be cellular microorganisms, biological particles or multicellular parasites; however, the vast majority are harmless and are fundamental to environmental, animal and human health. In humans, normal microbial flora play integral roles in maintaining health although they may cause disease in circumstances where the usual defence mechanisms are disrupted or where there is a disruption in the normal microbial flora. For example, immunosuppressive drugs, such as steroids or antimicrobial therapeutics, can result in opportunistic infections from natural microbiota such as the yeast *Candida albicans*, causing thrush.

In Australia, pathogens that are significant to human health are formally identified and managed in accordance with a range of public health legislation and regulation. A notifiable disease is one that must be reported to state and territory health departments. Table 3.1 lists notifiable infections in Australia from 2009–19, not including infections from COVID-19 which emerged in late 2019. Over this time, the most prevalent infections were influenza, *Chlamydia* and campylobacteriosis.

The epidemiology of infections varies according to local and regional, environmental and population, and societal factors. For example, the warmer conditions of Australia's tropical north predispose it to mosquito-borne infections such as malaria and dengue. Aboriginal and Torres Strait Island peoples experience disproportionately higher rates of infection and disease than the non-Indigenous population due to inequities such as poverty derived from centuries of systemic privilege and racism.[1]

As noted in Table 3.1, the majority of notifiable infections in Australia are bacterial and viral, and reflect their importance in human health. These pathogens infect via a number of routes that include the gastrointestinal tract, respiratory system, sexual transmission, contact with animals and humans, and bites from insects and blood (e.g. sharing needles) (see 3.4 Transmission of pathogens). The epidemiology of these and other infections is influenced by a range of complex, interconnected factors that span prevention, such as vaccine reluctance, to control, such as modifying risk-based behaviours, to treatment, including empiric and targeted therapeutics.

3.1 Pathogenic microorganisms

Generally speaking, microorganisms are unicellular cells that are too small to be seen by the naked eye and whose visualisation requires the use of a microscope. Although organisms such as fleas and mites are small, these are multicellular organisms that contain cells as part of tissues and detailed body plans and are not defined as microorganisms. In this chapter we will briefly cover some of these multicellular parasites, due to their clinical importance.

Pathogenic microorganisms can be prokaryotic or eukaryotic and are defined as 'living' as they are capable of self-replication if provided with appropriate nutrients. Prokaryotic cells are simpler than eukaryotic cells and differ in a variety of ways including their size and sub-cellular structures (Fig 3.1). Typically, eukaryotic cells are about five to ten times larger than prokaryotic cells and contain a variety of membrane-bound structures called organelles, with the nucleus containing the DNA being most notable. As we will learn later, differences in sub-cellular structures between these cell types are important in the effectiveness of chemotherapeutics used to treat bacterial infections. Prokaryotic cells include bacteria and archaea; however, as there are no known human or animal archaeal pathogens, these will not be discussed here. In the context of eukaryotic cells, fungi and protozoa cause infections in humans and animals.

3.1.1 Prokaryotic cellular pathogens

Many of the important pathogens affecting humans, particularly in clinical environments, are bacterial. These microorganisms are diverse in structure with bacillus (rod-shaped) and coccus (sphere-shaped) shapes being the most common. Most bacteria can be subdivided into Gram negative or Gram positive on the basis of a staining procedure called the Gram stain that differentiates bacterial cells according to their envelope structure and which has important historical roots in diagnostics (Fig 3.2). Gram-positive cells stain purple due to their thick cell wall (20–80 nm) made of a polymer called peptidoglycan positioned outside of the cytoplasmic membrane, whereas Gram-negative cells stain pink due to a thin peptidoglycan cell wall (2–7 nm) in between the cytoplasmic and outer membranes. Some bacterial pathogens lack a cell wall, including *Mycoplasma* and *Chlamydia* species. *Mycobacteria* species, which includes the bacterium responsible for tuberculosis, contains a modified peptidoglycan cell

TABLE 3.1 Main notifiable infectious diseases affecting Australians from 2009–19

Disease	Main route of infection	2009	2010	2011	2012	2013	2014	2015	2016	2017	2018	2019	Average
All		239,475	214,260	242,391	249,127	230,067	278,891	338,372	345,076	519,103	328,762	593,055	325,325
Bacterial													
Campylobacteriosis	Gastrointestinal	16,106	16,994	17,723	15,704	14,689	19,938	22,551	24,241	28,698	32,133	35,869	22,241
Listeriosis	Gastrointestinal	92	71	70	93	76	80	70	85	71	73	52	76
Paratyphoid	Gastrointestinal	61	86	69	77	74	70	76	79	68	80	117	78
Salmonellosis	Gastrointestinal	9,400	11,777	12,166	11,120	12,667	16,191	16,886	18,014	16,376	14,149	14,682	13,948
Shigellosis	Gastrointestinal	617	552	493	548	537	1,035	1,037	1,410	1,748	2,508	3,157	1,240
STEC	Gastrointestinal	128	80	95	112	180	115	136	341	497	562	655	264
Typhoid fever	Gastrointestinal	115	96	135	122	150	117	114	104	144	176	202	134
Legionellosis	Respiratory	297	307	356	382	507	425	364	368	387	449	431	388
Meningococcal disease (invasive)	Respiratory	256	226	241	223	147	167	181	252	380	281	206	233
Tuberculosis	Respiratory	1,307	1,362	1,386	1,315	1,262	1,339	1,249	1,362	1,436	1,436	1,520	1,361
Chlamydial infection	STI	63,193	74,367	81,081	83,238	83,837	86,818	86,420	94,627	101,244	104,796	102,514	87,467
Gonococcal infection	STI	8,269	10,321	12,087	13,963	15,062	15,692	18,478	23,874	28,371	30,889	34,317	19,211
Syphilis	STI	1,285	1,097	1,243	1,532	1,763	2,063	2,791	3,376	4,415	5,080	5,795	2,767
Haemophilus influenzae type b*	Respiratory	19	23	13	16	20	21	16	17	16	18	22	18
Pertussis*	Respiratory	30,185	34,832	38,752	24,093	12,376	11,892	22,572	20,120	12,236	12,583	12,024	21,060
Pneumococcal disease (invasive)*	Respiratory	1,554	1,640	1,883	1,824	1,553	1,563	1,498	1,664	2,050	2,031	2,131	1,763
Brucellosis	Zoonosis	32	21	37	31	14	17	19	18	19	28	9	22
Leptospirosis	Zoonosis	141	133	214	105	85	84	72	130	146	142	85	122
Ornithosis	Zoonosis	63	58	89	76	47	41	16	22	21	9	21	42
Q fever	Zoonosis	317	338	359	371	491	474	605	560	478	513	563	461

Data sourced from: Infectious and communicable diseases – Australian Institute of Health and Welfare (aihw.gov.au).

Viral

Disease	Category												
Hepatitis B (newly acquired)	Blood-borne	248	231	192	194	176	180	150	176	146	137	163	181
Hepatitis C (newly acquired)	Blood-borne	400	384	620	705	668	710	820	738	620	615	787	642
Hepatitis D	Blood-borne	65	52	53	47	73	66	49	71	65	79	70	63
Hepatitis A	Gastrointestinal	564	267	145	166	190	231	179	145	217	434	246	253
Hepatitis E	Gastrointestinal	33	37	41	32	34	58	41	43	48	39	52	42
Barmah Forest virus infection	Vectorborne	1,472	1,465	1,865	1,728	4,236	741	628	329	448	343	255	1,228
Dengue virus infection	Vectorborne	1,404	1,228	821	1,539	1,838	1,721	1,714	2,238	1,136	932	1,462	1,458
Flavivirus infection (unspecified)	Vectorborne	4	14	13	6	16	20	11	116	17	8	11	21
Ross River virus infection	Vectorborne	4,739	5,120	5,129	4,678	4,312	5,310	9,544	3,734	6,930	3,139	2,961	5,054
Influenza (laboratory confirmed)*	Respiratory	59,040	13,457	27,213	44,539	28,303	67,686	100,583	90,884	251,290	58,869	313,428	95,936
Measles*	Respiratory	104	70	194	199	158	339	74	99	81	103	285	155
Mumps*	Respiratory	166	97	153	201	217	186	645	804	812	634	171	371
Rotavirus*	Gastrointestinal	1,820	3,918	3,331	3,797	3,208	3,022	4,136	2,733	7,266	3,163	6,173	3,870
Rubella*	Respiratory	27	44	58	35	25	16	17	17	10	9	22	25
Varicella zoster (chicken pox)*	Direct touch	1,798	1,797	2,103	1,991	2,134	2,112	2,489	3,030	3,172	4,600	4,386	2,692

Protozoal

Disease	Category												
Cryptosporidiosis	Gastrointestinal	4,624	1,482	1,811	3,142	3,852	2,408	4,064	5,421	4,695	3,011	2,678	3,381
Malaria	Vectorborne	504	404	419	344	423	325	234	305	364	408	379	374

STI: sexually transmitted infection; *: vaccine-preventable disease.
Data sourced from: Infectious and communicable diseases. Australian Institute of Health and Welfare. Available: https://aihw.gov.au. 1 Sep 2022.

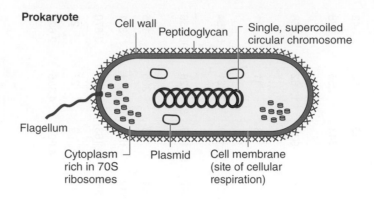

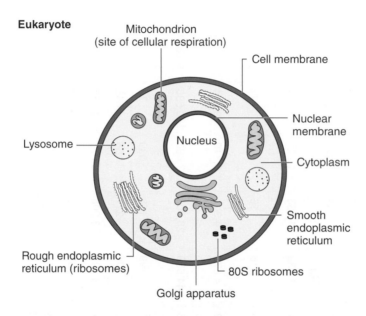

FIGURE 3.1 Prokaryotic and eukaryotic cellular structure. Generally, prokaryotes are 0.5–2 μm in size consisting of a rigid peptidoglycan cell wall and membrane-enclosed cytoplasm containing cellular DNA and other sub-cellular structures including chromosomal DNA, 70S ribosomes and sometimes a plasmid(s) of which the functions are summarised in Table 3.2. Eukaryotic cells are approximately 5–10x larger than prokaryotic cells and more complex containing a membrane-bound nucleus where the DNA resides, 80S ribosomes and diverse organelles that fulfil important cellular roles (see text for details)
Source: George, A., & Charleman, J. E. (2017). Elsevier's Surgical Technology Exam Review. Elsevier.

wall with mycolic acids covalently bound, giving the cell surface a waxy finish.

In addition to the cell wall, bacteria are differentiated from eukaryotic cells with their ribosomes being smaller (i.e. 70S versus 80S) and having a different composition of proteins and RNA. They contain a variety of cellular structures that are important in virulence, some of which are summarised in Table 3.2 and further discussed in Section 3.5 Host–pathogen interactions. Of note is the ability of some bacterial pathogens to form spores, dormant structures that are highly resistant to general

methods of pathogen control, such as chemical disinfection. They can survive for long periods of time without nutrition and have the ability to convert back into a growing state when conditions improve. Some pathogens, such as *Bacillus anthracis* (anthrax), *Clostridium tetani* (tetanus) and *Clostridium botulinum* (botulism), are spore formers. For example, *C. botulinum* spores are widely found in soil and water and, if ingested or enter a wound, produce a toxin that causes muscle paralysis and possibly death. On the positive side, botulinum toxin has been repurposed in multiple medical procedures, including

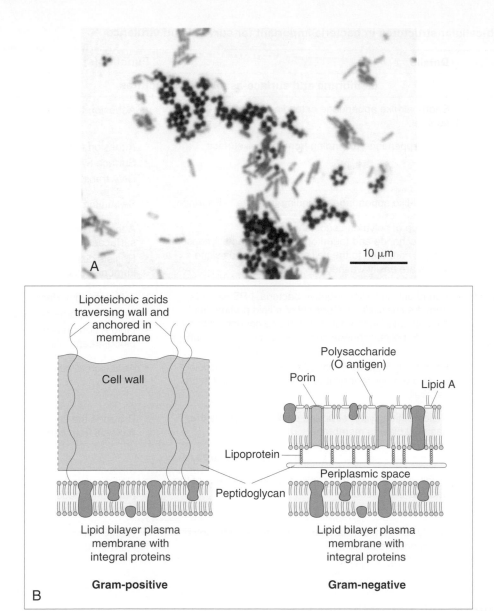

FIGURE 3.2a and b Gram stain of a mixture of the Gram-negative bacillus *Escherichia coli* and the Gram-positive coccus *Staphylococcus aureus* staining pink and purple respectively: (a) Envelope structure of Gram-positive cells (left) and Gram-negative cells (right). Gram-positive cells contain a cytoplasmic membrane (plasma membrane) and a thick cell wall with teichoic acids and lipoteichoic acids sometimes anchored in the cell wall and cytoplasmic membrane respectively (b). Gram-negative cells contain a cytoplasmic membrane, an outer membrane and a periplasmic space in between where a thin cell wall resides. The outer membrane in Gram-negative bacteria is the site for LPS

Source: (a) Godbey, W. T. (2022). Biotechnology and its applications: using cells to change the world. Elsevier.
(b) Bassert, J. M. (2022). McCurnin's Clinical Textbook for Veterinary Technicians and Nurses. Elsevier.

controlling migraines, excessive sweating, muscle spasticity and in cosmetic procedures (i.e Botox). To avoid foodborne botulism, the canned vegetable food industry must take precautions, including high temperature treatment, to ensure the destruction of *C. botulinum*

spores. Additionally, there are concerns regarding the weaponisation of bacterial spores, such as in the 2001 Anthrax attacks in the United States of America where a series of letters were sent containing anthrax spores in the form of a powder resulting in five deaths.

TABLE 3.2 Sub-cellular structures in bacteria important for survival and virulence

Structure	Details	Function(s)
Membrane and surface-associated structures		
Fimbriae	Short hair-like appendage extending from the cell surface	• Adhesion to surfaces
Pilus	Short appendage extending from the cell surface	• Adhesion to surfaces • Surface twitching motility • DNA transfer (conjugation)
Flagellum	Thread-like appendage extending from the cell surface	• Swimming motility
Capsule/ slime layer	Made up of polymeric substances such as polysaccharide and found on the cell surface. A capsule is tightly adhered to the cell surface, whereas slime layers are easily washed off	• Adhesion and biofilm formation to surfaces • Resists desiccation and phagocytosis by immune cells
Lipopolysaccharide (LPS)	Found only in Gram-negative bacteria, LPS extends from the cell surface. Consists of a lipid portion (lipid A) embedded in the outer membrane connected to a variable polysaccharide component called the O antigen	• Adhesion to surfaces • Creates a permeability barrier • Lipid A portion is highly inflammatory in bloodstream. Also called endotoxin
Teichoic acids	Found only in some Gram-positive bacteria, teichoic acids are a phosphorylated polyalcohol present in the cell wall	• Adhesion to surfaces
Cell wall	Rigid peptidoglycan structure positioned outside the bacterial plasma membrane	• Provides the cell with integrity and protects from osmotic stress
Internal structures		
Plasmid	Small, circular DNA that replicates independently of the bacterial chromosome	• Can move between bacteria and transfer genetic traits such as antibiotic resistance and virulence genes
Spores	Highly resistant dormant structure produced by some Gram-positive bacteria	• Highly resistant to environmental stress. Hard to destroy

3.1.2 Eukaryotic cellular pathogens

Eukaryotic microorganisms are more complex than prokaryotic microorganisms and are therefore substantially more structurally diverse. Figure 3.1 illustrates the general characteristics of a eukaryotic cell shown with a series of labelled organelles holding important cellular roles. Mitochondria are involved in energy (i.e. adenosine triphosphate [ATP]) production. The endoplasmic reticulum (ER) are flattened, enclosed membrane sacs that are involved in the synthesis and modification of multiple cellular products such as lipids and proteins. Rough ER is so named due to its appearance in having ribosomes attached to it and is therefore important in protein and glycoprotein synthesis, whereas smooth ER is important for the synthesis of lipids, phospholipids and steroids. The golgi apparatus transports ER-produced products and the lysosome contains enzymes that digest proteins, fats and polysaccharide for reuse. In addition, eukaryotic microorganisms can harbour flagella and cilia that are involved in motility. Compared to flagella, cilia are much shorter and tend to coat the cell and move synchronously.

Of the eukaryotic microorganisms, the members of fungi and protozoa are human pathogens. Microscopically, fungi can appear as unicellular cells called yeast, or as moulds that are long, branched filaments of cells called hyphae forming a mass called mycelium (Fig 3.3). Fungi may also produce spores that aid in dispersion and are organised into elaborate structures that are useful in diagnostic microscopy. Fungi possess cell walls that are usually made of chitin although some may produce cell walls of other polysaccharides, such as cellulose. Importantly, some fungi are dimorphic and can morph between a mould and yeast form, including pathogens such

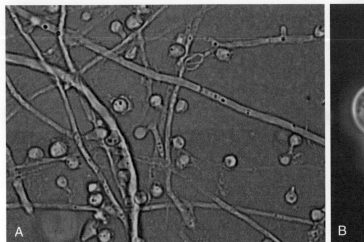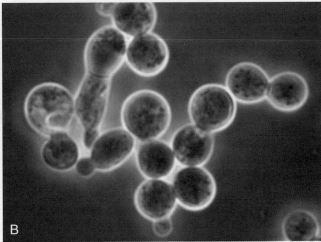

FIGURE 3.3 Microscopic images of *Blastomyces dermatitidis* in mould (a) and yeast (b) forms. As a mould, long cells called hyphae are observed. Sacs called conidia containing spores branching from the hyphae. In yeast form, cells are thick-walled and oval-shaped

Source: Images courtesy of Bruce Klein, University of Wisconsin.

as *Blastomyces dermatitidis* that convert to a yeast form at a human body temperature of 37°C (Fig 3.3).

Pathogenic protozoa are responsible for some important human diseases, and these include malaria and trypanosomiasis caused by species of the *Plasmodium* and *Trypanosoma* genera respectively. Protozoa are unicellular eukaryotes that feed on organic material and in this state they are called trophozoites (Fig 3.4a). Many protozoa are capable of encystment, a process where the trophozoite becomes simpler and converts into a cyst that is marked by a low metabolic rate and the formation of a cell wall (Fig 3.4b). Cysts are more resistant to environmental stress and in pathogenic protozoa are important in transmission between human and animal hosts. Protozoa covert back into a trophozoite state in favourable conditions in a process called excystment.

3.1.3 Horizontal gene transfer in bacteria

An important behavioural feature of bacteria is their ability to share DNA in a process called horizontal gene transfer (HGT) which has been pivotal in the emergence of many problematic pathogens and antibiotic-resistant pathogens.[2] There are three mechanisms of HGT: i) conjugation; ii) transformation; and iii) transduction (Fig 3.5). Conjugation requires cell-to-cell contact and through a pilus, DNA (usually a plasmid) is transferred. Transformation is the uptake of naked DNA and requires the bacterium to change physiology and become competent, a state where DNA

uptake is possible. Transduction is DNA transfer from one bacterial cell to another with a bacterial virus (bacteriophage) being the intermediate.

Except for plasmids which can self-replicate, transferred DNA must integrate into the chromosome or a residing plasmid in order to be replicated and be passed on to progeny during cell division. There are multiple ways by which transferred DNA may integrate that go beyond the scope of this chapter; however, a common method is homologous recombination where a natural cellular process recombines DNA with high homology.

All mechanisms of HGT are common and there are numerous examples of each driving the evolution of pathogens and antibiotic resistance. For example, *Escherichia coli* are natural inhabitants of the gastrointestinal tract of humans and animals; however, some are capable of causing diarrhoeal disease and urinary tract infections of which horizontally acquired genes are often identified as being involved in disease.[3] Important to infection prevention and control is antibiotic resistance and many bacterial pathogens show evidence of horizontally receiving plasmids and other genetic elements that provide them with resistance to multiple antibiotics.[4]

3.1.4 Koch's postulates

Traditionally, infectious diseases were investigated as a single pathogen causing disease and formed the basis for Koch's postulates, a series of logical truths designed by the microbiologist Robert Koch that are applied to

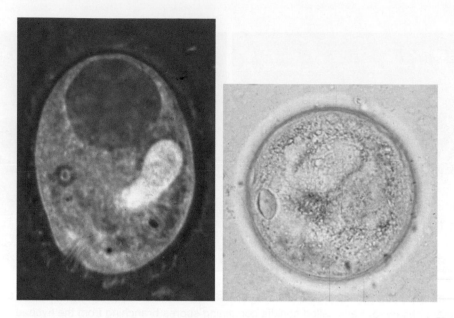

FIGURE 3.4 Parasitic intestinal pathogen *Balantidium coli* in trophozoite (left) and cyst (right) form. Infection occurs through oral consumption of cysts that excyst into trophozoites. Trophozoites multiply in the intestine and are passed out in faeces where they encyst as the faeces dry out

Source: Sirois, M. (2020). Laboratory Procedures for Veterinary Technicians. Elsevier.

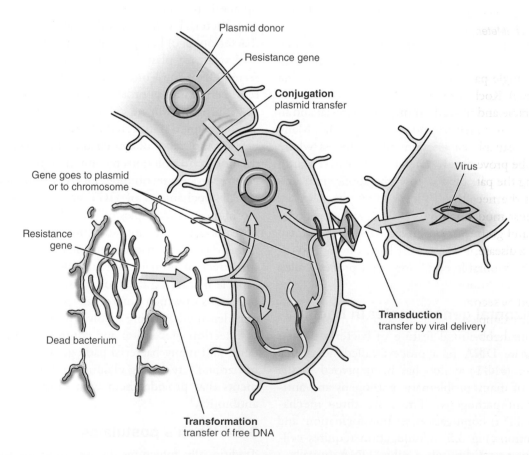

FIGURE 3.5 Horizontal gene transfer in bacteria can occur through transformation, conjugation or transduction. Transformation is the uptake of free DNA sources from a lysed bacterium. Conjugation requires cell-to-cell contact and the transfer of DNA (usually a plasmid) through a pilus. Transduction is transfer of DNA from one bacterial cell to another through a bacterial virus (bacteriophage) intermediate

Source: Zachary, J. F., & McGavin, M. D. (Eds.). (2012). Pathologic Basis of Veterinary Disease. Elsevier.

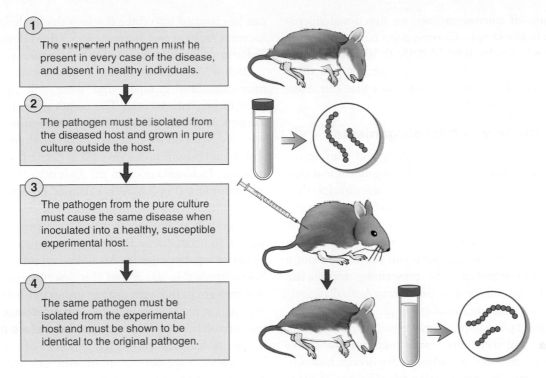

1. The suspected pathogen must be present in every case of the disease, and absent in healthy individuals.

2. The pathogen must be isolated from the diseased host and grown in pure culture outside the host.

3. The pathogen from the pure culture must cause the same disease when inoculated into a healthy, susceptible experimental host.

4. The same pathogen must be isolated from the experimental host and must be shown to be identical to the original pathogen.

FIGURE 3.6 Koch's postulates used for proving a single pathogen is responsible for an infectious disease
Source: VanMeter, K. C., Hubert, R. J. & VanMeter, W. (2010). Microbiology for the healthcare professional. Elsevier.

prove that a single pathogen is responsible for a single disease (Fig 3.6). Koch's postulates require that a pathogen be culturable and that a host model system be available for infection experiments, and where this is not possible, the postulates cannot be applied. Nevertheless, causality can be proved with a variety of techniques that allow tracking the pathogen within the infected human host without the need for cultivating the pathogen or infecting a host model. Additionally, some diseases can be complex and go beyond a single pathogen being responsible for a disease, making it difficult to apply Koch's postulates. The human immunodeficiency virus (HIV) is a pathogen that diminishes host immunity, but disease is often caused by secondary infection with other pathogens. Another example is dental diseases that are caused by complex microbial communities adhered to the teeth and gums. Other diseases are opportunistic and only infect when the host conditions change, such as a disruption of the host microbiome (see 3.1.5 Microbiomes) or host immune system. Due to these complexities, research increasingly examines how host microbiome and immunity changes affect susceptibility to, or the severity of, an infectious disease.

3.1.5 Microbiomes

Microorganisms are found in almost every niche on Earth and play essential roles in global nutrient cycling.

They are involved in numerous interactions that support the growth and health of higher organisms. As a collective, these microorganisms are known as the microbiome. Microorganisms are naturally found in most parts of the human body including skin, gastrointestinal tract, nose, mouth and vagina, and combined these are referred to as the 'human microbiome'. If referring to the microorganisms associated with a part of the body, then we refer to them as the 'human gut microbiome' or 'human skin microbiome'. The human microbiome is estimated to hold about 100 times more genes than those in the human genome, with research supporting important roles in digestion of nutrients, synthesis of vitamins, protection from pathogens, and immune stimulation and regulation.[5] If we consider the colon, the number of bacteria can number 10^{11}–10^{12} per gram of contents, and imbalances in microbiome composition are linked to a variety of gastrointestinal conditions that include inflammatory bowel syndrome and inflammatory bowel disease. Identifying the exact mechanism(s) by which the gut microbiome might influence disease is complex and remains elusive. Studies into microbiome composition largely utilise DNA-based techniques that require extraction of DNA from an environment (e.g. faeces) and this is called metagenomic DNA. Metagenomic DNA is then subjected to other DNA sequencing techniques that identify the composition of microorganisms or functional microbial genes in the sample. Comparisons between healthy and diseased samples help identify those microorganisms or genes that correlate with disease; however, there is substantial inter-individual variation that can make identifying trends tricky.

3.1.6 Taxonomy of microorganisms

Taxonomy is the science of classifying and naming organisms using defined criteria. Microorganisms in a classification group will share more characteristics than those outside of the group, and so classifying a microorganism provides the advantage of ascribing what we know about a microorganism in a group to others within that group. In this way, decisions can be made about a microorganism whether it be prescribing appropriate treatment for an infection or protecting Australia's agriculture industry through quarantine procedures.

Historically, phenotypic characteristics such as cellular morphology and metabolism were used in classification and are still useful today in pathogen diagnostics; however, genetic-based methods comparing the sequence of a taxonomic marker gene(s) or the entire microbial genome are becoming commonplace and have the benefit of reflecting the phylogenetic relationships that microorganisms have with one another. A useful gene in taxonomy and phylogeny is the single subunit ribosomal RNA (SSU rRNA) gene that is found in all cells and encodes an RNA molecule required for the protein synthesis function of ribosomes. Based on SSU RNA sequences, all cells

can be classified into three domains that include the prokaryotes Archaea and Bacteria, and a third domain called Eukarya which is made up of the eukaryotes (Fig 3.7).

Below 'domain' are further subclassifications, and the microorganisms grouped into these will progressively share more characteristics. The names given to microorganisms (and all organisms) follow the binomial naming system developed by Carolus Linnaeus where the genus and species classifications are used to derive the name. For example, *Escherichia coli* is in the *Escherichia* genus and *coli* species groups (Fig 3.8). What defines a species is sometimes controversial and there is much discussion and debate about how best to classify a microorganism into a species. In general, a 2–3% divergence in the SSU rRNA sequence separates species. An additional subclassification below 'species' is 'strain' and this describes microorganisms that are in the same species group but have a different phenotypic characteristic(s). These differences are often derived from HGT events (see 3.1.3 Horizontal gene transfer in bacteria) and so the genomes of microorganisms within a species group are said to contain a core genome and a pan genome. A core genome are all those genes that are common among all strains within a species, whereas a pan genome are those genes that are uncommon and are often derived from HGT.

3.2 Pathogenic biological particles

In addition to cellular pathogens there are pathogenic biological particles which are incapable of self-replication.

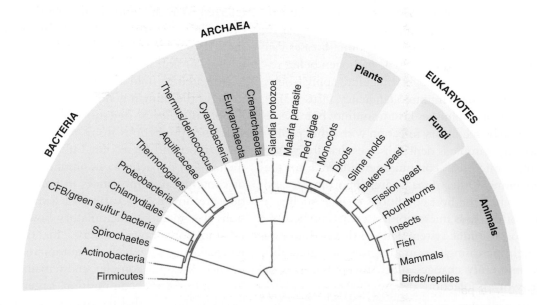

FIGURE 3.7 Tree of life derived from the SSU rRNA sequence of all cells showing three clades that classify all into the three domains of Bacteria, Archaea and Eukarya

Soltis, D., & Soltis, P. (2019). The great tree of life. Academic Press.

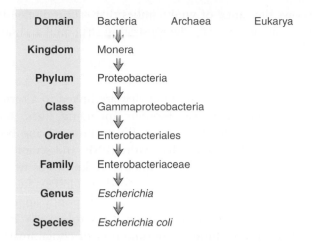

Domain	Bacteria	Archaea	Eukarya
Kingdom	Monera		
Phylum	Proteobacteria		
Class	Gammaproteobacteria		
Order	Enterobacteriales		
Family	Enterobacteriaceae		
Genus	*Escherichia*		
Species	*Escherichia coli*		

FIGURE 3.8 The binomial system developed by Carolus Linnaeus is used to name organisms including microorganisms. On the left are the various classifications and the names of the genus and species groups are used to derive the name of the organisms which in this instance is *Escherichia coli*

Source: VanMeter, K. C., & Hubert, R. J. (2022). Microbiology for the Healthcare Professional. Elsevier.

They are intracellular obligate parasites that must infect a living cell and use the host's cellular machinery for their reproduction. Human pathogenic biological particles include viruses and prions. Viruses are defined as nucleic acid (DNA or RNA) enclosed within a protein coat, although some may also contain a membrane envelope. Prions are infective protein particles.

3.2.1 Viruses

Viruses are important pathogens responsible for devastating pandemics in humans including influenza virus causing flu, severe acute respiratory syndrome coronavirus 2 (SARS-CoV-2) causing COVID-19, and HIV causing acquired immune deficiency syndrome (AIDS). Viruses are very small and range from approximately 20–400 nm in size with a single viral particle known as a virion. A virion, at minimum, consists of a nucleocapsid which is nucleic acid surrounded by a protein coat (Fig 3.9). The capsid acts to protect the nucleic acid although it may also aid in adhesion to a host cell. Capsid structures are mostly icosahedral or helical, with other shapes known as 'complex'.

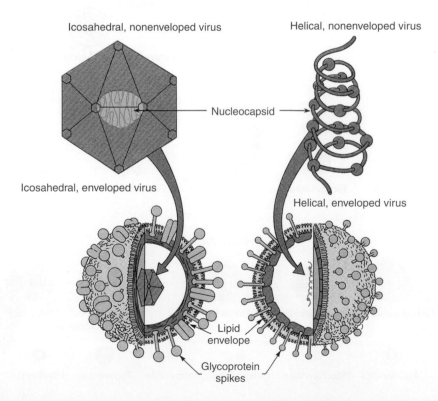

FIGURE 3.9 Viral particles. The capsids of both enveloped and non-enveloped virions mostly have an icosahedral or helical shape and act to protect the nucleic acid. Many eukaryotic viruses are enveloped with the membrane derived from the host cell nuclear or plasma membrane during infection. The envelope contains glycoprotein spikes (sometimes called peplomers) that are important for adhesion to the host cell which initiates the infectious process

Source: Tille, P. (2022). Bailey & Scott's diagnostic microbiology. Elsevier.

Many eukaryotic viruses contain a membrane envelope surrounding the nucleocapsid which is acquired from the host nuclear or plasma membrane during infection. The viral protein contains proteins called spikes or peplomers that are required for host cell adhesion, a critical step in infection (see 3.5.4 Viral pathogens). The viral nucleic acid may be double- or single-stranded DNA (ssDNA or dsDNA) or RNA (ssRNA or dsRNA) and will encode genes that are required for host cell infection and for virion replication and synthesis.

Taxonomy of viruses is mostly based on virion structure, type of nucleic acid, mode of replication, host cell range and the kind of disease it causes. Figure 3.10 shows the range of viral families that causes disease in humans and animals, demonstrating structural and nucleic acid diversity.

3.2.2 Prions

Prions are infective proteins that are linked to a series of neurodegenerative disorders including kuru and variant Creutzfeldt-Jakob (vCJD) in humans, and bovine spongiform encephalopathy (BSE) and scrapie in sheep.[6] These diseases are collectively known as transmissible spongiform encephalopathies (TSEs) due to their effect on the brain resulting in a spongy appearance when brain slices are observed histologically. Prions are spread through consumption of contaminated

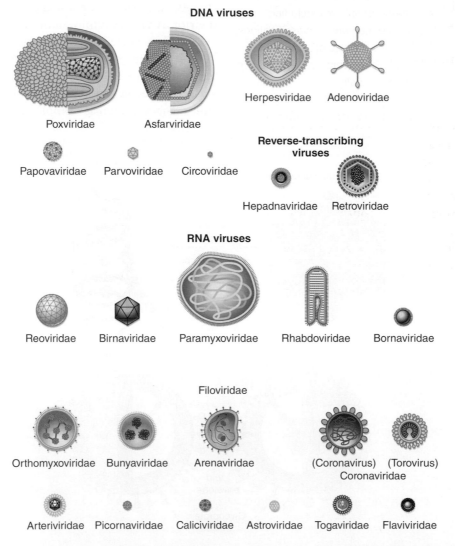

FIGURE 3.10 Shapes and sizes of viral families that infect humans and animals. In this figure, virions are grouped according to their nucleic acid type and in some, a cross-section of capsid and envelope is shown. Artistic licence has been used in representing viral structures

Source: Cann, A. J. (2016). Principles of molecular virology. Academic press.

meat containing the infectious protein that is thought to force a conformational change of a normal protein in brain cells, presumably affecting its normal function. vCJD emerged in the 1990s and was linked to the consumption of beef sourced from cattle suffering from BSE or 'mad cow disease' as it was colloquially known. Kuru affected specific tribes in Papua New Guinea due to a cannibalistic ritual where tribe members would consume body parts of a deceased family member. TSE pathology usually takes years to develop post exposure. There are no effective therapies and prions are highly resistant to standard methods of infection control.

3.3 Multicellular parasites

Beyond unicellular pathogens and biological particles that detrimentally affect humans are multicellular parasites that include helminths (worms) and ectoparasites, which are arthropods living on the surface of the human body.

3.3.1 Helminths

Worm infections are common in parts of the world where access to clean drinking water is limited and where there is poor sanitation. They tend to cause intestinal infestations leading to gut symptoms such as diarrhoea; however, some can migrate to other parts of the body causing more serious complications. Although worm infections are rarely fatal, a high worm load in the intestine can deprive a person of substantial nutrition and in a child can lead to growth and mental retardation. On the other hand, *Schistosoma* is a flatworm that kills approximately 200,000 people per year, with 230 million requiring treatment. Long periods of infection by this worm lead to severe inflammatory immune reactions in organs where eggs have been deposited. In Australia, worm infections are rare; however, remote Indigenous communities are particularly affected by a worm infection called *Strongyloidiasis* where it migrates to the lungs and then the gut, causing a cough or wheeze and a variety of gut-related symptoms such as abdominal pain and diarrhoea. Additionally, hookworm is prevalent in Australian Indigenous communities.

There are three types of helminths that cause disease in humans, namely cestodes (tapeworms), trematodes (flukes) and nematodes (roundworms) (Fig 3.11). Table 3.3 provides a list of worm-related infections in humans. Tapeworms are segmented containing a head (celled scolex) that is used to latch onto the host's intestinal wall and then consists of segments called proglottids that grow from the neck of the head. The proglottids contain male and female gonads that produce thousands of eggs that are shed into faeces as mature proglottids. Tapeworms have no digestive tracts and rely on absorption of nutrients from the host intestine. Flukes are non-segmented flattened worms that have an incomplete digestive system consisting of a mouth and a digestive tract but no anus. They are muscular suckers which allows attachment to tissue. Nematodes are non-segmented cylindrical worms with tapered ends. They are coated in a chitinous cuticle and have a

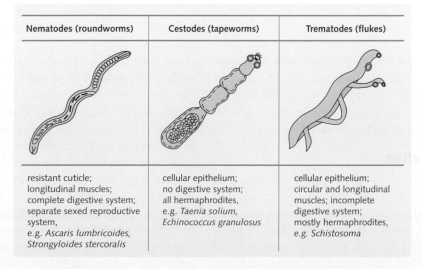

Nematodes (roundworms)	Cestodes (tapeworms)	Trematodes (flukes)
resistant cuticle; longitudinal muscles; complete digestive system; separate sexed reproductive system, e.g. *Ascaris lumbricoides, Strongyloides stercoralis*	cellular epithelium; no digestive system; all hermaphrodites, e.g. *Taenia solium, Echinococcus granulosus*	cellular epithelium; circular and longitudinal muscles; incomplete digestive system; mostly hermaphrodites, e.g. *Schistosoma*

FIGURE 3.11 Main groups of helminths affecting humans
Source: Xiu, P. (2016). Crash Course Pathology. Mosby Ltd.

TABLE 3.3 Examples of helminth infections

Helminth	Disease and symptoms	Transmission
Tapeworms		
Taenia saginata	Larvae attach to intestinal gut and mature into adult worms. May be asymptomatic but high worm loads in the gut may result in weight loss and other gut-related symptoms such as abdominal pain and diarrhoea	Consumption of undercooked beef containing larvae
Hymenolepsis nana	Eggs hatch in intestine maturing into adult worms. May be asymptomatic but high worm loads in the gut may result in weight loss and other gut-related symptoms such as abdominal pain and diarrhoea	Consumption of eggs
Flukes		
Schistosoma species	Schistosomiasis occurs when larvae invade skin, migrating through blood to liver and urinary bladder, maturing into worms in blood vessels. Complications occur from eggs becoming trapped in tissues causing severe inflammatory reactions	Exposure to water environments containing larvae
Fasciola hepatica	Excystation in duodenum then burrow through the lining of the intestine and migrate to the bile ducts causing inflammation and blockage	Consumption of cysts
Nematodes		
Wuchereria bancrofti	Filariasis occurs when larvae in the bloodstream enter tissues and mature into adults. The worms reside in the lymph system causing blockages and fluid accumulation, possibly leading to lymphedema and elephantiasis	Transmitted from the bite of a mosquito
Strongyloides stercoralis	Larvae migrate through blood to lungs where they are coughed up and swallowed into the digestive tract where they develop into adults. Symptoms are gut-related with infection in children affecting growth and mental retardation	Larvae in soil penetrate through skin
Ancylostoma duodenale and *Necator americanus* (hookworm)	Similar disease and symptoms to *S. stercoralis*	Larvae in soil penetrate through skin

complete digestive tract including a mouth and anus. While nematodes only produce worms of male or female sex, tapeworms and flukes are capable of hermaphrodism where one worm contains both sets of gonads and is capable of self-fertilisation.

3.3.2 Ectoparasites

Ectoparasites are arthropods that colonise the surface of the skin where they feed and reproduce causing skin irritation and allergic reactions. The main ectoparasites affecting humans are scabies (a mite), fleas, lice, bedbugs and ticks (Fig 3.12). Table 3.4 provides a summary of these ectoparasites and their effect on humans. Ectoparasites are not lethal; however, they can be vectors for

other pathogens or produce an environment for secondary infections. For example, fleas are the vector for the bacterium *Yersinia pestis* responsible for bubonic plague and the human body louse (*Pediculus humanus*) is a vector for the bacterium *Rickettsia prowazekii* that causes typhus. Ticks are also carriers of bacterial pathogens including *Rickettsia* species and in North America, *Borrelia burgdorferi* causing Lyme disease. Of particular importance are scabies which is endemic in Australia's northern Indigenous communities but is also common in urban areas where there is human crowding. Extensive scratching from scabies may cause serious secondary infections such as staphylococcal and group A streptococcal bacterial infections.

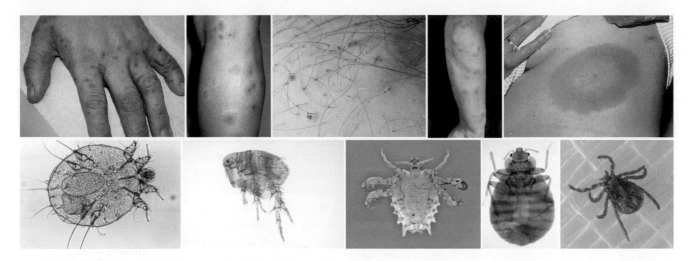

FIGURE 3.12 The effect of bites or colonisation by ectoparasites (in order from right to left scabies, flea, crab louse, bedbug, tick) on human skin surfaces (above) and images of the ectoparasites (below). Most ectoparasites produce minor irritation at site(s) of bite or colonisation. The upper tick bite image shows radiating redness from the bite site as a result of a bacterial infection by *B. burgdorferi* causing Lyme disease

Source: Kaji, A., & Pedigo, R. A. (2021). Emergency Medicine Board Review. Elsevier; Micheletti, R. G., James, W. D., Elston, D., & McMahon, P. J. (2021). Andrews' Diseases of the Skin Clinical Atlas. Elsevier; Ko, C. J. (2021). Dermatology: Visual Recognition and Case Reviews. Elsevier; Micheletti, R. G., James, W. D., Elston, D., & McMahon, P. J. (2021). Andrews' Diseases of the Skin Clinical Atlas. Elsevier; Chintamani, M., & Mani, M. (Eds.). (2021). Lewis's Medical-Surgical Nursing, Fourth South Asia Edition. Elsevier; Paller, A. S., & Mancini, A. J. (2020). Paller and Mancini-Hurwitz Clinical Pediatric Dermatology. Elsevier; Chambers, J. A. (2021). Field Guide to Global Health & Disaster Medicine. Elsevier; Micheletti, R. G., James, W. D., Elston, D., & McMahon, P. J. (2021). Andrews' Diseases of the Skin Clinical Atlas. Elsevier; Hendrix, C. M., & Robinson, E. D. (2022). Diagnostic parasitology for veterinary technicians. Elsevier; Paller, A. S., & Mancini, A. J. (2020). Paller and Mancini-Hurwitz Clinical Pediatric Dermatology. Elsevier.

TABLE 3.4 Summary of ectoparasites affecting humans

Ectoparasite	Disease and symptoms	Transmission
Scabies (*Sarcoptes scabei*)	Female mite burrows under skin to lay eggs causing irritation. May occur anywhere on the body but tends to affect hands and forearms	Direct contact with infected individuals or by coming into contact with their bedding or clothing
Fleas (Siphonaptera)	Minor irritation from bite	Contact with animals, usually pets, that carry fleas

Lice
    Head louse (*Pediculus humanus capitis*)
    Body louse (*Pediculus humanus corporis*)
    Crab louse (*Phthirus pubis*)
	Bite causes irritation. Different lice affect different parts of the body including head (head louse), body (body louse) and pubic (crab louse) regions	Direct contact with affected individuals or coming into contact with their bedding or clothing

Bedbugs (*Cimex lectularius*)	Intense itching and irritation from bite which may develop into a painful welt	Bedbugs do not live on human skin. Instead, they infest unhygienic environments, mainly coming out at night to feed on the blood of sleeping individuals
Ticks (Ixodidae)	Minor irritation from bite	Live in humid bush areas and colonise passing humans

3.4 Transmission of pathogens

When discussing transmission of pathogens, it is important to note that some are capable of human-to-human transmission and others are not. Arguably, pathogens that spread between humans are more problematic but depending on the source, pathogens that do not spread between humans can still have a major impact. The mass production of food means that contaminated food sources can be the major cause of infectious outbreaks without human-to-human transmission. Infection proceeds through six interconnected steps called the 'chain of infection' that describes the transmission of a pathogen from its natural reservoir, through a portal of exit, and transmission to a susceptible host through an appropriate portal of entry (Fig 3.13). Breaking one or more of the links connecting the steps helps prevent further infection.

3.4.1 Reservoirs

Settings where pathogens naturally grow are called reservoirs and this includes humans, animals or the environment. Although a reservoir may be where an infectious agent is naturally found, it may not be the source

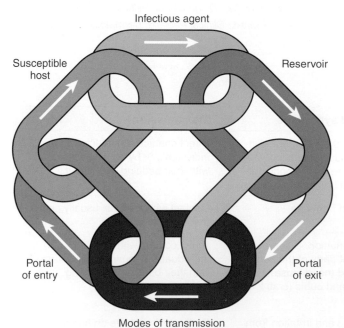

FIGURE 3.13 The chain of infection describes a series of events that leads to a susceptible host becoming infected with a pathogen. Any break in the link may prevent further spread

Source: Leifer, G., & Keenan-Lindsay, L. (2019). Leifer's Introduction to Maternity & Pediatric Nursing in Canada. Elsevier.

of an infection. For example, the bacterium causing Legionnaire's disease is naturally found in freshwater environments; however, it is when cooling tanks that are using contaminated water aerosolise the pathogen through air-conditioning systems that lung infections occur. Another example is spores of *C. botulinum*, which are naturally present in soil, but improperly canned vegetables is the source of infection. Where humans are the only reservoir, infectious agents may be eradicated through vaccination, for example smallpox, although this is rare. Human reservoirs may be controlled if a person who is aware they are infectious isolates themselves. Importantly, some people do not show symptoms and are unaware they are infectious and in these circumstances, transmission may occur more freely.

Many infections that affect humans come from animal reservoirs in a process called 'zoonosis'. Many diseases that are endemic now are thought to have originated from animals, including smallpox, measles, tuberculosis and malaria. Importantly, 70% of new infectious diseases arise from zoonosis. COVID-19 is a likely zoonosis, although the exact reservoir is unknown. It is largely accepted that the SARS-CoV-2 virus, like SARS-CoV-1, emerged from an animal reservoir, probably bats. Other examples include new strains of influenza (pigs and birds), HIV (non-human primates) and Ebola virus (bats). In the environment, plants, soils and water are reservoirs. Many pathogenic *Vibrio* species such as *V. cholerae* (cholera diarrhoea), *V. parahaemolyticus* (diarrhoea) and *V. vulnificus* (wound infections) are naturally present in marine and estuarine environments. Additionally, many fungal pathogens originate from soil environments. In the case of animal and environmental reservoirs, infectious agents can be consistently reintroduced into the human community despite being cleared.

3.4.2 Portals of exit

Portals of exit define the method by which the infectious agent leaves its reservoir. In humans, the main portals of exit are: the upper respiratory tract, from saliva or respiratory droplets from sneezing, coughing and breathing; blood; the gastrointestinal tract, from vomit, diarrhoea/faeces; the urogenital tract, from urine or genital fluids; and the skin, from wounds containing infectious discharge and mucous membranes. For animal reservoirs, the portals of exit are largely the same. For environmental reservoirs, the portal of exit is dependent on the environment. If we consider pathogenic *Vibrio* bacteria found in marine/estuarine waters, the portal of exit is water and its movement or contact with humans or human food and drinking water sources.

3.4.3 Modes of transmission

Modes of transmission are subdivided into direct and indirect. Direct transmission refers to the infectious agents directly transferring from a reservoir to a host and this may occur through direct contact, droplet spread or vertical transmission. For human reservoirs, direct contact may occur through skin-to-skin contact, kissing and sex (Fig 3.14). Animal bites or contact with animal faeces and contact with environmental water, soil or plants may facilitate transfer from animal and environmental reservoirs, respectively. Droplet spread refers to short-range aerosols containing the infectious agent generated from coughing, singing, talking and breathing that is then spread to others nearby. The effectiveness of droplet spread is dependent on conditions such as distance between people and ventilation. Vertical transmission is the transfer of an infectious agent from mother to unborn child.

Indirect transmission refers to the transfer of infectious agents from a reservoir to a host via an intermediary and include suspended air particles, inanimate objects (fomites) and animate intermediaries (vectors).

Infectious agents suspended on air particles facilitate airborne transmission and unlike droplet spread, can be carried over longer distances on air currents (e.g. measles virus). This may include infectious agents on dust particles or dried residue called droplet nuclei of less than 5 microns. Inanimate objects or fomites include food and drinking water or contaminated items such as bedding, surgical equipment, dental equipment or syringes. Technology can also be an efficient transmitter of diseases such as Legionnaire's disease, which is spread through evaporative condensers and air-conditioners. Vectors are arthropods such as mosquitoes and fleas that carry the infectious agent and deliver it to a host, usually through a bite. Many dangerous pathogens, such as those causing malaria and the plague, are vectorborne.

3.4.4 Portals of entry

The portal of entry is the method by which a pathogen enters a susceptible host. Pathogens generally infect specific tissues, and so for an infection to take hold, the portal of entry should provide appropriate access. For

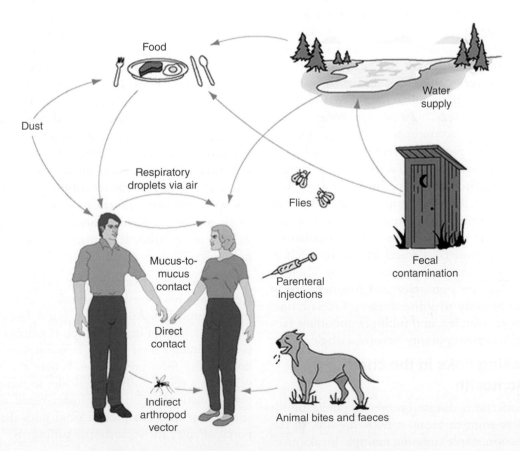

FIGURE 3.14 Modes of transmission for infectious disease

Source: Quah, S. R. & Cockerham, W. C. (2017). International encyclopedia of public health. Academic Press.

the most part, the portals of exit and portals of entry are the same and include the gastrointestinal, respiratory and urogenital tracts. Consumption of contaminated food and drinking water with faecal material from a portal of exit is often the portal of entry for many gastrointestinal pathogens and typifies the faecal-oral route. Respiratory infections are mostly spread through droplets, and sexual contact often facilitates transmission of disease affecting the urogenital tract. Human behaviours such as intravenous drug use and sharing of needles, or medical procedures such as blood transfusions, may spread blood-borne pathogens such as hepatitis viruses or HIV. Skin wounds permit entry of pathogens from direct contact with reservoirs (e.g. environment or other humans) or fomites. Some pathogens, such as hookworms, are capable of penetrating directly through skin and others enter through mucous membranes such as the eye (e.g. SARS-CoV-2 or Ebolavirus).

3.4.5 Susceptible host

Host susceptibility to an infection is an important link in the chain of transmission and is governed by a series of complex factors such as host genetics and host microbiome, age, pregnancy, use of medications, health status (e.g. malnutrition or dehydration) and underlying health conditions (e.g. diabetes). If we consider age, the very young have immature immune systems, increasing their vulnerability to infectious diseases whereas the very old harbour decreased immunity and generally accumulate more comorbidities such as high blood pressure, placing them at higher risk of disease complications. Factors such as nutrition, stress or environmental pollutants can reduce immune responses. Specific genetic conditions can adversely affect immunity whereas genetics generally dictate the variable response observed by populations to disease. Some modern medical treatments such as medications (e.g. immunosuppressants) or chemotherapy can dampen immunity and pregnancy may increase susceptibility to some diseases. Overall, host susceptibility is complex, and multiple colluding factors increase host susceptibility beyond a single factor.

3.4.6 Breaking links in the chain and public health

In battling infectious disease outbreaks, public health officials will attempt to break at least one link in the chain of infection, while targeting multiple breaks gives better outcomes. However, which link(s) to target is often dependent on the infectious disease and may be

limited by cost or sociocultural barriers (e.g. human behavioural and cultural practices).

Controlling reservoirs or eliminating pathogens at source: In the context of medical health, infectious people are isolated or treated to eliminate the reservoir. In society, extensive testing can help identify human reservoirs for isolation and treatment. Where the source is a fomite, then effective waste disposal, disinfection or sterilisation methods such as washing bedding and cleaning dirty surfaces and equipment is key. Where the reservoir is animal or environmental, avoiding the reservoir is one strategy but in the case of food-producing animals, this may not be possible. For example, to control outbreaks of influenza in birds, extreme measures such as culling have been used to prevent spread. Outbreaks from contaminated food sources must first be identified and then controlled by closing the source and issuing alerts to those exposed.

Protecting portals of entry and disrupting transmission: Standard precautions and personal protection equipment is important in medical health. Standard precautions are designed to minimise risk of transmission to healthcare workers when engaging with patients. For example, strict precautions are in place when handling syringes to avoid accidental needlestick injuries. Face masks and gloves prevent transmission but also protect a portal of exit and have the additional benefit of minimising transmission to patients. Hand hygiene is another key tool in infection prevention that controls infectious agents on hand surfaces to minimise transmission to patients or common-touch surfaces. For some airborne infections, modifying ventilation or air pressure and air filtration can also be effective in preventing airborne transmission within a hospital.

In society, effective treatment and disposal of human faecal waste has played a major role in disrupting faecal-oral transmission. Additionally, good hygiene such as regular washing of hands disrupts transmission between people through direct touch or fomites or contamination during food preparation. Where the transmissive vehicle is a vector, using insecticides to control the vector population is common. Insect repellents, clothing and bed netting can protect from bites that provide a portal of entry for vectorborne pathogens.

Increasing host defences: The treatment or control of underlying diseases or prophylactic treatment with antimicrobials are options. Patients may be given postoperative antimicrobials to decrease the likelihood of developing an infection; however, the rise of antimicrobial resistance requires prudent use of this approach. The most effective host defence-boosting intervention is vaccination. Vaccination of a population can dramatically decrease the transmission of an infectious agent and if rates are sufficiently high, can facilitate herd immunity, forcing the outbreak to burn out and thus protecting those who cannot be vaccinated or who are unable to mount an immune response in response to the vaccine.

3.5 Host–pathogen interactions

This section gives an overview of the diverse methods that pathogens use to cause infection and disease, and an overview of host immunological responses to infection.

3.5.1 Bacterial pathogens

Bacterial strategies in infection are highly diverse and research into the methods by which bacterial pathogens cause disease is extensive. With that said, there are common themes that can be teased out. Exposure of the pathogen to its target tissue is critical and this is discussed in 3.4 Transmission of pathogens. However, it is important to note that some pathogens are opportunistic and only cause disease if the circumstances are

right. Autoimmune conditions, disruptions in the microbiome or other bodily changes may allow commensal bacteria to opportunistically infect. Additionally, normal flora in one part of the body may cause infection if accidentally relocated to another part of the body. For example, faecal bacteria are commonly implicated in urinary tract infections.

Adhesion of the bacterium to host tissue is an important first step that helps the pathogen to establish a discrete focal point of infection. Without adhesion, a bacterium may be easily removed through natural bodily processes such as peristaltic motion of the intestine, passage of urine through the urethra, coughing or sneezing. A variety of cell surface structures are important in adhesion including fimbriae, pili, flagella and capsular polysaccharide and there is most often a specific interaction between the bacterium and a host tissue. There are multiple examples of adhesins such as fimbriae and pili used by certain strains of *E. coli* in adhesion to the urinary tract or the pilus used by diarrhoeal-causing strains of *Vibrio cholerae* in adherence to the intestine.

Following adhesion, bacteria use diverse strategies that assist in adjacent spread and invasion of tissue and/or spread into the bloodstream or other tissues. Secretion of toxins (exotoxins) is one strategy (see Table 3.5 for a representative list). Toxins are substances that disrupt the normal function of the host and include enzymes that break down polymeric substances holding

TABLE 3.5 Examples of toxins produced by bacteria and mechanism of action

Bacterium	Disease	Toxin	Mechanism of action
Secreted toxins			
Clostridium botulinum	Botulism	Neurotoxin	Blocks excitation of muscles causing flaccid paralysis
Clostridium tetani	Tetanus	Neurotoxin (tetanus toxin)	Prevents inhibition of motor neurons blocking relaxation of muscles
Corynebacterium diphtheriae	Diphtheria	Diphtheria toxin	Inhibition of protein synthesis
Listeria monocytogenes	Listeriosis	Listeriolysin	Lysis of multiple host cells
Shigella dysenteriae	Dysentery (Bloody diarrhoea)	Shiga toxin	Inhibition of protein synthesis. Mainly affects blood vessels
Vibrio cholerae	Cholera diarrhoea	Enterotoxin (cholera toxin)	Disrupts ion flow in the intestine causing massive water loss and diarrhoea
Injectosome delivered toxins			
Salmonella enterica Typhimurium	Inflammatory gastroenteritis	Multiple effector proteins delivered to intestinal cells by a Type III secretion injectosome system	Induces entry into host cell and manipulates multiple host cell pathways involved in actin arrangement, cytokine production and apoptosis

tissues together such as connective tissue, collagen and mucin, or substances that have specific impacts on host cells such as cell lysis, protein synthesis inhibition, interference with or inhibition of neurotransmitters or interference of host cell regulatory chemicals. Toxins are often named depending on the cell types they attack. Toxins that affect multiple host cell types are referred to as cytotoxic whereas toxins that attack specific host cell types are named accordingly, such as neurotoxin (nerve cells), hepatotoxin (liver cells), cardiotoxin (heart cells) or enterotoxin (enteric cells). Toxins may also be named according to the disease they cause (e.g. cholera toxin and tetanus toxin), activity or biochemical properties (e.g. heat-stable toxin). In some instances, people can be impacted by bacterially produced toxins without infection. Food intoxication occurs when food is consumed containing a toxin secreted by a bacterium such as staphylococcal intoxication, causing nausea and vomiting, or botulism, a severe paralysis disease caused by *Clostridium botulinum*-produced neurotoxin. Some toxins are directly injected by bacteria into host cells through injectosome needle-like secretion systems and these toxins are referred to as effector proteins. The lipid A portion of LPS in Gram-negative bacteria is often referred to as endotoxin and has inflammatory effects in the bloodstream. LPS may slough in small amounts but if released in large amounts from lysis due to phagocytosis or chemotherapeutic activity, may cause dangerous endotoxic shock.

Some bacteria grow on host tissue forming a slime layer called a biofilm which is defined as bacteria adhered to a surface in multi-layered communities encased in an extracellular polymeric matrix that is rich in polysaccharide. Biofilms can form on animate or inanimate surfaces and is a natural process that is widely considered the normal mode of bacterial growth rather than planktonic growth in a liquid medium (Fig 3.15). Biofilms have multiple advantages in infection including the coordinated and regulated efforts of a bacterial population to cause tissue damage and the polymeric matrix acting as a physical barrier to host immune cells and chemotherapeutics. As such, biofilms are often involved in chronic infection such as *Pseudomonas aeruginosa* infections in the lungs of cystic fibrosis sufferers or periodontal diseases. Implants such as hip joints or heart valves are prone to biofilm formation that often must be removed from the patient to clear the infection.[7] Temporarily implanted medical devices such as catheters are also prone to biofilm formation, increasing the risk of infection. Beyond infection, biofilms are important on hospital surfaces and within the water pipe infrastructure by acting as reservoirs of pathogens and antimicrobial resistance genes. Bacteria within biofilms are more resistant to disinfectants and the close cell-to-cell contact facilitates horizontal gene transfer processes that spread antimicrobial resistance genes, degrading options for treating bacterial pathogens (see Box 1 Resistance plasmids are everywhere!).

Some bacterial pathogens are adept at invading host cells, enabling evasion from the immune system and creating an intracellular replicative niche. Some intracellular pathogens are obligate, such as *Chlamydia trachomatis* spp. (*Chlamydia*) and *Mycobacterium tuberculosis* (tuberculosis), and can only replicate within a host cell whereas others are facultative, such as *Salmonella* typhi (typhoid), *Legionella pneumoniae* (Legionnaire's disease) and *Yersinia pestis*

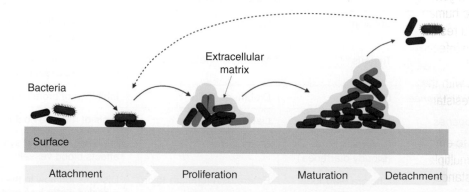

FIGURE 3.15 Biofilm formation in bacteria is initiated by adhesion of bacterial cells to a surface. Proliferation and maturation occur through cellular growth and the production of an extracellular matrix that encases the bacteria and helps protect them from immune cells, chemotherapeutic agents and disinfectants. Cells can detach from the biofilm and travel to other sites to reinitiate the process

Source: Costa, P., Costa, C. M., & Lanceros-Méndez, S. (Eds.). (2021). Advanced Lightweight Multifunctional Materials. Woodhead Publishing.

(plague) and can replicate inside and outside of a host cell. Intracellular lifestyle strategies are diverse, with some pathogens being internalised by phagocytosis whereas other pathogens induce host cells to uptake them. Intracellular bacterial pathogens use a number of virulence factors to subvert and control normal cellular functions including escaping destruction within immune cells and manipulating host actin to move directly from cell to cell.

BOX 3.1 Resistance plasmids are everywhere!

Bacteria can naturally evolve resistance to antimicrobials through mutation; however, many of the most problematic hospital pathogens acquire resistance from plasmids. Plasmids are circular pieces of DNA that replicate independently of the chromosome, with many containing conjugative genes (called conjugative plasmids) that facilitate transfer to other bacterial cells through a protein bridge called a pilus.

Due to the extensive use of antimicrobials in humans and animals, and their presence in waste streams, there is selective advantage for bacteria to acquire and keep a resistance plasmid. Additionally, waste streams are important in the dissemination of resistant bacteria and DNA including plasmids into the environment which are thought to re-enter into the community through water consumption or the food chain. As a result, resistance plasmids are not only common in pathogens but also in commensal and environmental bacteria, and these act as a source for pathogens. In fact, carriage of resistant plasmids in the human gut comes with a higher risk of developing a resistant infection due to possible transfer into an infecting pathogen.[8] Importantly, the passage of plasmids across different bacteria provides them with the opportunity to acquire novel antimicrobial resistance genes from the vast bacterial metagenome.

It is important to emphasise that resistance plasmids often contain multiple resistance genes thus providing resistance to multiple classes of antimicrobials. This means that a single conjugative transfer event into a pathogen can significantly limit treatment options for an infection. Therefore, effective infection prevention and control also includes the control of nefarious genetic material such as resistance plasmids.

3.5.2 Fungal pathogens

Despite being widely spread among humans, a small number of fungal species infect humans with very few causing life-threatening infections. Environmental fungi can infect humans if they are able to penetrate protective barriers such as skin, survive host immune defences, lyse tissue(s) and grow at human body temperature. With advancements in treatments that have allowed patients to survive where normally they would have succumbed, severe fungal infections have become more common in the immunocompromised or those with underlying health conditions.

Superficial, cutaneous and subcutaneous mycoses: Dermatophytoses are common mycoses also known as ringworm or tinea caused by fungi that usually localise at the level of skin, hair or nails (*Microsporum canis*: tinea capitis and tinea corporis). They are common in tropical regions including in Australia. Many predisposing factors can favour infection in the host including environmental factors (humidity, temperature), immunological and general health status of the host, and socio-economic factors. Recently, mask tinea was described in India and was linked to the use of masks for protection against COVID-19 infection.[9]

Dermatophytoses usually present as circular red scaly lesions on skin. Infected nails may be separated from the nail bed after discoloration, thickening and desquamation. Cutaneous infection may lead to invasive infections in immunocompromised patients, leading to ulcers and abscesses. Overall, these infections trigger a host inflammatory response at the level of the skin. Development of dermatophytosis includes three main steps: adherence, penetration and maintenance. Fungal cells attach to keratinised tissues via adhesins that connect it to the skin—this is often linked to a change in local skin pH which prevents the action of protective host enzymes that work better in acidic conditions. To penetrate the tissue, the fungal pathogen secretes several types of enzymes including keratolytic proteases. Once in the tissue, the fungus maintains itself by using nutrients from the host tissue and adapting to host metabolic changes. Dermatophytes are also able to produce biofilms which could explain why some infections are difficult to treat.

Systemic opportunistic fungal infections: Most severe to life-threatening fungal infections are systemic and occur in the immunocompromised. Fungi such as *Candida* spp., *Cryptococcus* spp. or *Aspergillus* spp. are major causes of systemic infections with high mortality rates when they cannot be cleared by the host defence system. This evolution from asymptomatic to systemic is usually linked to a host's immune status. Individuals suffering from HIV/AIDS or treated with immunosuppressants for transplants or cancer are most at risk of developing these systemic diseases after being infected by an opportunistic fungus that would normally have caused a benign, subclinical infection in an otherwise healthy individual.

Both *Aspergillus* spp. and *Cryptococci* spp. can enter the lungs as spores. In invasive pulmonary aspergillosis, the pathogen enters the lung, then invades and damages the tissues before entering the blood, leading to a systemic infection allowing the dissemination of the infection to other organs such as the brain. Cryptococcosis is particularly severe in patients with low CD4 T-lymphocytes (see 3.6 Immunological responses) counts, making it a major cause of AIDS-related deaths, with the pathogen being able to spread to several organs with a high affinity for the central nervous system. *Candida albicans* is part of the microbiome that colonise humans; however, this colonisation can evolve into infection, notably among hospitalised patients in intensive care. Bloodstream infection occurring during disseminated candidiasis has a high mortality rate and this opportunistic infection occurs not only in immunocompromised patients but particularly in patients who present rupture of anatomical barriers after catheterisation or surgery in addition to broad-spectrum antibacterial therapy.

Through evolution, fungi have lost their flagella and use other means to invade a host. The hyphae (long tube-like structure branching from the main body of the fungus) in *Candida albicans* for instance is a highly polarised structure that helps the fungus to propel itself within the human body by penetrating epithelial and endothelial cells, causing damage by releasing hydrolytic enzymes, allowing access to the bloodstream and being responsible for systemic infections such as candidiasis. *Candida* spp. and more particularly pathogenic *C. albicans* and *C. glabrata* possess a wide range of adhesins on their surface that allow them to firmly attach to host cells (endothelium, epithelium) via molecules such as fibronectin and glycans, and abiotic surfaces such as glass or plastic, helping them to form biofilms. Some of these adhesins are also found in *Aspergillus fumigatus* and *Cryptococcus neoformans*. Airborne spores produced by fungi such as *Aspergillus* spp. are transported passively into the host and then germinate as hyphae, where they can produce large mycelial lesions in the lungs. In *Cryptococcus* spp. desiccated yeasts are an infectious form that can

propagate the infection. After adhesion, to allow invasion, these fungi secrete various digestive enzymes able to dissolve host tissues and provide substrate for survival. Some invasive *Aspergillus* spp. secrete elastases that degrade elastin in the lung alveoli. *Cryptococci* secrete multiple enzymes such as ureases that facilitate the passage through the blood–brain barrier or a metalloprotease also required for central nervous system invasion. *C. albicans*, *A fumigatus* and *Cryptococcus* spp. secrete phospholipases that enhance their virulence by increasing their adhesion to respiratory epithelial cells.

3.5.3 Parasitic pathogens

Intestinal protozoan parasites: Intestinal protozoan parasites are some of the main causes of foodborne infections following the ingestion of contaminated water or food. The most common and relevant to human infections are *Giardia lamblia*, *Cryptosporidium parvum* and *Entamoeba histolytica*. The clinical presentation of the infection caused by these parasites can vary from persistent diarrhoea with loose stools, fatigue, abdominal cramps (*G. lamblia*); mild to acute diarrhoea with nausea, vomiting, abdominal pain and low-grade fever (*C. parvum*); to bloody mucoid diarrhoea with abdominal pain, fever, liver abscesses and life-threatening infection with dissemination to organs other than the gastrointestinal tract (*E. histolytica*).

The overall biological cycle of *Giardia* spp. and *Entamoeba* spp. starts with the ingestion of an infectious cyst via the faecal-oral route (e.g. contaminated water or food). Due to the changes in their environment when reaching the stomach, the parasites emerge from the cyst in a stage known as excystation and transform into trophozoites. These trophozoites, considered as the disease-causing stage, attach to the intestinal epithelial cells where they proliferate. Interaction with the intestinal epithelial cells triggers multiple changes, including surface and attachment-associated proteins such as adhesins and lectins as well as metabolic enzymes, that help source energy and fight host immunity. As the parasite is transported further into the gastrointestinal tract towards the small intestine, it converts back into a cyst (encystation stage), enabling it to survive outside the host for weeks once it is excreted in the faeces. In the case of *Entamoeba histolytica*, the trophozoites colonise the colon. In a large majority of cases the colon is not invaded and individuals remain asymptomatic or present mild symptoms. However, if the colon barrier is breached, the trophozoites may spread to surrounding tissues and cause local tissue damage such as necrosis and ulcers through the production of cytolytic molecules. If the parasites reach the liver and the lungs via the bloodstream, life-threatening amebiasis may result.

Cryptosporidium hominis is the main cause of cryptosporidiosis in humans in Australia, and in the 1980s it was an AIDS-defining illness. *Cryptosporidium* spp., unlike other apicomplexan parasites such as *Plasmodium* and *Toxoplasma*, completes its life cycle within the gastrointestinal tract of its single host. When the host ingests oocysts, they undergo excystation and release sporozoites, and as for *Giardia* spp., excystation is triggered by environmental factors such as temperature, pancreatic enzymes and bile salts. The sporozoites move across the epithelial cells, invading them. While moving over the host cells, the parasite secretes various proteins involved in attachment and later invasion, leading to its encapsulation in a host-membrane derived vacuole called the parasitophorous vacuole (PV). The cycle continues by a sexual stage multiplication and the formation of cysts that are shed into the environment, allowing propagation of the infectious cycle. Although not fully invasive and confined at the level of the host cell plasma membrane, *Cryptosporidium* spp. are able to disturb the function of the intestinal epithelium.

Also transmitted by ingestion of cysts, *Toxoplasma* parasites, mainly *Toxoplasma gondii*, cause few gastrointestinal symptoms but are responsible for severe pathologies, both acute and chronic, ranging from flu-like to lymphadenopathy, encephalopathy, abortion, stillbirth or congenital abnormalities. Parasites contained in the ingested cysts are released and invade the intestinal epithelial cells where they transform and multiply intracellularly within a PV. *Toxoplasma* uses what has been described as an 'invasion machinery'. This machinery contains proteins needed for cell invasion and manipulation of the host cell. Within the PV, the rapid multiplication leads to the rupture of the cell and invasion of the neighbouring cells. At this stage, depending on the response of the host, parasites can either be eliminated (most common case in immunocompetent hosts) or form a cyst. Many cells can be invaded by the parasite which likely uses this advantage to disseminate to other tissues, notably via infiltrating immune cells but also endothelial cells, through what can be described as a 'Trojan horse' type of invasion. These cysts can therefore be found in areas of low immune surveillance such as the eye or muscles. Parasites can also use this means of invasion to cross the blood–brain barrier and reach the brain.

Protozoan parasites acquired from insect bites:
Whether the insect vector is present in Australia or not, cases of insect-transmitted protozoan infections are frequently diagnosed. Two of the major ones are classified as imported, with malaria caused by *Plasmodium*, and American trypanosomiasis or Chagas disease caused by *Trypanosoma cruzi*. The latter is now considered an emerging disease in Australia. Malaria is caused by the *Plasmodium* species and five strains are known to infect humans—*P. falciparum*, *P. vivax*, *P. malariae*, *P. ovale* and *P. knowlesi*—with the first being the most virulent and the last being defined as a zoonosis as it historically infected monkeys.

The life cycles of *Trypanosoma cruzi* and *Plasmodium* spp. are complex and involve several hosts, vectors, life cycles and parasite stages specific to each part of the overall cycle. In both cases the parasite is taken up from the infected host through the bite of the vector during a blood meal, i.e., the Anopheles mosquito (malaria) or the triatome bug (trypanosomiasis). In malaria, the parasite is directly injected into a new host during the vector's next blood meal, while in trypanosomiasis the parasite is deposited in the vector's faeces during a blood meal and enters the host via neighbouring mucous membranes or directly via the bite site. From there the parasites penetrate various tissues and multiply in target organs.

Uncomplicated malaria is defined by the occurrence of non-specific flu-like symptoms (fever, chills, body aches) and the presence of parasites in the blood but can evolve into severe or complicated malaria. This occurs mainly in children under the age of five or non-immune individuals, i.e., individuals who have never encountered the parasite or have lost their immunity against the parasite. Severe malaria is mostly associated with *P. falciparum* infection and can clinically present as a neurological syndrome with coma and seizures, a severe anaemia or multi-organ failure. During malaria infection, after being injected into the dermis of the host, the parasites which are motile need to reach the liver by traversing capillaries and being transported to hepatic sinusoids, cross the endothelial cells and enter the hepatic parenchyma. Very much like *Toxoplasma*, *Plasmodium* sporozoites release the contents of invasive organelles to allow for hepatocyte invasion and folding of the plasma membrane to form a PV where the parasite will live and perform its cycle. From the liver, the parasites then migrate to the blood where they start the erythrocytic cycle which is associated with malaria symptomology. The cycle starts when the parasites are released from the ruptured hepatocytes and then invade erythrocytes. The erythrocytes will be used as a protective vehicle and source of energy and will undergo significant remodelling, including export to the erythrocyte membrane of hundreds of proteins from the PV via a network of conduits. One family of these exported proteins is the *P. falciparum* erythrocyte membrane protein 1 (PfEMP1) family. Each PfEMP1 protein has a defined adhesive domain that allows it to bind to specific receptors within different vascular beds including the brain and the placenta. This binding to endothelial cells (blood vessels) or syncytiotrophoblasts (placenta) allows infected erythrocytes to sequester into the tissues, escape splenic clearance and be an integral part of the pathogenesis of severe malaria forms such as cerebral and placental malaria.

American trypanosomiasis presents in two phases—acute (up to 2 months) and chronic (up to several years/decades). The acute phase is associated with the presence of parasites in the blood together with non-specific symptoms such as fever, headache, enlarged lymph glands, muscle pain or no symptoms. During that time the parasite multiplies in organs such as the heart and the gastrointestinal tract. Patients can stay asymptomatic (~70%) but others will develop organ-associated symptoms such as chest pain, cardiomyopathy, neurological alterations or enlarged oesophagus or colon. When the parasite enters the host it will invade cells, usually of the mucous membrane of the nose, conjunctiva or any fragile surface, and will transform into amastigotes (intracellular stage of the parasite that has lost its flagella). These forms will then multiply before they burst out of the cells and enter the bloodstream to invade new cells and propagate the infection to tissues such as the heart and the gastrointestinal tract. The parasite uses various virulence factors while interacting with the host. These factors not only allow the parasite to resist host defence mechanisms and evade the immune response but also promote cell adhesion and invasion. The parasites express enzymes that can inhibit the defence mechanism from macrophages. The parasite is also able to avoid lysis by blocking the complement pathways using complement-regulating factors. To allow adhesion and invasion of the host cells, *T. cruzi* expresses at its surface molecules such as transsialidases (specific to the parasite), mucins, mucin-associated surface glycoproteins and phospholipases.

Multicellular parasites: Humans and helminth parasites have coexisted and co-evolved for millennia. In Australia, infections caused by roundworm (strongyloidiasis caused by *Strongyloides stercoralis*), hookworm (*Ancylostoma duodenale*), tapeworm (echinococcosis) and soil-transmitted helminthiases can disproportionately affect Indigenous populations. Although helminth infections can be associated to severe comorbidities, they rarely cause lethal infections, suggesting that the hosts have learnt to tolerate the parasites and develop a disease tolerance leading to limited damage to both host and parasite. Some of these parasites' life cycles are simple, involving humans as the definitive host (i.e. host where the parasite completes its sexual stage). In the case of taeniasis, humans become infected by ingesting raw or undercooked meat from infected cattle (*Taenia saginata*) or pigs (*Taenia solium*). Once in the animal, the ingested parasite eggs hatch and invade the intestinal wall and migrate to the striated muscles to form cysts. In the case of *Ancylostoma duodenale*, larvae penetrate the skin, are carried via blood vessels to the heart and lungs, penetrate the pulmonary alveoli, ascend the pharynx and are either coughed up or swallowed by the host. To penetrate the skin, the parasite secretes enzymes that facilitate migration through tissue. While migrating through the body the parasites not only trigger direct tissue damage but also release inflammatory mediators, typically through the shedding of their outer chitin layer during moulting and also via the release of excretory–secretory products including proteases, protease inhibitors, lectins, allergens and glycolytic enzymes. In the case of strongyloidiasis, one of the severe forms is the dissemination of the infection outside the gastrointestinal tract, which can occur in immunocompromised patients where the parasite is able to infiltrate organs such as the lungs, kidneys, liver or central nervous system.

3.5.4 Viral pathogens

Viral infections all follow a generalised cycle that is summarised in Figure 3.16.

1. *Attachment:* Adhesion is the first step and is a very specific interaction between the virus and host cell. The spike proteins facilitate adhesion by binding to host cell receptors. If the receptor is common then the virus may infect a range of host cells. For example, the Ebolavirus is capable of infecting multiple cell types due to the commonality of its host receptor. On the other hand, HIV adheres only to receptors on human immunity CD4+ cells. Some viruses like rabies can

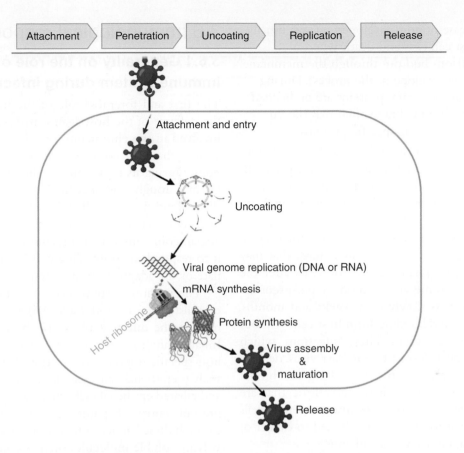

Attachment | Penetration | Uncoating | Replication | Release

Attachment and entry

Uncoating

Viral genome replication (DNA or RNA)

mRNA synthesis

Host ribosome

Protein synthesis

Virus assembly & maturation

Release

FIGURE 3.16 The general viral replication strategy. A eukaryotic virus will attach to a host cell and enter via endocytosis or membrane fusion. Upon entry, the virion is uncoated allowing release of the nucleic acid. The nucleic acid is replicated and mRNA is produced using host ribosomes to make viral proteins required for viral assembly and maturation. The viral particle then exits the host cell via lysis or budding. Modified from ElBagoury M, et al 2021

Source: Modified from ElBagoury, M., Tolba, M. M., Nasser, H. A., Jabbar, A., Elagouz, A. M., Aktham, Y., & Hutchinson, A. (2021). The find of COVID-19 vaccine: Challenges and opportunities. Journal of infection and public health, 14(3), 389-416.

infect multiple animal species due to the presence of an interspecies receptor.

2. *Penetration:* The virus penetrates the cell and this occurs by one of two processes, endocytosis or fusion. Endocytosis is a natural process that eukaryotic cells use to bring in substances, and examples of both enveloped and non-enveloped viruses using this method of entry exist. Some enveloped viruses fuse their membrane with the host cell membrane allowing entry of the nucleocapsid into the host cell.

3. *Uncoating:* Depending on the virus, different mechanisms exist for uncoating that facilitate the entry of the nucleic acid into the cytoplasm.

4. *Replication:* The viral nucleic acid dictates the nucleic acid replication strategy. The virus often brings in or

produces its own enzyme for nucleic acid replication. Production of viral mRNA is key and host ribosomes drive synthesis of viral proteins that take over the host cell and then synthesise the virion. Viral DNA locates to the nucleus where mRNA is synthesised and transported out into the cytoplasm for protein synthesis. Synthesised proteins are transported into the nucleus for virion assembly. Viral RNA remains in the cytoplasm where synthesised mRNA directs protein synthesis and assembly proceeds. HIV is an RNA retrovirus that converts its RNA genome into DNA and inserts it into the host cell genome in the nucleus using a specialist viral enzyme called reverse transcriptase. From this position, it produces mRNA, which also acts as the viral genome, to drive synthesis of proteins allowing assembly to proceed in the cytoplasm.

5. *Release:* Release of non-enveloped virions usually results in host cell lysis and death whereas enveloped virions bud out through the membrane, acquiring their envelope in the process. During the replication stage, viral proteins are embedded into the host cell membrane, such that the viral envelope contains virus-specific proteins.

Different animal virus infections have different outcomes that are defined as acute, latent, persistent or oncogenic. Acute infections such as influenza or COVID-19 are rapid (days to weeks) resulting in death of infected cells. Latent infections such as lip or genital sores caused by herpes simplex viruses initiate as an acute infection but enter into a latent stage that may revert into an acute phase months or years after the original infection. Some viruses produce persistent infections that progress slowly over weeks and months, slowly replicating and budding from host cells without necessarily destroying them. These infections, which include the glandular fever Epstein–Barr virus, deprive their host of energy, sometimes resulting in chronic fatigue. Finally, oncogenic viruses are those that are capable of transforming host cells into cancerous cells such as the human papilloma virus linked to cancer of the cervix, vulva, vagina, penis and anus.

3.6 Immunological responses

3.6.1 Generality on the role of the immune system during infection

The first and foremost role of the immune system is the defence of the host against pathogens but it is also involved in the elimination of toxic or allergenic substances that can come in contact with or enter the body. During its development, the immune system has learnt through tolerance mechanisms to differentiate the self and the non-self and therefore to not eliminate host cells or to avoid responses that would destroy beneficial, commensal microorganisms. This ability allows it to respond to an invading pathogen through the innate or the adaptive immune responses.

The immune system is composed of a large variety of cells (Fig 3.17 and Table 3.6) which have specific roles in the different phases of the immune response. Innate immunity can be defined as an immediate and non-specific response to infection that involves barriers such as epithelial cells (e.g. skin, mucosa, mucous layers and ciliated epithelial cells) that are all able to physically prevent entry of pathogens. If a pathogen breaks through these barriers, other protective mechanisms involving soluble molecules such as complement system

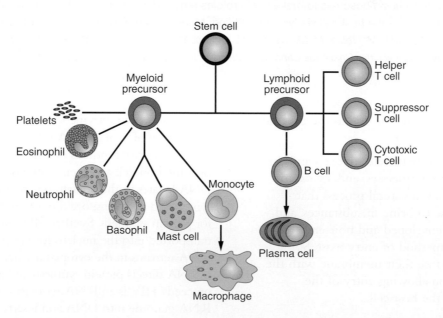

FIGURE 3.17 Cells of the immune system arise from a common haematopoietic stem cell in the bone marrow that will differentiate and mature into two different cell lineages, myeloid and lymphoid. From these precursors, the major cells of the immune response will mature, themselves being able to further differentiate into more specialised cells, such as plasma cells. Table 3.6 describes these cells and their roles
Source: McCuistion, L. E., Yeager, J. J., Winton, M. B., & DiMaggio, K. V. (2021). Pharmacology. Elsevier.

TABLE 3.6 **Main cells of the immune system, their role and location**

Cell type	Main role	Location
Polymorphonuclear eosinophils	Release toxins that can kill bacteria and parasites	Blood vessels and can migrate to tissue during infection
Polymorphonuclear neutrophils	Ingest and kill microorganisms (mainly bacteria and fungi). First responders at the site of infection. Release molecules that attract other immune cells at the site of infection	Blood vessels and can migrate to tissue during infection
Polymorphonuclear basophils	Defence against parasites. Release molecules that can participate to the expulsion of an extracellular parasite	Blood vessels and can migrate to tissue during infection
Mast cells	Release molecules involved into the destruction of pathogens	Connective tissue, mucous membranes
Monocytes	Phagocytic cells that can engulf pathogens and cells and later differentiate into macrophages once they have left the blood circulation and entered a tissue	Blood vessels and can migrate to tissue during infection
Macrophages	Phagocytic cells that can engulf pathogens and release molecules stimulating other immune cells	Migrate from blood vessels into infected tissues
T-lymphocytes (Helper)/ CD4 T helper cells	Specialised T-lymphocytes helping other T and B-cells perform their functions by interacting directly with them or releasing soluble molecules. Express CD4 antigen	Blood vessels and can migrate to tissue during infection
T-lymphocytes (Suppressor)	Specialised T-lymphocytes (also called regulatory T-cells) that suppress various cellular and humoral mechanisms of the immune response. Express CD4 antigen	Blood vessels and can migrate to tissue during infection
Cytotoxic T-lymphocytes/ CD8 Cytotoxic T-cells	Kill infected cells. Express CD8 antigen	Blood vessels and can migrate to tissue during infection
B-lymphocyte	Sub-type of lymphocyte that can present foreign antigens to other immune cells, secrete soluble molecules and produce antibodies when differentiated	Blood vessels and can migrate to tissue during infection
Plasma cell	Differentiated B-lymphocytes that produce antibodies	Blood vessels and can migrate to tissue during infection
Natural killer cells	Kill mainly virus-infected cells	Blood vessels and can migrate to tissue during infection
Dendritic cells	Initiate antigen-specific immune responses	Resident cells of the skin, lung and digestive tract. Migrate to lymph nodes after activation by a pathogen

proteins, defensins, mediators of inflammation, reactive free radical species and cytokines and chemokines can take over (the humoral part of innate immunity). Innate immunity is able to recognise general classes of pathogens such as bacteria, fungi, viruses and parasites but will not be able to make fine distinctions within each of these. The innate immunity will attempt to immediately destroy the pathogens and if unable, will contain the infection until the more powerful adaptive immune system acts (Fig 3.18).

Adaptive immunity can be defined as a delayed and very specific response that is able to recognise each unique type of foreign antigen. It is slower to respond,

with effector cells produced within a week and the whole response occurring within two weeks. Contrary to innate immunity which will mount the same response upon repeated exposure to the same pathogen, adaptive immunity develops a memory of a specific pathogen and will respond upon re-exposure in a faster or more potent manner. Both B- and T-lymphocytes are major cells of the adaptive immunity and are responsible for the specific immune recognition of pathogens. The adaptive immunity combines a humoral immunity defined by the production of antibodies (Fig 3.19) by differentiated B-cell lymphocytes (called plasma cells) and a cell-mediated immunity involving T-lymphocytes that will mature into

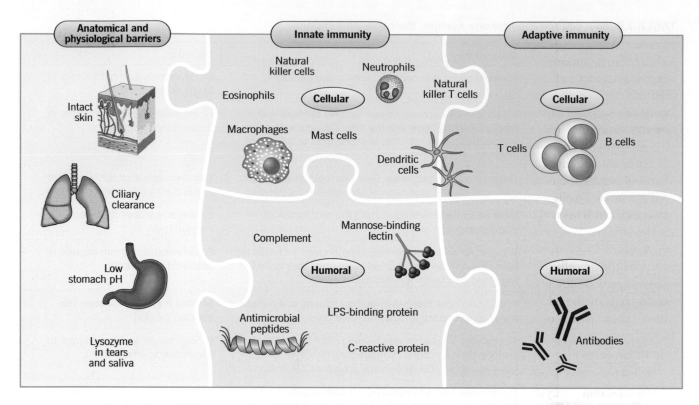

FIGURE 3.18 Innate and adaptive immune responses. The human microbial defence system can be simplistically viewed as consisting of three levels: 1) anatomical and physiological barriers; 2) innate immunity; and 3) adaptive immunity. Both innate and adaptive immunity can be further subdivided into cellular and humoral. The innate cellular immunity involves specific cell types such as macrophages or polymorphonuclear cells (eosinophils and neutrophils) that have non-specific antimicrobial responses while adaptive cellular immunity involves highly specialised T- and B- lymphocytes. Cells such as natural killer cells or dendritic cells are part of both types of cellular responses and are considered as the interface between the two responses. Humoral immunity will involve soluble molecules, proteins or peptides; in the case of innate humoral response these proteins, peptides or other molecules will non-specifically target pathogens while antibodies, part of the adaptive humoral response, will recognise specific epitopes on pathogens
Source: Malamed, S. F. (2022). Medical Emergencies in the Dental Office. Elsevier.

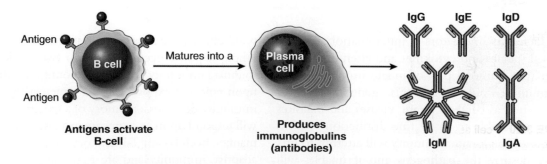

FIGURE 3.19 Production of immunoglobulin by B-cells. When an antigen activates a B-cell, they mature into a plasma cell and that then produces immunoglobulins (antibodies). The first classes of immunoglobulins produced are the IgM and IgD produced by mature B-cells. Following activation by specific signal, the plasma cells switch the production of immunoglobulins to classes IgE, IgA and IgG. See Table 3.7 for main roles of immunoglobulin classes
Source: Chabner, D. E. (2022). Medical Terminology: A Short Course. Elsevier.

effector helper cells (CD4 T–lymphocytes) and cytotoxic T–cells (CD8 T–lymphocytes) (Table 3.6). Adaptive immunity can be summarised by the following sequence of events: a CD4 T–cell encounters an antigen–presenting cell (dendritic cell) and gets activated via the engagement of receptors on its surface. The CD4 T–cell then releases molecules (cytokines) that will either activate B–cells that will in turn produce antibodies and engage the humoral response, or stimulate cytotoxic CD8 T–cells that will engage the cell–mediated response. Plasma cells and cytotoxic T–cells are called effector cells as their involvement ends up with the destruction of the pathogen or the infected host cell.

A critical link between innate and adaptive immunity is the dendritic cells which phagocytose pathogens that have entered tissues, process them and present antigens to the cells of the adaptive system (CD4 and CD8)—hence their name of professional antigen–presenting

cells. Dendritic cells express at their surface pattern recognition receptors (PRR) such as toll–like receptors that recognise pathogen associated molecular patterns (PAMPs) on pathogens.

The immune system therefore responds to different microbes in specialised ways that are best to eliminate them. Broadly, the adaptive immune response can be separated into a pro–inflammatory or an anti–inflammatory response depending on the type of pathogen involved and the type of soluble molecules (cytokines and chemokines) secreted to regulate the recruitment, differentiation and activation or inhibition of immune cells. A T–helper cell type 1 (Th1) response is characterised by the overall production of pro–inflammatory molecules while a T–helper cell type 2 (Th2) is associated with the presence of anti–inflammatory molecules (Fig 3.20). To eliminate pathogens that require internalisation to survive, such as intracellular parasites, viruses or some intracellular bacteria,

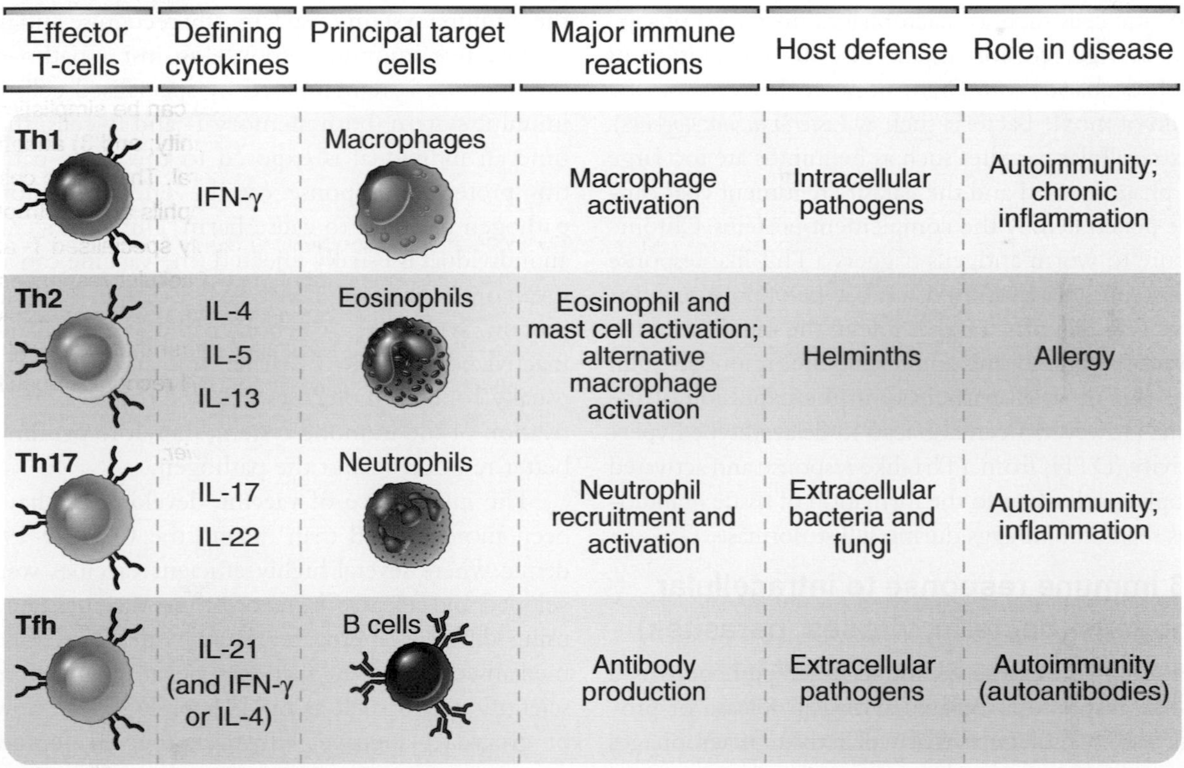

Effector T-cells	Defining cytokines	Principal target cells	Major immune reactions	Host defense	Role in disease
Th1	IFN-γ	Macrophages	Macrophage activation	Intracellular pathogens	Autoimmunity; chronic inflammation
Th2	IL-4 IL-5 IL-13	Eosinophils	Eosinophil and mast cell activation; alternative macrophage activation	Helminths	Allergy
Th17	IL-17 IL-22	Neutrophils	Neutrophil recruitment and activation	Extracellular bacteria and fungi	Autoimmunity; inflammation
Tfh	IL-21 (and IFN-γ or IL-4)	B cells	Antibody production	Extracellular pathogens	Autoimmunity (autoantibodies)

FIGURE 3.20 T-cell subsets and Th responses. Naïve CD4+ T-cells (have never been exposed to the foreign antigen) can differentiate into subsets of effector cells following interaction with an antigen or in response to cytokines. These Th responses are associated with a panel of cytokines that will in turn activate target cells that will have a specific role in the response to different pathogens. Th1 cells produce interferon-γ (IFN-γ), which activates macrophages to kill intracellular microbes. Th2 cells produce cytokines (interleukins, IL) that stimulate immunoglobulin E production and activate eosinophils in response to parasitic infection. Th17 cells secrete IL-17 and IL-22 that play an important role in responses to fungi. Tfh cells produce IL-21 and provide help to B-cells for antibody production

Source: Townsend, C. M. (2016). Sabiston textbook of surgery. Elsevier.

a Th1 polarised response is usually necessary. Conversely, for large extracellular parasites such as helminths, a Th2 response is usually present and is considered protective.

3.6.2 Immune response to extracellular pathogens (bacteria, yeasts, parasites)

The immune response to various types of pathogens will vary depending on how accessible they are to immune cells and molecules. The innate immunity is effective on pathogens that are not inside cells, whether they are strict extracellular pathogens or have an extracellular stage in their life cycle. This includes extracellular bacteria, worms, fungi, protozoa or viruses that can be found in interstitial spaces, blood, lymph or at the surface of epithelial cells. In these sites, pathogens can be targeted by antibodies (Table 3.7) such as immunoglobulin type A (IgA) that can block viral adherence and cell entry, immunoglobulin type M and G (IgM, IgG) that can activate the complement system and directly lyse pathogens and enveloped viruses, or they can be engulfed by phagocytic cells such as macrophages (increased phagocytosis is triggered, for instance, by the recognition of lipopolysaccharide on Gram-negative bacteria or the flagellin of motile bacteria such as *Listeria monocytogenes*).

Extracellular parasites such as helminths are too large to be phagocytosed and the parasite tegument coat cannot be penetrated by the complement proteins. Chronic exposure to worm antigens triggers a Th2-like response which results in activation of a sub-type of polymorphonuclear cells that play a major role in the innate immune response, the eosinophils and release of immunoglobulin type E (IgE) that all participate in the expulsion of the parasite. However, it can also lead to delayed type hypersensitivity (DTH) from a Th1-like response and activated macrophages, leading to the formation of tissue granulomas as seen around eggs during schistosomiasis.

3.6.3 Immune response to intracellular pathogens (bacteria, viruses, parasites)

The immune response to intracellular pathogens is a Th1-like response associated with the release of pro-inflammatory molecules that will activate macrophages

and other antigen presenting cells. When the pathogen is digested, peptides are presented via the Major Histocompatibility Complex I and CD8 cytotoxic T-cells are activated in order to kill the infected cell. Natural killer cells may also be involved. This is the common response to most viruses. In addition, for pathogens such as *Legionella* spp., mycobacteria or *Cryptococcus neoformans* that have developed ways to survive inside vesicular structures of macrophages (legionella containing vacuoles [LCV], phagolysosomes) the immune system will need to activate further macrophages to reverse the changes triggered by the pathogen. In the case of tuberculosis for instance, the mycobacterium has developed a way to inhibit the antimicrobial responses of macrophages and survive within the phagolysosome.

3.6.4 Vaccines

Vaccination is a way to provide long-term protection against specific pathogens. A vaccine trains the cells of the immune system to specifically recognise and mount a protective immune response against a pathogen. As the response is remembered by specialised cells of the immune system (both memory T- and B-cells) the next time an individual is exposed to this same pathogen, this protective response can be effective before the pathogen has time to cause harm. During vaccination, an individual is usually injected (the vaccine can also be given orally or nasally) with part (peptide, toxin, surface protein, synthetic) or whole pathogen (weakened or inactivated) together with an adjuvant. This adjuvant usually contains molecules that will trigger a strong activation of the immune system, therefore priming it to better respond against the pathogen.

The importance of vaccine development has never been more realised than during the COVID-19 pandemic where several highly efficient vaccines were developed and released in record time. Vaccines generated using different approaches were widely discussed and mediatised in a way that was never seen before and scientific terms such as mRNA or PCR are now part of everyday language. However, the development of

TABLE 3.7 **Main classes of immunoglobulins and their roles**

Immunoglobulin class	IgM	IgG	IgE	IgA
Main function	Complement activation	Bind to pathogen and increase phagocytosis by recognition of its receptor by the phagocytic cell; complement activation	Immunity against helminths	Mucosal immunity: transport of IgA through epithelia to form a barrier and take up foreign antigens

vaccines is not always this successful. Looking at the different vaccines available to prevent human infections it is easy to see that they cover mostly viruses and bacteria. Although a vaccine against the HIV virus has been in development for decades and many candidates are in the pipeline, so far none has proved successful. There is also no known vaccine against human parasites. Only very recently, an anti-malaria vaccine, decades in the making, was released (RTS,S/AS01) and offered only to a very select population of children at risk of severe malaria in Africa. The hope, in the vaccine developers' community, is that the progress made to develop the COVID-19 vaccine will be able to be transferred to other infections.

There are several types of vaccines, from inactivated vaccines, live-attenuated vaccines, messenger RNA (mRNA) vaccines and subunit/recombinant/polysaccharide/conjugate vaccines to toxoid vaccines. Each type of vaccine uses a different approach to trigger a protective immune response:

- Inactivated vaccines use a killed form of the pathogen and are used to protect against hepatitis A, the flu, polio and rabies.

- Live-attenuated vaccines use the same pathogen that causes the disease but in a weakened form. They are used against measles, mumps, rubella (combined into the MMR vaccine), rotavirus, smallpox, chicken pox and yellow fever and often necessitate regular booster shots.

- Subunit/recombinant/polysaccharide/conjugate vaccines are designed to create a response against a specific protein or sugars from the pathogen. They are used against *Haemophilus influenzae* type b, hepatitis B, human papilloma virus, whooping cough, pneumococcal disease, meningococcal disease and shingles.

- Toxoid vaccines trigger a response that is directed against a toxin released by the pathogen instead of the pathogen itself. It is used against diphtheria and tetanus.

- Messenger-RNA vaccines (mRNA) are the most recent type of vaccine to be used in human health. These vaccines contain mRNA encoding a pathogen protein that is encapsulated in a lipid bubble that when delivered onto the host, is translated to produce the protein that will trigger an immune response. This technique bypasses the need to manufacture and purify pathogen proteins and considerably shortens the development time. Although studied for decades, and with several pathogens in the pipeline (HIV, flu, cytomegalovirus), the vaccine against COVID-19 is the only one that has been commercialised for humans.

3.6.5 Strategies used by pathogens to evade the immune system

Unsurprisingly, some microorganisms have evolved mechanisms to resist and evade host immunity; these mechanisms are important virulence determinants of various infectious agents.

Anatomical seclusion: Some pathogens live intracellularly, therefore avoiding both the innate and adaptive immune responses. Infected cells are not recognised by the immune cells unless they present foreign proteins on their surface. Viruses such as *Varicella zoster* (chicken pox) can hide from the immune system by invading neurons where they can remain for years, re-emerging if the defences of the host are lowered. Bacteria such as *Borrelia burgdorferi* (Lyme disease) and *Burkholderia pseudomallei* (meliodosis) can also remain hidden, with patients presenting symptoms years after the initial infection. During their life cycle, *P. vivax* and *P. ovale* produce a specific stage of the parasite (hypnozoite) that remains hidden in the liver and can start a new parasite cycle months or years after the initial mosquito bite and exposure to the parasite. The radical cure used to treat *P. vivax* infections must kill both the blood stages of the parasite as well as liver hypnozoites. By residing in immunologically privileged sites, i.e., where little immunosurveillance by immune cells occurs, such as the eye or the brain, helminths can also avoid the immune response.

Antigenic variation: This strategy has been adopted by many pathogens and allows them to change the molecules expressed at their surface, making it difficult for the immune system to mount specific responses that adapt to the changes. Some key examples are given below:

- *Plasmodium* spp. expresses different antigens (hundreds of variants) at different stages of its life cycle and the switch between each variant is very fast.

- *Giardia* spp. expresses one variant surface protein (VSP) at a time but has a repertoire of 190 VSPs and can spontaneously switch to a different variant.

- African trypanosomes have one glycoprotein (VSG) that covers the entire surface of the parasite and is immunodominant for antibody responses, but gene cassettes of VSGs (2000 genes involved) allow regular switching between the genes.

- Bacteria such as *Neisseria meningitidis* or *Streptococcus pneumoniae* are capable of capsule switching (there are 84 known *S. pneumoniae*, each with a different polysaccharide capsule, i.e., serotype). *Neisseria gonorrhoeae* is also capable of antigenic variation at the level of its pilin protein pilE by altering the sequence of the *pilE* gene, generating variability affecting the pilus function and allowing it to evade immune surveillance.

Molecular mimicry: Bacteria and parasites such as helminths can express surface proteins that are similar to host proteins, therefore avoiding being recognised as 'non-self' by the immune system. *Neisseria meningitidis* or some strains of *E. coli* have a capsule containing polysaccharides that are structurally similar to polysaccharides on the surface of mammalian cells. Although this pathway provides the pathogen with a survival advantage, the host immune system still has other ways to recognise the presence of the pathogen. In addition, molecular mimicry is not all advantageous for the pathogen as firstly, maintaining the production of the mimic protein can be energetically costly for the pathogen, and secondly, molecular mimicry has been associated with autoimmunity. This occurs because the immune response mounted against the pathogen can also target molecules from the host that have a similar structure therefore triggering a response against the self, also called autoimmunity. On the other hand, according to the 'hygiene hypothesis', there is an inverse association between exposure to pathogens such as parasites and the onset of autoimmune diseases, which means that the increase in occurrence of autoimmune diseases may be associated with less infections.

Manipulation of immune responses: A classic example of this strategy is the ability of helminth parasites, such as *Schistosoma* spp. or *Ascaris* spp., to inhibit the activation of innate immune cells, induce the production of T- and B-regulatory T-cells (characteristic of an immunotolerant phenotype) instead of effector T-cells (CD4 helper T-cells and CD8 cytotoxic T-cells) and antibody-producing plasma cells. One particularity of these helminths is the release of secretory molecules or helminth-derived products that are powerful modulators of inflammation. They can modulate toll-like receptor signals and trigger the production of anti-inflammatory mediators that prevent the expulsion of the parasite and allow its survival.

3.7 Diagnosis of pathogens

Accurate disease diagnosis and therefore pathogen identification are important as they help determine the course of treatment and patient outcome. In general, a sample is required and this is usually taken from where in the body the pathogen is causing disease. For example, nasal or throat swabs are often taken for respiratory infections, urine for urinary tract infections, faecal samples for gastrointestinal infections, cerebrospinal fluid for meningitis, pus for wounds or a blood sample for systemic infections. Diagnosis can be made directly on the appropriate specimen using a variety of techniques but in some cases may require culture of the pathogen to allow identification and test for susceptibility to antimicrobial drugs. Depending on whether the disease is in an acute or a chronic phase, different approaches can be taken to either identify the pathogen itself or the level of the immune response through the titration of specific immunoglobulins/antibodies. The latter approach, however, may not be indicative of current infection. The type of immunoglobulin detected can provide some information regarding the time of the infection, as immunoglobulins type M appear two to four weeks after infection while immunoglobins type G takes about four to six weeks to be detectable in the blood.

Direct microscopy of a specimen, whether it is a blood smear, a wet mount of urine, stools or a cerebrospinal fluid, remains the definitive diagnostic criteria for many infections, notably parasitic (malaria, trypanosomiasis, schistosomiasis, giardiasis) but also bacterial or fungal infections. Microscopic examination of a specimen can confirm the presence, quantity and identity of the type of organism and, in some cases, differentiate between species and therefore inform the appropriate treatment (e.g. *P. falciparum* vs *P. vivax*). However, notably in the case of parasitic infections, it is time consuming, and an experienced microscopist is essential in order to obtain the right diagnosis.

Microscopy is therefore often paired with faster and easier approaches, including the use of molecular techniques such as Quantitative Polymerase Chain Reaction (qPCR). This method amplifies a specific pathogen nucleic acid sequence (typically <500-bp) in a sample and is sensitive enough to detect very low levels. It is routinely used to detect and quantify viral, bacterial and parasitic pathogens. The method can target the DNA, or RNA in the case of many viruses, using Reverse Transcriptase qPCR (RT-qPCR) that allows conversion of RNA to DNA before qPCR. The use of qPCR and RT-qPCR to identify a pathogen in CSF can dramatically improve the outcome for patients by allowing identification within a few hours rather than the 24–48 hours needed to culture a bacterial pathogen, for instance. In the case of parasitic infections such as malaria, qPCR is the only definitive diagnostic method accepted outside direct microscopy.

Advanced methods such as matrix–assisted laser desorption/ionisation–time of flight (MALDI–TOF) mass spectrometry (MS) are routinely used in diagnostic laboratories to identify bacteria or fungi (Bruker or Biomerieux). This simple and rapid method uses a protein fingerprint to identify pathogens down to the strain level if the instrument contains the appropriate library. Its sensitivity and specificity also allows identification of pathogens within a specimen such as blood or urine, therefore removing the need to culture the pathogen and significantly shortening the identification time and consequently the start of an appropriate treatment.

Immunological methods relying on the detection of antigens by ELISA (enzyme-linked immunosorbent assay), rapid detection tests (RDT, also called rapid antigen test, RAT) or card agglutination test (CAT) can be used to identify the presence of pathogen antigens in the bodily fluid tested (blood, serum, saliva, urine, CSF). They use the same principle where a major antigen from the pathogen is captured by a specific antibody immobilised on a plastic plate (ELISA), a nitrocellulose membrane (RDT) or on latex beads (CAT). The reaction can then be revealed by a colorimetric enzymatic method or the development of aggregates visible to the naked eye (Figs 3.21 and 3.22). ELISA are

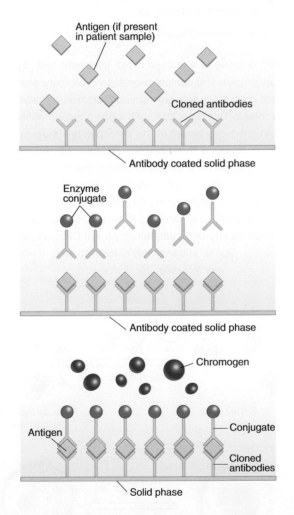

FIGURE 3.21 ELISA principle (a). An antibody specific for a pathogen antigen is coated on a surface. A suspension (patient plasma, serum, other bodily fluid or tissue lysate) containing (or not) the pathogen antigen is incubated with the coated antigen (top image). A second antibody (identical to the coated one or targeting another epitope of the pathogen antigen) is then added. This secondary antibody is conjugated with a signal molecule (middle image). This signal molecule is then recognised by a chromogen that allows the visualisation of the reaction (bottom image). A typical conjugate/chromogen is the enzyme-linked antibody to which is added a substrate, for instance horseradish peroxidase-conjugated antibody + hydrogen peroxide which will result in a brown colour. A standard curve performed with a synthetic form of the antigen allows the quantification of levels of antigen in the patient plasma.

Continued

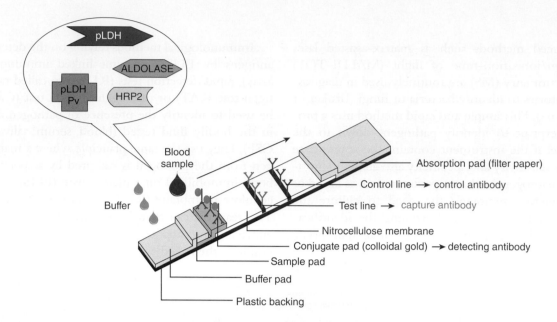

FIGURE 3.21 (cont'd) Schematic drawing of a malaria rapid diagnostic test (b). Blood and buffer are applied, respectively, to the sample and buffer pad. The content migrates via capillary action through the pad where it first encounters the conjugate pad, which contains a detection antibody against a Plasmodium antigen, such as PfHRP2, Pf-pLDH, Pv-pLDH, pan-pLDH or aldolase. This detection antibody is a mouse-antibody conjugated to colloidal gold. If present in the sample, the Plasmodium antigen is bound to this detection antibody-conjugate. Next, the antigen-antibody-conjugate complex migrates further until it is bound to the capture antibody, which binds to another site of the Plasmodium target antigen. As the capture antibody is applied on a narrow section of the strip, the complex with the conjugated signal is concentrated and the colloidal gold becomes visible as a coloured line. The excess of detection antibody-conjugate that was not bound by the antigen and the capture antibody moves further until it is bound to an anti-mouse antibody (control antibody), thereby generating a control line *PfHRP2: Plasmodium falciparum* histidine-rich proteins 2; *Pv-pLDH:* P. vivax-specific parasite lactate dehydrogenase; *pan-pLDH:* pan-parasite lactate dehydrogenase
Source: Maltha, J., Gillet, P., & Jacobs, J. (2013). Malaria rapid diagnostic tests in travel medicine. Clinical Microbiology and Infection, 19(5), 408-415.

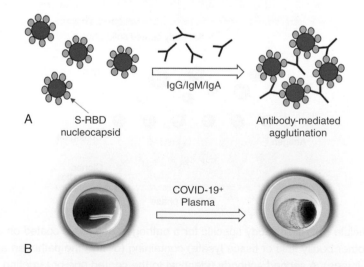

FIGURE 3.22 Illustration of the principle of agglutination assay for SARS-CoV-2 antibody testing. (A) Latex particles or red blood cells (RBCs) are coated on their surface with a SARS-CoV-2 antigen, S-RBD, or nucleocapsid. Incubation with plasma containing antibodies against the antigen will induce agglutination of the latex particles or RBCs. (B) Representative image of a positive agglutination assay using latex beads coated with S-RBD
S-RBD: SARS-CoV-2 receptor binding domain
Source: Esmail, S., Knauer, M. J., Abdoh, H., Voss, C., Chin-Yee, B., Stogios, P., ... & Li, S. S. C. (2021). Rapid and accurate agglutination-based testing for SARS-CoV-2 antibodies. Cell reports methods, 1(2), 100011.

widely employed in epidemiology where they can be used for high throughput testing of samples, while RDTs are useful for suggestive diagnostic criteria giving rapid results (usually 15–30 min). Due to their capacity to give false positives or negatives in a minority of cases, they usually need verification by qPCR. The COVID-19 pandemic has seen the use of RDTs increase significantly to allow the general public to punctually self-test, or to perform large screening of populations as seen prior to HSC exams in Australia. RDTs also exist for malaria where they can detect antigens common to all *Plasmodium* species or specific to either *P. falciparum* or *P. vivax*. CAT is often used in low-income countries to perform mass screening of populations for trypanosomiasis, for instance. However, agglutination tests are widely used in microbiology to discriminate between different pathogens to discriminate between pathogens of the same genus (beta-haemolytic *Streptococci* via Lancefield grouping, *Staphylococci* via coagulase test), to determine the serotype of pathogens (*Staphyloccoci*, *Salmonella*) or to identify a pathogen within a CSF among the main causative agents of meningitis (CSF test).

As mentioned above, accurate pathogen identification and disease diagnosis will inform the appropriate treatment; however, another parameter needs to be entered into the equation due to antimicrobial resistance (AMR): antimicrobial susceptibility. This often requires culturing the pathogen and can be performed manually using techniques such as the EUCAST (European Committee for Antimicrobial Susceptibility Testing) method that is widely used in Australia. These methods are time consuming, detect sensitivity to selected antimicrobials and cannot identify all resistant strains. Instruments such as the VITEK 2 (Biomerieux) combines high throughput identification and antimicrobial sensitivity testing. The system records simultaneously fluorescence, turbidity and colorimetric signals and can provide minimum inhibitory concentrations (MICs) for all antibiotics tested. A possible future alternative is next generation sequencing (NGS) such as Illumina, PacBio and Nanopore sequencing technologies that are fast becoming cheap.[10] These allow samples to be whole genome sequenced and the sequence interrogated for pathogens and any AMR genes they harbour using bioinformatics (the science of analysing complex biological data such as nucleic acid sequences). Importantly, the presence of an antimicrobial resistance gene does not tell you anything about the MIC like culture-based methods possibly excluding an antimicrobial that may be effective.

Beyond AMR, NGS techniques are becoming highly valuable in investigating infectious disease outbreaks. Comparison of pathogen genomes is highly useful in identifying possible sources and reservoirs. Tied with databases comprising of clinical and environmental samples from around the globe, the movement of pathogens and specific genetic elements (e.g. plasmids) can be tracked. During the COVID-19 outbreak, genome sequences identified multiple variants and was useful in tracking their movement. At a fine scale, genome sequencing could be used to determine if a viral infection was locally acquired or acquired from another geographic area, thus helping to identify transmissive pathways (e.g. leaks from quarantine facilities).

3.8 Therapies for pathogens

By and large, the bulk of therapies for pathogens are antimicrobial chemotherapeutics that target the pathogen; drugs that target toxins produced by the pathogen; or drugs that modify the immune response the pathogen elicits. Where there are no chemotherapeutics, symptom management is used.

3.8.1 Antimicrobial chemotherapeutics

Simply, these are chemicals used in medicine to kill or inhibit the growth of pathogens. Antimicrobials can be subdivided into categories depending on the microorganism/virus they are active against, such as antibacterials, antivirals, antifungals or antiprotozoals. Often, the term 'antibiotic' is used which, historically, is defined as a chemical produced by a microorganism to kill or inhibit the growth of another microorganism and which, in nature, is used by microorganisms to outcompete each other. For the most part, antimicrobial chemotherapeutics are antibiotics and have simply been repurposed for medical therapy. These chemicals have been chemically modified to create newer antibiotics (semi-synthetic antibiotics) that have altered characteristics allowing oral administration, broadening their spectrum of activity or to overcome resistance. It is important to note that as most antibiotics are antibacterial, the term 'antibiotic' has become synonymous with 'antibacterial'.

Key to the success of chemotherapeutic antimicrobials is selective toxicity, an important feature that requires the drug to selectively kill or inhibit the pathogen at a concentration that does not adversely affect host cells. Additionally, the drug must be capable of reaching a concentration at the site of infection that will have activity. Antimicrobials can be delivered topically, orally or intravenously. Topical or oral delivery are ideal as they can be self-administered by the patient; however, some antimicrobials cannot be delivered in this manner for reasons such as being destroyed by the acidic pH of the stomach or not reaching the desired concentration at the site of infection and these therefore require intravenous delivery. Some antimicrobial drugs are narrow spectrum, meaning they only attack certain microorganisms, whereas broad spectrum drugs will attack a wider range. Generally, narrow spectrum drugs are less likely to drive antimicrobial resistance due to the lesser selection pressure they impose.

A greater range of antibacterial chemotherapeutics exist than antifungals, antiprotozoals and antivirals, arguably due to the number of sites that are distinct between bacterial and eukaryotic host cells. As fungi and protozoa are eukaryotic, identifying drug targets that are non-toxic to host cells is more challenging, particularly for systemic infections. Superficial mycoses are easier to treat using topical treatments. Being intracellular obligate pathogens, viruses use host cell machinery for viral replication and so antivirals tend to target specific nucleic acid viral replicative enzymes or other processes unique to the viral life cycle, such as blocking adhesion or entry into the host cell or blocking uncoating. In bacteria, antibacterial chemotherapeutics target five main mechanisms: peptidoglycan cell wall synthesis; protein synthesis; nucleic acid synthesis; function of the cell membrane; and metabolic pathways. Bacterial resistance to these drugs is from one or more of the following mechanisms: reduced permeability to the drug; drug inactivation; alteration of drug target; modification of a metabolic pathway; or effective efflux of the drug.

3.8.2 Bacteriophage therapy

Bacteriophage therapy uses viruses that infect bacteria (called bacteriophage) to treat infection. Although bacteriophage therapy is not new, it has only recently been welcomed into Western medicine due to rising rates of antimicrobial resistance.[11] The therapy relies on cultivating and purifying bacteriophages that are active against a bacterial pathogen and administering it to an infected patient. They have the benefit of multiplying as they infect and kill their target, thus not requiring as many doses as antibacterials and, as they are very specific to their target bacteria, they do not disrupt the host microbiome. The disadvantage of this specificity is that it is difficult to isolate single bacteriophage that are active against all strains of a pathogen. Additionally, resistance to the bacteriophage can develop. As a result, multiple bacteriophages are usually delivered to minimise the likelihood of resistance developing and to cover a variety of pathogenic strains.

3.8.3 Monoclonal antibody (MAb) therapy

Monoclonal antibody (MAb) therapy potential has been studied for many years and is increasingly promising for treatment of infectious diseases. Several of these MAbs are currently in clinical trials or approved, notably to target bacterial toxins such as the bezlotoxumab for *C. difficile* TcdB or MEDI4893 to neutralise the haemolysin of *Staphylococcus aureus* and prevent invasion. More work is underway to produce MAbs against outer membrane surface proteins notably involved in bacterial adhesion or immune evasion or against polysaccharides. In 2020, approval was given by the US Food and Drug Administration for a co-administration of casirivimab and imdevimab (Regen-Cov) to treat mild to moderate COVID-19 in adults and paediatric patients. In August 2021, the Australian Therapeutic Goods Administration (TGA) granted provisional approval for the use of sotrovimab that was shown to reduce the risks of COVID-19 disease progression.

3.8.4 Other therapies

In some instances, tissue injury and disease may be caused both by the host response to the microbe and the infectious agent itself. Therefore, eliminating the pathogen is important but limiting or controlling the host response is also primordial. To that effect, adjunctive therapies are administered at the same time as the antimicrobial treatment. For instance, during a septic shock, treatment is given to maintain blood pressure and during meningitis corticosteroids can be administered to prevent excessive brain oedema. In cases of diphtheria or tetanus, anti-toxins are used to block the deleterious effects of the toxins produced by the bacteria.

Useful websites/resources

- Pathology Tests. The Royal College of Pathologists. https://www.rcpa.edu.au/Manuals/RCPA-Manual/
- Pathology-Tests Test Reference Manual. QML Pathology. https://www.qml.com.au/clinicians/testreference-manual/
- The Australian Society of Microbiology. https://www.theasm.org.au/
- The Australian Virology Society. https://www.avs.org.au/

References

1. Duke DLM, Prictor M, Ekinci E, Hachem M, Burchill LJ. Culturally adaptive governance—building a new framework for equity in Aboriginal and Torres Strait Islander health research: theoretical basis, ethics, attributes and evaluation. Int J Environ Res Public Health. 2021;18(15): 7943.

2. Partridge S, Kwong SRM, Firth N, Jensen SO. Mobile genetic elements associated with antimicrobial resistance. Clin Microbiol Rev. 2018;31(4):e00088-17.

3. Leimbach A, Hacker J, Dobrindt U. E. coli as an all-rounder: the thin line between commensalism and pathogenicity. In Dobrindt U, Hacker J, Svanborg C, eds. Between pathogenicity and commensalism. Current topics in microbiology and immunology. Berlin, Heidelberg; Springer, 2013.

4. Iredell J, Brown J, Tagg K. Antibiotic resistance in Enterobacteriaceae: mechanisms and clinical implications. BMJ. 2016;352:h6420.

5. Gomaa EZ. Human gut microbiota/microbiome in health and diseases: a review. Antonie van Leeuwenhoek, 2020; 113(12):2019-2040.

6. Venneti S. Prion diseases. Clin Lab Med. 2010;30(1): 293-309.

7. Arciola CR, Campoccia D, Montanaro L. Implant infections: adhesion, biofilm formation and immune evasion. Nat RevMicrobiol. 2018;16(7):397-409.

8. Gorrie CL, Mirčeta M, Wick RR, Edwards DJ, Thomson NR, Strugnell RA, et al. Gastrointestinal carriage is a major reservoir of Klebsiella pneumoniae infection in intensive care patients. Clin Infect Dis. 2017; 15;65(2):208-215.

9. Agarwal A, Hassanandani T, Das A, Panda M, Chakravorty S. 'Mask tinea': tinea faciei possibly potentiated by prolonged mask usage during the COVID-19 pandemic. Clin Exp Dermatol. 2021;46(1):190-193.

10. Gu W, Miller S, Chiu CY. Clinical metagenomic next-generation sequencing for pathogen detection. Ann Rev Pathol: Mechanisms of Disease. 2019;14:319-338.

11. Kortright KE, Chan BK, Koff JL, Turner PE. Phage therapy: a renewed approach to combat antibiotic-resistant bacteria. Cell Host Microbe. 2019;25(2):219-232.

CHAPTER 4

Infection prevention and control programs and plans

PROFESSOR RAMON Z. SHABAN[i-iv]

Dr DEBOROUGH MACBETH[v]

Dr CATHERINE VIENGKHAM[i]

Chapter highlights

- The formally documented and sanctioned infection prevention and control (IPC) programs and plans that are essential to the prevention and control of HAIs in Australia
- The characteristics and contexts of IPC programs and plans across different levels of the Australian governments, including current differences between states and territories
- Challenges regarding IPC programs and plans in Australia

i   Susan Wakil School of Nursing and Midwifery, Faculty of Medicine and Health, University of Sydney, Sydney, NSW

ii Sydney Infectious Diseases Institute, Faculty of Medicine and Health, University of Sydney, Sydney, NSW

iii Public Health Unit, Centre for Population Health, Western Sydney Local Health District, Westmead, NSW

iv New South Wales Biocontainment Centre, Western Sydney Local Health District, Westmead, NSW

v   Gold Coast Hospital and Health Service, Southport, QLD

Introduction

The successful implementation and regular evaluation of infection prevention and control (IPC) programs and plans is critical to preventing healthcare-associated infections (HAIs) and controlling the spread of communicable diseases within healthcare facilities. This chapter provides an overview of how these plans are developed and implemented across the different levels of the Australian government. Effective infection prevention guidelines and strategies for the control and prevention of HAIs are required for all health contexts and settings, from large hospitals to independent home and practice settings. Every facility will require programs and procedures that are tailored to accommodate their size and function, but the core infection prevention principles remain the same across all healthcare settings.

4.1 Infection prevention, control and management

4.1.1 Infection prevention and control (IPC) programs

Infection prevention and control programs are formal and coordinated structures and processes that aim to prevent and contain the transmission of infection and infectious diseases using evidence-based and evaluated infection prevention and control strategies. In any healthcare setting, ranging from small home practices to large, multi-storey hospital complexes, IPC programs are an essential component of providing safe and high-quality healthcare services. The development and implementation of IPC programs has grown exponentially, catalysed by the vast improvements in the understanding of infections and infectious disease transmission at the turn of the 20th century. Hand hygiene is one of the oldest methods of infection prevention and, to this day, is still a critical practice that is rigorously taught and monitored for effective implementation and compliance across all healthcare settings. Presently, IPC programs continue to evolve with continued progress in research and in adaptation to new issues, such as antibiotic-resistant microorganisms.

Programs are typically developed by individual healthcare facilities and incorporate different IPC principles and strategies specific to their healthcare context and requirements, as mandated by their jurisdictions (if any). That said, a successful IPC program should include all six of the following elements (see Fig 4.1):

1. surveillance

2. quality improvement, monitoring and review

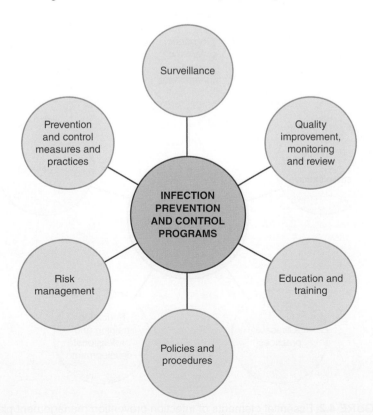

FIGURE 4.1   Essential elements of infection prevention and control programs

3. education and training

4. policies and procedures

5. risk management

6. prevention and control measures and practices.

4.1.2 Infection control management plans (ICMP)

An infection control management plan is a formal set of procedures and protocols that guide the actions of healthcare workers and facilities at the local level in the prevention, reduction and control of HAIs and communicable diseases. They are in place to ensure the provision of safe and high-quality healthcare and, importantly, they should be formally documented by the facility providing the health service, and regulated and evaluated by a governing body. For example, in Queensland, the ICMP for each healthcare facility is approved by the Communicable Diseases Branch on behalf of the Chief Health Officer. The plan ensures that institutions are held accountable and that they can meet their IPC obligations. Furthermore, the ICMP must also take into consideration the overall strategic plan of the organisation and the context of the facility,

factoring in characteristics such as the demographics of the population served by the facility, the epidemiology of infection, the availability of resources and the interests of key stakeholders.

Effective ICMPs rely on five key elements (Fig 4.2). These are:

1. corporate governance and management

2. consultancy

3. education, training and professional development

4. clinical practices

5. research and surveillance.

Strong management and leadership are critical to ensure stakeholder buy-in. The ICMP is typically helmed by a dedicated Infection Control Committee (ICC) which is responsible for setting short- and long-term objectives, as well as developing the appropriate performance measures and evaluative processes for demonstrating the effectiveness of ICMPs in terms of cost and service benefits. Consultancy with ICP experts is essential to address any gaps in the knowledge of the local managing party. This allows governing bodies to resolve issues and develop solutions based on the most up-to-date and rigorously tested evidence. Most states and

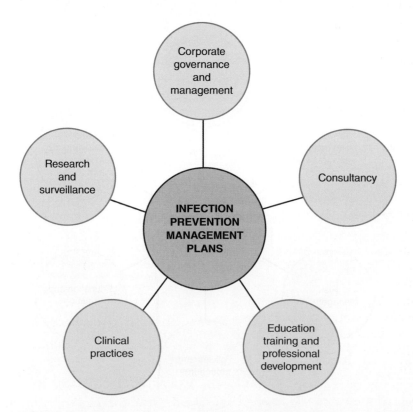

FIGURE 4.2 Essential elements of infection prevention management plans

territories in Australia require the appointment of either an IPC professional or a multidisciplinary committee that can coordinate and monitor local IPC activities, as well as to report and make actionable recommendations based on the outcome of these activities to a higher managing board.

Surveillance involves the ongoing collection, analysis and interpretation of data on incidents related to infections and HAIs. Plans must include establishing systems of surveillance for such issues as HAIs, multidrug-resistant strains of microorganisms and notifiable diseases, occupational body fluid exposures and other environmental issues, such as water quality management. Surveillance aids in the early detection of infection, which is crucial for swift intervention and the prevention of further spread. However, ongoing surveillance is also critical to monitor infection trends and for research initiatives, serving to provide benchmarks to monitor and evaluate the effectiveness of interventions and, subsequently, to aid the development of new ones. Furthermore, monitoring the uptake, understanding and correcting the performance of IPC interventions by healthcare workers is essential for the process of review and improvement in the quality of healthcare services provided.

Infection control management plans must ensure that effective and practical education, training and professional development opportunities are available and readily accessible to all staff. The distribution of information regarding policies, procedures and actions must be thoroughly documented and proofed for cohesiveness and consistency. Interventions should be easy for workers to adopt and integrate into their regular routines, and have objective measures of compliance and effectiveness so they can be efficiently evaluated and audited. Ideally, these procedures should be made available in multiple formats and modalities (e.g. print, online, signage and seminars) and with multiple ways to access them, to ensure workers are able to locate them in any situation. Furthermore, systems must be in place to monitor completion of training by staff, with regular checks to ensure that competency is maintained. Education and training inform clinical practice, and shape the core activities that ensure the minimisation of all infection risks. These include requirements for standard and transmission-based precautions, such as: hand hygiene; environmental and equipment sanitation; protocols for the correct donning and doffing of personal protective equipment; appropriate sharps safety and waste disposal; aseptic technique; and antimicrobial stewardship.

4.2 Commonwealth IPC programs and plans

In Australia, although formally documented IPC programs and plans are a relatively new endeavour, they have been operating in some form or capacity in hospitals since the 1960s. More formal and nationally coordinated approaches, including accreditation programs, did not begin until 1974 when the Australian Council on Healthcare Standards (ACHS) required hospitals to appoint an infection control nurse and establish an infection surveillance and control program. The ACHS later published *Fundamentals for Infection Control Services*, in 2001, which provided national recommendations for activities and strategies for hospitals to incorporate into their IPC programs.

In 2006, the Australian Commission on Safety and Quality in Health Care (ACSQHC) was officially formed for the purposes of developing a national approach to improving the safety and quality of healthcare. This led to the release of the first edition of the National Safety and Quality Health Service (NSQHS) Standards ('the Standards'), against which the assessment of health service organisations officially began in 2013.[1] The second edition of the Standards was released in 2017 and used in formal assessment in 2019. This edition later received an update in 2021 to include lessons learnt from the SARS-CoV-2 (COVID-19) response and remains the most recent version of the Standards at time of writing.[2] The Standards were developed in collaboration with the Australian Government, states and territories, private sector providers, clinical experts, patients and carers. The current publication is comprised of eight standards that together aim to 'protect the public from harm and to improve the quality of health service provision'. Among these is the Preventing and Controlling Infections Standard, which is driven by four criteria:

1. clinical governance and quality improvement systems to prevent and control infections and support antimicrobial stewardship and the sustainable use of IPC resources
2. infection prevention and control systems
3. reprocessing reusable equipment and devices
4. antimicrobial stewardship.

Each criterion is further described in Table 4.1. The Australian Guidelines for the Prevention and Control of Infection in Healthcare[3] ('the Guidelines') was co-funded by the ACSQHC and the National Health and

TABLE 4.1 Criteria of the NSQHS Preventing and Controlling Infections Standard

1) Clinical governance and quality improvement systems	This criterion requires systems to be in place that: • establish multidisciplinary teams for the identification and management of risks pertaining to infections using the hierarchy of controls and IPC systems, as well as the promotion of antimicrobial stewardship • ensure the workforce has access to training and the necessary skills and resources to implement IPC systems and antimicrobial stewardship • monitor and implement strategies to improve and report on the performance of IPC systems and antimicrobial stewardship to all relevant groups • collect, monitor and report surveillance data pertaining to infections and antimicrobial use to all relevant groups • support and monitor the safe and sustainable use of IPC resources • plan for public health and pandemic risks • ensure all the above are performed in line with the Clinical Governance Standard and Partnering with Consumers Standard (when actively involved with patients and sharing information).
2) Infection prevention and control systems	The health service organisation has processes (i.e. training, testing, monitoring, auditing, improving) to apply: • standard and transmission-based precautions • hand hygiene • aseptic technique • invasive medical devices • clean and safe environment • workforce screening and immunisation • infection control in the workforce.
3) Reprocessing of reusable equipment and devices	When reusable equipment and devices are used, the health service organisation has: • processes for reprocessing that are consistent with relevant standards and manufacturers' guidelines • a traceability process that can identify the patient, the procedure and the equipment, instruments and devices that were used • processes to plan and manage reprocessing requirements • controls for novel and emerging infections.
4) Antimicrobial stewardship	The health service organisation has an antimicrobial stewardship program that: • includes an antimicrobial policy • provides access to, and has antimicrobial formulary that is informed by the most current evidence-based Australian therapeutic guidelines and resources • reviews and reports antimicrobial prescription and use based on surveillance data and audits, and uses this to inform and improve future antimicrobial programs.

Source: Adapted from https://www.safetyandquality.gov.au/publications-and-resources/resource-library/nsqhs-standards-2021-preventing-and-controlling-infections-standard

Medical Research Council (NHMRC) and released in 2019. The Guidelines are directly referenced and linked by the Standards and serve as a national foundation for healthcare to develop comprehensive IPC procedures and protocols they can adapt to their local contexts.

In Australia, all public and private hospitals, day procedure services and most public dental practices must be accredited (see Chapter 12). The Commission coordinates national accreditation processes via the Australian Health Service Safety and Quality Accreditation (AHSSQA) Scheme. Healthcare organisations are assessed by external agencies (approved by the ACSQHC)

to show they meet the requirements of the NSQHS Standards. Healthcare organisations that fail to meet the Standards and are unable to demonstrate improvements within 60 business days will have various sanctions applied, such as loss of licence and funding.

4.3 State and territory IPC programs and plans

While both the NSQHS Standards and the Guidelines are nationally formulated initiatives, the implementation and enforcement of the Standards is conducted at state and territory levels—more specifically, overseeing the accreditation scheme content, receiving relevant accreditation data and escalating responses where the NSQHS Standards are not met is the responsibility of state and territory governments. Ultimately, it is these governments, and the active legislation within each jurisdiction, that decide which healthcare services and organisations need to be assessed against the Standards.

While the Standards and Guidelines provide a broad foundation for ICMPs, states and territories must ensure they are appropriately adapted to the healthcare landscape of their jurisdiction and that appropriate state-level legislation and infrastructure are in place to enforce and regulate these plans. Moreover, healthcare facilities must be aware that statutory requirements of the jurisdiction take precedence when differences exist (unless otherwise stated). State and territory governments also provide a range of resources and support materials to healthcare facilities and services, many of which are localised versions of national Guidelines. Furthermore, they are responsible for providing policy and good practice guidance to health services and for maintaining a state-wide perspective to ensure an equitable distribution of resources.

Additionally, healthcare services are now extending beyond hospitals and into community contexts, such as smaller, office-based practices. The risks of HAIs do not attenuate in these settings, as many practices still involve some degree of skin penetration, invasive procedures or the exchange of bodily fluids. In these contexts, the implementation of effective IPC programs remains just as critical. The Commission's Standards and Guidelines were primarily developed for hospital-based healthcare services, and the accreditation of hospitals, with specific caveats made for day procedure services and public dental practices. However, the national Standards do not automatically extend towards non-hospital-based health services, and the responsibility of assuring the adequate implementation of IPC systems in these settings is determined by state and territory legislation.

4.3.1 Comparison of ICMP requirements across Australian states and territories

The requirement and regulation of IPC plans across different healthcare settings varies between jurisdictions and some states have additional IPC policies that operate simultaneously with the national accreditation Standards. Table 4.2 provides a state-by-state comparison of the bodies that oversee hospital accreditation;

whether independent IPC plans or policies are active; whether these plans explicitly extend beyond hospital contexts; and whether any active legislation exists to enforce the plans and the regulating bodies.

Queensland: In Queensland it is required by law that 'declared health services' have an ICMP. This requirement is enforced under the *Public Health Act 2005* (Qld)[4] and establishes the precedent for corrective actions and penalties to be applied in response to inadequate or unsafe infection control practices by healthcare professionals. The Act specifically defines declared health services as 'intended to maintain, improve or restore the person's health; and ... involves the performance of an invasive procedure or an activity that exposes the person ... to blood or another bodily fluid'.[4] These include, but are not limited to, public sector hospitals, medical practices, dental practices, acupuncture clinics, midwifery services and blood banks, and includes mobile premises associated with the facility, such as ambulances, as well as home-based services and services supporting the healthcare facility, like laundry and cleaning. ICMP templates are provided for both hospital and non-hospital settings. Exemptions to this law include general practices (which are already accredited against the Standard for General Practice), local government-owned healthcare facilities that perform immunisation services, private health facilities (which are separately regulated by the *Private Health Facilities Act 1999*)[5] and aged care services.

The act defines an ICMP for a healthcare facility as a 'documented plan to prevent or minimise the risk of infection, in relation to a declared health service'. Furthermore, the developed ICMP is required to state:
- the infection risks associated with the health service
- the measures taken to prevent or minimise infection risks
- the process for monitoring and reviewing the implementation and effectiveness of measures
- the provision of training in relation to the ICMP for employees or engaged persons
- how often the ICMP is reviewed; and
- the name of any person responsible for providing advice about and monitoring the effectiveness of the ICMP.

Additionally, the facility must ensure that the ICMP is easily understood and accessed by relevant personnel and that it is reviewed and amended regularly to

TABLE 4.2 State and territory infection control management plans and associated legislation

State	NSQHS Standards Accreditation Body	ICMP	ICMP Title	Non-hospital settings?	Required by law?	Acting Legislation	Governing Body
ACT	Health Protection Service (all)	Yes	Public Health (Health Care Facility) Code of Practice 2021 (No 1)[14]	Yes	Yes	Public Health Act 1997 (ACT)[15]	Minister for Health
NSW	Clinical Excellence Commission (public, DPS, DS), Private Health Care Unit (private)	Yes	Infection Prevention and Control Policy[6]	No	Yes	Health Services Act 1997,[7] Private Health Facilities Regulation 2017,[8] Health Practitioner Regulation National Law Act (NSW) No 86[18]	NSW Ministry of Health
NT	Department of Health (all)	No	–	–	–	–	–
QLD	Patient Safety and Quality Improvement Service (public, DPS), Private Health Regulation (private, DPS)	Yes	Infection Control Management Plan[4,19]	Yes	Yes	Public Health Act 2005 (Qld),[4] Public Health Regulations 2018[20]	Chief Health Officer, Communicable Diseases Branch
SA	Safety and Quality (public, DPS, DS), Health Licensing Unit (private, DPS)	Yes	Healthcare Associated Infection Prevention Policy Directive[10,11]	No	Yes	South Australian Public Health Act 2011,[21] Health Care Act 2008[22]	Chief Executive of Department of Health and Wellbeing
TAS	Department of Health Regulation (all)	Yes*	–	–	–	Health Service Establishments Regulations 2021[23]	Tasmanian Department of Health
VIC	Commissioning, Performance and Regulation (public), Dental Health Services (DS), Private Hospitals, Health Service Performance and Programs (private, DPS)	Yes*	–	–	–	Health Services (Health Service Establishments) Regulations 2013[24]	Chief Quality and Safety Officer
WA	Licensing and Accreditation Regulatory Unit (all)	No	–	–	–	–	–

*For day procedure services and private hospitals; DPS: day procedure services; DS: dental services; PHO: public health organisation; LHN: local health network.

accommodate newly identified risks and prior to providing new health services.

Compliance is monitored by the Communicable Diseases Branch on behalf of the Chief Health Officer of Queensland which has the power to report contraventions to a relevant entity, such as a health ombudsman, a board established under the Health Practitioner Regulation National Law ('the National Law') or another entity that has the power under state or Commonwealth legislation.

New South Wales and South Australia: Both New South Wales (NSW) and South Australia (SA) operate similar policy directives that specifically mandate the development and implementation of IPC programs in the states' healthcare facilities. In both states, the operation and evaluation of the programs is overseen by the chief executive of each local health district or network and apply to both acute and non-acute healthcare services. Health organisations in NSW are required to comply with the Infection Prevention and Control Policy.[6] This is a policy directive that outlines the mandatory IPC requirements for NSW Public Health Organisations (PHOs) and is enforced under the *Health Services Act 1997*.[7] Additional requirements for written ICMPs for private health facilities are enforced under the Private Health Facilities Regulation 2017.[8]

In NSW, PHOs encompass local health districts, statutory health corporations and affiliated health organisations. The policy operates in tandem with the *NSW Infection Prevention and Control Practice Handbook* and closely complements the actions set out in the NSQHS Standards.[9] Each NSW PHO is required to appoint an executive 'at the highest level within the organisation' that is responsible for leading the infection control program and reporting to the highest management level within the organisation. Specifically, PHOs in NSW are responsible for:

* assigning leadership, personnel and resources to implement and comply with the policy
* working with the directors of clinical governance, as well as clinical and senior leaders, to ensure that the policy is clearly communicated to managers and healthcare workers
* ensuring that systems to implement and evaluate infection prevention and control programs are in place; and
* seeking additional advice, where knowledge is limited, from experts or an ICC.

Overall, the policy requires the development of a risk management framework or risk plan which specifies the protocols for improving and measuring the performance of tools and strategies for HAI prevention and risk management. This risk plan must be reviewed and endorsed by the PHO's ICC and incorporated in the broader plans of the organisation. Furthermore, the policy briefly outlines the minimal training and education requirements for healthcare workers pertaining to HAIs, risk identification and risk mitigation requirements, including the thorough adoption and compliance with standard and transmission-based precautions. Additional requirements outlined in the policy include strategies for the prevention and management of HAI caused by multidrug-resistant organisms and communicable diseases, quality monitoring and surveillance, outbreaks, and the handling of animals as patients.

Similarly, SA has the Healthcare Associated Infection Policy Directive,[10,11] to which SA Health employees, or persons who provide health services on behalf of SA Health, must adhere. These directives complement the objectives of the SA Health and Wellbeing Strategy 2020–2025.[12] Furthermore, SA Health has developed a number of resources, including a suite of audit tools, to assist healthcare facilities to comply with Standard 3.[13] The primary roles and responsibilities in the policy are distributed between the CE and the local health network (LHN) governing boards. The CE must ensure that all healthcare facilities have an active IPC program and that all healthcare staff have access to the relevant SA Health policies and procedures. A checklist for HAI management plans for both acute and non-acute health services is provided in the appendices of the policy directive.

Australian Capital Territory: In the Australian Capital Territory (ACT), healthcare facilities are required to implement and maintain an ICMP under the Health Care Facility Code of Practice 2021,[14] which is enforced by the *Public Health Act 1997*.[15] Specifications pertaining to the ICMP are described under Standard 3 – Infection Control within the Code of Practice, including the required appointment of qualified IPC staff to coordinate the plan. The Standard provides a list of factors to be considered for inclusion in the ICMP including, but not limited to, surveillance, standard and transmission-based precautions, environmental risks, equipment processing, personal protective equipment, quality management and pest control. Under the Code of Practice, the ICMP must be made available for inspection and revision at the request of an authorised public health officer and the Minister for Health. Adherence to the Code of Practice and its Standards is required for the licensing of all hospitals and day procedure centres.

The ACT also provides separate infection prevention and control policies for community-based healthcare services that involve any skin penetration procedures—defined as 'any process involving the piercing, cutting, puncturing or tearing of a living human body but do not include the cutting, shaving or dyeing of a person's hair, or closed ear piercing or the use of test equipment'.[16] The ACT Health Infection Control for office practices and other community based services Code of Practice 2005[17] ('the Code') is enforced under the *Public Health Act 1997* (ACT)[15] for the purpose of 'minimising the risk of transmission of blood borne and other infections associated with skin penetration and other infection risk procedures'. The Code covers health services such as dental practices, diagnostic clinics, pharmacies and acupuncture clinics, as well as personal services, such as beauty therapists, tattoo studios, piercing businesses and mobile practitioners.

4.4 Developing an infection control management plan

The primary goal of an infection control management plan (ICMP) is to:
* take a systematic approach to identifying all the possible infection risks associated with the provision of the health service;
* develop a range of strategies to mitigate each of those risks; and
* develop mechanisms to evaluate the effectiveness of the risk mitigation strategies.

There is no universal structure or process for the development of an ICMP. Whatever the format, all ICMPs share common goals. They must:

1. identify the context in which the care is provided. This must be detailed and include the health status and challenges of patients and residents, case mix, staffing profile and other matters including the built environment

2. identify the HAI and communicable diseases risks of the setting that are largely foreseeable and preventable. Both active and passive surveillance systems to identify emerging HAI and communicable diseases threats must be included

3. identify the interventions used to identify, prevent, control and mitigate the risk of HAI and communicable diseases, and in doing so, clearly specify the delegates and teams that are responsible

4. document how these interventions are monitored and evaluated, and importantly the frequency and veracity of the systematic review and feedback mechanisms.

In doing so, ICMPs address the series of questions listed in Box 4.1.

Responsibility for the development of an ICMP usually falls to the ICP in the first instance. The draft plan is then presented to a range of stakeholders, representing the entire health service. This should be achieved by having the ICC, or equivalent, review and ratify the plan if the committee is truly representative of the organisation. Finally, the ratified plan should be

---

BOX 4.1 Infection control management plan (ICMP): development guiding questions

* What are the contextual characteristics of the setting that the ICMP applies to?
* Who is responsible for infection prevention and control (IPC) and antimicrobial stewardship (AMS)?
* What are the organisation's infection and AMS risks?
* How are each of these risks mitigated?
* Who will decide on the appropriateness of the mitigation strategies?
* How will mitigation strategies be implemented?
* How will mitigation strategies be communicated to all staff?
* How will the success of the mitigation strategies be measured?
* What does success look like?
* How will members of the organisation know their role and responsibility?
* How will new risks be identified?
* Do all the risks identified apply to all areas within the organisation? If not, how will inclusion or exclusion of services be determined and documented in the ICMP?
* How often will the ICMP be reviewed, by whom, and against what criteria?

endorsed by the highest level of governance in the organisation, such as the chief executive who is ultimately responsible for the safety of the organisation. Involvement of the chief executive also helps to ensure the allocation of the resources necessary to implement the program.

There are a range of possible structures for an ICMP. One method is to use the elements of the Preventing and Controlling Healthcare-associated Infection Standard within the NSQHS Standards. An example is provided in Table 4.3.

Each element of the ICMP should be assessed in terms of a risk rating based on whether the risk has been mitigated (low risk), partially mitigated (medium risk) or is unmitigated (high risk). The element should also be considered with respect to the service to which it applies. In a large organisation, there may be a combination of acute facilities (hospitals), community-based facilities, long-term care facilities or home-based services. Links to supplementary material, such as policy or procedure documents, training materials, reports or surveillance plans, can be included in the ICMP. The benefit of using NSQHS Preventing and Controlling Infections Standard as the framework for the ICMP is that it also serves to collect the evidence required when the surveyors assess the organisation for accreditation. The plan must specify an implementation date, a date for review, and the consultation, review and approval processes and

TABLE 4.3 Governance element of an ICMP using the NSQHS Standards

Category:	Governance
Criteria:	Integrating clinical governance
Prescribed actions. 3.01 The workforce uses the safety and quality systems from the Clinical Governance Standard when:	a) implementing policies and procedures for healthcare-associated infections (HAI) and antimicrobial stewardship (AMS) b) identifying and managing risks associated with infection c) implementing policies and procedures for AMS d) identifying and managing antimicrobial stewardship risks.
Summary of evidence:	a) New or revised state-wide policies, standards and protocols are brought to the attention of the Infection Control Committee (ICC) to undertake an organisational impact analysis prior to implementation. There is a local process in place for rescinding and unpublishing superseded documents. All infection control procedures include an audit strategy and audit results demonstrate the procedure is followed (e.g. environmental audit reports, hand hygiene audit reports, practice audits). Antimicrobial stewardship uses a similar approach with governance via the AMS Sub-committee. AMS Sub-committee procedures are audited using National Antimicrobial Prescribing Survey (NAPS) and AMS weekly unit audits. b) New or uncontrolled infection risks are identified through incident reports, surveillance activities (e.g. occupational body fluid exposure surveillance, surgical site surveillance, practice and environmental audits), pathology results (e.g. unusual pathogen) and notification through health departments, other national bodies and the World Health Organization. c) Antimicrobial prescribing and management procedure is available at (provide hyperlink to procedure). d) Antimicrobial stewardship risks are identified through the results of audit and benchmarking data and are managed using procedures, audit reports and feedback of results to prescribing clinicians.
Prescribed actions. 3.02 The health service organisation:	a) establishes multidisciplinary teams to identify and manage risks associated with infections using the hierarchy of controls in conjunction with IPC systems b) identifies requirements for, and provides the workforce with access to, training to prevent and control infections c) has processes to ensure that the workforce has the capacity, skills and access to equipment to implement systems to prevent and control infections d) establishes multidisciplinary teams, or processes, to promote effective antimicrobial stewardship e) identifies requirements for, and provides access to, training to support the workforce to conduct AMS activities f) has processes to ensure that the workforce has the capacity and skills to implement AMS g) has plans for public health and pandemic risks.

Continued

TABLE 4.3 Governance element of an ICMP using the NSQHS Standards—cont'd

Summary of evidence:	a) The ICC is a multidisciplinary team responsible for identifying and managing risks associated with infections using the hierarchy of controls in conjunction with IPC systems as outlined in this ICMP. Risk mitigation strategies are implemented for each infection risk identified. The effectiveness of the mitigation strategies is determined on the basis of a range of surveillance initiatives. b) Infection control training is considered essential for all new employees and is therefore included in orientation programs and via learning-on-line modules. Completion of an annual refresher provided online is required for clinical staff and support service staff. Training in aseptic technique is required for all clinical staff who insert, manage or access invasive devices or perform invasive procedures. Compliance with training requirements is monitored. c) Compliance monitoring regarding IPC procedures is undertaken through audits (hand hygiene, practice and environmental) and review of incident reports pertaining to infection risks. The audits and reports identify any deficits in training, non-compliance and new risks for investigation and/or rectification. d) Multidisciplinary teams involving doctors and pharmacists perform consult and virtual rounds using the AMS Sub-committee dashboard. The AMS Sub-committee uses reports from the National Antimicrobial Prescribing Survey (NAPS), the National Antimicrobial Utilisation Surveillance Program (NAUSP) and local AMS key performance indicators (KPI) to monitor its effectiveness. Summary data is reported to the governance committee. e) The AMS Sub-committee provides constant training and supports to prescribers through mandatory induction training, support and education to prescribers, pharmacists and nurses and formal presentations. f) Access to the Therapeutic Guidelines, antimicrobial prescribing and management procedure (hyperlink) and antimicrobial formulary equip staff with skills to implement AMS. The AMS Sub-committee reports antibiograms, NAPS results and antibiotic use data to the Clinical Governance Committee. Antibiograms and NAPS results are published on the AMS Sub-committee website for all staff to view. g) The pandemic plan is reviewed every two years by the ICC and the Emergency Response Committee and amended as required.

Adapted from: https://www.safetyandquality.gov.au/publications-and-resources/resource-library/nsqhs-standards-2021-preventing-and-controlling-infections-standard

those involved. The plan could be developed by changing the questions in Box 4.1 into sub-headings within the plan and then providing the answers along with the supporting materials—reports, meeting minutes, training materials, surveillance plans—either as appendices or hyperlinks. Importantly, a clear governance pathway needs to be described, ensuring the overall responsibility for the ICMP rests with the highest level of governance within the organisation. A variety of historical templates is available to download via the Elsevier Companion Website Evolve®.

4.5 Challenges for infection prevention and control (IPC) programs

Most healthcare facilities and organisations that provide healthcare services will likely have an IPC program in place. However, the legislation attached to this obligation is still relatively underdeveloped in Australia and ICMP practices remain highly varied and inconsistent across Australian states and territories. The Standards introduced by the Commission in 2011 and the subsequent accreditation scheme were a considerable influence in facilitating a national approach to managing HAIs. While their adoption across all Australian states and territories is encouraging, their limited scope and primary application to public and private hospital settings ignores the extensive range of health services that are being provided in community and office-based practices. Some states (at time of writing Queensland and the ACT) have taken the initiative to ensure that these services have a legal duty to develop and maintain ICMPs. However, this requirement is not yet consistent across all of Australia.

Furthermore, the expanding contexts in which healthcare services are provided will continue to introduce new issues and unforeseen potential for HAIs. Different healthcare services and settings have vastly different risks, capabilities and resources. For example, community-based health services include the delivery of healthcare by nurses in home settings, which is highly advantageous for certain patient populations that are less mobile and where this provision of care is less disruptive to their regular routines. Infections and HAIs will remain a potent issue regardless of where healthcare services are provided and will only be exacerbated in such novel and unpredictable environments where the guidelines offered by current IPC standards are underdeveloped and limited. However, the diversification of care provision outside of hospital settings will continue to grow as the needs of the population shift and change. Legislation is slow to change; therefore, coordinated IPC programs and plans must be responsive and able to continue to adapt and evolve to address these changes in an ever-dynamic healthcare landscape.

Conclusion

Healthcare-associated infections will continue as long as health services are being provided. It is the responsibility of governing bodies across all levels of the Australian health system to ensure effective IPC programs and plans are in place to best minimise the incidence of HAIs and ensure that the safest and highest quality of care is provided to its patients. Accreditation via the NSQHS Standards holds health services accountable to their IPC obligations. While the Standards introduced a nationally consistent framework, current governance of this process and the extent to which the Standards are applied to non-hospital healthcare settings are dependent on state and territory laws. The practice of requiring all healthcare facilities to develop ICMPs has been introduced by some states, for example Queensland which, by law, also requires these plans to be regularly amended and formally approved by an acting authority. Infection prevention and control programs and plans are dynamic and will continue to evolve and develop in response to new research and best practice, as well as adapt to changes in the avenues in healthcare provision and health legislature across Australia.

Useful websites/resources

- Queensland Health. Infection control management plans. https://www.health.qld.gov.au/clinical-practice/guidelines-procedures/diseases-infection/infection-prevention/management-plans-guidance/icmp
- Australian Commission on Safety and Quality in Health Care. Infection prevention and control systems. https://www.safetyandquality.gov.au/standards/nsqhs-standards/preventing-and-controlling-healthcare-associated-infection-standard/infection-prevention-and-control-systems

References

1. Australian Commission on Safety and Quality in Health Care (ACSQHC). National safety and quality health service standards (NSQHS). 1st ed. Sydney: ACSQHC, 2011.
2. Australian Commission on Safety and Quality in Health Care (ACSQHC). National safety and quality health service standards (NSQHS). 2nd ed. Version 2. NSQHS. Sydney: ACSQHC, 2021.
3. National Health and Medical Research Council (NHMRC) and Australian Commission on Safety and Quality in Health Care (ACSQHC). Australian guidelines for the prevention and control of infection in healthcare. Canberra: NHMRC, ACSQHC, 2019.
4. Public Health Act 2005 (Qld).
5. Private Health Facilities Act 1999 (Qld).
6. Clinical Excellence Commission. Infection Prevention and Control Policy. Sydney: Clinical Excellence Commission, 2017.
7. Health Services Act 1997 No 154 (NSW).
8. Private Health Facilities Regulation 2017 (NSW).
9. Clinical Excellence Commission. Infection prevention and control practice handbook. Sydney: Clinical Excellence Commission, 2020.
10. Government of South Australia. Healthcare Associated Infection Prevention Policy Directive. Adelaide: SA Health, 2020.
11. Government of South Australia. Healthcare Associated Infection Surveillance Clinical Directive. Adelaide: SA Health, 2020.
12. Government of South Australia. South Australian Health and Wellbeing Strategy 2020-2025. Adelaide: SA Health, 2020.
13. Government of South Australia. Preventing and controlling healthcare associated infection: Audit Tools. Adelaide: SA Health, 2022.
14. Public Health (Health Care Facility) Code of Practice 2021 (No 1) (ACT).
15. Public Health Act 1997 (ACT).
16. ACT Government: ACT Health. Infection control Canberra: ACT Health, 2021 [cited 19 April 2022]. Available from: https://www.health.act.gov.au/businesses/infection-control.
17. Infection control for office practices and other community based services: Code of Practice 2005, (2005).
18. Health Practitioner Regulation National Law Act (NSW) No 86 (NSW).
19. Queensland Health. Infection control management plans Queensland: Queensland Health, 2019 [cited 2022 19 April]. Available from: https://www.health.qld.gov.au/clinical-practice/guidelines-procedures/diseases-infection/infection-prevention/management-plans-guidance/icmp.
20. Public Health Regulation 2018 (Qld).
21. South Australia Public Health Act 2011 (SA).
22. Health Care Act 2008 (SA).
23. Health Service Establishments Regulations 2021 (Tas).
24. Health Services (Health Service Establishments) Regulations 2013 (Vic).

CHAPTER 5

The role of the infection control professional

Dr DEBOROUGH MACBETH[i]

PROFESSOR RAMON Z. SHABAN[ii-v]

Chapter highlights

- A description of the evolution of the role of the infection control professional
- An overview of the knowledge, skills and attributes required for the contemporary role of infection control professional
- A set of case studies applying the principles described in the chapter on Evolve

i   Gold Coast Hospital and Health Service, Southport, QLD
ii Susan Wakil School of Nursing and Midwifery, Faculty of Medicine and Health, University of Sydney, Sydney, NSW
iii Sydney Infectious Diseases Institute, Faculty of Medicine and Health, University of Sydney, Sydney, NSW
iv Public Health Unit, Centre for Population Health, Western Sydney Local Health District, Westmead, NSW
v   New South Wales Biocontainment Centre, Western Sydney Local Health District, Westmead, NSW

Introduction

In the 1950s, hospitals in the United States, Europe and the United Kingdom experienced outbreaks of staphylococcal infection that led to renewed interest in infection control and the establishment of infection control programs. This also provided the impetus for establishing the role of the infection control professional (ICP).[1,2] Antibiotic resistance in microorganisms was recognised soon after the introduction of penicillin and the problem of antibiotic resistance continued to grow, compounding the risk of poor patient outcomes.[3] Infection control as a specialised nursing practice commenced in England in 1960 and the first infection control nurse (ICN) was appointed at Stanford University Hospital in the United States in 1963.[1] Simultaneously, the Centers for Disease Control and Prevention (CDC) in the United States began to recommend that healthcare facilities undertake nosocomial (hospital–acquired) infection surveillance, and to gather data as a basis for monitoring infection and implementing rational control measures. The original intention was that a physician with specialised training in hospital epidemiology should undertake the surveillance; however, by the 1970s the results of a number of studies demonstrated that a nurse with specialised infection control training would be more appropriate.[4]

In the same decade, concerns that competing fiscal priorities might bring an end to the fledgling specialty led the CDC to initiate a study to determine whether, and to what extent, infection control programs and the role of the infection control nurse were effective in preventing and controlling infection. The Study on the Efficacy of Nosocomial Infection Control (SENIC) was the hallmark study that provided the evidence that hospitals with established infection control programs had infection rates 32% lower overall than hospitals without such programs.[4] Evidence from the SENIC not only ensured the longevity of the established programs of the day, it also resulted in the widespread establishment of infection control programs across the United States and around the world.

Although the role of the ICP was originally limited to surveillance, at the time of SENIC, the role had evolved to include both surveillance and control activities. The role of the ICP has continued to evolve since its inception, and this evolution and the forces shaping it, are discussed in this chapter.[4-6] A specific focus is the various iterations of the ICP in the contemporary Australian context.

5.1 The healthcare context

Significant changes in the context in which healthcare is delivered have occurred over time and have impacted directly on the role of the ICP.[7] In general, patients admitted to hospital now have a much higher acuity than those admitted when the role was originally established. The concept of the 'hospital without walls' has been introduced, and as a consequence some patients are discharged from hospital but continue to receive complex care, such as intravenous antibiotics, total parenteral nutrition, wound care and other therapies, in their own homes.[8] This change has reduced the length of hospital stay for patients, allowing them to return to the comfort of their home where the care delivery continues, and it also frees up beds for new patients.

Delivery of in-home care has meant that invasive devices such as intravenous access devices remain in the patient after discharge so therapy can continue; however, these devices not only require care but can become the portal of entry or focus for infection. Thus, the ICP focus on nosocomial infection has had to broaden to consider all infections that occur as a result of healthcare intervention, whether they occur inside the hospital or as a consequence of ongoing care following discharge. The term 'nosocomial' has largely been replaced by the term 'healthcare-associated infection' (HAI). The role of the ICP has had to expand to incorporate surveillance activities that include infections associated with healthcare provided in the home.

Another change in the way care is delivered is the introduction of day surgery, where patients having relatively minor surgical procedures present on the day of surgery, have the procedure and then go home, all on the same day. This has resulted in a reduction in bed requirements, such that surgical beds are now reserved for more complex surgical procedures and emergency and traumatic injuries. Even patients undergoing complex elective surgical procedures are commonly admitted to hospital on the day of the procedure, via a surgical admitting unit where they are met, assessed and reviewed immediately prior to transfer to the operating theatre for the procedure and then to the inpatient unit postoperatively. These changes have resulted in significant increases in throughput in the operating theatres, but with less preoperative hospitalisation which reduces the risk of colonising with a multiresistant bacteria preoperatively.

Technological advances have also impacted the healthcare context, the delivery of care and the role of the ICP. Where once only the most seriously ill patients or those having surgery would have an intravenous device, now most patients will have an intravascular device inserted, either on admission to hospital or at some point during their stay. As previously mentioned, some patients have intravascular devices still in place when they are discharged from hospital and many, such as those who are reliant on haemodialysis or are undergoing a course of chemotherapy or antibiotics, have intravascular access devices for weeks, months or even years.

Bypass machines used during cardiac and thoracic surgery, mechanical ventilators and endoscopic instruments all represent advances in treatments that save, prolong and improve lives but each has an associated infection risk. The ICP needs to understand these risks and be able to respond appropriately.

5.1.2 Governance and quality

In the early 1990s a number of studies were published on the quality of healthcare, based on the incidence of adverse outcomes including infection.[9] In Australia, this work identified that 5.5% of patients included in the study developed a hospital-acquired infection or sepsis.[10] The results of this study saw a mobilisation of government resources designed to prevent adverse outcomes associated with healthcare provision and eventually resulted in the establishment of the Australian Commission on Safety and Quality in Health Care (ACSQHC). Established in 2006, the Commission was responsible for 'leading and coordinating national improvements in the safety and quality of health care'.[11] The ACSQHC was given permanent status through the *National Health and Hospitals Network Act 2011*.

Preventing and controlling HAI was one area of focus for the ACSQHC, and its ability to influence clinical practice was achieved by the development and publication of the National Safety and Quality Health Service (NSQHS) Standards and their incorporation into the hospital accreditation process.[12] Failure to meet the NSQHS Standards may result in loss of accreditation of a healthcare facility or service, resulting in the facility or service being unable to continue operation. There are eight Standards in the NSQHS Standards, and the Preventing and Controlling Infections Standard is the standard for infection prevention and control.[13] This Standard has 16 sections, and the healthcare facility or service must provide evidence that all elements of each section are being met in order to meet the requirements for accreditation. Overall responsibility for the performance and outcomes of healthcare rests with the chief executive and associates; however, for the purposes of accreditation

against the NSQHS Standards, responsibility for ensuring the appropriate evidence is available to meet the Preventing and Controlling Infections Standard often rests with the ICP.

The context has been established to consider the contemporary role of the ICP in Australia. Such consideration requires recognition of the changes in the way healthcare is delivered, the increased acuity of the patients admitted to hospital, the technologies used in the delivery of healthcare, and the governance framework that drives and supports quality and accountability for the prevention and control of HAI.

According to the NHMRC's Guidelines, ICPs require the 'skills, experience and qualifications relevant to their specific clinical setting and must be able to:
- develop, manage and evaluate governance of infection prevention and control systems, related programs and services
- provide expert infection prevention consultancy and strategic direction to the healthcare facility and external agencies'.[14]

This chapter provides an outline of the elements of the role. While surveillance and education remain core activities associated with the role of the ICP, the nature and extent of these has changed and expanded over the years, and additional responsibilities have become either fleetingly or permanently part of the role.[15] These activities and responsibilities can be organised as follows and each will be discussed separately: surveillance; education; consultation; governance; staff health; planning and professionalism; and knowledge generation.

5.2 Surveillance

Surveillance has been described as the cornerstone of infection prevention and control (IPC), as case-finding postoperative surgical site infections (SSI) and nosocomial infections caused by antibiotic-resistant bacteria were the primary focus of the ICP when the role was originally established. Over subsequent decades, additional surveillance activities have been added to the role.

In Australia, the role of the ICP varies in relation to a range of circumstances including: whether the hospital is privately or publicly funded; the type of hospital—rural, regional or metropolitan; the size of the hospital and the services provided; and whether there are other members of the infection prevention and control team.[16] These considerations determine the specific surveillance activities that are undertaken by the ICP. However, if we consider the wider range of surveillance activities that could be included, the ICP might require knowledge, expertise and skill in: surgical site infections, bacteraemia; hand hygiene compliance; occupational blood and body fluid exposures; multi-antibiotic resistant and significant organisms; outbreak detection; and a range of environmental risk mitigation activities.

5.2.1 Surgical site surveillance

The ICP must have a clear understanding of the definitions associated with each surveillance activity and, wherever possible, access to and knowledge of a complex web of systems to support the surveillance initiatives.[17] Surgical site infection surveillance requires the ability to identify the patients who are having the specific operative procedures that are under review so that prospective surveillance can be conducted. Access to information about the patient's underlying medical conditions, the procedure that was performed, whether antibiotic prophylaxis was warranted perioperatively and if so, was administered, are all required in order to interpret the eventual outcome. Access to pathology results, postoperative inpatient and outpatient appointment medical records and notifications of unplanned readmissions are all necessary to assist the ICP to determine whether an infection event has occurred postoperatively, and equally importantly, what contributed to the infection so that risk mitigation strategies can be identified and implemented.

5.2.2 Bloodstream infection surveillance

Bacteraemia surveillance may be limited to those healthcare-associated bloodstream infections (BSI) caused by *Staphylococcus aureus*, which is currently the only HAI rate data published and available to the Australian public through the MyHospitals website.[18] Alternatively, a health service or facility may include all episodes of healthcare-associated bacteraemia in the surveillance program, irrespective of the specific organism. Again, the ICP will need a sound knowledge of the definitions for healthcare-associated bacteraemia and access to systems that identify all possible episodes of BSI, as well as inpatient and outpatient medical records and pathology results.

5.2.3 Hand hygiene compliance

The Preventing and Controlling Infections Standard of the NSQHS requires each organisation to have a hand hygiene program consistent with the national hand hygiene initiative to monitor hand hygiene compliance and address non-compliance.[13,19] The role of the ICP has been extended to include responsibility

for monitoring and reporting hand hygiene compliance and addressing poor compliance (Fig. 5.1). The extent of the involvement of the ICP will depend on the size and type of organisation, but the role may require the ICP to collect, analyse and report all hand hygiene compliance data, and to address poor performance. Alternatively, the ICP may be responsible for training hand hygiene auditors to audit compliance across the service, thereby delegating some data collection responsibility but retaining the collation and reporting responsibilities as well as identifying improvement opportunities and activities.

5.2.4 Occupational blood and body fluid exposure

The management of occupational exposure to blood and body fluids may not be the responsibility of the ICP in many facilities; however, it is usual for the ICP to have some analysis and reporting responsibilities for these incidents. This is particularly important when considered in light of other ICP responsibilities, which include evaluating new products, developing procedures to ensure safe practice, educating others about preventing exposure, and managing staff immunisation records and programs.[14]

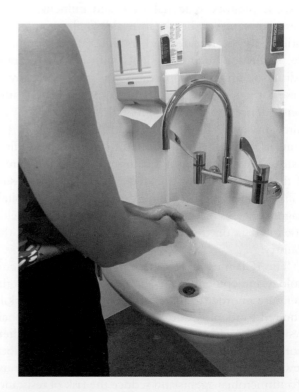

FIGURE 5.1 Hand hygiene is essential for infection prevention

5.2.5 Multi-antibiotic resistant and significant organisms

Since its inception, the role of the ICP has included responsibility for case-finding multi-antibiotic resistant organisms. While methicillin-resistant *Staphylococcus aureus* (MRSA) was the pathogen of concern initially, both the development and use of new antimicrobial agents and the corresponding increase in antimicrobial resistance seen in microorganisms has led to an ever-increasing expansion of organisms of significance and concern.

Resistance has not only been seen in Gram-positive bacteria (*Staphylococcus aureus* and Enterococci) but has become problematic in Gram-negative bacteria (carbapenamase-producing *Enterobacteriaceae*)[20,21] and fungi (*Candida auris*).[22] Multi-drug resistance has been an unwelcome development in diseases such as tuberculosis (MDRTB), leading not only to increased morbidity and mortality in the community but to occupational transmission to healthcare workers, resulting in their death in some countries including the United States.[23] Australia has been spared from the spread of MDRTB; however, isolated cases have been imported.[24]

Other organisms of significance added to the list of concerns for the ICP include *Clostridium difficile*, norovirus, respiratory syncytial virus and influenza. All of these can cause outbreaks in health facilities, infecting patients and healthcare workers alike.[25,26] In a vulnerable population such as patients with chronic comorbidities or immunosuppression, infection with any of these pathogens can have serious and possibly terminal consequences. Hypervirulent strains of *C. difficile* resulted in severe disease and death in hospitalised patients in the United Kingdom, Europe and the United States.[27] Concern about the introduction and spread of these strains in Australian hospitals led to the surveillance and national submission of data on hospital-diagnosed cases of *C. difficile* for a short time to develop baseline data on the incidence of the organism in this country.[28]

The ICP must have some understanding of microbiology and epidemiology and remain current with the literature in order to maintain the knowledge and skills required to identify and manage any new risks associated with resistant and significant organisms. Furthermore, since the widespread introduction of antibiotic stewardship programs, designed to ensure prudent use of antimicrobial agents and reduce the risk of resistance developing, the ICP role will often incorporate some responsibility for antimicrobial stewardship (AMS).[29]

Based on the history to date, it is likely that this element of the ICP role will continue to expand and evolve to meet the new challenges yet to present themselves.

5.2.6 Outbreak management

Outbreak management is included in surveillance because without routine surveillance to establish endemic rates of resistant organisms or infectious diseases it can be difficult to identify an outbreak. Conversely, a single presentation of an illness or infection may represent an outbreak if it is not usually seen in the facility or service. In recent years, norovirus has been the cause of many outbreaks in hospitals and facilities, and both patients and healthcare workers have been affected.[30] Norovirus provides a good example of the role of the ICP in outbreak management.[25] The ICP needs to know when there is one case of norovirus in the facility but will also be reviewing the patient's record to determine whether the patient had the infection on admission or became infected after admission. In either case, the ICP must ensure infection control strategies are in place including: patient isolation; the use of appropriate personal protective equipment (PPE); adequate cleaning regimes for both the environment and equipment; heightened awareness among staff regarding the need for strict hand hygiene compliance; and early reporting of gastrointestinal symptoms in any other patients or staff. Development of case definitions, early reporting and escalation processes, rapid testing where available, and clear communication pathways to staff, patients, visitors and the executive are all within the purview of the ICP. If further cases are identified, the ICP may need to convene an outbreak management team to assist in controlling the outbreak and ensure all relevant stakeholders are aware of the issues and the role their respective team has in managing the outbreak.[14]

5.2.7 Environmental surveillance

The role of the physical environment in infection prevention and control has been demonstrated over the decades largely through investigations into the sources of various outbreaks. Apart from the cleanliness of the physical environment the ICP has a role to play in water quality management and air handling.[31]

The ICP is involved in, or consulted on, the cleaning and disinfectant products and regimes used in the facilities, and must establish some form of auditing and feedback regarding the cleanliness of the facilities.

Knowledge of air-handling systems, especially relating to negative or positive pressure isolation and high-efficiency particulate air (HEPA) filters used in theatres and other areas throughout the facility, is also required. A basic understanding of how the negative pressure system works to protect staff, patients and visitors outside the isolation room helps the ICP ensure the rooms are correctly designed and functioning.[31] Where negative pressure rooms are used, the ICP needs some system of assurance that they are functioning appropriately. To a lesser extent, knowledge of the purpose and functioning of positive pressure rooms is important to ensure patients with infection transmitted via the airborne route are not mistakenly placed in positive pressure isolation rooms.

The importance of water quality management in preventing and controlling infection has been recognised by ICP for decades. In particular, the water towers used in air-conditioning systems are a recognised reservoir for *Legionella* spp. as well as the thermo-mixing valves used to prevent scalding at handbasins, sinks and showers that provide a consistent low temperature of water which is more amenable to the growth of bacteria, especially when the flow of water through the pipes and outlets is not regular. The chlorine in the water that helps to control microbial growth deteriorates quickly and may no longer be present in water left to stagnate for a period of time. Regular maintenance of cooling towers and air-handling systems, as well as regular sampling of water throughout the facility and microbiological testing is managed by other services within the health facility; however, the ICP must know that the testing is being undertaken and must know the results of sampling, especially if there are any positive *Legionella* spp. results or high bacterial counts.[32,33] Water quality is also important in relation to haemodialysis and steam sterilising.

More recently water used on other equipment has been implicated in infection transmission. Heater-cooler units used in cardiac bypass surgery have been identified as the source of infection with a specific pathogen *Mycobacterium chimera*.[34] It appears that aerosols containing contaminated water from these machines have made their way into sternal wounds intraoperatively; however, because the organism is slow-growing, it can take some time before the infection is declared. Environmental surveillance of these machines through water sampling has been added to the environmental surveillance responsibilities of the ICP.

The ICP may include environmental audits in the infection control program. These audits generally involve a visit to the areas audited, where a review is undertaken to check the general state of cleanliness and repair of the area, as well as compliance with basic infection control principles such as the availability and accessibility of PPE, hand hygiene products, appropriate storage of sterile stock, and the safe use and disposal of sharps.

Surveillance has always been the cornerstone of the role of the ICP and over the years the amount and type of surveillance has increased, placing additional demands on the ICP in terms of knowledge and skills required to conduct, coordinate, analyse, interpret and report the various results of surveillance activities in a timely and meaningful way.[16] Surveillance data can identify what is happening and whether there is a problem but feedback of the surveillance results to key stakeholders is required to address any issues identified. Surveillance remains a key component of the ICP role to monitor care outcomes, identify problems and provide a sound basis for the development and implementation of mitigation strategies. Of course, ongoing surveillance is required to measure the effectiveness of the strategies that have been implemented.

5.3 Education

The inclusion of education as an element of the ICP role early in this discussion demonstrates its importance to the role. Even before a facility is built and healthcare service commences, the organisation needs assurance that the people providing the service are competent and able to provide a safe service.[15,35] The ICP needs to ensure that staff entering the organisation are aware of, and able to practise, in accordance with basic infection control principles, so infection control education is always a component of any orientation program. At a minimum, this education includes: the five moments for hand hygiene; safe sharps use and disposal; standard and transmission-based precautions; asepsis; and some elements of staff health, such as immunisation requirements or occupational body fluid exposure management processes, as well as how and where to locate local infection control procedures and other resources.[14]

Once the service is underway, the results of surveillance activities identify what is working well, and if and where any infection risks remain uncontrolled. A key component of any risk mitigation strategy is education. If bacteraemia surveillance results indicate a problem with intravenous cannulae remaining in situ unnecessarily, the ICP may undertake an education and awareness campaign. Education may be targeted if specific wards or departments or specific staff groups are identified as needing education, or a more general awareness campaign may be implemented if the problems appear to be more widespread.

Newly identified pathogens, such as emerging antibiotic resistance in specific bacteria, would require education for the staff likely to be dealing with any patients who are colonised or infected by this pathogen. Antibiotic resistance is a topic that requires regular education to ensure that staff are aware not only of any new resistance issues, but are reminded of challenges not yet conquered.

The COVID-19 pandemic brought home to us all the lack of competence among healthcare workers in relation to the donning and removal of PPE. The equipment has been widely used in healthcare for decades; however, when healthcare workers were required to don and remove it during the pandemic, the lack of knowledge and competence led to increased anxiety and potentially to infection transmission. This experience demonstrates the need to revisit and reinforce previous education.[36]

Various aspects of the education the ICP is required to provide present specific challenges. The first is that the target audience is usually adult healthcare workers, so principles of adult learning need to underpin the education strategies used.[37] Often, the ICP is presenting the same message to reinforce or update previous education, and for this reason the ICP will need to find new and meaningful ways to impart the information so that it becomes more than theoretical knowledge and is instead applied and embedded in practice.

Education needs to illuminate and be practical. The information needs to be presented in such a way as to engage the target audience, provide them with a 'light-bulb moment' so that the theory they may have already heard becomes real, tangible, relevant and applicable in everyday practice. Achieving this level of education requires real skill where the ICP is authentic, credible, compelling and communicates in a manner that is meaningful and understandable to the audience, something they can grasp and use.[38]

The ICP may decide to undertake education needs analysis to determine what the knowledge deficits are, and among which groups they exist. A range of skills including presentation, communication, marketing, technical knowledge and the ability to be creative in education delivery are all needed, in addition to the ability to evaluate the outcomes of any education both in terms of how it was received by the participants on the day, and whether and to what extent the theory has become embedded into practice which is the real measure of success.[39,40]

5.4 Consultation

Every element of the ICP role involves consultation of some kind. As already discussed in the surveillance section, feedback of surveillance data is as important as the data collection and analysis. Without feedback of the results and discussion of the implications there will be no change. Excellent communication skills are vital to the success of the ICP. The broad nature of the scope of the role requires the ICP to engage and communicate with people at every level within the organisation, and the way the ICP communicates must be relevant and appropriate to the specific group during each interaction.[5,35] Recently the response to the SARS-CoV-2 pandemic has demonstrated the need to expand the circles of consultation to include engineers with knowledge and expertise in air handling systems, and has also forged and strengthened ties between the hospital-based ICP and the Public Health teams to collaborate on issues such as hotel quarantine.

Consultation can relate to the management of patients known or suspected to have infectious diseases or conditions. In a large healthcare organisation, this type of consultation will likely be a daily occurrence. Consultation might be frequent and built into the program of work such as the regular meetings the ICP attends. These will include some form of committee responsible for overseeing the work of infection control. Other regular meetings in which the ICP participates could include a committee that reviews new products for introduction into the organisation; any group involved in planning or overseeing a building or refurbishment project; or any group involved in the various elements of the Preventing and Controlling Infections Standard of the NSQHS. The number and type of committees and other groups the ICP meets with regularly will depend on the type and size of the organisation or service.[14]

No matter the meeting group, the ICP must be a valued member, and that can only be achieved if the ICP understands the infection control principles that apply in the specific circumstances and is able to succinctly and clearly articulate the relevant information to the rest of the group. The most meaningful interaction for all involved is where the ICP addresses the issues or concerns of any member of the group and provides evidence-based guidance on the topic. A solid knowledge of the relevant Australian Standards, guidelines and legislative requirements, as well as of the local circumstances and situation, is required.

One of the most important elements of the ICP's role is the development of successful relationships with other members of the healthcare team. These relationships provide a safety net for the ICP when challenges seem insurmountable, and when forged through the fire of adversity, they are likely to develop into life-long colleagues and allies. These longstanding relationships can expedite the implementation of strategies when faced with challenging situations that require immediate action, such as infection outbreaks or a pandemic response. In these situations, these colleagues already know and trust the ICP and are generally ready to roll up their sleeves and help rather than argue the point and waste time. Therefore, time spent cultivating these relationships is time well spent.

5.5 Governance

The ICP and their associated program is subject to context-specific governance processes. The specific place of the infection control team in the organisational structure will depend on the facility or organisation. As previously indicated, the Infection Control Committee or equivalent body usually has some authority over the infection control program and can assist the ICP to set and achieve goals, address challenges and, if functioning correctly, support and promote the infection control agenda within the areas of responsibility of the individual members.[41]

Another governance function of the role of the ICP is the development, implementation and evaluation of specific governance documents. These include infection control policies, or procedures which operationalise national guidelines or standards at a local level. The ICP is required to review various documents, including procedures developed by others, and local work instructions. Any policy or procedure developed will require some form of audit process to determine whether it has been implemented and whether it is fulfilling its purpose. If not, the ICP must undertake additional work to identify barriers and develop strategies to manage them, revise the document, and then review again. The development and refinement of these documents also requires communication and education, so staff know what is required.[14]

Health facilities and organisations also have responsibilities to external agencies. Some of these responsibilities, relating to infection control, are described in the NSQHS Standards, some are embodied in Australian Standards, and some require data collection and submission to jurisdictional health departments. The ICP is required to participate in some way, if not shoulder the main responsibility, for ensuring these responsibilities and obligations are met.[12,13]

5.6 Staff health

The inclusion of staff health as an element of the ICP role is somewhat controversial. Requirements vary from state to state, and also between organisations and facilities, depending on the size of the organisation and available resources. Arguably, though, the health of staff is important to the ICP and it is integral to both the functioning of the health service and the safety of patients and staff.[13]

As discussed in 5.2 Surveillance, the ICP will undoubtably be interested in the incidence of occupational body fluid exposure. Analysis of such exposure incidents provides the ICP with valuable information to assist with product evaluation, educational priorities, clinical workflow and the efficacy of policies and procedures. Also of importance in relation to occupational exposures is demonstrating hepatitis B virus immunity amongst staff. This is very helpful when managing an occupational exposure and hepatitis B immunisation is generally a condition of employment for staff who may be occupationally exposed to blood and body fluids.

Evidence of immunisation against a range of vaccine-preventable diseases including measles, mumps, rubella, varicella and pertussis is commonly required for employment in the health system (Fig. 5.2), although it

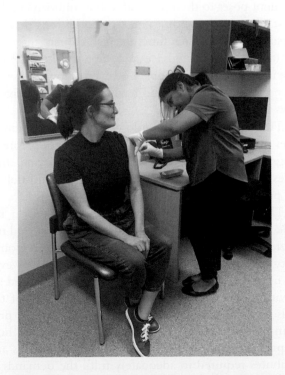

FIGURE 5.2 Immunisation against vaccine-preventable diseases protects healthcare workers

has not always been a requirement. Therefore, it is entirely possible that staff employed for many years in the same organisation may not have been immunised against some of the vaccine-preventable diseases mentioned, or they may require booster doses of vaccine to maintain immunity. Screening for tuberculosis is also commonly a requirement for new employees. Some ICP roles have a greater level of responsibility for these components of staff health than others. Many ICPs have some responsibility for the annual staff influenza vaccination program and there are many reports in the literature regarding strategies to improve uptake.[42-44]

Staff will often seek advice from the ICP about whether they should attend work if they or members of their household have various infectious diseases or conditions. Knowledge of these infectious diseases, their modes of transmission, and the risks of transmission to other staff and patients is required to provide sound advice. Staff may also seek advice and support from the ICP in relation to dermatitis, especially if it is considered to be related to hand hygiene products or other products and substances within the organisation.

Staff expect to be safe from infection when at work and the ICP must be knowledgeable, accessible and able to clearly articulate the information required in a range of situations. Pregnant healthcare workers often seek advice from the ICP as to the risks the work environment poses to themselves and their unborn child, as do staff members with a range of conditions that can impair their immune function. Of course, there are limitations to what advice and support the ICP can provide in these situations; however, knowing where your responsibilities lie and having clear referral pathways is important.

This discussion of the role of the ICP, including a brief overview of the elements of the infection control program, has identified the knowledge, skills and attributes required for the ICP to coordinate and deliver the program. These are summarised in Table 5.1.

The knowledge, skills and attributes listed in the table below do not represent an exhaustive list, and not all elements of the program listed will be the responsibility of the ICP in a specific organisation. However, the table identifies a range of knowledge, skills and attributes required for each element, and many of the skills and attributes listed will apply to multiple program elements. The question now is, where and how do prospective ICP develop the knowledge, skills and attributes required to adequately fulfil the demands of the role? The answer is discussed in terms of how the ICP develops and maintains their own professional

practice, and also, how they contribute to the professional development of those coming after them. These constitute other elements of the role: planning and professionalism, and knowledge generation.

5.7 Planning and professionalism

The ICP responsible for a team of people has administrative duties associated with staffing, rostering and succession planning. In addition, this ICP will have responsibility—possibly shared—for planning the program and ensuring it meets the needs of the health service or facility and is aligned with the organisation's strategic goals. Ongoing professional development is a requirement for the ICP, as is the need to assist in the professional development of other members of the team and colleagues in the broader infection control community.[14]

5.7.1 Strategic planning

The ICP must consider the program priorities for the year ahead, develop a plan that will address them, and wherever possible, contribute to the advancement of the program for the years to come. This constitutes strategic planning and can be the difference between struggling to react to a new requirement suddenly imposed, and having the foresight to undertake small, incremental steps so that by the time a new requirement is imposed it is already an accepted and functioning part of the program.

5.7.2 Internal

Internal strategic planning involves first, reviewing the program from the previous year; second, identifying any deficits or gaps; and third, rectifying them in the plan for the coming year. Goals and priorities are to be established and a review of available resources is required. To make a case for additional resources the ICP must demonstrate how the resources will enable the organisation to meet legislative or accreditation requirements, ensure compliance with relevant standards and guidelines, and align with the organisation's strategic goals and priorities. The ICP will also need to explain why the goals of the resource increase cannot be achieved within current resource allocation.

5.7.3 External

Effective strategic planning requires a clear vision of the goal to be achieved and this vision cannot be developed in isolation. For the purposes of infection control, the development of a vision requires immersion in the

TABLE 5.1 Knowledge, skills and attributes required for the infection control professional role

Role element	Knowledge	Skills	Attributoo
Surveillance	Accepted infection definitions	Data collection, entry and analysis	Diligence and precision
	Appropriate sources of information and evidence	Report writing and presentation	Confidence and assurance
	National benchmarks, relevant Australian Standards, Legislative requirements	Interpretation and application of standards and legislative requirements	
	Appropriate control measures	Conflict resolution and collaboration	Reassuring, pragmatic
	Microbiology	Interpretation of laboratory results	
Education	Adult learning principles	Education needs analysis development and implementation	Open communication style
	Infection control principles	Presentation development and delivery	Engaging and interactive
	Evidence base underpinning principles and practice	Application of evidence	Messaging and delivery appropriate to target audience
	Evaluation methodology	Interpretation of evaluation results	Reflective and improvement focused
Consultation	Elements of design, air, water and environmental systems and services	Reading and interpreting building and renovation plans	Reliability and credibility
	Disease transmission and control methods	Risk stratification for efficient use of available resources	Meaningful engagement with stakeholders
	Contact tracing	Case definition development and investigation	Coordination of people and resources
	Reprocessing of reusable medical devices	Product evaluation	
Governance	Relevant standards, policies, guidelines and legislation	Operationalise standards, policies and legislative requirements	
	Organisational priorities and strategic goals	Demonstrate alignment of program priorities and goals to organisation	Systematic approach to risk identification
	National and jurisdictional benchmarks and reporting requirements	Evaluate compliance with policies and procedures	
Staff Health	Immunisation schedules and vaccine cold chain management	Data management and cold chain audit and assurance	
	Interpretation of serology results		Consultation and referral as needed
	Disease incubation periods		
	Occupational blood and body fluid exposure management principles	Pre- and post-test counselling for blood-borne virus testing	

subject through reading journal articles, attending seminars and conferences, and actively participating in the activities and work of the professional organisation. The ICP must take a long view, scan the horizon to see what is coming and prepare in advance. As Australia is an island nation and relatively geographically isolated, it often has the advantage of a delay between the emergence of new pathogens or more resistant bacteria identified in other parts of the world, such as Europe, the United States and the United Kingdom, and by maintaining currency with reports in the scientific literature, attending conferences and remaining connected to professional organisations, the ICP can identify future challenges for Australia and prepare for them.

Where and how do the people with these attributes develop? The various elements that constitute the role have been considered; however, the ICP is also responsible for their own ongoing professional development, and for the professional development of others. The ICP responsible for leading a team of other ICPs to deliver a program is also responsible for helping other members of the team to grow and develop. Even the ICP who constitutes a team of one needs someone to relieve them when they take leave, so developing that person or a few people to share the load is important. It would be irresponsible to be concerned for the program only while you are in the team; someone must take up the challenge if, and when, you leave temporarily or permanently.

5.7.4 Education and credentialling

In the same way that the role of the ICP has evolved over time, the need for specific specialist training for the role and the opportunities for such preparation have also evolved. While there are no specific educational requirements for ICPs within most countries, including Australia, in the United States a credentialling process has been established by the Certification Board of Infection Control and Epidemiology (CBIC). According to the CBIC website, certification is awarded based on 'an objective measurement of standardised current knowledge' and the measurement is based on the score achieved by the candidate who undertakes a written examination.[45] If successful, the candidate is certified as competent for a period of five years, after which time the candidate must re-certify at five-yearly intervals. Certification is a voluntary process and is not necessarily a requirement for appointment as an ICP. The Association of Professionals in Infection Control and Epidemiology (APIC) offers educational courses, workshops and conferences to support the development

of Infection Preventionists (IP) and recommends certification to its members.[46]

Australia has taken a different approach. For many years there were no formal postgraduate courses designed to prepare ICPs for their role. The Australian Infection Control Association (AICA) which was the precursor to the current Australasian College of Infection Prevention and Control (ACIPC), as the peak professional body for ICP in Australia, recognised the need to develop a credentialling process. The original credentialling process was designed to credential experts in infection prevention and control, those who had been working for many years in the field and were recognised as experts by their peers before the advent of formal tertiary infection control courses.[47,48] The credentialling process was developed by AICA in recognition that self-regulation is the hallmark of a profession. It was established as a peer-review process, requiring the applicant to submit a professional portfolio demonstrating their expertise and experience and supported by professional references.[49] Around the same time the credentialling process was launched, some Australian universities began offering formal tertiary infection control courses and it was noted that graduates of these courses were applying to AICA for credentialling. Those who completed the tertiary courses clearly valued peer recognition of their expertise. The credentialling process evolved in response and incorporated tertiary qualifications in infection control into the credentialling process so that the higher the qualification held by the applicant, the less reliance on the professional portfolio, although support from professional colleagues through references and demonstration of ongoing professional development, active employment in the discipline, and evidence of reflective practice were still required.

In January 2012, ACIPC ('the College') was founded, bringing the existing state and territory infection control associations together and replacing them in one entity.[50] The College recognised the importance of the credentialling process as a mechanism to ensure professional practice, to identify a community of experts and guide ICP development. The credentialling framework was revised in 2016 to provide a career pathway for ICP from novice, through advanced and finally to expert practice. Based on the success of the original framework, the three-tiered framework includes practice and educational requirements as well as critical reflection designed to encourage the applicant to identify opportunities for further professional development and growth, and to consider how to contribute back to the profession as appropriate at advanced and expert level.[51] Each applicant requires the support of a reference from professional colleagues and the application is reviewed by a panel of ICP peers who assess the application against a range of criteria and make a recommendation to the ACIPC Board.[51]

The credential is awarded for a period of three years, at which point the ICP can apply for recredentialling at the same level or apply for credentialling at a higher level. Recredentialling requires the applicant to demonstrate ongoing professional development, current practice in infection prevention and control, critical reflection, good standing through references from professional colleagues, registration with the relevant professional registration authority and knowledge generation as appropriate. Recredentialling is required every three years.[51]

Education and credentialling are closely connected due to the educational requirements associated with credentialling at each level, as well as the requirement to demonstrate ongoing professional development when applying for recredentialling. Australian universities now offer specific infection control qualifications from Graduate Certificate to Masters' level and an increasing number of ICP are undertaking doctoral programs of research in their field, thereby contributing to the evidence that underpins practice. In response to the needs of novice ICPs, the College has developed and offers a foundation course in infection prevention and control, thereby providing a base level of education for those new to the discipline and those aspiring to be ICPs. The College also offers a range of professional development opportunities in the form of workshops, webinars and an annual scientific conference.[52] Other specific ICP educational opportunities are offered through the Australian Commission on Safety and Quality in Health Care. The ACSQHC website has links to a number of online education modules and also coordinates the national hand hygiene initiative (NHHI) including hand hygiene auditor training and other useful resources.[13,19]

Despite the development and evolution of both credentialling and educational opportunities, neither is required to hold a position as an ICP in Australia. However, there is growing acceptance of the benefits of both, and credentialling and formal tertiary qualifications are increasingly included in the preferences for ICP positions vacant.[49,53]

A significant change in the recognised role of the ICP occurred with the release of the three-tiered ACIPC credentialling framework.[51] This new framework recognised the importance of providing support, education and credentialling for people not previously considered ICPs. This expanded view of the ICP recognised the infection control components of roles such as beauticians, tattooists and sterilisation technicians as well as a One Health approach to include veterinarians and others (see Chapter 2). This chapter has focused on HAIs and the role of the ICP, so the less traditionally recognised ICP roles have not been discussed, and readers are referred to the ACIPC website for additional information if required.

5.8 Knowledge generation

Some very experienced and well-educated ICP have moved into research and teaching roles and continue to support the discipline by contributing new evidence, helping to prepare new ICPs, and supporting those who are already in the profession and are working to augment their experience with formal qualifications. It is critical that these expressions of the ICP role are valued and included in our credentialling framework, so that our evidence base continues to grow and future generations of ICP are assured. However, the responsibility for generating new knowledge and preparing the next generation of ICPs does not rest solely with academics and researchers. All ICPs at advanced and expert level have a responsibility to recognise and embrace opportunities to undertake research.

The most useful model for this is a partnership between experienced researchers and academics and ICPs working in, or coordinating, infection control programs. Such a partnership is symbiotic in that the academic partner has access to the clinical context where the need for solutions to new challenges arise, and the clinical ICP has access to the research experience of their academic colleague. Such a partnership ensures that the research undertaken is rigorous, organised and ethically approved while also ensuring it is clinically relevant and applicable. These partnerships are more likely to see the outcomes of the project published or presented at scientific meetings, so the work is shared, and findings contribute to the body of science that underpins our practice. Research undertaken by partnerships like this often attracts research grant funding, so the research is supported by the human and material resources required to do it well.

A further advantage to academic and clinical partnerships is that the clinician has the opportunity to learn about research methods and design, and develop skills and experience in this specialised area. Attracting research grant funding is a special skill in its own right and competition is fierce, so any opportunity to learn the skills required for successful grant applications should be embraced.

Generation of new knowledge is the responsibility of all members of the infection prevention and control community and is explicitly identified as a key requirement for those ICPs who are considered experts in the field.[54]

Conclusion

This chapter has described the evolution of the ICP role over the past five decades and how this evolution is related to new and emerging pathogens, increasing antimicrobial resistance, new medical technologies, and changes in the way and context in which healthcare is delivered. The role has expanded significantly since it was originally established and, in many ways, ICPs have had to embrace and respond to the changes as they arise. The ongoing need for research and the role of formal education for the ICP continues to challenge the profession and it is largely left to the individual ICP to pursue and fund. Accepted staffing levels vary and fail to allow for outbreak management, pandemic planning and response, or for any real innovation in the roles and programs.

There is a distinct lag between the career pathway expressed in the ACIPC credentialling framework, from novice to advanced and finally expert level, and the staffing models for infection control programs in Australian health facilities. There is an inherent element of risk in the staffing models in that an ICP who may only be able to demonstrate the requirements for credentialling at novice level, may be responsible for the infection control program of a facility or service, with no advanced or expert ICP mentor to assist or advise. It is unclear whether, and to what extent, this risk is recognised by health executives.

The one constant element of the ICP role is change, and yet it seems that some things never change because we are still battling to achieve high levels of hand hygiene compliance. The recent pandemic has again identified the lack of knowledge and expertise in basic infection control practices, such as the appropriate use of PPE and the role of environmental cleaning. It has been fascinating to see the terms 'hand hygiene', 'social distancing' and 'personal protective equipment' become part of the everyday vernacular among the media and the general public. Now may be the most opportune time for ICPs to take control and direct the course of the profession for the future rather than continuing to be buffeted by the winds of change and external forces.

Despite its challenges, the role of the ICP is pivotal in ensuring the delivery of safe and effective patient care; the maintenance of safe work environments through environmental design, staff training and education; and the ongoing monitoring and feedback of data collected through surveillance initiatives. The importance of the role has been clearly demonstrated through research such as the SENIC project; its evolution in response to changes in healthcare services and contexts; and more recently, the response to the SARS-CoV-2 pandemic has revealed the prominence of the role to health executives, government agencies and the general public.[4]

Useful websites/resources

- National Health and Medical Research Council. Australian Guidelines for the Prevention and Control of Infection in Healthcare (2019). https://www.nhmrc.gov.au
- Australian Commission on Safety and Quality in Health Care. https://www.safetyandquality.gov.au/infection-prevention-and-control

References

1. Wenzel K. The role of the infection control nurse. The Nursing Clinics of North America. 1970;5(1):89-98.
2. Larson E. A retrospective on infection control. Part 2: twentieth century—the flame burns. Am J Infect Control. 1997;25(4):340-349.
3. Cohen FL, Tartasky D. Microbial resistance to drug therapy: a review. Am J Infect Control. 1997;25(1):51-64.
4. Haley RW, Culver DH, White JW, Morgan WM, Emori TG, Munn VP, et al. The efficacy of infection surveillance and control programs in preventing nosocomial infections in US hospitals. Am J Epidemiol. 1985;121(2):182-205.
5. Manning ML, Borton DL, Rumovitz DM. Infection preventionists' job descriptions: do they reflect expanded roles and responsibilities? Am J Infect Control. 2012;40(9):888-890.

6. Pogorzelska-Maziarz M, Gilmartin H, Reese S. Infection prevention staffing and resources in U.S. acute care hospitals: results from the APIC MegaSurvey. Am J Infect Control. 2018;46(8):852-857.

7. Gray J, Oppenheim B, Mahida N. The journal of hospital infection - a history of infection prevention and control in 100 volumes. J Hosp Infect. 2018;100(1):1-8.

8. Keller S, Salinas A, Williams D, McGoldrick M, Gorski L, Alexander M, et al. Reaching consensus on a home infusion central line-associated bloodstream infection surveillance definition via a modified Delphi approach. Am J Infect Control. 2020;48(9):993-1000.

9. Institute of Medicine Committee on Quality of Health Care in A. In: Kohn LT, Corrigan JM, Donaldson MS, eds. To err is human: building a safer health system. Washington (DC): National Academies Press (US). National Academy of Sciences, 2000.

10. Wilson RM, Runciman WB, Gibberd RW, Harrison BT, Newby L, Hamilton JD. The Quality in Australian Health Care Study. Med J Aust. 1995;163(9):458-471.

11. Australian Commission on Safety and Quality in Health Care. About us 2020 [Internet] Sydney: ACSQHC, 2020 [cited March 2021]. Available from https://www.safetyandquality.gov.au/.

12. Australian Commission on Safety and Quality in Health Care. The NSQHS Standards 2021 [Internet]. Sydney: ACSQHC, 2021. Available from: https://www.safetyandquality.gov.au/standards/nsqhs-standards.

13. Australian Commission on Safety and Quality in Health Care. Preventing and Controlling Infections Standard, 2021. Sydney; ACSQHC; 2021. Available from: https://www.safetyandquality.gov.au/publications-and-resources/resource-library/national-safety-and-quality-health-service-standards-second-edition.

14. National Health and Medical Research Council. Australian guidelines for the prevention and control of infection in healthcare (2019). Canberra: NHMRC, 2019.

15. Hall L, Halton K, Macbeth D, Gardner A, Mitchell B. Roles, responsibilities and scope of practice: describing the state of play for infection control professionals in Australia and New Zealand. Healthcare Infection. 2015;20(1):29-35.

16. Mitchell BG, Hall L, Halton K, MacBeth D, Gardner A. Time spent by infection control professionals undertaking healthcare associated infection surveillance: a multi-centred cross sectional study. Infection, Disease and Health. 2016; 21(1):36-40.

17. Australian Commission on Safety and Quality in Health Care. Approaches to surgical site infection surveillance 2019 [Internet] Sydney: ACSQHC, 2019. Available from: https://www.safetyandquality.gov.au/publications-and-resources/resource-library/approaches-surgical-site-infection-surveillance.

18. Australian Institue of Health and Welfare. MyHospitals 2020 [Internet]. AIHW, 2020. Available from: https://www.aihw.gov.au/reports-data/myhospitals.

19. Australian Commission on Safety and Quality in Health Care. National hand hygiene initiative 2019 [Internet]. ACSQHC, 2019. Available from: https://www.safetyandquality.gov.au/our-work/infection-prevention-and-control/national-hand-hygiene-initiative.

20. Australian Commission on Safety and Quality in Health Care. Recommendations for the control of carbapenemase-producing Enterobacteriacae (CP) - a guide for acute care health facilities. 2019 [Internet]. ACSQHC, 2019. Available from: https://www.safetyandquality.gov.au/publications-and-resources/resource-library/recommendations-control-carbapenemase-producing-enterobacteriaceae-cpe-guide-acute-care-health-facilities.

21. Wilson AP, Livermore DM, Otter JA, Warren RE, Jenks P, Enoch DA, et al. Prevention and control of multi-drug-resistant Gram-negative bacteria: recommendations from a joint working party. J Hosp Infect. 2016;92 Suppl 1:S1-44.

22. Short B, Brown J, Delaney C, Sherry L, Williams C, Ramage G, et al. Candida auris exhibits resilient biofilm characteristics in vitro: implications for environmental persistence. J Hosp Infect. 2019;103(1):92-96.

23. Gosch ME, Shaffer RE, Eagan AE, Roberge RJ, Davey VJ, Radonovich LJ, Jr. B95: a new respirator for health care personnel. Am J Infect Control. 2013;41(12):1224-1230.

24. Cheung YM, Van K, Lan L, Barmanray R, Qian SY, Shi WY, et al. Hypothyroidism associated with therapy for multi-drug-resistant tuberculosis in Australia. Intern Med J. 2019; 49(3):364-372.

25. Steele MK, Wikswo ME, Hall AJ, Koelle K, Handel A, Levy K, et al. Characterizing norovirus transmission from outbreak data, United States. Emerg Infect Dis. 2020;26(8):1818-1825.

26. Rubin LG, Kohn N, Nullet S, Hill M. Reduction in rate of nosocomial respiratory virus infections in a children's hospital associated with enhanced isolation precautions. Infect Control Hosp Epidemiol. 2018;39(2):152-156.

27. Pires RN, Monteiro AA, Saldanha GZ, Falci DR, Caurio CFB, Sukiennik TCT, et al. Hypervirulent clostridium difficile strain has arrived in Brazil. Infect Control Hosp Epidemiol. 2018; 39(3):371-373.

28. Australian Commission on Safety and Quality in Health Care. Surveillance of Clostridium difficile infection 2019 [Internet]. Sydney: ACSQHC, 2019. Available from: https://www.safetyandquality.gov.au/our-work/healthcare-associated-infection/consultation-on-clostridium-difficile.

29. Australian Commission on Safety and Quality in Health Care. Antimicrobial stewardship 2019. [Internet]. Sydney: ACSQHC, 2019. Available from: https://www.safetyandquality.gov.au/our-work/antimicrobial-stewardship.

30. Schulz-Stübner S, Reska M, Schaumann R. Affected healthcare workers during outbreaks: a report from the German consulting center for infection control (BZH) outbreak registry. Infect Control Hosp Epidemiol. 2019;40(1):113-115.

31. Committee HICPA. Environmental infection control guidelines 2003 [Internet]. Available from: https://www.cdc.gov/infectioncontrol/guidelines/environmental/index.html.

32. Health Q. Legionella, legionellosis and Legionnaires' disease 2019 [Internet]. Available from: https://www.health.qld.gov.au/clinical-practice/guidelines-procedures/diseases-infection/diseases/legionnaires.

33. Muzzi A, Cutti S, Bonadeo E, Lodola L, Monzillo V, Corbella M, et al. Prevention of nosocomial legionellosis by best water management: comparison of three decontamination methods. J Hosp Infect. 2020;105(4):766-772.

34. Garvey MI, Bradley CW, Walker J. A year in the life of a contaminated heater-cooler unit with mycobacterium chimaera. Infect Control Hosp Epidemiol. 2017;38(6):705-711.

35. Bubb TN, Billings C, Berriel-Cass D, Bridges W, Caffery L, Cox J, et al. APIC professional and practice standards. Am J Infect Control. 2016;44(7):745-749.

36. Kuhn L, Lim ZJ, Flynn D, Potter E, Egerton-Warburton D. Safety briefing and visual design key to protecting health care personnel during the COVID-19 pandemic. Am J Infect Control. 2020;48(9):1122-1124.

37. Taylor DC, Hamdy H. Adult learning theories: implications for learning and teaching in medical education: AMEE Guide No. 83. Med Teach. 2013;35(11):e1561-1572.

38. Read ME, Olson AJ, Calderwood MS. Front-line education by infection preventionists helps reduce Clostridioides difficile infections. Am J Infect Control. 2020;48(2):227-229.

39. Le AB, Buehler SA, Maniscalco PM, Lane P, Rupp LE, Ernest E, et al. Determining training and education needs pertaining to highly infectious disease preparedness and response: a gap analysis survey of US emergency medical services practitioners. Am J Infect Control. 2018;46(3):246-252.

40. Lim K, Kilpatrick C, Storr J, Seale H. Exploring the use of entertainment-education YouTube videos focused on infection prevention and control. Am J Infect Control. 2018;46(11):1218-1223.

41. Halton K, Hall L, Gardner A, MacBeth D, Mitchell BG. Exploring the context for effective clinical governance in infection control. Am J Infect Control. 2017;45(3):278-283.

42. Corace KM, Srigley JA, Hargadon DP, Yu D, MacDonald TK, Fabrigar LR, et al. Using behavior change frameworks to improve healthcare worker influenza vaccination rates: a systematic review. Vaccine. 2016;34(28):3235-3242.

43. To KW, Lai A, Lee KC, Koh D, Lee SS. Increasing the coverage of influenza vaccination in healthcare workers: review of challenges and solutions. J Hosp Infect. 2016; 94(2):133-142.

44. Oguz MM. Improving influenza vaccination uptake among healthcare workers by on-site influenza vaccination campaign in a tertiary children hospital. Hum Vaccin Immunother. 2019;15(5):1060-1065.

45. Certification Board of Infection Control and Epidemiology, Inc. About CBIC 2019 [Internet]. Vancouver: CBIC, 2019. Available from https://www.cbic.org/CBIC/Marketing-Toolkit/AbouttheCIC.pdf.

46. Association for Professionals in Infection Control and Epidemiology, Inc. CIC Certification 2020 [Internet]. Vancouver: APIC, 2020. Available from: https://apic.org/education-and-events/certification/.

47. Gardner G, Macbeth, D. Credentialling the infection control practitioner. Australian Infection Control. 1997;2(4):19-20.

48. Macbeth D. Pathway to credentials. Australian Infection Control. 1999;4(4):21-23.

49. MacBeth D, Hall L, Halton K, Gardner A, Mitchell BG. Credentialing of Australian and New Zealand infection control professionals: an exploratory study. Am J Infect Control. 2016;44(8):886-891.

50. Australasian College for Infection Prevention and Control. About ACIPC 2020 [Internet]. Hobart: ACIPC, 2020. Available from: https://www.acipc.org.au/abput-acipc/.

51. Australasian College for Infection Prevention and Control. ACIPC Credentialling 2020 [Internet]. Hobart: ACIPC, 2020. Available from: https://www.acipc.org.au/credentialling/.

52. Australasian College for Infection Prevention and Control. Education and Professional Development 2020 [Internet]. Hobart: ACIPC, 2020. Available from: https://www.acipc.org.au/professional-development/.

53. Mitchell BG, Hall L, Halton K, MacBeth D, Gardner A. Infection control standards and credentialing. Am J Infect Control. 2015;43(12):1380-1381.

54. Australasian College of Infection Prevention and Control. ACIPC Credentialling 2020 [Internet]. Hobart: ACIPC, 2020. Available from: https://www.acipc.org.au/credentialling/.

CHAPTER 6

Governance, accreditation and standards in infection prevention and control

PROFESSOR RAMON Z. SHABAN[i-iv]

Dr DEBOROUGH MACBETH[v]

Dr CATHERINE VIENGKHAM[i,ii]

Chapter highlights

- Describes the importance of clinical governance and its purpose in the context of ensuring effective infection prevention and control
- Provides an overview of the organisational structure and the interconnected roles and responsibilities of the governing body, chief executive officer, infection control committee and infection control team in ensuring good IPC practice and its continued impact on healthcare outcomes
- Recounts the 100-year-old history of healthcare accreditation in Australia and how it eventually led to the Australian Health Service Safety and Quality Accreditation Scheme and the release of national healthcare standards
- Summarises the present healthcare accreditation process, schedule and outcomes
- Provides a brief overview of the current edition of Australia's healthcare standards, including the Preventing and Controlling Infections Standard

i   Susan Wakil School of Nursing and Midwifery, Faculty of Medicine and Health, University of Sydney, Sydney, NSW
ii Sydney Infectious Diseases Institute, Faculty of Medicine and Health, University of Sydney, Sydney, NSW
iii Public Health Unit, Centre for Population Health, Western Sydney Local Health District, Westmead, NSW
iv New South Wales Biocontainment Centre, Western Sydney Local Health District, Westmead, NSW
v   Gold Coast Hospital and Health Service, Southport, QLD

Introduction

Governance systems are necessary to ensure the establishment and maintenance of effective infection prevention and control (IPC) programs and are essential for the safety of patients, staff and visitors in healthcare. Every healthcare institution is unique and has different needs, resources, staffing and healthcare users, and this affects how these systems are developed and implemented. This chapter provides an overview of how clinical governance requirements have been characterised and presented in the current IPC healthcare standards in Australia. It also highlights the key components needed for effective IPC governance, and summarises the general expertise, roles, functions and activities these systems should involve. In this chapter we synthesise the broad function of ICP programs and plans, as well as the role of the IPC professional, introduced in Chapters 4 and 5. Finally, we briefly describe the current standards for IPC accreditation across Australia.

6.1 Defining clinical governance

6.1.1 What is clinical governance?

This section discusses the recommendations for governance systems for IPC provided by national and international literature and guidelines. Specifically, these include the National Health and Medical Research Council (NHMRC) and Australian Commission on Safety and Quality in Health Care's (ACSQHC) Australian Guidelines for the Prevention and Control of Infection in Healthcare,[1] and the ACSQHC's National Safety and Quality Health Service (NSQHS) Preventing and Controlling Infections Standard.[2]

The ACSQHC defines clinical governance as 'the set of relationships and responsibilities established by a health service organisation between its department of health (for the public sector), governing body, executive, clinicians, patients, consumers and other stakeholders to ensure good clinical outcomes'.[3] In short, the responsibility for safe and high-quality patient care falls on people across all levels of the healthcare system. As described in Chapter 4, effective and efficient infection prevention and control requires a facility-wide programmatic approach, where responsibilities and obligations are delegated and documented, and clinical outcomes are routinely monitored. The data that is subsequently collected then continuously feeds back into the cycle of improving clinical care.[1]

6.1.2 Clinical governance and infection prevention and control

Preventing and controlling the transmission of infectious disease should be a vital component of any clinical governance system. It is important to realise that effective systems of IPC practice cannot occur in isolation, and the larger the healthcare organisation, the more effort that needs to be made to thoroughly integrate good IPC practice into its culture and function. The introduction of the national healthcare standards, and most pertinently, standards targeting infectious disease and antimicrobial usage, has been paramount in ensuring that all healthcare systems are adequately equipped with systems and structures to prevent and control adverse infection-related incidents, including healthcare-associated infections, outbreaks, increasing antimicrobial resistance and the emergence of novel, pandemic-level infectious diseases. Ultimately, good clinical governance is critical in ensuring the short- and long-term success of IPC practice; how well it is implemented and received by the healthcare organisation; how effectively it is continuously developed and improved upon; and the overall impact it has on the health outcomes of patients and the preparedness of the workforce.

The role of clinical governance in the context of infection prevention and control may include, but is not limited to:

- ensuring the governing body and highest office of the organisation is strongly engaged in IPC processes, strategies and outcomes, and that good IPC practice is incorporated within the overarching mission of the organisation and the culture of the workforce
- establishing multidisciplinary committees and teams to identify and manage risks associated with infections, and to develop, implement and report on the effectiveness of IPC systems and practices
- identifying IPC deficits or weaknesses in the healthcare system and workforce, and subsequently providing the appropriate training and resources, as well as ensuring these provisions remain up to date and are regularly evaluated
- ensuring systems and protocols are in place to respond to public health and pandemic risks
- establishing a surveillance strategy for infections and antimicrobial use that incorporates data from national and jurisdictional databases and internal surveillance systems; reporting this data to relevant

bodies within the organisation; and using the data to inform IPC practices and measure the effectiveness of implemented IPC strategies on health outcomes over time

- providing an accessible feedback and complaints management system that seeks input from both patients and the workforce, and integrating this input into improving safety and quality systems
- evaluating the performance of key IPC groups, such as the infection control committee (ICC) and infection control team (ICT), by establishing performance and health outcomes and objectives, and conducting regular reviews to confirm whether these objectives have been satisfied
- maintaining processes for facilitating and implementing evidence-based practice and new IPC programs and practices.

6.2 Roles in clinical governance

Addressing IPC issues requires a multi-component, facility-wide program and it is everybody's responsibility. As the size of the healthcare organisation changes, so do the processes used to govern infection prevention and control. Similarly, the roles involved in the clinical governance of IPC, as well as the responsibilities attached to those roles, will also vary from facility to facility. The following section describes several roles and bodies that are typically found in a general healthcare setting, like a hospital. While the titles may differ across organisations, each healthcare facility must ensure that there is at least one person, or body of people, to carry out the listed responsibilities to ensure effective IPC.

6.2.1 The governing body

Most Australian healthcare organisations are governed by bodies, such as a board of directors, that are generally responsible for its corporate governance. This includes clinical governance but also encompasses financial, risk and other governance responsibilities that keep the organisation functioning smoothly. Importantly, the components of corporate governance are heavily intertwined, and decisions that affect one will inevitably affect the others. Their roles differ from the responsibility held by managerial positions. The National Model of Clinical Governance Framework distinguishes this by suggesting that where management has an operational focus, governance has a strategic focus. Managers run organisations, whereas their boards ensure that organisations are run well and in the right direction.[3] The governing body holds the authority to conduct

the business of the organisation and make large financial and organisational decisions. It is its responsibility to ensure that good governance systems (clinical and otherwise) are established and to be accountable for the outcomes and performance of the organisation, as well as to the external shareholders. Additionally, one of the key roles of the governing body is to appoint the position of the chief executive officer (CEO), supporting them to lead the organisation and evaluating their performance.

6.2.2 Chief executive officer

The responsibility for ensuring the safe delivery of healthcare and associated IPC measures belongs to the highest office in the healthcare organisation. For the purposes of this chapter, this position will be referred to as the CEO.

The CEO is appointed by the governing body and must ensure that all appropriate IPC systems and strategies are in place, functional and meet accreditation standards. These responsibilities may be delegated by the CEO to another person, but the CEO still retains ultimate responsibility for IPC outcomes. There should be clearly established channels of information flow, reporting and communication between IPC specialists, IPC outcomes and the CEO. Depending on the size and structure of the organisation, the CEO may sit directly on a dedicated IPC committee or appoint an appropriate representative. Alternatively, IPC information and outcomes may be reported by an appointed IPC representative, or another intermediary body that holds broader responsibilities in clinical governance and quality control, on the same board or subcommittee as the CEO.[4] The frequency and information reported during these meetings should be well established between all attending parties and documented. A summary of the general responsibilities of the CEO is presented in Table 6.2.

6.2.3 The infection control committee (ICC)

The establishment of a formal infection control committee (ICC) is paramount for ensuring that the healthcare facility meets, and continues to improve upon, their IPC standards. The ICC should engage a multidisciplinary membership that involves input from both IPC specialists, as well as healthcare providers like clinicians and nurses (Table 6.1). They should be responsible for the development, implementation, evaluation and resource allocation for all matters relating to IPC.[4] Activities undertaken by the ICC are to be reported on a regular basis to the relevant governing bodies. The ICC may also work with other administrative bodies and healthcare

TABLE 6.1 The core and optional members within an infection control committee

Core membership[1]	Optional members[4]
• The CEO or a designated representative • An executive member with the authority to allocate resources and take remedial action as needed • An infection control professional • A medical practitioner, preferably with qualifications in clinical microbiology and/or infectious disease	• An infection control nurse (ICN) • The director of nursing or a designated representative • An occupational health physician • Representatives from the major clinical specialties or departments (e.g. microbiology, pathology, pharmacy, surgery, medicine, housekeeping, food preparation)

staff within the healthcare organisation when promoting and ensuring the appropriate implementation of IPC plans and programs.[4] As a result, ICC membership should also ideally involve representatives from a range of clinical services and departments, including those responsible for cleaning, sterilisation and food preparation.

The broad responsibilities of the ICC are summarised in Table 6.2. The ICC is required to meet on a regular schedule determined by such factors as the size of the facility, its case-mix complexity and infection risks.[1] All standard administrative processes apply, including the proper documentation, storage and dissemination of correspondence and decisions resulting from each meeting. The ICC is also responsible for formal reports, whether annual or otherwise, that describe a predetermined number of quality and performance indicators relating to IPC, as well as how these indicators fall within the broader goals and standards set for that period.[4] The committee's activity is to be measured against an operational plan and its set priorities and targets. These plans and targets must be regularly reviewed and take into consideration patients' and healthcare workers' experiences and feedback. On a day-to-day level, the committee should have an established avenue for everyday management and reporting activities, including a clear strategy for reporting and escalating significant infection-related incidents, such as an outbreak, to the relevant authorities both within and outside the healthcare organisation.

6.2.4 The infection control team (ICT)

The infection control team is a vital component of clinical governance in IPC and provides an integral link between the organisation's governance structures and its workforce and consumers. The ICT is responsible for the day-to-day, onsite operation of IPC programs and protocols within the healthcare organisation, and it reports activities and outcomes regularly to the ICC.[4] Establishing an ICT has been reported to reduce the incidence of HAIs by up to 33%.[5,6] Infection control teams are comprised of infection control professionals who have skills, experience and qualifications to develop, implement and evaluate IPC systems, practices and programs, and provide expertise on all other matters relating to IPC. Additionally, many of these professionals hold qualifications in other roles, such as within a specific clinical practice or in nursing.[1] The general responsibilities of the ICT are outlined in Table 6.2. A brief description of the roles and responsibilities of various ICT members is provided in the following section. For a more detailed overview of IPC professionals, see Chapter 5.

Director of IPC: The director of IPC is usually a nursing or medically qualified senior staff member with expertise in IPC. This could be a specialist nurse, microbiologist, epidemiologist or infectious diseases physician. Regardless of background, it is imperative that the director has special interest, knowledge and experience in different aspects of IPC. The director takes a leading role in managing and directing the ICT, acting as a central and authoritative point of correspondence for all team members. They are heavily involved in setting quality standards, surveillance and audits with regard to IPC. They also typically act as the designated representative of the ICT on the ICC and may also function as the committee's chair. The position on the ICC allows for a two-way communication channel between the committee and the members of the ICT. As the link between both practice and governance, their expertise and onsite experience is critical in informing and preparing the plans, policies and long-term IPC programs and strategies for both the ICC and at higher organisational levels.

Infection control professional (ICP): An infection control professional (ICP) is a person with specialised qualifications or training in both the academic and

TABLE 6.2 Summary of the roles and responsibilities of the governing bodies, chief executive officer, infection control committee and infection control team in the clinical governance of IPC

Role	Responsibilities
Governing bodies	• Establish a strategic framework that is routinely reviewed • Set priorities for the provision of safe and high-quality healthcare and communicate these to all levels of the organisation and the community • Appoint a CEO, delegate the CEO's responsibilities, support them in leading the organisation and monitor and evaluate their performance • Ensure that all roles and responsibilities are clearly defined for staff across all levels of the organisation • Develop a culture of safety and quality improvement within the organisation • Monitor the performance of the organisation and ensure that there is a focus on continuous progress and improvement on safety and quality performance • Approve budgets and make other major financial and organisational decisions • Ensure that major risks are identified and managed • Evaluate reports and review feedback, suggestions and complaints • Ensure partnership, communication and accountability to patients, carers and consumers, as well as to other internal and external stakeholders • Ensure that the organisation is properly managed, that services exceed minimum standards and compliance obligations are met

Chief executive officer	• Establish IPC outcomes as a key performance indicator
	• Establish clear reporting and communication channels with a dedicated IPC committee, such as:
	  ◦ regularly attending or appointing a representative to attend IPC committee meetings
	  ◦ appointing an IPC representative to attend and report on a clinical governance or quality control board or committee that the CEO also attends
	• Endorse the appointment of dedicated IPC roles, leadership responsibilities and accountabilities for staff
	• Ensure that IPC professionals have full access to required resources, such as workspace, technology, equipment, access and information, to achieve accreditation requirements and meet performance goals
	• Ensure the facility has an established IPC program that is fully resourced with equipment and staff, and is supported, monitored and regularly revised
	• Establish and commit to an IPC program which details the IPC objectives, priorities and targets within a given period. Goals should be specific and measurable and developed jointly with IPC professionals and other relevant stakeholders
	• Authorise IPC professionals to implement IPC program recommendations and to intervene when practices pose infection risks
	• Facilitate remedial action when IPC measures are compromised
	• Support an organisational culture that promotes individual responsibility for IPC among staff and that highlights the value of IPC to the safety of patients, healthcare workers and others

Continued

TABLE 6.2 Summary of the roles and responsibilities of the governing body, chief executive officer, infection control committee and infection control team in the clinical governance of IPC—cont'd

Role	Responsibilities
Infection control committee	• Establish a multidisciplinary team that includes members who have the expertise and the executive authority to inform and implement effective IPC systems and strategies • Review and approve the IPC plans and policies on a regular schedule • Assess and promote improved IPC practice at all levels of the facility • Ensure staff training in IPC • Direct and support the infection control team and other IPC professionals and ensure they have access to all required resources, supplies, data, information and access to address problems that are identified • Ensure availability of appropriate supplies needed for IPC • Review epidemiological surveillance data and identify areas for intervention • Review infection risks associated with new technologies and monitor risks of new devices and products, prior to their approval for use • Review and provide input into the process of conducting an outbreak investigation • Review and approve construction/renovation projects regarding infection prevention • Communicate and cooperate with other committees with common interests or in which IPC practices are integral
Infection control team	• Monitor and evaluate the day-to-day activities designed to prevent infection and ensure 24-hour access to IPC staff for advice on all aspects of IPC • Identify problems in the implementation of IPC activities that need to be solved or addressed by the ICC • Investigate outbreaks and use these incidents as opportunities to evaluate practice and identify areas for improvement • Organise regular meetings between all team members at least several times a week, and establish a reliable communication channel and documentation system • Develop a training plan to train and educate all levels of staff in IPC policy, practice and procedures relevant to their own areas • Ensure the facility-wide dissemination of IPC information and protocols, as well as regulations, rules and recommendations • Develop an annual plan with clear objectives, as well as formal policies and procedures, and design, coordinate, implement and continuously evaluate these plans and policies • Participate in audit activities, as well as compliance with accreditation, licensing, policy or regulatory requirements • Ensure the availability of supplies and equipment needed for IPC • Monitor the efficacy of sterilisation and disinfection measures • Collaborate with pharmacy and antibiotic committees to supervise antibiotic prescription and use • Obtain approval from the ICC to implement programs and to support and participate in research and assessment programs • Organise epidemiological surveillance data for infectious diseases, HAIs and antimicrobial use, and submit the data to relevant organisational bodies • Communicate with and submit regular reports on activities and outcomes to the ICC • Inform facility construction and design, patient placement ratios (e.g. single rooms, negative pressure rooms), environmental assessments and equipment and product evaluation • Seek and assimilate feedback from healthcare workers and consumers • Review team performance at least annually and ensure adequate opportunities for individual professional development are provided

practical components of IPC. The ICP is often a registered nurse. They operate as an advisor in all matters regarding IPC, are responsible for the day-to-day IPC activities and provide specialist input in the identification, prevention, monitoring and control of infection. They are heavily involved in the development, implementation and monitoring of IPC policies and procedures. Additionally, they participate in surveillance and outbreak investigation activities; identify and investigate hazardous practices; conduct training and educational programs; prepare documents related to service and quality standards; and are active members on committees where expert IPC advice is required.

Infection control link nurse or practitioner: Infection control link nurses and practitioners work closely with ICPs to ensure adequate IPC practices and education within other healthcare departments. Essentially, link nurses operate as an established point of contact between ICPs and the link nurses' own wards. The ICP helps the link nurse to identify problems in existing IPC practice, and to implement strategies and goals for improvement. Link nurses are subsequently responsible for monitoring, facilitating and encouraging good IPC practice among other ward staff, including activities like hand hygiene, PPE use and aseptic technique. The link nurse may take greater initiative and responsibility in attending to infection-related incidents, such as reporting infection; initiating patient isolation/precautions; ordering cultures of specimens from patients; identifying signs of infectious disease; and ensuring the adequacy of IPC supplies within the ward.

6.3 Accreditation

6.3.1 What is accreditation?

Accreditation is the process of ensuring that a service meets a set of standards. In healthcare, accreditation involves the review of the quality and safety of care and services provided, and is conducted by an independent reviewer on a three-year cycle. In addition to assessment, accreditation is also performed for the purpose of improving the quality and effectiveness of healthcare organisations and to publicly recognise that the organisation meets national quality standards.

6.3.2 A brief history of accreditation in Australia

Formal systems of accreditation were introduced in the United States (US) in the early 20th century to regulate the quality of hospital environments as suitable places to practise medicine and to establish structures for the maintenance of medical records.[7] Interest in the accreditation of healthcare soon followed in countries like Canada and Australia, with the Australian Medical Association (AMA) requesting funding from New South Wales, Victoria and New Zealand to conduct a study that sought to introduce a similar accreditation program in both countries.[8] However, this early initiative did not gain enough traction and further attempts to introduce accreditation in Australia did not begin until after World War II.

The Australian Hospital Association (AHA) was established in 1946 with the primary purpose of ensuring higher standards of healthcare and improved conditions for patients. Early objectives included establishing a medical record training program and, again, introducing a hospital grading system similar to what was used in the US. To emulate the progress in the US, the AHA invited the Royal Australasian College of Physicians (RACP) and the Royal Australasian College of Surgeons (RACS) to cooperate in developing the accreditation scheme. While a form of the accreditation process was implemented, it was voluntary and very few hospitals agreed to be graded and this initiative also dwindled.[8]

Beginning in 1959, independent strides to advance hospital accreditation were made by both the NSW AMA Committee and the Victorian AHA Committee. The NSW Branch of the AMA had successfully formed a conjoint board, which included representatives from the RACS, RACP and other medical colleges. The NSW AMA Committee developed a point scoring accreditation system for NSW hospitals, which was approved by the federal AMA Council to be trialled in selected teaching and city hospitals. At the same time, the Victorian AHA Committee established a subcommittee for accreditation, which was tasked with preparing recommendations for the implementation of hospital accreditation on a national scale. Joint action between the Victorian AHA Committee and the NSW AMA Committee led to the first standards for Australian hospitals to be drafted in 1963 and finalised in 1964.

A national joint steering committee on hospital accreditation with equal representation from both the AMA and AHA was established in 1968. This committee would later be renamed the Australian Hospital Standards Committee in 1972. Between 1973-74, financial support was secured from the federal government, which enabled the appointment of an executive director, and which gave further momentum to the accreditation program. Requests for the cooperation of all statutory health authorities in Australia in the accreditation program yielded lengthy negotiations pertaining to the composition of the national body and state representation. The Australian Council on Healthcare Standards (ACHS) was formally established in 1974, and remains one of several independent, national accrediting agencies operating to this day.

Sustained development in the accreditation process within Australia has occurred since the 1970s, evolving from a voluntary process of participation to a requirement for licensing healthcare services. Throughout this evolution, the requirements on health services have become increasingly more prescribed until the national standards were produced, and preexisting accreditation organisations were approved to assess the health service organisations in terms of their compliance with the standards. The introduction of national standards was most prominently catalysed following the release of the seminal results of the Quality in Australian Health Care Study (QAHCS) in 1995, which reported that up to 51% of the adverse events in hospital admissions were considered preventable.[9]

This swiftly led to the establishment of the Taskforce on Quality in Australian Health Care and the introduction of a number of recommendations, although many of them were not fully implemented. This was then followed by the National Expert Advisory Group on Safety and Quality in Australian Health Care in 1998, which recommended 10 national actions, and then the Australian Council for Safety and Quality in Health Care in 2002.[10] The Council became the Commission (ACSQHC) at the end of its original five-year term and was given a further five years before being established as a permanent entity under the *National Health and Hospitals Network Act 2011* and the *National Health Reform Act 2011*. In the same year, the Australian Health Ministers approved the Australian Health Service Safety and Quality Accreditation (AHSSQA) Scheme, which mandated that all Australian hospitals and day procedure centres needed to be accredited. In September 2011, the first edition of the Commission's NSQHS Standards was submitted and approved, and formal accreditation against these standards began in 2013. The NSQHS Standards are described in more detail in the final section of this chapter.

As of present day, all public and private hospitals, day procedure services and most public dental practices in Australia must be accredited. Other healthcare facilities not mandated may also voluntarily choose to be

accredited to be accountable for the quality of services they provide. The formal accreditation process is described in the following section.

6.3.3 How healthcare organisations are accredited

Healthcare organisations are assessed by external agencies to show they meet the requirements of the NSQHS Standards. Healthcare organisations that fail to meet the Standards, and that are unable to demonstrate improvements within 60 business days, are subject to various sanctions, such as loss of licences and funding. Table 6.3 summarises the government bodies that regulate accreditation within each state and territory.

Overall, to become accredited, a health service organisation must:
• implement the actions in the NSQHS Standards in their organisation
• routinely conduct self-assessment processes to determine if each of the actions in the NSQHS Standards are being met
• participate in an onsite assessment conducted by an independent accrediting agency, approved by the Commission; and

TABLE 6.3 The state and territory government bodies that regulate accreditation, as provided by the ACSQHC[11]

State	NSQHS Standards Accreditation Body
ACT	Health Protection Service (all)
NSW	Clinical Excellence Commission (public, DPS, DS), Private Health Care Unit (private)
NT	Department of Health (all)
QLD	Patient Safety and Quality Improvement Service (public, DPS), Private Health Regulation (private, DPS)
SA	Safety and Quality (public, DPS, DS), Health Licensing Unit (private, DPS)
TAS	Department of Health Regulation (all)
VIC	Commissioning, Performance and Regulation (public), Dental Health Services (DS), Private Hospitals, Health Service Performance and Programs (private, DPS)
WA	Licensing and Accreditation Regulatory Unit (all)

Source: Based on Australian Commission on Safety and Quality in Health Care. State and territory health department contact details Sydney: ACSQHC; [cited 5 Sep 2022]. Available from: https://www.safetyandquality.gov.au/standards/nsqhs-standards/assessment-nsqhs-standards/state-and-territory-health-department-contact-details.

- take steps to address shortcomings in cases where the accrediting agency has found actions related to specific NSQHS Standards that have not been met.

Approved accreditation agencies: Accreditation assessments are conducted by independent accrediting agencies, approved by the Commission, as part of the AHSSQA Scheme. The Commission approves accrediting agencies to assess health services against the NSQHS Standards under the Australian Health Service Safety and Quality Accreditation Scheme. Health service organisations need to engage an approved accrediting agency to conduct their assessment against the NSQHS Standards. As of January 2023, the following agencies are approved to assess health service organisations to the specified sets of standards.[12]

- Australian Council on Healthcare Standards (ACHS)
- Certification Partner Global (CPG)
- Global-Mark Pty Ltd

- HDAA Australia Pty Ltd
- Institute for Healthy Communities Australia Certification (IHCAC) Pty Ltd
- Quality Innovation Performance (QIP) Limited.

Prior to initiating the assessment process, accrediting agencies must ensure several requirements are met. These include establishing an effective assessment process by appointing a lead assessor, who is qualified and able to manage and coordinate the assessment process. All assessors must be adequately trained and equipped with assessment methodologies, including *PICMoRS* (Process; Improvement; Consumer participation; Monitoring; Reporting; and Systems) (Table 6.4), the Commission's technical tools and resources, and documentation protocols. They must also regularly participate in and complete the accreditation agency's relevant courses and training. The context and scope of the healthcare facility being assessed should also inform the size and mix of the assessors that are appointed, such as those who have experience working in the area, as well as to identify the patient groups and key safety and quality systems involved.[13,14]

TABLE 6.4 The PICMoRS method assessors use to structure and standardise the accreditation process

Abbreviation		Description
P	Process	The assessor seeks an explanation of the process being reviewed. This information enables an assessor to determine if actual practice matches the practice as described in the policy and procedures. This information allows the assessor to: • identify the person/s involved in the process and who should be interviewed • understand the multiple elements of a process • identify where the process is being applied and documented • understand how the workforce is kept up to date on changes to the process
I	Improvement strategies	The assessor determines if the organisation has reviewed the effectiveness of the process and whether any improvements have been implemented. Where improvements have been introduced, an assessor seeks to clearly establish: • the rationale for change • how the workforce has been made aware of changes • the implementation strategies used • how effective the strategies and changes are. Where no improvements have been made, the assessor determines: • if the process is effective • if monitoring is in place to ensure it is still fit for purpose • if the organisation is not aware of the process or need for change
C	Consumer participation	The assessor evaluates consumer participation in safety and quality systems and processes, including their own care. Participation will vary depending on the safety and quality process evaluated. In the context of the Clinical Governance Standard, this may involve engaging with consumers in the design, monitoring and evaluation of services within a program, department or the organisation. It may involve being a full member of a quality improvement and redesign team, or providing input through focus groups, feedback mechanisms, surveys or social media

Continued

TABLE 6.4 The PICMoRS method assessors use to structure and standardise the accreditation process—cont'd

Abbreviation		Description
Mo	Monitoring	The assessor examines the extent and type of monitoring a health service organisation conducts on its safety and quality processes and considers how this information is used to plan, deliver and improve patient care. Effective monitoring enables health service organisations to: • evaluate the effectiveness of existing safety and quality processes and the effectiveness of changes that are introduced • identify areas of under-performance and high-performance • prioritise areas for improvement • measure changes over time. Information gained allows the assessor to understand: • what monitoring occurs • the frequency, sample size, scope and currency of data collection • who is involved in these processes
R	Reporting	The assessor determines where and how collected information is reported. Reporting processes may be internal, occurring to and from a service area, direct line managers or committees, and executives and the governing body. It may also involve external reporting to consumers, the community and other health services. Information gained allows the assessor to determine: • where the information on the process is reported and where it is documented • the frequency of reporting • the population the information is reported to • whether feedback is provided on the information reported
S	Safety and quality systems	The assessor examines the efficacy and efficiency of safety and quality systems. Processes, such as collecting outcomes data, should inform other relevant systems, such as policy and training systems. The assessor should understand: • how the information from one process is being used to change, inform and/or improve other processes • how the connectedness between systems is being documented

Furthermore, the accrediting agency must ensure that no conflicts of interest exist between the assessors, the agency and the healthcare organisations. Contracts with healthcare organisations should explicitly allow for Commission staff to observe onsite assessments, confirm submission of data to the Commission and provide public reporting of accreditation outcomes. Assessors should only assess standards that are approved for assessment concurrently with the NSQHS Standards. Any other standards that are assessed must be completed after assessment of the NSQHS Standards. Upon arrival for onsite assessment, accrediting agencies must ensure that at least 60% of assessment time is spent in clinical practice and operational areas, and that no longer than 30 minutes is spent during the introductory meeting prior to starting the assessment.[14]

Accreditation schedules: From 1 January 2019 to time of writing, the revised AHSSQA Scheme introduced the second edition of the NSQHS Standards, as well as two accreditation pathways:

• *Planned assessment:* one assessment every three years by an approved accrediting agency of all NSQHS Standards; and

• *Short notice assessment:* three short notice assessments are performed by an approved accrediting agency within the three-year cycle and all NSQHS Standards will be assessed within the three-year cycle, with no more than two assessments in any given year. Each assessment reviews three or four NSQHS Standards and up to four may be assessed more than once during the cycle. Healthcare organisations are to receive at least 48 hours' notice of the pending assessment date and which NSQHS Standards are to be assessed.

Accreditation assessment process: Under the planned assessment pathway, the assessment process occurs once every three years and is conducted over a period of one to four months. This involves an initial assessment, as well as a final assessment in cases where a healthcare organisation does not meet all the actions during the initial assessment.

An accreditation assessment involves an onsite visit by assessors who look for evidence that each action in the Standards has been implemented. During an accreditation assessment, assessors use a well-defined method of reviewing each safety and quality process described in the NSQHS Standards. Assessors examine evidence of actual performance by reviewing hospital performance data, documentation and records, observing clinical practice, inspecting resources, testing high-risk scenarios and interviewing the workforce, patients and consumers. Assessors use the *PICMoRS* method to ensure a structured, standardised assessment process. All six parts of the *PICMoRS* method must be completed to conduct a comprehensive assessment of the safety and quality processes being examined.

Assessors rate the NSQHS Standards actions implemented by health service organisations using a standardised rating scale of 'Met', 'Not Met' and 'Met with Recommendations' (Table 6.5). Under certain circumstances, it may also be appropriate to apply ratings of 'Not Applicable' and 'Not Assessed'.

Assessment outcomes: Following the initial assessment, accreditation is awarded based on whether the healthcare organisation has met all the actions in the Standards. The healthcare organisation is provided with a final report of assessment outcomes, at which time they may engage in an appeal process and submit the necessary documents

TABLE 6.5 Each action on the NSQHS Standards is assessed and then rated using the rating scale described

Rating	Description
Met	All requirements are fully met
Met with recommendations	The requirements of an action are largely met across the health service organisation, with the exception of a minor part of the action in a specific service or location in the organisation, where the additional implementation is required
Not met	Part or all of the requirements of the action have not been met
Not applicable	The action is not relevant in the service context being assessed. The Commission's advisory relating to 'not applicable' actions for the health sector needs to be taken into consideration when awarding a 'not applicable' rating and assessors must confirm the action is not relevant in the service context during the assessment visit
Not assessed	Actions that are not part of the current assessment process and therefore not reviewed

to the accrediting agency. If a health service organisation has shown it meets all the NSQHS Standards (or more specifically, that less than 16% of actions are not met, or less than eight actions from the Clinical Governance Standard are not met), accreditation is awarded, and the healthcare organisation will be assessed at the next scheduled assessment in three years. Healthcare organisations that are accredited typically display a certificate or accreditation award at the front entrance of the facility or a public waiting area. The certificate states that the organisation has been assessed against, and successfully meets, the requirements of the NSQHS Standards.

However, if the healthcare organisation has actions that are not met after the initial assessment, it is given a remediation period to address the safety and quality issues and to implement appropriate strategies to meet these actions. These are then reviewed by assessors at the final assessment and if sufficient change has been made, accreditation is awarded. If at the final assessment the action is still not met, the health service organisation is not awarded accreditation. Various sanctions apply depending on the extent and type of actions that have not been met. These sanctions may include administrative oversight by the regulator, loss of licences and/or loss of funding. Any healthcare organisation that does not achieve accreditation must undergo a reassessment to all eight NSQHS Standards within 12 months to be allowed to continue to operate.

6.4 Infection prevention and control standards

The ACSQHC was officially established by the Council of Australian Governments in 2006 to coordinate national improvements in the safety and quality of healthcare. As previously mentioned, this led to the release of the first edition of the NSQHS Standards in 2011, and the beginning of the formal accreditation of healthcare organisations in 2013.[15] The Standards were developed in collaboration with the Australian Government, states and territories, private sector providers, clinical experts, patients and carers. The second and current edition of the Standards was released in 2017 and began formal assessment in 2019. This edition was later updated in 2021 following the COVID-19 pandemic to incorporate specific measures for responding to infectious disease outbreaks, epidemics, pandemics and the emergence of novel pathogens.[16] The current publication is comprised of eight standards that together aim to 'protect the public from harm and to improve the quality of health service provision' (Table 6.6).

TABLE 6.6 The eight National Safety and Quality Health Service Standards (2nd ed)

Standard	Scope
Clinical governance[17]	Ensuring the implementation of a clinical governance framework so health service organisations can better maintain and improve the reliability, safety and quality of healthcare and improve health outcomes
Partnering with consumers[18]	Establishing systems for person-centred healthcare that ensures patients and consumers are involved in their own care and decision making
Preventing and controlling infections[2]	Reducing the risk of acquiring preventable infections to patients, consumers and the workforce, effectively managing the infections that do occur, and promoting appropriate antimicrobial use and stewardship
Medication safety[19]	Ensuring that clinicians safely prescribe, dispense and administer medication and that consumers understand their own medicine needs and risks
Comprehensive care[20]	Integrating screening, assessment and risk identification processes for developing a care plan to minimise risk of harm to patients and ensuring care is aligned with the patient's expressed goals and healthcare needs
Communicating for safety[21]	Ensuring effective and timely communication and documentation between patients, clinicians and the wider healthcare organisation across all stages of care
Blood management[22]	Improving patient outcomes through the safe and effective care of patients' blood and the appropriate administration of blood supplies/products
Recognising and responding to acute deterioration[23]	Responding promptly and effectively to physical, mental or cognitive deterioration

The Preventing and Controlling Infections Standard[2] is the most relevant in the context of IPC, and comprises four main criteria:

1. clinical governance and quality improvement systems to prevent and control infections and support antimicrobial stewardship and sustainable use of IPC resources
2. infection prevention and control systems
3. reprocessing reusable equipment and devices; and
4. antimicrobial stewardship.

Additionally, the Clinical Governance Standard[17] and Partnering with Consumers Standard[18] also play important roles and both are incorporated within the Preventing and Controlling Infections Standard. This Standard was originally named the Preventing and Controlling Healthcare-Associated Infection Standard in the first edition of the publication, as well as in the original release of the second edition. The name was changed to its current form following the 2021, post-pandemic revision.

The Preventing and Controlling Infections Standard is to be used in tandem with the Australian Guidelines for the Prevention and Control of Infection in Healthcare,[24] which is a comprehensive, evidence-based national infection prevention and control guideline released by the NHMRC and the ACSQHC in 2019. These guidelines are directly referenced and linked by the Standards and serve as an invaluable foundation for

healthcare organisations to inform and develop effective IPC procedures and protocols. The adequate implementation of a number of items within the Preventing and Controlling Infections Standard, such as the use of standard and transmission-based precautions and invasive medical devices, relies heavily on these guidelines.

See Table 6.7 for a detailed summary of each criterion and item listed in the Preventing and Controlling Infections Standard.[2]

Conclusion

The effective implementation of IPC plans and programs, as well as the consistent and correct practice of IPC protocols, cannot occur in isolation without individual clinicians and healthcare workers. This issue becomes increasingly pertinent as the size of a healthcare organisation increases, leading to more staff, more patients and more opportunities for poor IPC adherence and an increased risk of infection and outbreaks. Clinical governance and the establishment of dedicated IPC structures, systems and roles are essential in ensuring that IPC programs are effective at preventing healthcare-associated infections and the spread of infectious disease. Good IPC should underpin action and practice at all levels of the healthcare system, from the person holding the highest office, to the clinicians, nurses and auxiliary hospital staff who attend and interact with patients on a day-to-day basis.

TABLE 6.7 Summary of the NHQHS Standards: Preventing and Controlling Infections Standard[2]

Criteria	Aim	Item	Action	Summary
1. Clinical governance and quality improvement systems are in place to prevent and control infections, and support antimicrobial stewardship and sustainable use of infection prevention and control resources	To ensure clinical governance and quality improvement systems exist for the specific purpose of infection prevention and control and antimicrobial stewardship	Integrating clinical governance	3.01	Use the safety and quality systems from the Clinical Governance Standard[17] when: • implementing IPC policies and procedures and antimicrobial stewardship • identifying and managing IPC risks and antimicrobial stewardship
			3.02	The health service organisation: • establishes multidisciplinary teams to identify and manage IPC risks and antimicrobial stewardship • identifies requirements for, and provides workforce with the training, capacity, skills and resources, for IPC and antimicrobial stewardship • plans for public health and pandemic risks
		Applying quality improvement systems	3.03	Apply the quality improvement system from the Clinical Governance Standard[17] when: • monitoring the performance of IPC systems and the effectiveness of antimicrobial stewardship • implementing strategies to improve IPC systems and antimicrobial stewardship outcomes • reporting to all relevant stakeholders on the performance of IPC systems and antimicrobial stewardship outcomes • supporting and monitoring the use of IPC resources
		Partnering with consumers	3.04	Use the organisational processes consistent with the Partnering with Consumers Standard[18] when assessing risks, implementing IPC and antimicrobial stewardship systems to: • involve patients in their own care • meeting patients' information needs • share decision making
		Surveillance	3.05	Has a surveillance strategy for infections, infection risk and antimicrobial use that: • incorporates national and jurisdictional information in a timely manner • collects organisational-level HAI, infection and antimicrobial use data, using this data to reduce infection risks, to report to relevant stakeholders and to monitor responsiveness to risks

Continued

TABLE 6.7 Summary of the NHQHS Standards: Preventing and Controlling Infections Standard—cont'd

Criteria	Aim	Item	Action	Summary
2. Infection prevention and control systems	To ensure that evidence-based systems have been adopted and implemented to facilitate effective IPC	Standard and transmission-based precautions	3.06	Has processes to apply standard and transmission-based precautions that are consistent with the Australian Guidelines for the Prevention and Control of Infection in Healthcare,[1] jurisdictional requirements, laws and policies, and work health and safety laws
			3.07	Has processes for: • the assessment and communication of infection risks to patients and the workforce • IPC systems to reduce transmission of infections • the appropriate use and implementation of personal protective equipment • monitoring and responding to changes in knowledge about infections, relevant national or jurisdictional guidance, policy and legislation • auditing compliance, assessing workforce competence in and improving compliance with standard and transmission-based precautions
			3.08	Members of the workforce apply standard precautions and transmission-based precautions whenever required, and consider: • patients' risks • existing or a preexisting colonisation or infection with organisms of local or national significance • patient accommodation needs to prevent and manage infection risks • risks to the wellbeing of patients in isolation • environmental control measures to reduce risk • precautions required when a patient is transferred internally or externally • the need for additional environmental cleaning or disinfection processes • the type of procedure being performed • equipment required for routine care
			3.09	Has processes to: • review and respond to infections in the community that may affect patients and/or the workforce • communicate details of a patient's infectious status during an episode of care, and at transitions of care • provide relevant information to a patient, their family and carers about their infectious status, infection risks and the nature and duration of precautions to minimise the spread of infection
		Hand hygiene	3.10	Has a hand hygiene program incorporated in its IPC program and: • is consistent with the current National Hand Hygiene Initiative and jurisdictional requirements • addresses non-compliance with national hand hygiene benchmarks • reports on the results of hand hygiene compliance audits and subsequent action to relevant stakeholders • uses audits to improve hand hygiene compliance

Criteria	Aim	Item	Action	Summary
		Aseptic technique	3.11	Has processes for aseptic technique that: • identify the procedures in which aseptic technique applies • assess the competence of the workforce in performing aseptic technique • provide training to address gaps in competency • monitor compliance with the organisation's policies on aseptic technique
		Invasive medical devices	3.12	Has processes for the appropriate use and management of invasive medical devices that are consistent with the Australian Guidelines for the Prevention and Control of Infection in Healthcare[1]
		Clean and safe environment	3.13	Has processes to maintain a clean, safe and hygienic environment, consistent with the Australian Guidelines for the Prevention and Control of Infection in Healthcare[1] and jurisdictional requirements, to: • respond to environmental risks • require using products listed on the Australian Register of Therapeutic Goods, consistent with manufacturers' instructions and frequencies • provide training on cleaning processes for routine and outbreak situations • audit the effectiveness of cleaning practice and compliance with environmental cleaning policy • use audits to improve environmental cleaning processes and compliance
			3.14	Has processes to evaluate and respond to infection risks for: • new and existing equipment, devices and products used • clinical and non-clinical areas, and workplace amenity areas • maintenance, repair and upgrade of buildings, equipment, furnishings and fittings • handling, transporting and storing linen • novel infections, and risks identified as part of a public health response or pandemic planning
			3.15	Has a risk-based workforce vaccine-preventable diseases (VPDs) screening and immunisation policy and program that: • is consistent with the Australian Immunisation Handbook • is consistent with jurisdictional requirements for VPDs • addresses specific risks to the workforce, consumers and patients
			3.16	Has risk-based processes for preventing and managing infections in the workforce that: • are consistent with the Australian Guidelines for the Prevention and Control of Infection in Healthcare[1] and jurisdictional regulations • align with jurisdictional requirements for workforce screening and exclusion • manage risks to the workforce and patients • promote non-attendance at facilities when infection is suspected or actual • monitor and manage the movement of staff between clinical areas, care settings, amenity areas and healthcare organisations • manage and support isolation and quarantine practices following exposure • provide for outbreak monitoring, investigation and management • ensures ongoing service provision during outbreaks and pandemics

Continued

TABLE 6.7 Summary of the NHQHS Standards: Preventing and Controlling Infections Standard—cont'd

Criteria	Aim	Item	Action	Summary
3. Reprocessing of reusable equipment and devices	To ensure that the reprocessing of reusable equipment meets current best practice	Reprocessing of reusable equipment and devices	3.17	Has processes for: • reprocessing that are consistent with relevant national and international standards, and with manufacturers' guidelines • tracing the use of critical and semi-critical equipment, instruments and devices that are capable of identifying ◦ the patient ◦ the procedure ◦ the reusable equipment, instruments and devices that were used for the procedure • planning and managing reprocessing requirements, and additional controls for novel and emerging infections
4. Antimicrobial stewardship	To ensure that systems are in place for the safe and appropriate prescribing and use of antimicrobials	Antimicrobial stewardship	3.18	Has an antimicrobial stewardship program that: • includes an antimicrobial stewardship policy • provides access and promotes the use of current evidence-based Australian guidelines and resources on antimicrobial prescribing • has an antimicrobial formulary that is informed by current evidence, restriction rules and approval processes • incorporates core elements, recommendations and principles from the current antimicrobial stewardship clinical care standard[25] • uses audits to promote continuous quality improvement
			3.19	The antimicrobial stewardship program: • reviews antimicrobial prescribing and use • uses surveillance data to support appropriate prescribing • evaluates performance of the program, identifying areas for improvement and taking action to improve • reports to relevant bodies on: ◦ compliance with policy ◦ areas of action for antimicrobial resistance ◦ areas requiring improvement, based on current evidence and resources ◦ performance over time for use and appropriateness of use

Good governance structures not only ensure effective IPC practice, but that systems are in place to continuously monitor, develop and improve the quality of existing practice, as well as identify potential infection-related issues and risks before they can happen. It also ensures the recognition and integration of feedback from all levels and areas of the workforce and from consumers, and the seamless adoption and implementation of research and evidence based strategies. The demonstration of effective clinical governance is a prerequisite for hospitals to receive accreditation—a now mandatory requirement that is enforced by national legislation and which holds hospitals accountable for the quality and safety of the services they provide.

Useful websites/resources

- National Health and Medical Research Council. Australian Guidelines for the Prevention and Control of Infection in Healthcare. https://www.nhmrc.gov.au
- Australian Commission on Safety and Quality in Health Care. Preventing and Controlling infections standard. https://www.safetyandquality.gov.au/infection-prevention-and-control

References

1. National Health and Medical Research Council. Australian guidelines for the prevention and control of infection in healthcare. Canberra: Australian Government, 2019.
2. Australian Commission on Safety and Quality in Health Care. National safety and quality health service standards 2nd ed. Preventing and controlling infections standard. Sydney: ACSQHC, 2021.
3. Australian Commission on Safety and Quality in Health Care, editor. National model clinical governance framework. Sydney: ACSQHC, 2017.
4. Rasslan O. Organisational structure. In: Friedman C, Newsom W, eds. IFIC basic concepts of infection control, 3rd ed. Portadown: International Federation of Infection Control, 2016.
5. Halton K, Hall L, Gardner A, MacBeth D, Mitchell BG. Exploring the context for effective clinical governance in infection control. Am J Infect Control. 2017;45(3):278-283.
6. Hogg S, Baird N, Richards J, Hughes S, Nolan J, Jones A, et al. Developing surgical site infection surveillance within clinical governance. Clinical Governance: An International Journal. 2005.
7. McPhail R, Avery M, Fisher R, Fitzgerald A, Fulop L. The changing face of healthcare accreditation in Australia. Asia Pacific Journal of Health Management. 2015;10(2):58-64.
8. Duckett S. Assuring hospital standards: the introduction of hospital accreditation in Australia. Australian Journal of Public Administration. 1983;42(3):385-402.
9. Wilson RM, Runciman WB, Gibberd RW, Harrison BT, Newby L, Hamilton JD. The quality in Australian health care study. Med J Aust. 1995;163(9):458-471.
10. Smallwood RA. The safety and quality of health care: from council to commission. Med J Aust. 2006;184(S10): S39-S40.
11. Australian Commission on Safety and Quality in Health Care. State and territory health department contact details [Internet]. Sydney: ACSQHC, 2022 [cited 5 Sept 2022]. Available from: https://www.safetyandquality.gov.au/standards/nsqhs-standards/assessment-nsqhs-standards/state-and-territory-health-department-contact-details.
12. Australian Commission on Safety and Quality in Health Care. Approved accrediting agencies contact details [Internet]. Sydney: ACSQHC, 2022, [cited 5 Sept 2022]. Available from: https://www.safetyandquality.gov.au/standards/nsqhs-standards/assessment-nsqhs-standards/approved-accrediting-agencies-contact-details.
13. Australian Commission on Safety and Quality in Health Care. Fact Sheet 12: Assessment framework for safety and quality systems. Sydney: ACSQHC, 2020.
14. Australian Commission on Safety and Quality in Health Care. Responsibilities of your accrediting agency. Sydney: ACSQHC, 2020.
15. Australian Commission on Safety and Quality in Health Care (ACSQHC). National safety and quality health service standards (NSQHS). 1st ed. Sydney: ACSQHC, 2011.
16. Australian Commission on Safety and Quality in Health Care (ACSQHC). National safety and quality health service standards. 2nd ed. Version 2. NSQHS. Sydney: ACSQHC, 2021.
17. Australian Commission on Safety and Quality in Health Care. National safety and quality health service standards. 2nd ed. Clinical governance standard. Sydney: ACSQHC, 2021.
18. Australian Commission on Safety and Quality in Health Care. National safety and quality health service standards. 2nd ed. Partnering with consumers standard. Sydney: ACSQHC, 2021.
19. Australian Commission on Safety and Quality in Health Care. National safety and quality health service standards. 2nd ed. Medication safety standard. Sydney: ACSQHC, 2021.
20. Australian Commission on Safety and Quality in Health Care. National safety and quality health service standards. 2nd ed. Comprehensive care standard. Sydney: ACSQHC, 2021.
21. Australian Commission on Safety and Quality in Health Care. National safety and quality health service standards. 2nd ed. Communicating for safety standard. Sydney: ACSQHC, 2021.
22. Australian Commission on Safety and Quality in Health Care. National safety and quality health service standards. 2nd ed. Blood management standard. Sydney: ACSQHC, 2021.
23. Australian Commission on Safety and Quality in Health Care. National safety and quality health service standards. 2nd ed. Recognising and responding to acute deterioration standard. Sydney: ACSQHC, 2021.
24. National Health and Medical Research Council (NHMRC) and Australian Commission on Safety and Quality in Health Care (ACSQHC). Australian guidelines for the prevention and control of infection in healthcare. Canberra: Australian Government, 2019.
25. Australian Commission on Safety and Quality in Health Care. Antimicrobial stewardship clinical care standard. Sydney: ACSQHC, 2020.

CHAPTER 7

Risk assessment and management in infection prevention and control

Dr DEBOROUGH MACBETH[i]

PROFESSOR DALE DOMINEY-HOWES[ii]

Chapter highlights

- Risk is defined in terms of both its likelihood and impact
- The application of risk management principles to infection prevention and control (IPC) is described and demonstrated
- The Risk Assessment and Management Framework is both an *approach* and a *tool*
- Risk assessment and management is a whole-of-organisation responsibility but the culture of risk management should be set by and led from the Executive
- All members of an organisation have a role in, and responsibility for, risk management

i   Infection Control, Gold Coast Hospital and Health Service, Southport, QLD
ii School of Geosciences, The University of Sydney, Sydney, NSW

Introduction

The infection control professional (ICP) role exists to prevent and control infection in healthcare services. This can only be achieved if the infection risks are identified, and rational control measures are implemented. The effectiveness of control measures must be monitored and reviewed so that gaps and deficits can be identified, and strategies revised and refined.

According to the Australian Standard Risk Management Guidelines, risk is defined as 'the effect of uncertainty on objectives'.[1] Risk is everywhere and is associated with all manner of activities, situations and challenges. Risk has accompanied humanity on our species' journey through history and while, undoubtedly, risk to human life is problematic, risk itself need not be overwhelming. Risk is the companion to advancement, modernity and the technologies and opportunities of the modern age.[2] At a broader level and well understood within the wider risk sciences, risk can never be zero. Zero risk is virtually impossible to achieve for a variety of reasons, but in reality, one of the most significant barriers is cost. It can be prohibitively expensive to reduce risk to near zero. While it is conceptually important to understand this fundamental point, an inability to reduce risk to zero is not of itself problematic.

Risk assessment and management is a mechanism to identify and control the risk of harm or deviation from the desired or expected outcome of an activity. In Australia, risk experts have come to agree on a standard structure and approach to risk assessment and management.[1] It is sufficiently simple in form but robust enough that it is used in all manner of industries, organisations, sectors and systems, and is applied to a wide range of 'risks' to life as diverse as natural and technological hazards (e.g. earthquakes and motor vehicle accidents) as well as to health-related issues, such as infection, in both humans and animals. It is both an 'approach' and a 'tool' that has application to risk problems in all domains of interest.

In human and animal health it is used to identify risks and develop control measures designed to mitigate them. One important application is to provide a systematic approach to the prevention and control of healthcare-associated infection (HAI). Inherent in its use for infection prevention and control (IPC) are policy and procedure development; staff training and education; and monitoring and reporting the outcomes of implemented risk management strategies.[3]

Like many technical areas, depending on your training, perspective, roles and responsibilities, a concept like 'risk' can be contested. Broadly speaking though, in the wider family of 'risk sciences', risk has two separate and interconnected definitions and meanings. First, risk is considered in terms of the mathematical or statistical probability of something, an event, occurring—for example an infection. Therefore, we define risk as a probability. For example, there is a 1:5 chance/probability (or 20% chance/probability) that a patient will contract a specific infection. The other, equally valid definition of risk relates to 'impact', or the consequences of a risk event of a specific magnitude. That is, in relation to that infection risk is a consequence—for example, mortality or morbidity. For major events, such as the COVID-19 pandemic, risk consequence ripples out across connected, health socio-economic systems to include such impacts as loss of individual income or a nation's gross domestic product, unemployment, increases in stress and poorer mental health, or increasing family violence.

Having noted these two interconnected definitions and meanings of risk, here and for the rest of this chapter, risk is defined as the 'effect of uncertainty on objectives' and can be expressed as 'risk sources, potential events, their consequences, and their likelihood'.[1] Risk management refers to activities designed to control the effect of uncertainty in order to achieve a desired outcome.

According to the Australian Risk Management Guidelines, risk assessment and management must incorporate the following specific elements to be effective:

- integration and customisation of risk management throughout an organisation
- involvement of all relevant stakeholders
- adaptability to meet changing needs and challenges
- consideration of human and cultural factors
- continuous improvement; and
- a structured approach.[1]

These elements are shown in Figure 7.1. In relation to IPC in human health, risk assessment and management requires a comprehensive, context-specific IPC program or plan that is designed to:

1. identify the infection risks inherent in the delivery of the healthcare service
2. develop and implement strategies and activities to mitigate the risks; and
3. evaluate the outcomes to determine whether, and to what extent the risk mitigation strategies have been successful.

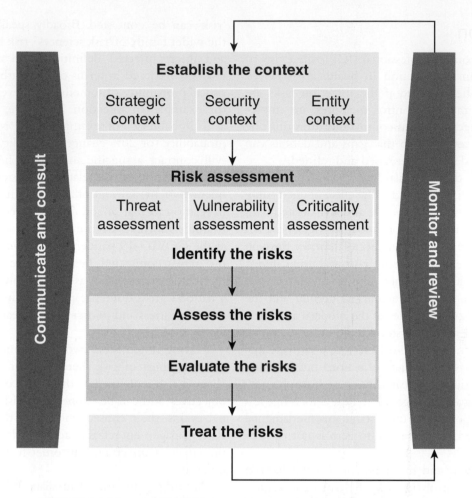

FIGURE 7.1 The simplified risk assessment and management framework
Source: Australian Government, 2014[4]

This entire process is iterative and cyclical, and re-quires continuous communication between all relevant stakeholders and ongoing adjustment as more is learnt about the risk as responsible stakeholders work through this process.

The remainder of this chapter describes and provides examples of the application of risk assessment and man-agement principles to the mitigation of infection risks in the delivery of healthcare in Australia. While the focus is on Australia (in line with this publication), the principles discussed apply equally in other countries.

7.1 The healthcare context

Healthcare in Australia is delivered in a range of settings including office-based practices (dental and general practice clinics); day surgery hospitals; rural, regional and metropolitan hospitals both publicly and privately funded; residential aged care facilities; community clinics;

onsite occupational health clinics; and in patients' homes. Infection risk is not only dependent on the healthcare setting but also on the acuity and comorbidities of the patient and the skill and knowledge of the healthcare provider, as well as a range of other factors.[3]

Healthcare is delivered within the boundaries of service accreditation, legislative requirements, and national standards and guidelines. Australia benefits from a rigorous set of national standards provided by the National Safety and Quality Health Service (NSQHS) (see Useful websites/resources at the end of this chapter). From an infection control perspective, accreditation of a service or facility is based on the ability to demonstrate compliance with a range of cri-teria described in the NSQHS Preventing and Con-trolling Infections Standard (Fig 7.2).[5] This Standard provides a risk management approach to IPC and can be used as a basis for developing a comprehensive program.

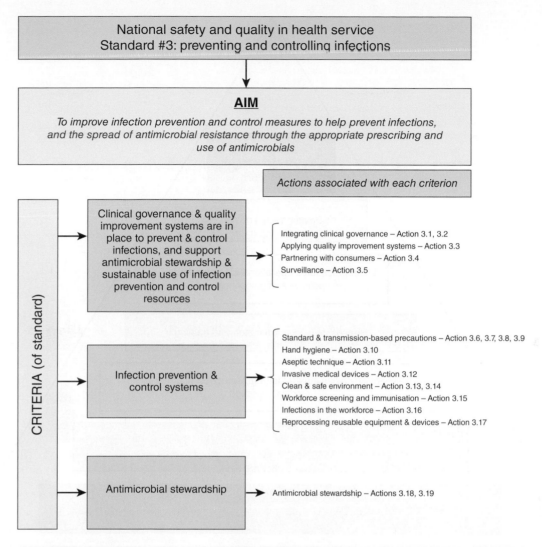

FIGURE 7.2 A schematic of the NSQHS Preventing and Controlling Infections Standard

Source: Based on Australian Commission on Safety and Quality in Health Care. Preventing and Controlling Healthcare-Associated Infection Standard 2019. Available from: https://www.safetyandquality.gov.au/standards/nsqhs-standards/preventing-and-controlling-healthcare-associated-infection-standard.

7.1.1 Potential infection risks

Infection has been identified as one of the potential adverse outcomes of healthcare.[6] In the course of delivering healthcare services there are multiple potential sources of infection. The primary focus of any healthcare service is the patient, and the patient is at risk of infection through:

- invasive procedures performed and devices inserted during the healthcare encounter
- environmental factors
- contact with healthcare providers who may themselves be the source of infection
- fomites, i.e. an inanimate object or surface that can act as a contaminated source of infection and

which has contact with the susceptible host—or any other object not sterilised but present in the healthcare setting that comes into contact with the patient.[7-10]

Patient factors, such as decreased immunity due to a disease process or therapy, specific patient behaviours or poor infection control knowledge, may also contribute to the risk of infection. However, healthcare-acquired infection, by definition, requires the infection to be the result of some healthcare intervention.

Consequently, to assist all relevant stakeholders working and participating in the healthcare setting where patients are present, a hierarchical structure is in place. This includes policies, plans and procedures from the national

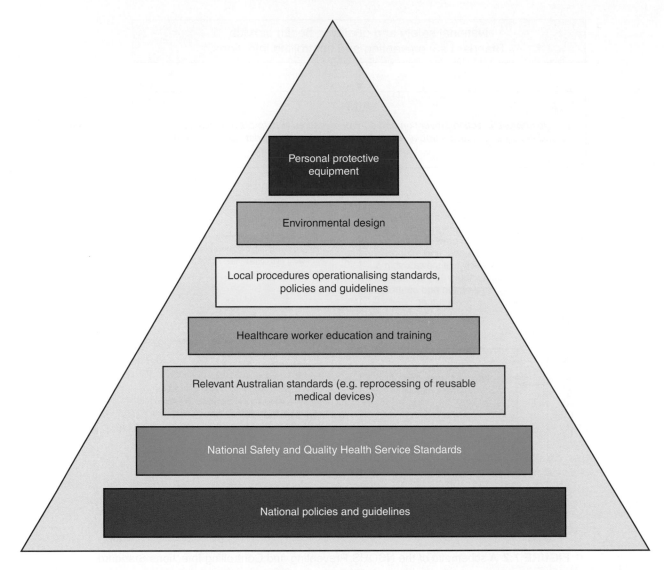

FIGURE 7.3 Risk pyramid of infection prevention and control with indicative risk management strategies listed at each level

level down to infection control plans inside individual wards that are designed and scaffolded together to facilitate IPC via a risk assessment and management process using a 'risk pyramid' (Fig 7.3). This approach aims for a plan that is customised, inclusive, dynamic and based on the best available information. The plan will incorporate cultural and human factors and focus on continuous improvement.

7.2 Governance

In accordance with the principles of risk assessment and management, integration of the IPC program must encompass the entirety of the organisation's health service. While ultimate responsibility for the safety of the service and the quality of care provided rests with the Executive of the organisation, it is incumbent on the Executive to ensure all members of the organisation are aware of their responsibility for identifying and managing risks. The governance system in which responsibility and accountability for minimising risks and continuously improving the quality of care is shared among all, is one that ensures integration of the program into the organisational culture.[11] To achieve this level of integration, the Executive must mandate the importance of the program as a key component of an organisational culture of safety, provide the resources required to implement the program, ensure everyone in the organisation is aware of their personal responsibilities, and provide appropriate training and skills development to deliver infection control outcomes.[3]

7.2.1 Mandating safety

Active promotion of the IPC program by the Executive is a clear demonstration of the organisation's commitment to infection risk assessment and management and a call to action for the rest of the organisation. The organisation may require the Executive to endorse the infection control plan, which not only authorises the implementation of the strategies detailed in the plan but also acts as an assurance that the necessary resources will be provided. Executive commitment is considered essential to effective risk management.[12]

In an acute care hospital setting, responsibility for the development and coordination of the IPC program will likely rest primarily with an infection control professional (ICP) and be overseen by a multidisciplinary committee. For the purposes of discussion, this committee will be referred to as the Infection Control Committee (ICC) although it may have various titles and be incorporated into an overall safety program.

The role of the Infection Control Committee (ICC): The ICC is responsible for endorsing the infection control program and evaluating its success by reviewing surveillance data and other evidence. Depending on the specific context, surveillance data may include postoperative wound infections; bloodstream infections resulting from the presence of an invasive device such as an intravenous cannula used to deliver fluids or medication directly into the bloodstream; or occupational exposures to blood and body fluid through needlestick injuries. Other sources of evidence include the results of audits, such as hand hygiene audits, or environmental audits where the facility is inspected to ensure the physical environment supports infection control principles and practice, for example, whether sterile stock is stored correctly, personal protective equipment is available and accessible to all staff, and the physical environment is clean and well maintained.

The composition of the ICC is critical to the success of the program because members need to represent all stakeholders in the organisation and assess the proposed program elements from the perspective of the areas for which they have responsibility (hence the various arrows back and forth, and the two side bars representing 'Communicate and Consult' and 'Monitor and Review' in Fig 7.1). ICC members must also have the position and authority to promote the program and its implementation to the people and areas they represent. Thus, the role of the ICC includes communication and consultation as well as monitoring and review. Both leadership and strong organisational

support are necessary for the integration of the program throughout the organisation and essential for continuous improvement—the never-ending, iterative cycle requiring constant reflection and reappraisal.[11]

The ICC is also responsible for the development and endorsement of policies and procedures that guide practice and assure safety for staff, patients and visitors. Policies and procedures must be based on the best available evidence and be reviewed regularly. Compliance also needs to be evaluated, along with all the other elements of the program, and this is also the responsibility of the ICC. Data from infection control surveillance activities and investigation of incidents reported through the incident management system are two mechanisms regularly used to assess compliance with policies and procedures and the success of prevention strategies.[13] Regular feedback of performance and outcome data throughout the organisation to staff and the Executive is essential to improve poor performance and sustain positive outcomes, rewarding staff for 'best practice'.

Since all members of the organisation must be aware of their responsibilities right from the point of entry to the organisation, IPC education is an essential component of all induction programs. This awareness must also be maintained, such as through annual training and awareness programs and campaigns.[1]

7.2.2 Allocation of resources

Executive support for infection risk assessment and management includes the allocation of resources, both human and material, to implement the IPC program.[1,3,12] Resources required for a comprehensive and effective program include:

- an infection control team with an appropriate skill mix
- access to information technology systems for systematic data collection and analysis
- access to specialist expertise; and
- adequate financial resources.[11]

The expertise of the ICP leading the program is likely to influence program outcomes, with evidence suggesting that programs led by ICPs with formal postgraduate infection control qualifications and who are credentialled deliver better program outcomes.[14-16] The skills mix of the infection control team should meet the current needs of the organisation and also include novice ICPs, so they can be supported and their development encouraged and overseen by more experienced ICPs. This model allows for succession planning. The team also needs access to specialist expertise, such as infectious disease physicians, medical microbiologists and hospital engineers.

The resources required to mitigate the infection risks associated with healthcare are many and varied and extend to every facet of the organisation. Examples include:

- provision and access to hand hygiene products and facilities
- personal protective equipment (PPE)
- appropriate facility design and engineering controls, such as negative pressure isolation rooms to accommodate patients with diseases transmitted via the airborne route
- filtered air under positive pressure in the operating room to protect the sterile field and the operative site
- systems and processes to ensure water quality is managed and monitored
- information technology systems that facilitate infection data collection and analysis; and
- education that is practical, accessible, targeted to the relevant audience and mandated.

7.2.3 Assigning responsibility

Responsibility for risk management rests with every member of the organisation. Examples of the allocation of responsibilities relating to IPC include:

- the Executive of the organisation—has overall responsibility
- the ICC—has oversight responsibility for identifying infection risks and designing and implementing mitigation strategies
- all staff—are required to comply with the safe work practices described in the organisation's policies and procedures, and to recognise and report infection risks and take action to mitigate the risk identified.

Applying these principles to the infection risk associated with surgical procedures, the responsibility is shared as follows:

- the Executive is responsible for ensuring the facilities are appropriately designed, and suitably qualified and experienced staff and resources are allocated to perform the procedures safely
- the facility's management personnel are responsible for ensuring the engineering controls are in place and maintained in working order[17]
- the operative team is responsible for ensuring the patient's skin at the operative site is prepared with antiseptic, the antibiotic prophylaxis is administered at the appropriate time and dose,

the instruments used are sterile, the sterile field is established and maintained, and asepsis is upheld throughout the procedure

- the ICC is responsible for monitoring outcomes through surgical site surveillance reports and acting where appropriate to investigate negative trends[17]
- the central sterilising department is responsible for reprocessing reusable medical instruments; and
- the Environmental Services staff are responsible for maintaining a clean physical environment.

To monitor the efficacy of risk mitigation strategies the organisation needs a systematic method for reporting infection risks. These reports must be analysed, contributing factors identified and mitigation strategies implemented, and their success evaluated (see feedback loops, Fig 7.1).[18]

A more generalised infection risk is the transmission of blood-borne viruses associated with the use of sharps including needles and syringes, scalpels and other sharp objects. The measures to mitigate this risk include:

- mandatory vaccination against hepatitis B for at-risk staff
- documented policies and procedures regarding the safe use and disposal of sharps, and the action required in the event of an injury
- elimination of sharps where possible or the use of safety-engineered devices such as retractable needles to minimise the risk of injury
- appropriate sharps disposal units available as close as practicable to where the sharp is generated and used
- staff education to ensure they understand the safety protocols and what to do in the event of an exposure; and
- review of incidents reported to identify further opportunities for improvement.[19,20]

(See risk pyramid, Fig 7.3.)

While responsibility for preventing occupational exposure to blood and body fluids is shared across the organisation, the role of the ICP may involve:

- establishing safe work processes through the development and publication of policies and procedures
- reviewing immunisation records of new staff to ensure hepatitis B immunity
- educating staff about sharps safety
- collecting, analysing and reporting data on occupational sharps injuries.

The responsibilities associated with infection risk mitigation must be clearly assigned to the relevant personnel, and each member of the organisation must be aware of their responsibilities and have the necessary training and resources to meet these obligations.

7.3 A structured and comprehensive approach

The allocation of adequate resources and assignment of responsibility for infection risk assessment and management can only be undertaken when all the risks have been identified and mitigation strategies developed and implemented (see Fig 7.1). The IPC plan or program should be both structured and comprehensive, but developing such a plan from the beginning is quite a daunting prospect. Fortunately, in Australia at least, the NSQHS Preventing and Controlling Infections Standard can be used as the guide for a risk assessment plan. Note that other, similar standards exist in other countries.[5,21-23]

Each of the criteria in the Standard represents a potential infection risk and, using this as a guide, the ICP can consider what strategies are in place to mitigate the risk represented by each criterion. Consideration should also be given to the evidence available to demonstrate the success of the mitigation strategy. Where the available evidence suggests the strategy is unsuccessful, or only partially successful, further investigation is warranted to identify contributing factors and tailor strategies to control them, or to identify new mitigation strategies and then implement and evaluate those.

One example to illustrate this is hand hygiene, which is considered the simplest and most effective infection prevention strategy. The NSQHS Preventing and Controlling Infections Standard requires the health service to have an established hand hygiene program that aligns with the National Hand Hygiene Initiative (NHHI) and addresses non-compliance.[24] The IPC plan must include hand hygiene training and education, as well as hand hygiene compliance auditing and reporting. Evidence that hand hygiene facilities are available and accessible will need to be provided. Compliance data must be collected, analysed and reported, and a documented process for dealing with poor performance needs to be available and in use.[5] Hand hygiene auditors must be trained in accordance with the requirements of the NHHI to ensure inter-rater reliability of the national data set.[24] The plan must address all of these points, and evidence of implementation and evaluation, including improvement strategies, is required.

An ICP starting work at a new facility, and who is responsible for an IPC program, could evaluate the established infection control plan against the criteria from the NSQHS Preventing and Controlling Infections Standard as a means of assessing its effectiveness or otherwise.

7.3.1 Customised

The assessment of infection risks will be tailored to the specific organisation or facility and its potential infection context. While some infection risks and their associated mitigation strategies will apply to all health service delivery, such as the need to comply with hand hygiene requirements and the appropriate use of PPE, other risks only apply to some services. For example, a day surgery unit will have risks associated with the use of reusable medical devices, their transport, cleaning, reprocessing and storage, and the plan for that facility will include significant detail about appropriate risk management strategies. In contrast, a residential aged care facility may make limited use of medical devices and use only disposable items, and therefore only needs to include a policy or procedure stating that only single-use items will be used and they must not be reprocessed or reused.

7.3.2 Inclusive

The success of any risk assessment and management program relies in equal measure on Executive leadership and stakeholder engagement. Including the appropriate members on the Infection Control Committee (ICC) is key to ensuring adequate representation from all areas, and assists in disseminating information and implementing the program at every level.[3]

Consultation needs to encompass more than just the ICC if risks are to be identified and controlled. The purchase of new clinical equipment and consumables may present a range of infection risks, ranging from an inability to correctly reprocess the item to the purchase of materials that do not meet Australian Standards. Therefore, ICP representation on product evaluation committees and involvement in the assessment of specific items such as PPE is important.

The overlap between IPC in matters such as employee vaccination, management of occupational blood and body fluid exposures, and the appropriate use of PPE means it is prudent to include a member of the Workplace Health and Safety team on the ICC and the ICP on the Workplace Health and Safety Committee (see the 'Communicate and Consult' side bar in Fig 7.1). This ensures a regular flow of relevant information between the two areas, provides the opportunity for collaboration on projects and campaigns of mutual interest, and prevents duplication of effort.[3]

It is imperative to have ICP input into any building and refurbishment projects to ensure the design phase considers the infection risks associated with dust and debris caused by renovation and construction, and how these risks are to be mitigated. In addition, the detailed plans must consider appropriate workflow, use materials that are easy to clean, and allow adequate and appropriate storage of equipment and stock, especially sterile stock. Failure to include ICP advice in the planning stage can result in significant rectification costs and further work after the project is completed.[3]

These are just some examples that demonstrate the importance of an inclusive approach to infection risk assessment and management.

7.3.3 Dynamic and responsive

A risk assessment and management approach must be dynamic, especially in relation to infection control (see Iterative and cyclical nature of framework, Fig 7.1). New risks to human life and wellbeing are emerging and old ones re-emerge, including antimicrobial resistance in pathogens, new mechanisms of infection transmission, disease outbreaks and pandemics. Some examples of these are discussed below.

Antimicrobial resistance: Until the early 20th century, infectious pathogens claimed untold human lives and caused considerable morbidity, suffering and loss. The discovery of penicillin, and its antimicrobial properties, saw an explosion in the investigation, identification and subsequent manufacture of a suite of antimicrobial agents, including antibiotics to treat bacteria, antivirals for viruses and antifungals for fungi. Following their widespread application—especially in wealthier, western countries (note that the history of antimicrobials is not one of global equal access)—deaths and morbidity associated with microbial infections fell dramatically.[25] However, from the later part of the 20th century onwards, the widespread and ubiquitous use of antimicrobials has driven a natural evolutionary response—a selection pressure—to favour microorganisms that possess resistance to antimicrobials. Put simply, the more antimicrobials we have used, the more antimicrobial resistance has emerged and spread. If you kill most microorganisms, the ones left are usually the ones with resistance. These are the ones that then multiply and spread.

The issue of the emergence and spread of antimicrobial resistance is a wicked problem and a so-called 'One Health' issue (see Chapter 2). However, put simply, human health is intimately intertwined with the health of the planet, its ecosystems and animals—wild, companion and livestock. Since microbial pathogens can be zoonotic—emerging in one species (say a bat) and jumping to another animal host and then humans, or direct from a host wild animal to a human through the consumption of bushmeat or habitat encroachment—IPC has to be seen as a One Health system problem. Quantitatively, more antimicrobials are used in the treatment and care of animals than in humans, and excess antimicrobials from the animal sector 'leak' into natural environments such as rivers, lakes and seas and can be picked up or consumed by humans, thereby selecting for microorganisms on and in those new human hosts. The potential implications for subsequent IPC are profound and demonstrate the utility of the risk assessment and management process for tackling the risk associated with antimicrobial resistance.[26]

The challenge associated with antimicrobial resistance is the 'increased' risk associated with the reduction in effectiveness of antimicrobial agents to which common pathogens are susceptible. The mitigation strategies applied to this risk include the implementation of antimicrobial stewardship (AMS) programs aimed at ensuring antimicrobial agents are only used when necessary and are targeted at the specific pathogen causing the infection. This has required a multifaceted approach using education and training for prescribers, awareness programs targeting the health consumer, the establishment of guidelines for prescribing, and surveillance programs aimed at monitoring resistance to determine both the success of the strategies and the emergence of new resistance patterns. The risk of antimicrobial resistance is ongoing, which is why the mitigation strategies need to be both dynamic and responsive.

Clusters/outbreaks: Intermittently, new sources of infection are identified, and these risks must also be managed and mitigated. One example is the recognition that deep sternal wound infections presenting long after cardiac surgery were associated with heater-cooler units used for blood bypass during surgery.[27] The organism causing the infections, *Mycobacteria chimera*, is thought to have originated as a contaminant in the heater-cooler units at the point of manufacture and enters the surgical wound at the time of surgery via aerosols disseminated by the fan at the rear of the unit. Research into the cause of the infections eventually identified the mechanism of transmission, and now these heater-cooler units undergo regular cleaning and disinfection as well as microbiological sampling of the water to ensure the effectiveness of the interventions.[27]

The early identification and management of infection outbreaks must be a component of any risk management approach. While the aim of the IPC plan is to prevent infection and especially outbreaks, they do occur, and the surveillance systems that are part of the plan should provide early warning and allow rapid intervention to minimise impact. These events can arise from unexpected sources such as an outbreak that involved an organism called *Burkholderia cenocepacia*.[28] Routine surveillance of healthcare-associated bloodstream infections identified a number of patients with bacteraemia caused by this unusual organism. Investigations were undertaken and it soon became apparent that the portal of entry was the central line insertion site (see Fig 7.4). It was expected that the reservoir for this organism was a fluid of some description so multiple fluids associated with central line insertion and maintenance, and the fluids administered via the line, were sampled and cultured. Eventually the source of infection was found to be contaminated gel used in the ultrasound guidance for line insertion. The gel was contaminated at the factory where it was produced. This dynamic response and collaboration with colleagues at a range of facilities and using professional networks identified the source and prevented further infection globally.[28]

Pandemics: While outbreaks and novel sources cause infection in a discrete number of patients, pandemics challenge infection control on a different level altogether. While pandemics are considered relatively rare events, the commonplace nature of international travel means that infection can spread across the planet very quickly. The past two decades have seen a number of potential pandemics—avian influenza, severe acute respiratory syndrome (SARS-CoV) and Ebola virus disease (EVD); we have also experienced two pandemics: H1N1 influenza in 2009 and a new form of SARS (SARS-CoV-2) in 2019.[29-31] It is the requirement of a comprehensive response for such a sustained period of time that is so challenging. There is first a need to respond rapidly to a pandemic in its early stages where the disease is unfamiliar and much is unknown, and then to modify the response as the epidemiology of the disease is increasingly understood and to ensure the response is measured, sustained and comprehensive. Although pandemics are rare events, recent history has demonstrated how important it is to have a pandemic plan as a risk mitigation strategy to ensure there is capacity to respond rapidly. The lessons learnt during the H1N1 influenza pandemic were used to refine Australia's existing pandemic plans which have been further refined during the SARS-CoV-2 response.

Debriefing sessions associated with the SARS-CoV-2 response can only assist those responding to pandemics in the future. An example of the benefits of debriefing and using the knowledge gained through experience with one pandemic to better prepare for the next is provided in Case study 1. The establishment of fever clinics during the H1N1 pandemic proved very useful in preventing the spread of infection within the hospital setting; however, it had not been done previously and had to happen quickly. Debriefing after the H1N1 pandemic and using that experience as the basis for refining the pandemic plan meant that there was clear, detailed and precise information available to assist in the rapid establishment of fever clinics in the SARS-CoV-2 response.

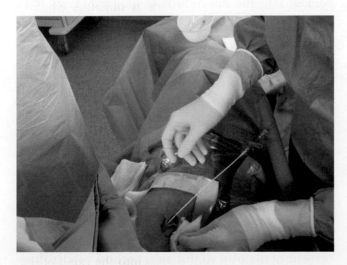

FIGURE 7.4 Peripherally inserted central catheter (PICC) insertion

CASE STUDY 1

Pandemic planning

The lessons learnt responding to the H1N1 pandemic were used to inform the subsequent pandemic plan. One of the elements that was found to be very successful was the early establishment of a 'fever clinic' where patients presenting with symptoms of H1N1 could be seen in a stand-alone clinic so that they did not mix with other patients presenting to the emergency department (ED) and potentially overwhelm the ED or act as a source of infection for other patients normally presenting to ED.

The establishment of the fever clinic required a range of resources both human and material.

Staff: to manage patients and visitors from the point of entry to the point of exit: administration, triage, assessment, testing, treatment, transfer or discharge. Those required included security, administrative, nurses, medical officers, cleaners, porters, radiographers, pharmacists and food services.

Supplies: stationery, medication, clinical equipment such as stethoscopes, emergency trolleys, wheelchairs, desks, chairs, thermometers, disposable cups, food to be taken with medication, scales to weigh children to determine medication dosage, swabs, waste receptacles and liners, linen and linen skips, hand hygiene products, PPE, cleaning supplies and so much more.

Communications: signage to direct patients and visitors, telephones, computers networked to the hospital system for pathology results and patient registration, a range of documentation to provide for the patients about their care, isolation requirements, result notification, how to access further assistance, printers, label makers, photocopiers and scanners.

At the conclusion of the H1N1 response, the local pandemic plan was written to incorporate detailed information, such as the requirements for the establishment of a fever clinic. When the SARS-CoV-2 response was initiated, and a fever clinic needed to be established, the plan was used and the people responsible for establishing it used the information in the pandemic plan to guide the allocation of all the resources required. Consequently, on the day the decision was made to establish a fever clinic, the decision was made at 9.00 am and the fever clinic was established and receiving patients by midday the same day.

7.3.4 Best available information

A dynamic response to outbreak events is reliant on the ICP having the best available information and evidence. The development of a robust and effective infection prevention and management plan is only possible if it is based on current evidence and therefore the ICP

requires access to relevant information including standards, guidelines and research results.

To achieve this awareness, ICPs should link into professional networks in Australia such as the Australasian College of Infection Prevention and Control (ACIPC), as well as other relevant colleagues, who will assist the ICP to remain current with new initiatives and provide access to a range of resources, including the ACIPC journal *Infection, Disease and Health*, educational initiatives—online workshops and courses—and current research endeavours and findings through the annual conference. ICPs should also make use of the wide range of peer-reviewed and professional journals available. In other countries, similar professional colleges, organisations and associations provide parallel expertise.

Membership of ACIPC enables the ICP to remain connected to professional colleagues and have access to ready advice through online forums and to participate in committees and working groups. The professional connections developed through participating in these activities are invaluable when the individual is faced with difficult and challenging situations. The opportunity to reach out to a colleague who understands the situation and may have faced something similar in the past, can provide the ICP with a source of advice on what steps to take, and also identify potential pitfalls based on previous experience.[32]

Ongoing research in the field of IPC contributes to the evidence base on which the guidelines and standards of practice are predicated. Access to journals, guidelines and Australian Standards is required for the ICP to ensure new knowledge and evidence is incorporated into the infection risk mitigation plan. ICPs also have a responsibility to engage in research initiatives as participants and investigators and to contribute to the evidence base.

7.3.5 Human and cultural factors

The infection prevention and management plan must consider the specific human and cultural factors inherent in the organisation. The most comprehensive plan will not succeed if it does not align with the organisation's goals and priorities.[3]

Effective implementation of risk mitigation strategies requires two-way communication. The plan must be communicated to all members of the organisation, but members should have been consulted in the development of the plan so that any potential barriers have been identified and addressed before the plan is published and implemented.[33,34] The ICC can provide the opportunity for two-way communication as well as any other consultative processes in which the ICP is engaged. Actively listening to members of the organisation, reviewing reports of infection risks and incidents, and the results of audits are all mechanisms that can assist in the two-way communication process.

Face-to-face education sessions also offer the opportunity for direct feedback from participants. The ICP may be there to deliver education and impart knowledge on a specific topic but the questions posed by participants can provide insight into any barriers to the practical application of the information in the workplace. Working through issues such as these in the education session engages the participants, helps them apply the knowledge and information in a practical sense, and fosters a sense of ownership in implementing the practice at a local level.

Engagement with members of the organisation at every level assists in ensuring the IPC plan remains relevant and fits comfortably within the organisational culture. Where the fit is obviously difficult, an assessment of the problem must be undertaken to determine whether the plan needs to be modified or the culture needs to change. Adjusting the plan is much easier than changing the culture.

Marketing the work of IPC and the various elements of the plan maintains awareness across the organisation of the expectations and responsibilities each member must contribute to the safety of all. Since the message remains largely unchanged, the challenge in marketing the program elements is to find new ways to communicate the program such that each member recognises their own unique role and accepts their responsibility. Marketing requires a specific skill set and it is rare for an IPC plan to include any marketing initiatives or to have access to marketing resources. Nevertheless, focusing on one or two specific aspects of the plan and running awareness campaigns can result in positive outcomes. Evidence of the influence of marketing can be seen in annual staff influenza vaccine uptake rates.[35,36]

In all these aspects the ability to connect on a human level and make the IPC plan resonate with the individual as something worthwhile and important is necessary for effective implementation and to achieve the positive outcomes required.

7.3.6 Continuous improvement

The IPC plan must be a living document—it requires regular review and evaluation of the mitigation strategies it embodies, giving it an iterative, cyclical and never-ending nature. Data derived from surveillance initiatives provide evidence of the plan's success or otherwise. Compliance audits, incident reports, feedback from surveys and education initiatives all provide useful information to assist in reviewing and refining mitigation strategies.

Policies and procedures must incorporate an audit strategy to determine compliance, and data from these audits can identify whether further action is required and what would be most effective. Additional education may be required in specific areas, or in relation to specific issues.

7.4 Risk assessment

Risk assessment—one of the risk assessment and management process elements illustrated in Figure 7.1—uses a systematic and comprehensive approach to identify, mitigate, monitor and review, and report outcomes.[1] As discussed earlier, one framework for a systematic and comprehensive approach to the assessment of infection risks associated with healthcare delivery is the NSQHS Preventing and Controlling Infections Standard (Fig 7.2).[5] This Standard directs the ICP's attention to the infection risks, including staff health, communicable diseases management, AMS, environmental risks, the appropriate use of PPE, safe use and disposal of sharps, and reprocessing of reusable medical devices (RMD). The Standard also prescribes some of the mitigation strategies including staff education, the development of safe work practices expressed in policies and procedures, surveillance initiatives, consumer engagement and Executive support and oversight.

An example of the application of risk identification, assessment, mitigation and review is provided in Case study 2.

CASE STUDY 2

Example of occupational body fluid exposure risk assessment and mitigation

A nurse reported an occupational body fluid exposure and was to be followed up in the staff clinic. In the clinic the nurse described the incident as follows:

1. A patient presented to a facility seeking help due to a significant bleed resulting in haematemesis, leading to collapse and cardiac arrest.

2. While waiting for the ambulance to arrive and transport the patient to an emergency department, the nurse commenced cardiopulmonary resuscitation (CPR).

3. The room in which this lifesaving treatment was being administered did not contain any PPE, so the nurse had no gloves or protective eyewear.

4. Other staff rallied to assist, bringing an emergency trolley which did contain PPE but despite repeated requests from the nurse, no one stepped in to relieve so that PPE could be applied.

5. These circumstances were all documented on the incident form submitted by the nurse in question. At the staff clinic, the nurse complained that she was made to feel like a 'trouble-maker' for highlighting the deficits, and to date no remediation had been undertaken.

Discussion

Appropriate assessment and treatment of the affected staff member is the first priority, along with reassurance that the nurse acted responsibly and appropriately in reporting the incident and identifying the deficits so the situation could be addressed. A review was undertaken of the management of the situation with the other staff involved, especially the most senior staff member supervising the response. The importance of assuring the safety of the staff as well as managing the emergency for the patient was highlighted. A supply of PPE was placed in the room where the patient had been managed and regular reviews through environmental audits were undertaken to ensure the PPE supply was maintained. The incident was used (with modification to protect the confidentiality of the staff member) in education sessions to clearly illustrate the importance of ensuring PPE supplies are maintained and staff use the PPE as appropriate.

Evaluation of the success of the strategies implemented is necessary for continuous improvement. Monitoring the availability of PPE in the area on an ongoing basis through environmental audits, and reviewing incident reports to ensure no recurrence of exposure will provide evidence that the strategies have been successful. However, if unsuccessful, further investigation and a review and revision of mitigation strategies and ongoing review would be required.

This incident demonstrates how various sources of information can be used to improve a system or environment to prevent the recurrence of an infection risk. The remainder of this chapter explores the elements of risk assessment: risk identification, risk mitigation, monitoring and reviewing mitigation strategies, and recording and reporting risks, mitigation and outcomes.

7.5 Risk identification

The identification of infection risks associated with healthcare delivery may be determined by asking the following questions:

* Who is at risk of infection?
* What are the potential sources of infection?
* How can infection be transmitted?

Patients, visitors and staff are all potentially at risk where healthcare is delivered. Patients are at risk of infection as a direct result of the healthcare provided through invasive procedures and devices that bypass the normal defence mechanisms of the human body. Patients may also be placed at increased risk of infection because the healthcare treatment reduces their ability to defend themselves against infection, such as immunosuppressive therapy administered to organ transplant patients to prevent the body rejecting the new organ, or due to the immunocompromised state caused by chemotherapy.

Visitors to the healthcare facility may be at risk of infection if infection risks are not identified and managed effectively. Healthcare workers themselves may be at risk of infection when they are exposed to infectious patients, visitors or colleagues, or they may be exposed to infection from the environment, contaminated equipment or through injuries resulting from contaminated sharps such as needles and scalpels.

Infection may be transmitted through direct or indirect contact with droplets of body fluids or secretions that gain entry to the body through mucous membranes or non-intact skin, or are inhaled or ingested. Infection can be transmitted through the air if it is contaminated with pathogens small enough to remain suspended in the air and move on air currents (Fig 7.5).

The number of people within a healthcare organisation who are potentially at risk of infection, the variety of sources of infection and the mechanisms of infection must all be considered when developing mitigation strategies. The risks must be analysed to determine the likelihood and frequency of the specific risk occurring, and the magnitude of the consequences which can be achieved using a basic risk matrix (Fig 7.6). Based on these parameters, the level of risk associated with each possibility can be measured and the control strategies prioritised. A risk that has major consequences and is likely to occur would be rated as more significant than

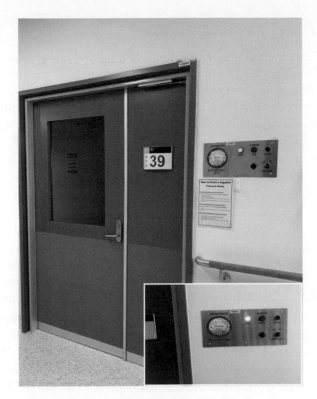

FIGURE 7.5 Doorway into negative pressure anteroom. Inset: Control panel on the right side of the image indicates the pressure is within the appropriate range and the negative pressure is functioning
Source: Author photo

breakdown of the health system, resulting in infection transmission to patients, healthcare providers and others. This has been clearly demonstrated during the response to COVID-19, where failure to accurately assess risks and implement appropriate risk management strategies has resulted in multiple outbreaks in residential aged care facilities.[37] The development and implementation of mitigation strategies without ongoing monitoring and review has also resulted in infection transmission and community outbreaks arising from sources within the quarantine hotels designed specifically to prevent such incidents (Case study 3).[38]

one that would have minor consequences and be very unlikely to occur. Priority for risk mitigation is given to the highest risk with consideration given to any existing controls.[3]

It is worth noting that a failure to identify potential risks and plan mitigation strategies can lead to a complete

CASE STUDY 3

Infection control breaches associated with COVID-19 transmission in hotel quarantine and residential aged care facilities in Australia

The risk mitigation strategies outlined above are provided as examples. At the time of publication, a Commission of Enquiry is being conducted into COVID-19 infections associated with a 'second wave' in Victoria that originated from hotel quarantine breaches and which resulted in deaths among elderly people resident in residential aged

Likelihood	Consequence				
	Insignificant	Minor	Moderate	Major	Severe
Almost certain	Medium	High	High	Extreme	Extreme
Likely	Medium	Medium	High	Extreme	Extreme
Possible	Medium	Medium	High	High	Extreme
Unlikely	Low	Medium	Medium	High	High
Rare	Low	Low	Medium	High	High

FIGURE 7.6 Simplistic risk matrix showing likelihood and consequence. The higher the probability and the more serious the consequences, the more extreme the risk

care homes in a number of Australian states. Thus, it is important to provide examples of how these strategies can break down, and the recent experience in Australia in response to COVID-19 has provided many well recognised examples of failure.

Residential aged care facilities (RACF) across Australia have been shown to be desperately unprepared to manage infection risks such as those associated with COVID-19. A lack of plans, staff training, PPE and other resources combined with the need for workers to work across multiple facilities to make a living, all contributed to the disaster that ensued. These problems were exacerbated by a cripplingly slow response, with staff complaining that they had no access to PPE long after the issues were highlighted.

Similar issues occurred in quarantine hotels in Victoria where security staff were given responsibility for maintaining infection control standards and practices without sufficient training and education. Breaches also occurred in quarantine hotels in other Australian states, leading to community transmission. Ongoing work to address identified problems continues, such as investigations into hotel air-handling systems that were implicated as a contributing factor, especially when guests were using nebulisers and continuous positive airway pressure (CPAP) machines.

7.6 Risk mitigation

The development of infection risk mitigation strategies builds on the identification and stratification of the risks. The same questions that are asked when identifying risks can be considered during strategy development with minor adjustment. The approach is one of control:

* How can those at risk of infection be protected?
* How can the sources of infection be eliminated or controlled?
* How can infection transmission be prevented?

Responses to these questions should also consider the hierarchy of controls as depicted in the diagram in Figure 7.7 and then choose the most effective risk mitigation strategies available.

7.6.1 Strategies aimed at protection

Patients can be protected through immunisation against vaccine-preventable diseases. Other forms of protection can include:

* well-documented policies and procedures directing safe work processes that maintain asepsis and prevent the introduction of infection through invasive devices or procedures
* education of healthcare workers regarding safe care, hand hygiene and appropriate use of PPE, and

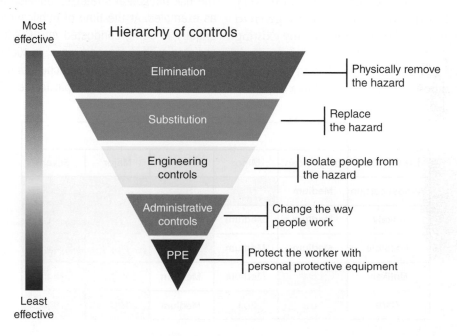

FIGURE 7.7 Hierarchy of controls
Source: NIOSH, 2015[39]

- well-designed workflows and working environments that support the desired practice, such as ensuring PPE is available and accessible and there is ample opportunity for hand hygiene. Visitors can be protected by:
- clear and repeated messaging about hand hygiene
- not coming to visit patients when they are ill themselves; and
- ensuring their own immunisations are current and complete.

Healthcare workers can be protected through education about infection risks and their own health. Healthcare worker immunisation is now usually a condition of employment in most healthcare organisations and influenza vaccination programs are held at hospitals and health services annually. Intact skin acts as a barrier against infection for the healthcare worker, so education about hand care is an important component of hand hygiene compliance initiatives. Education and training for healthcare workers on the appropriate use of PPE can assist in improving compliance with PPE use and ensure it is used correctly and therefore provides the protection it is designed to provide.

7.6.2 Strategies aimed at controlling infection

Environmental sources of infection can be controlled through thoughtful design to ensure the environment can be cleaned and maintained (Fig 7.8). Design should incorporate appropriate storage and mechanisms of

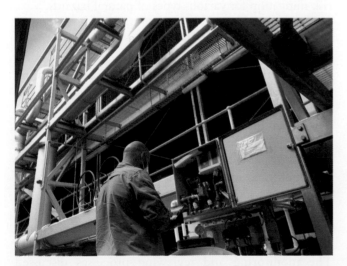

FIGURE 7.8 Control box associated with cooling tower monitoring demonstrating the importance of careful design and review processes
Source: Author photo

transport for reusable medical devices and associated equipment to ensure the packaging is not damaged or exposed to heat, water, dust or humidity.

Food supplied to patients must be managed within the required temperature range so it is delivered safely. Similarly, refrigerated medications and vaccines must be stored at appropriate temperatures so they are effective when administered to patients.

Patients with infectious diseases or conditions must be identified quickly so the appropriate controls can be instituted, such as single room accommodation and prompts to ensure those entering the room are wearing the correct PPE. Unless the condition is self-limiting, there must be mechanisms to identify the risk should the patient re-present to the facility following discharge.

7.6.3 Strategies aimed at preventing infection

Engineering controls are used where possible to mitigate or remove risk. Special air-handling and ventilation systems such as high-efficiency particulate air (HEPA) filters are used in operating rooms to filter air coming into the room over the operative site, ensuring it is clean and not a potential source of infection. Conversely, negative pressure ventilation systems are used to remove air contaminated with minute particles that contain pathogens. These systems do not allow recirculation of the contaminated air but exhaust it separately into a safe space.

Engineering controls have also been incorporated into the design of some sharp implements, such as needles and intravenous cannulae, so that the sharp is retracted before it can be the source of a sharp injury to the healthcare worker and a means of transmission of blood-borne pathogens. This is an example of how infection transmission can be prevented. If the sharp is eliminated after it is contaminated but before it can cause harm, transmission has been interrupted. Engineering controls usually require the healthcare worker to initiate them, so education is important so the healthcare worker can contribute to their own safety and the safety of others.

7.7 Monitoring and reviewing

Identifying infection risks and developing and implementing mitigation strategies alone may not achieve the anticipated results. Systems that monitor outcomes and the effectiveness of the interventions are also necessary. For the ICP, the infection surveillance program provides some assurance that the strategies have been effective and the risks managed. Most infection surveillance systems will include surgical site infections (which may be targeted to specific procedures); healthcare-associated bacteraemia; occupational body fluid exposures; and the incidence of significant and multi-antibiotic resistant microorganisms (MRO). Surveillance of MRO will be linked to AMS programs.[13]

Additional information that assists in monitoring the effectiveness of mitigation strategies includes hand hygiene compliance audits, practice audits, vaccine-preventable diseases status of new employees on commencement, annual staff influenza vaccination uptake, environmental audits, and microbiological sampling where specific environmental risks have been identified, such as air-conditioning cooling towers, tap water chlorine levels, and heater-cooler units used in cardiac bypass surgery.[40]

Systematic collection of data over time provides the ICP, the ICC and the Executive with baseline data that allows early identification of infection increases and facilitates a rapid response. A sudden increase in the number of needlestick injuries reported would warrant investigation. It might be that the safety devices are not being used, and education and an awareness campaign might be required to improve sharps safety. The increase may be related to a specific procedure and investigation might reveal that new equipment is being used that does not have a safety-engineered component or a change in practice may be required.

Monitoring and review are key components of the continuous improvement cycle. New technologies are developed and released, and new products and procedures find their way into organisations, and the ICP is not always aware of the changes until investigation of an increase in infection or other risk uncovers the change.

7.8 Recording and reporting risks

The infection control management plan (ICMP) should encapsulate all the infection risks associated with the healthcare service and serves as a method of recording the risks and mitigation strategies. Additional recording and reporting are required when new risks arise, when the risk cannot be managed within the existing resources or frameworks, or when unexpected events, such as outbreaks, occur.

7.8.1 New risks

Refurbishment of an existing building, or building a new facility, presents new opportunities but also new infection risks. These risks need to be identified, quantified and mitigated. Stakeholder consultation and the development of a plan that includes specific actions, deadlines and allocation of responsibilities is required. The plan must be disseminated for comment to allow stakeholders to identify any gaps and to ensure shared ownership of the plan.

7.8.2 Unmanageable risks

Sometimes a risk cannot be managed within existing resources and the nature of the risk and its consequences, as well as proposed mitigation strategies and associated costs, need to be communicated to the Executive of the organisation. The Executive will consider the issue against competing priorities and decide what level of risk is acceptable and allocate resources accordingly. One example might be the delivery of the annual staff influenza vaccination program. If the organisation is providing the vaccine for staff, the Executive has already made a commitment to the program, the health and wellbeing of the staff, and the safety of the patients. If the uptake of the program is limited by accessibility to the vaccine because it is only offered at certain times on specific days, additional resources may be required. If there is no capacity to reallocate existing resources, a case would need to be made for an increase in resources to improve access and therefore uptake. As noted in the opening paragraph of this chapter, rarely is it possible to reduce risk to zero. What may be more appropriate is to address risk so that it becomes as 'low as reasonably practical'—an approach adopted, for example, in relation to risk mitigation for various types of natural hazards.

7.8.3 Unexpected risks

Although the IPC program aims to control infection risks, sometimes it is not possible to foresee a risk. One example is the emergence of a new pathogen or an outbreak of a previously controlled infection. The emergence of a new pathogen can herald a pandemic, or its effect might be limited to a small area or a discrete number of countries. The COVID-19 pandemic has provided many examples of the poor outcomes associated with lack of resources, training and review (see Case study 3).

Locally, more circumscribed outbreaks can occur and cause significant disruption to the organisation. The monitoring and reviewing processes discussed should assist in identifying an outbreak when it occurs, but controlling the outbreak will require the ICP to rapidly marshal resources and implement control measures. Once the outbreak has been controlled, a comprehensive review of the event is worthwhile to identify any factors that contributed to the outbreak, strategies that impacted positively or negatively, and what could be done differently in future. Reports such as this help to prevent future outbreaks; develop tools and processes that will assist in the event of another outbreak; and illustrate to the broader healthcare team all of the elements that are required to bring an outbreak under control.

Conclusion

As demonstrated throughout the chapter, the ICP role exists to prevent and control infection in healthcare services. This can only be achieved if the infection risks are identified, and rational control measures are implemented. The effectiveness of control measures must be monitored and reviewed so gaps and deficits can be identified, and strategies can be refined and revised.

The context of healthcare is dynamic, encompassing new technologies and facing new challenges. The infection control program must be equally dynamic in its risk identification and response.

Communication and engagement with all stakeholders are required to test the pragmatism and fit of the plan into every part of the organisation and to foster local ownership. The success of the plan is dependent on the degree to which all members of the organisation accept their responsibility for its implementation and for contributing to the safety of patients, healthcare workers and visitors.

Useful websites/resources

- National Safety and Quality Health Service Standards. https://www.safetyandquality.gov.au/standards/nsqhs-standards

References

1. Standards Australia. AS ISO 31000: 2018 Australian standard risk management - guidelines. SAI Global Pty Limited, 2018.
2. Adams J. Risk. London: UCL Press, 1995.
3. National Health and Medical Research Council. Australian guidelines for the prevention and control of infection in healthcare. Canberra: Australian Government, 2019. Available from: https://www.nhmrc.gov.au/about-us/publications/australian-guidelines-prevention-and-control-infection-healthcare-2019#block-views-block-file-attachments-content-block-1
4. Australia Council for the Arts. Risk management framework policy. In: Arts ACft, editor. 2014.
5. Australian Commission on Safety and Quality in Health Care. Preventing and Controlling Infections Standard, 2021. Sydney; ACSQHC; 2021. Available from: https://www.safetyandquality.gov.au/publications-and-resources/resource-library/national-safety-and-quality-health-service-standards-second-edition.
6. Wilson RM, Runciman WB, Gibberd RW, Harrison BT, Newby L, Hamilton JD. The quality in Australian health care study. MJA. 1995;163(9):458-471.
7. Kobayashi K, Imagama S, Kato D, Ando K, Hida T, Ito K, et al. Collaboration with an infection control team for patients with infection after spine surgery. Am J Infect Control. 2017;45(7):767-770.
8. Robertson J, McLellan S, Donnan E, Sketcher-Baker K, Wakefield J, Coulter C. Responding to Mycobacterium chimaera heater-cooler unit contamination: international and national intersectoral collaboration coordinated in the state of Queensland, Australia. J Hosp Infect. 2018;100(3):e77-e84.
9. Guspiel A, Menk J, Streifel A, Messinger K, Wagner J, Ferrieri P, et al. Management of risks from water and ice from ice machines for the very immunocompromised host: a process improvement project prompted by an outbreak of rapidly growing mycobacteria on a pediatric hematopoietic stem cell transplant (Hsct) unit. Infect Control Hosp Epidemiol. 2017; 38(7):792-800.
10. Brown CK. A call for improved occupational surveillance for measles in the United States. Am J Infect Control. 2019;47(12): 1519-1520.
11. Halton K, Hall L, Gardner A, MacBeth D, Mitchell BG. Exploring the context for effective clinical governance in infection control. Am J Infect Control. 2017;45(3):278-283.
12. Safe Work Australia. Model code of practice: how to manage work health and safety risks 2020. Canberra: Australian Government, 2020. Available from: https://www.safeworkaustralia.gov.au/doc/model-code-practice-how-manage-work-health-and-safety-risks.
13. Mitchell BG, Hall L, Halton K, MacBeth D, Gardner A. Time spent by infection control professionals undertaking healthcare associated infection surveillance: a multi-centred cross sectional study. Infection Disease and Health. 2016;21(1):36-40.
14. MacBeth D, Hall L, Halton K, Gardner A, Mitchell BG. Credentialing of Australian and New Zealand infection control professionals: an exploratory study. Am J Infect Control. 2016;44(8):886-891.
15. Mitchell BG, Hall L, Halton K, MacBeth D, Gardner A. Infection control standards and credentialing. Am J Infect Control. 2015;43(12):1380-1381.

16. Hall L, Halton K, Macbeth D, Gardner A, Mitchell B. Roles, responsibilities and scope of practice: describing the 'state of play' for infection control professionals in Australia and New Zealand. Healthcare Infection. 2015;20(1):29-35.

17. Parvizi J, Barnes S, Shohat N, Edmiston CE, Jr. Environment of care: is it time to reassess microbial contamination of the operating room air as a risk factor for surgical site infection in total joint arthroplasty? Am J Infect Control. 2017;45(11): 1267-1272.

18. Bert F, Giacomelli S, Amprino V, Pieve G, Ceresetti D, Testa M, et al. The "bundle" approach to reduce the surgical site infection rate. J Eval Clin Pract. 2017;23(3):642-647.

19. Smith DR, Mihashi M, Adachi Y, Shouyama Y, Mouri F, Ishibashi N, et al. Organizational climate and its relationship with needlestick and sharps injuries among Japanese nurses. Am J Infect Control. 2009;37(7):545-550.

20. Bush C, Schmid K, Rupp ME, Watanabe-Galloway S, Wolford B, Sandkovsky U. Blood-borne pathogen exposures: difference in reporting rates and individual predictors among health care personnel. Am J Infect Control. 2017;45(4): 372-6.

21. World Health Organization GRC, Integrated Health Services. Guidelines on core components of infection prevention and control programs at the national and acute health care facility level, 2016. WHO, 2016. Available from: https://www.who.int/publications/i/item/9789241549929.

22. National Institute for Health and Care Excellence. Healthcare-associated infections: Quality Standard (QS113), 2016. Available from: https://www.nice.org.uk/guidance/qs113.

23. Healthcare Infection Control Practices Advisory Committee. Core infection prevention and control practices for safe healthcare delivery in all settings - recommendations of the HICPAC 2017. CDC, 2017. Available from: https://www.cdc.gov/hicpac/recommendations/index.html#anchor_1555353663.

24. Australian Commission on Safety and Quality in Health Care. National hand hygiene initiative 2019. Sydney: ACSQHC, 2019. Available from: https://www.safetyandquality.gov.au/our-work/infection-prevention-and-control/national-hand-hygiene-initiative.

25. Michael CA, Dominey-Howes D, Labbate M. The antimicrobial resistance crisis: causes, consequences, and management. Front Public Health. 2014;2:145.

26. Dominey-Howes D, Bajorek B, Michael CA, Betteridge B, Iredell J, Labbate M. Applying the emergency risk management process to tackle the crisis of antibiotic resistance. Front Microbiol. 2015;6:927.

27. Stewardson AJ, Stuart RL, Cheng AC, Johnson PD. Mycobacterium chimaera and cardiac surgery. Med J Aust. 2017;206(3):132-135.

28. Shaban RZ, Maloney S, Gerrard J, Collignon P, Macbeth D, Cruickshank M, et al. Outbreak of health care-associated Burkholderia cenocepacia bacteremia and infection attributed to contaminated sterile gel used for central line insertion under ultrasound guidance and other procedures. Am J Infect Control. 2017;45(9):954-958.

29. Weber DJ, Rutala WA, Fischer WA, Kanamori H, Sickbert-Bennett EE. Emerging infectious diseases: focus on infection control issues for novel coronaviruses (Severe Acute Respiratory Syndrome-CoV and Middle East Respiratory Syndrome-CoV), hemorrhagic fever viruses (Lassa and Ebola), and highly pathogenic avian influenza viruses, A(H5N1) and A(H7N9). Am J Infect Control. 2016; 44(5 Suppl):e91-e100.

30. Schwartz RD, Bayles BR. US university response to H1N1: a study of access to online preparedness and response information. Am J Infect Control. 2012;40(2):170-174.

31. Wee LEI, Sim XYJ, Conceicao EP, Aung MK, Tan KY, Ko KKK, et al. Containing COVID-19 outside the isolation ward: the impact of an infection control bundle on environmental contamination and transmission in a cohorted general ward. Am J Infect Control. 2020;48(9):1056-1061.

32. Australasian College of Infection Prevention and Control. [Internet] Home page 2020. Available from: https://www.acipc.org.au/.

33. O'Donovan R, Ward M, De Brún A, McAuliffe E. Safety culture in health care teams: a narrative review of the literature. Journal of Nursing Management. 2019;27(5):871-883.

34. Peter D, Meng M, Kugler C, Mattner F. Strategies to promote infection prevention and control in acute care hospitals with the help of infection control link nurses: a systematic literature review. Am J Infect Control. 2018;46(2):207-216.

35. Yue X, Black C, Ball S, Donahue S, De Perio MA, Laney AS, et al. Workplace interventions associated with influenza vaccination coverage among health care personnel in ambulatory care settings during the 2013-2014 and 2014-2015 influenza seasons. Am J Infect Control. 2017;45(11): 1243-1248.

36. Kwok KO, Li KK, Lee SS, Chng PHY, Wei VWI, Ismail NH, et al. Multi-centre study on cultural dimensions and perceived attitudes of nurses towards influenza vaccination uptake. J Hosp Infect. 2019;102(3):337-342.

37. Pagone G, Briggs L. Aged care and COVID-19: a special report. In: Safety RCiACQa, ed. Oct 2020. Available from: https://agedcare.royalcommission.gov.au/publications/aged-care-and-covid-19-special-report.

38. Thorne L. Victorian coronavirus hotel quarantine staff became infected in community, not at work, CHO says: Australian Broadcasting Network [Internet], 2020. Available from: https://www.abc.net.au/news/2020-10-02/dhhs-details-on-victoria-coronavirus-hotel-quarantine-staff/12724594.

39. National Institute of Occupational Health and Safety. Hierarchy of Controls. Atlanta, USA: NIOSH, 2015. Available from: https://www.cdc.gov/niosh/topics/hierarchy/default.html.

40. Uguen M, Daniel L, Cosse M, Cabon S, Canevet M, Le Grand A, et al. Influence of risk assessment inspection on the prevention of nosocomial infection. J Hosp Infect. 2016;93(3):315-317.

CHAPTER 8

Infection prevention and control for One Health

PROFESSOR DALE DOMINEY-HOWES[i]

ASSOCIATE PROFESSOR MAURIZIO LABBATE[ii]

Chapter highlights

- A detailed explanation of the concept of 'One Health', explaining where and how it originated; its various definitions, advantages and limitations; and an exploration of its utility in designing interventions for infection prevention and control
- An outline of the range of indicative One Health factors that shape disease outbreaks, demonstrating how these factors span the human-animal-environment domains
- An exploration of antimicrobial resistance, influenza and legionellosis, in case studies on Evolve showing how to use One Health both conceptually and practically
- Professional practice tips for health practitioners when thinking in a 'One Health' way

i   School of Geosciences, The University of Sydney, Sydney, NSW
ii School of Life Sciences, Faculty of Science, University of Technology Sydney, Ultimo, NSW

Introduction

This chapter defines and explores the concept of 'One Health' in the context of infection prevention and control. After reading this chapter, the reader should be able to:

1. understand the 'One Health' nature of infectious diseases and that human, animal, and environmental systems (also referred to as 'domains') are interconnected such that pathogens can emerge in any one system/domain and move into the others

2. understand that a wide range of environmental and anthropogenic factors influence the emergence of pathogens, their movements between One Health domains, and the severity of infectious outbreaks; and

3. take this new One Health understanding of diseases and articulate it into interventions that can be developed and employed to influence infection prevention and control (IPC).

Like many concepts, One Health is broadly defined, somewhat contested, and thought of in different ways by different experts or stakeholders. This chapter explores why and how the concept of One Health is important to clinicians working in human health settings, and specifically to infection prevention and control. It charts the origins of the concept of One Health—embedded as it was in the early work of pioneers of human and animal medicine—and briefly acknowledges the criticisms of One Health but then flips these to illustrate its power and usefulness. The indicative range of factors that influence the One Health nature of infectious diseases is outlined, demonstrating the complex nature of the concept. Antimicrobial resistance, influenza and legionellosis are used as case studies to enforce One Health concepts and to understand the value of using One Health as a conceptual tool for thinking about infection prevention and control. The chapter concludes with a brief exploration of practice tips for clinicians that can be derived from the case studies.

8.1 One Health: its origins and importance to infection prevention and control

Essentially, the concept of One Health is very simple and can be defined and understood in the following statement: *the health of humans, animals and the environment is interconnected, interdependent and interrelated.* While conceptually easy to grasp, the challenge to professional practice is that human, animal and environmental systems—also referred to as 'domains'—are highly complex systems, and that is even before considering the numerous links that exist between them. For example, human susceptibility to infectious disease is influenced by a myriad of factors that includes genetics, environment, lifestyle, diet, interaction with other humans, education, food security, government policy, geography, income levels and technology—among others. The interrelationships between animals and their environments—meaning human contact with wild, companion and food-producing animals and the environmental ecosystems of which they are a part—may expose humans to infectious diseases, both known and novel.

In relation to environments, it would be hard if not impossible to find a natural environment that has not been affected by anthropogenic activity, and in many instances natural environments have been modified according to the needs and desires of humans. Land clearing to create human habitat or agricultural land and industrialisation has led to massive ecosystem change, including the extinction of many animals and other organisms. Most of the human population lives in urbanised environments that are very different to a 'natural' ecosystem. That said, experts who study urban and human systems often refer to urban environments as having their own, unique, 'ecosystems' that include interconnected human, animal and environmental elements. Therefore, for the purposes of this chapter the environmental domain includes anthropogenically modified and urbanised environments as well as more pristine natural environments. Urbanised environments may drive infectious disease outbreaks. For example, rainwater can pool in natural hollows or artificial vessels or tanks, providing a perfect habitat for mosquito reproduction. Mosquitoes carry important human diseases, such as malaria and dengue. Additionally, sewage and water pipes provide perfect reservoirs for pathogenic microorganisms and so the pathogenic potential of urban environments goes on.

Numerous factors within each One Health domain increase exposure and disease risk and/or facilitate the flow of pathogens between the domains, including climate change, land clearing, travel and food production and distribution. The complexity of One Health should by now be obvious. The idea that the health and wellbeing of humans is interconnected with that of the wider global ecosystem has emerged in the broader health sciences in recent years and has acquired the pithy, contemporary title of 'One Health'. However, switched-on readers will quickly recognise that this concept is not new at all—just a repackaging, or rebranding, of an idea that has been around for quite some time.

8.1.1 Origins

Atlas[1] provides a succinct overview of the origins, status and future of One Health. Atlas notes that the concept of One Health is important since it attempts to reconcile and build on the linkages between human, animal and environmental health 'by cutting across the boundaries' that exist in the—often siloed—study of the health of these systems. This is significant because many infections in humans (e.g. cat scratch disease, rabies, Lyme disease, etc) are acquired from animals (referred to as 'zoonoses') and many infections in animals are acquired from the environments in which they live.[2] Humans can also pick up pathogens directly from the environments they live in, travel through or visit. These ideas are unpacked shortly, but the take-home message is that all three systems or domains are intrinsically interconnected.

Conceptually and practically, One Health owes its origins to the research and practice of the early pioneers of modern human and animal medicine in the late 19th and early 20th centuries. Leading microbiologists Louis Pasteur and Robert Koch, and the architects of medical education and practice Rudolph Virchow and William Osler, all worked collaboratively with human and animal health colleagues on a variety of human and animal disease types and infections. This included the *overlap* between infections in animals and humans—a quintessential One Health approach. For example, Atlas[1] eloquently explains how Pasteur took such an approach in the 1880s in his work to identify and produce a vaccine to treat rabies. First, Pasteur infected rabbits with canine rabies. He then took those infected rabbits, opened their spinal cords to the atmosphere and transferred the infection from one rabbit to another. He continued this process, infecting one new rabbit at a time every two weeks, and slowly attenuated the virulence of the rabies virus. In the last step, he took the virus with reduced virulence derived from the rabbit experiments and gave this back to dogs. The dogs did not subsequently develop rabies when exposed to the wild-type virus and Pasteur thus showed he had developed a successful preventive vaccine. In continuing to demonstrate his One Health credentials, Pasteur went on to experiment with the post-exposure vaccination of humans, stepping across the animal–human health chasm, and there you have it—a One Health approach in action!

While it is an impressive effort, and one that is still responsible for the widespread vaccination of dogs in the developing world today, it is vital to understand that Pasteur did not solely work on rabies as a case, and nor was he alone. Many other notable human and animal clinicians and researchers were taking similar approaches and making equivalent advances for a wide range of infections. Thus, the foundations of One Health were made early and clearly.

8.1.2 Some definitions

Having noted the origins of the concept of One Health, let us return to its definition. The basic, simple definition provided at the beginning of this section holds true. But as was also indicated, the idea is somewhat contested and articulated in different ways by different organisations and stakeholders. Some leading stakeholders and experts provide a more nuanced overview.

On its global website (at the time of publication), the World Health Organization (WHO) defines One Health as:

> '... an approach to designing and implementing programmes, policies, legislation and research in which multiple sectors communicate and work together to achieve better public health outcomes. The areas of work in which a One Health approach is particularly relevant include food safety, the control of zoonoses (diseases that can spread between animals and humans, such as flu, rabies and Rift Valley fever), and combatting antimicrobial resistance [when microorganisms change after being exposed to chemotherapeutic antimicrobials and become more difficult to treat]'.[3]

The WHO argues we need a One Health approach because humans and animals are often infected by the same microorganisms and these microbes reside in our shared ecosystems or environments. Consequently, unless experts from each of these areas, and more, work collaboratively it will be very difficult, if not impossible, to solve many health challenges.

In Australia, there is no single organisation tasked with coordinating a One Health approach. However, at the Commonwealth level, One Health has been recognised as a critical conceptual and practical tool for approaching and solving numerous interrelated health challenges. Specifically, the antimicrobial resistance (AMR) initiative of government (see Case study 1 on Evolve) cuts across human, animal and environmental health, takes a One Health approach, and coordinates policy development, and strategic and action plans.

It also involves collaboration between human and animal as well as other experts.

The Australian Government defines a One Health approach as: '... when we coordinate actions across human, animal and ecosystem health'.[4]

The Public Health Association of Australia (PHAA) has a Special Interest Group (SIG) devoted to One Health that defines it as:

> 'the collaborative effort of multiple disciplines working locally, nationally and globally "to attain optimal health for people, animals and the environment". The One Health movement has had a focus on infectious diseases and particularly on emerging and re-emerging infectious diseases. About 75% of emerging infectious diseases arise in animals, including food animals and wildlife. Understanding and responding to these diseases requires contributions from the medical profession, from animal health experts, from wildlife specialists and ecologists, and from environmentalists, economists, and social scientists. The One Health approach is also applicable to non-infectious diseases and in addressing broader issues such as food safety and food security. Using a One Health approach is relevant to research, to operational activities (such as prevention, preparedness and response), and to policy development'.[5]

Last, there are specialist organisations in Australia set up and funded to examine and respond to various threats to human, animal and environmental health and one of the most significant (at the time of writing) is the National Centre for Antimicrobial Stewardship or NCAS—funded by the Australian federal and Victorian governments and the National Health and Medical Research Council (NHMRC) Fund. NCAS defines One Health as:

> '... a concept that recognises that the health of humans, animals and the environment are all unified and interconnected. This approach utilises multidisciplinary expertise and resources in a coordinated and collaborative manner, addressing, with regard to antimicrobial stewardship, the regulation and registration of antibiotics, and the use of guidelines for infection control and the prudent use of antibiotics, with the ultimate aim of reducing the threat of antimicrobial resistance in all sectors. There are several bodies within Australia that promote One Health approaches to research and policy-making, including the Australian Veterinary Association (AVA) and Public Health

Association of Australia (PHAA), which have established special interest groups for this topic'.[6]

It is worth summarising the key take-home messages here, which are that One Health:

1. focuses on the health of humans, animals and the environment

2. necessitates the inclusion of experts from multiple fields—not just in health sciences but including disciplines such as social sciences, decision making, economics, geography, microbiology, political science, law, food supply, ethicists, nursing and pharmacy

3. takes a multi-scalar approach from micro, local levels to the macro global. To examine a specific issue (say in Queensland, Australia) through a One Health lens, it is essential to look beyond the local, since all places, processes and things are interconnected in complex webs of feedback loops and actions

4. has a temporal dimension. Taking a One Health approach allows us to see linkages in actions, processes, impacts and consequences through time, and to devise strategies and plans at various stages before, during and after a specific event (e.g. the outbreak of a novel disease such as COVID-19). This is critical in relation to thinking about the value of infection prevention and control.

So, what might One Health look like diagrammatically? Figure 8.1 presents one graphical representation of One Health but there are many (just Google One Health and select 'images').

8.2 One Health: a concept by another name

It is interesting to note that even within human and animal medicine and other discipline fields, One Health can be referred to by several other names. For example, the term 'planetary health' has recently begun to swirl with increasing attention—clearly articulated in 2014 in *The Lancet* in a landmark article, 'From public to planetary health: a manifesto'[7] and in the subsequent Rockefeller Foundation-Lancet Commission report[8] on sustaining human health as a part of a wider need for planetary health. The Rockefeller Foundation-Lancet Commission sees this idea as vital as we move forward into a destabilised world impacted by rapid population growth, increasing urbanisation, loss of ecosystems and global environmental and climate change.[9,10]

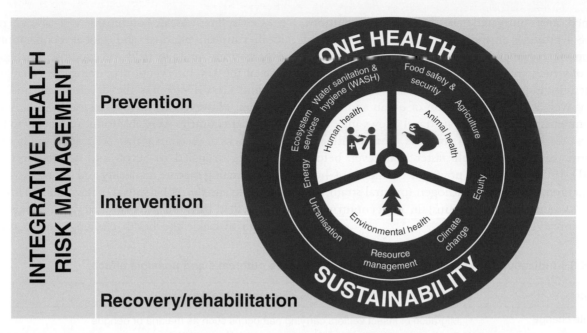

FIGURE 8.1 A diagrammatic representation of the One Health concept. This version was selected because it places the constituent elements of One Health in relation to the requirements of 'prevention, intervention and recovery/rehabilitation' that are useful when thinking about the application of One Health to infection prevention and control. For example, that is, we can *prevent* infections from arising/occurring in the first place if we adopt a One Health approach

Source: Ammann, W.J., Colbert, M., Rechkemmer, A. One Health: Summary and Outlook, in Colbert M, Stiffler M, Ammann WJ (Eds.). GRF One Health Summit 2012 – One Health – One Planet – One Future: Risks and Opportunities, Extracts from the Proceedings, OECD- GRF Davos, p. 115–120.

Elsewhere, geography, earth sciences, environmental studies, urban studies and sustainability sciences have been discussing the interlinkages between ecosystem/ environmental, human, animal and the more-than-human health for many decades using a variety of terms and concepts—all of which are akin to the idea of One Health (see, for example, ideas about one/planetary health and wellbeing in the overview given in Castree, 2014[11]).

Last, even the broad concept of Gaia (as in the Gaia hypothesis) developed by Lovelock and Margulis in the early 1970s is, at its core, a hypothesis that states the entire planet Earth is a single, living system comprised of many interconnected parts (e.g. ecosystems, the Earth itself and all living things). Thus, the health of the Earth is inevitably dependent on the health of all its constituent parts.

8.3 Challenges or critiques of One Health

As noted by Atlas,[1] critiques of One Health include that as a concept it is not well defined, it is hard to implement and might be construed to mean the holistic nature of One Health demeans, devalues, lessens or diminishes the detailed study of specific sub-disciplines of health (human or otherwise). But in our view these critiques are unjustified—it is, in fact, the *strength* of One Health that it builds upon and extends the detailed, conceptual and practical knowledge of many experts across numerous disciplines to achieve global health outcomes that go far beyond the capability and capacity of individual health sub-fields or sub-disciplines. As an example, if we consider human health—the role of a general practitioner does not demean or devalue the expertise of specialists (e.g. cardiologists, dermatologists, microbiologists, veterinarians). They work together to achieve the best outcome for individual patients as well as the wider society.

8.4 Factors within One Health driving infectious disease outbreaks

Infectious disease outbreaks are driven by multiple factors, and these may span one or more of the One Health domains. It is important to appreciate these factors to better understand how outbreaks are initiated, sustained and mitigated via different interventions. Table 8.1 provides an indicative, non-exhaustive list of common factors that drive infectious disease outbreaks, many of which are directly caused or enhanced by human activity, including personal, social and civil behaviours as well as the manipulation of urban and natural environments. For example, air travel allows infectious diseases to cross national borders and continents far more easily and much faster than ever before. COVID-19 has provided powerful examples of how the emergence of a viral pathogen (or viral strain, e.g. the Delta and Omicron strains) in one country can rapidly spread globally.

Controlling disease outbreaks will always require local, national, regional and global cooperation and experts from multiple fields of expertise. For example, one of the key intervention or mitigative strategies for tackling COVID-19 was the development and use of vaccines. However, access to vaccines is not universal. Wealthier countries were able to move quickly to buy up large stocks of vaccines as they were approved but poorer countries struggled to access and administer vaccines, demonstrating vaccine inequality and setting the stage for outbreaks and the global spread of new strains. This clearly means that this intervention (vaccines) alone is not enough to tackle the health challenges of COVID-19.

TABLE 8.1 Indicative list of factors driving infectious disease outbreaks and possible effects

Factor	Exemplar effects on infectious disease outbreaks
Climate change	• Migration of insect vectors carrying pathogens such as malaria or dengue • Destruction of habitat resulting in movement of animals into urban areas carrying pathogens • Displacement of people resulting in dense and unsanitary conditions facilitating spread of disease
Urbanisation	• Dense cities facilitating rapid spread of disease • Transport systems allowing movement of pathogens as 'passengers' riding along with humans
Land clearing	• Destruction of habitat resulting in movement of animals into urban areas carrying pathogens
Global air travel	• Rapid spread of pathogens across international borders and between continents
Trade	• Spread of insect vectors carrying pathogens • Contaminated food increases the reach of the pathogen across international borders
Technology	• Some technologies can provide a niche and mechanism of spread for pathogens such as *Legionella pneumophila* in cooling tanks feeding air-conditioning units in buildings • Drinking water pipes can harbour pathogens
Human behaviour	• Drug use, sexual practices, etc can drive infectious disease outbreaks • Consumption of exotic meats and food products bringing humans into contact with 'exotic' pathogens • Cultural practices, including handling the dead, that might allow infection of new patients
Human demographics	• Ageing population is more susceptible to infectious disease • Education and income levels may affect susceptibility to disease as individuals do not understand basic principles of infection control and hygiene, or lack economic resources to buy basic medicines
Institutional culture/ procedures	• A lack of health safety culture or detailed safe working methods can facilitate disease in clinical health environments • Poor practices in abattoirs can allow pathogens to contaminate meat
Poverty and social inequity	• Poorer countries lack resources and well-developed healthcare systems and are less prepared for dealing with infectious disease outbreaks, impacting their severity
Politics	• Conflict, including war, displaces people resulting in dense and unsanitary conditions that facilitate the spread of disease • Fear of sanctions means some countries have withheld information about emerging diseases • Politicisation of public health measures such as lockdowns and mask-wearing impacts social adherence

Of course, some factors are outside human control, and disasters triggered by natural and human processes (e.g. earthquakes, tropical cyclones, technological failures and war) causing human displacement or the destruction of water and sewerage infrastructure can trigger disease outbreaks (see, for example, the review by Suk et al 2020[12] that examines disease outbreaks in Europe following flood and earthquake disasters). But even in these circumstances global cooperation can lessen the severity.

One Health helps us to shift our thinking about infectious disease from a traditional approach centred on reacting to outbreaks (and responding to just the patient in front of us now and needing our care) towards one centred on developing interventions that lessen the risk or impacts of outbreaks, and which places a specific disease pathogen and outbreak into the wider 'complex systems web' of which it is a part. In the long run, this approach costs less, saves lives and reflects the notion of 'prevention is better than cure'. It also reminds us that the decisions we make have consequences, and these consequences can ripple out across human-animal-environment systems at scales from the local to the global, and through time. Traditional reactionary approaches, while useful and often successful, have limitations in a world where microorganisms are quick to evolve, adapt and infect a densely populated planet. Consider antimicrobial resistance (AMR) (see Case study 1 on Evolve)—the very drugs that we use to fight a plethora of infectious diseases are losing their effectiveness because we have failed to appreciate how their use, often unnecessarily, in multiple human and animal settings and their pollution of natural environments has driven the evolution of resistant pathogens. As we will learn, many of the reasons for AMR are related to human behaviour, policy development and decision making. One Health forces us to think about the entire journey of a pathogen, from where it emerges to its eventual movement into the human domain, thus helping us think about how our behaviours and systems—such as land management or agriculture—can be modified to reduce the risk of an infectious disease outbreak occurring. This is imperative if we consider how COVID-19 has brought the world to its knees by shutting down the global economy, affecting livelihoods and soaking up the resources needed to treat and manage other important health-related issues (e.g. HIV, malaria, malnutrition and poverty). The economic costs and loss of life have gone beyond the immediate effect of the virus in causing disease.

The case studies on Evolve draw upon the factors described in Table 8.1 to show, using the One Health

concept, how they contribute to the emergence and spread of infectious diseases or significant health problems. A sound understanding of the links between these factors and the One Health domains allows for the design and development of interventions at the local level (e.g. the local professional practice setting, hospital or local health network), as well as the national or global level, thus reducing the risk of an infectious disease outbreak, or reducing its severity once one has occurred. The aim is to help healthcare workers cultivate a holistic view of infectious disease and to recognise that treating infections in an outbreak is the end point of a pathogen's journey that has likely been brewing for months to years, supported by the collusion of multiple factors in one or more of the One Health domains.

PRACTICE TIP 1

Depending on the nature of a pathogen, disease outbreak or health issue/context a human health clinician might be asked to address, the range of 'practice tips' that might be appropriate are almost endless. However, in reflecting on the broader One Health nature of this chapter and the material covered, human health clinicians should consider the following basic professional practice tips:

- when treating an individual patient in front of you, consider whether you have enough detailed information about the infection, pathogen, disease outbreak or health context to make informed decisions. If you are in any way unsure, seek more information from a range of other specialists or colleagues. Be mindful that your decisions may have downstream, ripple effects in the interconnected domains of human, animal and environmental health. Try to be mindful of the big picture and the longer-term consequences of your decision making

- try to avoid feeling overwhelmed or paralysed from decision making, action and treatment—there are a lot of options open to you

- the source and consequences of those kinds of infections or health issues we have examined are not necessarily healthcare or hospital-based, but they rapidly become problems for those contexts and the wider community so think about the options with an open mind and a view towards the longer-term possible consequences

- to the best of your ability, commit to a program of life-long learning and continuous professional development, reading widely and learning to see how your expertise and role fits into a larger 'jigsaw picture' of global health and wellbeing. Know that your expertise sits alongside that of a wide range of interconnected experts and stakeholders

- do not be frightened to challenge dogma, established ways of doing work in your context or the views and decisions of older, more experienced colleagues. No one has a monopoly on knowledge and good/better ideas and practice. By asking questions and speaking up you may allow space for more reflective, better decision making; and

- develop a practice of critical self-reflection. When time permits, reflect on your professional practice: what lessons have you learnt; and how can your experiences help you shape future better professional practice?

Conclusion

Clinicians, together with other healthcare professionals, are at the sharp end of caring for individual patients and entire populations. They carry a significant burden of responsibility. In exercising their professional duty of care and clinical practice, clinicians and healthcare professionals must balance a wide range of contextual factors and competing priorities. While acknowledging

these challenges, this chapter has drawn attention to the wider 'complex web', to help professionals understand that their decisions for treatment can and do have impacts and effects that ripple out far beyond the patient in front of them.

Supporting the health and wellbeing of individual people and entire populations is critical but the health of humans is connected to the health of animals and the environment—that is, all things are interconnected in One Health. Understanding the One Health nature of a specific infection, disease outbreak or complex health issue (such as antimicrobial resistance) provides clinicians and other healthcare professionals with a sophisticated awareness of their place in a wider context of ensuring the long-term health of all things. It also equips healthcare professionals with the knowledge and skills to interact with other experts, and to design and implement interventions to manage IPC, both downstream and upstream, of an individual patient or event.

Finally, it is important to recognise that things are always changing, and the local, state and Commonwealth arrangements regarding One Health may have changed from those described here. This is okay! The point is you now have the knowledge and skill to continue your reading and learning, and to familiarise yourself with the current definitions of One Health and the policies relevant to your professional practice. You will also be able to search for, identify and connect with organisations, groups and bodies that support a One Health approach to your professional practice.

Useful websites/resources

- National Centre for Antimicrobial Stewardship – One Health. https://www.ncas-australia.org/one-health
- Public Health Association Australia (PHAA) One Health Special Interest Group. https://www.phaa.net.au/about-us/SIGs/one-health-sig
- Indo-Pacific Centre for Health Security. https://indopacifichealthsecurity.dfat.gov.au/one-health
- One Health Organisation. https://onehealthorganisation.org/
- Journals
    - One Health. https://www.journals.elsevier.com/one-health
    - International Journal of One Health: https://www.onehealthjournal.org/
    - One Health Outlook. https://onehealthoutlook.biomedcentral.com/
    - One Health & Implementation Research. https://ohirjournal.com/

References

1. Atlas RM, One Health: its origins and future. In: Mackenzie JS et al, eds. One Health: the human-animal-environment interfaces in emerging infectious diseases: the concept and examples of a One Health approach. Berlin: Springer, 2013.
2. Cross AR et al. Zoonoses under our noses. Microbes Infect. 2019;21(1):10-19.
3. World Health Organization. One Health. Geneva: WHO, 2017 [cited 28 Jan 2022]. Available from: https://www.who.int/news-room/questions-and-answers/item/one-health.
4. Australian Government. Antimicrobial resistance: about this initiative. Canberra, 2017 [cited 28 Jan 2022]. Available from: https://www.amr.gov.au/about-us/about-this-initiative.
5. Public Health Association Australia. One Health SIG. [cited 28 Jan 2022]. Available from: https://www.phaa.net.au/about-us/SIGs/one-health-sig.
6. National Centre for Antimicrobial Stewardship. One Health. 2020 [cited 28 Jan 2022]. Available from: https://www.ncas-australia.org/one-health.
7. Horton R et al. From public to planetary health: a manifesto. Lancet. 2014; 383(9920):847.
8. Hatosy SM, Martiny AC. The ocean as a global reservoir of antibiotic resistance genes. Appl Environ Microbiol. 2015;81:7593-7599.
9. Dominey-Howes D. Hazards and disasters in the Anthropocene: some critical reflections for the future. Geoscience Letters. 2018;5(1):7.
10. Independent Group of Scientists appointed by the Secretary-General. Global sustainable development report 2019: The future is now – science for achieving sustainable development. New York: United Nations, 2019.
11. Castree N. Geography and the Anthropocene II: current contributions. Geography Compass. 2014;8(7):450-463.
12. Suk JE et al. Natural disasters and infectious disease in Europe: a literature review to identify cascading risk pathways. European Journal of Public Health. 2020;30(5):928-935.

CHAPTER 9

Public health and infection prevention and control

Dr CATHERINE VIENGKHAM[i]

Dr BENJAMIN SILBERBERG[ii]

Dr SHOPNA BAG[ii,iv]

ASSOCIATE PROFESSOR STEPHEN CORBETT[iii]

PENELOPE CLARK[ii]

PROFESSOR RAMON Z. SHABAN[i,ii,iv,v,vi]

Chapter highlights

- An overview of public health systems and structures in Australia
- Explores the intersection between public health and infection prevention and control (IPC) in Australia
- Examines contemporary challenges for public health and IPC in Australia

i Susan Wakil School of Nursing and Midwifery, University of Sydney, Sydney, NSW

ii Centre for Population Health, Western Sydney Local Health District, North Parramatta, NSW

iii Western Sydney Clinical School, The University of Sydney, Sydney, NSW

iv Sydney Institute for Infectious Diseases, Faculty of Medicine and Health, University of Sydney, Sydney, NSW

v Public Health Unit, Centre for Population Health, Western Sydney Local Health District, NSW

vi New South Wales Biocontainment Centre, Western Sydney Local Health District, Westmead, NSW

Introduction

The implementation of public health interventions, supported by both surveillance intelligence and research, has seen the substantial decline and in some cases eradication of several infectious diseases over the last century. The ongoing development and application of public health policies continues, striving to improve the safety and quality of healthcare, prevent and control healthcare-associated infections, and prepare timely and effective strategies to mitigate new and emerging IPC challenges in Australian healthcare.

9.1 Defining public health

The definition of 'public health' has evolved over time and differs from country to country. The World Health Organization (WHO) defines public health as the practice of 'preventing disease, prolonging life and promoting health through the organised efforts of society'. Alternatively, public health can also refer to the actual state of health of the people and the population as a whole. Public health interventions broadly describe initiatives, programs and campaigns that aim to improve some aspect of population health (Table 9.1). These interventions may aim to prevent the occurrence of certain diseases by promoting prophylactic activities like regular hand hygiene or introducing standards to regulate the quality of food and water. They may facilitate access to care services for people who are experiencing acute illness and require diagnosis and treatment or provide long-term support for those who experience chronic disabilities. Public health has played, and continues to play, a critical role in infectious disease prevention efforts in Australia. Public health initiatives are organised and implemented by a wide range of bodies and are often collaborative efforts between state and federal governments, public, private, commercial and not-for-profit (NFP) organisations, research institutions and universities.

9.2 A brief history of public health: from Europe to Australia

The application of public health interventions to suppress infection and effect disease control can be traced back to ancient civilisations. Concepts of good cleanliness, hygiene and sanitation were frequently linked with religious beliefs and practices across many societies, which incentivised the deliberate construction of infrastructure to provide clean water and drain sewerage.[2] Despite this, the periods that followed, broadly known as the Middle Ages (500–1500), were particularly perilous times. The movement of large groups of people for trade, together with the propagation of domesticated animals and ongoing crusades across Europe, facilitated the rapid and unchecked spread of infectious diseases such as leprosy, smallpox, cholera, measles and the devastating bubonic plague.

The 18th century marked the beginning of the Industrial Revolution, which saw the introduction of modernised, machine-powered tools and immense

TABLE 9.1 Levels of public health interventions and their aims for different aspects of population health and disease

Levels of intervention	Aim	Examples
Primary prevention	Preventing a disease before it has the chance to occur.	• Campaigns to promote exercise and regular physical activity • Education initiatives to teach nutrition and the practice of a well-balanced diet • Sun protection advertisements promoting the use of sunscreen, hats and sunglasses to protect against skin cancer • Immunisation programs against vaccine-preventable diseases like measles and influenza
Secondary prevention	Reducing the impact of a disease that has already occurred, through early detection and providing treatment to inhibits disease progress, shortens disease duration or prevent additional complications.	• Screening programs for disease like bowel cancer and breast cancer • Medicare-subsidised access to primary care services such as general practitioners, specialists, tests and operations • National network of emergency services
Tertiary prevention	Managing the impact of ongoing disease, by mitigating long-term impairments and improving function and quality of life with the disease.	• Rehabilitation and long-term care facilities to support patient physical and/or mental recovery • Support groups that bring together people with similar health issues to share experiences and strategies for living well

advances and innovation in technology and architecture. Improvements in agricultural production methods reduced the demand for rural workers and facilitated the exponential growth of urban centres across Great Britain, Europe and the United States. Rapid increases in the population saw urban centres overwhelmed with issues such as overcrowding, poor sanitation and polluted water and food. These conditions exacerbated epidemics of disease, such as cholera, typhoid and tuberculosis, and infectious diseases remained one of the greatest causes of morbidity and mortality during this period. The same diseases were brought to Australia following British colonisation in 1788 and were particularly devasting to the country's Indigenous population, who had no prior exposure to or defences against the novel diseases. The early 19th century saw an influx of free settlers from Great Britain, followed by European, Chinese and US immigrants during the Australian gold rushes that started in 1851. Large urban settlements were soon established to accommodate the increasing population where similar issues of overcrowding, poor sanitation and disease spread prevailed.

The rise of public health policies and organised health reform was, in no small part, catalysed by the endeavour to combat infectious diseases. The informally termed 'sanitary revolution' was initiated in the mid-19th century and largely driven by the work of Edwin Chadwick. Following a series of outbreaks in the 1830s, Chadwick strongly championed environmental (or 'miasma') theories of disease spread and pushed for sanitary reform. In 1842, he published the Report on the Sanitary Conditions of the Labouring Population of Great Britain, which argued that poverty, poor sanitation and living conditions were the causes of disease. The report recommended interventions such as clean water, improved drainage systems and ventilation that would improve health and productivity and reduce the need for 'poor relief' and expenditure on welfare.

While the miasma theory was eventually superseded by the now accepted germ theory of disease, the improved sanitation measures implemented were ultimately effective and established the link between sanitary conditions and the spread of disease. Further work facilitated by John Snow, Louis Pasteur and Robert Koch towards the end of the 19th century saw the recognition of microorganisms as the cause of disease and highlighted the importance of epidemiology in informing public health policies and understanding how infectious diseases may be controlled. The wider adoption of sanitary measures, better hygiene and other prophylactic practices greatly reduced the burden of infectious diseases, both in the general public and in healthcare. Following this, significant advances were made with the discovery of penicillin and antibiotics for the treatment of infections in the early 20th century and the mass development and systemic dissemination of vaccinations. The last 100 years has witnessed the fall of infectious disease from being one of the greatest causes of human mortality to accounting for approximately 2.0% of the total disease burden in Australia today.

9.3 Public health infrastructure in Australia

Australian public health structures and policies closely emulated those established in Great Britain and subsequently, the United States. The Australian federal government was established in 1901, and the first public health act, the Quarantine Act, was enacted in 1908. This act saw the Commonwealth responsible for maritime and interstate quarantine, the collection of public health information and infectious disease research. The inaugural Department of Health was established in 1921 and the National Health and Medical Research Council (NHMRC) in 1936. The actions of the Commonwealth were critical in several health events that occurred from the turn of the 20th century onwards, from the influenza pandemic of 1918 to the subsequent influenza, poliomyelitis, HIV/AIDS and COVID-19 outbreaks, as well as the introduction of publicly funded universal healthcare towards the latter end of the century.

Today, the importance of public health programs in reducing the incidence of disease and healthcare-associated infections is recognised across all levels of government. Public health initiatives are frequently facilitated through a wide range of collaborators, including universities, research institutions, non-government, not-for-profit (NFP) and professional organisations, as well as the healthcare industry and primary care workforce. The development and implementation of an effective public health program requires multidisciplinary teams that involve individuals with specialist expertise in the areas of proposed change, members with regulatory powers to enact the change at systemic levels and agencies who are able to monitor the short- and long-term effects of the intervention. The following section summarises the contributions of government bodies, research institutions, NFP and professional organisations, and the primary care workforce in public health interventions.

9.3.1 Commonwealth, state and territory and local governments

While historically the role of the Commonwealth was limited to overseeing matters of quarantine (Quarantine

Act 1908), its role has since broadened significantly to include the development of national health policies, guidelines and standards; the financing of access to medical and public health services; the funding of health and medical research; and the regulation of pharmaceuticals and therapeutic devices. State and territory governments are responsible for the management and provision of public health services and the regulation of health facilities and their workers, as well as the implementation of disease prevention and control activities (e.g. immunisation, screening). Each jurisdiction establishes its own public health programs, priorities, labour divisions and organisational arrangements.

Within each state and territory a large number of local government bodies perform a variety of public health service functions. These functions differ between jurisdictions, as determined by their respective Health Acts and Local Government Acts. In general, local governments contribute at the service level, having a central role in public health surveillance and action. Local councils also vary with respect to their location (rural or metropolitan), the role they play, and the extent to which they respond to local needs. Some responsibilities are shared across all levels of government under national agreements, such as the

Council of Australian Governments (COAG). These include the funding of public hospitals, the registration and accreditation of health professionals, improving the quality of healthcare services and programs, and responding to national health emergencies.[3] The primary roles of each level of government are summarised in Table 9.2.

9.3.2 Universities and research institutions

Universities and dedicated research institutions are key sources of public health research and education. While health and medical research may be funded by a range of government and non-government organisations, the Australian Government remains the major funder, contributing $4.4 billion (78% of total funding) in 2017–18. This is followed by state and territory governments and non-government organisations, which contributed $0.8 and $0.4 billion in 2017–18, respectively.[3] The Australian Government funds health and medical research through the NHMRC and the Medical Research Future Fund (MRFF), which are both highly competitive and rigorously peer reviewed. The Australian Government also contributes grant funding to both public and private research institutions and organisations that play important roles in public health research efforts, such as the Commonwealth

TABLE 9.2 Primary public health roles and responsibilities of different levels of the Australian Government[1]

Level	Primary roles
Federal	• Development and implementation of national public health policies and programs • Planning, monitoring, reporting, training and evaluation of public health activities • Development of nationally consistent standards, legislation and regulation, workforce competencies, environmental protection, disease prevention and outbreak control methods • Financing innovation in population health programs and advocating for a population health constituency with key players and the public • Consulting with partners and Australia's international responsibilities and obligations in public health
State and territory	• Identifying state-wide public health issues through epidemiological surveillance • Timely intervention and monitoring of health outcomes • Policy development in relations to communicable diseases, environmental health, health promotion, immunisation, workplace risk and emergency management • Organising preventive and early detection programs • Supporting population health literacy and health-promoting behaviour • Developing strategies for emerging health problems • Give government the power to act quickly in public health emergencies • Collaborate with other government and non-government public health sectors and authorise to address public health issues and provide for a competent workforce
Local	• Coordinate with higher government bodies in implementing public health service functions with respect to local needs • Interacts with public health activities involving environmental management, economic development, public safety, maintaining roads, cultural and recreation development, land use and provision of community services • This is particularly important for Australians living in rural and remote Australia who have poorer access to healthcare and worse health outcomes than those in urban and metropolitan areas

Source: Lin V, Smith J, Fawkes S, Robinson P, Gifford S. Public health practice in Australia: the organised effort. 2nd ed. London: Routledge, 2020.

Scientific and Industrial Research Organisation (CSIRO), Cancer Australia and national centres that focus on HIV/AIDS, immunisation and drugs and alcohol.[5]

The allocation of funds is also determined by pre-established research priorities. Every three years, the *National Health and Medical Research Council Act 1992* (NHMRC Act) requires the CEO to review the nation's major health priorities and to identify the health challenges and emerging issues where national capacity or capability in health and medical research is most needed.[6] The NHMRC's health priorities reflect broad, rather than specific, diseases. For the 2021–24 triennium, these priorities included:

- strengthening resilience to emerging health threats and emergencies, including environmental change, pandemics and antimicrobial resistance
- improving the health of Aboriginal and Torres Strait Islander peoples, including through research that addresses health inequities
- building capacity and innovation in the effective translation of research into quality health policy, services and care
- preventing and managing multimorbidity and chronic conditions
- identifying emerging technologies in health and medical research and in healthcare, and promoting their safe, ethical and effective application.

9.3.3 Non-government, not-for-profit and community organisations

Non-government organisations play a critical role in promoting health and facilitating public health initiatives in communities. This sector boasts a diverse scope of services and interests, and may be funded from a variety of government, non-government and community sources. Many organisations focus on a specific health issue (e.g. heart disease, asthma, diabetes, cancer) or target specific at-risk population groups (e.g. Aboriginal and Torres Strait Islander peoples, people with HIV/AIDS, children and older Australians). Other organisations may have broader and more dynamic public health objectives that shift with national health priorities and the overarching health landscape. For example, the Public Health Association of Australia (PHAA) is a non-government, NFP organisation for public health in Australia with members and branches located across each state and territory. The PHAA's campaigns target a wide range of public health interests, with the most recent priorities including increasing investments in preventive health, preventing chronic disease, closing the gap on Indigenous youth health, and protecting the natural environment.

The PHAA also operates several special interest groups (SIGs) that direct initiatives in more targeted health areas. As with most NPF organisations, the PHAA is funded through a combination of membership fees, events, donations and government subsidies. NFP and non-government organisations are founded upon an informed understanding and care of the issues faced by their targeted communities and often boast strong relationships with key community members and spokespeople.

9.3.4 Primary healthcare and healthcare providers

The Australian Institute of Health and Welfare (AIHW) defines 'primary healthcare' as the entry level into the health system. Primary healthcare encompasses an individual's first encounter with the health system and may involve a range of activities and services, from health promotion and prevention to treatment and management of acute and chronic conditions.[7] The backbone of the community-based primary healthcare system is the general practice, where general practitioners (GPs) are the most commonly accessed source for information and advice on health issues, reducing or preventing health risks and providing health education. Pharmacists, nurses and other allied health professionals, such as dentists and physiotherapists, are also examples of primary healthcare providers.

Primary healthcare is typically provided in community settings, where it is ideally positioned to serve many important public health functions and is integral in facilitating and advocating for public health initiatives. These may include encouraging the greater use of one-to-one clinical consultation opportunities, operating screenings, organising group education activities, promoting preventive healthcare, and facilitating broader community development strategies and population-based policy. In Australia, Primary Health Networks (PHNs) are independent organisations that coordinate primary healthcare in designated areas and operate closely with state and territory local hospital networks. PHNs aim to improve the efficiency and effectiveness of health services for people, in particular for those at risk of poor health outcomes, as well as improve the coordination and accessibility of these services.

9.4 Intersections of public health and infection prevention and control

Over the last century, Australia has implemented numerous national public health interventions and strategies aimed at controlling, preventing and eliminating infectious disease (Table 9.3). These interventions have

ment Quarantine

TABLE 9.3 Historical overview of successful infectious disease control activities[3,9]

Year	Primary public health interventions
1908	The first federal public health legislation, the *Quarantine Act 1908*, was passed
1930–40	Improvements in sanitation and drinking water reduced waterborne diseases
1932	National vaccination program for diphtheria in children introduced
1941	Penicillin developed
1942	Vaccination program for pertussis introduced
1947	Effective treatment for tuberculosis discovered
1948–51	Tuberculosis Screening and Treatment Program initiated Australian WHO Collaborating Centre for Reference and Research on Influenza established
1956	Vaccination program for poliomyelitis introduced
1963	WHO guidelines on drinking water quality released
1966	Oral poliomyelitis vaccine introduced
1970–71	Measles vaccination introduced Rubella vaccination for schoolgirls introduced
1972	NHMRC issued guidelines on drinking water quality in Australian capital cities based on WHO guidelines
1983	Australia certified malaria-free by the WHO
1987	'Grim Reaper' HIV/AIDS campaign launched
1989	First National HIV/AIDS Strategy published Communicable Diseases Control Network established (later CDNA) Measles-mumps-rubella vaccine released for all infants at 12 months
1992	National Water Quality Management Strategy launched
1995	The Cooperative Research Centre for Water Quality and Treatment established
1996	Australian Childhood Immunisation Register (ACIR) established
1999	National Influenza Vaccine Program for Older Australians commenced
2000	Australia declared polio-free Hepatitis B vaccine for infants introduced National food safety standards developed. OzFoodNet established
2003	High-risk food industry sectors required to implement food safety programs based on Hazard Analysis and Critical Control Point methods
2004	NHMRC issued further Australian drinking water guidelines to incorporate framework for management of drinking water quality
2005	National Pneumococcal Vaccine Program for Older Australians commenced Varicella vaccine introduced for children NHMRC guidelines for managing recreational water introduced
2006	National guidelines of water recycling issues, focusing on the treatment of sewage and greywater
2007	Rotavirus vaccine introduced Human Papilloma Virus (HPV) vaccine introduced for school-aged girls
2018	Australia declared rubella-free by the WHO

Source: Australian Institute of Health and Welfare. Health system overview, 2020; Gruszin S, Hetzel D, Glover J. Advocacy and action in public health: lessons from Australia over the twentieth century, 2012.

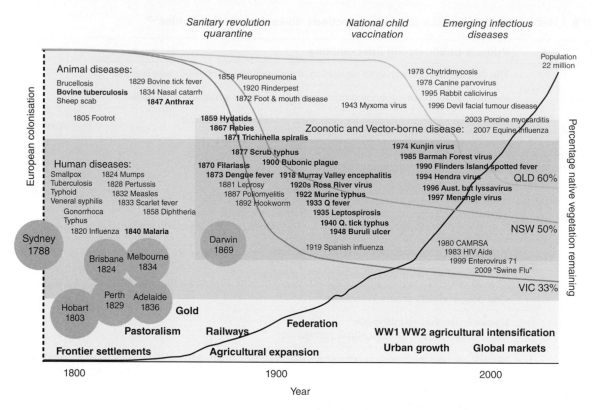

FIGURE 9.1 History of infectious disease emergence in Australia, 1788–2009,
with key developments and public health events
*Source: McFarlane, S. (2016). Australian Institute of Health and Welfare (AIHW).
Primary health care in Australia. Canberra, Australia.*

evolved over time to integrate new developments made in medicine and medical technology and in response to novel disease threats. This section describes the various public health measures that have been taken to combat infection and infectious diseases since the start of the 20th century (Fig 9.1).

9.4.1 Quarantine

Introduced in official federal legislation under the Commonwealth *Quarantine Act 1908*, quarantine was one of the earliest public health strategies put in place to combat infectious diseases in Australia. However, even prior to the establishment of the act, quarantine strategies had been employed in response to most known infectious disease outbreaks in the country, most notably smallpox, measles and the plague. Historically, quarantine served to prevent the entry of diseases into Australia via infected travellers arriving by ship. The act also extended to cover the importation of animal and plant diseases. Maritime arrivals with confirmed or suspected infections were quarantined at sea for a period of several weeks prior to entry. These

strategies proved to be effective to a point, notably having successfully delayed the introduction of the H1N1 influenza A virus, which caused the 1918–19 global pandemic, to the Australian population for several weeks. However, breaches in quarantine were to become a major issue, and failures to identify all infected cases eventually saw the novel influenza strain circulate across all states and territories in the country. Moreover, viruses and pathogens carried by animals, such as the bubonic plague, were also near impossible to manage and control once the ship had docked.

Nevertheless, quarantine remains a widely implemented public health strategy for controlling the spread of infectious disease in the present day. The *Quarantine Act 1908* was superseded more than 100 years later by the *Biosecurity Act 2015*, which was vigorously tested during the recent SARS-CoV-2 (COVID-19) pandemic. The development of modern transport infrastructure and increased accessibility to cars and air travel have made quarantine an increasingly difficult strategy to implement and regulate. Modern travellers are now more mobile than ever before, capable of traversing across the entire world within 24 hours. The rapid spread of SARS-CoV-2 starkly highlights how easily a novel infectious disease can take advantage of human mobility to spread from country to country.

9.4.2 Hygiene, water sanitation and food safety

Similar to the conditions of cities in Britain and Europe, the major settlements of Australia by the beginning of the 20th century were fraught with poor sanitation, deteriorating building structures and overcrowded living conditions. The lack of proper infrastructure combined with high density living led to the accumulation of human waste, which contaminated both living and working environments. Urban centres were prime conduits for disease epidemics, such as smallpox, typhoid and the bubonic plague. By this time, the sanitary revolution and the reforms had already begun in Britain. Public health efforts implemented to 'remove noxious exhalations' by improving sanitation and introducing proper drainage and ventilation systems, also incidentally removed the actual cause of disease: microorganisms. Increased scientific understanding of the causes of disease subsequently led to the introduction of environmental health policies, particularly those pertaining to the safety and quality of food and water.

Water sanitation: Initiatives to provide clean drinking water and to separate main water pipelines from being contaminated with raw sewage and human waste marked some of the first public health reforms across Australian states and territories. Public health

policies to improve water sanitation can be traced as far back as 1850 in Sydney, which introduced the initial legislation 'for the better sewerage, cleansing and draining of the City of Sydney'.[10] Furthermore, water shortages caused by frequent droughts and mounting public anxiety about water supplies led to the appointment of a Royal Commission in NSW in 1867 to investigate methods of reliably supplying water to the rapidly growing city and its surrounding suburbs.

The result was the development of the Upper Nepean Scheme, which saw the collection of water on the Southern Highlands that would then be channelled down and stored in a reservoir in Prospect. Construction was completed in 1888, and by this stage approximately 85% of Sydney's population was connected to the water supply (Fig 9.2). The original infrastructure also lent itself to progressive expansion, as four new dams were added between 1888 and 1935 to accommodate the growing population and several periods of drought. This scheme remains a major landmark in the history of public health in Sydney, and continues to supply 20–40% of the city's water today.[11] Subsequent initiatives in water quality came with the introduction of chlorination in the 1930s and 1940s, where processes of filtration and disinfection were recognised for their purpose in eliminating microorganisms and preventing waterborne disease outbreaks such as dysentery, typhoid and cholera. Since then, many water treatment methods have been developed, and regulating the supply of clean, high-quality drinking water remains an important public health endeavour to the present day.[12]

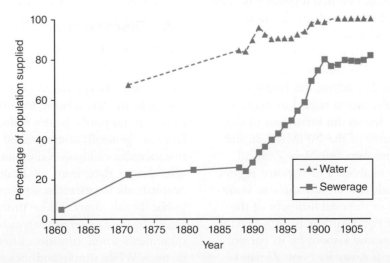

FIGURE 9.2 Proportion of Sydney population served by water and sewerage connections, 1860–1906

Source: de Looper, M. W., Booth, H., & Baffour, B. (2019). Sanitary improvement and mortality decline in Sydney, New South Wales, 1857–1906: drinking water and dunnies as determinants. The History of the Family, 24(2), 227-248.

At the same time, public health initiatives targeting the management of sewage and waste disposal were also in effect. In the 1850s, attempts to construct an underground drainage system to channel both stormwater and raw sewage into Sydney Harbour were ultimately ineffective at dispersing the sewage, leading to the serious pollution of waterways.[13] By the 1870s, less than 50% of households were connected to sewers and most people were still relying on cesspits and surface drainage systems. The Sydney Sewerage Board reported that 4700 of the city's 5400 toilets were contaminating the city's drinking water mains with sewage.[10] This led to the construction of two gravitation sewers in 1889 by the Public Works Department, which included a northern sewer discharging to the ocean near Bondi and a southern sewer draining to a sewerage farm at Botany Bay. By 1906, more than 75% of Sydney's population was connected to the new sewerage system. Similar construction in other Australian cities followed.

Food safety: Food safety is a key public health responsibility overseen by all states and territories. Foodborne diseases can occur as a result of bacteria, parasites, toxins and viruses, most of which lead to the presentation of acute diarrhoeal disease and may occasionally develop into more serious illness. The first law for regulating food was introduced in Victoria in the form of the *Victoria Public Food Act 1854*, which allowed the Board of Health to inspect, seize and destroy unwholesome foods. Following federation at the beginning of the 20th century, food legislation became the prime responsibility of individual state and territory governments. The heterogeneity of food laws across states created issues with interstate trade, leading to a series of Commonwealth/state conferences throughout 1910 to 1927 to institute uniform food standards.[14] The establishment of the NHMRC in 1936 served to advise the Department of Health on food regulations in regard to matters of public health, which led to the formation of the Food Standard Committee of the NHMRC in the 1950s. By 1996, the Australian and New Zealand governments agreed to establish a bi-national regime to develop food standards that would apply in both countries. This resulted in the establishment of the Australia New Zealand Food Authority (ANZFA) in 1996, which in 2002 became known by its current name: the Food Standards Australia New Zealand (FSANZ). FSANZ is an independent statutory authority that develops food standards and regulates the use of ingredients, additives, vitamins and minerals, as well as food composition, labelling requirements and recall protocols.

The primary sources of foodborne disease have shifted significantly over the last century. In the early 1900s, most foodborne disease outbreaks originated in the home as a result of undercooked or improperly prepared family meals or home preserved goods. However, the modern era has introduced mass food importation as well as a greater culture for consuming food outside of the home. In the present day, foodborne diseases are more likely to be contracted as a result of dining out, with restaurants in Australia accounting for 46% of all foodborne outbreaks and 37% of all reported cases. In 2016, approximately 4.1 million people were infected by foodborne diseases in Australia annually, costing an estimated $1.2 billion.[15] Campylobacteriosis and salmonellosis, both typically originating from the consumption of undercooked poultry products, were the most frequently notified infections and comprised up to 95% of total notifications.

Currently, foodborne diseases are monitored by OzFoodNet, which was established in 2000 by the Australian Government Department of Health and is represented within the CDNA. OzFoodNet works in collaboration with FSANZ, the Department of Agriculture, Water and the Environment, state and territory food authorities and the Public Health Laboratory Network. The surveillance system publishes quarterly and annual reports summarising the incidence and epidemiology of foodborne outbreaks over the specified reporting period. Reports are published independently for national data and for each Australian state and territory.[15]

9.4.3 Disease surveillance and notifiable diseases

Disease surveillance is the ongoing, systematic collection, analysis and interpretation of health data. Surveillance is crucial in matters relating to communicable disease and in informing public health action. Two types of surveillance are generally distinguished: passive and active. Passive surveillance involves the routine collection of notifiable disease data from all healthcare sources, such as hospitals, clinics, specialist services, laboratories and other public health units. These procedures are usually enforced by state or territory legislature and hence, the requirements for notification often differ between jurisdictions. While simple and inexpensive, the data may be incomplete or have irreconcilable inconsistencies, depending on where it was collected. Active surveillance is used for active case-seeking, such as during an outbreak of a specific disease, and usually involves the employment of staff to regularly contact healthcare providers for information. This strategy will provide more specific case definitions, resulting in more complete data but at a greater cost of resources.[16]

There have been significant improvements in national and state-based surveillance of infectious diseases through mandatory notification and other alert and control systems over the last 20 years. The National Notifiable Diseases Surveillance System (NNDSS) is a passive surveillance system established in 1990 under the CDNA that records and publishes fortnightly national data of the incidence of selected diseases across all Australian states and territories.[17] Health practitioners, laboratories and hospitals are responsible for alerting local, state and Commonwealth authorities upon detecting a notifiable disease, so that the appropriate protocols and procedures can be implemented to prevent the potential spread of the infection within the larger community. The current list of nationally notifiable diseases in Australia is presented in Table 9.4.

TABLE 9.4 Nationally notifiable diseases in Australia[5,18]

Anthrax	Malaria
Australian bat lyssavirus	Measles
Avian influenza in humans (AIH)	Meningococcal infection (invasive)
Barman Forest virus infection	Middle East respiratory syndrome coronavirus (MERS-CoV)
Botulism	Monkeypox
Brucellosis	Mumps
Campylobacteriosis	Murray Valley encephalitis virus infection
Chikungunya	Paratyphoid
Chlamydial infection	Pertussis (whooping cough)
Cholera	Plague
Creutzfeldt-Jakob disease (CJD)	Pneumococcal disease (invasive)
Creutzfeldt-Jakob disease–variant (vCJD)	Poliovirus infection
Cryptosporidiosis	Psittacosis (Ornithosis)
Dengue virus infection	Q fever
Diphtheria	Rabies

TABLE 9.4 Nationally notifiable diseases in Australia—cont'd

Donovanosis	Respiratory syncytial virus (RSV) laboratory-confirmed
Flavivirus infection	Ross River virus infection
Gonococcal infection	Rotavirus
Haemolytic uraemic syndrome (HUS)	Rubella
Haemophilus influenzae serotype b (Hib)	Rubella (congenital)
Hepatitis A	Salmonellosis
Hepatitis B (newly acquired or unspecified)	Severe acute respiratory syndrome (SARS)
Hepatitis C (newly acquired or unspecified)	Shiga toxin-producing *Escherichia coli* (STEC)
Hepatitis D	Shigellosis
Hepatitis E	Smallpox
Hepatitis B (not elsewhere classified)	Syphilis (congenital OR infectious <2 years duration OR >2 years or unknown duration)
Human immunodeficiency virus (HIV; individuals <18 months old OR newly acquired OR unspecified individuals >18 months old)	Tetanus
Human coronavirus with pandemic potential (COVID-19)	Tuberculosis
Influenza (laboratory-confirmed)	Tularaemia
Invasive Group A Streptococcal (iGAS) disease	Typhoid
Japanese encephalitis virus infection	Varicella zoster (chicken pox)
Legionellosis	Varicella zoster (shingles)
Leprosy (Hansen's disease)	Varicella zoster (not elsewhere specified)
Leptospirosis	Viral haemorrhagic fever (quarantinable)
Listeriosis	West Nile/Kunjin virus infection
Lyssavirus (not elsewhere classified)	Yellow fever

Source: Australian Institute of Health and Welfare. Health and medical research, 2020; Communicable Diseases Network Australia. Australian national notifiable diseases and case definitions, 2021

9.4.4 Disease screening

Screening programs are effective for the early detection of infectious diseases, allowing for swift intervention to prevent spread and reduce morbidity and mortality. Historically, a number of national health screening programs have been organised and conducted to great success, reducing both the incidence and subsequent burden of diseases such as tuberculosis (TB).

Today, public health programs provide important screening services in antenatal healthcare for the early detection of infectious diseases transmitted from mother to baby before or during pregnancy, such as rubella, syphilis, hepatitis B and HIV.[19] Timely detection allows for the administration of effective treatment and improved outcome of the pregnancy. While recent programs for screening in the general population have largely shifted to the detection of more chronic diseases and cancer, the advent of multiple infectious disease outbreaks, including the COVID-19 pandemic at the start of 2020, highlight the continued need for disease screening and surveillance, particularly when such diseases are able to traverse longer distances than ever before.

The Australian Tuberculosis Campaign (1950–76)

Tuberculosis is a contagious bacterial disease that is spread through respiratory air droplets and primarily attacks the lungs. It was a major cause of mortality, particularly in infants, in the early 20th century. While improvements in living standards and nutrition saw a general decline of TB case numbers in the early 1900s,

approximately 4000 cases were still notified annually between 1917 and 1950. This led to the establishment of the Division of Tuberculosis within the Department of Health in 1927. Efforts to tackle TB began in earnest following World War II, facilitated by the work of Dr Harry Wunderly and Dr Cecil Eddy who developed an x-ray apparatus that allowed for mass screenings of TB in Australian troops. The plan was to extend this screening process to the general Australian population in an extensive attempt to eliminate the disease altogether (Fig 9.3).

A national campaign against TB was launched with the passing of the *Tuberculosis Act 1945*, and its successive amendment in 1948 by the Commonwealth Government. The aptly named Australian Tuberculosis Campaign (ATC) offered free tuberculosis screening and was steered by a council of medical experts. It was steadily launched across all Australian states and territories between 1950 and 1963. Although some states, such as Victoria and NSW, already provided x-ray services, this was the first nationally coordinated and widely advertised campaign that promoted the procedure to the greater population in tandem with activities that aimed to reduce the stigma and fear associated with the disease (Fig 9.4). Importantly, the campaign was also nationally funded, which allowed the service to be provided to citizens free-of-charge. Additional costs such as those associated with medical care, an allowance for citizens unable to work, and the maintenance of infrastructure required for the tests were also covered nationally. In return, states needed to ensure that notifications for all forms of TB were reported and that compulsory x-raying was conducted for all people

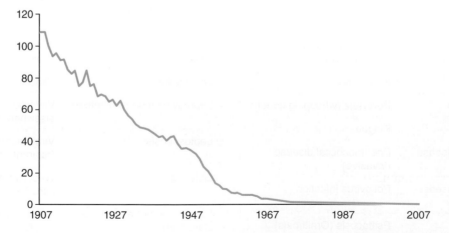

FIGURE 9.3 Age-standardised death rate from tuberculosis (per 100,000 persons)

Source: History of tuberculosis control in Australia. NHMRC: https://www.nhmrc.gov.au/about-us/resources/impact-case-studies/history-tuberculosis-control-australia

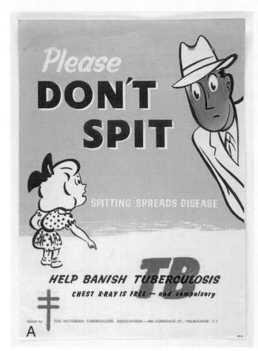
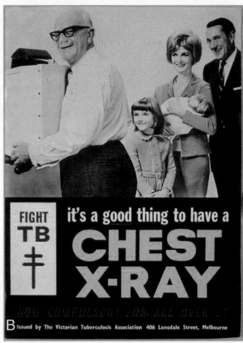

FIGURE 9.4a and b Tuberculosis campaign posters circulated during the Australian Tuberculosis Campaign (1950–76) in Victoria

Source: Museums Victoria. https://collections.museumsvictoria.com.au/articles/16869.

over 14 years of age, as well as all contacts and suspects. The ATC operated for almost 30 years and, in conjunction with the introduction of a vaccination and antibiotics, facilitated the near-eradication of TB in Australia.

The campaign ended in 1976, and since then Australia has maintained a low incidence of approximately 5–6 cases per 100,000 and a case fatality rate of 1%.[20] Efforts in controlling TB have continued in recent years and are overseen by the National Tuberculosis Advisory Committee, which was established in 1999 as an advisory committee to the CDNA. The rate of TB in Australia is low by global standards and sets the precedent for the complete eradication of the disease in the country. Despite the success of earlier efforts, there has arguably been little progress made to continue the decrease of TB in recent decades and the prevalence of the disease persists, with infected individuals migrating from countries with greater TB burden as well as in specific, vulnerable sub-populations in Australia; for example, in Indigenous communities, case numbers are up to six times higher compared to the non-Indigenous population (Fig 9.5).

At the time of writing, *The Strategic Plan for Control of Tuberculosis in Australia, 2016–2020: Towards Disease Elimination* is the most recently published national plan for TB control in Australia.[21] The plan outlines the strategy milestone of achieving <10 cases per million population by 2035 and highlights additional key short-term goals, such as reducing TB incidence by 10% on average per annum and reducing the disparity between Indigenous and non-Indigenous populations. Screening measures continue to be implemented to detect cases of TB as migration from high-incidence countries continues to be the most challenging source of TB in Australia, comprising up to 85–90% of cases.[20] The 2016–2020 Strategy highlights the need for pre- and post-migration screening and for the provision of culturally and linguistically appropriate care and access to treatment.

9.4.5 Vaccines and mass immunisation

Vaccination and inoculation against infectious diseases has been successfully implemented at moderate scales since the mid-1800s. At the time, diseases like smallpox were particularly prevalent, and testing of the effectiveness of inoculation first began in Great Britain. Practices were subsequently imported to the colonies in Australia; however, records of the numbers and uptake of immunisation are sparse. Since then, national immunisation programs have been implemented where vaccines have been made available. The first instances of community vaccination began in 1932 with the

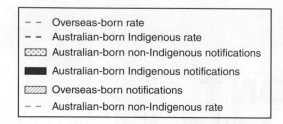

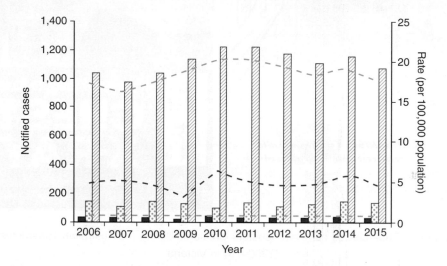

FIGURE 9.5 Notified cases and rates of tuberculosis, Australia, 2006–15, by population subgroup
Source: National Tuberculosis Advisory Committee. (2018). The strategic plan for control of tuberculosis in Australia, 2016–2020: towards disease elimination. The National Tuberculosis Advisory Committee for the Communicable Diseases Network Australia Communicable Diseases Intelligence, 2019(43), 1–19.

introduction of school-based immunisation programs that administered the diphtheria toxoid vaccine to children. Diphtheria, a bacterial infection of the nose and throat, was a top cause of mortality in infants at the beginning of the 20th century, and accounted for over 4000 deaths between 1926 and 1935.[22] Routine vaccination against diphtheria has continued with the Australian National Immunisation Program (NIP). Nowadays, diphtheria is exceedingly rare, with three deaths having been reported between 1997 and 2016,[23] and most reported cases imported from overseas.

Australia's response to poliomyelitis: Polioviruses are human enteroviruses, transmitted person-to-person via the faecal–oral route. Ninety-five percent of primary infections cause a transient viraemia without symptoms; however, paralysis occurs in one in 150 infections.[24] Australia was struck with several polio epidemics from the late 1930s to 1960s which resulted in up to 1000 annual cases and over 100 deaths across multiple outbreaks.[25,26] However, the disease itself had been described as early as 1887 and had caused several smaller outbreaks across several states

and territories at the beginning of the 20th century, becoming a notifiable condition in 1922. The last polio epidemic lasted from 1949 to 1956 and saw a nationwide case count of over 10,000, with record numbers in NSW, Queensland and South Australia.[25,26]

An immunisation program was initiated in 1955 in the wake of the official announcement of the Salk inactivated polio vaccine (IPV) by Dr Jonas Salk earlier that year. The mass immunisation process began in mid-1956 (Fig 9.6). Vaccine was manufactured at the Commonwealth Serum Laboratories (CSL) in Melbourne and states were directed to independently organise immunisation campaigns that kept prioritised sub-populations in mind. Vaccination rollout began for all persons under 14 years of age, pregnant women and those in high-risk groups. The oral polio vaccine (OPV) was subsequently developed by Dr Albert Sabin in 1961 and was adopted by Australia in 1966 where it eventually replaced the IPV as it was easier to administer. Both vaccines provided individuals with protection against all three poliovirus serotypes; however, OPV

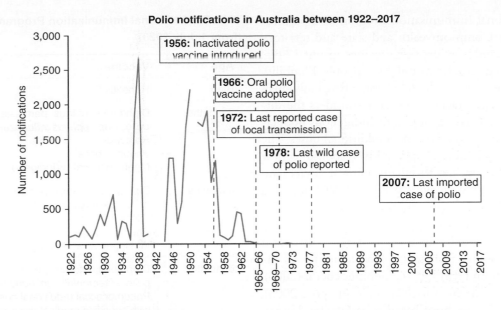

FIGURE 9.6 Notifications of poliomyelitis in Australia, 1922–2007, with all major public health milestones labelled

Source: AIHW (2019). Vaccine-preventable diseases fact sheets [Dataset]

was observed to occasionally (though rarely) become virulent and cause vaccine-associated paralytic polio-myelitis (VAPP). Additionally, some vaccine strains were circulated through excretions, and the resulting cases were known as vaccine-derived poliovirus (cVDPV). By the turn of the 21st century, cases of cVDPV would outnumber cases of wild polio glob-ally.[27,28] Global strategies in recent years have evolved to combat this issue with a gradual transition to IPV.

The immunisation program against polio was a great success, both in Australia and globally. Reported polio cases had reduced to one by 1966, with the last case of wild polio reported in 1978. Australia, along with 36 other countries, was declared polio-free by the World Health Organization in October 2000.[29] IPV continues to be recommended and administered to infants and children on a four-dose schedule at two, four and six months and four years of age. The contin-ued efforts towards the eradication of polio in Australia and around the world are contingent on rigorous ad-herence to vaccination schedules and the public health systems that make the benefits of this process widely understood and accessible. The importance of herd im-munity should also not be understated as there are still countries where polio is endemic, and travel to and from these countries carries a high risk of causing out-breaks in Australia. At time of writing, the last case of imported polio in Australia was reported in 2007 when an overseas student returned from Pakistan and was admitted to hospital upon a diagnosis with polio.

Sufficiently high levels of immunisation will ensure that if polio cases do re-emerge, that outbreaks can be more effectively contained and eliminated.

The National Immunisation Program (NIP): The elimination of polio highlights the effectiveness of mass immunisation as a public health strategy to protect the population from, and potentially eliminate, infectious diseases. The first national vaccination schedules for diphtheria, tetanus, pertussis and measles were established in 1975. Prior to this, the ages at which infants and children received specific vaccine doses varied slightly between jurisdictions. After 1975, new recommendations were periodically added to the national schedule as new vaccines were introduced and funded. Data from the 1989–90 National Health Survey showed an approximate full immunisation coverage (i.e. children that had received adequate vaccine doses for diphtheria, tetanus, pertussis, polio, measles and mumps) rate of 53%.[30]

The first National Immunisation Strategy was initi-ated in 1993, which was followed by the Australian Childhood Immunisation Register (ACIR) in 1994 and the National Immunisation Program (NIP) in 1997. The ACIR expanded to become the Australian Immunisation Register (AIR) in 2016, which maintains the records of vaccines administered to people of all ages in Australia, as well as continuing to provide comprehensive reports of immunisation coverage to the present day.

The National Immunisation Program is a partnership between Commonwealth and state and territory governments, and provides free vaccines against 17 diseases (including shingles) for eligible people. Eligibility for certain vaccines is scheduled for when individuals enter specific age brackets, and also considers the different needs of at-risk groups and Indigenous populations for earlier immunisation or additional doses. The immunisation schedule is updated in response to new research and public health efforts, clinical advice and the adoption of new vaccines. When the NIP launched in 1997, it provided vaccinations for nine diseases. The most notable vaccination appointments that have been added to the schedule since the program's inception include the funding of hepatitis B vaccines for all infants starting from birth (2000), meningococcal (2003), pneumococcal (2005), varicella (chicken pox; 2005), rotavirus (2007), a school-based schedule for human papillomavirus (2007, 2013) and shingles (herpes zoster; 2016). At the time of writing, the most recent change made was in July 2020, to introduce the meningococcal B vaccine for Aboriginal and Torres Strait Islander infants at two, four and 12 months of age—with an additional dose at six months for those with specified medical risk conditions.[31] The current national vaccination schedule is presented in Table 9.5. States and territories are also authorised to include additional vaccination appointments, which are typically informed by the prevalence or burden of diseases that are specific to their location.

Over the last 20 years, immunisation programs targeted at protecting individuals starting from infancy and through to adulthood have been highly effective at controlling vaccine-preventable diseases (VPD). The evolution and nationwide dissemination of vaccines against measles, mumps and rubella is particularly illustrative of the congruence between vaccination research and a well-founded public health structure. Vaccines for measles, rubella and mumps were registered and released independently in 1968, 1969 and 1980, respectively.[32] The combined measles-mumps (MM) vaccine was introduced in 1982 and was then replaced by the measles-mumps-rubella (MMR) vaccine shortly after in 1989.[32] Elimination of endemic measles in Australia was endorsed by the World Health Organization in 2014 and this was followed by rubella in 2018 (Fig 9.7).[33,34]

The immunisation of children at one, two and five years of age for all recommended vaccines has increased considerably over the last two decades (Fig 9.8).[35,36] As of December 2021, 94.61% of one-year-old and 94.98% of five-year-old children are

TABLE 9.5 National Immunisation Program schedule (from 1 July 2020)*

Age	Vaccine
Birth	Hepatitis B
2 months	Diphtheria, tetanus, pertussis, hepatitis B, polio, *Haemophilus influenzae* type b (Hib) Rotavirus Pneumococcal Meningococcal B (Indigenous children)
4 months	Diphtheria, tetanus, pertussis, hepatitis B, polio, *Haemophilus influenzae* type b (Hib) Rotavirus Pneumococcal Meningococcal B (Indigenous children)
6 months	Diphtheria, tetanus, pertussis, hepatitis B, polio, *Haemophilus influenzae* type b (Hib) Pneumococcal (additional dose for children with specified medical risk conditions) Pneumococcal (Indigenous children living in WA, NT, SA, QLD) Meningococcal B (Indigenous children with specified medical risk conditions)
12 months	Meningococcal ACWY Measles, mumps, rubella Pneumococcal Meningococcal B (Indigenous children)
18 months	*Haemophilus influenzae* type b (Hib) Measles, mumps, rubella, varicella (chicken pox) Diphtheria, tetanus, pertussis Hepatitis A (Indigenous children in WA, NT, SA and QLD)
4 years	Diphtheria, tetanus, pertussis, polio Pneumococcal (additional dose for children with specified medical risk conditions) Pneumococcal (Indigenous children living in WA, NT, SA, QLD) Hepatitis A (Indigenous children in WA, NT, SA, QLD)
12–13 years	Diphtheria, tetanus, pertussis Human papillomavirus (HPV)
14–16 years	Meningococcal ACWY
> 50 years	Pneumococcal (Indigenous adults)
> 70 years	Pneumococcal (non-Indigenous adults)
70–79 years	Shingles (herpes zoster)
Pregnant women	Pertussis

* Additional doses are indicated in pink and marked for either Indigenous children or adults; and blue for children with specified medical risk conditions
Source: Australian Government Department of Health and Aged Care. Data from https://www.health.gov.au/topics/immunisation/when-to-get-vaccinated/national-immunisation-program-schedule

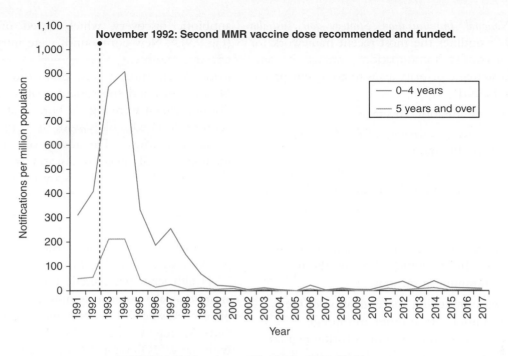

FIGURE 9.7 Measles notifications, 1991–2017

Source: Data from AIHW (2019). Vaccine-preventable diseases fact sheets [Dataset]

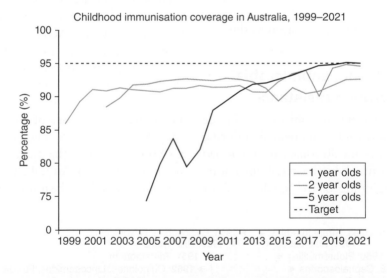

FIGURE 9.8 Childhood immunisation coverage of 1-, 2- and 5-year-old children from 1999–2021. This represents the proportion of children that have received 'full immunisation', which includes vaccination against hepatitis B, diphtheria, tetanus, pertussis, *Haemophilus influenzae* type b (Hib), polio, measles, mumps, rubella, pneumococcal, varicella and meningococcal C

Source: Data from: https://www.health.gov.au/topics/immunisation/immunisation-data/childhood-immunisation-coverage/historical-coverage-data-tables-for-all-children

fully immunised. Immunisation coverage for two-year-old children, while substantially greater compared to rates in the 1980s, has plateaued in recent years and currently lags behind other age groups with a coverage rate of 92.6%. Comparatively, coverage for one- and two-year-old Aboriginal and Torres Strait Islander children is also lower, at 92.42% and 91.38% respectively. However, coverage for five-year old children has surpassed the national immunisation target and is currently the highest of any age group.[35,36]

The *National Immunisation Strategy for Australia 2019–2024*[37] outlines the most recent framework for efforts to maximise immunisation coverage. It comprises eight strategic priority areas to complement and strengthen the NIP:

1. Improve immunisation coverage

2. Ensure effective governance of the National Immunisation Program

3. Ensure secure vaccine supply and efficient use of vaccines for the National Immunisation Program

4. Continue to enhance vaccine safety monitoring systems

5. Maintain and ensure community confidence in the National Immunisation Program through effective communication strategies

6. Strengthen monitoring and evaluation of the National Immunisation Program through assessment and analysis of immunisation register data and vaccine-preventable disease surveillance

7. Ensure an adequately skilled immunisation workforce through promoting effective training for immunisation providers

8. Maintain Australia's strong contribution to the region.

9.4.6 Curative medicine, antimicrobial drugs and antimicrobial resistance

The discovery of the first antimicrobial drugs in the form of salvarsan, sulphonamides and penicillin during the early 20th century was revolutionary for the broad treatment of diseases caused by bacterial infections. The 1940s saw the beginning of the 'golden era' for antibiotic discovery, which lasted until the 1960s (Fig 9.9).[38] New compounds were introduced for the effective treatment of osteomyelitis, empyema, rheumatic fever, tuberculosis, gonorrhoea and syphilis. Notifications and subsequent deaths caused by these diseases, which were a great burden at the start of the century, declined rapidly with the wide dissemination of the new drugs.[39] The advent of antibiotics carried the hope that all infectious diseases would eventually be eliminated. However, the discovery of new antibiotics has stalled in recent times. Additionally, there has been an alarming increase in antimicrobial resistance where the misuse and overuse of antimicrobials have led to the emergence of drug-resistant pathogens, which present a significant threat to human health.

Health strategies aimed at resisting the spread of antimicrobial resistance is now a key national health priority. Australia's First National Antimicrobial Resistance Strategy was released in 2015 and solely aligned with the WHO's Global Action Plan on Antimicrobial Resistance.[40] The Strategy offered a national framework for coordinating a cross-sectoral response, which included the creation of a central online repository for trusted information, the Antimicrobial Use and Resistance in Australia (AURA) Surveillance System, and significant investments into antimicrobial research via government-funded grants. The subsequently released 2020 Strategy[40] presents a 20-year plan, which broadens the original scope to include food, the environment and other classes of antimicrobials, such as antifungals and antivirals. The Strategy was endorsed by COAG, indicating the necessary combined involvement of all levels of Australian government in achieving the objective of this health initiative.

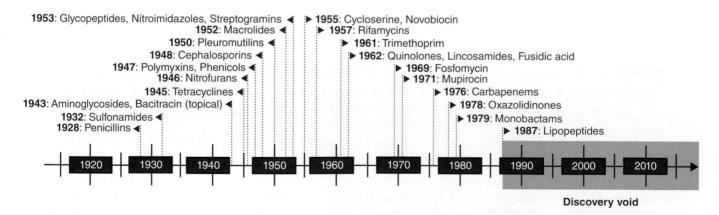

FIGURE 9.9 Timeline of the discovery of antibiotics

Source: Adapted from Silver L L. Challenges of antibacterial discovery. Clin Microbiol Rev. 2011;24:71–109.

9.4.7 Health protection

Health protection is overseen by both the Commonwealth and state and territory governments, and can be broadly defined as 'the prevention and control of threats to health from communicable diseases and the environment'.[41] Health protection is achieved through the collaboration of an extensive array of activities involving multiple people and agencies. At the national level, the Australian Health Protection Principal Committee (AHPPC) is responsible for advising on emerging health threats, including on infectious diseases. The AHPPC works closely with state and territory Chief Health Officers to ensure a consistent application of health policies and standards. It is advised by several specialised committees, including the Communicable Diseases Network Australia (CDNA), which currently surveys and records all notifiable disease events in Australia.

Health protection within states and territories replicates this general structure one level down. For example, Health Protection NSW comprises one of the branches within the Population and Public Health Division of the Ministry of Health, which coordinates the 'strategic direction, planning, monitoring and performance of population health services across the state'.[42] The major factors that protect a population's health, as highlighted by Health Protection NSW, are listed in Table 9.6. Health Protection NSW's Communicable Disease and Environmental Health branches work in tandem with public health units (PHUs) in local health districts, clinicians, government agencies, local government and communities. Additionally, other centres within the same division have overlapping interests,

TABLE 9.6. Factors that protect a population's health (NSW Ministry of Health)

• Clean drinking water • Housing that is safe and not overcrowded • Safe disposal of waste • Clean recreational water • Safe food • Clean air	• Vaccination • Education about safe behaviours including hygiene and safe sex • Sterile equipment used for procedures that penetrate the skin • Effective medicines for the treatment and prevention of infectious diseases • Built environments that are conducive to good health

Source: NSW Ministry of Health. Data from https://www.health.nsw.gov.au/about/ministry/Pages/hpnsw.aspx

such as the State Preparedness and Response Branch, responsible for state-level preparedness to critical clinical incidents and emergencies, as well as the Centre for Population Health, which aims to improve the health and reduce the burden of those infected with viruses like HIV and hepatitis B and C.

Regular reports are published which highlight notifiable disease statistics such as vaccine-preventable diseases, blood-borne viruses, STIs, enteric diseases and influenza, as well as immunisation coverage in comparison to national benchmarks and new vaccination campaigns.[41] The reports also provide updates on the development, progress and achievements of implemented programs, services and infrastructure, particularly those related to air quality and safe drinking water, waste and sewerage facilities, housing projects and Aboriginal and Torres Strait Islander health initiatives.

9.5 Contemporary challenges for public health and IPC in Australia

9.5.1 COVID-19: A new nexus for public health and IPC

COVID-19 is a disease caused by the SARS-CoV-2 virus, from a family of viruses called the coronaviruses. It causes mild to moderate febrile and respiratory symptoms in most people who are infected, such as fever, cough, lack of energy and muscle aches and pains. In some individuals, particularly older people or those with underlying medical conditions, the illness can develop to cause a severe pneumonitis or inflammation of the lungs, as well as inflammation of the heart muscle and other complications, and in some cases can be fatal. COVID-19 is highly infectious, and transmission occurs primarily from person to person via respiratory droplet or aerosol transmission.

The exact origin of the SARS-CoV-2 virus has not yet been established, but most experts consider it to be a zoonotic infection. The original infections may have occurred in bats, as was found to be the case with the SARS-CoV-1 and MERS-CoV viruses, and transmitted via an intermediate species to humans. Reverse/backwards zoonotic transmission of SARS-CoV-2 has also been observed, with humans having transmitted the SARS-CoV-2 virus to mink and white-tailed deer, among others.[43,44]

The first cases of COVID-19 were identified in the city of Wuhan in China in December 2019, after a cluster of unusual cases of pneumonia was reported.

Following this, the virus spread rapidly around the globe through person-to-person transmission and was declared to be a global pandemic by the World Health Organization (WHO) in March 2020.

The first case in Australia was confirmed in January 2020, in a man who had recently arrived from Wuhan. More cases were identified in returned travellers until March 2020 when the first case of local community transmission was reported.[45] In line with WHO advice, the Australian Health Protection Principal Committee (see Chapter 11) recommended quarantine of contacts of individuals with COVID-19 for a period of 14 days. Both in these initial stages and throughout most of the response to COVID-19 in Australia, broader public health measures were supported by a comprehensive and coordinated system of contact tracing, interviewing individuals with COVID-19 to identify their close contacts and directing these individuals to quarantine.

As case numbers rose globally, incremental regulatory measures were introduced in Australia through March 2020, with restrictions on large gatherings, targeted travel restrictions and instructions for international arrivals to self-isolate. On 19 March 2020,[46] the Australian Government took the unprecedented step of closing Australia's borders to all non-citizens and non-residents and in the following week announced that a system of managed quarantine in hotels would be coordinated where returning individuals would be required to quarantine for 14 days. Broader restrictions on movement, business and social activities domestically were also introduced through the first half of 2020, including the closure of non-essential industries, recommendations to work and study from home and domestic travel restrictions. These restrictions were underpinned by the enforcement of emergency orders, issued under existing public health legislation in Australian states and territories.[47]

These initial control measures were centred on the restriction of movement, to reduce the number of people with COVID-19 who were entering the Australian community while infectious and to remove the risk of onward transmission in those individuals already in the community. In terms of infection control principles, the focus of these interventions—systematically applied at the level of the entire population—was to break the chain of infection and eliminate any community COVID-19 transmission in Australia.

The global significance and rapid spread of COVID-19, as well as the need to implement whole-of-government and whole-of-society control measures, necessitated a defined emergency management framework to structure the response. This framework enabled inter- and intra-agency cooperation at various levels of government, industry and the wider community and provided governance arrangements to support the intensity of the surge response.

Over the course of the first year, more evidence emerged on how the SARS-CoV-2 virus spread, how it could be prevented and how the disease it caused progressed and could be treated. The importance of aerosols in transmitting the infection through even fleeting face-to-face contact, even in individuals without significant symptoms, was recognised. The use of non-pharmaceutical interventions increased, such as mask-wearing and social distancing, as disease control measures became more widespread in response to this changing understanding.

As the worldwide response to the COVID-19 pandemic flexed and adapted, so did the virus itself and a novel development in the response to this pandemic was the use of whole genome sequencing and genomic surveillance to characterise the evolution of the SARS-CoV-2 virus. New viral variants were assessed by the WHO to determine their likely impact on the development of the pandemic, and if required were designated *variants of interest* or *variants of concern*.[48] Labels were given to *variants of concern* based on the Greek alphabet, from the Alpha variant first detected in the UK in September 2020, to the Omicron variant currently dominant worldwide at the time of writing in January 2023.

This viral evolution had profound implications for the public health management of COVID-19 in Australia. As a public health emergency, the response to COVID-19 went well beyond business-as-usual. Critical to this was the extension and translation of non-pharmaceutical control interventions into the community at a mass scale level, such as the required application of public health and IPC principles across a diversity of settings (e.g. warehouses, offices, community settings). All of these settings required different foci of priority based on context and risk profile, all of which were enabled by legislation and its enforcement. Additional restrictions applied to high-risk settings (e.g. hospital, aged care, disability care) to limit exposure to the disease of the most vulnerable, especially at the start when there were no other therapeutic interventions available and the impact of COVID-19 disease was unknown.

Establishing and implementing a single, united strategy across Commonwealth, state and territory governments has been challenging, especially in the early phase of the outbreak.[49] A range of goals had been coined and espoused including, but not limited to, 'slowing the spread', 'flattening the curve', 'stopping the spread', 'aggressive suppression' and 'zero community transmission',[49] Fundamentally, all public health prevention and control interventions were, and are, aimed to prevent, control and contain the spread of COVID-19, however termed or coined. The activities and measures deployed by Australian governments at both state and federal levels—physical distancing, restrictions on gathering and movement, mandatory quarantine and isolation, and national and international travel restrictions—have been successful at preventing outbreaks of COVID-19, or containing outbreaks when they occurred, such as Victoria's second wave in 2020. Through the latter part of 2020, while international border restrictions remained in place, much of the restriction on internal movement and activities was relaxed as local case numbers decreased and COVID-19 was effectively eliminated from the Australian community. Sporadic and localised outbreaks did occur but were controlled with targeted measures. This changed with the introduction of the Delta variant of SARS-CoV-2 into Australia in June 2021. The increased transmissibility of this variant led to an exponential increase in the number of people infected, which stretched and then exceeded the capacity of the public health system to effectively eliminate COVID-19 and a change in strategy was required.

Underlying this change, and arguably the most important result of the global research effort in response to COVID-19, was the development of several highly effective vaccines, taking advantage of existing technology, such as adenovirus vector and protein subunit vaccines, as well as expanding the use of novel approaches such as mRNA vaccines for the first time. These vaccines, along with other developments including monoclonal antibody therapies and antiviral medications, paved the way for a change in emphasis in the public health response to COVID-19. A population-wide COVID-19 vaccination campaign was mounted in Australia, with over 41 million doses of COVID-19 vaccine administered between April and December 2021.[50] Against this background, the objectives of the COVID-19 response shifted from eliminating the infection to mitigating the risks of serious illness and death, particularly for the most vulnerable in society. In terms of infection control principles, the focus changed to reducing the susceptibility of everyone in the population in order to control case numbers and protect against severe illness.

Despite this change in strategy, there remained high-risk settings where more direct interventions were implemented to control disease transmission and protect the most vulnerable members of society from infection and disease. These settings could be defined both as those at high risk of uncontrolled transmission (including childcare centres, boarding schools and prisons) and those at high risk of severe consequences of disease (including hospitals, rural Aboriginal communities, group homes and particularly residential aged care facilities). The response to COVID-19 outbreaks in these settings was grounded in longstanding experience in the use of health protection strategies to control outbreaks in closed settings, including norovirus, gastroenteritis and influenza. This built on existing collaboration between public health and infection control professionals and focused on the principles of outbreak investigation, infection prevention and disease control. The targeted implementation of the same measures initially applied to control the spread in the general population—namely the selective use of testing, contact tracing, isolation, quarantine, personal protective equipment (PPE) and vaccination—was applied to interrupt the chain of transmission.

9.5.2 Environmental factors and climate change

Natural fluctuations in the environment and climate, in addition to human-caused climate change, will become increasingly relevant and unpredictable influences on infections and infectious diseases, both in the present and the near future. Between 2030 and 2050, climate change is expected to cause approximately 250,000 additional deaths per year from malnutrition, malaria, diarrhoea and heat stress alone.[51] Pressingly, climate change is already impacting human health in many ways. Extreme weather events, such as heatwaves, storms and floods, have both directly and indirectly increased illness and mortality. Climate and weather conditions are critical for the necessary survival, reproduction and transmission of disease pathogens, vectors and hosts.[52] Extreme weather conditions create opportunities for disease outbreaks in unexpected places. For example, heavy rains and floods across large areas on the eastern coast of Australia in 2022 led to outbreaks of water- and vectorborne diseases, such as Japanese encephalitis. These weather effects also predict the rise of zoonoses, foodborne diseases, and mental health issues.[51]

9.5.3 At-risk populations

Aboriginal and Torres Strait Islander peoples: The 1960s was a decade of major social change for First

Nations peoples, which also catalysed the introduction of health and research programs by state and territory governments. During this time, Aboriginal and Torres Strait Islander mortality primarily resulted from infections and neonatal deaths caused by a combination of poor access to adequate healthcare services, poor nutrition and sanitation. While certain infectious diseases such as pneumonia, gastroenteritis and syphilis were on the decline in the general population, they still imposed significant health threats to the Indigenous population well into the 1990s.

In general, while infectious disease is no longer a leading cause of disease burden, it still remains higher in Indigenous Australians compared to the general population.[53] Infectious diseases like trachoma (a chronic eye infection), tuberculosis, skin infections and certain sexually transmitted infections (STIs) all present at a higher rate. A further disparity is access to healthcare services, which is exacerbated by the higher proportion of the Indigenous population living in rural and remote areas compared to non-Indigenous Australians. Some progress has been made to ensure healthcare systems and policies are developed to consider the unique interests, characteristics and health issues of Aboriginal and Torres Strait Islander peoples. However, disparities in socio-economic and health outcomes persist and the long-lasting impacts of colonisation, displacement, erasure and disruption of cultural practices, customs and languages, intergenerational trauma and racial discrimination are still strongly felt (see Chapter 36).[54]

Aboriginal Community Controlled Health Organisations (ACCHOs) are specifically designed for Aboriginal people and provide holistic, culturally sensitive and high-quality healthcare and health education services. ACCHOs and Aboriginal Community Health Services (ACCHSs) are funded nationally under the Indigenous Australians' Health Programme (IAHP). The IAHP funds work under four themes: 1) primary healthcare services such as immunisation; 2) improving access to primary healthcare; 3) targeted health activities; and 4) capital works, such as buying, leasing, building and upgrading infrastructure.

Conclusion

Public health initiatives have been greatly influential in the prevention, control and elimination of infectious diseases in Australia over the last 200 years. Initial progress began with improvements in sanitation, hygiene, general living conditions and providing access to clean drinking water. This was further catalysed with new advances in medicine and medical technology, which saw the introduction of antimicrobial drugs and vaccines, and the subsequent implementation of mass screening programs and comprehensive immunisation schedules. Today, promoting high vaccine coverage and good infection prevention and control practices in the community continues to be a key strategy for ensuring that the incidence and spread of infectious disease remains low. Despite considerable successes in reducing, and even eradicating, certain diseases in the country, new issues pertaining to infectious disease continue to emerge—many of which demand timely public health action. In recent years, issues such as the COVID-19 pandemic and the alarming increase of antimicrobial resistance, have prompted the need for a comprehensive, full-system response across all levels of government. Strong public health strategies will play an integral role in preparing the healthcare system and the wider community to face these new challenges.

Useful websites/resources

- Australasian College for Infection Prevention and Control. https://www.acipc.org.au/
- Australasian Faculty of Public Health Medicine. https://www.racp.edu.au/about/college-structure/australasian-faculty-of-public-health-medicine
- Public Health Association of Australia. https://www.phaa.net.au/
- World Health Assembly. https://www.who.int/about/governance/world-health-assembly

References

1. Lin V, Smith J, Fawkes S, Robinson P, Gifford S. Public health practice in Australia: the organised effort. 2nd ed. London: Routledge, 2020.
2. Tulchinsky TH, Varavikova EA. A history of public health. In: The new public health. 3rd ed. Elsevier, 2014.
3. Australian Institute of Health and Welfare. Health system overview. Canberra: AIHW, 2020 [cited 21 Jun 2022]. Available from: https://www.aihw.gov.au/reports/australias-health/health-system-overview.
4. Australian Government Department of Health. The Australian health system. Canberra: Australian Government, 2019 [cited 21 Jun 2022]. Available from: https://www.health.gov.au/about-us/the-australian-health-system.

5. Australian Institute of Health and Welfare. Health and medical research. Canberra, Australia: AIHW, 2020 [cited 21 Jun 2022]. Available from: https://www.aihw.gov.au/reports/australias-health/health-and-medical-research.

6. National Health and Medical Research Council. NHMRC health priorities 2021–2024 Australia. Canberra: NHMRC, 2021 [cited 21 Jun 2022]. Available from: https://www.nhmrc.gov.au/research-policy/research-priorities/nhmrc-health-priorities.

7. Australian Institute of Health and Welfare. Primary health care in Australia. Canberra: AIHW, 2016.

8. McFarlane RA, Sleigh AC, McMichael AJ. Land-use change and emerging infectious disease on an island continent. Int J Environ Res Public Health. 2013;10(7):2699-2719.

9. Gruszin S, Hetzel D, Glover J. Advocacy and action in public health: lessons from Australia over the twentieth century. South Australia: Public Health Information Development Unit, The University of Adelaide, 2012.

10. de Looper MW, Booth H, Baffour B. Sanitary improvement and mortality decline in Sydney, New South Wales, 1857–1906: drinking water and dunnies as determinants. The History of the Family. 2019;24(2):227-248.

11. Water NSW. The Upper Nepean Scheme. Sydney, Australia: Water NSW [cited 22 Jun 2022]. Available from: https://www.waternsw.com.au/supply/heritage/water-schemes/upper-nepean-scheme-anniversary.

12. National Health and Medical Research Council. National Water Quality Management Strategy: Australian Drinking Water Guidelines 6. Canberra: NHMRC, 2011.

13. Wong A. Colonial sanitation, urban planning and social reform in Sydney, New South Wales 1788-1857. Australasian Historical Archaeology. 1999;17(1999):58-69.

14. Boisrobert C, Stjepanovic A, Oh S, Lelieveld H. Ensuring global food safety: exploring global harmonization. Cambridge MA: Academic Press, 2009.

15. The OzFoodNet Working Group. Monitoring the incidence and causes of disease potentially transmitted by food in Australia: annual report of the OzFoodNet network, 2016. In: Department of Health, ed. Canberra: Communicable Diseases Intelligence, 2021.

16. Nsubuga P, White ME, Thacker SB, Anderson MA, Blount SB, Broome CV, et al. Public health surveillance: a tool for targeting and monitoring interventions. In: Disease control priorities in developing countries. 2nd ed. Washington (DC): The International Bank for Reconstruction and Development/ The World Bank, 2006.

17. Australian Government Department of Health and Aged Care. Introduction to the National Notifiable Diseases Surveillance System 2015 [cited 28 Mar 2022]. Canberra: Australian Government, 2015. Available from: https://www.health.gov.au/internet/main/publishing.nsf/Content/cda-surveil-nndss-nndssintro.htm.

18. Communicable Diseases Network Australia. Australian national notifiable diseases and case definitions. Canberra: Australian Government Department of Health, 2021 [cited 28 Mar 2022]. Available from: https://www1.health.gov.au/internet/main/publishing.nsf/Content/cdna-casedefinitions.htm.

19. Australian Government Department of Health and Aged Care. Population-based health screening Canberra: Australian Government, 2021 [cited 11 Apr 2022]. Available from: https://www.health.gov.au/initiatives-and-programs/population-based-health-screening.

20. Bright A, Denholm J, Coulter C, Waring J, Stapledon R. Tuberculosis notifications in Australia, 2015–2018. In: Department of Health, ed. Canberra: Communicable Diseases Intelligence, 2018.

21. The National Tuberculosis Advisory Committee. The Strategic Plan for Control of Tuberculosis in Australia, 2016–2020: Towards Disease Elimination. Commun Dis Intell. 2018;43.

22. Feery B. One hundred years of vaccination. NSW Public Health Bull. 1997;8:61-63.

23. Australian Institute of Health and Welfare. Diphtheria in Australia. Canberra: AIHW, 2018.

24. Nathanson N, Kew OM. From emergence to eradication: the epidemiology of poliomyelitis deconstructed. Am J Epidemiol. 2010 Dec 1;172(11):1213-1229.

25. Hall R. Notifiable diseases surveillance, 1917 to 1991. Commun Dis Intell. 1993;17:226-236.

26. Australian Institute of Health and Welfare. Polio in Australia. Canberra: AIHW, 2018.

27. Badizadegan K, Kalkowska DA, Thompson KM. Polio by the numbers—a global perspective. J Infect Dis. 2022 Oct 15; 226(8):1309-1318.

28. Burgess MA, McIntyre PB. Vaccine-associated paralytic poliomyelitis. Commun Dis Intell. 1999 Mar 18;23:80-81.

29. Watson C, D'Souza RM, Kennett M. Australia declared polio free. Quarterly report. Commun Dis Intell. 2002; 26(2).

30. Australian Bureau of Statistics. 1989-90 National health survey children's immunisation survey, Australia: ABS, 1992. (Cat. no. 4379.0.)

31. Australian Government Department of Health and Aged Care. Clinical update: National Immunisation Program (NIP) schedule changes from 1 July 2020 – advice for vaccination providers. Canberra: Australian Government, 2020 [cited 12 Apr 2022]. Available from: https://www.health.gov.au/news/clinical-update-national-immunisation-program-nip-schedule-changes-from-1-july-2020-advice-for-vaccination-providers.

32. National Centre for Immunisation Research and Surveillance. Significant events in measles, mumps and rubella vaccination practice in Australia. 2019.

33. World Health Organization. Third Annual Meeting of the Regional Verification Commission for Measles Elimination in the Western Pacific, Seoul, Republic of Korea, 18-21 March 2014: report.

34. Australian Government Department of Health and Aged Care; The Hon Greg Hunt MP. Rubella officially eliminated from Australia [press release], 2018. Canberra: Australian Government, 2018.

35. Public Health Association of Australia. Top 10 public health successes over the last 20 years. Canberra: Public Health Association of Australia, 2018.

36. Australian Government Department of Health and Aged Care. Historical coverage data tables for all children. Canberra, Australia: Australian Government, 2022 [cited 12 Apr 2022]. Available from: https://www.health.gov.au/topics/immunisation/immunisation-data/childhood-immunisation-coverage/historical-coverage-data-tables-for-all-children.

37. Australian Government Department of Health. National Immunisation Strategy for Australia 2019-2014. Canberra: Australian Government, 2018.

38. Hutchings MI, Truman AW, Wilkinson B. Antibiotics: past, present and future. Curr Opin Microbiol. 2019;51:72-80.

39. Conly J, Johnston B. Where are all the new antibiotics? The new antibiotic paradox. Can J Infect Dis Med Microbiol. 2005;16(3):159-160.

40. Australian Government. Australia's national antimicrobial resistance strategy: 2020 and beyond. Canberra: Australian Government, 2019.

41. NSW Ministry of Health. Health Protection Report NSW. Sydney: NSW Health, 2017.

42. NSW Ministry of Health. Our structure. Sydney: NSW Health, 2022 [cited 13 Apr 2022]. Available from: https://www.health.nsw.gov.au/about/ministry/Pages/structure.aspx.

43. Oude Munnink BB, Sikkema RS, Nieuwenhuijse DF, Molenaar RJ, Munger E, Molenkamp R, Van Der Spek A, Tolsma P, Rietveld A, Brouwer M, Bouwmeester-Vincken N. Transmission of SARS-CoV-2 on mink farms between humans and mink and back to humans. Science. 2021 Jan 8;371(6525):172-177.

44. Palmer MV, Martins M, Falkenberg S, Buckley A, Caserta LC, Mitchell PK, Cassmann ED, Rollins A, Zylich NC, Renshaw RW, Guarino C. Susceptibility of white-tailed deer (Odocoileus virginianus) to SARS-CoV-2. J Virol. 2021;10;95(11):e00083-21.

45. Shaban RZ, Li C, O'Sullivan MVN, Gerrard J, Stuart RL, Teh J, et al. COVID-19 in Australia: our national response to the first cases of SARS-CoV-2 infection during the early biocontainment phase. Intern Med J. 2021;51(1):42-51.

46. Campbell K, Vines E. COVID-19: a chronology of Australian Government announcements (up until 30 June 2020). In: Department of Parliamentary Services, ed. Canberra: Parliamentary Library; 2021.

47. Storen R, Corrigan N. COVID-19: a chronology of state and territory government announcements (up until 30 June 2020). In: Parliament of Australia, ed. Canberra: Australian Government, 2020.

48. World Health Organization. Tracking SARS-CoV-2 variants. Geneva: WHO, 2022. [updated 7 Jun 2022.] Available from: https://www.who.int/activities/tracking-SARS-CoV-2-variants.

49. Duckett S, Clay K. Go for zero: how Australia can get to zero COVID-19 cases. Melbourne: Graham Institute, 2020.

50. Australian Government. COVID-19 vaccine roll-out. In: Operation COVID Shield, ed. Canberra: Australian Government, 2021.

51. World Health Organization. Climate change. Geneva: WHO [cited 22 Jun 2022]. Available from: https://www.who.int/health-topics/climate-change.

52. Wu X, Lu Y, Zhou S, Chen L, Xu B. Impact of climate change on human infectious diseases: empirical evidence and human adaptation. Environ Int. 2016;86:14-23.

53. Australian Institute of Health and Welfare. Australian burden of disease study: impact and causes of illness and death in Aboriginal and Torres Strait Islander people 2018 – summary report. Canberra: AIHW, 2022.

54. Osborn E, Ritha M, Macniven R, Agius T, Christie V, Finlayson H, et al. No one manages it; we just sign them up and do it: a whole system analysis of access to healthcare in one remote Australian community. Int J Environ Res Public Health. 2022;19(5):2939.

CHAPTER 10

Epidemiology and surveillance

PROFESSOR PHILIP L. RUSSO[i-ii]

Chapter highlights

- This chapter outlines the basic principles of epidemiology that are relevant for those working in infection prevention and control
- A variety of healthcare-associated infection (HAI) surveillance methods can be used to inform infection control programs
- HAI data must be reported back to those who need to know
- The use of administrative coding data alone for HAI surveillance should be avoided
- The increasing use of automated surveillance systems is improving surveillance efficiency

i   School of Nursing and Midwifery, Monash University, Frankston, VIC
ii Cabrini Research, Malvern, VIC

Introduction

Epidemiology and surveillance are intricately linked within healthcare-associated infection (HAI) prevention programs. It is crucial that those involved in infection prevention and control (IPC) programs have a basic understanding of the principles and concepts of epidemiology to structure meaningful surveillance programs. Likewise, it is crucial that surveillance programs are in place that will provide meaningful data to inform and structure an IPC program.

Epidemiology is defined as the study of the occurrence and distribution of health-related event, states and processes in specified populations, including the study of the determinants influencing such processes, and the application of this knowledge to control health problems.[1]

In exploring the three components of frequency, distribution and determinants further, we can see the importance of epidemiology in healthcare. Frequency involves the quantification of the existence or occurrence of a condition. Distribution relates to the who, when and where of the condition's occurrence. These two components then inform the third component, determinants, which involves forming and testing a hypothesis regarding risk factors for the disease.[2,3]

Surveillance programs are designed to provide basic epidemiological descriptive data, such as the time, place and person involved in the particular event under observation. Such basic information enables the monitoring of the event over time.[4]

Surveillance can be viewed as an information cycle, typically commencing with recognition of an event, data collection, data analysis, interpretation and importantly, dissemination of results to enable action.[4] It is this action which differentiates surveillance from simply monitoring events.[5]

The purpose of HAI surveillance is to provide quality data that can act as an effective monitoring and alert system and reduce the incidence of preventable infections.[6,7]

This chapter provides a broad overview of common epidemiological and surveillance principles and methods specific to HAI. While terminology in epidemiology can be very broad, for the purposes of this chapter, specific infection prevention terminology will be used to explain definitions and in examples.

10.1 Epidemiology

Epidemiology is the study of the occurrence and distribution of health-related diseases or events in specified populations, including the study of determinants influencing such states, and the application of this knowledge to control the health problem.[1]

Epidemiology is a critical element of all HAI prevention programs, and when used correctly, provides the foundation for infection prevention guidelines and policy. Broadly speaking, epidemiology can be categorised into two types, descriptive and analytic.

10.1.1 Descriptive epidemiology

Descriptive epidemiology aims to accurately describe and understand the distribution of a disease. One of the purposes of descriptive epidemiology is to generate a hypothesis that can be tested. Before this can be done, a detailed understanding of 'time, place and person' is required. To do this, it is common to undertake a cross-sectional or descriptive study. This may be in the form of a survey of people who have been affected by the disease, to collect some basic data. In an IPC context, this could be collecting basic data on patients who have a specific HAI.

Time: Health conditions change over time and can also be seasonal. Being able to describe a condition in relation to time provides important information in understanding whether something unusual is happening. For example, an increase in upper respiratory infections over winter may not be considered unusual. However, an increase in upper respiratory infections over summer may indicate an unusual event. In IPC, if there is suspicion of an unusual increase in infections, it is common to generate a chart to observe the trend over time. In Figure 10.1 it can be clearly seen that there has been an unusual spike in infections during the months of May to September in the second year compared to the previous year.

Place: Placing a geographical context to disease events is often very insightful. This could be a hospital ward, operating room, outpatient clinic, or at a broader level, a shopping centre, suburb and so on. Identifying the location of acquisition can provide important information on potential causes and transmission pathways. The classic illustration of this is the cholera epidemic in London in 1954 when an anaesthetist, John Snow, linked cases of cholera to a water pump in Broadway by mapping out where victims had obtained their water.[8] Similar mapping out of cases is frequently done when investigating potential outbreaks of gastroenteritis in hospital settings. Noting that patients from the same ward or in a shared room are developing signs and symptoms

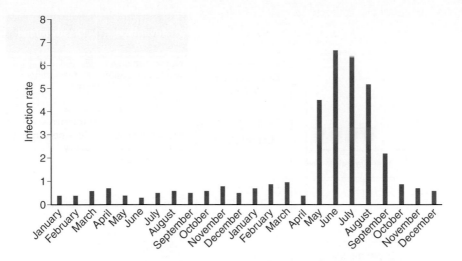

FIGURE 10.1 Infection rate over time

of gastroenteritis will indicate a likely person-to-person mode of transmission, and inform where interventions need to occur.

Person: Analysing demographic data of cases adds further important information in the epidemiological investigation. Commonly, data on age and gender are analysed, but other important data also include preexisting health conditions (immunocompromised status), lifestyle factors (smoking), and place of residence, all of which may reveal certain risk factors for the acquisition of certain diseases.

By organising data using the above categories, potential explanations may emerge in relation to the cause of the event and related risk factors. It is at this stage that analytical epidemiology plays an important role.

10.1.2 Analytic epidemiology

Analytic epidemiology aims to test a hypothesis about causal relationships, and to search for cause and effect. For example, if a cross-sectional study identifies a potential risk factor for an infection, then analytic techniques can be used to test if this is true. It is unlikely that epidemiology will be able to prove a cause and effect, but it may provide measurements of association that will facilitate control and prevention interventions.

Studies used to assist this process are either observational or experimental. Observational studies which are generally more common and feasible include cohort or case control studies, which explore the exposure and outcome status of participants. Experimental studies determine the exposure status of an individual and then follow up to determine the effects of the exposure.

Experimental studies tend to be more resource intensive and take longer to conduct, which is not always practical in a healthcare outbreak stetting.

Which type of study is best used will depend on a number of factors. Study types will be explored further in 10.1.3 Common study designs. (See also Chapter 12.)

10.1.3 Common study designs

Various study designs are available to test hypotheses and assist in outbreak investigations (Fig 10.2) but not all study types provide a strong level of evidence, and which type of study is used will depend on several factors, including resource availability and the time required to undertake the study. The study types listed below all provide varying levels of strength and rigour, with the least informative being a case series, through to the strongest level of evidence, a randomised controlled trial (RCT). Each is described briefly below.[2] (See also Chapter 12.)

Case series: A case series is simply a report of one or more patients affected by similar events. For example, it may be a description of three patients who all developed an infection after bowel surgery. There may be some similar characteristics, but there is no comparison group and it is often based on a sample of convenience. Case series are subject to strong bias and confounding and are unable to provide any causal inferences, though they may generate a hypothesis.[1,2]

Cross-sectional study: A cross-sectional study is an observational study of a sample of the population that gathers information about the disease (infection) and

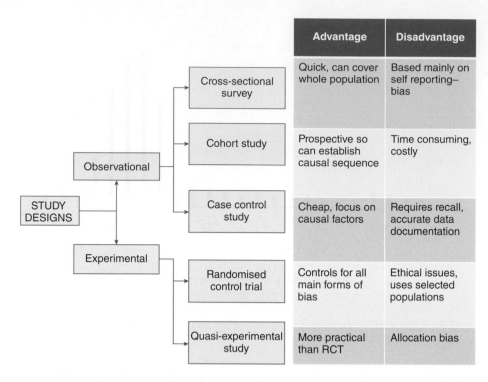

FIGURE 10.2 Summary of study types and their advantages and disadvantages

other factors of interest that may or may not increase risk. Cross-sectional studies are usually inexpensive and able to be conducted at short notice; however, they are subject to selection bias, and potential associations must be interpreted with care. This is because they are often unable to distinguish temporal associations, such as which came first—the potential risk factor or the outcome.[2,9] An example of an infection-prevention-related cross-sectional study is an online survey of dentists' knowledge, preparedness and experience during the COVID-19 pandemic in Australia.[10]

Case control study: A case control study involves studying those who have the outcome of interest (infection) and comparing them with a similar group who have not developed the outcome of interest (a comparison group).[1] Case control studies are always retrospective, and careful consideration is required when selecting the appropriate comparison group to ensure they are adequately representative of the group who developed the outcome.[2]

Allowance for potential confounders must also be made during the analysis with various statistical techniques.[9] While case control studies will identify potential associations of risk factors, they cannot generate a relative risk of a risk factor.[2] An example of

an infection-prevention-related case control study is a recent exploration of factors associated with the acquisition of VRE.[11]

Cohort: Unlike a case control study, where participants are selected on the presence or not of the outcome of interest, a cohort study includes participants based on the presence or not of the exposure (risk factor) who are then compared to determine if they develop the outcome of interest (infection). Cohort studies may be conducted prospectively or retrospectively, depending on when the outcome of interest occurs.[2] Although cohort studies may be considered more informative than case control studies because they can generate incidence and relative risk, and more than one outcome can be examined, they are often highly resource-intensive and may take a long time to conduct, particularly if they are prospective and the outcome of interest is rare. An example of an infection-prevention-related retrospective cohort study was a recent exploration of hospital contact tracing for COVID-19.[12]

Quasi-experimental studies: Quasi-experimental studies are commonly used in infection prevention and are able to evaluate associations between an intervention and its outcome. Often referred to as 'before and after', or 'pre and post' studies, they can be used to measure the effect of large-scale interventions on longitudinal measurements, such as monthly infection rates [13] Quasi-experimental studies require fewer resources and do not invite the ethical complexities of randomised controlled trials. A broad variety of quasi-experimental studies differ on the use, or not, of control groups, or the timing of interventions between the control and study groups. They are also favoured in infection prevention because they are considered to be pragmatic and often more representative of real-world effectiveness.[13]

Randomised control trials (RCTs): Randomised controlled trials are experimental studies in which participants are randomly allocated into groups, usually a study and control group, to either receive or not receive an experimental treatment.[1] Randomised controlled trials provide the highest level of evidence; however, in infection prevention they are uncommon as they are generally expensive and are often accompanied by complex ethical issues.[2]

Bias and confounding: Potential bias and confounding must be considered when undertaking any study. Bias needs to be addressed at the time of study design. One common bias error is selection bias, such as not selecting the correct participants for the study. Once this is done, bias cannot be corrected for in the analysis, and interpretation of the results will be severely limited.

Confounding occurs when a factor is associated with both the exposure and the outcome of interest. However, statistical methods used in the analysis can usually limit the influence of confounders on the interpretation of the results if the confounders are correctly identified.[2]

10.1.4 Measures of disease frequency

The first step in understanding the true situation of a potential infection issue is to establish whether or not something unusual is occurring. It is therefore crucial to accurately and correctly measure the event. This is commonly done by calculating the incidence and/or prevalence of a certain condition.

Incidence: Incidence is defined as the number of instances of a new health event occurring during a given period in a defined population.[1] In IPC it is commonly expressed as a rate. For example, during this month, if 25 patients underwent hip replacement surgery, and two developed post surgical site infection, then this month's infection rate for surgical site infection (SSI) for hip replacement surgery would be expressed as 8 per 100 patients (i.e. 2/25*[100]).

Prevalence: The other measurement commonly used is that of prevalence. Prevalence is defined as the number of individuals with a particular condition at a particular time divided by the number of individuals at risk of having that condition.[1] Generally in infection prevention there are two types of prevalence measurements used, point prevalence and period prevalence. Point prevalence refers to the proportion of patients with a specific condition at a specific point in time (e.g. how many patients with gastroenteritis at midday on a 30-bed ward). Whereas period prevalence refers to the proportion of patients with the condition at any time over a defined period.

10.1.5 Measures of effect and association

Relative risk and odds ratio: Relative risk, also called the risk ratio, compares the risk of an outcome in one group with the risk of the same outcome in another group. The groups are usually characterised by different attributes, often a demographic factor (e.g. age, gender) or by an exposure to a potential risk factor.[14] A simple example may be the risk of developing a bloodstream infection (BSI) among those who had a central line versus the risk of developing a BSI among those who did not have a central line. The relative risk is calculated by dividing the incidence of BSI in those with a central line by the incidence of BSI in those without a central line. A relative risk greater than 1.0 indicates a positive association, meaning the central line is associated with a BSI. A relative risk of less than 1.0 indicates a negative association, meaning that the central line may be protective against a BSI. Relative risk is often used in cohort and randomised controlled studies.

Another measurement of association is the odds ratio. The odds ratio is used in a case control study, because the population size from which the cases are selected is unclear. The odds ratio is interpreted as an approximation of the relative risk, which is particularly useful when the outcome is rare (Fig 10.3).

P value: The p value refers to a statistical test that provides an indication as to probability of whether or not a particular outcome could occur by chance. The p stands for probability. Typically, a p value of less than 0.05 (i.e. $p<0.05$) leads investigators to conclude that the result is statistically significant as this means the likelihood it occurred by chance is less than 5%.

		Infection	
		Present (cases)	Absent (controls)
Factor	Present (exposed)	A	B
	Absent (not exposed)	C	D

Relative Risk
Risk of infection among exposed persons = A/(A+B)
Risk of infection among unexposed persons = C/(C+D)
Relative risk = [A/(A+B)]/[C/(C+D)]

Odds Ratio
Odds of exposure, given infection = A/C
Odds of exposure, given no infection = B/D
Infection odds ratio = [A/C]/[B/D] = AD/BC

FIGURE 10.3 Calculations for relative risk and odds ratio

The p value has been commonly used in medicine for many years. Held in high esteem, it is suggested that a p value of statistical significance was the major determining factor in getting studies published, sometimes leading to less than ethical behaviour.[15] It is important to understand that p values are influenced by the sample size and the magnitude of the difference between two groups. In recent years there has been robust debate as to how to interpret the p value, and questioning of its use in healthcare and statistics overall. The increasing consensus is that the p value must not be interpreted in isolation, but should be considered along with sample sizes, means, standard deviations, confidence intervals and effect sizes.[15-17]

Confidence intervals: In light of the above shortcomings of the p value, arguably the next most useful estimate to inform decision making is the confidence interval. Confidence intervals provide the parameters within which the real value lies. They should always accompany relative risk, odds ratios and proportions. The closer the confidence intervals are to each other, the more certain we are of the estimate.

A common example is the provision of an infection rate, which should be accompanied by a 95% confidence interval.

For example, if we see the following data:

SSI rate for Surgeon X

16 patients with an SSI from 763 patients = SSI rate of 2.1 per 100 patients. (95% CI 1.2–3.4)

This means that we are 95% certain that the true SSI rate for this surgeon is between 1.2 and 3.4. This gives confidence to the reported rate of 2.1.

However, confidence intervals are influenced by the sample size and number of events. Note the difference in the following example:

SSI rate for Surgeon X

9 patients with an SSI from 98 patients = SSI rate of 12.2 per 100 patients. (95% CI 6.4–20.4)

The confidence intervals are now much wider and tell us that the true SSI rate for this surgeon lies somewhere between 6.4 and 20.4. So in reality, the true rate may be as low as 6.4 per 100 patients, or as high as 20.4 per 100 patients. This highlights the importance of accompanying infection rates with confidence intervals.

Confounding and bias: Two other important concepts that must be considered are those of confounding and bias. Confounding is defined as when all or part of an observed effect is due to factors other than the primary exposure of interest.[14] A confounder is associated with both the exposure and the outcome of interest. There are many potential confounders in healthcare research but these can be controlled for either in the design stage of the study or in the analysis. However, if it is to be controlled for in the analysis, it is crucial that data is collected about it during the study.[18] Either way, it is crucial that confounders are identified so they can be controlled for.

Bias is an error in the conception and design of a study, or in the collection, analysis, interpretation and reporting of data that leads to incorrect results or conclusions.[1] There are many different types of bias in epidemiology. Two common categories of bias are selection bias and information bias. Selection bias is an error introduced when the study population does not appropriately represent the target population. This can be caused by inadequate definitions of the population under study or lack of an appropriate sampling frame. Selection bias can be controlled when the variables influencing selection are measured on all study subjects.[19]

Information bias occurs at the time of data collection. A common type is misclassification bias which includes detection bias, observer/interviewer bias, recall bias and reporting bias. Some of these biases can be controlled through blinding of participants. Another type of bias well known in infection prevention is that which occurs via the Hawthorne effect.[19] Commonly described in the hand hygiene compliance research, the Hawthorne effect is where an outcome is affected because participants are aware they are being observed.[20,21]

10.2 Surveillance

It is commonly stated that the cornerstone of any IPC program is surveillance.[22,23] Without knowing how many healthcare-associated infections are occurring in any given setting, it is impossible to know whether or not an IPC program is effective.

The foundations of HAI surveillance are found in Vienna in the mid-19th century due to the work of physician Ignaz Semmelweis.[24] Semmelweis collected data on maternal death rates and compared the difference between those women cared for by physicians and students, and those cared for by midwives. He found that the maternal death rate of those cared for by physicians and students was 10%, and those cared for by midwives was 3%. Through a series of observational studies he noted that medical students and physicians conducted autopsies while midwives did not, and hypothesised that 'cadaveric material was the cause of death'. He introduced a handwashing intervention for all staff on entry to the delivery room which resulted in a significant decrease in mortality rates.[24]

More recently, a landmark study conducted in the USA by Robert Haley in the 1980s clearly demonstrated the benefits of a surveillance program. After evaluating multiple hospital infection control programs over a 10-year period that reviewed surgical site, bloodstream and urinary tract infections as well as ventilator-associated pneumonia, Haley identified four essential components of an effective IPC program:

1. a structured surveillance program
2. one infection prevention nurse per 250 beds
3. an infection prevention physician; and
4. a system for reporting infection rates to surgeons.

Different combinations of these factors had varying effects on the four types of infections, but only surveillance was present for each type of infection.[25,26]

These days it is expected that every healthcare setting in Australia will have some type of surveillance program. Standard 3 of the National Safety and Quality Health Service Standards (NSQHS) established by the Australian Commission for Safety and Quality in Health Care (ACSQHC) is listed in Box 10.1.

In Australia, it is these criteria that are used for hospital accreditation.

Although HAI surveillance is crucial, it is also resource intensive. A cross-sectional study undertaken across 152 hospitals in 2014 estimated the mean full

---

BOX 10.1 Action 3.05 states

The health service organisation has a surveillance strategy for infections, infection risk, and antimicrobial use and prescribing that:

- Incorporates national and jurisdictional information in a timely manner
- Collects data on healthcare-associated and other infections relevant to the size and scope of the organisation
- Monitors, assesses and uses surveillance data to reduce the risks associated with infections
- Reports surveillance data on infections to the workforce, the governing body, consumers and other relevant groups
- Collects data on the volume and appropriateness of antimicrobial use relevant to the size and scope of the organisation
- Monitors, assesses and uses surveillance data to support appropriate antimicrobial prescribing
- Monitors responsiveness to risks identified through surveillance
- Reports surveillance data on the volume and appropriateness of antimicrobial use to the workforce, the governing body, consumers and other relevant groups.[27]

time equivalent (FTE) infection prevention nurses per 100 beds to be 0.66, or 1 FTE per 152 beds, and remained relatively constant when stratified by hospital size. From the same study, infection prevention nurses estimated they spent 36% of their time undertaking surveillance activities, of which 56% was spent on collecting data.[28,29]

10.2.1 Purpose and objectives of HAI surveillance

Purpose: By its very existence, the science of 'infection prevention' implies that HAIs are preventable. Exactly what proportion of HAIs are preventable is unclear and difficult to establish due to limitations with study designs. It is generally agreed that a significant proportion, and probably the majority, of HAIs are preventable.[30,31]

The purpose of HAI surveillance is to provide quality data that can act as an effective monitoring and alert system and reduce the incidence of preventable infections.[6,7]

Thinking back to the previous sections on epidemiology, HAI surveillance systems are used to provide the descriptive information about when, where and who is acquiring HAIs, essentially the time, place and person—the basic epidemiology parameters.

Surveillance systems generally comprise several stages: data collection; data validation and analysis; and interpretation and dissemination (Fig 10.4). Crucial to any surveillance program is feedback and dissemination of the data to 'those who need to know'.[32] This means there is no point in collecting surgical site infection data if you do not tell the surgeon what their infection rates are. Data needs to be used for action, and if the surgeon does not know how many of their patients acquire an infection, how can they possibly take any action to prevent them?

Objectives: Not all HAI surveillance programs are the same. Much will depend on the patient population and resources. A surveillance program designed for a large acute care hospital is unlikely to be suitable for a small, regional healthcare facility. So it is important to be clear about the purpose and objectives of the surveillance program (See Box 10.2.).

10.2.2 Key elements of surveillance programs

A common error when establishing a surveillance program is to attempt to collect as much data as possible, even though its immediate purpose may not be clear. If data is not used for action, then it should not be collected. Collecting data that is not required wastes scarce resources, and the complexity of the data collected needs to be balanced between information needs and available resources.[4]

There are two essential elements in any surveillance program.[4] First, the case definition of the event under

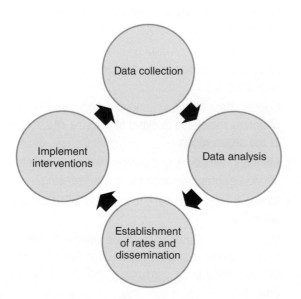

FIGURE 10.4 The surveillance cycle

BOX 10.2 Common objectives of HAI surveillance programs[6,26]

- Establish baseline and endemic rates of infections
- Detect clustering in time and space and potential outbreaks
- Alert key personnel of the existence of a problem
- Assess the effectiveness of IPC measures
- Generate hypotheses concerning risk factors
- Provide data to be used for quality improvement activities
- Guide treatment and/or prevention strategies
- Meet regulatory requirements
- Conduct research
- Provide data for education of healthcare workers
- Make comparisons within and between hospitals or networks
- Benchmark outcomes
- Reduce the incidence of healthcare-associated infections

surveillance needs to be standardised and applied consistently to ensure accurate measurement of the event.[26,33] The more complex a definition of HAI is, the less likely it is to be applied consistently. The second element is clearly defining the population under surveillance. In the case of HAI surveillance, it may mean all patients in a particular ward (e.g. ICU) or all patients having a particular type of procedure (e.g. hip replacement).

A successful HAI surveillance program must be epidemiologically sound and balance attributes such as accuracy, timeliness, usefulness, consistency and practicality.[34] A summary of these attributes is listed in Table 10.1.

Hospital-wide and targeted surveillance: HAI surveillance can be categorised into two strategies: hospital-wide surveillance and targeted surveillance. Hospital-wide surveillance involves prospective and continuous surveillance of all areas of the hospital. While comprehensive, it is resource intensive and costly. Although still requiring substantial resources, more efficient is targeted surveillance, which also includes surveillance by objective or priority. Typically this involves targeting high-risk patients, or areas, for prospective surveillance at the risk of missing clusters that may occur in other areas.[18,26]

A comparison of the two surveillance strategies is provided in Table 10.2.

Targeted surveillance is generally more common as it requires fewer resources and provides more meaningful data.[34] Furthermore, targeted surveillance allows for flexibility, in that more resources can be dedicated to areas of greater priority, rather than having to provide surveillance resources in areas where infections are uncommon or of little consequence.

The Australian Guidelines for the Prevention and Control of Infection in Healthcare note that hospital-wide surveillance for all infections is not feasible, therefore surveillance programs should be targeted towards specific sites of infection (e.g. bloodstream), specific populations (e.g. neonates), specific organisms (e.g. multiresistant organisms), or specific locations (e.g. intensive care units).[22]

Passive and active surveillance: Surveillance can be either passive or active, or a combination of both. Passive surveillance generally involves using data already collected by other systems, such as

TABLE 10.1 Common attributes of an HAI surveillance program[34]

Attribute	Description
Accuracy	Aided by the use of case definitions and accurate denominator data by ensuring all those in the population under surveillance are at risk of acquiring the infection under surveillance. The presence and intensity of post discharge surveillance will strongly influence the numerator data
Timeliness	Prospective surveillance is recommended to enable quick identification and prompt investigation. Retrospective surveillance is best suited for issues that have little need for intervention due to the delay in data analysis
Usefulness	Surveillance resources should only be directed towards actionable issues
Consistency	Case definitions must be applied uniformly, surveillance methods and data sources should be consistent, and education of those involved in identifying cases should be uniform. Routine cross-checking of case determinations should be performed regularly
Practicality	Surveillance objectives must be achievable within the resources available

Source: Data from Allen-Bridson K, Morrell GC, Horan TC. Surveillance of Healthcare-Associated Infections. In: Mayhall CG, editor. Hospital Epidemiology and Infection Control. 4th ed. Philadelphia: Wolters Kluwer; 2012. p. 1329-43.

TABLE 10.2 Advantages and disadvantages of surveillance strategies

Strategy	Advantages	Disadvantages
Facility-wide	Provides data on all infections Establishes baseline infection rates Identifies clusters Recognises outbreaks early Identifies risk factors Raises profile of infection control Amendable to smaller facilities	Expensive, resource and time intensive Yields excessive data with little time to analyse Detects infections that are not preventable No defined objectives; interventions difficult Overall infection rates not comparable
Targeted	Concentrates limited resources to high-risk areas Responsive to finding of facility risk assessment Focus on high-risk patients/areas More efficient, less resource intensive	May miss clusters in other areas Collects data only for targeted patients/areas No baseline rates in other areas

Modified from [18,26,34]

microbiology data. Active surveillance involves collecting data that is not already captured by other systems, such as reviewing medical charts and wounds to determine if a patient has a surgical site infection. The advantage of passive surveillance is that it requires fewer resources when compared to active surveillance; however, it is dependent on input from other sources which may affect accuracy and timelines. Although active surveillance requires dedicated resources, it has the advantage of increasing the visibility of the IPC team, which can lead to increased case detection.[34]

Many surveillance programs involve both passive and active methods. For example, an unusual microbiology result noted by the IPC team may indicate a possible infection which can then be either confirmed or not by actively visiting the patient. This is also a common feature of newly developed automated surveillance programs, which are discussed below.

Process surveillance and outcome surveillance:
Process surveillance usually refers to a program that measures compliance with certain activities that are known to reduce infection. A well-known example of a process measure is the measurement of compliance with hand hygiene. Many hospitals use 'bundles' of prevention practices. Bundles are a combination of prevention activities aimed at reducing infection rates.[34] For example, a bundle to reduce surgical site infection could comprise the following factors: ensuring that the patient receives the correct preoperative antimicrobial at the right time and dose, appropriate hair removal, normoglycaemia and normothermia. Process surveillance would measure compliance with each of those activities to provide an understanding of adherence to best practice. The advantages of process surveillance are usually simple to define and measure, do not require risk adjustment, can predict outcome, and can be captured quickly.[22]

Outcome surveillance is focused on measuring the outcomes of care, often adverse events such as infection.[22,34] The value of outcome surveillance is dependent on rigorous method, reliability of data collection, and the application of definitions.[22,34] A major challenge in outcome surveillance in HAI surveillance programs is the variation that can occur. A 2015 Australian study of IPC staff who undertake surveillance found variation in correctly identifying an HAI when presented with several vignettes.[35] This finding supported earlier work conducted internationally that serves to highlight the many challenges of outcome surveillance HAI programs.[36-40]

Many surveillance programs are a combination of processing outcomes measures running side by side. For example, process measurement could be undertaken on compliance with a surgical care bundle for patients undergoing colon surgery, while at the same time undertaking outcome surveillance on the same patient cohort for surgical site infections. Finally, outcome surveillance can often be a trigger to review processes. A high bloodstream infection rate may indicate the need to undertake process surveillance activities on the interactions of intravenous catheters. This may identify poor compliance with aseptic technique, hence highlighting the need for further education.

Surveillance activities: Determining what type of surveillance activities to undertake, which HAIs to focus on, and in which populations to survey will vary between facilities and is also influenced by external agencies. In Australia, the only national HAI surveillance activity is annual reporting of *Staphylococcus aureus* bloodstream (SAB) infection rates which is considered a key performance indicator for acute care hospitals in Australia.[41] All acute care public hospitals are required to submit the number of patient episodes of SAB (see AIHW METeOR in Useful websites/resources at the end of this chapter) with the denominator being the number of patient days.[42] The lack of a national HAI surveillance program is somewhat surprising given it is a common element of most developed countries' IPC activities.[43] An Australian national study using a discrete choice experiment with over 120 key IPC leaders identified a strong preference for a national surveillance program with a mandatory core component using a standard surveillance protocol, and with public reporting of hospital-level data not associated with any financial penalty.[44]

Otherwise, some states and territories have mandatory surveillance requirements. Victoria's HAI surveillance program, Victorian Nosocomial Infection Surveillance System (VICNISS), has a range of performance indicators based on hospital size and whether the hospital is publicly or privately funded. For example, for large public hospitals (>100 acute beds) with an intensive care unit, continuous surveillance for central line-associated bloodstream infections (CLABSI) in intensive care units must be undertaken. If more than 50 hip arthroplasty procedures are undertaken annually, then continuous SSI surveillance for those undergoing hip arthroplasty must be performed. Common types of HAI surveillance activities across all hospitals are listed in Table 10.3.

TABLE 10.3 Common HAI surveillance activities

Surveillance activity	Type
Central line-associated bloodstream infection	Outcome
Peripheral line-associated bloodstream infection	Outcome
Catheter-related urinary tract infection	Outcome
Clostridiodies difficile infection	Outcome
Haemodialysis-associated bloodstream infection	Outcome
Staphylococcus aureus bloodstream infection	Outcome
Methicillin-resistant *Staphylococcus aureus* infections	Outcome
Surgical site infections	Outcome
Ventilator-associated pneumonia	Outcome
Vancomycin-resistant infections	Outcome
Hand hygiene compliance	Process
Surgical antimicrobial prophylaxis compliance	Process
Influenza vaccination rates among healthcare workers	Process
Healthcare worker hepatitis B immunity	Process

This list is not comprehensive

10.2.3 Data collection and analysis

Numerator data: A major challenge for IPC teams is the timely and accurate identification of HAIs. The uniform application of validated definitions is crucial. Many countries have national HAI surveillance programs that provide protocol and definitions for HAI surveillance.[45] Australia does not have a national HAI surveillance program; however, a 2015 study indicated that most use the HAI definitions established by the National Health and Safety Network (NHSN) in the Centers for Disease Control and Prevention (CDC) in the USA.[46] The NHSN HAI definitions use a number of infection criteria that involve clinical findings and diagnostic tests. Even though the NHSN definitions are well established, clinical finding could include direct patient observation or a review of patient records, and diagnostic test criteria involves the availability and undertaking of certain diagnostic tests.[34] This highlights the potential variation in application of definitions that may occur within and between facilities.

Another challenge in case finding is ascertaining acquisition. For an infection to be healthcare associated it must be related to a healthcare event. A general rule of thumb is that if a patient shows signs and symptoms of an infection within the first 48 hours of hospitalisation, it cannot be considered to be hospital acquired; however, it may still be healthcare associated if the patient was receiving healthcare outside of the hospital or was recently discharged from a healthcare facility.

Case finding: Case finding methodology varies depending on the purpose of the surveillance program, the healthcare setting and the resources available. Case finding methodology often involves a number of components, from full medical record review to scanning microbiology results for unusual patterns. An increased use in technology to assist data collection has lessened the burden of surveillance, and the rapid evolution of technology and implementation of electronic medical records offer the opportunity to drastically change surveillance methods. This issue will be further explored in automated surveillance systems. Case finding methods are summarised in Table 10.4.

Collecting data: Essential data in HAI surveillance programs will include some basic patient demographic data, data about the infection, microbiology data, and data about diagnostic test or operative procedures undertaken.[34] However, the extent of data to be collected will depend on the purpose of the surveillance program and the resources available.

The advent of electronic medical records (EMR) means that much of this data is accessible from the one source; however, in hospitals that have not fully implemented EMRs, data sources can be a combination of reviewing patient records, operation notes and microbiology data.

10.2.4 Data quality

Accuracy: Accurate data is crucial to any surveillance program. Determining the accuracy of HAI surveillance data is commonly done using three measures—sensitivity, specificity and the positive predictive value (PPV).[33] Sensitivity provides a measure of the proportion of people with true infection who are reported as having an infection, specificity refers to the proportion of people without an infection who are reported as not having an infection, and the PPV measures the proportion of people reported as having an infection who do have a true infection.[47]

TABLE 10.4 Summary of case finding methods

Method	Explanation	Points to consider
Total chart review	Involves the surveillance team reviewing healthcare worker notes for each patient on a regular basis (1–2 times per week)	Extremely time intensive Less common with introduction of electronic databases
Laboratory-based surveillance	Daily review of all microbiology results to observe for unusual pathogens or trends, e.g. a *Staphylococcus aureus* in a blood culture would prompt the surveillance team to review more closely the patient data to determine if it is an HAI	This process is dependent on sampling practices of the facility (not all wounds may be swabbed) and also assumes that all HAI will generate a positive microbiology result. This means it may be good for identifying healthcare-associated bloodstream infections, but not surgical site infections
Clinical ward rounds	The surveillance team visit all clinical areas on a regular basis (2–3 times per week) to speak to staff about any patients who may be suspected of developing an infection and may require further investigation	Time intensive but has the advantage of making the surveillance team highly visible, which can often lead to the identification of other infection prevention issues
Computer-based surveillance	Various types of commercial and in-house software programs have been developed to assist in surveillance. These are often linked to microbiology databases, admission and discharge databases to automate data collection`	Functionality often depends on the information technology environment of the facility. Can be expensive to develop and implement. Usually associated with maintenance costs

In practical terms, if a surveillance program reports a high sensitivity and a low specificity, this means that most patients with an infection are captured, but the low specificity means that many patients who do not have an infection will be reported as that they do have an infection. The PPV is influenced by the sensitivity and specificity, and the prevalence of the HAI. A low PPV will result in non-HAIs being investigated, meaning that surveillance resources are being wasted, and may also lead to the implementation of unnecessary interventions.[48]

It is recommended that independent, trained observers be engaged to measure the sensitivity, specificity and PPV of a surveillance program.[33] However, such validation studies are expensive to conduct, have inherent methodological difficulties, and often tend to focus on one aspect of data collection.[49]

Nevertheless, with the advent of public reporting, benchmarking, and the potential for HAI outcome data to be linked to hospital funding, the importance of validity and reliability of HAI data has increased.[50-52]

Emori[53] first measured the accuracy of reporting ICU HAIs to the National Nosocomial Infection Surveillance (NNIS) program of the CDC in 1998 and identified a sensitivity range of 30%–85% and a PPV range of 72%–87% for prospectively identified HAIs.[53] A good specificity of over 98% was reported for all HAIs. Their encouraging conclusion was that when an

ICU HAI is reported it is likely to be a true HAI— patients who do not acquire an HAI are identified accurately; however, because of the low sensitivity reported it is likely that some HAIs were not being identified. To address this Emori[53] recommended the training of data collectors to facilitate consistent application of infection criteria.

In a review of 14 validation studies on HAI surveillance, Fabry et al[49] noted large variation in designs, studies were often limited to one or a few facilities and were often focused on one aspect of surveillance. In the studies under review, many had similar findings to Emori,[53] with low to moderate sensitivity and high specificity. When PPV was estimated they were generally high.[49]

While large validation studies on national HAI programs are complex to conduct, in the USA several states have undertaken their own validation studies. Horan et al[54] from the NHSN reported that at May 2011, at least 15 states in the USA had conducted validation studies, but again with variable results, supporting findings from other similar validation studies.[55-57]

Comparable results can be found in Australian validation studies performed in two state-wide HAI surveillance programs.[58-60] In a review of SSI reported from over 4500 coronary artery bypass surgery procedures under surveillance as part of the VICNISS, Friedman et al[58] found a PPV of 96%, but a sensitivity of 55% and a specificity of 100%. When the review was limited to only those infections that occurred in the sternum (as opposed to sternum and graft site), the PPV was 91%, sensitivity 62% and specificity 100%.[58] These results implied that not all SSIs, particularly those not at the sternal site, are identified.

Another study conducted by researchers from VICNISS on ICU CLABSI surveillance estimated the sensitivity to be 35%, specificity 87% and PPV 59%.[59] These findings revealed poor accuracy and consistency from those participating in ICU CLABSI surveillance in the VICNISS program.[59]

In Western Australia, a review of all SAB events reported by public hospitals identified 164 that were classified as healthcare-associated events during 2008.[60] On review of the medical records of each notified case, researchers estimated that the overall sensitivity was 77% and specificity 100%, and in hospitals that did not have an on-site microbiology service, the sensitivity was only 40%.[60]

In a national study, when Australian IPC staff were presented with seven vignettes describing HAI scenarios, agreement on whether or not an HAI existed varied from 53% to 75%, and those who had been trained in surveillance and worked in larger teams were associated with a correct response.[35]

Method variation: There are other influences that can affect the quality of surveillance data, such as variation in methodology. In a review of HAI national surveillance programs in 10 countries and one multinational program (HELICS), in which all report using the CDC/NHSN definitions and methods, variation was identified in the type of surgical procedures under surveillance and length of time of follow-up.[61] Further differences were also found in data collection methods, category of staff performing surveillance, prospective and retrospective data collection methods, data sources, and the inclusion of routine post discharge surveillance as a routine part of case finding.[61] It was also noted that validation of data did not occur on a regular basis. This, together with the differences identified between the programs, contributes some uncertainty about the quality of the data and also limits the ability to make comparison of rates between different programs, despite being based on the same methodology.[61]

In a cross-sectional study of 126 hospitals designed to characterise variation in surveillance methods and application of HAI definitions, Keller et al[38] used a series of clinical vignettes to measure variation among IPC staff. Despite all sites participating in and following NHSN methods, only 61% of responses correctly identified an HAI. Interestingly, 24% of those collecting HAI data did not have a clinical background, which on multivariate analysis was an independent predictor of an incorrect application of the HAIs definitions.[38]

As mentioned earlier, in the review of the German surveillance program Krankenhaus Infektions Surveillance System (KISS) researchers recently demonstrated a sensitivity of 85.7% by measuring the sensitivity and specificity of 189 surveillance personnel through a series of clinical vignettes presented over a period of three years.[62] Accuracy was positively associated with surveillance experience and higher education levels.[62]

In a large ethnographic study across 17 ICUs all participating in the same HAI surveillance program, Dixon-Woods et al[36] illustrated broad variation in data collection systems and the application of infection criteria. Dixon-Woods et al[36] concluded that HAI data reported and used as hospital performance indicators clearly misrepresented real infection rates. Rather than any deliberate attempt to 'game' data, the study identified that those involved in surveillance occasionally disagreed with the standardised definitions and applied local interpretations largely because of inequity aversion, that is, a dislike of unfair outcomes.[36] This is an important finding, particularly if penalties are associated with infection rates.

In a cross-sectional survey of 106 hospitals participating in mandatory orthopaedic surgical site surveillance in the United Kingdom, Tanner et al[63] identified variation in a number of areas including definitions applied, and the extent of post discharge follow-up. Not surprisingly, it was noted that those who conducted inpatient surveillance alone, and those who conducted both inpatient surveillance and readmission surveillance, reported significantly lower SSI rates than those who also undertook post discharge surveillance.[63] Furthermore, the methods used to identify HAIs on readmission and through post discharge surveillance varied enormously, also affecting the reported rates.[63]

A national Australian study found that only 51% of IPC staff undertaking surveillance had been trained, and fewer than half performed prospective surgical site surveillance. Less than half reported risk-adjusted surgical site infection rates, and variation in HIA definitions was also identified.[46]

In an era of increased public reporting and performance measurement, validation studies highlight the limitations in interpreting HAI data, and despite participating in networked surveillance programs, variations in surveillance methods between facilities continue. It is reasonable to expect similar findings among Australian facilities, but studies are lacking that describe and measure this variation, and if such variation has any impact on reported HAI rates.

Data accuracy and surveillance methods play a major role in the reliability of a surveillance program. Misinterpretation of surveillance definitions and inconsistent surveillance methods are the primary reasons for the misclassification of infections.[64] Other factors that influence the quality of the data include: who collects it; who applies the definitions; the skill of those collecting it; the data sources; the intensity of case finding; and the activities under surveillance.

It remains unclear what level of accuracy is acceptable, and what level of resources and effort can be justified to provide high levels of accuracy.

10.2.5 Reporting outcome data

Critical to all surveillance programs is the dissemination of data. How data is reported is influenced by many factors, not the least the audience, and differing audiences will often require different reports. For example, data on the frequency of HAI that is reported to consumers will likely be fashioned as higher-level summary data, whereas data reported to funders may require very specific and detailed information. For the purposes of this section, the focus is on data reported within healthcare facilities for healthcare workers.

Healthcare-associated infection rates can be reported in a variety of ways, depending on whether or not the measurement is incidence or prevalence. Point prevalent surveys of HAIs are reported as the number of patients who had an infection on the day of the survey, and this is expressed as a proportion. For example, if all 570 patients in a hospital were surveyed, and 62 were found to have an infection, then the prevalence of HAI is expressed as $62/750$ $(\star 100) = 10.9$. The multiplier of 100 is used to facilitate easier interpretation, so we can say that almost 11% of all patients in hospital on that day had an HAI.

More commonly, IPC surveillance programs undertake incidence surveillance, that is, the number of new events over a given period of time, and this is expressed as a rate. Sometimes further layers of stratification are required to make the rate reported more meaningful. These can include a monthly rate as opposed to a yearly rate, and furthermore a rate per device-type used, a rate per location, a rate per operative procedure, a rate stratified by risk factors, and a rate per surgeon are some examples of how the data may be expressed.

Surgical site infection (SSI) rates: Surgical site infection rates are commonly reported as a rate per 100 patients. However, not all patients are at equal risk of developing a SSI, therefore it is important to apply some risk adjustment to the data. The most common risk adjustment method used for reporting SSI is the basic NHSN risk index.[65] This index categorises patients into different risk categories depending on the preoperative ASA score, whether the procedure is classified as clean, contaminated or dirty, and the duration of the procedure. This stratification allows for more reasonable comparison of infection rates as patients at similar risk of infection are able to be compared (see Table 10.5).

Device-associated infection rates: Device-associated infection rates are calculated by counting the number of device-related infections as the numerator and the number of device days as the denominator, and reporting per 1000 devices. For example, when reporting monthly CLABSI rates in an ICU, the number of patients who developed a new CLABSI for the month is divided by the number of central line devices days for that month, and multiplied by

TABLE 10.5 Surgical site infection rates by basic risk index

Risk category#	Number of patients with infection	Number of patients who had procedure	SSI rate	95% confidence interval
0	1	60	1/60 (*100) = 1.7	(0.0–0.9)
1	3	62	3/62 (*100) = 4.8	(0.1–13.3)
2	4	35	4/35 (*100) = 11.4	(3.2–26.7)
3	3	22	3/22 (*100) = 13.6	(2.9–34.9)

0: lowest risk; 3: highest risk

1000. Similar methods are used for urinary catheter-associated UTIs, ventilator-associated pneumonia, and less often, peripheral line-associated BSIs. For example:

6 patients in the intensive care unit developed a new CLABSI in May.

There were 5847 device days in the month in ICU. $6/5847 = 0.00103 (\star 1000) = 1.03$ CLABSIs per 1000 devices

Standardised infection ratio: The standardised infection ratio (SIR), while not commonly used in Australia, is a standard method for reporting HAIs in the NHSN USA.[66] The SIR is a useful summary measure that compares the actual numbers of HAI reported to the number of HAIs that are predicted using a large standard population adjusted for risk factors found to be associated with HAI. An SIR greater than 1.0 indicates that the number of HAIs is higher than what could be expected, and an SIR of less than 1.0 indicates fewer HAIS were reported than expected.

The NHSN has drawn upon its large national database and used logistic regression to central line-associated bloodstream infections (CLABSI), mucosal barrier injury laboratory-confirmed bloodstream infections (MBI-LCBI), catheter-associated urinary tract infections (CAUTI), surgical site infections (SSI), *Clostridioides difficile* infections (CDI), methicillin-resistant *Staphylococcus aureus* bloodstream infections (MRSA), and ventilator-associated events (VAE).[66]

Public reporting: Benchmarking has been defined as the 'process of making comparisons between organisations with the aim to identify and implement best practice and improve performance'.[45] The purpose of publicly reporting health data is to enable consumers to make informed choices about their healthcare, subsequently involving them in the benchmarking process.[45,67] It follows then that wherever public reporting of data is facilitated, so too is benchmarking.

Two common measures are used in healthcare for benchmarking purposes: process and outcome. Process measures determine compliance with evidence-based practice, while outcome measures determine if the desired results have been achieved.[68] Infection prevention-related examples of process measures used for benchmarking include hand hygiene, central line insertion practices and compliance with surgical antimicrobial prophylaxis. Common outcome measures include the incidence of SSI, BSI, CLABSI and ventilator-associated pneumonia.[45]

Benchmarking and public reporting of HAI-related process and outcome data is now well embedded in the USA, UK and many European countries.[45,69,70] In Australia, one HAI outcome measure and one process measure are now routinely reported. Following a broad consultative process, annual hospital-identifiable SAB rates have been publicly reported since 2012.[71] Hand hygiene compliance rates by hospitals are also reported publicly.[71] This process indicator data has become embedded in the Australian healthcare setting since commencing in 2009, and has been associated with a reduction of SAB.[72]

Public reporting of HAI data attracts contrasting opinions. Proponents argue it promotes transparency, motivates organisations to implement best practice, and ultimately improves patient outcomes.[73,74] It is also suggested that publicly reported HAI data can be used by consumers to make informed choices when deciding which hospitals to attend.[73] Although there is little evidence of a direct effect on improved patient outcomes, public reporting has been associated with organisational change and increased awareness of infection prevention.[45] Humphreys[75] argues that public reporting of national data as a benchmark not only drives down infection rates in hospitals within a country, but benchmarking between countries can also serve to drive improvements.

Opponents argue that mandatory public reporting, particularly of outcome data, is flawed due to the variability in measurements between hospitals, and the competition it creates between hospitals places undue pressure on infection control teams.[50,70]

In Australia, although reporting of SAB and hand hygiene compliance data are now considered routine, there has been criticism of the lack of validation and appropriate risk stratification of SAB data.[76] Further, the resources required to sustain the mandated volume of hand hygiene auditing has also been criticised.[77]

Aware of early concerns relating to public reporting of HAI data, in 2005 the Healthcare Infection Control Practices Advisory Committee at the CDC developed a series of recommendations for policy makers when considering state-wide public reporting of HAIs.[67] They included sound epidemiological methods and risk adjustment, and suggested using a combination of process and outcome data for the 'production of useful reports for stakeholders'.[67] Process measures are considered ideal for public reporting and hospital performance measurement as they do not require any risk adjustment.[67] Outcome measures require appropriate risk adjustment for comparison, without which they are prone to misinterpretation.[67]

In a review of public reporting across Europe, Martin et al[69] noted that debate continues about the utility of public reporting, and doubt as to whether the public can interpret HAI data appropriately. Kiernan[78] notes that even if public reporting is not particularly useful for the public, it captures the attention of politicians and organisations, which can then translate into action.

Given the momentum of public reporting HAI data internationally, it is reasonable to assume that it will also continue to expand in Australia. Therefore, the discussion now is not so much about whether or not HAI data should be publicly reported, but rather how it should be reported, and which HAI data are suitable to be used as a performance measurement. A recent study regarding consumer knowledge and attitudes in Australia identified that many consumers preferred not to be informed of hospital infection rates, and many were only mildly interested.[79]

In a survey of IPC leaders from 34 European member countries, despite general support for public reporting of HAI data and it being considered a major driver to strengthen infection prevention in hospitals, there was strong disagreement about the benefits of public reporting, as well as the type of data and format of the reports. The expert group conceded that benchmarking needed to be accompanied by standardised methods and validation, and preferred reporting of process indicators over outcome indicators.[69]

By comparison, a review of healthcare performance measures undertaken by Berenson, Pronovost and Krumholz[68] recommended moving from process measures to outcome measures. While acknowledging the many challenges of outcome measures as performance indicators, the authors state that process measures do not always predict outcomes, and often require resource-intensive, manual data collection.[68]

Acknowledging the concerns when using HAI data as performance indicators—namely lack of objectivity in applying infection definitions and insufficient risk adjustment—the Healthcare Infection Control Practices Advisory Committee has produced recommendations for public reporting of HAI data[70] as an adjunct to its 2005 recommendations.[67] While not specifically addressing which infections are suitable for public reporting, the recommendations highlight uniformity of definitions, acknowledge that the difference between surveillance and clinical definitions may result in discordance, and recommend that the final decision of determination must rest

with IPC teams. The recommendations then emphasise validation of reported data and recommend clear documentation of decision making in determining the presence of infection, external audit, and a review of any claims regarding potential under-reporting.[70]

In summary, the demand for public reporting of HAI data appears to be increasing. Regardless of any perceived informed decision making benefits for patients, their use as a hospital performance indicator will likely continue. This further emphasises the epidemiological surveillance principles for uniformity and standardisation, and appropriate risk adjustment, that are key to any good HAI surveillance program.

10.2.6 Surveillance in aged care facilities

Australia has over 2600 aged care facilities operated by not-for-profit and government organisations.[80] Full details are provided in Chapter 30. Residents of aged care facilities are particularly vulnerable to respiratory and urinary tract infections, as well as skin and soft tissue infections.

Not all surveillance activities that are undertaken in acute facilities can be undertaken in aged care facilities. This is because of the significant differences between long-term and acute care, including patient population, morbidities, healthcare activity, service providers and patient throughput. In addition, aged care facilities are generally considered to be social care settings rather than healthcare settings.[81] Surveillance requirements in aged care facilities are subject to state and territory programs. At a national level, since 2015, all facilities have been invited on an annual basis to participate in the Aged Care National Antimicrobial Prescribing Survey (acNAPS). acNAPS is an annual point prevalence survey that collects data on antimicrobial prescribing practices and infections. Standardised infection definitions are consistent with the McGeer criteria.[80,82] Data are collected by nurses, IPC professionals or pharmacists. In 2017, data from 292 facilities were reported.[83]

In Europe, the European Centre for Disease Prevention and Control (ECDC) supports undertaking point prevalent healthcare-associated infection surveillance in long-term care facilities. Definitions are also based on the McGreer criteria. The first large survey was undertaken in 2010, followed by another in 2013.[84] Data were collected during 2016–17, from 3062 long-term care facilities in 24 EU/EEA countries and two EU candidate countries participated in the point prevalence survey.[85]

The NHSN/CDC in the USA also has a surveillance component for long-term care facilities. Launched in 2012, long-term care facilities can contribute data on UTIs, multidrug-resistant organisms and *clostridioides difficile* infection, and compliance with hand hygiene and gown and glove use. Summary data from 2018 reported that 279 LTCFs contributed data between 2013-15.[86]

Apart from the acNAPs annual point prevalence survey, surveillance of HAIs in aged care facilities at a national level is largely lacking. The COVID-19 pandemic has highlighted many gaps in IPC in Australian aged care facilities and further supports the need for national surveillance activities.

10.2.7 Automated surveillance systems

While there is clear evidence that electronic surveillance systems are beneficial in relation to resources and case ascertainment,[87] an exciting development in surveillance is the development of automated surveillance systems. Traditional surveillance systems are not only highly resource intensive, they are also subject to large variation and lack standardisation.[35]

The increasing availability of electronic data provides an opportunity to develop automated processes that improve the efficiency of surveillance. Recent international studies have identified novel surveillance methods that are less intensive and more accurate than traditional methods.[88,89] The construction of algorithms based on a combination of data from microbiology, pharmacy, admission and discharge data sets has improved the accuracy of detecting HAIs and uses less resources. Dutch researchers demonstrated that the application of an algorithm identifying patients with a high probability of a SSI following knee and hip replacement surgery reduced the number of patient records that needed to be reviewed by the IPC team by 95%. This represents a dramatic reduction in workload.[90]

Algorithms have the potential to be applied uniformly across multiple facilities, making them ideal for performance measurement. Furthermore, researchers from the NHSN in the USA have demonstrated that the use of algorithms based on patient characteristics also improves the prediction of HAI, improving risk adjustment when comparing hospitals and benchmarking,[91] which would further strengthen the quality of HAI data.

Two types of automated surveillance have been described, semiautomated and fully automated. Semiautomated surveillance uses validated algorithms to identify patients with a high probability of having an HAI, but still requires confirmation of infection.[89] This greatly reduces the number of patient records that must be reviewed. Fully automated systems also use validated algorithms, but do not require any manual confirmation by a healthcare worker as the algorithm applies a predetermined and agreed definition of an HAI.

Automated surveillance systems are subject to the availability of accurate and reliable electronic data. The algorithms commonly use data from microbiology, pharmacy, operative, admission and discharge, and pharmacy databases. The gradual implementation of electronic databases and electronic medical records in Australia offers the opportunity to test automated surveillance systems in the local environment.

The introduction of automated surveillance systems has the potential to improve the quality and efficiency of HAI surveillance.[89] It would also facilitate undertaking broader surveillance activities on HAIs that are not normally targeted. As an example, the national Australian point prevalence survey undertaken in 2017 found that SSIs were the most common HAI; however, only 17% would have been part of a typical SSI surveillance program.[92] An automated surveillance system would allow surveillance across broader operative categories.

The use of automated surveillance systems may also require different HAI definitions to those currently used that often require some level of human application and interpretation. However, this would also need to be balanced against clinical acceptance of HAIs being reported without human input.[89]

Administrative coding data: Attempts to use administrative coding data (ACD) to identify HAIs continue to fail. The use of ACD is attractive because codes are often uniform across hospitals, are stored electronically and are therefore convenient for applying algorithms.[93] A 2014 systematic review found that in studies reporting the use of ACD for identifying HAIs, moderate sensitivity and high specificity was found when detecting *Clostridium difficile* infections (CDI) and orthopaedic SSIs.[93] Another systematic review found that sensitivity of administrative coding data to identify HAIs was modest at best, but particularly poor at identifying device-related infections.[94]

Despite this, the Australian Commission for Safety and Quality in Health Care (ACSQHC) developed a set of 16 hospital-acquired complications (HACs) for use in measuring patient safety and quality. Since 2018, HACs have been an element of the funding models of Australian public hospitals.

Within the 16 categories are the inclusion of various broad types of HAIs, including pneumonia, BSIs and SSIs. Data for the HACS are sourced from administrative coding data, specifically the International Statistical Classification of Disease and Related Health Problems, Tenth Revision, Australian Modification (ICD-10-AM) together with an insert flag.

A recent Australian study noted that while the positive predictive value for detection of pneumonia using the HAC data was higher than those reported from previous studies, sensitivity was not able to be reported.[95] In a review of BSIs over an 18-month period at a large acute care hospital, the sensitivity of the bloodstream HAC was reported as 31%, and the PPV was 38%.[96] Further research on the use of ACDs and the implications of using HACS in Australia is warranted. This may well also be influenced by the gradual implementation of electronic medical records. If the preference to use ACDs persists, research should also be directed to determine if they may have a role in HAI algorithms.[93]

Conclusion

It is often quoted that HAI surveillance is the cornerstone of IPC programs.[26] Surveillance and epidemiology are inextricably entwined, and a basic understanding of epidemiology is required to run a good HAI surveillance program. Without reliable HAI data, an IPC program cannot be tailored to meet the needs of the healthcare facility. Without reliable data, it is impossible to truly know the effect of the IPC program.

While many healthcare facilities will not be resourced to undertake robust studies, there are a variety of approaches using both process and outcome measures that will provide meaningful information.

It is crucial that HAI data collected are reported back to key stakeholders, particularly those who are in a position to authorise change and allocate resources so as to respond in a timely manner to any increases in HAI rates. Data should be disseminated widely without fear or favour, and HAI reports need to be tailored to meet the needs of the audience.

While traditional surveillance methods are resource intensive and are subject to variation, the advent of the electronic medical record and automated surveillance systems means that surveillance methods should become more efficient and accurate.

Useful websites/resources

- Centers for Disease Control and Prevention, National Healthcare Safety Network. https://www.cdc.gov/nhsn/index.html
- European Centre for Disease Prevention and Control, point prevalence survey database. https://www.ecdc.europa.eu/en/healthcare-associated-infections-acute-care-hospitals/surveillance-disease-data/database
- VICNISS. https://www.vicniss.org.au/
- Australian Commission on Safety and Quality in Health Care – HAI Surveillance. https://www.safetyandquality.gov.au/our-work/infection-prevention-and-control/hai-surveillance
- AIHW METeOR – Australian Institute of Health and Welfare. https://meteor.aihw.gov.au/content/725781

References

1. Porta MA, Greenland S, Hernan M, dos Santos Silva I, Last JM, eds. A dictionary of epidemiology. 5th ed. New York: Oxford University Press, Inc, 2014.
2. Lautenbach E. Epidemiologic methods in infection control. In: Lautenbach E, Preeti N, Malani PN, et al. Practical healthcare epidemiology. 4th ed. Chicago: The University of Chicago Press, 2010.
3. Hennekens CH BJ. Epidemiology in medicine. Maryent SL DR, ed. Boston: Little, Brown and Company, 1987.
4. Buehler JW. Surveillance. In: Rothman KJ, Greenland S, eds. Modern epidemiology. 3rd ed. Philadelphia, USA: Lippincott-Raven, 2008.
5. Garcia-Abren A, Halperin W, Danel I. Public health surveillance toolkit. The World Bank, 2002.
6. Wilson J. Surgical site infection: the principles and practice of surveillance: Part 2: analysing and interpreting data. Journal of Infection Prevention. 2013;14(6):198-202.
7. Damani N. Manual of infection prevention and control. 3rd ed. Oxford: Oxford University Press, 2012.
8. Tulchinsky TH. John Snow, cholera, the Broad Street pump; waterborne diseases then and now. Case Studies in Public Health. 2018;77-99.
9. Coggon D, Barker D, Rose G, Rose G. Epidemiology for the uninitiated. London: Wiley, 2009.
10. Sotomayor-Castillo C, Li C, Kaufman-Francis K, Nahidi S, Walsh LJ, Liberali SA, et al. Australian dentists' knowledge, preparedness, and experiences during the COVID-19 pandemic. Infect Dis Health. 2022;27(1):49-57.

11. Hughes A, Sullivan SG, Marshall C. Factors associated with vanA VRE acquisition in cardiothoracic surgery patients during an acute outbreak. Infect Dis Health. 2021;26:258-264.

12. Bailie CR, Leung VK, Orr E, Singleton E, Kelly C, Duising KL, et al. Performance of hospital-based contact tracing for COVID-19 during Australia's second wave. Infect Dis Health. 2022;27(1):15-22.

13. Schweizer ML, Braun BI, Milstone AM. Research methods in healthcare epidemiology and antimicrobial stewardship—quasi-experimental designs. Infect Control Hosp Epidemiol. 2016;37(10):1135-1140.

14. McBride KA, Ogbo F, Page A. Epidemiology. In: Liamputtong P, ed. Handbook of research methods in health social sciences. Singapore: Springer Singapore, 2019, p. 559-579.

15. Karpen SC. P value problems. Am J Pharm Educ. 2017; 81(9):6570.

16. Betensky RA. The p value requires context, not a threshold. The American Statistician. 2019;73(sup1):115-117.

17. Price R, Bethune R, Massey L. Problem with p values: why p values do not tell you if your treatment is likely to work. Postgrad Med J. 2020;96(1131):1-3.

18. Pottinger JM, Herwaldt LA, Perl TM. Basics of surveillance - an overview. Infect Control Hosp Epidemiol. 1997;18(7): 513-527.

19. Delgado-Rodriguez M. Bias. J Epidemiol Community Health. 2004;58(8):635-641.

20. Purssell E, Drey N, Chudleigh J, Creedon S, Gould DJ. The Hawthorne effect on adherence to hand hygiene in patient care. J Hosp Infect. 2020;106(2):311-317.

21. Wu K-S, Lee SS-J, Chen J-K, Chen Y-S, Tsai H-C, Chen Y-J, et al. Identifying heterogeneity in the Hawthorne effect on hand hygiene observation: a cohort study of overtly and covertly observed results. BMC Infect Dis. 2018;18(1).

22. National Health and Medical Research Council (NHMRC). Australian guidelines for the prevention and control of infection in healthcare. Canberra: Australian Government, 2019.

23. Burke JP. Infection control - a problem for patient safety. N Engl J Med. 2003;348(7):651-656.

24. LaForce MF. The control of infections in hospitals: 1750 to 1950. In: Wenzel RP, ed. Prevention and control of nosocomial infections. 2nd ed. Baltimore: Williams and Wilkins, 1993.

25. Haley RW, Culver DH, White JW, Morgan WM, Emori TG, Munn VP, et al. The efficacy of infection surveillance and control programs in preventing nosocomial infections in US hospitals. Am J Epidemiol. 1985;121(2):182-205.

26. Perl TM, Chaiwarth R. Surveillance: an overview. In: Lautenbach E, Woeltje KF, Malani PN, eds. Practical healthcare epidemiology. 3rd ed. London: University of Chicago Press, 2010.

27. Australian Commission on Safety and Quality in Health Care. National Safety and Quality Health Service Standards. 2nd ed. Sydney: ACSQHC, 2017.

28. Mitchell BG, Hall L, Halton K, MacBeth D, Gardner A. Time spent by infection control professionals undertaking healthcare associated infection surveillance: a multi-centred cross sectional study. Infect Dis Health. 2016;21(1):36-40.

29. Mitchell BG, Hall L, MacBeth D, Gardner A, Halton K. Hospital infection control units: staffing, costs, and priorities. Am J Infect Control. 2015;43(6):612-616.

30. Harbarth S, Sax H, Gastmeier P. The preventable proportion of nosocomial infections: an overview of published reports. J Hosp Infect. 2003;54(4):258-266.

31. Umscheid CA, Mitchell MD, Doshi JA, Agarwal R, Williams K, Brennan PJ. Estimating the proportion of healthcare-associated infections that are reasonably preventable and the related mortality and costs. Infect Control Hosp Epidemiol. 2011;32(2):101-114.

32. Gaynes R, Richards C, Edwards J, Emori TG, Horan T, Alonso-Echanove J, et al. Feeding back surveillance data to prevent hospital-acquired infections. Emerg Infect Dis. 2001;7(2):295-298.

33. Arias KM. Surveillance. In: Carrico R, ed. APIC text of infection control and epidemiology. 3rd ed. Washington DC: APIC, 2009.

34. Allen-Bridson K, Morrell GC, Horan TC. Surveillance of healthcare-associated infections. In: Mayhall CG, ed. Hospital epidemiology and infection control. 4th ed. Philadelphia: Wolters Kluwer, 2012.

35. Russo PL, Barnett AG, Cheng AC, Richards M, Graves N, Hall L. Differences in identifying healthcare associated infections using clinical vignettes and the influence of respondent characteristics: a cross-sectional survey of Australian infection prevention staff. Antimicrob Resist Infect Control. 2015;4(29):1-7.

36. Dixon-Woods M, Leslie M, Bion J, Tarrant C. What counts? An ethnographic study of infection data reported to a patient safety program. Milbank Q. 2012;90(3):548-591.

37. Haut ER, Pronovost PJ. Surveillance bias in outcomes reporting. JAMA. 2011;305(23):2462-2463.

38. Keller SC, Linkin DR, Fishman NO, Lautenbach E. Variations in identification of healthcare-associated infections. Infect Control Hosp Epidemiol. 2013;34(7):678-686.

39. Mayer J, Greene T, Howell J, Ying J, Rubin MA, Trick WE, et al. Agreement in classifying bloodstream infections among multiple reviewers conducting surveillance. Clin Infect Dis. 2012;55(3):364-370.

40. Schröder C, Behnke M, Gastmeier P, Schwab F, Geffers C. Case vignettes to evaluate the accuracy of identifying healthcare-associated infections by surveillance persons. J Hosp Infect. 2015;90(4):322-326.

41. Australian Commission for Safety and Quality in Health Care. Surveillance for Staphylococcus aureus bloodstream infection (SABSI). Sydney: ACSQHC, 2022. Available from: https://www.safetyandquality.gov.au/our-work/infection-prevention-and-control/hai-surveillance/surveillance-staphylococcus-aureus-bloodstream-infection-sabsi.

42. Australian Institute for Health and Welfare. National Healthcare Agreement: PI 22–Healthcare associated infections: Staphylococcus aureus bacteraemia, 2021: AIHW, 2021. Available from: https://meteor.aihw.gov.au/content/725781.

43. Russo PL, Cheng AC, Mitchell BM, Hall L. Healthcare associated infections in Australia – tackling the "known unknowns"! Aust Health Rev. 2018;42(2):178-180.

44. Russo PL, Chen G, Cheng AC, Richards M, Graves N, Ratcliffe J, et al. Novel application of a discrete choice experiment to identify preferences for a national healthcare-associated infection surveillance programme: a cross-sectional study. BMJ Open. 2016;6(5):e011397.

45. Haustein T, Gastmeier P, Holmes A, Lucet J-C, Shannon RP, Pittet D, et al. Use of benchmarking and public reporting for infection control in four high-income countries. The Lancet Infect Dis. 2011;11(6):471-481.

46. Russo PL, Cheng AC, Richards M, Graves N, Hall L. Variation in health care-associated infection surveillance practices in Australia. Am J Infect Control. 2015;43(7):773-775.

47. Akobeng AK. Understanding diagnostic tests 1: sensitivity, specificity and predictive values. Acta Pædiatrica. 2007;96(3): 338-341.

48. German RR, Lee LM, Horan JM, Milstein RL, Pertowski CA, Waller MN, et al. Updated guidelines for evaluating public health surveillance systems: recommendations from the

Guidelines Working Group. MMWR Recomm Rep. 2001;
50:1-35.

49. Fabry J, Morales I, Metzger M-H, Russell I, Gastmeier P.
    Quality of information: a European challenge. J Hosp Infect.
    2007;65, Supplement 2(0):155-158.

50. Fridkin SK, Olmsted RN. Meaningful measure of performance:
    a foundation built on valid, reproducible findings from
    surveillance of health care-associated infections. Am J Infect
    Control. 2011;39(2):87-90.

51. Klazinga N, Fischer C, Ten Asbroek A. Health services
    research related to performance indicators and
    benchmarking in Europe. J Health Serv Res Policy.
    2011;16 Suppl 2:38-47.

52. Perla RJ, Peden CJ, Goldmann D, Lloyd R. Health care-
    associated infection reporting: the need for ongoing
    reliability and validity assessment. Am J Infect Control.
    2009;37(8):615-618.

53. Emori TG, Edwards JR, Culver DH, Sartor C, Stroud LA,
    Gaunt EE, et al. Accuracy of reporting nosocomial infections
    in intensive-care-unit patients to the National Nosocomial
    Infections Surveillance System: a pilot study. Infect Control
    Hosp Epidemiol. 1998;19(5):308-316.

54. Horan TC, Arnold KE, Rebmann CA, Fridkin SK. Network
    approach for prevention of healthcare-associated infections.
    Infect Control Hosp Epidemiol. 2011;32(11):1143-4.

55. Backman LA, Melchreit R, Rodriguez R. Validation of
    the surveillance and reporting of central line-associated
    bloodstream infection data to a state health department.
    Am J Infect Control. 2010;38(10):832-838.

56. Kainer MA, Mitchell J, Frost BA, Soe MM, eds. Validation of
    central line associated blood stream infection [CLABSI] data
    submitted to the National Healthcare Safety Network
    [NHSN]: a pilot study by the Tennessee Department of
    Health [TDH]. 5th Decennial International Conference on
    Healthcare-Associated Infections: 2010 March 3; Atlanta, GA.

57. Soe MM, Kainer MA, eds. Sustainable, cost-effective internal
    data validation of healthcare associated infections surveillance
    reported to the National Healthcare Safety Network
    [NHSN]. 5th Decennial International Conference on
    Healthcare-Associated Infections: 2010 March 3; Atlanta, GA.

58. Friedman ND, Russo PL, Bull AL, Richards MJ, Kelly H.
    Validation of coronary artery bypass graft surgical site infection
    surveillance data from a statewide surveillance system in
    Australia. Infect Control Hosp Epidemiol. 2007;28(7):812-817.

59. McBryde ES, Brett J, Russo PL, Worth LJ, Bull AL, Richards
    MJ. Validation of statewide surveillance system data on
    central line-associated bloodstream infection in intensive
    care units in Australia. Infect Control Hosp Epidemiol.
    2009;30(11):1045-1049.

60. VanGessel H, McCann RL, Peterson AM, Goggin LS.
    Validation of healthcare associated Staphylococcus aureus
    bloodstream infection surveillance in Western Australia.
    Healthc Infect. 2010;15:21-25.

61. Grammatico-Guillon L, Rusch E, Astagneau P. Surveillance
    of prosthetic joint infections: international overview and
    new insights for hospital databases. J Hosp Infect.
    2015;89(2):90-98.

62. Schröder C, Behnke M, Gastmeier P, Schwab F, Geffers C.
    Case vignettes to evaluate the accuracy of identifying
    healthcare-associated infections by surveillance persons. J
    Hosp Infect. 2015;90(4):322-326.

63. Tanner J, Padley W, Kiernan M, Leaper D, Norrie P, Baggott R.
    A benchmark too far: findings from a national survey of
    surgical site infection surveillance. J Hosp Infect. 2013;
    83(2):87-91.

64. Rich KL, Reese SM, Bol KA, Gilmartin HM, Janosz T.
    Assessment of the quality of publicly reported central

line-associated bloodstream infection data in Colorado, 2010.
Am J Infect Control. 2013;41(10):874-879.

65. Culver DH, Horan TC, Gaynes RP, Martone WJ, Jarvis WR,
    Emori TG, et al. Surgical wound infection rates by wound
    class, operative procedure, and patient risk index. National
    Nosocomial Infections Surveillance System. Am J Med.
    1991;91(3b):152s-157s.

66. Centers for Disease Control and Prevention (CDC). The
    NHSN Standardised Infection Ratio (SIR), updated April
    2022. CDC, 2022. Available from: https://www.cdc.gov/
    nhsn/pdfs/ps-analysis-resources/nhsn-sir-guide.pdf.

67. McKibben L, Horan T, Tokars JI, Fowler G, Cardo DM,
    Pearson ML, et al. Guidance on public reporting of
    healthcare-associated infections: recommendations of the
    Healthcare Infection Control Practices Advisory Committee.
    Am J Infect Control. 2005;33(4):217-226.

68. Berenson RA, Pronovost PJ, Krumholz HM. Achieving the
    potential of health care performance measures. Urban
    Institute, 2013 [cited 19 Dec 2015]. Available from: http://
    www.rwjf.org/en/library/research/2013/05/achieving-the-
    potential-of-health-care-performance-measures.html?cid=
    xem_hcpm5-21-13A&cid.

69. Martin M, Zingg W, Hansen S, Gastmeier P, Wu AW, Pittet
    D, et al. Public reporting of healthcare-associated infection
    data in Europe. What are the views of infection prevention
    opinion leaders? J Hosp Infect. 2013;83(2):94-98.

70. Talbot TR, Bratzler DW, Carrico RM, Diekema DJ, Hayden
    MK, Huang SS, et al. Public reporting of health care-
    associated surveillance data: recommendations from the
    healthcare infection control practices advisory committee.
    Ann Intern Med. 2013;159(9):631-635.

71. Australian Institute for Health and Welfare. MyHospitals
    [Internet]. Canberra: Australian Government, 2022.
    Available from: https://www.aihw.gov.au/reports-data/
    myhospitals.

72. Grayson ML, Stewardson AJ, Russo PL, Ryan KE, Olsen KL,
    Havers SM, et al. Effects of the Australian National Hand
    Hygiene Initiative after 8 years on infection control practices,
    health-care worker education, and clinical outcomes:
    a longitudinal study. Lancet Infect Dis. 2018;18(11):
    1269-1277.

73. Hibbard JH, Stockard J, Tusler M. Does publicizing hospital
    performance stimulate quality improvement efforts? Health
    Affairs (Project Hope). 2003;22(2):84-94.

74. Werner RM, Asch DA. The unintended consequences of
    publicly reporting quality information. JAMA. 2005;293(10):
    1239-1244.

75. Humphreys H, Cunney R. Performance indicators and the
    public reporting of healthcare-associated infection rates. CMI.
    2008;14(10):892-894.

76. Worth LJ, Thursky KA, Slavin MA. Public disclosure of
    health care-associated infections in Australia: quality
    improvement or parody? Med J Aust. 2012;197(1):29.

77. Page K, Barnett AG, Campbell M, Brain D, Martin E,
    Fulop N, et al. Costing the Australian national hand hygiene
    initiative. J Hosp Infect. 2014;88(3):141-148.

78. Kiernan MA. Public reporting of healthcare-associated
    infection: professional reticence versus public interest. J Hosp
    Infect. 2013;83(2):92-93.

79. Russo PL, Digby R, Bucknall T. Consumer knowledge and
    attitudes toward public reporting of health care–associated
    infection data. Am J Infect Control. 2019.

80. Bennett N, Imam N, James R, Chen C, Bull A, Thursky K,
    et al. Prevalence of infections and antimicrobial prescribing
    in Australian aged care facilities: evaluation of modifiable
    and nonmodifiable determinants. Am J Infect Control.
    2018;46(10):1148-1153.

81. Mitchell BG, Shaban RZ, MacBeth D, Russo P. Organisation and governance of infection prevention and control in Australian residential aged care facilities: a national survey. Infect Dis Health. 2019;24(4):187-193.

82. Stone ND, Ashraf MS, Calder J, Crnich CJ, Crossley K, Drinka PJ, et al. Surveillance definitions of infections in long-term care facilities: revisiting the McGeer criteria. Infect Control Hosp Epidemiol. 2012;33(10): 965-977.

83. Bennett NJ, Imam N, Ingram RJ, James RS, Buising KL, Bull AL, et al. Skin and soft tissue infections and current antimicrobial prescribing practices in Australian aged care residents. Epidemiol Infect. 2019;147:e87.

84. Control ECfDPa. Protocol for validation of point prevalence surveys of healthcare-associated infections and antimicrobial use in European long-term care facilities - 2016–2017 version 1.1. Stockholm: ECDC, 2016.

85. Suetens C, Latour K, Kärki T, Ricchizzi E, Kinross P, Moro ML, et al. Prevalence of healthcare-associated infections, estimated incidence and composite antimicrobial resistance index in acute care hospitals and long-term care facilities: results from two European point prevalence surveys, 2016 to 2017. Eurosurveillance. 2018;23(46).

86. Palms DL, Mungai E, Eure T, Anttila A, Thompson ND, Dudeck MA, et al. The national healthcare safety network long-term care facility component early reporting experience: January 2013-December 2015. Am J Infect Control. 2018;46(6):637-642.

87. Russo PL, Shaban RZ, Macbeth D, Carter A, Mitchell BG. Impact of electronic healthcare-associated infection surveillance software on infection prevention resources: a systematic review of the literature. J Hosp Infect. 2018; 99(1):1-7.

88. Lin MY, Woeltje KF, Khan YM, Hota B, Doherty JA, Borlawsky TB, et al. Multicenter evaluation of computer automated versus traditional surveillance of hospital-acquired bloodstream infections. Infect Control Hosp Epidemiol. 2014;35(12):1483-1490.

89. van Mourik MSM, Perencevich EN, Gastmeier P, Bonten MJM. Designing surveillance of healthcare-associated infections in the era of automation and reporting mandates. Clin Infect Dis. 2018;66(6):970-976.

90. Sips ME, Bonten MJM, van Mourik MSM. Semiautomated surveillance of deep surgical site infections after primary total hip or knee arthroplasty. Infect Control Hosp Epidemiol. 2017:1-4.

91. Anderson DJ, Chen LF, Sexton DJ, Kaye KS. Complex surgical site infections and the devilish details of risk adjustment: important implications for public reporting. Infect Control Hosp Epidemiol. 2008;29(10):941-6.

92. Russo PL, Stewardson A, Cheng AC, Bucknall T, Mitchell BG. The prevalence of healthcare associated infections among adult inpatients at nineteen large Australian acute-care public hospitals: a point prevalence survey. Antimicrob Resist Infect Control. 2019;8(114).

93. Goto M, Ohl ME, Schweizer ML, Perencevich EN. Accuracy of administrative code data for the surveillance of healthcare-associated infections: a systematic review and meta-analysis. Clin Infect Dis. 2014;58(5):688-696.

94. van Mourik MSM, van Duijn PJ, Moons KGM, Bonten MJM, Lee GM. Accuracy of administrative data for surveillance of healthcare-associated infections: a systematic review. BMJ Open. 2015;5(8).

95. Bartley D, Panchasarp R, Bowen S, Deane J, Ferguson JK. How accurately is hospital acquired pneumonia documented for the correct assignment of a hospital acquired complication (HAC)? Infect Dis Health. 2021;26(1):67-71.

96. Herson M, Curtis SJ, Land G, Stewardson AJ, Worth LJ. Performance of a hospital-acquired complication algorithm using administrative data for detection of central line-associated bloodstream infections: experience at an Australian healthcare facility. J Hosp Infect. 2021;112:116-118.

CHAPTER 11

Outbreak management

PROFESSOR RAMON Z. SHABAN[i-iv]

Dr DEBOROUGH MACBETH[v]

Dr CATHERINE VIENGKHAM[iii]

Chapter highlights

- A brief overview of the history of healthcare-associated outbreaks in Australia
- A detailed account of the procedures and guidelines Australia has put in place at the national, state and territory levels to manage outbreaks
- A comprehensive description of the outbreak investigation process, with a real-world case study

i   Sydney Infectious Diseases Institute, Faculty of Medicine and Health, University of Sydney, Sydney, NSW

ii Public Health Unit, Centre for Population Health, Western Sydney Local Health District, North Parramatta, NSW

iii Susan Wakil School of Nursing and Midwifery, Faculty of Medicine and Health, University of Sydney, Sydney, NSW

iv New South Wales Biocontainment Centre, Western Sydney Local Health District, Westmead, NSW

v   Gold Coast Hospital and Health Service, Southport, QLD

Introduction

Generally speaking, an outbreak is defined as an incident of a disease occurring in two or more individuals linked by a similar time and place and which exceeds the expected rate of the disease for that population. In the case of a rare or unusual disease that is not usually reported in Australia, or that has long been eradicated, even the detection of a single case can constitute an outbreak. Infectious disease outbreaks can be dangerous and have the potential to become a national-level threat.

Healthcare facilities are highly vulnerable to disease outbreaks and must be ready to face them from two directions of attack. First, healthcare systems must be prepared for community-acquired disease outbreaks, including diseases that have permeated the Australian population from overseas. Epidemic events, such as those caused by smallpox, influenza and most recently COVID-19, have detrimentally impacted countless Australian lives. Second, healthcare systems must also be prepared to respond to internal disease events or healthcare-associated outbreaks. These outbreaks are particularly insidious, as they may spread between already unwell patients or potentially lead to a community outbreak if proper control measures are not rapidly implemented.

It is the responsibility of the public health system to protect the population from infectious disease outbreaks and to prevent diseases from spreading. An outbreak management plan requires a multidisciplinary, evidence-based approach that provides appropriate guidance on the handling of communicable diseases across different populations and settings. This includes being prepared to:

1. recognise the outbreak of an infectious disease
2. identify and eliminate the source
3. stop further spread
4. prevent recurrence; and
5. ensure effective communication between all public health agencies.

This chapter covers the principles, overall approaches and responsibilities of different Australian health agencies in responding to outbreaks.

11.1 The history of outbreaks in Australia

Although the burden of infectious diseases in Australia is relatively small (2.0% of total burden), infectious diseases outbreaks have the potential to cause significant morbidity and mortality and to disrupt the life of Australians, both socially and economically.[1] Some organisms responsible for infectious diseases have developed resistances to antimicrobial agents, increasing the risk of more lengthy and complex treatment and poor health outcomes.[2]

Fortunately, Australia has made considerable progress over the last century in the detection and suppression of infectious diseases (Table 11.1). Mortality resulting from infectious disease (not including respiratory diseases like influenza) has decreased—from accounting for approximately 13% of all deaths at the end of the 19th century to 1.3% at the start of the 21st century.[3,4] While from afar this triumph appears positively decisive, closer inspection reveals that the war on infectious disease is far from conclusive. It is notable that in recent years mortality rates due to infectious disease have begun to exhibit a slight upwards trend.[3] Although many of the diseases that have previously plagued the population, such as smallpox, have been eradicated, emerging and re-emerging HAIs and infectious diseases such as multidrug-resistant organisms, HIV/AIDS and hepatitis remain ongoing concerns.[5]

11.1.1 Outbreaks from the 18th to the early 20th century

The first disease outbreaks in post-settlement Australia are generally regarded to have been caused by smallpox. The two outbreaks that occurred along the eastern coast of Australia at the turn of the 18th century adversely affected the First Nations peoples and was estimated to have killed as many as three-quarters of the population.[6-8] Throughout the 19th century new infectious diseases continued to arrive, with the opening of overseas trade and increased migration leading to outbreaks of measles, scarlet fever and bubonic plague.[9-11] However, most of these outbreaks paled in comparison to the 1918 H1N1 influenza A epidemic, which spread rapidly worldwide before documenting its first Australian case in January 1919.[12,13] This strain of the influenza virus was characterised by standard influenza symptoms such as high fevers, coughs, aches and extreme fatigue, but was coupled with additional pneumonia-like complications and rapid deterioration. This virus was particularly deadly, and uniquely targeted healthy young adults between the ages of 20 to 40 years old in addition to the usual at-risk age groups of infants and those over 65 years of age. It was estimated to have infected over 2 million Australians and killed between 12–15,000 over the course of the year.

The epidemic in Australia eventually came to an end by late 1919; however, it became clear that Australia was

TABLE 11.1 Selected outbreaks and epidemics of significance in Australia, 1789–2023

Year	Disease	Affected states	Estimated deaths
2022–present	Mpox	NSW, VIC, QLD, WA, SA, ACT	0
2020–present	COVID-19	All	12 639 (as of January 2023)
2009	Influenza (H1N1 influenza A virus)	All	191
2009	Dengue fever	QLD	1
2008–09	Hendra virus	OLD	2
1994	Hendra virus	QLD	2
1968–69	Influenza (H3N2 influenza A virus)	All	1000
1957–58	Influenza (H2N2 influenza A virus)	All	800
1937–60	Poliomyelitis	All	150
1918–19	Influenza (H1N1 influenza A virus)	All	12,000–15,000
1918–28	Encephalitis lethargica	All	600
1900–25	Bubonic plague	All	535
1875	Scarlet fever	NSW, VIC, SA	8000
1867	Measles	NSW	748
1857	Smallpox	VIC	Unknown
1828	Smallpox	NSW, VIC	19,000
1789	Smallpox	NSW	Unknown

ill prepared for controlling such large-scale outbreaks of disease. While initial control measures, which included the maritime quarantine of returning troops, were successful in delaying the virus from reaching the domestic population, plans that had been put in place to respond to the first internally detected cases disintegrated before ever being implemented.[13] Upon becoming aware of the virus in November 1918, the Commonwealth, states and territories had agreed to a national, uniform response to the epidemic. However, due to jurisdictional disagreements, this plan collapsed by February 1919 and they began to independently enact their own plans, including quarantine measures, interstate travel restrictions and border closures.[14] Intrastate restrictions on mobility were also implemented, but with dubious success. Social restrictions were eased prematurely following a decrease in cases towards the end of April, only to lead to an even greater peak in infection in June and July later that year.[15]

The deadly influenza strain ultimately propagated across all Australian states and territories, including remote Aboriginal communities, due to the ineffectiveness of the measures imposed. Concern about future infectious disease outbreaks in Australia subsequently led to the establishment of the Commonwealth Department of Health in 1921.[16]

11.1.2 Outbreaks from the 20th century to the present

The remainder of the 20th century was headlined by three main diseases: polio, influenza and human immunodeficiency virus/acquired immunodeficiency syndrome (HIV/AIDS). Poliomyelitis (or polio) is a highly contagious viral infection characterised by muscle weakness, paralysis and potential fatality. Localised polio outbreaks occurred in Europe and the United States in the early 1900s, prior to the first Australian polio epidemic in 1937.[17] The disease primarily affected children, with more than 50% of cases affecting those under three years of age, and is estimated to have killed approximately 2000 people over multiple outbreaks between the 1930s and 1960s. Post-polio syndrome can also afflict survivors, who experience a return of paralytic symptoms as adults despite recovering from the disease as children. The initial waves of the epidemic were combated using similar strategies to the 1919 influenza epidemic—strict border closures and travel restrictions placed on children.[15] The epidemic in 1951 was the final surge, causing approximately 357 deaths, before the vaccine was introduced in 1956.[18]

Overlapping the polio epidemics were two new influenza strains which hit Australia in 1957 and 1968.[14] The H2N2 influenza A strain was first identified in East Asia in early 1957, with Australia detecting its first case by May the same year. While the disease was highly contagious it was milder than the H1N1 flu strain that caused the 1918 pandemic, and also led to comparably lower mortality worldwide and in Australia. Similarly, the H3N2 influenza A strain that emerged one decade later evolved directly from the H2N2 strain. Like the previous flu strain, the virus was highly contagious but relatively mild, leading to a high infection rate but low mortality rate. It is estimated that the two pandemics increased influenza-related mortality by two to five times compared to non-pandemic years.

The human immunodeficiency virus infection and acquired immunodeficiency syndrome (also known as HIV/AIDS) epidemic began in Australia in 1982.[19,20] HIV is a retrovirus and is primarily spread through unprotected sex, contaminated blood transfusions, hypodermic needles or through vertical transmission from mother to child. The virus targets the immune system, which may lead to the development of AIDS where the infected individual becomes increasingly prone to opportunistic infections and tumours. Cases of HIV peaked in the mid-to-late 1980s, reaching its highest annual case notification of 2773 in 1987. Diagnosis of AIDS peaked slightly later, with 954 cases in 1994.[21] Since then, new cases of HIV have decreased and stabilised at around 1000 new cases per year.[22] AIDS and AIDS-related deaths have also continued to decline following the introduction of antiretroviral drug treatments in 1987. While there is no official cure for HIV, antiretrovirals are a highly effective treatment for the infection. Antiretrovirals work by controlling the viral load and preventing replication of the virus. This prevents the virus from adversely affecting the immune system and inhibits the subsequent development of AIDS. Individuals receiving treatment are likely to have a near-normal life expectancy.[23] In Australia, HIV/AIDS has been successfully kept under control through widespread education and preventative measures. While the disease continues to propagate within the population to the present day, the country has maintained an extremely low infection and mortality rate.[22]

From the 1960s onwards, mortality resulting from infectious diseases has been largely limited through a combination of high living standards and the progressive adoption of vaccines and antimicrobial treatments and therapies, together with the adoption of universal healthcare and a robust public health system.[3] However, outbreaks have continued to occur sporadically in recent years, with another influenza (H1N1) A strain and COVID-19 (SARS-CoV-2) causing global pandemics in 2009 and 2020 respectively.[24,25] COVID-19 is now, and will continue to be, an endemic disease for decades to come in many countries around the world.

11.2 Outbreak management in Australia—government and health sector response frameworks

11.2.1 Australia vs the world

Australia has experienced fewer outbreaks of infectious disease in number and magnitude than other countries.[26-28] This is due to a number of contributing factors. For example, Australia has stable systems of government. It is a resource-rich, highly developed, mixed economy with high living standards. Furthermore, it is an island nation that is geographically isolated, particularly from countries where serious communicable or high-consequence infectious diseases, such as Ebola virus disease, are endemic. Australia has strong, well-developed and exercised systems for biosecurity and quarantine, and has a small population that is geographically dispersed across a large landmass. Moreover, it has well-developed public health systems based on the principles of universal healthcare, meaning that all people have access to the health services they need, when and where they need them, and without financial hardship. This includes the full range of essential health services, from health promotion to prevention, treatment, rehabilitation and palliative care.[29]

Measures, or states, of preparedness are directly dependent on the agility, responsiveness and adaptability of systems therein to respond to emerging circumstances. There is no single, universal health system to manage outbreaks of infectious diseases. Health systems globally comprise of a complex array of country and jurisdictional-level systems that interact or intersect to varying degrees. In aggregating countries or jurisdictions, the challenges of realising a coordinated, agile, responsive and adaptable health system for managing infectious diseases are significantly magnified. It is important to note that globally, health systems routinely operate in circumstances where demand well exceeds supply. In many countries, particularly low- and middle-income countries, the health and medical needs of individuals and populations are systematically unmet—and with little or no opportunity for these needs to be met, for a range of complex, interrelated reasons. Even health systems in high-income countries, such as Australia, routinely operate in circumstances where demand exceeds supply.

In 2019, the Global Heath Security (GHS) Index Report assessed and ranked the health security capabilities of 195 countries that comprise the States Parties to the International Health Regulations 2005.[30,31] The GHS examined each country's national health security across six categories, with each given a score out of 100. The overall score for each country was taken as the average across the six categories:

1. prevention (of the emergence or release of pathogens)

2. detection and reporting (for epidemics of potential international concern)

3. rapid response (to and mitigation of the spread of an epidemic)

4. health system (sufficient and robust enough to treat the sick and protect health workers)

5. compliance with international norms (commitments to improving national capacity and financing plans to address gaps); and

6. risk environment (and overall country vulnerability to biological threats).

The 2019 GHS Index Report ranked Australia fourth out of 195 countries. In order of rank, the five countries with the highest overall GHS scores were the USA (83.5), the UK (77.9), the Netherlands (75.6), Australia (75.5) and Canada (75.3). A second assessment was conducted in 2021 following the COVID-19 pandemic, which ranked Australia second behind the United States, with a score of 71.1.[32] It is important to realise that both reports explicitly noted that no country is fully prepared for an epidemic or pandemic and that even the highest ranked will have issues and weaknesses that need to be addressed.

11.2.2 Commonwealth vs state, territory and local governments

Australia is a federation comprised of six states and two territories. The Australian federal and state and territory governments share responsibility for funding, operating, managing and regulating the health system, which is established constitutionally.[33] When the Australian Government was established in 1901, it had limited involvement in public health issues pertaining to infectious disease and was largely only responsible for overseeing quarantine measures. Surprisingly, this has remained relatively unchanged, and state and territory governments are still the primary operators and major decision makers for the public health management of infectious diseases in their respective jurisdictions.[34]

In reality, the roles and responsibilities, as well as the relationship between the different levels of government, is dynamic and will adapt to the evolving nature of an emerging outbreak or disease event.

See Box 11.1 for a list of the health and health-related matters for which the Australian Government Department of Health has responsibility.[33]

BOX 11.1 Australian Government Department of Health's responsibilities[33]

- The Medicare Benefits Schedule (MBS)
- The Pharmaceutical Benefits Schedule (PBS)
- Supporting and regulating private health insurance
- Supporting and monitoring the quality, effectiveness and efficiency of primary healthcare services
- Subsidising aged care services, such as residential care and home care, and regulating the aged care sector
- Collecting and publishing health and welfare information and statistics through the Australian Institute of Health and Welfare (AIHW)
- Funding health and medical research through the Medical Research Future Fund and the National Health and Medical Research Council (NHMRC)
- Funding veterans' healthcare through the Department of Veterans' Affairs (DVA)
- Funding community-controlled Aboriginal and Torres Strait Islander primary healthcare organisations
- Maintaining the number of doctors in Australia (through Commonwealth-funded university places) and ensuring they are distributed equitably across the country
- Buying vaccines for the national immunisation program
- Regulating medicines and medical devices through the Therapeutic Goods Administration (TGA)
- Subsidising hearing services
- Coordinating access to organ and tissue transplants
- Ensuring a secure supply of safe and affordable blood products
- Coordinating national responses to health emergencies, including pandemics
- Ensuring a safe food supply in Australia and New Zealand
- Protecting the community and the environment from radiation through nuclear safety research, policy and regulation

> ### BOX 11.2 Australian state, territory and local governments' health and health-related responsibilities[33]
>
> - Managing and administering public hospitals
> - Delivering preventive services such as breast cancer screening and immunisation programs
> - Funding and managing community and mental health services
> - Public dental clinics
> - Ambulance and emergency services
> - Patient transport and subsidy schemes
> - Food safety and handling regulation
> - Regulating, inspecting, licensing and monitoring health premises

The individual Australian state, territory and local governments, health and health-related responsibilities are listed in Box 11.2.[33]

There is a range of legislative frameworks in place across Australia's federal, state and territory governments to respond to national health emergencies. These include the *National Health Security Act 2007*, signed by all levels of government in April 2008, which aims to ensure a coordinated approach between the nation and its states in the event of a public health event of national significance.[35] Other legislation includes the *Biosecurity Act 2015*, the *Therapeutic Goods Act 1989*, and Australia's international legislative obligations within the International Health Regulations (2005).[36,37]

States and territories hold and exercise a range of legislative powers which enable them to implement biosecurity, public health containment and emergency response measures alongside those of the Australian Government. For example, in NSW, provisions of the *Public Health Act 2010* were invoked from which public health orders were made to manage the COVID-19 outbreak.[38] The Commonwealth also shares responsibility with the states (via the Council of Australian Governments (COAG), which has been replaced by the National Cabinet and the National Federation Reform Council).[39,40] These other activities include:

- funding public hospital services
- implementing preventive services, such as free cancer screening programs including those under the National Bowel Cancer Screening Program

- registering and accrediting health professionals
- funding palliative care
- national mental health reform, and
- responding to national health emergencies.

11.2.3 Response plans to communicable disease incidents

Three levels of communicable disease incidents have been defined and at each increment, additional response plans are introduced to account for the increasing scale of the issue. These are:[41]

1. Level 1: incidents managed under jurisdictional arrangements
2. Level 2: incidents of national significance which require national health sector coordination
3. Level 3: incidents of national significance which require national coordination.

The Australian Health Protection Principal Committee (AHPPC) is the primary body for coordinating Australia's health sector response when an outbreak affecting multiple states or territories is identified. It is comprised of all state and territory Chief Health Officers and is chaired by the Australian Chief Medical Officer. The Committee works with states and territories to develop and adopt national health protection policies, guidelines and standards, and to ensure the alignment of plans. The AHPPC is supported by five subcommittees. Perhaps the most relevant of these is the Communicable Diseases Network Australia (CDNA), which is responsible for providing up-to-date information and developments in communicable diseases and ongoing surveillance reports on notifiable diseases. In addition are the Public Health Laboratory Network (PHLN) and the National Health Emergency Management Standing Committee (NHEMS) which inform on human health microbiology and disaster health infrastructure respectively.[41]

Level 1: The first level of a communicable disease incident is managed according to state and territory health sector emergency and communicable disease plans. It is coordinated by committees in the jurisdiction in collaboration with the AHPPC, and by associated health advisory bodies where needed. Essentially, states and territories are responsible for implementing the appropriate public health responses to an outbreak in their jurisdiction. They must also report incidences of disease to their respective health departments and work with local communities to recover from the crisis. Dedicated disease-specific resources and guidelines containing vital information regarding the nature of the disease, symptoms and transmission mode are made widely available to public health units, and provide comprehensive recommendations for protection, prevention and response. These act as a basic template from which customised guidelines should be prepared, tailored to the unique situation of the facility and its residents. New and updated guidelines are disseminated with the emergence of new diseases and health threats.

Level 2: The second level of incident activates when a communicable disease has the potential to overwhelm the capacity of the affected jurisdiction, affect multiple jurisdictions, is an emerging or re-emerging organism of high virulence, has a high likelihood to grow in scale and severity, or is a source of major public concern (usually if it has already caused international events and subsequent media coverage). At this level, two additional plans will be implemented in addition to those previously outlined. The Emergency Response Plan for Communicable Disease Incidents of National Significance (CD Plan), published in 2016, is specifically targeted at health sectors. Its purpose is to ensure rapid and coordinated action and to minimise morbidity and mortality, as well as burden on the healthcare system.[42] Additionally, the National Health Emergency Response Arrangements (NatHealth Arrangements) are also activated at this level.[43] Operations at this level are still largely overseen by the AHPPC.

Level 3: The third and final level of incident is triggered when a communicable disease event is predicted—or has already started—to cause major disruptions to Australian society. A nationwide epidemic (usually the consequence of a global pandemic) is a prime example of when a national response is required—one that involves careful collaboration between both the health sector and all levels of government. The Emergency Response Plan for Communicable Disease Incidents of National Significance: National Arrangements (National CD Plan) was introduced to operate in tandem with the CD Plan.[41] Its purpose is to ensure a coordinated national response across local, state, territory and federal governments. Additional government bodies are included at this level, such as the Australian Government Crisis Committee, the National Crisis Committee and the Inter-departmental Emergency Task Force. Furthermore, the Australian Government

Crisis Management Framework (AGCMF) details the structure through which government officials are equipped to support ministers in making appropriate decisions (Fig 11.1). At the time of writing, this plan was most recently activated in response to an outbreak of Japanese encephalitis in eastern Australian states.[44]

Overall, these plans exist to emphasise that clear communication between healthcare providers and government health officials is critical, both to ensure that healthcare facilities are aware and adequately prepared to receive and treat patients in the event of an external infection outbreak, but also to alert the appropriate authorities if infectious diseases and potential outbreaks are detected within healthcare settings. For example, during the COVID-19, the pandemic, the National Cabinet aimed to provide a coordinated response to COVID-19 across Australia's states and territories. While the National Cabinet made decisions designed to guide emergency responses to COVID-19, state and territory governments remained responsible for implementing these decisions using special powers available under their own emergency and public health legislation.[45]

Furthermore, as an outbreak event progresses, new and timely guidelines are also created in direct response to provide relevant and disease-specific information, such as the Australian Health Sector Emergency Response Plan for Novel Coronavirus (COVID-19) which included a national approach and operational plan that was published within weeks of the first detected case in Australia.[46] The strategic objectives of the guideline were to:

1. identify and characterise the nature of the virus and the clinical severity of the disease in Australia

2. minimise transmissibility, morbidity and mortality

3. minimise the burden on support health systems; and

4. inform, engage and empower the public.[46]

These further informed a range of prevention and containment measures, such as restrictions on gathering and movement, and on domestic and international travel, which were introduced at different times and to different degrees in response to the varying epidemiology of COVID-19 across Australia.

These plans are continuously maintained and revised so that they can be immediately and effectively implemented in future occurrences or to combat similar, emerging diseases that has yet to receive official protocols. For example, following the 2009 outbreak of

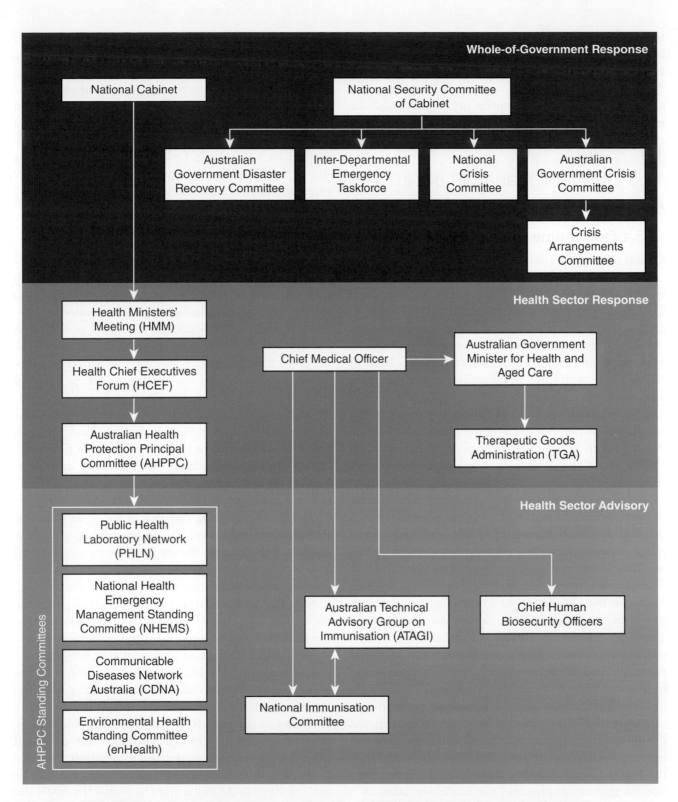

FIGURE 11.1 Whole-of-government, health sector and health advisory responses involved in the decision making for a public health emergency, such as a pandemic

human swine influenza (H1N1) in Australia and the lessons learnt from the H1N1 pandemic, the Australian Health Management Plan for Pandemic Influenza was developed.[47,48] This plan was revised and updated through to 2019 and key aspects of the plan remained relevant in managing the COVID-19 outbreak.[49]

11.3 Outbreak management in Australia—broad strategies

11.3.1 Quarantine

Quarantine is a restriction on the movement of people, animals and goods which is intended to prevent the spread of disease or pests. It is often used in connection to disease and illness, preventing the movement of those who may have been exposed to a communicable disease, yet do not have a confirmed medical diagnosis. Historically, in Australia quarantine has always been in the first line of defence to incoming viruses that were reported overseas. This was likely facilitated by its geographic location, far from most of the highly populated countries of the northern hemisphere. Additionally, Australia is an isolated island continent, surrounded on all borders by the ocean and for a long time was only reachable by sea travel.

Around the turn of the 19th century, the movement towards federation also facilitated the emergence of a national approach to public health, and one matter raised regularly was that a national government should have the power to make laws for quarantine.[50] The first federal quarantine legislation was introduced in 1908, known as the *Quarantine Act 1908*, which was later replaced by the *National Health Security Act 2007* and the *Biosecurity Act 2015*.[35,36] The act specifically targeted the likely infiltration of diseases at Australia's maritime ports. Such quarantine measures were initially effective in managing the 1919 influenza outbreak by delaying the virus's infiltration into the domestic population via returning maritime troops who were likely exposed during overseas operations. The first infected ship was intercepted in October 1918, three months earlier than the first reported domestic case. Continued interception of incoming ships and the implementation of a seven-day quarantine detected an additional 79 infected vessels out of 228 and a total of 2795 infected people over the course of seven months.[13,51]

Today, quarantine laws also extend to international air travel, which has since replaced sea travel as the primary mode of transport to Australia and has subsequently made travel to the country considerably more expedient and widely utilised. Unfortunately, air travel has allowed diseases a new avenue to spread even more rapidly from country to country, often passing through on asymptomatic passengers and infecting the domestic population with little detection. Nevertheless, quarantine remains a vital form of defence against disease and is still implemented on a mass scale for global outbreaks, including during the COVID-19 pandemic where for a period of time international travellers were required to undergo a 14-day hotel quarantine upon arriving in the country.[52]

11.3.2 Surveillance and notification

Disease surveillance is an epidemiological practice by which the spread of disease is monitored to establish patterns of progression. The purpose of surveillance is to predict, observe and minimise the harm caused by outbreak, epidemic and pandemic situations, as well as to increase our understanding of the factors that contribute to such circumstances. The early detection of infectious disease outbreaks can reduce the ultimate size of the outbreak, with lower overall disease-caused morbidity and mortality. Numerous approaches to the earlier detection of outbreaks exist in Australia, and methods have been developed to evaluate progress on timeliness.

In Australia, surveillance systems begin outside its borders through regular correspondence with international surveillance networks, such as the World Health Organization, ensuring Australia is aware of potential threats before they reach the country. Additionally, the role of communicable disease surveillance at a national level includes detecting outbreaks and emerging trends; guiding policy development and resource distribution; monitoring and evaluating disease control programs; coordinating national responses to outbreaks; describing rare diseases; and supporting quarantine activities.[53]

National coordination of surveillance activities occurs through the CDNA. Established in 1989, its membership includes Commonwealth and state government representatives, representatives from other countries in the region as observers, members of key organisations in the communicable diseases field and others with relevant expertise.[54] Members convene fortnightly to exchange information about communicable diseases in Australia and the region. In 2001, the CDNA began to revise and develop standard surveillance case definitions for all nationally notifiable diseases.[55] This group included members representing all jurisdictions and the Australian Government Department of Health, the Public Health Laboratory Network, OzFoodNet, the Kirby Institute, the National

Centre for Immunisation Research and Surveillance and other communicable disease experts. Case definitions were initially formed on a foundation of research conducted by the Public Health Laboratory Network and were continuously refined through a consensus approach over several years.

Communicable disease surveillance also operates at state and local levels. Legislation requires that each detected case is reported to state and territory health departments. State and territory health departments collect notifications of communicable diseases under their public health legislation. States produce a weekly surveillance report to provide a profile of influenza from a number of perspectives, including laboratory-confirmed notifications and hospitalisations due to influenza.[56] The notification system in Australia enables public health authorities to detect outbreaks and abnormal rates of infectious diseases. There are 73 Australian national notifiable diseases including blood-borne diseases, gastrointestinal diseases, listed human diseases, sexually transmissible infections, vaccine-preventable diseases, vectorborne diseases, zoonoses and other bacterial diseases.[57] Additionally, diseases such as Creutzfeldt-Jakob disease and HIV are under national surveillance performed by surveillance bodies other than the Department of Health and Aged Care.[58]

11.3.3 Restrictions on gathering and movement

Each state or territory is constitutionally responsible for enforcing public health measures, such as restrictions on gathering and movement, within their jurisdictions. Border closures and restrictions on interstate travel are independently enforced by different Australian states and territories. Border closures between states have been implemented as an outbreak containment strategy since the very first influenza epidemic in the 1900s.[12,59] States are responsible for organising the screening and quarantine measures of individuals travelling between borders, as well as the identification and tracing of potential high-risk individuals. In addition to limiting interstate travel, the state governments are also responsible for imposing restrictions on individual mobility within their state. These include placing limitations on mass gatherings, as well as on businesses and activities that promote heavy traffic and mass gatherings. This also includes isolation and lockdown measures that restrict individual movement to their place of residence when not travelling for essential services.[60] Overall, these restrictions act to limit the geographical spread of the disease by reducing the circumstances under which physical transmission can occur.

11.3.4 Vaccination

Immunisation is a critical strategy for outbreak management and vaccines have played a pivotal prophylactic role in preventing and suppressing disease outbreaks. Effective vaccines have been produced and distributed for nearly all of the diseases that have contributed to large outbreaks in Australian history, such as smallpox, measles and polio. While vaccines are largely voluntary and Australians reserve the right to choose whether or not they are vaccinated,[61] a strong and thorough dissemination of vaccines in response to previous epidemics has seen drastic reductions in infection and mortality rates. Mass vaccination programs have eradicated potentially deadly viruses like polio from the population, with Australia officially declared polio-free in 2000.[62] Prior to the introduction of the vaccine, polio cases had multiple, severe surges over a three-decade period.[17] As of 2017, 95% of one-year-old infants have been vaccinated for polio.[63] New cases remain incredibly rare and polio-related fatalities only continue to affect the survivors of previous infections.

Immunisation programs are governed by all levels of Australian government. The Australian Government will fast-track the assessment and approval of a customised vaccine should it become available; procure vaccines; develop a national vaccination policy and a national immunisation program; and communicate immunisation information on the program to the general public and health professionals. The state and territory governments are then responsible for distributing the vaccines; organising the infrastructure to facilitate distribution; and coordinating the appropriate resources, announcements and administrative systems to ensure a seamless process. Additionally, programs like the National Immunisation Program launched in 1997, continue to promote vaccinations and the maintenance of broad immunisation coverage across the country by providing accessible and structured vaccination plans from birth.[64] The plan implements a nationally consistent schedule for children to receive the necessary doses of specific vaccines to ensure they are best protected from many serious communicable diseases.

11.4 Outbreak management in and for healthcare settings

In addition to responding to outbreaks that occur in the wider Australia population, healthcare facilities must also be prepared for detecting and controlling disease outbreaks that occur internally. Patients and healthcare residents are highly vulnerable to new infections, which are likely to introduce additional complications to people who are already unwell and potentially immunocompromised. Additionally, visitors and healthcare workers are also susceptible to healthcare-associated infections and, at worst, are likely to unknowingly contribute to the spread of the disease both to other patients in the healthcare facility and to the wider population. Non-human transmitted diseases are also a prevalent issue and a common source of outbreaks, such as foodborne pathogens like salmonella that emerge as a consequence of inadequately heated food. At best, potential outbreaks can be detected and suppressed at the first sign of detection, and at worst the outbreak can propagate beyond the physical healthcare facility and become a multijurisdictional, or even a national, health issue.

11.4.1 Guidelines—SoNGs

Outbreak management and responses in a healthcare setting are informed by established national and state guidelines. The Series of National Guidelines (SoNGs) are guidelines developed by the Australian Government in consultation with the CDNA and AHPPC and are widely distributed by the CDNA.[65] These guidelines offer key disease-specific information for almost 30 communicable diseases (e.g. COVID-19, Ebola, HIV), in addition to notification criteria and broad procedures for outbreak management and control. The guidelines are designed specifically to target public health units for the purpose of delivering nationally consistent advice and guidance in responding to a notifiable disease event. SoNGs are produced in collaboration with subject matter experts, public health practitioners and other specialists and industry professionals.[66]

The guidelines draw upon existing knowledge and research efforts regarding the disease to ensure an informed and up-to-date profile of its characteristics. Furthermore, pre-existing guidelines produced by other nations, such as the USA, UK and New Zealand, as well as those produced by Australian states and territories, are also reviewed. Where applicable, these guidelines help inform the SoNG and also ensure there are no major discrepancies in suggestions at national and state levels.[67] Importantly, SoNGs explicitly encourage state and local governments to adapt the implementation of these guidelines where necessary.

11.4.2 Guidelines—state and territory governments

As noted previously, state and territory governments also commission their own *disease-specific* control guidelines which cover additional diseases not yet included in the SoNGs (e.g. anthrax, botulism, malaria).[68,69] These guidelines are thorough, including pertinent information regarding the disease, its transmission, symptoms and incubation period. Importantly, the guidelines also provide direct and clear outbreak management procedures including its notification status, steps for case identification, contact tracing and prophylactic measures. They also contain state-specific information such as what phone line to contact in the case of a notifiable disease.[70]

Some states also offer more general, *non-disease-specific* guidelines. For example, Queensland Health published the management of outbreaks of communicable disease in healthcare facilities in 2017 which provided comprehensive recommendations for best practice strategies aimed at hospital and health service employees.[71] The guideline describes the general steps in outbreak response and recruitment of an outbreak control team. It is also appended with a series of checklists and additional resources relevant to disease reporting in the state, and template logbooks.

More specific guidelines are typically created to manage particularly volatile combinations of outbreak and healthcare facility. In recent times, the COVID-19 outbreak has been particularly devastating to older Australians, which has led to a disproportionately high mortality rate in aged care facilities. In response, a number of both Commonwealth and state guidelines have been made available to outline the steps in approaching COVID-19 outbreaks in residential aged care facilities.[72-75]

While national and state guidelines exist to inform outbreak responses in healthcare settings, they alone are not sufficient to replace outbreak management plans. Ultimately, each state or territory health department and their respective public health units use these guidelines to create, test and implement their own outbreak protocols that are customised to the resources, administration and infrastructure unique to their facilities. Healthcare facilities must ensure that evidence-informed protocols are put in place to direct a rapid and effective response to the occurrence of an outbreak. This includes, but is not limited to, ensuring:

- immediately accessible places, expertise and resources are available for outbreak management
- staff are comprehensively educated and trained in the management of an outbreak
- staff knowledge is regularly updated and tested
- screening and preventive measures are ready to be implemented to contain the outbreak; and
- enough staff and health workers are available.

11.5 Outbreak investigation

This section describes in detail the steps of an outbreak investigation. Of course, not all outbreaks are the same—they vary in scale and severity—and not all will warrant investigators to follow these steps through to completion. However, each step is important and serves a specific purpose. Taken together, an outbreak investigation should be able to isolate the source of the outbreak, either eliminate that source or implement measures to control the spread of infection, reduce deleterious health impacts, and produce a comprehensive and evaluative report of the incident that provides informed and actionable recommendations to either prevent or manage future outbreaks.

The ten steps of an outbreak investigation are:

1. verify the existence of an outbreak
2. determine if there were changes in case findings or diagnostics
3. establish diagnosis of reported cases
4. case finding
5. characterise cases
6. formulate a hypothesis
7. test the hypothesis
8. implement control measures and follow-up
9. evaluate the efficacy of control measures
10. communicate and write the final report.

To provide a more comprehensive description of each step of the process we will compare these steps to the actions that were taken during a real outbreak of *Burkholderia cenocepacia* bacteria across four Australian hospitals in early 2017.[76]

11.5.1 Verify the existence of an outbreak

To begin an outbreak investigation, we first must confirm that an outbreak has occurred. Recall that outbreaks are defined as an excess level of a disease over what is expected within a geographic area. It is important to distinguish an outbreak of disease from the regular fluctuations of a disease that is simply endemic to a certain area. Investigators will compare the number of cases with the usual baseline incidence from previous months or years, which are usually obtained by searching for cases on local databases, or from national surveillance systems or research literature if local data is not available. Alternatively, detection of a disease that is highly unusual or uncommon and appears in two or more patients at the same place over a short period of time, may also be enough to constitute an outbreak. In the case of notifiable diseases, detection warrants immediate reporting to health department officials.

B. cenocepacia is a bacterium under the *Burkholderia cepacia* complex (BCC) of Gram-negative aerobic bacilli and is primarily an environmental organism, frequently found in plants, soil and moist environments. In the context of human infection, it is typically detected in the bloodstream, respiratory and urinary systems. BCC poses no major medical risks to healthy adults, although it has been previously linked to the acquisition of healthcare-associated pneumonia[77] and bronchiectasis.[78] However, in individuals that are immunocompromised, BCC is recognised as a severe threat, particularly to those with existing comorbidities and respiratory disorders, such as chronic granulomatous disease[79,80] and cystic fibrosis.[81-83] Infection in such cases can result in the diagnosis of Cepacia syndrome, which is characterised by fever, pneumonia, respiratory failure, leukocytosis, an increased erythrocyte sedimentation rate and a rapid clinical deterioration that is frequently fatal.[84,85]

The medical staff at the Gold Coast University Hospital first detected *B. cenocepacia* bacteria in the blood culture of a 64-year-old ICU patient (Patient 1). Patient 1 was admitted to ICU for pneumonia and was known to have a history of severe underlying lung disease prior to admission. Furthermore, they also had a similar bloodstream infection of *Pseudomonas aeruginosa* a few days earlier. However, over the span of six days, the same bacterium was detected in the blood culture of three additional ICU patients within the same hospital. Of these patients, none were diagnosed with, nor admitted for, respiratory or pneumonia-related illnesses. Indeed, as the detection of *B. cenocepacia* in blood culture is uncommon, unexpected, and occurring well above baseline level, investigators officially verified this incident as an outbreak.

11.5.2 Determine if there were changes in case findings or diagnostics

Medical technology and testing have improved substantially over the last century. These improvements allow us to test for, detect and identify cases more accurately and quickly than ever before. Part of determining an outbreak is to also establish a new baseline for disease and specifically to ensure that the increase in case findings is in fact an anomaly and not simply an incidental detection of a previously unmeasured occurrence. Furthermore, additional testing and clarification is an important cautionary step to rejecting the likelihood of false positives.

For example, in the *B. cenocepacia* outbreak, the bacteria were first detected in the patients' blood culture. However, prior to testing, a blood sample first needed to be taken from the patient and stored in a blood culture bottle. As part of an outbreak investigation, it is vital to examine and eliminate the possibility that *B. cenocepacia* was detected as a result of contaminated blood culture bottles (or any subsequent handling) and establish that infection already existed within the bloodstream prior to sample collection. Such external contamination events are not uncommon, as previous *B. cenocepacia* detections have been linked with sample contamination from collection equipment such as rubber stoppers,[86] anaesthetic spray bottles[87] and antiseptic solutions.[88]

To do this, the outbreak investigation team had other blood samples that were collected using the same batch of blood culture bottles across the hospital tested for the bacteria. All cultures returned a negative result for *B. cenocepacia*, thus ruling out the possibility that the external contamination of post-collection cultures was the source of the outbreak.

11.5.3 Establish diagnosis of reported cases

The next step is for the cases to be clinically described and a specific diagnosis to be formally established. To facilitate this, investigators will begin to obtain and organise all information relevant to the medical status of the patient. This includes identifying population risk factors pertaining to their age, race, sex and socio-economic status, as well as any existing clinical data, such as the onset of symptoms and the frequency and duration of clinical features associated with the outbreak. Additional biological samples and specimens may also be collected from affected cases for further laboratory analysis.

The outcome of this step should allow for important protocols to be established. Specifically, it should inform the criteria needed to precisely identify potential cases and on what basis they should be included or excluded. These should be specific and include objective and measurable information, such as a unit of time and place and specific biological and/or clinical criteria. The definition should allow medical practitioners to accurately gauge case count and to differentiate between finer nuances, such as the difference between infection and colonisation. Defining a graded criteria that categorises cases along a likelihood spectrum (e.g. 'definite', 'probable', 'possible') is also recommended, particularly for diseases that elicit more complex signs and symptoms.

11.5.4 Case finding

With the criteria defined, it is now critical to identify and document any additional cases that have yet to be detected. A case search is directed on the basis of information from a variety of sources such as laboratory reports, medical records, patient charts, physicians and nursing staff and public health data. Suspecting a multi-site outbreak, several modes of search were employed for the *B. cenocepacia* outbreak, including interrogation of the Queensland Health state-wide system and a number of national professional electronic medical forums. The former search identified three cases across two other Queensland-based hospitals, while the latter search yielded two interstate cases from Canberra Hospital, in the Australian Capital Territory (ACT). In sum, there were a total of nine BCC infection cases identified in four different hospitals across two states. New details may emerge from these cases which can be used to further expand and refine the criteria.

11.5.5 Characterise cases

Now with more cases being identified, we can begin to assemble and organise all available information for analysis. This information will elucidate the characteristics of the population that are most at risk by taking into consideration the timing, place and shared features of the people involved in the outbreak.

Investigators will place individual cases on a timeline to define the exact period of the outbreak. This timeline should also include information such as the likely period of exposure and the date of onset of illness for each case. At this stage, an *epidemic curve* is constructed, which usually takes the form of a histogram with time intervals plotted along the x-axis and the number of cases (defined by the onset of illness) on the y-axis. Epidemic curves are highly informative, as the shape of the curve allows us to establish specific and useful characteristics about the nature of the outbreak and the type of action that needs to be taken against it.

It can be used to inform several important statistics, such as the *incidence rate* of the outbreak, which measures the number of new cases occurring in the population during a specified period out of the number of people exposed to the risk of developing the disease during that period. Additionally, we can also determine the *attack rate* which measures the cumulative incidence rate of infection in a group over a period of an epidemic. The minimum and maximum incubation periods can also be defined and used to calculate the exposure period to the source of infection.

Furthermore, the shape of the epidemic curve allows investigators to determine whether the source of the infection was common, propagated or a combination of the two. A *common* infection source is characterised by an explosive increase in cases over a short duration of time, with a large number of people exposed concurrently and subsequently little variability in the overall incubation period. The epidemic curve of a common point exposure is usually U-shaped with a noticeable peak and then a gradual fall-off across the period of the outbreak. As the name suggests, this curve is typical in the case where many people are exposed to a single source of infection, and all exhibit an onset of illness simultaneously. For example, the 1976 Legionnaire's disease outbreak in Philadelphia infected almost 200 convention attendees and staff within a two-week period. This outbreak was caused by the bacteria *Legionella pneumophilia*, which was spread via the venue's air-conditioning system. A common source of infection can also be intermittent, where, instead of many people coming into contact with the source simultaneously, it is fewer people coming into contact over a longer period of time. This curve is defined by sporadic case numbers, usually with no single discernible peak.

On the other hand, a *propagated* infection source is continuous, where there is ongoing transmission of the infection from person to person. This type of curve is usually defined by a significant increase in the number of cases over a long period of time (usually a span of several weeks or more) and is typical for highly infectious and contagious disease outbreaks such as measles and chicken pox. Propagated infections are also more likely to generate secondary and tertiary cases, creating an epidemic curve with multiple peaks and intervals between peaks typically equivalent to the incubation period of the disease. Due to the mobility of the infection source, propagated infections are highly likely to spread exponentially if appropriate preventive and containment measures aren't effectively implemented.

The *places* and locations surrounding the outbreak also need to be carefully scrutinised to understand the geographical reach. Furthermore, important information may emerge through the identification of localised clusters or broader patterns, such as a common water pipeline or grocery supply chain. If most cases were centralised to a specific place, then it is highly likely that is where the source of the infections originated. For example, in case of the *B. cenocepacia* outbreak all infected patients had been residents of the Gold Coast University Hospital ICU.

Finally, the characteristics of the *people* infected need to be considered. These characteristics can be grouped into three categories:

1. *the patient*, which defines characteristics intrinsic to the person, such as broad demographics like age, sex and race, as well as the existence of underlying disease and comorbidities
2. *possible sources of exposure*, which encompasses sources both inside the healthcare facility, such as through medical and nursing staff and other patients, and outside the healthcare facility, such as through interaction within their occupation or leisure activities; and finally,
3. *therapy and treatment*, such as through the administration of invasive procedures, medications and antibiotics.

Let's examine the characteristics of the patients that were infected at the Gold Coast University Hospital. Patient 1 was a 64-year-old female patient with a high fever and a cough. She had several underlying illnesses, including lung disease, and had been admitted into ICU with pneumonia and bloodstream infection. Patient 2 was a 61-year-old male who was positively identified for *B. cenocepacia* in the bloodstream two days after Patient 1. Patient 2 also had a history of lung disease, including chronic obstructive pulmonary disease (COPD) which characterises a chronic inflammation of the lungs that obstructs airflow. His medical history also included sepsis, vasculopathy, rotten feet and thrombotic aorta and he was admitted into the ICU for generalised decline. Patient 3 and Patient 4 were both septic in ICU postoperatively and exhibited multiple comorbidities. All patients were critically unwell and required a central venous catheter (CVC) to be placed to administer medication and fluids.

11.5.6 Formulate hypothesis

By considering all available information and identifying the common factors, investigators must then formulate a hypothesis—an attempt at an explanation that will best account for the majority of observations in the situation. Importantly, the hypothesis needs to be falsifiable, meaning that investigators should be able to directly test and reject it if it fails to explain the outbreak. Upon reviewing the characteristics of the *B. cenocepacia* outbreak, investigators realised that all cases involved patients that were critically unwell enough to be admitted to the ICU and all patients had undergone a procedure where central lines were placed.

11.5.7 Test the hypothesis

Unfortunately for investigators, the ICU contains an abundance of equipment, fluids and surfaces that could be the potential source of infection. Furthermore, there were no comprehensive records that specifically detailed which products were used on the case patients. This eventuated in a large and time-consuming search which involved the careful analysis of all liquids, gels and fluids that were used in the ICU.

Often, the first hypotheses made may turn out to be incorrect. For the *B. cenocepacia* outbreak, initial suspicion rested on the intravenous fluids, non-sterile gels and equipment in the ICU which were collected and tested for the bacteria. However, none of these items returned a positive result. Under this circumstance, the tested equipment can be cleared, and investigators must return to the drawing board and use these findings to re-evaluate and propose new hypotheses.

In this case, investigators sourced further information from the staff and clinicians directly responsible for executing the CVC procedure on the infected patients. This investigation revealed that all procedures used a sterile wrapped CVC insertion 'kit' that contained several individually packaged items used for different parts of the procedure. The testing of items in this kit would reveal the point source culprit to be contaminated sachets of ultrasound gel from ultrasound probe cover kits. Three sachets were tested at the Gold Coast Hospital and another three at the Canberra Hospital and all specimens cultured heavy growth of *B. cenocepacia* bacteria. The investigators also needed to verify that the *B. cenocepacia* bacteria identified in these ultrasound gel sachets were indeed responsible for the infected patients. Since the bacteria also exists in the environment, this additional step was necessary to eliminate the possibility that the infections were caused by a different source of the same bacteria. Investigators achieved this using whole genome sequencing analysis and were able to confirm that the bacteria found in the sachets shared a considerably higher genetic relation to those found in patient blood cultures, in comparison to isolates of the bacteria found in unrelated cases and environmental samples.

11.5.8 Implement control measures and follow-up

Upon identifying the source of infection, healthcare and outbreak control professionals will implement a variety of IPC measures depending on the nature of the agent, the mode of transmission, the existing healthcare infrastructure and other relevant environmental and patient factors. Interventions to control an outbreak generally involve separating the people from the source of infection in some form or another. Sometimes the source of the infection is already contained or is largely immobile, such as salmonella existing within spoiled food or a contaminated surface. These pathogens can be directly eliminated through appropriate disposal or disinfection. Other times, the source of the pathogen is mobile, such as airborne and waterborne agents, or carried by other humans or animals. In these instances, protective and preventive measures need to be taken to limit people's exposure to these pathogens. Typically, multiple prophylactic measures will be implemented concurrently to reduce risk and ensure a safe outcome.

Investigators confirmed the contamination of *B. cenocepacia* was limited to the ultrasound gel sachets and all hospitals involved swiftly removed the gel kits from use. Alarmingly, the identification of the bacteria on the same gel packets across two different hospitals suggested that the product was not locally contaminated but more likely as a result of an oversight during the manufacturing process. Batches of these gel packets were likely still in circulation around Australian hospitals and investigators alerted the Therapeutic Goods Administration (TGA) who issued a notice of recall to the distributors and manufacturers within 24 hours of notification. As a result, 2500 ultrasound probe cover kits were recalled from 13 hospitals and distributors in QLD, ACT, NSW and WA.

11.5.9 Evaluate the efficacy of control measures

The efficacy of control measures needs to be astutely observed and evaluated from implementation. If cases cease to occur or return to an endemic level following the implementation of the control measures, then it may be safe to assume that these measures were effective in controlling the outbreak. However, if there is no decrease in the rate of infection (or worse, if the rate of infection increases), then existing measures will need immediate and ongoing revision until an effective strategy is found.

11.5.10 Communicate and write final report

Communication from the outbreak investigation team is vital both during and after the investigation. Throughout the investigation process, it is up to investigators to ensure up-to-date information is delivered to healthcare administrators and the appropriate authorities so that all affected parties can monitor and prepare for various potential outcomes of the evolving situation. Furthermore, outbreak investigations typically engage the expertise of professionals across multiple jurisdictions and is a highly collaborative process. The *B. cenocepacia* outbreak was resolved through the work of many individuals, from the technicians involved in detecting the infected blood culture and whole genome sequencing, to the clinicians recalling the use of packaged kits for CVC procedures and the investigators identifying related cases across state borders.

Investigators should also prepare and disseminate a written final report describing the outbreak and the effectiveness of the interventions. This report should also summarise the contribution of each team member who participated in the investigation. It should directly elucidate existing systemic issues and factors that may have led to the outbreak in the first place and, importantly, include recommendations to prevent outbreaks in the future. The report ultimately serves both as a record of the outbreak and as a guide for future investigators should a similar outbreak be detected.

After the *B. cenocepacia* outbreak, procedures towards the utilisation of ultrasound gel in central line insertion were called into question. While the report does detail the purpose of ultrasound gel in facilitating the success rate of the procedure, it also highlighted the potential risks and weaknesses in the process of doing so. For example, the sachets were inconsistently packaged from kit to kit and also lacked vital details such as a manufacturer, a lot number and an expiration date.

11.6 Challenges in outbreak management in Australia

Outbreak management extends beyond the role of public health and often requires communication and coordination across multiple sectors and countries. For example, the detection of zoonotic infectious diseases requires horizontal interaction between the agencies, departments and ministries responsible for public health, medical professions, veterinary services and the environment. Vertical interaction is also crucial for outbreak detection. As outbreaks start in communities, involving community members in this early phase could yield important information. While medical practitioners and healthcare professionals are required to contact

their state health authorities in instances of a notifiable disease, not all individuals in the community present for medical care and of the people who do, not all are tested or notified. As a result, infectious diseases and, in particular, infectious diseases that may have a long incubation time or involve cases who are asymptomatic, may propagate through the community unchecked and affect thousands before being detected. The number of notifications may be influenced by changes in testing practices (tendency to test for certain diseases or use more sensitive diagnostic tests). Finally, laws must consider the broader social context. The public have high expectations about the preservation of individual liberty and freedom of movement; therefore, dissatisfaction and disobedience should be expected responses to prevention and control measures.[34]

Conclusion

Disease outbreaks have the potential to cause great harm to Australians on both local and national scales. In addition to their negative impacts on human health and wellbeing, outbreaks can also cause wider social and economic disruptions. Therefore, careful outbreak planning and management is vital from the moment an unusual disease is detected or multiple cases are linked. Historically, Australia has endured a range of epidemics of varying severity and over the past century has built a relatively comprehensive framework of disease-related legislation, medical infrastructure and response guidelines in preparation for future occurrences.

Healthcare workers are one of the most affected groups in the instance of an outbreak and are intimately linked with the systems and protocols that direct the outbreak response. The Australian, state and territory governments are responsible for providing the most up-to-date information on a disease, and also for providing evidence-based management plans that are tailored to the disease and the local characteristics of their state. Furthermore, it is up to local healthcare facilities to remain up to date with these guidelines and to develop and enforce actionable protocols and infrastructure that can be realistically and efficiently implemented in the case of an outbreak.

Useful websites/resources

- Communicable Diseases in Australia. https://www.health.gov.au/topics/communicable-diseases/in-australia.
- Shaban RZ, Maloney S, Gerrard J, Collignon P, Macbeth D, Cruickshank M, et al. Outbreak of health care-associated *Burkholderia cenocepacia* bacteraemia and infection attributed to contaminated sterile gel used for central line insertion under ultrasound guidance and other procedures. Am J Infect Control. 2017;45(9): 954-958.

References

1. Australian Institute of Health and Welfare. Australian burden of disease study: impact and causes of illness and death in Australia, 2018. Canberra: AIHW, 2021.

2. Australian Bureau of Statistics. Causes of death, Australia. Canberra: Australian Government, 2021 [cited 05 Mar 2022]. Available from: https://www.abs.gov.au/statistics/health/causes-death/causes-death-australia/latest-release.

3. Australian Institute of Health and Welfare. Mortality over the twentieth century in Australia: trends and patterns in major causes of death. Canberra: AIHW, 2006.

4. Australian Government Department of Health. Communicable diseases. Canberra: Australian Government, 2022 [cited 08 Mar 2022]. Available from: https://www.health.gov.au/health-topics/communicable-diseases.

5. Dore GJ, Li Y, Kaldor JM, Plant AJ. Trends in infectious disease mortality in Australia, 1979-1994. MJA. 1998; 168(12):601-604.

6. Cousen N. "The smallpox on Ballarat": nineteenth-century public vaccination on the Victorian goldfields. Provenance: The Journal of Public Record Office Victoria. 2018(16).

7. Mear C. The origin of the smallpox outbreak in Sydney in 1789. Australia: The Free Library, 2008 [cited 09 Mar 2022]. Available from: https://www.thefreelibrary.com/The+origin+of+the+smallpox+outbreak+in+Sydney+in+1789.-a0180278188.

8. Poulter J. The smallpox holocaust that swept Aboriginal Australia - red hot echidna spikes are burning me. Australia: Can do better, 2014 [cited 08 Mar 2022]. Available from: https://candobetter.net/node/3720.

9. Cliff A, Haggett P, Smallman-Raynor M. Island epidemics. New York: Oxford University Press, 2000.

10. Tout-Smith D. Scarlet fever epidemics in Victoria. Victoria, Australia: Museums Victoria Collections, 2020 [cited 02 Mar 2022]. Available from: https://collections.museumsvictoria.com.au/articles/16828.

11. Curson P, McCracken K. Plague in Sydney: the anatomy of an epidemic. Sydney: University of New South Wales Press, 1989.

12. Curson P, McCracken K. An Australian perspective of the 1918–1919 influenza pandemic. N S W Public Health Bull. 2006;17(8):103-107.

13. Cumpston JHL. Influenza and maritime quarantine in Australia. Melbourne, Australia: Authority of the Minister for Trade and Customs, 1919.

14. Australian Government Department of Health. History of pandemics. Canberra: Australian Government, 2011.

15. Huf B, Mclean H. Epidemics and pandemics in Victoria: historical perspectives. Research paper No. 1, May 2020. Melbourne: Department of Parliamentary Services Parliament of Victoria, 2020.

16. Australian Government Department of Health. 100 years of health. Canberra: Australian Government, 2021 [cited 08 March 2022]. Available from: https://www.health.gov.au/about-us/100-years-of-health.

17. Hall R. Notifiable diseases surveillance, 1917 to 1991. Communicable Diseases Intelligence. 1993;17.

18. Australian Institute of Health and Welfare. Polio in Australia. Canberra: AIHW, 2018.

19. Gerrard JG, McGahan SL, Wills EJ, Milliken JS, Mathys JMJ. Australia's first case of AIDS?: pneumocystis carinii pneumonia and HIV in 1981. MJA. 1994;160(5):247-250.

20. Nakhaee F, Black D, Wand H, McDonald A, Law M. Changes in mortality following HIV and AIDS and estimation of the number of people living with diagnosed HIV/AIDS in Australia, 1981–2003. Sexual Health. 2009; 6(2):129-134.

21. McDonald AM, Li Y, Dore GJ, Ree H, Kaldor JM. Late HIV presentation among AIDS cases in Australia, 1992–2001. ANZJPH. 2003;27(6):608-613.

22. Holt M. Progress and challenges in ending HIV and AIDS in Australia. AIDS and Behavior. 2017;21(2):331-334.

23. Collaboration ATC. Life expectancy of individuals on combination antiretroviral therapy in high-income countries: a collaborative analysis of 14 cohort studies. Lancet. 2008; 372(9635):293-299.

24. Collignon PJ. Swine flu—lessons learnt in Australia. MJA. 2010;192(7):364.

25. Team C-NIRS. COVID-19 Australia: Epidemiology Report 57: Reporting period ending 16 January 2022. Communicable Diseases Intelligence (2018). 2022;46.

26. Vos T, Lim SS, Abbafati C, Abbas KM, Abbasi M, Abbasifard M, et al. Global burden of 369 diseases and injuries in 204 countries and territories, 1990–2019: a systematic analysis for the Global Burden of Disease Study 2019. Lancet. 2020;396(10258):1204-1222.

27. World Health Organization. The top 10 causes of death. Geneva: WHO, 2020 [cited 10 March 2022]. Available from: https://www.who.int/news-room/fact-sheets/detail/the-top-10-causes-of-death.

28. Michaud C. Global burden of infectious diseases. Encyclopedia of Microbiology. 2009:444.

29. World Health Organization. Universal Health Coverage. Geneva: WHO; 2021 [cited 07 Mar 2022]. Available from: https://www.who.int/health-topics/universal-health-coverage#tab=tab_1.

30. World Health Organization. International Health Regulations. Geneva: WHO, 2005.

31. Nuclear Threat Initiative, Johns Hopkins Center for Health Security, Johns Hopkins Bloomberg School of Public Health, The Economist Intelligence Unit. Global Health Security Index: Building Collective Action and Accountability, 2019.

32. Nuclear Threat Initiative, John Hopkins Center for Health Security, Johns Hopkins Bloomberg School of Public Health. Global health security index: advancing collective action and accountability amid global crisis. 2021.

33. Australian Government Department of Health. The Australian health system. Canberra: Australian Government, 2019 [cited 05 Mar 2022]. Available from: https://www.health.gov.au/about-us/the-australian-health-system.

34. Bennett B. Legal rights during pandemics: federalism, rights and public health laws—a view from Australia. Public Health. 2009;123(3):232-236.

35. National Health Security Act 2007 (Commonwealth).

36. Biosecurity Act 2015 (Commonwealth).

37. Therapeutic Goods Act 1989 (Commonwealth).

38. Public Health Act 2010 (New South Wales), 127.

39. Prime Minister of Australia The Hon Scott Morrison MP. Media Statement - National Cabinet. Canberra: Australian Government, 2020 [cited 08 March 2022]. Available from: https://www.pm.gov.au/media/advice-coronavirus.

40. National Federation Reform Council. Statement - cessation of the Council of Australian Governments (COAG). Canberra: Australian Government, 2020 [cited 08 Mar 2022]. Available from: https://pmc.gov.au/domestic-policy/national-federation-reform-council.

41. Australian Government Department of Health. The emergency response plan for communicable disease incidents of national significance: national arrangements

(National CD Plan). Canberra: Australian Government, 2018.

42. Australian Health Protection Principal Committee. The emergency response plan for communicable disease incidents of national significance (CD Plan). In: Department of Health, ed. Canberra: Australian Government, 2016.

43. Australian Health Protection Committee. National health emergency response arrangements (nathealth arrangements). In: Department of Health, ed. Canberra: Australian Government, 2011.

44. Australian Government Department of Health. Japanese encephalitis virus situation declared a communicable disease incident of national significance. Canberra: Australian Government, 2022.

45. McLean H, Huf B. Emergency powers, public health and COVID-19. Melbourne; Parliamentary Library and Information Service (Vic), 2020.

46. Australian Government Department of Health. Australian health sector emergency response plan for novel coronavirus (COVID-19). Canberra: Australian Government, 2020.

47. Australian Government Department of Health and Ageing. Review of Australia's health sector response to pandemic (H1N1) 2009: lessons identified. Canberra: Australian Government, 2011.

48. Overton K. The Australian public health response to the H1N1 pandemic. Australian Journal of Emergency Management. 2016;31(3).

49. Australian Government Department of Health. Australian health management plan for pandemic influenza. Canberra: Australian Government, 2019.

50. Kelsall H, Robinson P, Howse G. Public health law and quarantine in a federal system. Journal of Law and Medicine. 1999;7:87-95.

51. Paton R. Report on the influenza epidemic in New South Wales in 1919. Sydney: Department of Public Health, 1920.

52. Australian Government Department of Health. Getting ready for quarantine - a guide to the final step in coming home. Canberra: Australian Government, 2020.

53. World Health Organization. Priorities and areas of work. Geneva: WHO, 2021 [cited 08 Mar 2022].

54. Australian Government Department of Health. Communicable Diseases Network Australia (CDNA). Canberra: Australian Government, 2020 [cited 05 Mar 2022]. Available from: https://www1.health.gov.au/internet/main/publishing.nsf/Content/cda-cdna-index.htm.

55. Communicable Diseases Network Australia. Australian national notifiable diseases and case definitions. Canberra, Australia: Australian Government, 2021 [cited 08 Mar 2022]. Available from: https://www1.health.gov.au/internet/main/publishing.nsf/Content/cdna-casedefinitions.htm.

56. Communicable Diseases Network Australia. National notifiable diseases surveillance system - current CDNA fortnightly report. Canberra: Australian Government, 2022 [cited 08 Mar 2022]. Available from: https://www1.health.gov.au/internet/main/publishing.nsf/Content/cdnareport.htm.

57. Australian Government Department of Health. Australian national notifiable diseases by disease type. Canberra: Australian Government, 2021 [cited 08 Mar 2022]. Available from: https://www1.health.gov.au/internet/main/publishing.nsf/Content/cda-surveil-nndss-casedefs-distype.htm.

58. Australian Government Department of Health. Surveillance systems reported in Communicable Diseases Intelligence, 2016. Canberra: Australian Government, 2020 [cited 05 Mar 2022]. Available from: https://www1.health.gov.au/internet/main/publishing.nsf/Content/cda-surveil-surv_sys.htm.

59. Downes C, Mitchell S. Closed borders and broken agreements: Spanish Flu in Australia. Australia: National Archives of Australia, 2021 [cited 08 Mar 2022]. Available from: https://www.naa.gov.au/blog/closed-borders-and-broken-agreements-spanish-flu-australia#:,:text=On%201%20February%2C%20Queensland%20closed,and%20restrictions%20at%20land%20borders.

60. Storen R, Corrigan N. COVID-19: a chronology of state and territory government announcements (up until 30 June 2020). In: Parliament of Australia, ed. Canberra: Australian Government, 2020.

61. Australian Human Rights Commission. COVID-19 vaccinations and federal discrimination law. Australia: Australian Human Rights Commission, 2022 [cited 08 Mar 2022]. Available from: https://humanrights.gov.au/about/covid19-and-human-rights/covid-19-vaccinations-and-federal-discrimination-law.

62. Australian Government Department of Health. Polio (poliomyelitis). Canberra: Australian Government, 2022 [cited 05 Mar 2022]. Available from: https://www.health.gov.au/health-topics/polio-poliomyelitis.

63. Australian Government Department of Health. Childhood immunisation coverage. Canberra: Australian Government, 2022 [cited 08 Mar 2022]. Available from: https://www.health.gov.au/health-topics/immunisation/childhood-immunisation-coverage.

64. Australian Government Department of Health. National immunisation program schedule. Canberra: Australian Government, 2022 [cited 08 Mar 2022]. Available from: https://www.health.gov.au/health-topics/immunisation/when-to-get-vaccinated/national-immunisation-program-schedule.

65. Australian Government Department of Health. Series of national guidelines (SoNGs). Canberra: Australian Government, 2020 [cited 2022]. Available from: https://www1.health.gov.au/internet/main/publishing.nsf/Content/cdnasongs.htm.

66. Australian Government Department of Health. The process for developing and reviewing series of national guidelines (SoNGs). Canberra: Australian Government, 2018 [cited 05 Mar 2022]. Available from: https://www1.health.gov.au/internet/main/publishing.nsf/Content/cdna-song-development-reviewing.htm.

67. Australian Government Department of Health. The process for developing and reviewing series of national guidelines (SoNGs). Canberra: Australian Government, 2018 [cited 05 Mar 2022]. Available from: https://www1.health.gov.au/internet/main/publishing.nsf/Content/cdna-song-development-reviewing.htm.

68. New South Wales Health. Anthrax control guideline. New South Wales, Australia: New South Wales Health, 2016 [cited 08 Mar 2022]. Available from: https://www.health.nsw.gov.au/Infectious/controlguideline/Pages/anthrax.aspx.

69. New South Wales Health. Botulism control guideline. New South Wales, Australia: New South Wales Health, 2015 [cited 08 Mar 2022]. Available from: https://www.health.nsw.gov.au/Infectious/controlguideline/Pages/botulism.aspx.

70. Victoria State Government Department of Health. Notifiable infectious diseases, conditions and micro-organisms. Melbourne: Victoria State Government Department of Health, 2022 [cited 08 Mar 2022]. Available from: https://www.health.vic.gov.au/infectious-diseases/notifiable-infectious-diseases-conditions-and-micro-organisms.

71. Queensland Health. Management of outbreaks of communicable diseases in healthcare facilities. Brisbane: Queensland Government, 2017.

72. Communicable Diseases Network Australia. COVID-19 outbreaks in residential care: national guidelines for the prevention, control and public health management of COVID-19 outbreaks in residential care facilities. In: Department of Health, ed. Canberra: Australian Government, 2020, p.73.

73. New South Wales Health. Protocol to support joint management of a COVID-19 outbreak in a residential aged care facility in NSW. Sydney: New South Wales Health, 2020.

74. Queensland Health. Aged care sector. Brisbane: Queensland Government, 2021 [cited 08 Mar 2022]. Available from: https://www.health.qld.gov.au/clinical-practice/guidelines-procedures/novel-coronavirus-qld-clinicians/aged-care-sector.

75. Victoria State Government Department of Health. Residential aged care COVID-19 outbreak management toolkit. Melbourne: Victoria State Government Department of Health, 2022 [cited 08 Mar 2022]. Available from: https://www.health.vic.gov.au/covid-19/covid-19-residential-aged-care-outbreak-management-toolkit.

76. Shaban RZ, Maloney S, Gerrard J, Collignon P, Macbeth D, Cruickshank M, et al. Outbreak of health care-associated Burkholderia cenocepacia bacteremia and infection attributed to contaminated sterile gel used for central line insertion under ultrasound guidance and other procedures. Am J Infect Control. 2017;45(9):954-958.

77. Herkel T, Uvizl R, Doubravska L, Adamus M, Gabrhelik T, Htoutou Sedlakova M, et al. Epidemiology of hospital-acquired pneumonia: results of a Central European multicenter, prospective, observational study compared with data from the European region. Biomedical Papers. 2016;160(3):448-455.

78. Ledson M, Gallagher M, Walshaw M. Chronic Burkholderia cepaciabronchiectasis in a non-cystic fibrosis individual. Thorax. 1998;53(5):430-432.

79. Bottone EJ, Douglas SD, Rausen A, Keusch G. Association of Pseudomonas cepacia with chronic granulomatous disease. J Clin Microbiol. 1975;1(5):425-428.

80. Lacy D, Spencer D, Goldstein A, Weller P, Darbyshire P. Chronic granulomatous disease presenting in childhood with Pseudomonas cepacia septicaemia. Journal of Infection. 1993;27(3):301-304.

81. Holmes A, Nolan R, Taylor R, Finley R, Riley M, Jiang R-z, et al. An epidemic of Burkholderia cepacia transmitted between patients with and without cystic fibrosis. J Infect Dis. 1999;179(5):1197-1205.

82. Jones A, Dodd M, Govan J, Barcus V, Doherty C, Morris J, et al. Burkholderia cenocepacia and Burkholderia multivorans: influence on survival in cystic fibrosis. Thorax. 2004;59(11): 948-951.

83. Scoffone VC, Chiarelli LR, Trespidi G, Mentasti M, Riccardi G, Buroni S. Burkholderia cenocepacia infections in cystic fibrosis patients: drug resistance and therapeutic approaches. Front Microbiol. 2017;8:1592.

84. Coenye T, Vandamme P, Govan JR, LiPuma JJ. Taxonomy and identification of the Burkholderia cepacia complex. J Clin Microbiol. 2001;39(10):3427-3436.

85. Tablan OC, Chorba TL, Schidlow DV, White JW, Hardy KA, Gilligan PH, et al. Pseudomonas cepacia colonization in patients with cystic fibrosis: risk factors and clinical outcome. J Pediat. 1985;107(3):382-387.

86. Noskin GA, Suriano T, Collins S, Sesler S, Peterson LR. Paenibacillus macerans pseudobacteremia resulting from contaminated blood culture bottles in a neonatal intensive care unit. Am J Infect Control. 2001;29(2):126-129.

87. Zelencik S, Smith B, Wright M-O, Schora D, Das S, Harazin M, et al. A pseudo-outbreak of epidemiologically linked Burkholderia cepacia complex in clinical cultures at separate outpatient practices. Open Forum Infectious Diseases. 2015; 2(suppl_1).

88. Berkelman RL, Lewin S, Allen JR, Anderson RL, Budnick LD, Shapiro S, et al. Pseudobacteremia attributed to contamination of povidone-iodine with Pseudomonas cepacia. Ann Intern Med. 1981;95(1):32-36.

CHAPTER 12

Research in infection prevention and control

PROFESSOR RAMON Z. SHABAN[i-iv]

Dr DEBOROUGH MACBETH[v]

PROFESSOR BRETT G. MITCHELL[vi-viii]

PROFESSOR PHILIP L. RUSSO[viii,ix]

Dr CATHERINE VIENGKHAM[i,ii]

Chapter highlights

- A brief overview of the background and context for research, as well as current research priorities and challenges in infection prevention and control (IPC)
- An outline of the process of formulating and designing research questions to solve problems in IPC
- A discussion of the purpose of common study designs, how they allow researchers to answer research questions and the existing reporting guidelines
- The principles and importance of research ethics
- Case reports and the role of observational study designs in the context of outbreaks

i Susan Wakil School of Nursing and Midwifery, Faculty of Medicine and Health, University of Sydney, Sydney, NSW

ii Sydney Infectious Diseases Institute, Faculty of Medicine and Health, University of Sydney, Sydney, NSW

iii Public Health Unit, Centre for Population Health, Western Sydney Local Health District, Westmead, NSW

iv New South Wales Biocontainment Centre, Western Sydney Local Health District, Westmead, NSW

v Gold Coast Hospital and Health Service, Southport, QLD

vi School of Nursing, Avondale University, Lake Macquarie, NSW

vii School of Nursing and Midwifery, Monash University, Melbourne, VIC

viii Central Coast Local Health District, Gosford Hospital, NSW

ix Cabrini Health, Malvern, VIC

Introduction

Research is a systematic and rigorous process of inquiry that aims to acquire new knowledge or increase the body of knowledge in an existing area. It typically involves a process of information collection, organisation and analysis, which is then used to advance existing knowledge and understanding, inform overarching explanations and theories pertaining to certain phenomena, generate new ideas and re-evaluate old ones. Research is integral across all fields of health, science and medicine. In the context of this book, research facilitates a greater understanding of the distribution and causes of infectious disease and healthcare-associated infections (HAI), as well as the effectiveness of the systems and interventions we adopt to mitigate or eliminate these issues.

12.1 Background and context of infection prevention and control research

Our knowledge and existing practices in infection prevention and control (IPC) and HAI is informed by multiple overlapping and intrinsically integrated fields of research. The extent, variety and effectiveness of the prophylactic measures we take against infection and communicable diseases would be a trifling fraction of what they are today had it not been for the discovery and continued study of the pathogens and microorganisms that cause disease. The drastic decrease in the burden and deaths caused by infectious disease over the past century would not have been possible without the breakthroughs in antibiotics and the continued development, testing and refinement of curative medicines through clinical trials. The IPC programs implemented through the combined efforts of public health initiatives, education, surveillance and established systems of governance use the knowledge gained from the fields of sociology, epidemiology and nursing. Research is fundamental to increasing our understanding of existing issues in IPC, allowing us to objectively evaluate the effectiveness of applied interventions, as well as helping us to predict and tackle emerging issues like antimicrobial resistance and pandemics.

A review of the evidence underpinning infection control recommendations in guidelines globally has been undertaken.[1] The review indicates that the evidence used to make recommendations is, by and large, not strong. This reinforces the need for high-quality research in the area of IPC—and for it to be supported by funding agencies. An international panel of experts has identified global and national priorities, including improved coordination of services, accountability, and reporting nationally with stronger communication and greater engagement of networks.[2] Suggestions for further research include the identification and validation of innovative technologies to support IPC work; methodology to provide high-quality evidence demonstrating the cost-effectiveness of interventions; and investigating the role of patients and their families in infection control and notification processes.

12.1.1 Current research challenges

Surveillance of healthcare-associated infections:
Despite the frequent occurrence and seriousness of HAIs, the true burden globally and nationally remains unknown because of the difficulty of collecting reliable information to generate accurate and timely surveillance reports. Surveillance activities are key in characterising endemic trends, enabling timely identification of outbreaks or epidemics to implement appropriate IPC measures. However, HAI data are often complex and drawn from multiple sources, such as clinical records, patient observation charts, direct observation of wounds, line insertion sites, and discussion with the treating teams to clarify discrepancies or missing information. International research has identified high priority research areas for IPC to include the assessment of organisational, socioeconomic and behavioural barriers/facilitators for the implementation of IPC programs, evaluating and ameliorating the impact of overcrowding on the spread of infections, and the effect of infrastructure changes, at facility level, on the reduction of infections.[3]

Furthermore, the specificity and sensitivity of the findings vary depending on whether data are extracted retrospectively or prospectively. Retrospective surveillance typically has a low sensitivity because it is reliant on data extraction and coding of the medical records after the patient's discharge. It is limited by the quality of routinely recorded data and may lead to underreporting and misclassification. In Australia, HAI rates are collected and reported using two non-uniform data sets: administrative coded data and clinical surveillance data. National reports of the incidence of HAI are extracted retrospectively, identifying cases by diagnostic coding criteria.

However, coded data have been shown to poorly predict HAI incidences.[4-6] National surveillance data from 2015–2016 reported a rate of 60,037 HAIs,[7] contrasting with a yearly incidence of 83,096 HAIs described in a review of the peer-reviewed literature from 2010 to 2016.[8] HAI rates reported from these administrative data sets are lower than data retrieved prospectively. Prospective surveillance is typically performed by trained infection control professionals who actively monitor preselected indicators and seek evidence from a variety of data sources during the patient's hospitalisation. This method has a higher specificity and sensitivity but is more costly and resource intensive. When incomplete and missing data were accounted for, the likely incidence of HAIs from 2010 to 2016 increased to approximately 165,000 cases per year.[8]

Increasing the robustness and reliability of HAI surveillance data is a major priority and IPC researchers in Australia have called for a national consensus on definitions and reporting of surveillance methodology.[9] Priorities for the prevention and control of HAIs have been developed in Europe by experts and international panels, ranking prevention of surgical site infections, central line-associated infections, and the provision of information technology for early detection of outbreaks in healthcare facilities.[10] In Australia, a survey of staff working in infection control units in 152 hospitals revealed their highest-ranked priority was improved information technology.[11] This technology would facilitate prospective surveillance on HAIs during hospitalisation. These priorities focus attention on key areas that can inform the allocation of funds, for example translating research findings into clinical practice, and providing education and training to increase the capability of the workforce. However, currently there is no cogent published list of priorities for clinical research and practice in IPC in Australia.

Pandemics and COVID-19: COVID-19 has challenged the infection control practitioners both professionally and personally, as well as the science and practice of IPC like never before. The sustained and future effects of this once-in-a-century pandemic are only just emerging, with alarming international evidence that rates of HAIs increased during 2020 and 2021, particularly bloodstream infections. These discrepancies in surveillance data and systems, and the reporting of such data, suggest the need for research into IPC priorities in Australia. These may emulate existing consensus-based statements of priorities that have been developed by specialists in paediatric emergency medicine and emergency nursing.[12,13]

12.2 Solving problems in infection prevention and control

12.2.1 Designing research questions and the PICO framework

All good research must begin with a clear and well-defined question. This can be a challenging process, as research in many fields is exceptionally nebulous and an outcome, or a phenomenon of interest, may be impacted by overlapping and interconnected factors, many of which may be deserving of their own independent scrutiny and analysis. It is common for research to begin with a broad scope, and researchers typically benefit from gaining an understanding of the larger contexts and systems in which a topic of interest may exist. However, upon reaching the stage of developing and designing a research project, the scope of interest must be carefully narrowed and refined. The resulting research question should be:

- well informed
- supported by existing knowledge
- specific; and
- answerable using methods that are feasible and achievable.

The research question will inform many key components of the project, including its aims, hypotheses, design, methodologies and contributions to theoretical and practical knowledge.

The first step to developing a good research question is through a literature search: a systematic, purposeful and thorough collation of existing knowledge gained from research that has already been completed. The consideration of previous research is relevant across all stages of developing a research question, from the establishment of the broader contextual background and identifying gaps in existing knowledge, to posing and refining our own research questions. Ultimately, the literature search should be able to address the four fundamental questions posed in Table 12.1.

During the earlier stages, searches may be relatively free-form and undefined; however, as the scope of the topic of interest is narrowed, the restrictions and specificity placed on the literature search must increase. The advent of the internet and electronic databases have allowed researchers to gain access to an expansive array of research publications. Broad search terms often return an overwhelming excess of results, including publications which may only be tangentially related to the researcher's interests, or not remotely relevant at all. For example, the medical symptom 'anorexia' is used to describe a loss of appetite and is a frequent symptom of illnesses such as the common cold or a side effect of medications. However, the term is also commonly used as interchangeable shorthand for a particularly deleterious mental illness, *anorexia nervosa*—an eating disorder with a highly specific diagnostic criterion. A simple search of 'anorexia' in a database will return all results relating to both the medical symptom and the psychological disorder—a total of 1,130,000 results (Google Scholar, 2022).

TABLE 12.1 The Fundamental Four[14]

What do we know?	• What has already been written about the topic/issue of interest? • Has the issue of interest been investigated? If so, by whom, when and in what context? • Has the question already been answered?
What don't we know?	• Is this a new or emerging issue that has not been addressed previously? • Is there a gap in the research literature that makes this a new problem or issue? For example, has the problem or issue been investigated at a different time or in a different context?
What should we know?	• What is the specific gap that this study/literature review is going to address?
Why should we know it?	• Why is addressing that gap important? For patients? For families? For clinicians? For the broader health system?

Source: Considine, J., Curtis, K., Shaban, R. Z., & Fry, M. (2018). Consensus-based clinical research priorities for emergency nursing in Australia. Australasian Emergency Care, 21(2), 43-50.

TABLE 12.2 The four components of the PICO model[15]

Component	Description
Patient/population/problem	Describes the characteristics of the patient or population of interest, such as their demographics and health status as well as any primary health problem they may have
Intervention/exposure	What is the proposed intervention? This may include a treatment, procedure, diagnostic test and/or risk factors
Comparison/control	What is the intervention being compared to? This could be a control condition, an alternative intervention or an existing therapy/treatment
Outcomes	Describes the effect of the intervention in terms of what the researcher is hoping to achieve, such as a reduction in symptoms or an improvement in quality of life

Source: Sackett, D. L. (1997). Evidence-based medicine: Seminars in perinatology. Elsevier.

Researchers must have a system for defining and documenting search terms that will yield a search that is both sensitive and precise—exhaustively identifying all literature relevant to the research question and ignoring all irrelevant literature. The PICO framework is a well-established model for developing clear and answerable research questions. The framework consists of four components: patient (or population or problem), intervention (or exposure), comparison (or control) and outcome (Table 12.2). PICO can also be used as a tool for refining search strategies and developing terms to use during literature searches.[13,16,17] See Table 12.3, which demonstrates how the PICO framework can be used to define search terms for a literature search to determine the effectiveness of dialectical behavioural therapy in comparison to treatment-as-usual for patients with BPD.

You may notice that some terms are repeated in the BPD example. This is because alternative terms, spellings and phrasing must be considered to ensure a comprehensive search. Certain terms have localised variants and others may have changed slightly over time, such as diseases or treatments that are renamed. Moreover, depending on the topic of interest, a PICO search can generate many relevant keywords and phrases that should be included in a search. Fortunately, all databases accept Bool-

TABLE 12.3 PICO framework for defining search terms for a PICO question

Component		Terms
P	Patients diagnosed with borderline personality disorder (BPD)	Borderline personality disorder, BPD, borderline personality
I	Dialectical behavioural therapy (DBT)	Dialectical behavioural therapy, dialectical behavioral therapy, DBT, evidence-based treatment, EBT
C	Treatment as usual (TAU)	Treatment as usual, treatment-as-usual, TAU
O	Psychological outcomes, specifically the frequency and severity of self-harm and suicidal behaviour	Parasuicidal behaviour, suicidal behaviour, suicide ideology, suicide, self-injury, self-harm, hospitalisation, hospitalization

ean Operators and have methods for shorthand, which allow the inclusion of multiple terms in a search, as well as capturing various word combinations and spellings without having to individually type out all variations.

Boolean Operators are simple words (AND, OR, NOT) used to combine or exclude keywords in a search. Understanding the difference between these operators is critical, as they will return drastically different quantities of search results. For example, a search for different evidence-based treatments for BPD like 'dialectical behavioural therapy' OR 'mentalisation-based treatment' OR 'transference-focused psychotherapy' OR 'schema-focused therapy' will return 11,000 results on Google Scholar. In contrast, a search for 'dialectical behavioural therapy' AND 'mentalisation-based treatment' AND 'transference-focused psychotherapy' AND 'schema-focused therapy' will return 30 (Google Scholar, 2022). The difference is that the first search returns results that include any of the individually listed terms and the latter returns results in which all listed terms are included. The NOT operator excludes certain words or phrases in the search. In a previous example, the term 'anorexia' described both a symptom and a psychological disorder, and returns 1,130,000 results on its own. A researcher only interested in the symptom may exclude the term 'anorexia nervosa' using the NOT operator (in the case of Google Scholar '–' is used instead, so 'anorexia' – 'anorexia nervosa'), which will return approximately 700,000 results.

Truncation is a technique performed using the asterisk ($\star$) that returns words sharing the same root but with different endings. For example, hospital$\star$ will initiate a search of 'hospital', 'hospitals', 'hospitalisation', 'hospitalised' and so forth. The wildcard technique usually uses the question mark symbol (?) that can be substituted for zero or more characters in a word and is useful for words with different spellings. For example, behavio?r will return results for both 'behaviour' and 'behavior'. Not all databases use the same symbols for truncation so it is important to first establish what is used prior to starting a search. Finally, multiword terms must be entered using quotation marks to indicate a phrase ('dialectical behavioural therapy') otherwise an independent search will be performed on each singular word in the phrase ('dialectical', 'behavioural', 'therapy'). Additional inclusion and exclusion criteria not necessarily identified by search terms or functions may require the researcher to manually screen publications after they have been retrieved. As in previous steps, it is critical that such criteria are made transparent and are well documented by the researcher.

In addition to search terms, researchers must consider which databases to use for the literature search. A commonly used database in the field of health sciences is PubMed, which is one of the largest free-to-access repositories for abstracts and citations for research in biomedical and life sciences. PubMed encompasses both MEDLINE (the US National Library of Medicine's bibliographic database, including journals on medicine,

nursing, pharmacy, dentistry and healthcare) and PubMed Central (free full-text archive). The Cumulative Index for Nursing and Allied Health Literature (CINAHL) is another large database covering research in the areas of nursing, allied health, biomedicine and healthcare. Some databases offer more specific research emphasis, such as Embase for pharmacology and drug research, and PsycINFO for psychology and social sciences. The Cochrane Library is a collection of databases that contain high-quality information to inform decision making in healthcare. Notably, the Cochrane Reviews is a collection of over 7500 systematic reviews that synthesise and assess existing evidence on a particular healthcare issue or intervention. The flowchart in Figure 12.1 illustrates the steps of a literature search following the Preferred Reporting Items for Systematic Reviews and Meta-Analyse (PRISMA) reporting guideline.[18]

12.2.2 Descriptive epidemiology

Epidemiology is the study of the distribution and determinants of health-related states and disease events. Descriptive epidemiology largely pertains to the former aspect of the definition. So, in the context of IPC, it examines the patterns and distribution of infectious diseases, specifically those influenced by factors relating to people, place and time.

The incidence of a disease within a population may be dependent on the qualities of the individuals (the 'people'), such as their age, gender, socio-economic status, ethnicity and education level. For example, a simple examination of age of death and the leading causes of death in Australia in 2019 illustrates clear differences across age groups and genders.[19] Coronary heart disease was the leading cause of death in men that year, accounting for 12.1% of deaths, whereas dementia and Alzheimer's disease was the leading cause for women (11.9% of deaths).

'Place' refers to differences in geographic location. Examinations of place can range from a narrow, local scale, such as different rooms or wards within a healthcare facility, to massive global scales that examine patterns across different countries and continents. In Australia, overviews of health and disease events are frequently separated by states and territories, each of which covers wide areas of the continent's large and diverse landmass and where each jurisdiction independently enforces different legislation relating to health. However, other geographic factors like remoteness and rural living, defined by how far a group lives from main metropolitan areas, may have even larger effects on health outcomes. Those living in rural and remote areas typically indicate more limited access to primary healthcare and a greater burden of disease compared to those living in major cities.[20]

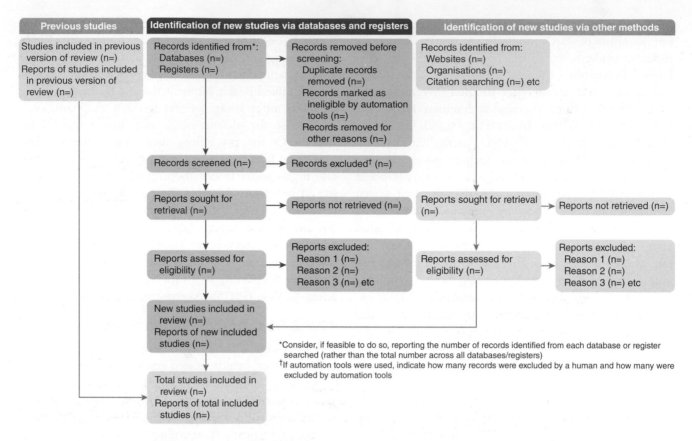

FIGURE 12.1 PRISMA (2020) flowchart template for systematic reviews[18]

Source: Adapted from M. Boers. Graphics and statistics for cardiology: designing effective tables for presentation and publication. Heart, 104 (2018), pp. 192-200, 10.1136/heartjnl-2017-311581 E. Mayo-Wilson, T. Li, N. Fusco, K. Dickersin, Muds investigatorsPractical guidance for using multiple data sources in systematic reviews and meta-analyses (with examples from the MUDS study).Res. Synth. Methods, 9 (2018), pp. 2-12, 10.1002/jrsm.1277 E. Stovold, D. Beecher, R. Foxlee, A. Noel-Storr. Study flow diagrams in Cochrane systematic review updates: an adapted PRISMA flow diagram. Syst. Rev., 3 (2014), p. 54, 10.1186/2046-4053-3-54.

The distribution and incidence of disease may also vary over time. Time trends are commonly distinguished into cyclic or secular trends. A cyclic trend captures recurrent increases and decreases in disease frequency within a year or over a period of years. A well-established example is the common cold, which closely follows annual seasonal cycles, where incidence increases during the winter and decreases as the weather warms. In contrast, a secular trend is one that characterises a gradual, typically monotonic, change over an extended timeframe. For example, the incidence of tuberculosis per 100,000 population in Australia has been on a steady, but slowing, decline over the last 100 years.[21,22]

In isolation, descriptive epidemiology is not a type of research design, but rather a means of collecting broad pieces of information across a wide range of variables which will subsequently inform research hypotheses that can be tested, confirmed or falsified. The role of analytical epidemiology is to propose potential determinants of specific health and disease events and establish the existence of a causal relationship between the two (Fig 12.2). The broad categories of analytic study designs are described in the following section, and some specific forms of descriptive studies related to outbreak investigations are highlighted later in this chapter.

12.3 Research designs

Following the formulation of a research question, the next step is to establish an appropriate study design. While there are many study designs available, the choice of design will depend on two questions:

1. Does this design allow the researcher to answer the research question exhaustively, or at the very least, satisfactorily?

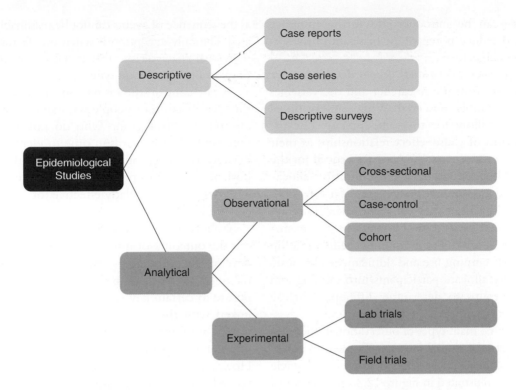

FIGURE 12.2 Broad overview of the branches comprising epidemiological studies
Source: https://s4be.cochrane.org/blog/2021/04/06/an-introduction-to-different-types-of-study-design/

2. What constraints exist to using this design and what are the necessary trade-offs/compromises?

Every well-formulated research question should have an optimal research design; however, research does not exist in a vacuum and the feasibility of the design will be affected by factors like limitations in existing knowledge, resources, timeframe and ethical considerations.

A comprehensive account and comparison of all research designs is beyond the scope of this chapter, although we do present a summary of some common design types in Table 12.3. That said, in this section we elaborate on some foundational frameworks through which most research designs in health sciences and IPC can be characterised.

12.3.1 Experimental vs observational designs

Health and disease research utilise both experimental and observational research designs. *Experimental studies* (also known as intervention studies) are perhaps the more powerful of the two, whereby researchers are able to directly observe the outcomes of interventions or manipulations they introduce under rigorously controlled conditions. Experimental studies are also frequently referred to as *clinical trials*. This is because the

design is often adopted for the purposes of evaluating *therapeutic interventions*, such as new drugs or surgical techniques, or *preventive interventions*, such as prophylactic activities and policies. Experimental designs emphasise the importance of appropriate controls—in a control condition, the intervention of interest is *not* applied in order to generate a separate set of outcomes from which the effectiveness of the intervention can be measured and compared. Participants in control conditions typically receive an existing standard of care, or alternatively a *placebo* when no existing treatments are available.

There are many varieties of experimental designs; however, most are differentiated by how the control condition is formed. *Randomised control trials* (RCT) are the gold standard for experimental research design, particularly in the context of clinical trials. Participants in these trials are randomly allocated to intervention or control conditions. Allocation by pure chance removes the potential influence of selection bias, which is a common issue in experimental designs where condition membership is self-selected or based on preexisting characteristics. Where viable, additional blinding protocols—in which both participants and experimenters are blind to condition membership during allocation, testing and data analysis—can be introduced to further improve robustness and reduce potential for biases from the experimenter or subject.

In contrast, *observational study designs* do not involve any intervention from the researcher and the variables of interest are purely observed. While observational designs do not allow for the same precise, one-to-one examination of cause–effect relationships as their experimental counterparts, they remain crucial for the study of health phenomena when condition allocation and selective intervention are simply not feasible. Commonly raised drawbacks of experimental studies are those imposed by its ethical limitations. For example, researchers interested in examining the relationship between indoor tanning use and skin cancer obviously cannot ethically allocate participants into tanning and non-tanning groups to determine differences in the incidence of skin cancer.

There are three main types of observational study designs. Cross-sectional studies are typically used to determine the prevalence of a variable of interest at a single point in time. As illustrated in Figure 12.3, cross-sectional studies are non-directional, as the factor of interest and the outcome are being assessed simultaneously, and because of this, isolated cross-sectional studies should not be used to infer cause-and-effect from simple association,

as the sequence of events cannot be reasonably differentiated. The only exception is when one factor involves an individual characteristic that is stable over time, such as one's ethnicity or blood type.

A case control study is retrospective, beginning with the identification of people with an outcome of interest and a control group who do not. The researcher then ventures backwards in time to identify differences between the two groups and determine the relative importance of various predictor variables to the outcome. This design is particularly effective for investigating the aetiology of rare diseases.

Cohort studies investigate a group of people without the outcome of interest and observe whether they develop the outcome over the period of study. The initial outcome-free group is also distinguished by its exposure to certain key variables that are predicted to be linked with the occurrence of the outcome. Cohort studies are typically prospective, with follow-up measurements happening at regular intervals as time passes. However, retrospective cohort studies are also possible whereby measurements are based on historical records.

12.3.2 Positivism vs naturalism

Positivism assumes a single objective reality, which is directly perceivable by the senses and measurable using

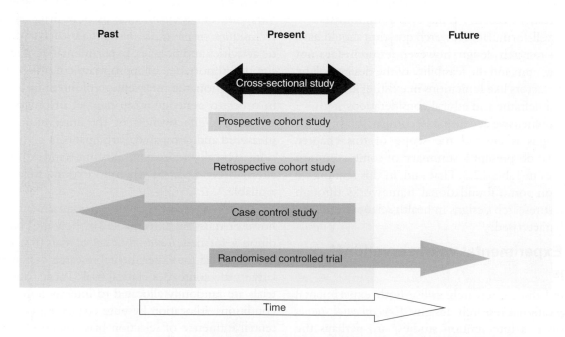

FIGURE 12.3 The direction of temporal observation of different observational study designs and randomised controlled trials[23]

Source: Von Elm, E., Altman, D. G., Egger, M., Pocock, S. J., Gøtzsche, P. C., & Vandenbroucke, J. P. (2007). The Strengthening the Reporting of Observational Studies in Epidemiology (STROBE) statement: guidelines for reporting observational studies. Bulletin of the World Health Organization. 85:867-72.

quantifiable methods. Researchers systematically observe and explain phenomena and human behaviour using objective and verifiable systems of measurement. In this sense, it also establishes human behaviour as a purely reactionary outcome to external forces and systems, which can be rigorously and methodically explained as more verifiable 'facts' are accrued. On the other hand, the *naturalism* approach emphasises how 'facts' are characterised by their meaningfulness to members of the social world. As opposed to assuming that singular realities exist and all individual action is the result of external forces, it assumes multiple realities, that are those constructed by individuals and their own interpretations of their perceptions and experiences.

These seemingly opposing schools of thought form the foundational arguments for the use of quantitative vs qualitative methodologies in research. Debates supporting and opposing either perspective were widespread throughout the 20th century; however, modern research generally sees the adoption of both quantitative and qualitative methodologies, depending on their appropriateness to the research question. The methods can be complementary, each allowing the researcher to capture unique facets of a phenomenon that cannot be attained using one method alone. Furthermore, different stages of the research process can benefit more from one methodology over the other. Qualitative techniques generate large quantities of rich and diverse data, which can efficiently provide broad perspectives and insights about relatively new or unknown topics. These insights allow the scope of the research enquiry to be narrowed and for more specific questions to be formulated. Quantitative techniques offer more direct, simple and reliable answers to these questions when most of the relevant parameters of interest are known and can be determined with an objective measure.

Quantitative methodologies: All data collected in quantitative research can be quantified or expressed as a numerical value. Quantitative data can be defined as either categorical or numerical. *Categorical data* operates like a label that classifies observations into distinct groups. Categorical data is *nominal* when there is no inherent order to the groups, and therefore no association between group identity and the numeric value. For example, the blood types A, B, AB and O can be assigned the numbers 1, 2, 3 and 4 respectively or in any other configuration. *Ordinal* categorical data assigns numeric value based on an inherent order in the variable. For example, an individual's income tax bracket may range from 1 to 5, where each

consecutively higher value designates the respective higher tax bracket. *Numerical data* presents a direct description of a count or measurement, where the number itself is meaningful to the variable being quantified, such as an individual's age, weight and height. Numerical data can be *discrete*, in which a unit can only be sensibly quantified in terms of integers, such as number of children. *Continuous* numerical data measures units to any degree of fractional specificity depending on the needs of the researcher and scale of variable being measured.

Quantitative data is examined using *descriptive* and *inferential statistics*. Descriptive statistics organise and summarise raw data points into a form that can be easily examined and interpreted. Categorical data is typically described in terms of the *frequency* and proportion of certain categories relative to other categories within the same variable. Numerical data is described using a measure of central tendency and a measure of spread. There are three measures of central tendency:

1. the *mean* or the average, which is calculated by the sum of numerical values divided by the count of numerical values
2. the *median*, which is the middle value when all numerical values are placed in an ordered list; and
3. the *mode*, which is the most common numerical value.

Measures of spreads are calculated based on the selected measure of central tendency. *Standard deviation* (SD) is the measure of the average distance between each value and the mean of the data set. Quartiles, which identifies the numeric value that cuts off the 25th, 50th and 75th percentile of an ordered data set, are used to illustrate the spread of data relative to the median (the median is equivalent to the 50th percentile). The *interquartile range* (IQR) is the difference between the values of the 25th and 75th percentile. Additionally, the difference between the smallest and largest number in the data set defines the *range*, which can also be an informative, descriptive measure of spread.

While descriptive statistics are useful, they do not allow researchers to make inferences from the sample and generalise to the greater population. Let's say a researcher wanted to determine the average weight of babies born in their state in the last month. They take a sample of babies from three local hospitals and calculate the average weight to be 3.31 kg. This average offers an estimate of the true population mean based on the sample, but how do we know how good this estimate is? A *confidence interval* (CI) provides us with a range of values around the sample means for which we assume, with a predetermined level of confidence, that the true population mean will fall. For example, the 95% CI for mean baby weight was [2.81, 3.81]. Based on this, the researcher can state that they are 95% confident that the true average weight of babies born in their state in the last month lies between 2.81 and 3.81 kg. The precision of the CI is akin to its width, which is determined by three factors: the level of uncertainty (a 90% CI calculated for the same data will always be narrower, and thus is the trade-off between uncertainty and precision), sample variability and sample size.

A *null-hypothesis statistical test* (NHST, also known as a null-hypothesis significance test) is a statistical procedure used for testing a null hypothesis (H_0), which predicts the absence of a relationship between the variables of interest. The outcome of the test is binary, leading to either a rejection of the null hypothesis or a failure to reject the null hypothesis. NHST begins with the assumption that the null hypothesis is true, and rejection occurs only when the likelihood of the observations happening, if there truly was no relationship, is acceptably low. 'Acceptably low' is numerically defined by a predetermined p-value, also known as a significance level (α). The most common p-values observed in research are .05, .01 and .001. If, for example, a researcher sets a p-value of .05 and calculates a test statistic for a set of observations to be .003, the researcher may reject the null hypothesis and declare a significant result. In general terms, this outcome indicates that there is a less than 5% probability of the observed results occurring if the null hypothesis was true. It should be noted that failure to reject the null hypothesis is not a confirmation of no relationship or no difference between variables, but simply a failure to detect a difference using the current method.

What happens when a researcher finds a significant result and rejects the null, but in reality, the null is true? By definition, when the level of significance is set to a value like .05, this indicates that there is a 5% probability that we will incorrectly reject a true null hypothesis. This is called a *Type I error* or a false positive, and the probability of making such an error is commensurate with α and is also known as the *Type I error rate*. On the other hand, when a researcher fails to reject a false null hypothesis (thus, concluding no difference between variables when there really is a difference) they have made a *Type II error*. The *Type II error rate* (β) is defined by the *power* ($1 - \beta$) of the statistical test being performed (Fig 12.4). Power is the probability of correctly

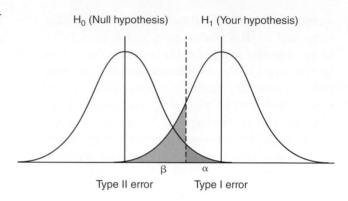

FIGURE 12.4 Type I and Type II errors
Source: https://vwo.com/blog/errors-in-ab-testing/

rejecting a false null hypothesis. The power of the study is determined by several factors: the predetermined value of α, the variability and size of the sample, and the effect size to be detected (δ).

Researchers will typically perform a power calculation during the design phase of the study to inform the parameters required to achieve a power of at least 80%. This calculation is particularly important in determining the size of the sample that needs to be recruited. The relationship between hypothesis, decision and error is summarised in Table 12.4.

Qualitative methodologies: Qualitative research methods attempt to describe phenomena in words rather than in numbers. Qualitative methodologies are usually flexible and highly responsive to the input being received. Unlike in quantitative research, researchers may freely adapt or redirect their research questions in response to new insights during the data collection and analysis processes, provided the changes are well rationalised and documented. This often results in data that is uniquely rich and that lends a comprehensive degree of understanding into the topic being investigated. Ideally, qualitative research allows researchers to access knowledge from

TABLE 12.4 Statistical errors

	True H_0	False H_0
Reject H_0	α Type I error (false positive)	$1 - \beta$ Power (correct decision)
Do not reject H_0	$1 - \alpha$ (correct decision)	β Type II error (false negative)

perspectives that are impossible to experience firsthand or elucidate using only quantitative methodologies. Qualitative research can be founded upon several methodological approaches, which are summarised in Table 12.5.

There are many techniques for collecting qualitative data including, but not limited to, observation, interviews (structured and unstructured), self-written accounts, focus groups, and historical and contemporary records and artifacts (Table 12.6). In the context of healthcare services and IPC, qualitative research is particularly important in the assessment and evaluation of interventions and systems of change, which typically involve highly complex contexts with multiple stakeholders and varying goals.[25,26] The rules and recommendations for organising and analysing qualitative data are broad and beyond the scope of this chapter.

TABLE 12.5 Major methodological approaches to qualitative research as listed by Dew[24]

Approach	Principles
Ethnography	Ethnography focuses on cultural beliefs and practices. This approach originated from anthropology and was used in the study of ethnicity and geographic location. However, the approach can be narrowed to the investigation of any healthcare organisation or setting. Ethnography heavily utilises participant observation where the researcher is integrated and active to some degree in the population they are observing
Phenomenology	Phenomenology centres its study on people's consciousness and subjective experiences. It asserts that people can be understood through their unique interpretations of the world and the society they live in. Insight is gained from lived experiences of diseases and interactions with healthcare systems
Grounded theory	Grounded theory involves a gradual and iterative process of theory building. Importantly, the theory must be based on data and observation. Research typically begins with a broad area of interest that is flexible to change. Core concepts are eventually identified and systematically refined, tested and verified as more data is collected
Discourse analysis	Discourse analysis studies the features of languages and the style of language and argumentation pertaining to specific issues and topics. Language is regarded as a tool people use to represent the world
Ethnomethodology	Ethnomethodology is the study of how societal organisation is achieved. Specifically, it elucidates how mutual awareness of engagement in certain behaviours, actions and speech by members of the same society, or within a particular setting, facilitates social order. Colloquially, it examines how 'common sense' informs behaviour and interpretations in everyday life
Action research	Action research involves the systematic and simultaneous application of both research and intervention. Problems and areas for improvement are identified and potential interventions are implemented. The impact and effectiveness of the intervention is continually evaluated and avenues for additional changes are developed

Source: Modified from Dew, K. (2007). A health researcher's guide to qualitative methodologies. Australian and New Zealand journal of public health, 31(5), 433-437.

TABLE 12.6 Summary of common qualitative research methodologies[27–30]

Methodology	Description
Observation	The gathering of data on a population or phenomena of interest through observation. Observation may be participative (researcher becomes directly involved in the population) or non-participative (researcher aims to be as unobtrusive as possible). It may be structured against a set of predetermined criteria or completely unstructured. Participants also may or may not know they are under observation. The settings can range from natural to in a laboratory, under controlled conditions or interventions

Continued

TABLE 12.6 Summary of common qualitative research methodologies—cont'd

Methodology	Description
Interviews	Interviews characterise a direct exchange between a researcher and a subject, where the researcher (interviewer) asks questions, and the subject (interviewee) responds accordingly. These exchanges are typically one-on-one but may also take place in a group setting (multiple interviewees). Interviews can range from a highly rigid question–answer format to a free-flowing conversation.[27] Conventionally, this has been distinguished into three categories: • *Structured*: typically designed to test a priori hypotheses involving fully standardised questions and analyses. Can generate data that is processed in a quantitative manner as interviewee responses are coded against predetermined criteria. This method aims to minimise biases and increase generalisability • *Semi-structured*: questions are guided by broader themes which help the interviewer direct the flow of conversation to topics of interest. Uses scheduled and unscheduled probes to encourage greater elaboration where necessary • *Unstructured*: purposely informal to replicate natural conversations that may happen in the field. Topics are driven by the interviewee and what they are willing to disclose at that time. Both semi-structured and unstructured interviews are useful in hypothesis-generation
Focus groups	Focus groups are a form of group interview in which group interactions are a key aspect of the method. Small groups ranging from four to eight participants are encouraged to interact and discuss interviewer questions with one another. This is driven by the idea that group processes and dynamics facilitate the clarification of views and can also serve to highlight contrary beliefs and attitudes based on differences in culture, priorities and lived experiences.[28] On the other hand, the opposite effect may also occur, where individual voices are inhibited depending on the composition of the group
Surveys and questionnaires	A series of closed and open-ended questions that subjects complete. These typically perform like structured interviews but are formatted so they can be easily distributed and data can be widely collected. Common formats include telephone and online surveys. They do not require a formal, face-to-face meeting between interviewer and interviewee. They have the advantage of being time-efficient and may provide insights into more sensitive topic areas due to the increased anonymity of the respondent[29]
Records, documents and artifacts	The collection and examination of historical or contemporary evidence and materials that already exist prior to researcher intervention. Depending on the topic area, these will come in many forms, such as diaries, journals, correspondence, reports, meeting notes, photographs and videos[30]

Source: DiCicco-Bloom B et al. The qualitative research interview. Med Educ, 2006; Kitzinger J. Qualitative research: introducing focus groups. BMJ, 1995; Braun V et al. The online survey as a qualitative research tool. Int J Soc Res, 2021; Bowen G. Document analysis as a qualitative research method. Qual Res J, 2009.

12.3.3 Research design reporting guidelines

International reporting guidelines have been published for many different study designs. The EQUATOR (Enhancing the Quality and Transparency of Health Research) Network is an international initiative that was established in 2006 with the aim of improving the reliability and robustness of published research through the systematic adoption of reporting guidelines. The Network operates centres worldwide to raise awareness and support good research reporting practices. The main reporting guidelines used for some common study designs are summarised in Table 12.7.

12.3.4 Hierarchy of evidence

Different research designs have different strengths and weaknesses, and as a result, some designs will present evidence of higher quality, weight and value compared to others. This is known as the hierarchy of evidence. When conducting literature reviews, researchers should consider the position of the described study design within the hierarchy to inform their appraisal and evaluation of the evidence relative to that of other available research.

Many variations of the hierarchy have been published, which implement different categorisation systems and letter–number grades. However, the general order of study designs along hierarchies is broadly consistent.

TABLE 12.7 Summary of main study types and the primary reporting guidelines used for each

Research design type	Description	Reporting guideline
Randomised trials (RCTs)	Involves the comparison of interventions between two or more groups, in which subjects have been randomly assigned. In an ideal experiment, all extraneous factors that may affect the measured outcomes are controlled between the groups, such that only the effect of the intervention is observed	CONSORT
Observational studies	Involves the study of an individual or cohort without any manipulation or intervention from the experimenter. This may involve the comparison of different groups (treatment vs no treatment), but the experimenter does not allocate individuals into these groups	STROBE
Systematic reviews	A systematic and reproducible method that uses a transparent and predefined eligibility criteria to identify, summarise and critically appraise all existing literature and research on a specific topic or question	PRISMA
Study protocols	A document outlining the overall organisation and timeframe of a study including, but not limited to, the study's objectives, design, methodology, planned analyses and expected outcomes. This document forms a template to guide the research process and may include more complex specifications for highly technical research	SPIRIT PRISMA-P
Diagnostic/prognostic studies	Involves studies that evaluate diagnostic and prognostic tests. Important measures include the accuracy, safety, effectiveness and predictive validity of these tests	STARD TRIPOD
Case reports	A detailed report of the symptoms, signs, diagnosis, treatment and follow-up of an individual patient. They usually follow unusual or novel occurrences	CARE STROBE
Clinical practice guidelines	A set of statements that include recommendations to optimise patient care. These should be founded upon systematically reviewed research evidence and assess the benefits and harms of alternative options	AGREE RIGHT
Qualitative research	Involves the collection and analysis of non-numerical data, typically in the form of first-hand accounts, interviews, questionnaires, focus groups, case studies and documents to describe and understand a subject's thoughts, opinions and experiences	SRQR COREQ
Animal pre-clinical studies	Involves the testing of novel therapeutic treatments and strategies on animals prior to human testing. This process allows researchers to gauge the potential efficacy and address any safety concerns associated with new interventions	ARRIVE
Quality improvement studies	Involves the collection of data for the purpose of improving the quality, safety and efficacy of processes, services and outcomes in a healthcare setting for both healthcare workers and patients	SQUIRE
Economic evaluations	Involves the assessment of healthcare interventions in terms of cost and outcomes. This informs how resources are allocated within the health sector. There are six commonly used forms of economic evaluation analyses: cost-minimisation, cost-effectiveness, cost-efficiency, cost-consequences and cost–benefit	CHEERS

Source: Adapted from https://www.equator-network.org/.

Figure 12.5 presents a framework published by Evans,[31] which distinguishes the evidence produced by various designs in four categories: poor, fair, good and excellent. Furthermore, each design is also evaluated on its ability to assess three parameters:

- effectiveness (Does this intervention work as intended?)

- appropriateness (Is this intervention appropriate for the intended recipient?); and
- feasibility (Can this intervention be implemented given any environmental constraints?).

In general, systematic reviews and meta-analyses of available information on a topic will offer the highest quality of evidence, particularly if research in that topic

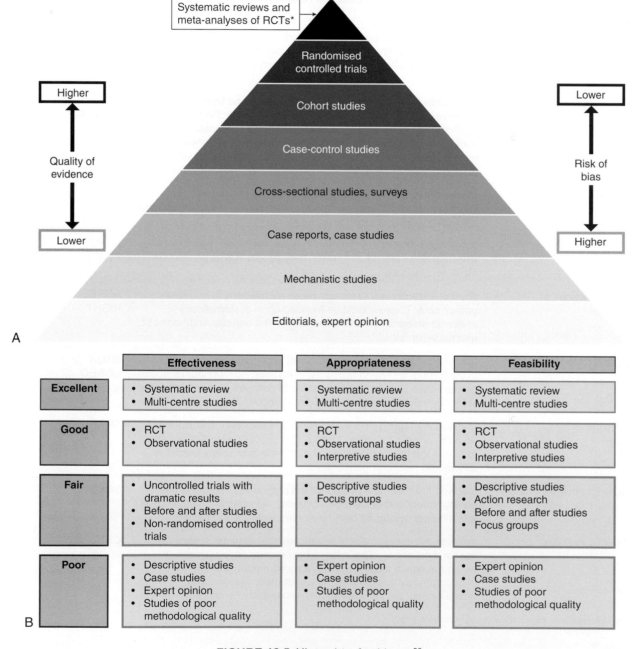

FIGURE 12.5 Hierarchy of evidence[30]

Source: Evans, D. (2003). Hierarchy of evidence: a framework for ranking evidence evaluating healthcare interventions. Journal of clinical nursing, 12(1), 77-84.

includes many randomised controlled trials—the highest ranked design in terms of singular studies. Experimental designs, such as non-randomised experimental studies, before-and-after studies and quasi-experimental studies are typically placed immediately under RCTs. This is followed by observational designs like cohort, case control and cross-sectional studies, which populate the middle of the hierarchy. Finally, case reports and case series provide the poorest quality of evidence. Other publications, such as expert opinion and personal communications, are also found here.

12.4 Research ethics

In Australia, the NHMRC's National Statement on Ethical Conduct in Human Research[33] is the active guideline for ethical human and animal research conduct, enforced under the *National Health and Medical Research Council Act 1992*.[34] All research activities must be guided by ethical principles. This is particularly pertinent in the field of medicine and health science, as it is the broad objective of these services to offer aid and treatment to the ill, injured and vulnerable.

Researchers interested in conducting human research must be approved by a Human Research Ethics Committee (HREC) prior to performing any research activities using human participants. These committees review research proposals to ensure they satisfy ethical

standards and guidelines. Approximately 200 HRECs have been established in Australia, and any major institution where research is conducted, such as universities and health districts, will have its own HREC and formal processes for application submission. The following sections highlight some of the ethical issues that researchers must consider in the context of health and IPC research, and which extend upon the broader ethical values highlighted in Table 12.8. Further information and more specific guidelines can be found by visiting the NHMRC website.

12.4.1 Informed consent

Respect for a person's autonomy is a central component of human research ethics. This involves recognising that each human being has value and the capacity to hold their own views and values, determine their own actions and make their own decisions. Hence, participation in a study must be under the individual's own volition and not under any form of coercion or deception. The NHMRC specifies two requirements for participation:

1. that consent must be a voluntary choice; and
2. it must be based on sufficient information and understanding of what the study will involve and any potential implications that result from participating in it.

TABLE 12.8 Basic values of ethical research conduct

Research merit and integrity	Research must have merit and be conducted with integrity. A study which has merit is one that is justifiable by its benefit in contributing to knowledge and potentially improving the lives and wellbeing in the relevant communities. It should be rigorously informed by existing knowledge or expertise and, where possible, its methods, facilities and human and non-human resources should be appropriate for optimal execution. Researchers are to carry out studies with integrity, understand that research is a search for knowledge and understanding, follow recognised principles of research conduct and be honest, and the work is to be communicated and readily scrutinised by the public, regardless of outcome
Justice	There are many inequalities across society and within the healthcare system. Regardless, researchers must ensure that all steps in the research process are reasonable, non-exploitative and fair to participants. For example, recruitment must be transparent in its selection, exclusion and inclusion processes, and no group should solely receive the benefits of participation or endure an unfair burden. Furthermore, access to the overall benefits of the research must be distributed fairly
Beneficence	Research must be conducted such that harm or discomfort to the participant is minimised and ensure that the benefit of the research will justify the risks of harm or discomfort to the participants. Benefits may be directly applicable to the participants, to the wider community or to both
Respect	Researchers must recognise that all humans have value and have 'regard for their welfare, beliefs, perceptions, customs and cultural heritage'. This also extends to respect for participants' privacy and confidentiality, and where relevant, sensitivity to their respective communities. Understanding autonomy and capacity for decision making is a fundamental aspect of informed consent

Source: Commonwealth of Australia. National Statement on Ethical Conduct in Human Research 2007 (Updated 2018); The National Health and Medical Research Council, the Australian Research Council and Universities Australia: Canberra, Australia, 2018.

Under no circumstance must researchers or health practitioners use their position of authority to manipulate, coerce or pressure a person into research participation. Where a person may lack the capacity to consent, such as infants and those with mental or intellectual disability, then an appropriate statutory body with lawful authority for the individual must be informed and decide based on the individual's best interests.

Sufficient information is specifically defined as an 'adequate understanding of the purpose, methods, demands, risks and potential benefits of the research'.[34] Consent is also an ongoing process and researchers must explicitly inform participants of their right to withdraw their consent and stop their participation in the study at any time. Renegotiating consent is also critical if the terms or expectations of a study changes from the point in time when consent was initially given. A list of the information that should be communicated to participants to establish informed consent is presented in Table 12.9. Most research institutions have preexisting templates that researchers populate with the specifics of their study; these are often submitted with ethics applications for approval by the institution's HREC.

In some instances, 'limited disclosure'—where not all of the study's aims and methods are fully disclosed to participants—may be necessary. This includes studies where some degree of concealment or deception is required to observe specific responses or behaviours. The same standards and processes apply to these studies, where researchers must obtain ethical approval via an HREC. However, additional justification must be provided for the purpose of limited disclosure, to state that such activities will not adversely affect participants in any way, and nor would they be likely to have changed their decision to participate in the study had they been fully aware.

12.4.2 Risk and benefit

A risk is a potential for harm, discomfort or inconvenience. Examples of harms, as specified by the NHMRC, include:

- physical harm (e.g. injury, illness, pain)
- psychological harm (e.g. distress, anger, embarrassment)
- devaluation of personal worth
- social harm (e.g. damage to social networks or relationships)
- economic harm (e.g. monetary costs); and
- legal harm (e.g. discovery and prosecution of criminal conduct).[34]

Discomfort is used to describe risks that are less serious than harms, such as minor side effects of medication or physical discomfort associated with a routine procedure. Inconveniences describe trivial risks, such as the time taken to participate in the research study. Research is 'low risk' where the only foreseeable risk is one of discomfort and 'negligible risk' where any foreseeable risk is no more than inconvenience. Risks to associated non-participants, such as family members, should also be identified and considered. Risk assessments involve the identification of potential risks, determining their

TABLE 12.9 Information to be communicated to participants to ensure informed consent

Components of informed consent	
Purpose of the study	Study methods
Study demands	Potential risks and benefits to the individual
Alternatives to participation	How the research will be monitored
Provision of services to participants adversely affected by the research	Contact details of researchers and person to receive complaints
How privacy and confidentiality will be protected	Participant's right to withdraw and associated implications (if any)
Sources and amount of funding	Financial or other relevant declarations of interests of researchers, sponsors, institutions, etc
Reimbursements	Likelihood and form of dissemination of research results (e.g. publications)
Expected benefits to the wider community	Any other research-specific information

Source: Commonwealth of Australia. National Statement on Ethical Conduct in Human Research 2007 (Updated 2018); The National Health and Medical Research Council, the Australian Research Council and Universities Australia: Canberra, Australia, 2018.

likelihood and severity, assessing the extent to which they can be minimised or managed, and evaluating whether the potential benefits of the research justify the risks. Risk assessment as it relates to IPC is described in detail in Chapter 7, though the broad process is applicable within research as well.

Researchers must consider whether the potential benefits of the planned study or intervention outweigh the risks involved. The nature of these benefits varies depending on the research but typically results in advances in knowledge and understanding, improvements for the welfare and quality of life for the represented population or participating members, and gains in skill and expertise for researchers.[34] Furthermore, benefits may not affect the study's participants directly, but rather the population the participants represent. Ultimately, it is up to ethical review bodies to approve studies based on this risk–reward evaluation. If approved, researchers are responsible for ensuring that potential participants understand the potential risks and rewards so that they are sufficiently informed in their decision to participate or not.

12.4.3 Privacy, confidentiality and data protection

All research generates data, which can take on many shapes and forms. This includes, but is not limited to, interview and focus group transcripts, digital video and audio recordings, responses to surveys and questionnaires, historical records, physical specimens, laboratory results and observations. Research is founded upon data collection, analysis and dissemination to inform our understanding of a specific research topic or question. A key risk that is applicable across all research arises from the management of data and the rights to privacy and confidentiality of individuals who created the data.

Privacy concerns arise when the proposed access to or use of the data does not match the expectations of the individuals from whom the data was obtained or to whom it related. For example, a participant may concede some privacy when granting researchers access to medical records for a specific research purpose. However, privacy is breached if commercial parties receive this information to use for purposes that were unauthorised and not consented to by the owner of the data. Confidentiality refers to the handling of data, particularly regarding data accessibility and identifiability. Precautions must be undertaken to ensure that data storage is secure, both physical and digital, depending on the format. Common strategies include physical containment within a facility that is only accessible by lock and key available to authorised persons, or on password-protected hard

drives or online data repositories. Ethical applications generally require a plan for data destruction, which usually occurs within a set period after results from the data are published. De-identification is also critical, involving the removal of personal identifiers so that data cannot be reasonably traced back to the person who produced it. This extends to when the data is published, shared or communicated in any form.

12.5 Outbreak investigation

12.5.1 Case reports and case series

Research relating to specific occurrences of outbreaks is usually reported in the form of case reports or case series. Case reports are a type of descriptive design that describes the characteristics and experiences of one individual. Case series are based on very small groups of patients or participants that shared similar medical histories, health events and disease presentation. These are typically conducted when an individual exhibits unique or unusual medical conditions, such as when an outbreak of a disease with potentially unknown aetiology occurs. These studies usually allow for a better understanding of:

• new hypotheses related to disease aetiology

• the situation, procedures and contexts that facilitate the occurrence of such outbreaks

• the characteristics of vulnerable patients

• the adverse effects of the disease under these exposures; and

• the effectiveness of any enacted interventions.

Case reports form a large proportion of literature in health sciences and, despite the considerable localised scope, can be used to identify or inform broader issues. Chapter 11 provides a detailed summary of an outbreak report for *Burkholderia cenocepacia*, which occurred across multiple Australian hospitals in 2017.

12.5.2 The ORION reporting guideline

The ORION (Outbreak Reports and Intervention studies Of Nosocomial Infection) statement is the current prevailing guideline for reporting outbreaks.[35] ORION was developed to 'raise the standards of research and publication in hospital epidemiology, to facilitate synthesis of evidence and promote transparency of reporting, to enable readers to relate studies to their own experience and assess the degree to which results can be generalized to other settings'.[35] It consists of a 22-item checklist, of which a simplified version relating specifically to outbreaks is presented in Table 12.10.

TABLE 12.10 ORION checklist. Reporting guideline for outbreak reports and intervention studies of nosocomial infections[35]

Section	Description
TITLE	
Title and abstract	Identifies paper as an outbreak report and provides a short description of main outcomes
Introduction	
Background	Provides scientific and clinical background, rationale and description of organism as epidemic, endemic or epidemic becoming endemic
Type of paper	If outbreak report, specifies the number of outbreaks
Dates	Start and finish dates of report
Objectives	Objectives for outbreak report
METHODS	
Design	Describe study design
Participants	Report number of patients and summarise relevant demographic and medical information, including length of stay and case definition
Setting	Description of the unit, ward or hospital, including the number of beds, the availability of an infection control team, etc
Interventions	Details of intervention
Culturing and typing	Details of culture media, use of selective antibiotics and local and/or reference typing. Where relevant, details of environmental sampling
Infection-related outcomes	Chart of duration of patient stay and date of organism detection
Economic outcomes	Description of resources used and cost breakdown (if relevant)
Potential threats to internal validity	Potential confounding variables are considered, recorded or adjusted for
Sample size	Details of power calculations (if relevant)
Statistical methods	Details of statistical analysis (if relevant)
RESULTS	
Recruitment	Details of recruitment process (if relevant)
Outcomes and estimation	Summary of main outcomes and appropriate graphical representation
Ancillary analyses	Subgroup analysis (where appropriate)
Adverse events	Describes and summarises any observed harms and adverse effects
DISCUSSION	
Interpretation	Consider clinical significance of observations and hypotheses generated to explain them
Generalisability	External validity of findings and to what extent they may be generalised to a broader population or setting
Overall evidence	General interpretation of results in context of current evidence

Source: Stone, S. P., Cooper, B. S., Kibbler, C. C., Cookson, B. D., Roberts, J. A., Medley, G. F., ... & Davey, P. G. (2007). The ORION statement: guidelines for transparent reporting of outbreak reports and intervention studies of nosocomial infection. Journal of Antimicrobial Chemotherapy, 59(5), 833-840.

Conclusion

Our modern understanding of infectious diseases and effective infection prevention and control practices has come about after centuries of rigorous research, discovery and advancement in science and medical technology. Research in this area is inherently multidisciplinary, examining everything from the microorganisms that cause diseases to informing the public health response to pandemic-level disease events on a global scale.

As such, this research also often takes on many forms, ranging from case studies of rare disease outbreaks to highly controlled randomised trials to large observational studies. Ensuring the continued suppression of infectious diseases and HAIs is an ongoing priority, as is informing new strategies for targeting increasing antimicrobial resistance and the emergence of novel, highly virulent diseases.

Useful websites/resources

- The Enhancing the QUAlity and Transparency Of health Research (Equator) Network. https://www.equator-network.org/
- Research Policy. National Health and Medical Research Council. https://www.nhmrc.gov.au/research-policy/ethics-and-integrity
- Infection Prevention and Control. World Health Organization. https://www.who.int/teams/integrated-health-services/infection-prevention-control

References

1. Mitchell BG, Fasugba O, Russo PL. Where is the strength of evidence? A review of infection prevention and control guidelines. J Hosp Infect. 2020;105(2):242-251.
2. Allegranzi B, Kilpatrick C, Storr J, Kelley E, Park BJ, Donaldson L. Global infection prevention and control priorities 2018–22: a call for action. Lancet Glob Health. 2017;5(12):e1178-e1180.
3. Lacotte Y, Ardal C, Ploy M-C, European Joint Action on Antimicrobial Resistance and Healthcare-assocaited Infections (EU-JAMRAI). Infection prevention and control research priorities: what do we need to combat healthcare-associated infections and antimicrobial resistance? Results of a narrative literature review and survey analysis. Antimicrob Resist Infect Control [Internet]. 2020; 24;9(1):142.
4. Mitchell BG, Ferguson JK, Anderson M, Sear J, Barnett A. Length of stay and mortality associated with healthcare-associated urinary tract infections: a multi-state model. J Hosp Infect. 2016;93(1):92-99.
5. Van Mourik MS, van Duijn PJ, Moons KG, Bonten MJ, Lee GM. Accuracy of administrative data for surveillance of healthcare-associated infections: a systematic review. BMJ Open. 2015;5(8):e008424.
6. Redondo-González O, Tenías JM, Arias Á, Lucendo AJ. Validity and reliability of administrative coded data for the identification of hospital-acquired infections: an updated systematic review with meta-analysis and meta-regression analysis. Health Serv Res. 2018;53(3):1919-1956.
7. Australian Commission on Safety and Quality in Health Care (ACSQHC). Healthcare associated infections (detailed fact sheet). 2018.
8. Mitchell BG, Shaban RZ, MacBeth D, Wood C-J, Russo PL. The burden of healthcare-associated infection in Australian hospitals: a systematic review of the literature. Infect Dis Health. 2017;22(3):117-128.
9. Russo PL, Cheng AC, Mitchell BG, Hall L. Healthcare-associated infections in Australia: tackling the 'known unknowns'. Aust Health Rev. 2018;42(2):178-180.
10. Dettenkofer M, Humphreys H, Saenz H, Carlet J, Hanberger H, Ruef C, et al. Key priorities in the prevention and control of healthcare-associated infection: a survey of European and other international infection prevention experts. Infection. 2016;44(6):719-724.
11. Mitchell BG, Hall L, MacBeth D, Gardner A, Halton K. Hospital infection control units: staffing, costs, and priorities. Am J Infect Control. 2015;43(6):612-616.
12. Deane HC, Wilson CL, Babl FE, Dalziel SR, Cheek JA, Craig SS, et al. PREDICT prioritisation study: establishing the research priorities of paediatric emergency medicine physicians in Australia and New Zealand. Emerg Med J. 2018;35(1):39-45.
13. Considine J, Curtis K, Shaban RZ, Fry M. Consensus-based clinical research priorities for emergency nursing in Australia. Australas Emerg Care. 2018;21(2):43-50.
14. Considine J, Shaban RZ, Fry M, Curtis K. Evidence based emergency nursing: designing a research question and searching the literature. Int Emerg Nurs. 2017;32:78-82.
15. Sackett DL, ed. Evidence-based medicine. Semin Perinatol. 21(1):3-5.
16. Eriksen MB, Frandsen TF. The impact of patient, intervention, comparison, outcome (PICO) as a search strategy tool on literature search quality: a systematic review. JMLA. 2018; 106(4):420.
17. Methley AM, Campbell S, Chew-Graham C, McNally R, Cheraghi-Sohi S. PICO, PICOS and SPIDER: a comparison study of specificity and sensitivity in three search tools for qualitative systematic reviews. BMC Health Services Research. 2014;14(1):1-10.
18. Page MJ, McKenzie JE, Bossuyt PM, Boutron I, Hoffmann TC, Mulrow CD, et al. The PRISMA 2020 statement: an updated guideline for reporting systematic reviews. BMJ. 2021;372:n71
19. Australian Institute of Health and Welfare. Deaths in Australia. Canberra: AIHW, 2021.
20. Australian Institute of Health and Welfare. Rural & remote health. Canberra: AIHW, 2019.

21. Bright A, Denholm J, Coulter C, Waring J, Stapledon R. Tuberculosis notifications in Australia, 2015-2018. In: Department of Health, ed. Canberra: Commun Dis Intell. (2018); 2020;44.

22. The National Tuberculosis Advisory Committee. The strategic plan for control of tuberculosis in Australia, 2016–2020: towards disease elimination. Commun Dis Intell. 2018;43.

23. Von Elm E, Altman DG, Egger M, Pocock SJ, Gøtzsche PC, Vandenbroucke JP. The Strengthening the Reporting of Observational Studies in Epidemiology (STROBE) statement: guidelines for reporting observational studies. Bull World Health Org. 2007;85:867-872.

24. Dew K. A health researcher's guide to qualitative methodologies. Aust N Z J Public Health. 2007;31(5):433-437.

25. Lamont T, Barber N, de Pury J, Fulop N, Garfield-Birkbeck S, Lilford R, et al. New approaches to evaluating complex health and care systems. BMJ. 2016;352.

26. Busetto L, Wick W, Gumbinger C. How to use and assess qualitative research methods. Neurol Res Pract. 2020;2(1):1-10.

27. DiCicco-Bloom B, Crabtree BF. The qualitative research interview. Med Educ. 2006;40(4):314-321.

28. Kitzinger J. Qualitative research: introducing focus groups. BMJ. 1995;311(7000):299-302.

29. Braun V, Clarke V, Boulton E, Davey L, McEvoy C. The online survey as a qualitative research tool. Int J Soc Res. 2021; 24(6):641-654.

30. Bowen G. Document analysis as a qualitative research method. Qual Res J. 2009;9:27-40.

31. Evans D. Hierarchy of evidence: a framework for ranking evidence evaluating healthcare interventions. J Clin Nurs. 2003;12(1):77-84.

32. Yetley E, MacFarlane A, Greene-Finestone L, Garza C, Ard J, Atkinson S, et al. Options for basing Dietary Reference Intakes (DRIs) on chronic disease endpoints: report from a joint US-/Canadian-sponsored working group. Am J Clin Nutr. 2016;105.

33. The National Health and Medical Research Council, The Australian Research Council, Universities Australia. National statement on ethical conduct in human research 2007 (Updated 2018). Canberra: Australian Government, 2007.

34. National Health and Medical Research Council Act 1992.

35. Stone SP, Cooper BS, Kibbler CC, Cookson BD, Roberts JA, Medley GF, et al. The ORION statement: guidelines for transparent reporting of outbreak reports and intervention studies of nosocomial infection. JAC. 2007;59(5):833-840.

SECTION 2

PRACTICE

CHAPTER 13

Standard precautions

Dr PETA-ANNE ZIMMERMAN[i]

DEBRA LEE[ii]

Chapter highlights

- Standard precautions are the principles and practices to be used during each and every interaction with a patient or client
- The aim of standard precautions is to protect patients/clients, staff and visitors from infectious disease transmitted primarily from blood and other body substances
- Maintaining asepsis in the provision of care prevents pathogens, such as bacteria, viruses and other microorganisms, from entering wounds and other susceptible areas via invasive medical devices and causing infection

i School of Nursing and Midwifery, Griffith University, Gold Coast, QLD
ii Office of Industrial Relations Queensland, Redcliffe, QLD

Introduction

Everyone can potentially be the source of infectious pathogens and therefore all blood and body substances must be considered to be potentially infectious. Standard precautions are practices designed to break the chain of infection and achieve a basic level of infection prevention and control (IPC). These practices aim to minimise the risk of transmission of disease-causing pathogens, particularly those caused by blood-borne viruses such as HIV, hepatitis B (HBV) and hepatitis C (HCV).[1]

This chapter introduces the principles of standard precautions and asepsis, with guidance to show how to use these in practice. These precautions aim to reduce the risk of transmission of blood-borne and other pathogens from both recognised and unrecognised sources. The chapter explores the key components of standard precautions and the principles of non-surgical asepsis while providing real-life examples of barriers to implementation as well as recommended methods.

13.1 Standard precautions overview

13.1.1 What we do for everybody, every day

Standard precautions are the minimum set of practices used in healthcare settings to prevent the transmission of infection from one person to another by providing protection from exposure to blood and body fluids (Fig 13.1).

Standard precautions apply to everyone, regardless of their known or presumed infectious disease status. Standard precautions must be used when there is contact—or potential contact—with:

- blood (including dried blood)
- all other body substances/fluids (excluding sweat), even if there is no visible blood
- non-intact skin
- mucous membranes.

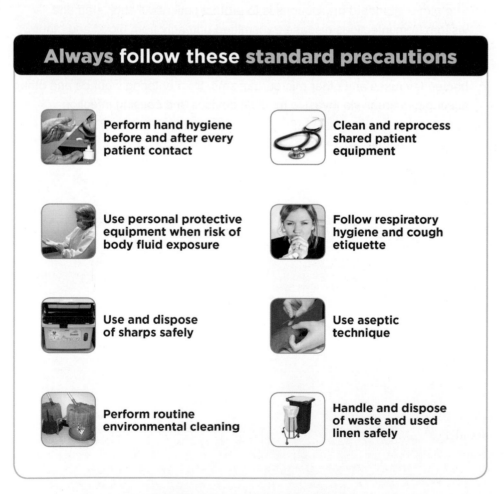

FIGURE 13.1 Standard precautions

Source: Reproduced with permission from Infection Prevention and Control Poster – Standard precautions poster, *developed by the Australian Commission on Safety and Quality in Health Care (ACSQHC). ACSQHC: Sydney 2022.*[2]

1. establishing the context
2. avoiding risks
3. identifying risks
4. analysing risks
5. evaluating risks; and
6. treating risks.[4]

To put this into practice consider Case study 1: Risk management.

CASE STUDY 1

Risk management

Situation: A patient has accidentally removed their peripheral intravenous cannula and a large amount of blood has soaked into the bedclothes and onto the floor. One of your colleagues attends to the patient and you offer to clean up the spill. Think about the risk management process above. How can you apply it in this situation?

Response: In this situation the process includes the following:

1. The context is a patient's room
2. In this scenario there is a body substance spill that must be cleaned up—it cannot be readily avoided
3. The identified risk is exposure to the blood as a potential source of infection to yourself and others
4. The risk has been identified as possible transmission of a blood-borne virus if it is not contained and handled correctly
5. This is evaluated to be a high risk and must be addressed immediately
6. The spill must be contained. Staff handling the spill must wear PPE that prevents exposure to the blood while containing and cleaning the spill. Where possible a spill kit should be used. The bulk of the spill must be soaked up with disposable absorbent materials and disposed of in the correct waste receptacle (check with local jurisdiction requirements) and then cleaned as per local policy. All PPE must be discarded appropriately after use and hand hygiene performed.

It is the HCW's responsibility to adhere to the workplace health and safety (WH&S) requirements of an institution by following relevant guidelines, attending training and us-

---

- Hand hygiene
- Respiratory hygiene and cough etiquette
- Selection and use of personal protective equipment (PPE)
- Maintaining a safe environment
- Safe handling of sharps
- Reprocessing reusable medical devices/equipment
- Environmental cleaning
- Safe handling of waste
- Safe handling of linen
- Asepsis
- Healthcare worker and employer responsibilities

Standard precautions are the foundation of all IPC practice, and if done well, may reduce or eliminate the need for further levels of precautions. The elements of standard precautions that are discussed in this chapter are detailed in Box 13.1.

After reading this chapter you will be able to describe and implement the necessary standard precautions for your work context.

13.1.2 Using a risk management approach to standard precautions

The selection and use of standard precautions to prevent the transmission of pathogens in the healthcare setting requires an assessment of the risk of exposure to blood and other body substances that may occur during interactions.[1] Each healthcare worker (HCW) must think ahead and prepare, to the best of their ability, for such exposures. By being prepared, unnecessary exposure can be avoided and transmission prevented. Healthcare facilities have a responsibility to provide facilities and consumable items such as hand hygiene stations, PPE, sharps containers and waste receptacles at point of use. Such availability helps HCWs to comply with standard precautions and to protect not only themselves but also their patients/clients and all visitors.[3] This risk assessment also includes identifying and containing potential sources of infection within the facility, such as providing masks to patients with respiratory symptoms and separating them from others in waiting rooms. In identifying what precautions are required, a risk management process can be applied through:

ing the equipment provided to protect themselves against exposure to pathogens and potentially infectious materials. For successful IPC and, in particular, the implementation of standard precautions, there must be cooperation between the facility management and the entire healthcare workforce. For further information see Chapter 7.

13.2 Hand hygiene

Since the time of Semmelweis, outcomes have been far better for HCWs and their patients due to a greater compliance with appropriate hand hygiene. Hand hygiene refers to cleansing hands by the use of either water and hand cleaning product (liquid soap/wash) or disinfectant solutions not requiring water—these are most commonly alcohol-based hand rubs

(ABHR).[5] It is best to avoid the use of bar soaps as these may harbour harmful organisms and transfer them from one user to another. The World Health Organization (WHO) advocates adherence to the 'Your 5 Moments for Hand Hygiene' program in Figure 13.2.

Good hand hygiene practices and compliance prevent the transmission of potentially pathogenic (harm-causing) microorganisms from: patient to patient, HCW to patient, patient to HCW, patient to themselves (i.e. into an invasive device), and from patient or HCW to the healthcare environment and equipment. This also protects any visitors that come into contact with the healthcare environment. Tangible reductions in healthcare-associated infections (HAIs) have been demonstrated where there are improvements in hand

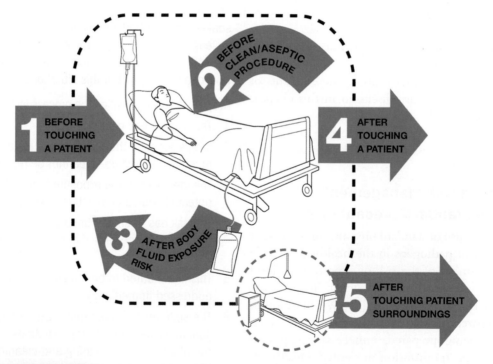

1	BEFORE TOUCHING A PATIENT	WHEN?	Clean your hands before touching a patient when approaching him/her.
		WHY?	To protect the patient against harmful germs carried on your hands.
2	BEFORE CLEAN/ ASEPTIC PROCEDURE	WHEN?	Clean your hands immediately before performing a clean/aseptic procedure.
		WHY?	To protect the patient against harmful germs, including the patient's own, from entering his/her body.
3	AFTER BODY FLUID EXPOSURE RISK	WHEN?	Clean your hands immediately after an exposure risk to body fluids (and after glove removal).
		WHY?	To protect yourself and the health-care environment from harmful patient germs.
4	AFTER TOUCHING A PATIENT	WHEN?	Clean your hands after touching a patient and her/his immediate surroundings, when leaving the patient's side.
		WHY?	To protect yourself and the health-care environment from harmful patient germs.
5	AFTER TOUCHING PATIENT SURROUNDINGS	WHEN?	Clean your hands after touching any object or furniture in the patient's immediate surroundings, when leaving – even if the patient has not been touched.
		WHY?	To protect yourself and the health-care environment from harmful patient germs.

FIGURE 13.2 Your 5 Moments for Hand Hygiene[6]

Source: World Health Organization. Your 5 Moments for Hand Hygiene. Geneva: WHO, 2009.

hygiene compliance rates.[7] Australia has led the way in demonstrating how a nationally coordinated multi-modal hand hygiene program can improve the rates of healthcare-associated bloodstream infections (BSI).[8,9]

Healthcare workers should be aware of how to perform hand hygiene correctly. Figure 13.3 illustrates how to handwash, and Figure 13.4 how to use an ABHR.

When performing hand hygiene, it is important to cover all hand and wrist surfaces with the cleansing product and to produce enough friction to dislodge any contamination. This is more effectively achieved when the hands and lower arms are free of clothing and jewellery, to allow contact of the hygiene products and prevent obstructions that harbour contamination. For this reason, many workplaces require staff to be 'bare below the elbows' while in the clinical care environment. If using ABHR, this must be allowed to dry naturally as it is the contact time with the skin that produces the disinfection action.

WASH HANDS WHEN VISIBLY SOILED! OTHERWISE, USE HANDRUB

Duration of the entire procedure: 40-60 seconds

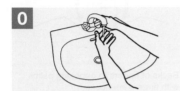

0 Wet hands with water;

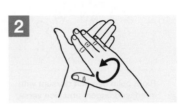

1 Apply enough soap to cover all hand surfaces;

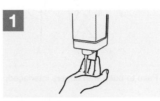

2 Rub hands palm to palm;

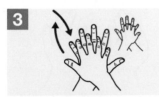

3 Right palm over left dorsum with interlaced fingers and vice versa;

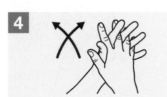

4 Palm to palm with fingers interlaced;

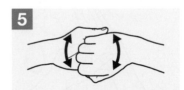

5 Backs of fingers to opposing palms with fingers interlocked;

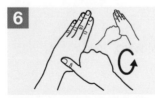

6 Rotational rubbing of left thumb clasped in right palm and vice versa;

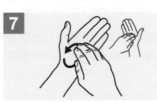

7 Rotational rubbing, backwards and forwards with clasped fingers of right hand in left palm and vice versa;

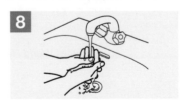

8 Rinse hands with water;

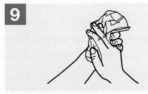

9 Dry hands thoroughly with a single use towel;

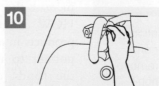

10 Use towel to turn off faucet;

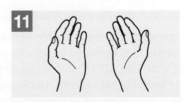

11 Your hands are now safe.

FIGURE 13.3 How to Handwash?[10]

Source: World Health Organization. How to Handwash? Geneva: WHO, 2009.

RUB HANDS FOR HAND HYGIENE! WASH HANDS WHEN VISIBLY SOILED

🕐 **Duration of the entire procedure: 20-30 seconds**

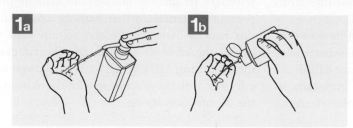

Apply a palmful of the product in a cupped hand, covering all surfaces;

Rub hands palm to palm;

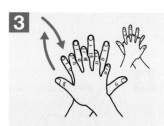

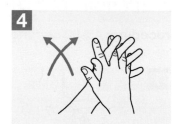

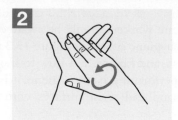

Right palm over left dorsum with interlaced fingers and vice versa;

Palm to palm with fingers interlaced;

Backs of fingers to opposing palms with fingers interlocked;

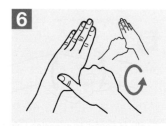

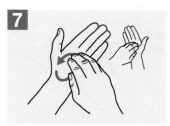

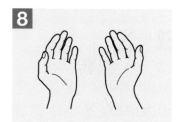

Rotational rubbing of left thumb clasped in right palm and vice versa;

Rotational rubbing, backwards and forwards with clasped fingers of right hand in left palm and vice versa;

Once dry, your hands are safe.

FIGURE 13.4 How to Handrub?[11]

Source: World Health Organization. How to Handrub? Geneva: WHO, 2009.

PRACTICE TIP 1

HAND HYGIENE

Where possible, if there is visible contamination on the hands, it is better to wash with water and cleanser than use ABHR. It is important to remove all debris from the hands and rubbing with non-water cleansers may not achieve that. Also, if there is potential for contamination with spore-forming organisms, such as *Clostridioides difficile*, it is important to wash hands because alcohol rubs are not effective against spores.[5]

It is essential that HCWs look after their hands and maintain their skin integrity as poor skin condition can increase the risk of infection transmission to both the HCW and their patients. Always use skin cleansing products in accordance with the instructions. It is important to use the correct amount of solution on the hands, enough to cover the hands adequately but not too much, as higher concentrations of solution may cause irritation. If washing, ensure the solution is effectively rinsed from the skin and gently pat the hands dry rather than rubbing harshly with a towel. Healthcare workers should also take the opportunity to moisturise their hands regularly, such as at the beginning and end of each shift, with a product that is compatible with the cleansers used.[1]

Gloves are not a replacement for appropriate hand hygiene. They should **not** be worn for routine care unless there is a risk of body fluid exposure and/or the patient is being cared for with additional transmission-based precautions (TBP) as described in Chapter 14. Certainly, they must be changed, and hand hygiene performed between patients and before and after procedures (Moment 2/3 in Fig 13.2). As with hands, if there is visible contamination on the gloves, it is time for hand hygiene: remove gloves, wash hands and don new gloves if required.

It is also important to purposefully include the patient and visitors in hand hygiene practices.[12] Provide patients with the opportunity to clean their hands before eating and after using the commode or bathroom. Likewise, if they are self-administering medications, such as insulin or eyedrops, or checking their own blood glucose levels, they should be encouraged to clean their hands before and after. Visual and conversational prompts can assist in visitors performing hand hygiene when they arrive and/or are assisting the patient with their activities of daily living (ADLs). Modelling safe practice by setting an example of good hand hygiene promotes trust and confidence for the patient and their visitors.

13.3 Respiratory hygiene and cough etiquette

Respiratory hygiene and cough etiquette are important practices, not only in healthcare facilities but as general practice in the community, by everyone. The principle behind these practices is to contain respiratory secretions and prevent exposure of others to these.[1] Covering the nose and mouth while coughing and sneezing prevents potentially infectious agents being dispersed into the air and/or falling to environmental surfaces that others could then touch. It is therefore recommended when coughing or sneezing to cover your nose with the inner aspect of your elbow or with a disposable tissue to contain secretions. If using a tissue, this must be disposed of immediately after use into a waste receptacle and hand hygiene performed. After any contact with respiratory secretions hand hygiene must be performed, and this includes coming into contact with frequently touched surfaces that may be contaminated with respiratory secretions (Fig 13.5).[1]

Healthcare workers must not attend work when experiencing symptoms of respiratory infection and should stay home until these are resolved. Equally, patients who attend health services with respiratory infection symptoms should be kept away from others when waiting to be seen and possibly provided with a disposable medical mask. During times of respiratory infection outbreaks, enhanced cleaning and increased regularity of cleaning of frequently touched surfaces should be put into place.[14]

13.4 Selection and use of personal protective equipment (PPE)

In the context of standard precautions, the appropriate selection and use of PPE in the clinical setting is largely based on the risk of exposure to blood and other body substances, as discussed in Section 13.1.2 above. Personal protective equipment should only be worn in clinical areas while performing clinical care or procedures. The wearing of PPE outside of these situations should be avoided, particularly after the equipment is contaminated, such as after patient contact.[15]

Table 13.1 provides examples of the type of PPE used with examples of clinical care provided. Remember to consider also any allergies, such as to latex, that may impact the selection of the PPE you use. If you have such an allergy, be sure to inform your manager/supervisor so that a safe alternative can be made available.[1] All PPE used in Australia must meet the relevant Therapeutic Goods Administration (TGA) criteria for listing on the Australian Register of Therapeutic Goods and must also meet the relevant Australian Standards.[1]

> **PRACTICE TIP 2**
> ## MASKS
>
> A mask in the context of standard precautions generally refers to a surgical or medical mask that is designed primarily to prevent transmission of pathogens via large droplets from the person wearing the mask. To meet the requirements of standard precautions—that is, preventing exposure of blood and other body substances to the wearer—these must be fluid resistant. These masks differ from particulate or filtering face piece respirator masks, which are covered in Chapter 14, in that they do not provide the high level of filtration required (at least 95% of airborne particles) for use in aerosol-generating procedures or in the care of patients suspected or confirmed to be infected with an airborne pathogen.[16]

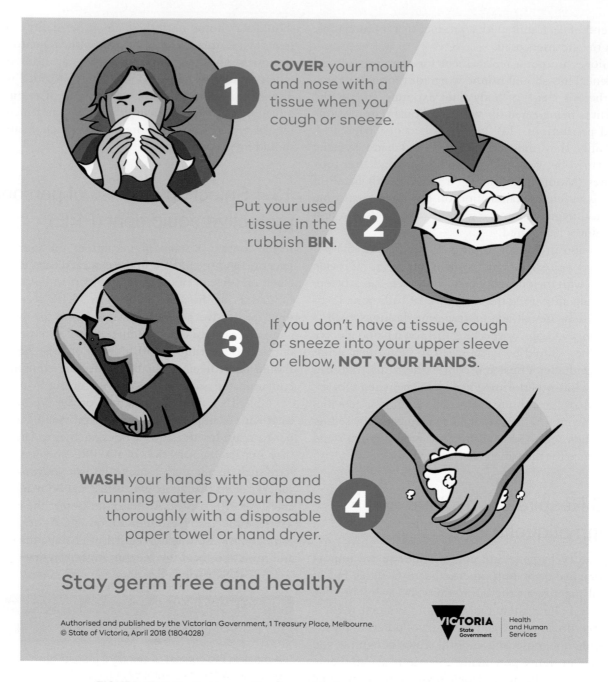

FIGURE 13.5 Protect yourself and your family: cover your cough and sneeze

Source: Victorian Government. Available from: https://www2.health.vic.gov.au/about/publications/policiesandguidelines/cover-your-cough-sneeze-poster

It is important to remember that you should always perform hand hygiene before and after removal of PPE. Wearing gloves, for example, does not mean that you do not need to perform hand hygiene. A number of reports in the literature indicate that clinicians often do not perform hand hygiene after the removal of gloves.[15,17-19]

Before putting on PPE always explain to the patient what you are doing and why. It is important that they understand that the use of PPE, like hand hygiene, is a normal part of the provision of care. Always put on your PPE before entering the patient care area and remove it before leaving to prevent contaminating the environment.

TABLE 13.1 Types of PPE and their purpose in the context of standard precautions

Type of PPE	Area protected	Examples
Gloves (non-sterile, medical, examination)	Hands/skin	Assisting with toileting Venepuncture Vaginal examination Cleaning a body Fluid spill
Eye protection/ face shield	Eyes and face (mucous membranes/ non-intact skin)	Emptying urinary drainage bag Dental procedures Suctioning
Mask (surgical, medical)	Mouth and nose (mucous membranes)	Aspiration Intubation Dental procedures
Fluid-resistant apron/gown	Clothing	Vomiting Possibility of sprays, spills or exposure to blood and body substances

Note: The above examples are in the context of standard precautions.

The general sequence for *putting on* PPE (Fig 13.6) is as follows:

1. perform hand hygiene
2. gown or apron
3. surgical mask (if required)
4. protective eyewear/face shield
5. gloves (covering cuff of gown if wearing one).

When removing PPE, it is important to do so in such a way that you do not contaminate yourself in the process. Remember not to touch the outside of any of your PPE when removing it, as these are contaminated surfaces.

The sequence for *removing* PPE, illustrated in Figure 13.7, is as follows:

1. gloves
2. perform hand hygiene
3. gown
4. protective eyewear/face shield
5. mask
6. perform hand hygiene.

The sequence of putting on and removing PPE may not be the same across jurisdictions or may change during an outbreak. The main points to remember are to perform hand hygiene before and after PPE removal, make sure your PPE is used as it was intended to be used, and be aware of any breaches you or your colleagues may make when using the PPE.

If at any time you feel you may have contaminated your hands while removing your PPE, perform hand hygiene.

PRACTICE TIP 3
PROTECTIVE EYEWEAR

If you wear spectacles for your vision, they do not replace the need for protective eyewear or a face shield. Spectacles are not protective equipment. If you require protective eyewear speak to your manager/supervisor about types that will fit over your spectacles safely and still provide protection.

13.4.1 Incorrect use of PPE

During standard precautions there is no need to wear gloves for care that does not involve exposure to blood or body fluids. If assisting a patient in routine activities of daily living, taking observations, or providing non-invasive care, PPE is not required. There is no need to wear gloves to change bedlinen that isn't soiled. Overuse of PPE can be as dangerous as not wearing it at all, so remember to assess the risk of exposure to blood and other body substances before you engage in a procedure or task.[1,20] Prolonged use of gloves can exacerbate skin irritation—so advocating correct glove use will reduce the risk of developing skin problems.[21]

13.5 Maintaining a safe environment

The challenges of healthcare delivery are many, and there are always competing demands for attention and time pressures. Often there are numerous clinicians and support staff in a space that is not necessarily adequate for the level of activity. Maintaining a hazard-free workplace within the clinical care environment is the responsibility of all workers. To achieve this, all must play their part in a coordinated and cooperative ap-

SEQUENCE FOR PUTTING ON PPE	
Put on PPE before patient contact and generally before entering the patient room	
1. PERFORM HAND HYGIENE • Wash hands or use an alcohol-based hand rub.	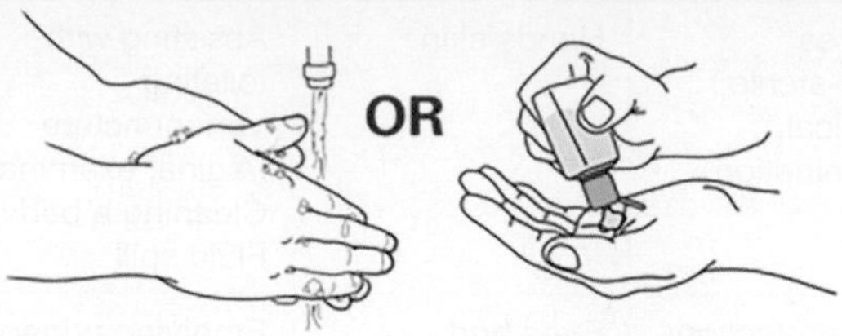
2. PUT ON GOWN • Fully cover torso from neck to knees, arms to end of wrists and wrap around the back. • Fasten at the back of neck and waist.	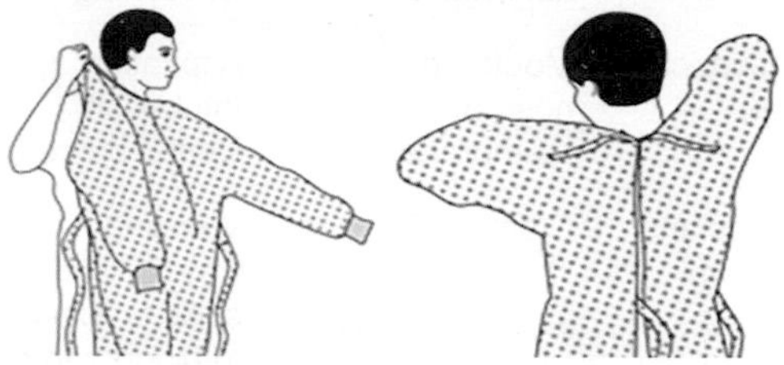
3. PUT ON MASK • Secure ties or elastic bands at middle of head and neck.	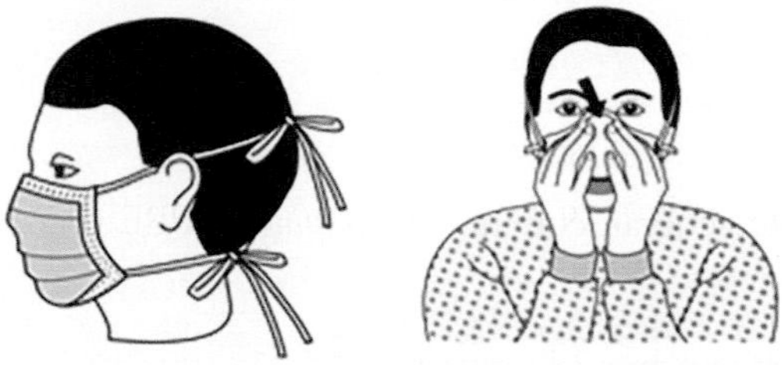
4. PUT ON PROTECTIVE EYEWEAR OR FACE SHIELD • Place over face and eyes and adjust to fit.	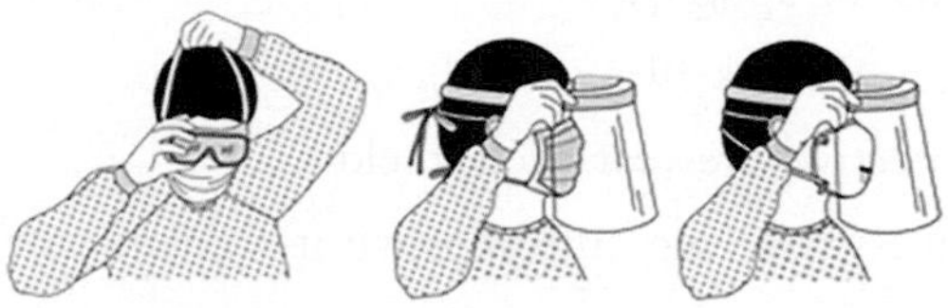
5. PUT ON GLOVES • Extend to cover wrist of isolation gown.	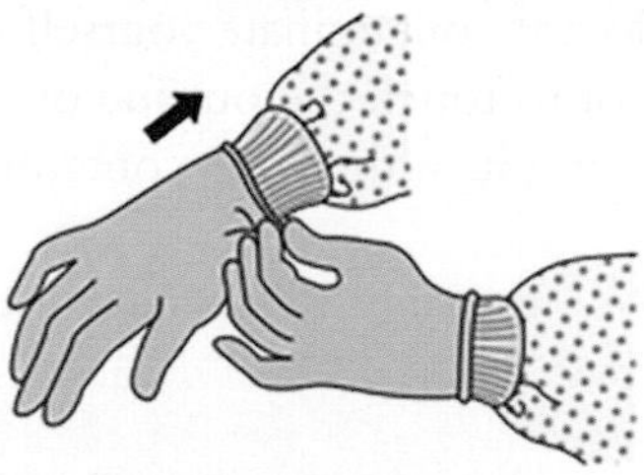

FIGURE 13.6 Sequence for putting on PPE

Source: NHMRC: Australian-guidelines-prevention-and-control-infection-healthcare-2019

SEQUENCE FOR REMOVING PPE

Begin PPE removal at the doorway or in the anteroom

1. REMOVE GLOVES

- Outside of gloves is contaminated!
- Grasp outside of glove with opposite gloved hand; peel off.
- Hold removed glove in gloved hand.
- Slide fingers of ungloved hand under remaining glove at wrist.
- Peel glove off over first glove.
- Discard gloves in waste container.

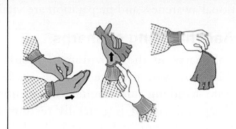

2. PERFORM HAND HYGIENE

- Wash hands or use an alcohol-based hand rub.

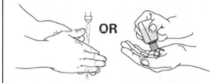

3. REMOVE GOWN

- Gown front and sleeves are contaminated!
- Unfasten ties.
- Pull away from neck and shoulders, touching inside of gown only.
- Turn gown inside out.
- Fold or roll into a bundle and discard.

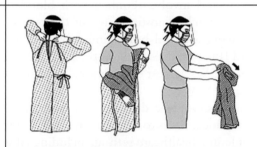

Alternatively gloves and gown can be removed as one step. Then perform hand hygiene.

4. REMOVE PROTECTIVE EYEWEAR OR FACE SHIELD

- Outside of eye protection or face shield is contaminated!
- To remove, handle by head band or ear pieces.
- Place in designated receptacle for reprocessing or in waste container.

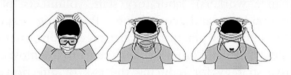

At a minimum, perform hand hygiene if the removed PPE is contaminated.

5. REMOVE MASK

- Front of mask is contaminated—DO NOT TOUCH!
- Grasp bottom, then top ties or elastics and remove.
- Discard in waste container.

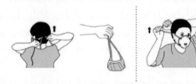

6. PERFORM HAND HYGIENE

- Wash hands or use an alcohol-based hand rub immediately after removing all PPE.

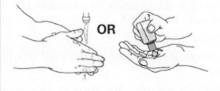

FIGURE 13.7 Sequence for removing PPE

Source: NHMRC: Australian-guidelines-prevention-and-control-infection-healthcare-2019

proach to ensuring the prompt and safe management of the environment. This includes waste, linen, sharps, routine and emergent cleaning, and the decontamination of reusable equipment and medical devices.

Situational awareness and preparation are vital.

13.5.1 Safe handling of sharps

The use of sharps in the provision of healthcare is unavoidable; however, practice can be made safer through safe handling and engineering controls to prevent sharps injuries. It is generally recommended that if using a sharp item, such as a scalpel, solid or hollow bore needle, trocars or the like, that you practise safely. This will help to prevent a sharp injury to yourself and/or others, thereby preventing occupational exposure to blood-borne pathogens via a penetrating injury.[22] Occupational exposure is defined as an incident that occurs during the course of a person's employment and involves contact with blood or body substances. Such exposure may put the person at risk of acquiring a blood-borne infection. Adherence to standard IPC practices remains the first line of protection for HCWs against occupational exposure to HIV, HBV and HCV.

Policies should be developed at national, jurisdictional and local levels to minimise the risk of injury for all people in a healthcare setting, including all staff and visitors such as clinical staff, non-clinical staff (e.g. administrators, housekeeping and laundry staff, maintenance workers), laboratory staff, volunteers, private contractors and consultants. Preventing exposure through safer practices, barrier precautions, safer needle devices and other methods remains the most effective strategy for reducing the risk of infection with HIV and other blood-borne pathogens in healthcare settings.[3,22]

Two significant prevention priorities are that all HCWs should be trained in, and be able to demonstrate competency in, standard precautions; and that staff should be provided with the necessary materials and protective equipment.[3]

The following measures aimed at reducing the incidence of occupational exposures related to the handling of sharps should be taken:[3]

- never recap needles
- where possible use safety-engineered needles and syringes
- do not disconnect needles from the syringe
- always transport (or pass to another person) sharp objects in a kidney dish or puncture-proof container

- sharps should be disposed of in puncture-proof containers (where possible at point of use).

Information on how to manage a sharps injury can be found in Chapter 26.

13.5.2 Reprocessing of reusable medical devices

Used instruments and equipment can be a reservoir for microorganisms and therefore spread infections to patients and staff. Procedures that prevent the spread of infection from reusable instruments and equipment are cleaning, disinfection and sterilisation.[22] Where reusable equipment, instruments and devices are used, the health service organisation must have:[1,3]

- processes for reprocessing that are consistent with relevant national and international standards, and in conjunction with manufacturers' guidelines
- a traceability process for critical and semi-critical equipment, instruments and devices that is capable of identifying the patient; the procedure; and the reusable equipment, instruments and devices that were used for the procedure.

In Australia, AS4187:2014 Reprocessing of Reusable Medical Devices in Health Service Organizations is the guiding Standard.[23] The Spaulding Classification system is used to identify the types of equipment used on patients and their risk of transmission of infection.[1]

Before disinfection and sterilisation can be achieved, all instruments must be cleaned and rinsed.[23] After cleaning, all instruments and other items used to touch tissue beneath the skin (such as during surgery or giving an injection) or to touch mucous membranes (such as during vaginal examination) should be sterilised or undergo high-level disinfection (HLD).

Sterilisation is the safest and most effective method for the final processing of instruments. When sterilisation of equipment is not available or not suitable, HLD is the only acceptable alternative.[23] Reprocessing of reusable devices, specifically disinfection and sterilisation, is explored in greater detail in Chapter 16, but the general principles of cleaning, which we are all responsible for, are described below. Table 13.2 provides a brief summary of the important aspects of reprocessing.

13.6 Cleaning

The aim of cleaning is to remove microbial, organic and inorganic soil. Ideally, cleaning is performed using an automated washer/disinfector.[1,23] The way in which

TABLE 13.2   Instruments and equipment by application and sterilisation method[1,23]

Category	Application	Type of processing	Example of items
Critical	Sterile tissues in the body	Sterilisation	Surgical instruments, diagnostic catheters, dental instruments, bronchoscopes, cystoscopes
Semi-critical	Non-sterile tissues in the body	Disinfection	Respiratory therapy equipment, dental impressions and other prosthetic appliances, gastroscopes, colonoscopes, endoscopes
Non-critical	Instruments that come in contact with intact skin	Cleaning	Bed pans, ECG leads, thermometers, stethoscopes, beds, bedside tables

Source: National Health and Medical Research Council (2019). Australian Guidelines for the Prevention and Control of Infection in Healthcare. Canberra: Australian Government; Standards Association of Australia. AS/NZS 4187. (2014). Reprocessing of reusable medical devices in health service organisations. Australia: SAI Global Professional Services.

this is done varies with the material composition of the equipment as well as its design.

Thorough cleaning of all instruments and equipment is an essential prerequisite in disinfection and sterilisation processes. Care must be taken that the cleaning process does not add to the bioburden. Cleaning methods shall be appropriate to the design of the instruments and equipment being cleaned and documented.[1,23]

It is imperative that cleaning protocols are devised for the cleaning of all instruments and equipment, particularly those made of various materials (polymers and metals). Cleaning should ensure the removal of adherent protein, soil and biofilm. After cleaning, the instruments should be free from any chemical residue.

The cleaning process is very important because:

- cleaning with neutral detergent and water removes protein, blood and other body fluids, oils and grease
- disinfection and sterilisation will not destroy microorganisms trapped in small particles of blood or protein. Thorough cleaning must be done to remove these particles
- when sterilisation facilities are not available, effective cleaning is the only way to protect patients from pathogenic spores (HLD may be an alternative).

13.6.1 Choosing a detergent for cleaning instruments and equipment

Using a hospital-grade neutral detergent is important for effective cleaning because water alone will not remove protein, oils and grease. Bleach powder without a detergent should not be used. Alcohol preparations likewise should not be used as they will coagulate blood

or body fluids and not remove them. Hand soap should not be used because it is made from fat (lard) and will leave a film or scum on instruments. Microorganisms can become trapped in the scum and will not be destroyed during sterilisation or disinfection.[1,22,23]

The cleaning solution must be appropriate for the type of equipment or instrument. Enzymes, usually proteases, are added to solutions to neutralise the PH solutions to aid in removing organic material such as blood and pus. Additionally, lipases (enzymes to act on breaking down fats) and amylase enzymes (to act on breaking down starch) are added to solutions.[1,22,23] Enzymes are not disinfectants and should be rinsed off instruments or equipment. Do not use abrasive cleaners because they can scratch the surfaces of equipment and instruments. Scratches are places where microorganisms can become trapped, and scratches increase metal corrosion (rusting).

13.6.2 Routine cleaning of used instruments and equipment

Routine cleaning of instruments and equipment removes many microorganisms and should be done at point of use where possible.

The items needed for the routine cleaning of instruments and equipment include:

- neutral detergent
- clean water
- brush or lint-free cloth
- gloves (utility gloves are best).

The procedure is as follows:

1. put on gloves and other PPE as per standard precautions
2. disassemble items if indicated by the manufacturer's cleaning instructions

3. using detergent and water and brush, completely remove all blood, tissue and dirt

4. thoroughly rinse with water because detergent can interfere with the disinfection or sterilisation process

5. air-dry equipment because moisture can interfere with the sterilisation or disinfection process

6. instruments and equipment are now ready for sterilisation or disinfection.

It is important to note that some products have a combined cleaning and disinfection action and should be used according to the manufacturers' instructions. These products reduce the number of steps needed to decontaminate equipment during reprocessing.[1]

13.6.3 Evidence of best practice

Reprocessing of reusable equipment, instruments and devices must be consistent with relevant current standards and meet current best practice. These aspects are discussed further in Chapter 16. Evidence of best practice in an IPC program and management plan is illustrated in Box 13.2.

13.7 Environmental cleaning

Basic principles in 'housekeeping' are fundamental to reducing risk of accidents and infection in the workplace. Avoiding clutter, returning items to their correct locations, prompt management of spills, and routine cleaning of equipment and the clinical workspace are essential in providing harm-free care and ensuring the safety of both patients and HCWs. Think of a teenager's room. Often clothing items have to be washed multiple times because if they are 'stored on the floor', it is impossible to tell which is clean and which isn't. So too in healthcare—the more equipment, stock and 'stuff' around the patient, the more that will require cleaning or disposal if there is a spill, contamination during care or at discharge. It saves time, effort, energy and resources to routinely keep the area tidy.

Microorganisms, if not removed, are capable of surviving on surfaces for extended periods of time.[24] It is therefore crucially important to regularly and completely remove them. A fundamental part of ensuring a safe working environment, and preventing cross-contamination between patients and staff, is cleaning the common touch surfaces and all equipment and furniture used for patient care, even if there is no *visible* contamination.

Simple detergents used with an adequate amount of friction are effective for cleaning in most circumstances, but if there is soiling or contamination with blood or body fluids, or if the patient was/is under additional TBP, a disinfectant process should also be used. It is important to note that some disinfectants do not include a detergent. The surfactant properties of detergent are necessary to remove the 'bioburden' and the disinfectant properties are required to inactivate the microbe with either biocidal or biostatic functions or both.

There is a growing body of evidence to suggest that residual contamination, either via uncleaned surfaces or microbiological biofilm residue,[25] contributes to an increased risk of healthcare-associated colonisation or infection with multiresistant organisms, particularly if the previous room inhabitant was positive.[26] Figure 13.8 summarises some of the benefits of environmental cleaning in the healthcare environment.

BOX 13.2 Evidence of best practice in an IPC program

---

1. Policy documents about reprocessing reusable equipment, instruments and devices

2. Policy documents about tracing critical and semi-critical reusable equipment, instruments and devices

3. Lists of critical and semi-critical equipment, instruments and devices used in the health service organisation

4. Committee and meeting records in which reprocessing and tracing of reusable equipment, instruments and devices are discussed

5. Audit results of the traceability system

6. Training documents about reprocessing and tracing of reusable equipment, instruments and devices

---

PRACTICE TIP 4

PATIENT-SHARED EQUIPMENT

Patient-shared equipment—such as shower chairs, observation machines, hoists and therapy equipment—is a potential source of cross-contamination. Therefore, appropriate and thorough cleaning should be performed between each patient. Think of it as another set of hands and clean this equipment just as frequently!

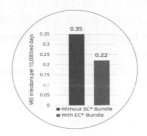

Reduction in the incidence of vancomycin-resistant enterococcus infections[1]

Thorough cleaning and disinfection inactivates organisms such as coronavirus, *Staphylococcus aureus* and multidrug-resistant organisms on environmental surfaces

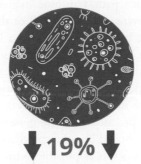

↓19%↓

Reduction in *Staphylococcus aureus* bacteraemia infections[1]

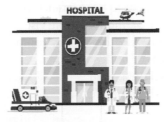

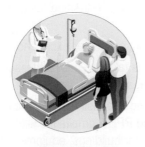

↓ ↓ ↓

Reduction in treatment costs and length of stay[2]

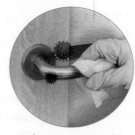

↑22%↑

Improvement in cleaning of high touch points in patient rooms and bathrooms when a comprehensive cleaning bundle approach was used[1]

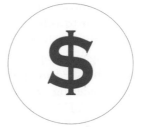

Cost-effective intervention ($2,500 per 10,000 occupied bed days)[2]

FIGURE 13.8 Benefits of environmental cleaning
Source: www.safetyandquality.gov.au

Keeping the general environment clean reduces the likelihood of HCW hand contamination and carriage from one patient or area to another. It also reduces the likelihood of patients and visitors encountering harmful pathogens as they negotiate their way around the space.

Specific information regarding the recommendations for cleaning schedules and products can be found in Chapter 15.

13.7.1 Safe handling of waste

Healthcare generates a significant amount of waste. Most of this is general or 'harmless' rubbish that will not subject others to the risk of exposure to blood and body fluids or other sources of infection. However, there is also waste that does carry that risk. As described in the 'sharps' section above, anything which could cause a penetration injury should be discarded carefully. Waste can also include non-sharp waste, such as used dressings, drainage bags, incontinence pads, feminine hygiene products, and disposable gowns and gloves. All of these items, plus many more, may be considered to be a high risk of infection carriage and are often referred to as 'clinical waste' (or contaminated, infectious or medical waste—jurisdiction dependent). Safe handling and disposal practices must be observed to manage their removal.

Where practicable, waste generated in the delivery of healthcare should be segregated according to its risk and discarded as soon as possible. Most healthcare providers have a system for waste segregation to reduce the cost of disposal, as waste that is considered a high risk due to contamination with blood or other body substances will require more cost and/or effort to process safely.

Methods of disposal of high-risk waste include incineration or burial. Regulations, technical or industrial availability and capacity will determine the frequency and method for local processing. It is of utmost importance that 'clinical' waste is not discarded with general waste, which could put handlers and the public at risk of exposure.[1,3]

13.7.2 Safe handling of linen

Linen used in healthcare, like waste, can be a potential source of infection to others and must be segregated and handled appropriately. As part of standard precautions, a risk management approach is used to determine how it is sorted, handled and processed. In Australia, the processing or laundering of healthcare linen must meet the requirements of Standard AS/NZS 4146:2000 Laundry Practice.[28] These requirements include that used linen must not be rinsed or sorted in patient care areas or washed in domestic-grade washing machines. Processed linen must be stored in a clean, dry location, free of vermin or risk of contamination, away from used linen.

All linen must be handled carefully so as not to disperse potential pathogens into the environment. Examples of poor handling include placing used linen on the floor, flicking sheets in the air, carrying used linen close to the body (which can contaminate your clothing) or carrying new linen close to the body. Wherever possible, linen bags mounted on trolleys should be brought to where used linen is being changed and PPE should be used when handling used linen when at risk of exposure to blood and other body substances. Linen that has not been contaminated with blood, other body substances, or used in the care of a patient who requires transmission-based precautions (see Chapter 14) can be placed together with general linen. Linen that is heavily contaminated with blood or other body substances should be placed in a leak-proof

laundry bag and labelled as such. PPE should be used if handling linen that is contaminated with blood or other body substances. Hand hygiene must always be performed after handling used linen.

As we have seen, the healthcare environment has a significant role to play in preventing HAI. See Box 13.3 for evidence of preventive strategies in relation to the healthcare environment.

13.7.3 The environment and managing risk

By using a risk management approach, you will quickly determine if you require contaminated linen bags, or sharps containers or rubbish bags prior to starting your activity, reducing the likelihood of having to race off mid-task and inadvertently putting yourself or someone else at risk. Consider Case study 2: Managing your environment safely, and reflect on how these real-life

---

BOX 13.3 Evidence of preventive strategies in relation to the healthcare environment

1. Documentation relating to training about the use of specialised PPE
2. Survey results from consumer experience surveys
3. Records of actions taken to deal with issues identified regarding cleaning and disinfection
4. Audits on: cleaning and disinfection practices; the use of specialised PPE; compliance with maintenance schedules for buildings, equipment, furnishings and fittings; and the handling, transport and storage of linen
5. Contracts with external linen providers that outline the requirements for managing clean and used linen to minimise infection risks; and with external cleaning providers that outline the requirements for cleaning and disinfection
6. Documented organisational policy on: maintaining a clean and hygienic environment; and evaluating and responding to the risks associated with linen, equipment, devices, products, buildings, furnishings and fittings
7. Schedules and records of completion for: cleaning and disinfection that meet the requirements outlined in jurisdiction requirements; and the maintenance of buildings, equipment, furnishings and fittings
8. Documentation of committee meetings relating to cleaning and disinfection

events could have been averted through managing the environment safely.

Managing your environment safely

Situation A: Imagine for a moment that you have entered a resident's room and you notice a pile of linen on the floor. Not seeing any of your colleagues around, you decide to pick it up so that no one trips ... only to find your hands and forearms covered in faeces.

Prevention:
- Bring a linen skip to the linen
- Wear PPE (gloves) when handling items potentially contaminated with blood or other body substances

Situation B: You are assisting in a resuscitation and the medical officer coordinating the management of the patient hands you a blood gas syringe with needle and instructs you to 'Get these results as soon as you can!'. You are racing towards the blood gas analyser and round a corner only to literally run into a colleague, stabbing them in the arm with the exposed syringe needle.

Prevention:
- Place the exposed sharp into a container for transportation
- Discuss with medical officer that sharps safety is their responsibility and the nurse has the right to refuse to accept the sharp (at an appropriate time)

Situation C: When cleaning tissues from your patient's/ resident's table you feel a sting. You examine the area to notice your finger is bleeding. Carefully peeling apart the tissues, you find a blood sugar lancet (or insulin pen needle) which is the source of the puncture in your finger.

Prevention:
- Wear PPE (gloves) when handling items potentially contaminated with blood or other body substances
- Sharps should be disposed of at point of use

Situation D: You are about to perform a bladder scan on a patient you suspect has urinary retention. As you pick up the probe to use it, you notice that your hand is now covered in gel that you have not yet added to the probe ... there are also several wiry pubic hairs stuck in the gel.

Prevention:
- All equipment should be cleaned after each patient use and stored clean and dry
- Wear PPE (gloves) when handling items potentially contaminated with blood or other body substances

13.8 Asepsis overview

Asepsis is defined as the absence of harm-forming microorganisms.[22] Aseptic technique protects patients during invasive clinical procedures by minimising, as far as practicably possible, the introduction and contamination of pathogenic organisms. When undertaken correctly and routinely, aseptic technique processes help prevent infections related to healthcare activities such as the insertion and management of peripheral intravenous cannulae and catheter-associated urinary tract infections (CAUTI).

In the simplest terms, no direct contact should be made between (a) any sterile items that will enter the patient, encounter non-intact skin (wounds) or their invasive devices, and/or (b) the HCW's hands or the surrounding environment such as clothing, bedding or bedside table.[22] All needles, needleless injection devices, syringes, dressings and other similar items must remain covered/protected until the moment they are used. Any time a circuit is entered, such as draining an indwelling urinary catheter or injecting a medication into an intravenous line or bung, it is essential to have clean hands, clean equipment, and avoid touching or contaminating any part of a device that is entering that system.

Aseptic techniques include two main types: *standard* and *surgical*. Both require the use of an aseptic field to protect the items which are to be used from contamination by the surrounding environment. Standard technique fields may be as small as a medication tray, or larger, such as the drape provided by a dressing pack, as long as all the sites remain protected until use during the procedure.

Standard aseptic technique is used when there are a small number of sites or items that need to be protected, such as administration of medication via a peripheral intravenous cannula. This consists of medication syringe(s), connector, cleansing swab and tray to provide a safe field or area within which to conduct the procedure.

Surgical aseptic techniques are employed when multiple and/or large items are being used, such as a central venous line insertion or laparoscopic procedure. This may require multiple surfaces to be covered with sterile drapes to provide adequate protection from environmental contact. These normally occur in an operating room or dedicated procedural environment.

Health services must have processes in place for aseptic technique that:[1,3]

- identify the procedures where aseptic technique applies
- assess the competence of the workforce in performing aseptic technique
- provide training to address gaps in competency; and
- monitor compliance with the health service's policies on aseptic technique.

13.8.1 Aseptic technique risk matrix

The use of standard aseptic technique is a risk-based approach. The Australian Commission on Safety and Quality in Health Care (ACSQHC) in conjunction with the National Safety and Quality Health Service (NSQHS) Standards have developed the Aseptic Technique Risk Matrix which can be used to assist health service organisations to prioritise competency assessments, and identify clinical areas and/or procedures of high risk.

How do we then best address gaps in HCW competency? Research by Gould and colleagues (2018) explored what nurses knew of the principles of aseptic technique.[29] Within their results they found:

'... 65% of nurses described aseptic technique in terms of the procedure used to undertake it, and 46% understood the principles of asepsis. The related concepts of cleanliness and sterilization were frequently confused with one another. Additionally, 72% reported that they had not received training for at least 5 years; 92% were confident of their ability to apply aseptic technique; and 90% reported that they had not been reassessed since their initial training. Qualitative analysis confirmed a lack of clarity about the meaning of aseptic technique.'[29]

It is with this in mind that training for HCWs on asepsis is necessary and requires careful thought. See Box 13.4 for evidence of asepsis and safe use of invasive devices. Case study 3: Success in asepsis training illustrates the level of thought required to achieve asepsis compliance with clinicians.

BOX 13.4 Evidence of asepsis and safe use of invasive devices[3]

Documentation and processes must be available to confirm safe practices in relation to aseptic technique and the use of invasive medical devices:

1. Policy documents that identify clinical procedures and activities for which aseptic technique is required; and about the selection, insertion, maintenance and removal of invasive medical devices. This includes:
   - *lists of all procedures* undertaken in the health service organisation that require aseptic technique; invasive clinical procedures included in the aseptic technique assessment; and invasive medical devices in use in the health service organisation and where they are used
   - *records of actions* taken to reduce identified risks associated with aseptic technique and to manage identified risks with the selection, insertion, maintenance and removal of invasive medical devices

2. Evidence of training and assessment. This includes:
   - the assessment of workforce competence in performing aseptic technique
   - skills appraisals and record of competencies of contractor, locum and agency workforce for aseptic technique
   - training documents about aseptic technique, including training to reduce gaps in competence

3. Audit results of:
   - compliance with aseptic technique procedures
   - workforce compliance with processes for the selection, insertion, maintenance and removal of invasive medical devices

4. Committee and meeting records in which use of invasive medical devices was discussed

5. A review of infection surveillance data about invasive medical devices

Source: Beaumont, K., Wyland, M., & Lee, D. (2016). A multidisciplinary approach to ANTT implementation: what you can achieve in 6 months. Infection, Disease & Health, 21(2), 67-71.

Success in asepsis training

Situation: Anecdotally it has been observed that many clinicians learn their aseptic technique practice from their colleagues at the time they are inducted into the workforce. This leads to significant variation in practices, many of which are unsafe and/or outdated and have not adapted to the changes in technology or the evidence base. The ACHS Standard 3 requirements for aseptic technique articulate the need for an assessment program and recording of compliance for clinical staff undertaking invasive procedures or managing invasive devices.

Response: In response to this, one facility embarked on a global retraining and reassessment program in order to standardise practice across the organisation and provide a baseline for future compliance auditing. By using an instructor and champion model, more than 1000 clinical staff were trained and assessed for competency in a 6-month period. This translated into increased compliance across all wards and departments and clinical professional groups, and also potentially contributed to an improvement in the facility hand hygiene compliance rate during that period.[30]

Further information about the specific requirements of surgical asepsis can be found in Chapter 33.

13.9 Healthcare worker and employer responsibilities for standard precautions

It is the responsibility of the HCW to integrate IPC principles into practice and this is largely linked to facility engagement in the provision of safe quality care and WH&S requirements.[1,3] We do, however also have our own personal responsibilities that help us to stay safe in our workplace while protecting patients and visitors.

Healthcare workers are at risk of exposure to blood and body substances, and to infectious diseases. Implementation of preventive measures by employers against infectious diseases, and managing occupational exposure to blood and body substances, will assist in the maintenance of staff health.[1] Chapter 26 covers these issues in greater detail.

The following preconditions support the minimisation of risk of bodily injury and/or infection in HCWs and should be addressed by healthcare facility leaders and managers to ensure that all HCWs adhere to evidence-based guidelines.[1,3,31]

Infrastructure/system change: access to the right equipment and supplies including PPE, and an environment that is designed and planned to facilitate patient and HCW safety. This includes immunisation programs.

Training and education: a program of routine WH&S education and training and periodic retraining for all personnel.

Monitoring, evaluation and feedback: Pre-employment health evaluation of HCWs (such as vaccine-preventable disease status) and the establishment of protocols for surveillance and management of job-related illnesses and exposures to infectious diseases.

Awareness raising/promotion: Prevention practices are reinforced through awareness raising such as use of posters displayed across healthcare facilities and regular education sessions.

Safety culture: Managers and leaders at every level of the healthcare setting show their visible support for HCW safety to help develop and reinforce a culture of patient safety. This includes counselling services for personnel regarding infection risks related to employment or special conditions and the development, review and revision of policies and procedures and their ready availability. Maintenance of confidential employee health and injury records is important.

13.9.1 Employer duties and responsibilities

Employers are required to:
- ensure a healthy and safe working environment for all employees
- provide employees with appropriate orientation, training and supervision on safety procedures
- have standard operating procedures and guidelines which include WH&S principles readily available to staff
- assess and manage any identified risks (e.g. investigate accidents and illnesses)
- document and report worker injury or illness while addressing confidentiality of the HCW
- ensure best practices for HCW safety and IPC
- have a process for worker feedback on safety issues.

**BOX 13.5 Recommendations to improve compliance with procedures
and eliminate the risk of occupational injuries or HAI**

The following recommendations are intended to improve compliance with procedures and eliminate the risk of occupational injuries or HAI:[1]

1. Establish appropriate engineering controls (controls are used to remove/reduce a hazard or place a barrier between the worker and the hazard in healthcare facilities)

2. Make available and use:
   - appropriate supplies and equipment
   - readily accessible hand hygiene facilities and materials
   - puncture-resistant, leak-proof, labelled or colour-coded sharps containers that are located as close as possible to their places of use
   - leak-proof containers for specimens and other regulated wastes that are properly labelled or colour-coded
   - easily accessible first-aid kit in all departments

3. Implement controls for work practices:
   - prohibit eating, drinking, smoking, applying cosmetics, and handling contact lenses in the work areas and on work surfaces that carry an inherent potential for contamination

- do not store food and drink in refrigerators, freezers or cabinets where blood or other potentially infectious material is stored. Such storage equipment should be clearly labelled to prevent this possibility
- wash hands and other skin surfaces that become contaminated with blood or other potentially infectious materials immediately and thoroughly with soap and running water
- thoroughly wash (flush) with water mucous membranes that become contaminated
- prohibit HCWs with open wounds or weeping skin rashes from all direct patient care, potentially hazardous laboratory procedures, and handling patient-care equipment until recovery
- cuts or abrasions should be protected with a waterproof dressing and gloves prior to performing any procedure that involves contact with blood and other potentially infectious material

4. Adequately staff healthcare facilities
5. Provide information and training
6. Record, investigate, monitor and report exposures to blood and body fluids
7. Monitor and maintain surveillance of work practices.

Source: NHMRC, 2019[1]

The recommendations in Box 13.5 are intended to improve compliance with procedures and eliminate the risk of occupational injuries or HAI.[1]

13.9.2 Healthcare worker practices

Healthcare workers are required to:

1. follow safe work practices at all times in line with jurisdiction and setting guidance
2. be familiar with written departmental policies
3. know the potential health and safety hazards of the job and protective measures by participating in appropriate WH&S training programs
4. use PPE as trained and report any changes in personal medical condition that would require a change in status as to wearing PPE
5. know how to report unsafe working conditions

6. report any work-related injury or illness to supervisor
7. participate in accident and injury investigations
8. know what to do in an emergency
9. participate in health and safety committees (when available)
10. practise 'bare below the elbows' to ensure good hand hygiene compliance
11. exclude themselves from the workplace when unwell
12. wear closed-in shoes in clinical settings
13. ensure hair is tied back and off the shoulders
14. wear clean clothes or uniform each shift as they can become contaminated with a variety of pathogens. Wash these separately from other items.

13.9.3 Pre-employment health evaluations (such as vaccine-preventable disease status)

When personnel are initially appointed or are reassigned to different jobs or areas, a pre-employment evaluation can be used to ensure that persons are not placed in jobs that would pose undue risk of infection to them, other personnel, patients or visitors. This can include determining a health worker's immunisation status and obtaining a history of any conditions that may predispose the HCW to acquiring or transmitting infectious diseases and ensuring that staff follow exposure-prone procedure protocol.

13.9.4 Personnel health and safety education

Personnel are more likely to comply with an IPC program if they understand the rationale; thus, HCW safety education should be a central focus, with:

- clearly written policies, guidelines and procedures to ensure uniformity, efficiency and effective coordination of activities
- training that is designed to cover all levels of staff, including doctors, nurses, clinical officers, laboratory workers, non-medical workers and support staff. Training should be matched to the roles/responsibilities of each group; and
- orientation/induction and in-service training programs for new employees, as well as in-service refresher training (e.g. yearly) for existing employees. This is the responsibility of all healthcare facilities to develop and implement.

13.10 Implementation of standard precautions

The efficiency of standard precautions in mitigating the risk of pathogen transmission and HAI acquisition depends on how effectively they are instituted within a healthcare facility and the level of compliance by HCWs, whereby meticulous observance of standard precautions is warranted for every patient encounter to reduce transmission rates.[32] We do, however, see a lack of compliance that is attributed to individual, psychosocial and institutional factors, in addition to insufficient knowledge and a lack of understanding of the underlying principles.[33] While standard precautions are a requisite for best practice, there is a tendency for HCWs to choose whether to adhere to them in practice, with aberrant behaviour compromising both HCW and patient safety.[34] It has been suggested that the intention for clinicians to behave in a particular way, for example adherence to IPC precautions, consists of three facets: attitudes and beliefs; subjective norms; and perceived behavioural control.[20] If long-lasting changes are to be instigated to improve adherence to standard precautions, then it becomes paramount to discern the crucial aspects of HCW behaviour that are responsible for non-compliance.[35]

13.10.1 Consumer involvement in standard precautions

How much could/should we include the 'consumer'? Health literacy is arguably at an all-time low since the beginning of the 20th century. Many consumers have access (via the internet) to a vast amount of information but still lack knowledge in the essentials. A simple search provides a deluge of information, but how does the average consumer evaluate what is real or misleading, when even skilled healthcare professionals have difficulty weighing the evidence for validity? It is important to include the consumer, patient/client and visitor/relative in preventing infection.

Every HCW has an obligation to provide instruction on required behaviours, particularly within acute healthcare, to assist in preventing infection. Instructions on hand hygiene before and after eating, after toileting and so on, as well as respiratory etiquette, device and waste management are essential in enabling the consumer and their support persons to participate in safe care. 'Fact sheets' can only do so much. Healthcare workers and support staff providing advice may be more helpful to communicate key messages to patients and consumers.

Consumer partnerships in healthcare are now viewed as integral to the development, implementation and evaluation of health policies, programs and services.[1] Patient and consumer partnerships are also a pillar of person-centred care—that is, care that focuses on the relationship between a patient and a clinician, and recognises that trust, mutual respect and sharing of knowledge are needed for the best health outcomes.

Patient and consumer partnerships should take many forms, at many levels. Different types of partnerships with patients and consumers exist within the healthcare system. These partnerships are not mutually exclusive and are needed at all levels to ensure that a health service organisation achieves the best possible outcome for all parties. Partnerships with patients and consumers comprise many different, interwoven practices that reflect the three key levels at which partnerships are needed:[1,3]

Individual: Partnerships relate to the interaction between patients and clinicians when care is provided. This involves providing care that is respectful; sharing information in an ongoing way; working with patients, carers and families to make decisions and plan care; and supporting and encouraging patients in their own care and self-management.

Service, department or program of care: Partnerships relate to the organisation and delivery of care within specific areas. Patients, carers, families and consumers participate in the overall design of the service, department or program. They could be full members of quality improvement and redesign teams, including participating in planning, implementing and evaluating change.

Health service organisation: Partnerships relate to the involvement of consumers in overall governance, policy and planning. This level overlaps with the previous level in that a health service organisation is made up of various services, departments and programs. Consumers and consumer representatives are full members of key organisational governance committees in areas such as patient safety, facility design, quality improvement, patient or family education, ethics and research. This level can also involve partnerships with local community organisations and members of local communities.

Supporting effective consumer partnerships means supporting multiple mechanisms of engagement. Meaningful methods of engagement range from representation on committees and boards, to contributions at focus groups, to feedback received through surveys or social media. When selecting methods of consumer participation, consider the diversity of the consumer population that uses, or may use, the services. Consumer partnerships add value to healthcare decision making.[1,3] Consumer involvement in the development, implementation and evaluation of healthcare contributes to:

- appropriately targeted initiatives
- efficient use of resources
- improvement in the quality of care provided by a health service.

There is growing acceptance that practices supporting partnerships at the level of the individual—from communication and structured listening, through to shared decision making, self-management support and care planning—can improve the safety and quality of healthcare, improve patient outcomes and experience, and improve the performance of health service organisations.

As consumer partnership becomes more embedded in the healthcare system, there is an increasing need to monitor and evaluate its impact. Monitoring, measuring and evaluating consumer partnerships—through mechanisms such as recording patient experience and patient-reported outcome measures—are vital to ensure that the partnerships are meeting the needs of the community and consumers.

Consumer partnerships should be meaningful and not tokenistic. To maximise the contribution of partnerships, consumers need to be seen and treated as people with expert skills and knowledge. In the same way that clinicians and other organisational partners are respected for their areas of expertise, consumer partnerships need to be recognised and valued for their unique perspective on the patient experience.[1,3]

Conclusion

As the multiple different topics in this chapter have demonstrated, there is much more to 'standard precautions' than just washing your hands. Infection prevention and control principles are founded on many different basic practices developed to disrupt the 'chain of infection'. By observing these fundamental, core principles much of the potential transmission of infection is mitigated. Do the basics well and there will be a solid foundation for all healthcare. Do it poorly and there will be a need to escalate precautions and actions to counteract the consequences. The simple things in life are often the best.

Useful websites/resources

- World Health Organization. Standard precautions in health care Aide Memoire (2007). https://www.who.int/docs/default-source/documents/health-topics/standard-precautions-in-health-care.pdf
- Australian Guidelines for the Prevention and Control of Infection in Healthcare (2019). https://www.nhmrc.gov.au/about-us/publications/australian-guidelines-prevention-and-control-infection-healthcare-2019
- Australian Commission on Safety and Quality in Health Care. https://www.safetyandquality.gov.au/infection-prevention-and-control

References

1. National Health and Medical Research Council. Australian Guidelines for the Prevention and Control of Infection in Healthcare. Canberra: NHMRC, 2019.

2. Australian Commission on Safety and Quality in Health Care (ACSQHC) Infection Prevention and Control Poster – Standard precautions poster. ACSQHC: Sydney 2022.

3. Australian Commission on Safety and Quality in Health Care. National Safety and Quality Health Service Standards. 2nd ed. Sydney: ACSQHC, 2017.

4. Standards Association of Australia. AS ISO 31000: 2018 Risk Management Guidelines. Australia: SAI Global Professional Services, 2018.

5. World Health Organization. WHO Guidelines on Hand Hygiene in Health Care: First Global Patient Safety Challenge Clean Care is Safer Care. Geneva: WHO, 2009.

6. World Health Organization. Your 5 Moments for Hand Hygiene. Geneva: WHO, 2009.

7. Sickbert-Bennett E, DiBiase L, Willis T, Wolak E, Weber R, Rutala W. Reduction of healthcare-associated infections by exceeding high compliance with hand hygiene practices. Emerg Infect Dis. 2016;22(9):1628-1630.

8. Grayson L, Russo P, Cruickshank M, Bear J, Gee C, Hughes C, et al. Outcomes from the first 2 years of the Australian National Hand Hygiene Inititiative. MJA. 2011;195(10):615-619.

9. Grayson L, Stewardson A, Russo P, Ryan K, Olsen K, Havers S, et al. Hand Hygiene Australia and the National Hand Hygiene Initiative. Effects of the Australian National Hand Hygiene Initiative after 8 years on infection control practices, health-care worker education, and clinical outcomes: a longitudinal study. Lancet Infect Dis. 2018; 18(11):1269-1277.

10. World Health Organization. How to Handwash? Geneva: WHO, 2009.

11. World Health Organization. How to Handrub? Geneva: WHO, 2009.

12. Butenko S, Lockwood C, McArthur A. Patient experiences of partnering with healthcare professionals for hand hygiene compliance. JBI Database System Rev Implement Rep. 2017;15(6):1645-1670.

13. Health and Human Services Victoria State Government. Cover your cough and sneeze. Melbourne: State of Victoria, 2018.

14. Barratt R, Shaban RZ, Gilbert G. Clinician perceptions of respiratory infection risk; a rationale for research into mask use into routine practice. Infect Dis Health. 2019;24:169-176.

15. Jain S, Clezy K, McLaws M-L. Glove: use for safety or overuse? Am J Infect Control. 2017;45(12):1407-1410.

16. Bradford Smith P, Agostini G, Mitchell JC. A scoping review of surgical masks and N95 filtering facepiece respirators: learning from the past to guide the future of dentistry. Saf Sci. 2020;131:104920.

17. Barr N, Holmes M, Roiko A, Dunn P, Lord B. Self-reported behaviors and perceptions of Australian paramedics in relation to hand hygiene and gloving practices in paramedic-led health care. Am J Infect Control. 2017;45(7):771-778.

18. Gillespie BM, Walker R, Lin F, Roberts S, Eskes A, Perry J, et al. Wound care practices across two acute care settings: a comparative study. J Clin Nurs. 2020;29(5-6):831-839.

19. Lin F, Gillespie BM, Chaboyer W, Li Y, Whitelock K, Morley N, et al. Preventing surgical site infections: facilitators and barriers to nurses' adherence to clinical practice guidelines—a qualitative study. J Clin Nurs. 2019;28(9-10):1643-1652.

20. Ward DJ. The application of the theory of planned behaviour to infection control research with nursing and midwifery students. J Clin Nurs. 2013;22(1-2):296-298.

21. Hand Hygiene Australia. Hand care issues. Canberra: HHA, 2020. Available from: https://www.hha.org.au/hand-hygiene/what-is-hand-hygiene/hand-care-issues.

22. Lee G, Bishop P. Microbiology and infection control for health professionals. 6th ed. Melbourne: Pearson Australia, 2016.

23. Standards Association of Australia. AS/NZS 4187:2014 Reprocessing of reusable medical devices in health service organisations. Australia: SAI Global Professional Services, 2014.

24. Kramer A, Schwebke I, Kampf G. How long do nosocomial pathogens persist on inanimate surfaces? A systematic review. BMC Infect Dis. 2006;6:130.

25. Ledwoch K, Dancer SJ, Otter JA, Kerr K, Roposte D, Rushton L, et al. Beware biofilm! Dry biofilms containing bacterial pathogens on multiple healthcare surfaces; a multi-centre study. J Hosp Infect. 2018;100(3):e47-e56.

26. Mitchell BG, Dancer SJ, Anderson M, Dehn E. Risk of organism acquisition from prior room occupants: a systematic review and meta-analysis. J Hosp Infect. 2015;91(3):211-217.

27. Australian Commission on Safety and Quality in Health Care. Benefits of environmental cleaning. Sydney: ACSQHC, 2020.

28. Standards Association of Australia. AS/NZS 4146:2000 Laundry Practice. Australia: SAI Global Professional Services, 2000.

29. Gould DJ, Chudleigh J, Purssell E, Hawker C, Gaze S, James D, et al. Survey to explore understanding of the principles of aseptic technique: qualitative content analysis with descriptive analysis of confidence and training. Am J Infect Control. 2018;46(4):393-396.

30. Beaumont K, Wyland M, Lee D. A multi-disciplinary approach to ANTT implementation: what you can achieve in 6 months. Infect Dis Health. 2016;21(2):67-71.

31. Safe Work Australia. Safe Work Australia. Canberra: Australian Government, 2020. Available from: https://www.safeworkaustralia.gov.au/.

32. Colet PC, Cruz JP, Alotaibi KA, Colet MKA, Islam SMS. Compliance with standard precautions among baccalaureate nursing students in a Saudi university: a self-report study. J Infect Public Health. 2017;10(4):421-430.

33. Cheung K, Chan CK, Chang MY, Chu PH, Fung WF, Kwan KC, et al. Predictors for compliance of standard precautions among nursing students. Am J Infect Control. 2015;43(7):729-734.

34. Bouchoucha S, Moore K. Standard precautions but no standard adherence. Aust Nurs Midwifery. 2017;24(8):38.

35. Shah N, Castro-Sánchez E, Charani E, Drumright LN, Holmes AH. Towards changing healthcare workers' behaviour: a qualitative study exploring non-compliance through appraisals of infection prevention and control practices. J Hosp Infect. 2015;90(2):126-134.

CHAPTER 14

Transmission-based precautions

Dr LYNETTE BOWEN[i]

Prof MARTIN KIERNAN[ii]

Chapter highlights

- Transmission-based precautions (TBPs) are used in addition to standard precautions
- Transmission-based precautions are required when specific pathogens are suspected or confirmed and relate to the associated modes of transmission
- A risk-based approach to TBPs supports the healthcare worker to identify measures within the hierarchy of control, including engineering and administrative controls as well as relevant personal protective equipment (PPE)
- The patient and family experience, including ethical considerations and education around relevant TBPs, is an important consideration for the quality and safety of care

i   School of Nursing, Avondale University, Lake Macquarie, NSW
ii Richard Wells Research Centre, University of West London, London, UK

Introduction

Transmission-based precautions are used in addition to standard precautions when a specific route of transmission poses a risk to others. This chapter outlines the principles of TBPs and PPE. Adopting a safety-risk approach, the types of TBPs are detailed, with emphasis on key attributes, and requirements for each type of precaution. A detailed explanation of the types of PPE and practices for donning and doffing follow. Finally, some controversies and other considerations appropriate to the implementation and practice of TBPs will be explored.

14.1 Historical segregation practices

Long before we understood how infection was transmitted, there was recognition that segregation had some effect in reducing spread of disease. However, historical attempts were often entwined with moral and religious overtones or superstition.

Religious and secular writings identified conditions considered to be unclean and therefore required separation from the rest of the community. Leprosy in its various forms was one such example. Initially the medieval approach was separation, later evolving into isolation in specifically established leper houses.[1]

At a similar time, various outbreaks of plague (*Yersinia pestis*) were becoming problematic. Households and people suffering plague were regularly segregated or quarantined (meaning 40 days). As well, civil authorities would attempt to protect healthy communities by closing transport routes, increasing sanitation and removing waste.[1] The concept of segregation and protection was the focus of management, but how plague was spread was attributed to evil spirits or miasma (unhealthy gases that spread disease).

Pulmonary tuberculosis, historically referred to as consumption, appeared sometime around the 16th century. Again, transmission was poorly understood, but segregation in sanitoriums was one approach for those who could afford it.[2]

The key feature of these historical examples was that they all included some type of segregation or confinement. However, scholars did not understand the concept of infection (contagion) or recognise that a microorganism caused the disease. Therefore, there was no knowledge of how it was transmitted.

14.2 Transmission of infection

Our understanding of the process by which infection is transmitted from a source to another person is addressed in detail in Chapter 3. The links in the chain that must occur for infection to be transmitted are:

- a reservoir, the normal habitat for the infectious agent, most frequently a human

- a portal of exit, being the route by which the infectious agent leaves the reservoir. Typical routes are respiratory tract, blood, skin lesions, urine and faeces

- the mode of transmission by which the infectious agent is transmitted to a susceptible host. This includes direct or indirect modes. Direct modes include direct contact aerosol (droplet/airborne) spread, while indirect modes include aerosol (droplet/airborne) spread, vehicle-borne or vectorborne spread

- a portal of entry that provides an avenue for the infectious agent to enter the susceptible host. The portal of entry is often the same avenue as was the portal of exit from the reservoir

- a host, the final link in the chain. Several factors influence the susceptibility of the host to the infectious agent, including health, genetic makeup, specific immunity, age and lifestyle factors.[3]

There is only one link in the chain that can be broken to interrupt infection. That link is transmission. This is the premise on which TBPs are designed. The use of hand hygiene, personal protective equipment, patient-dedicated equipment, and the segregation of patients with infectious disease, are strategies to reduce the transmission of infection.

14.3 Overview of transmission-based precautions

As outlined in the previous chapter, standard precautions are required in all situations and at all times. It is the principal approach to reducing the risk of healthcare-associated infection (HAI). However, as identified above, infectious agents can be transmitted by one or more routes, resulting in the need for further precautions to prevent transmission of infection. Therefore, recognising how an infectious disease is transmitted is paramount in responding to an infection risk. Transmission-based precautions are used when a person is confirmed or suspected (using relevant clinical and epidemiological data) of having an infectious disease.

14.3.1 A risk-based approach to transmission-based precautions

Identifying and assessing risk of contamination should apply when implementing any type of TBP. Each situation and context remains unique, even after identifying the route of transmission and therefore, the appropriate precautions. Risk factors to consider are identified and clustered together as patient factors or healthcare worker–patient interaction factors.[4] They are outlined in Box 14.1.

Therefore, awareness for risk of contamination needs to be factored into all activities undertaken within the context of TBPs.

Some emerging evidence suggests that the length of time spent with a patient being managed with TBPs and the number of activities may also impact the risk of transmission.[5] In another study, nurses' workflow was observed, finding that care activities were batched together when supporting someone in TBPs. This resulted in errors in contact with the patient and environment, without performing hand hygiene between activities.[6-8] Therefore, it is important to take a risk-based approach to the delivery of all aspects of healthcare when TBPs apply, as well as on entry and exit

from the area. Changing of gloves between procedures and hand hygiene remain relevant, regardless of the type of precautions in place.[5] For a more detailed discussion of risk assessment and management, refer to Chapter 7.

14.3.2 Practices applicable to all transmission-based precautions

Transmission-based precautions are dependent on the mode of transmission. They have been developed and adopted in response to our understanding of the spread of infection and are used in addition to standard precautions. The types of precautions are outlined in Box 14.2, noting that dissemination between droplet and airborne transmission is less clear. These should be considered a continuum and not an arbitrary dichotomy.

All types of TBPs require the use of PPE.[9] The type and components of PPE required will depend on the risk of transmission. Each category of TBPs outlined below includes a table identifying the recommended PPE to use.

Another consideration when applying any type of TBPs is to designate equipment to be used for the specific patient for the duration of TBPs.[9] This includes equipment for physical assessment, infusion pumps and mobility aids. Setting aside patient equipment reduces the risk of transmission of pathogens that could otherwise be carried on the equipment.[10,11] When precautions conclude, all equipment needs to be decontaminated.

Cleaning and disinfecting the patient care area is essential, both during the precautions and when they cease. Cleaning is addressed in detail in Chapter 15; however, in Australia, the NHMRC[9] recommends when a person is being cared for under TBPs, that surfaces are physically cleaned with a detergent solution followed by a hospital-grade disinfectant or cleaned with a combined 2-in-1 detergent disinfectant, approved by the Therapeutic Goods Administration (TGA).[9] Further detail on the TGA and the Australian

---

BOX 14.1 Risk factors for potential contamination

Patient factors:

- pathogen shedding and microbial burden
- respiratory (cough, sneeze, breath)
- antibiotic exposures
- situations such as patient wounds and/or urinary/bowel incontinence.

Healthcare worker–patient interactions that are high risk:

- contact with body waste and fluids
- changing wound dressings
- supporting hygiene activities
- managing endotracheal tubes.

Healthcare worker–patient interactions that are low risk:

- blood glucose monitoring
- medication administration.[4]

BOX 14.2 Types of transmission-based precautions

- Contact precautions
- Droplet precautions (aerosol)
- Airborne precautions (aerosol)

regulatory framework for medical devices, sterilants and disinfectants is provided in Chapter 16.

Movement of patients being managed with TBPs should be avoided where possible.[9] This supports a risk-based approach, minimising the risk of transmission of infection.

14.4 Specific transmission-based precautions

The following section outlines each precaution, identifying when it is used, what is entailed in the precaution, and highlights important considerations identified through research studies.

14.4.1 Contact precautions

Contact precautions are applied in addition to standard precautions. They are used in situations where the route of transmission of infection is by direct or indirect contact, which is the most common mode of transmission.[12] The difference between the two modes of transmission is that direct contact is the transfer of microorganisms from one infected person to another person, without a contaminated intermediate object or person, while indirect contact is the transfer of the infectious agent through a contaminated object or person.[12] Hand hygiene and decontamination of patient equipment are acknowledged as two strategies to reduce indirect transmission in the healthcare context;[10,11,13] however, these strategies need further strengthening by the addition of contact precautions.

Thus, contact precautions play an important role in infection prevention and control. They are particularly important in minimising transmission of infections such as *Clostridioides difficile* and multidrug-resistant organisms (MROs), such as methicillin-resistant *Staphylococcus aureus* (MRSA), vancomycin-resistant enterococcus (VRE), and carbapenemase-producing *Enterobacterales* (CPE).[14]

Contact precautions consist of some core elements:
- use of a single room (or cohorting)
- use of specific PPE
- enhanced cleaning (discussed in Chapter 16)
- considerations around use of equipment
- patient transfer considerations.

Single room: Contact precautions require a single room wherever possible (or, alternatively, cohorting). The single room ideally should include an ensuite bathroom and, where possible, an anteroom where donning and doffing of PPE will occur. The single room has the potential to reduce the transmission of MROs, improve compliance with hand hygiene and appropriate use of PPE, along with improved cleaning and decontamination.[9] However, a number of studies raise concerns about healthcare worker adherence to hand hygiene and PPE requirements.[15-18] It is imperative that a risk-based approach is adopted, identifying the risk of contamination, and creating a virtual demarcation between clean and contaminated zones in the individual healthcare worker's mind.[19]

Specific personal protective equipment (PPE): The PPE required for contact precautions always includes gloves and impervious apron/gown. Where there is a risk of splash of blood or body fluid, safety glasses or a face shield should also be included as part of standard precautions. The purpose of the apron/gown is to protect the healthcare worker's clothing from contamination. Gaps in gown coverage can be problematic,[17,18] as they expose the healthcare worker's own clothes to potential contamination. Therefore, correct donning and wearing of gowns will reduce the risk of transmission. As well, healthcare workers should be aware of potential breaches, such as placing hands under the gown to retrieve items such as pens or phones.[18] Details on how to don and doff these items and the recommended order are provided below in 14.5 Personal protective equipment.

Hand hygiene is an extremely important aspect of contact precautions. It is necessary before donning PPE, and during removal of PPE, but can be overlooked.[20] It may also be necessary to remove gloves between procedures while attending a patient on contact precautions. Hand hygiene must be performed again before donning the clean pair of gloves.[9] If a patient is known or suspected of being infected with *Clostridioides difficile* (CDI) or a non-enveloped virus, handwashing is the recommended approach for hand decontamination. Table 14.1 provides a summary of the requirements for contact precautions.

Equipment: Single use or patient-dedicated equipment should be used when caring for a patient on contact precautions. If there is limited equipment that cannot be dedicated to the contact precautions area, then the risk of transmission needs to be considered and cleaning performed as per the manufacturer's instructions, before the equipment is removed to the corridor.[9,17]

TABLE 14.1 Summary of requirements for contact precautions

Elements	Required	Instructions
Hand hygiene	✓	When donning/doffing PPE—locate at entry/exit point
Gloves	✓	Don on entry, change between procedures, remove on exit
Gown	✓	Don on entry, remove on exit
Mask	✓	Not required
Face protection	✓	Procedures with risk of splash/spray of blood/body substances
Signage	✓	Contact precaution signage at entry point
Single room	✓	With ensuite bathroom, close door. May consider cohorting
Equipment	✓	Single use or dedicated to patient. Clean before removal
Patient notes		Keep outside room
Patient transfer	Limit	Cover infected or contaminated areas of patient's body

Note: These are always in addition to standard precautions

Transfer: If it is necessary to move a patient, the NHMRC advises to cover or contain the infected or colonised areas. The healthcare worker should then carefully remove and dispose of contaminated PPE before moving the patient. On arrival at the new location, the healthcare workers should don clean PPE before assisting the patient.[9]

Other considerations: Signage is an important reminder for healthcare workers and visitors and improves adherence to precaution requirements.[14] The signage needs to provide clear instructions on requirements. Signage may differ slightly between jurisdictions; however, it should advise the type of precautions, requirements for entering and exiting the room and include pictures to support visitors who are unfamiliar with donning and doffing procedures for PPE. An example of a contact precautions sign is provided in Figure 14.1.

14.4.2 Droplet precautions

Droplet precautions are used in addition to standard precautions when the mode of transmission for an infection is via the droplet route. It is used when large particles, arbitrarily and historically defined as more than 5 microns in size, are generated through coughing, sneezing or speaking.[9] The definition of 'droplets' is under debate and defining size is problematic. Aerosols are small particles suspended in the air. These could range from larger particles which are less likely to transmit over long distances (historically more

aligned to the 'droplet' transmission route), to very small particles which would be considered airborne.

The larger droplets can also be created during some procedures such as suctioning, endotracheal intubation, cardiopulmonary resuscitation and some physiotherapy procedures.[12] The larger particles are heavier, unable to be suspended for long distances and, therefore, are likely to cause transmission in situations where contact is closer. Particles may also contaminate surfaces where they land; therefore, droplet precautions are technically also contact precautions.[12] This explains why contact and droplet precautions are often used together and have strong similarities.

If a droplet dries out, the remaining droplet nuclei is a much smaller particle and has been implicated in some incidents as creating airborne transmission.[12] This is concerning in confined spaces and our understanding of this phenomenon has been enhanced through research following the first SARS outbreak in 2003.[21] It is now thought to be a plausible explanation for unusual incidents of transmission of COVID-19, such as choir practice and hotel venues. Most importantly, the ability for a droplet nuclei to become an airborne particle reinforces the need for appropriate use of PPE, effective decontamination of surfaces and vigilant hand hygiene.[9]

Typically, droplet precautions will be implemented for influenza, mumps, norovirus, pertussis, meningococcus and some forms of pneumonia.[9,12] Other infections that may require droplet precautions for a short period of time, that is, until effective treatment has been

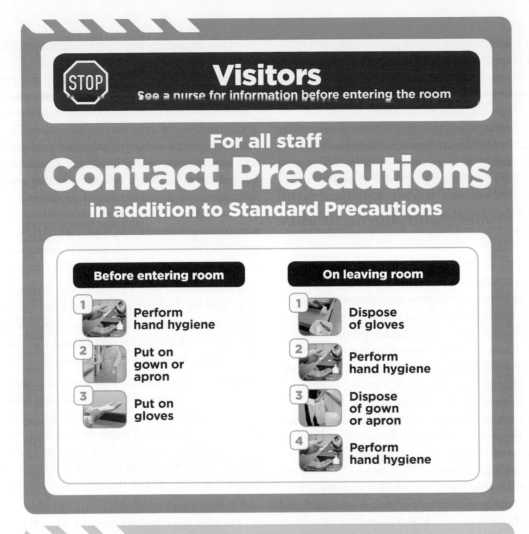

FIGURE 14.1 Example of contact precautions signage

Source: Reproduced with permission from Infection Prevention and Control Poster – Standard precautions poster, developed by the Australian Commission on Safety and Quality in Health Care (ACSQHC). ACSQHC: Sydney 2022.

in place for at least 24 hours, include some streptococcal and staphylococcal infections.[9]

Droplet precautions consist of some core elements:

- use of a single room (or cohorting)
- use of specific PPE
- enhanced cleaning (discussed in Chapter 16)

- considerations around use of equipment
- patient transfer considerations.

Single room: Creating a physical barrier is an important part of managing respiratory infections transmitted by droplets, as the purpose is to protect from transmission through close respiratory or mucosal contact.[12]

Therefore, a single room is best practice, with direct access to an ensuite bathroom. Droplet precautions do not require any special air-handling system, such as a negative pressure room, but the door to the room should be kept closed, apart from healthcare workers entering and leaving the room. If there is a shortage of single rooms, then a risk approach should be adopted. Single rooms should be allocated to patients with excessive coughing and sputum production.[9] Patients unable to be allocated a single room should be educated to follow cough etiquette and hand hygiene, and where possible cohorting should then be practised.[9]

Specific personal protective equipment: In addition to gown and impervious apron/gloves, the PPE required for droplet precautions includes a fluid-impervious surgical mask to protect nasal and oral mucosa.[9] Where there is risk of splash, aerosols or bodily fluid coming in contact with the eyes, eye protection is also recommended. PPE is donned on entry to the room or patient area. This includes the surgical mask, which has been shown to be effective with most respiratory viruses where transmission is by droplet.[9,22] The surgical mask should be donned following the gown and before gloves.[9] Once tied in place, it is important to ensure that it is moulded to fit around the nose and cheeks to improve its effectiveness as a barrier. When doffing, the mask is the last item of PPE to be removed—avoid touching the front of the mask and dispose of it immediately. Hand hygiene should then follow. Further details on donning and doffing procedures are provided in 14.5 Personal protective equipment.

Hand hygiene is an important strategy in droplet precautions. As previously mentioned, droplet precautions can be thought of as an extension of contact precautions;[12] therefore, contaminated surfaces, gloves, gowns and masks can increase the risk of self-contamination. Hand hygiene is an effective strategy to prevent transmission of viral pathogens associated with droplet precautions and respiratory transmission.[9] Soap and water for handwashing and alcohol-based hand rub should be readily available within the room and at the point of donning and doffing PPE. Hand hygiene is required before donning and after removing gloves, including when gloves are changed between procedures for the same person.[9] Table 14.2 provides a summary of droplet precaution requirements.

Equipment: Whenever possible, equipment should be dedicated to the specific patient. Like contact precautions, there is a risk that equipment may be contaminated; therefore, equipment should be decontaminated following manufacturers' guidelines.

Transfer: If it is necessary to move a patient on droplet precautions then, to avoid transmission by coughing or sneezing, the patient should wear a fluid-resistant surgical mask during transfer. As well, they should be instructed on respiratory hygiene and how to perform cough etiquette.[9] Education is important as it cannot be assumed a patient will know how to perform cough etiquette.[23]

Droplet precautions should also be practised in primary care type settings when patients present with frequent or excessive coughing. They should be segregated from others in waiting room areas, provided with

TABLE 14.2 Summary of requirements for droplet precautions

Elements	Required	Instructions
Hand hygiene	✓	When donning/doffing PPE—locate at entry/exit point
Gloves	✓	Don on entry, change between procedures, remove on exit
Gown	✓	Don on entry, remove on exit
Mask	✓	Surgical mask
Face protection	✓	Procedures with risk of splash/spray of blood/body substances
Signage	✓	Droplet precaution signage at entry point
Single room	✓	With ensuite bathroom, close door. Only cohort with patients with same pathogen
Equipment	✓	Single use or dedicated to patient. Clean before removal
Patient notes		Keep outside room
Patient transfer	Limit	Patient to wear surgical mask, respiratory hygiene/cough etiquette

Note: These are always in addition to standard precautions

facial tissues and a supply of alcohol-based hand rub and a waste bin should be available. Instructions on respiratory hygiene and cough etiquette (see Chapter 14) should also be provided.[9]

Other considerations: Signage outside the room or patient area provides guidance to staff and visitors about additional precautions required. The signage should be clearly visible and the directions on the sign should be easy to follow. An example of signage for droplet precautions is provided in Figure 14.2.

Another important consideration, when droplet precautions apply, is the approach to aerosol-generating

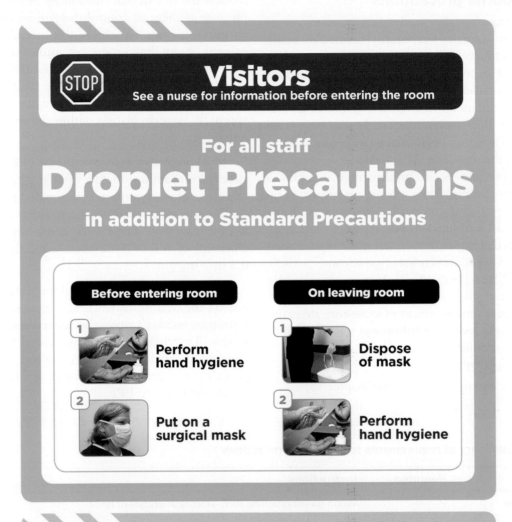

FIGURE 14.2 Example of droplet precautions signage

Source: Reproduced with permission from Infection Prevention and Control Poster – Droplet precautions, in addition to standard precautions poster, developed by the Australian Commission on Safety and Quality in Health Care (ACSQHC). ACSQHC: Sydney 2022.

procedures (AGPs) such as suctioning and endotracheal intubation. For such procedures, the level of precaution should be increased to airborne precautions for the duration of the procedures. If the patient is cohorting with others, then it is also advised to perform the procedure in a treatment room to reduce risk of transmission.[9]

14.4.3 Airborne precautions

Airborne precautions are used when transmission of infection is by particles—arbitrarily defined as being smaller than 5 microns. This can include airborne droplet nuclei that occurs from desiccation of infectious droplets. The smaller infectious particle is lighter and can travel over distance while remaining infectious. The resultant risk is that respiratory particles can be carried on air currents and may be inhaled by someone without encountering the source of the infection.[12]

Airborne precautions are implemented in addition to standard precautions when a patient is suspected of, or confirmed to be infected with, Mycobacterium tuberculosis, measles or chicken pox. As well, some cases of disseminated shingles (herpes zoster), smallpox, avian influenza A, severe acute respiratory syndrome (SARS), SARS-CoV-2 infection and monkeypox virus require airborne precautions.[9]

Airborne precautions consist of some core elements:
- use of a single room (or cohorting) with specific ventilation requirements
- use of specific PPE
- enhanced cleaning (discussed in Chapter 15)

- considerations around use of equipment
- patient transfer considerations.

Single room: Airborne precautions require a single room with, wherever possible, special negative pressure air handling and ventilation. This is referred to as a Class N room.[24] A negative pressure room reduces the risk of transmission by using a negative pressure gradient to control the airflow, only drawing air into the room. To achieve this, an independent exhaust system draws a greater amount of air from the room than is delivered to the room.[24,25] Where an independent exhaust system is not available, HEPA filters must be used for recirculated air.[24] For either approach, air recirculating within the room or to the outside, the door must remain closed.[9]

Personal protective equipment: The PPE required for airborne precautions includes gown, gloves and respirator. However, the recommended respirator for routine care of patients requiring airborne precautions is a P2 respirator.[9] The P2 respirator must have a filter efficiency of at least 94% when tested for particles at 0.2 to 2 microns.[9]

However, efficient filtering alone is not sufficient to protect the healthcare worker. It must seal around the healthcare worker's nose, cheeks and mouth to be effective. Therefore, it must be correctly fitted and checked to provide maximum protection.[9] Table 14.3 provides an overview of airborne precaution requirements and required PPE.

TABLE 14.3 Summary of requirements for airborne precautions

Elements	Required	Instructions
Hand hygiene	✓	When donning/doffing PPE—locate at entry/exit point
Gloves	✓	Don on entry, change between procedures, remove on exit
Gown	✓	Don on entry, remove on exit
Mask	✓	P2/N95 respirator, fit tested and fit checked
Face protection	✓	Procedures with risk of splash/spray of blood/body substances
Signage	✓	Airborne precaution signage at entry point
Single room	✓	With ensuite bathroom, close door. Negative pressure room, if available
Equipment	✓	Single use or dedicated to patient. Clean before removal
Patient notes		Keep outside room
Patient transfer	Limit	Patient to wear correctly fitted surgical mask, respiratory hygiene/cough etiquette. Cover skin lesions (e.g. chicken pox)

Note: These are always in addition to standard precautions

Transfer: If a patient on airborne precautions is required to leave the room, they should be asked to wear a surgical mask. Instructions on how to wear the mask should be provided and they should be assisted with donning the mask. As well, instructions on respiratory hygiene and cough etiquette should be provided. If a patient has lesions associated with the infection (e.g. chicken pox/shingles), the lesions should be covered to minimise risk of transmission. Where a child is on

airborne precautions, and if they need to leave the room, they need to have a correctly fitted mask and oxygen saturation levels should be monitored.[9]

Other considerations: Signage should be placed outside the room that advises airborne precautions are in place. The signage should include details of precautions required. An example of airborne precaution signage is provided in Figure 14.3.

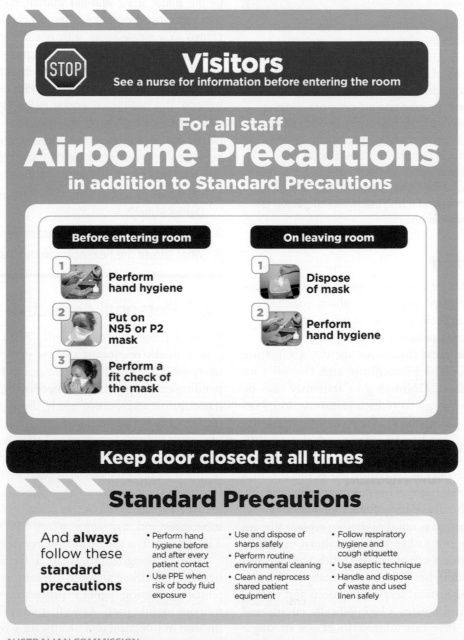

FIGURE 14.3 Example of airborne precautions signage

Source: Reproduced with permission from Infection Prevention and Control Poster – Airborne precautions poster, developed by the Australian Commission on Safety and Quality in Health Care (ACSQHC). ACSQHC: Sydney 2022.

Ideally, healthcare workers should have immunity to the infection. This can be confirmed using a vaccination history or serology. Where immunity is not known or staff are not immune, extreme care must be taken to ensure PPE fits and is correctly worn.[9]

PRACTICE TIP 1
CONSIDERING TRANSMISSION-BASED PRECAUTIONS

The manner in which transmission-based precautions are traditionally presented—as either contact, droplet or airborne—can present challenges. These three types of transmission-based precautions should not be considered in isolation. This is particularly so with droplet and airborne precautions, which use largely arbitrary measures to differentiate. There are also situations where a combination of these precautions is required. In this chapter, we have presented transmission-based precautions in these three groups for ease of explanation and for consistency with national and international guidelines at the time of publication.

14.4.4 Cohorting

For most TBP, a single room is used. In some situations, it may be appropriate to cohort patients together. Cohorting is the term used when confining to one area a group of patients who are all colonised or infected with the same infectious agent.[12] Cohorting still requires standard precautions and the relevant TBPs to be applied. Cohorting of staff may also be considered as a strategy to reduce transmission of infection.[26] An important consideration when cohorting is to still perform hand hygiene and change PPE *between* patients.[26]

An alternative option to cohorting is the use of a temporary isolation room. This commercially available alternative can be used for contact precautions and droplet precautions. It is not designed to replace the use of a single room, but rather to be an alternate option when a single room is not available.[27] Although it is not suitable for providing healthcare to critically ill patients, mainly due to the limited size of the room and visibility of equipment, it creates a biomedically engineered alternate option that can address shortages in single rooms. However, for the patient it may be less comfortable, being warmer than the outside area, and give a sense of confinement not experienced in the open ward area.[27]

CASE STUDY 1

Recognising and applying transmission-based precautions

Deidre Butler, a 72-year-old woman, has been diagnosed with vancomycin-resistant enterococci (VRE). She has been placed in a single room with ensuite facilities as she is suffering with diarrhoea and has experienced some faecal incontinence. You observe a fellow healthcare worker walk into the room without wearing any PPE or performing hand hygiene. The healthcare worker helps Deidre to sit up in bed, then their mobile phone rings. They withdraw the mobile phone from their pocket and take the call. After finishing the call, they return to the doorway, grab a pair of gloves and put them on as they return to the room.

1. What type of precautions should be implemented for Deidre Butler?
2. List the errors that the healthcare worker made.
3. What should the healthcare worker have done?

14.5 Personal protective equipment

Personal protective equipment (PPE) includes gloves, gowns, masks/respirators and eye protection (goggles or safety shield). Various combinations of PPE are used, depending on the potentially infectious agent, the route of transmission and, consequently, the type of precautions implemented. The required PPE has previously been identified for each category of TBPs. Personal protective equipment is also used with standard precautions, as outlined in the previous chapter. The difference is that, for standard precautions, the healthcare worker needs to identify potential risks of exposure to blood and body substances and use appropriate PPE. However, with TBPs, the PPE is specific to the mode of transmission.[28]

PPE is designed to form a barrier between the healthcare worker and the contaminated item or potentially infectious agent,[12] protecting skin, airways and mucous membranes.[9] As well, it serves to prevent transmission of infection to a healthcare worker's hands, skin and clothing,[9] and to patients and others.

A quick glance at the hierarchy of hazard controls (Fig 14.4) demonstrates that PPE is a weak hazard control measure, but the other options are not all appropriate

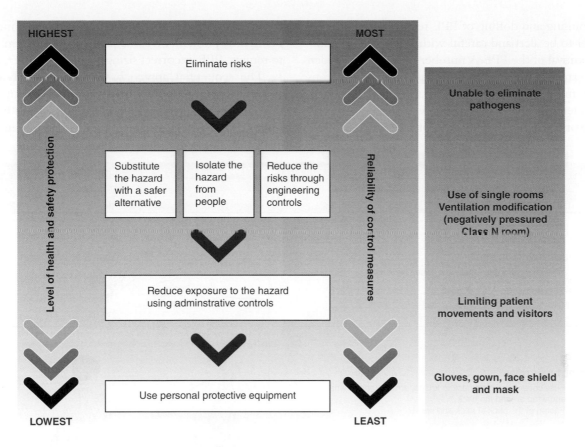

FIGURE 14.4 Hierarchy of hazard controls

Source: Safe Work Australia . Available from: https://www.safeworkaustralia.gov.au/system/files/documents/1901/code_of_practice_-_how_to_manage_work_health_and_safety_risks_1.pdf

when managing people with infectious diseases. Therefore, a combination of controls is the best option. It would not be possible to eliminate the hazard; consequently, alternate control measures, though less effective, need to be considered. As previously discussed, engineering controls such as single rooms to isolate a patient or ventilation modification are adopted. As well, limiting patient movements and visitors provides some administrative control.[4] PPE is effective when correctly used, but is a weak hazard control measure;[29] vigilance is required to ensure it provides an effective barrier.

Recognising when to wear PPE and which forms of PPE to use is essential for personal protection and prevention of transmission of infection. Previous studies have shown that healthcare workers are likely to miss some elements of PPE[30] and a suitable approach to reduce the likelihood of omitting items is to take a risk-based approach.[31]

The NHMRC[9] identifies the following risk factors to guide decisions about PPE:

- the probability of contamination by blood, body substances, secretions and excretions

- the specific body substance involved
- the probable type and probable route of transmission of the infectious agents.

Issues to consider include correct choice of protection, correct wearing and correct removal (doffing) of the PPE. Contingency plans in the event of a PPE failure, such as a glove perforation,[32] also need to be considered. Immediately following the specific purpose for which the PPE was used, it should be removed before leaving the area and discarded to prevent transmission.[9]

14.5.1 Putting on and removing PPE

There is a sequence of putting on (donning) and removing (doffing) PPE that will depend on the PPE required, determined by the risk of exposure to blood or body substances or the transmission of infection. It is important to check local policies and guidelines, as the order for putting on and removing PPE can vary slightly. However, the goals of applying and removing PPE remain unchanged, being to apply the appropriate PPE to ensure it protects you and then to remove it, without risk of contamination.

Donning and doffing of PPE requires the healthcare worker to be alert and careful with both the application and removal of the PPE. A number of studies have identified errors in the perception of risk, proper choice, use and donning of PPE.[31,33,34] Similarly, significant errors were identified when doffing PPE, resulting in healthcare worker self-contamination of clothing and hands from PPE.[28,34-37] Factors that influenced errors included being time poor, incorrect sequencing, insufficient room to remove PPE, incorrect sizing, and the level of training.

The sequential approach to donning and doffing PPE is designed to reduce errors and risk of contamination. The order for donning and doffing is outlined in Figure 14.5 and follows the sequence recommended by

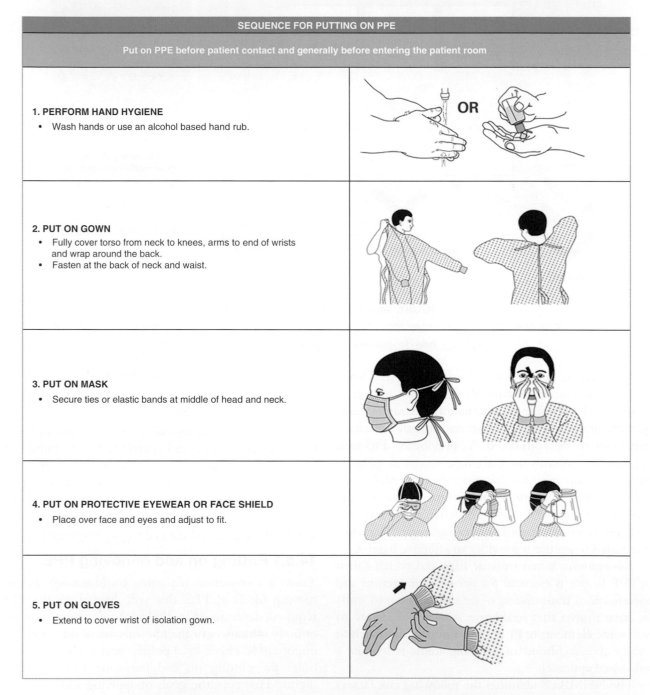

SEQUENCE FOR PUTTING ON PPE

Put on PPE before patient contact and generally before entering the patient room

1. PERFORM HAND HYGIENE
- Wash hands or use an alcohol based hand rub.

2. PUT ON GOWN
- Fully cover torso from neck to knees, arms to end of wrists and wrap around the back.
- Fasten at the back of neck and waist.

3. PUT ON MASK
- Secure ties or elastic bands at middle of head and neck.

4. PUT ON PROTECTIVE EYEWEAR OR FACE SHIELD
- Place over face and eyes and adjust to fit.

5. PUT ON GLOVES
- Extend to cover wrist of isolation gown.

FIGURE 14.5 Example of sequence for donning and doffing personal protective equipment
Source: National Health & Medical Research Council. Australian Guidelines for the Prevention and Control of Infection in Healthcare (2019). pp. 130–131.

the NHMRC.[9] The NHMRC also recommends that PPE be donned before patient contact and before entering a patient's room. Sequencing may differ slightly, dependent on the required PPE and local guidelines.

PPE should be removed at the doorway to the patient's room or in the anteroom, if available.[9] Importantly, there should be sufficient space to be able to remove the PPE without self-contamination[36,38] and hand hygiene needs to be observed in the correct sequencing.[28,34,37] To reduce doffing errors, a buddy system where staff can observe and identify potential errors has been encouraged and proven effective in some contexts.[39,41]

A closer look at each item of PPE follows. The discussion will highlight its application to TBPs and important considerations related to each item.

14.5.2 Gloves

The purpose of gloves is to provide a barrier to protect healthcare workers' hands. As well, gloves serve as a barrier to protect patients from transmission of pathogens on healthcare workers' hands. Gloves are normally single use, appropriate for the purpose and used when:

- they could encounter blood or body fluid, mucous membrane, non-intact skin, or other potentially infectious substances
- performing invasive procedures or contacting sterile sites
- providing direct contact to patients requiring any type of TBP
- handling or touching patient care equipment or environmental surfaces that are potentially or visibly contaminated.[9,12]

The choice of glove is important. First, it must be appropriate for the planned task. *If the task is an invasive procedure or involves contact with a sterile site, then choose sterile gloves.* Otherwise, non-sterile single use gloves should be used. Second, consider the glove material. Most often, gloves are made with natural rubber latex; however, some healthcare workers or patients can have latex sensitivity. Alternate synthetic materials should then be used.[9] Third, gloves should be close-fitting around the wrist,[12] correctly sized for hands[31,36] and nails should be short, fingers without rings to avoid glove perforation.[42] This avoids the risk of hands being contaminated, either during the procedure due to perforation or due to self-contamination on removal.[31,36,42]

Before applying gloves, or any other PPE, hand hygiene must be performed. It must be repeated again, immediately after removal of gloves.[9] When wearing gloves, they need to be changed between procedures and exposure to body substances for the same patient, an action that is frequently overlooked.[43,44] They need to be changed between patients and before touching any portable equipment, such as a computer keyboard, before it is moved to another location.[9]

When removing gloves, ensure there is a disposal receptacle at hand and be mindful that gloves are contaminated,[45,46] and removal of gloves can lead to self-contamination. Accidentally touching the outside of a glove with bare hands is a commonly reported mistake.[34,36] Box 14.3 outlines the procedure for removing disposable gloves.

14.5.3 Gowns/aprons

After gloves, gowns or aprons are the most frequently used PPE. Their purpose is to protect the clothing and arms of healthcare workers from blood and body fluids, along with contaminated surfaces.[9,12]

Gowns are used for all types of TBPs. The choice of gown or apron (see Table 14.4) will depend on the planned activity, but for TBPs, the gown should be single use and impervious to fluid.[9]

The gown is the first piece of PPE to be donned, regardless of the type of TBPs, prior to entering the patient's room or patient care area. Gowns should cover the torso from neck to mid-thigh as well as the arms.[9,12] Correct size is important to prevent contamination;[36,47] therefore, a range of sizes should be available. They are tied at the neck and waist[9] to avoid risk of contamination, an action sometimes overlooked.[17,18,48]

The sequence for removal of the gown will depend on the type of transmission-based precaution and PPE

BOX 14.3 Removal of disposable gloves

1. With one gloved hand, pinch up the outside of the glove near the wrist on the alternate hand, and carefully peel off
2. Hold the removed glove in the remaining gloved hand
3. Slide fingers of the un-gloved hand under the remaining gloved hand at the inner aspect of the wrist
4. Peel the glove back over itself, folding the first glove inside the second glove
5. Discard in waste receptacle
6. Perform hand hygiene.[9,12]

TABLE 14.4 Gown and apron uses and recommendations

Type	Recommended use
Plastic, single use aprons	General use to protect from possibility of spray, spills or exposure to blood or body substances for low-risk procedures During contact precautions when patient contact is likely
Impervious single use gown	Protection of healthcare worker's exposed body areas and prevention of contamination of clothing with blood, body substances or potentially infectious materials
Full long-sleeved, impervious single use gown	Worn when risk of healthcare worker contacting a patient's broken skin, extensive skin-to-skin contact, risk of contact with uncontained blood and body substances
Sterile gown	Worn for procedures that require a sterile field

being used. If the PPE includes safety glasses as well as gloves, then the gown is the last piece of PPE to be removed. Where a mask is also worn, it will be removed before the mask.[9]

The front and sleeves of the gown should be treated as contaminated.[45,46] Avoid touching the front of the gown with your un-gloved hands, a common error when doffing a gown.[18,33] Gowns should be untied at the neck and waist, then touching the inside only, carefully pulled away from the neck and shoulders, turning the gown inside out (see Fig 14.4). Still touching the inside of the gown, fold or roll it into a small bundle and dispose of it immediately.[9]

14.5.4 Eye and face protection

Earlier in this chapter, we reviewed the chain of transmission. The mucous membrane of eyes, nose and mouth are a portal of entry for pathogens.[3] Therefore, creating a barrier, when there is a risk of splash or spray of blood or body substances, is an element of standard precautions. Examples of situations when splash or spray may occur include coughing, sneezing, vomiting or procedures such as suctioning airways, dental procedures and surgery.[49] As well, it applies to TBPs, where the risk of contamination is equal. Unfortunately, eye protection is often the most overlooked element of PPE,[30,50] thus putting the healthcare worker at risk of contamination.

Eye and face protection are provided by face shields or safety glasses that can be disposable or non-disposable. The protection may also include a surgical mask, discussed below. The type of protection chosen is determined against the risk of contamination; therefore, the task to be performed will guide the decision.[9,49]

When choosing a face shield, it should be full face length from forehead to chin and wrap around the face to the ears. Ideally, there should be sufficient space

under the shield to accommodate a mask and optical glasses, if required.[9,12,49]

Advantages of face shields include the ease of donning and doffing, less fogging than with safety glasses, covers a large portion of the face, and is able to be worn with facial hair. As well, being transparent, patients can observe facial expressions and lip movements; however, some face shields create glare and they do not provide a seal around the face.[49]

If wearing a mask, face shields or safety glasses are donned after the mask, otherwise after donning the gown. The sequence for removal of the face shield or safety glasses is immediately after hand hygiene, which follows removal of gloves. As with all PPE, the outside of the safety glasses or face shield is contaminated.[9] Therefore, only touch the ties, headband or earpieces. Carefully place the face shield or safety glasses in the container for reprocessing or, if disposable, in the waste receptacle.[9,12]

Non-disposable face shields and safety glasses need to be cleaned following the manufacturer's instructions, then allowed to dry before being stored. If they require higher level disinfection, a Therapeutic Goods Administration (TGA) approved sterilant should be used, or alternatively, medical device disinfectant—low level, or follow AS/NZS 4187: 2014 if heat is needed.[9]

14.5.5 Face masks and respirators

As with any other piece of PPE, there are some important considerations to achieve effective protection. The mask should not be removed until outside the patient care area. It should be immediately disposed of in a closed receptacle.[9] Hand hygiene must be performed immediately after disposal of mask.

Facial hair can be an issue in attempting to create an adequate seal. The NHMRC advises that a powered air-purifying respirator (PAPR) should be used when facial hair prevents establishing a seal,[9] as they only filter inhaled air.

As with other pieces of PPE, the outside of the mask can potentially be contaminated.[38] Therefore, the following practice points need to be followed:

1. Always change masks between patients
2. Change masks as soon as they become soiled or wet
3. Once the mask is removed, discard. Do not reuse it
4. Never leave the mask hanging around the neck
5. Do not touch the front of the mask while wearing it
6. Perform hand hygiene if the mask is touched or immediately after discarding.[9]

When applying a mask/respirator in conjunction with other PPE, it is usually donned after the gown (see Fig. 14.5). Place it over the face and tie or secure the bands at the middle of the head and neck. Some masks/respirators may have elastic that loops around the ears. Press the mask/respirator over the bridge of the nose to improve the fit and protection.[9]

When removing the mask/respirator, it is the final piece of PPE to be removed.[9] Remember, the front of the mask/respirator is contaminated,[38] so do not touch it. Think of it as a vacuum filter, where all the contaminants are caught on the outside, so it is extremely contaminated. Therefore, carefully grasp the bottom, then top tie or elastic and remove away from the face. Discard in the waste receptacle, touching only the ties. Immediately perform hand hygiene.[9]

Another consideration is the choice of respiratory protection. This should be considered within the context of its use and the type of TBPs in effect. A variety of masks/respirators are outlined below, with details on their usage.

Surgical masks: Surgical masks are technically face protection, providing protection to the mucosal lining of the mouth and nose. They are part of the range of PPE used for standard precautions. As well, they are used when droplet precautions are in place, protecting the healthcare worker from respiratory secretions[9] and the potential for respiratory infection.[30] However, due to the design of the mask, being more loose fitting, they do not protect healthcare workers from inhalation of aerosol particles.[31] Therefore, surgical masks are only suitable for droplet precautions, not airborne precautions.

Surgical masks may be provided to coughing patients as part of the approach to respiratory hygiene.

The purpose is to reduce dissemination of potentially infectious respiratory droplets.[12] Where a surgical mask is required by a child, it needs to be a mask specifically designed for children. As well, the child's oxygen saturation needs to be monitored.[9]

There are three levels of surgical mask, determined by the effectiveness of the mask as a barrier. They are categorised as follows:

- *Level 1 mask*—routinely used to protect healthcare workers and/or patients from the risk of droplet transmission. They are not recommended when there is a risk of blood or body splash
- *Level 2 mask*—used in dentistry, in emergency departments, and where there is minimal risk of blood droplet exposure, such as when changing dressings on small or healing wounds
- *Level 3 mask*—used for all surgical procedures or in any area where the healthcare worker is at risk of blood or body fluid splashing in their face. This includes first aid in major trauma situations. The level 3 mask provides the most protection from blood and body fluid.

Therefore, choice of mask should match the risk and the required purpose.

Particulate filter respirators (P2/N95): There is a range of N95/P2 respirators and respirator styles. This is because they are used beyond healthcare as PPE in industry where a worker may be exposed to fine dust particles. In healthcare, that same purpose is to protect the healthcare worker from small airborne particles and droplet nuclei.[9] The P2 respirator is required to meet standards outlined in the AS/NZS 1715: 2009 and has 4–5 layers, including central layers that are electrostatic. Air drawn through the respirator is filtered through mechanical impaction and electrostatic capture. It is important to consider size and style, as fit is important. The P2 respirator is removed by grasping hold of the tapes at the back of the head and carefully removing without touching it.

The fit test: There are two types of fit test checks—one is qualitative, and the other is quantitative. The quantitative test is described in AS/NZS 1715:2009 Standard and requires a trained operator with special equipment. The purpose of the fit test is to assess for any leakage of air into the respirator and is described as a pass/fail result, generated by the response to the test agent.[51] An annual review of the fit test is required, and it assumes that the same respirator is consistently used.

The qualitative testing is subjective and influenced by the wearer.[9,51] It requires special solutions and equipment but is a much quicker process. The commercial solution contains 45% sodium saccharin and 95% water.[51] The healthcare worker applies the P2 respirator then the solution is sprayed towards them at varying angles. A failure occurs when the healthcare worker can taste the slightly sweet solution. The respirator is deemed to be an acceptable fit when the healthcare worker is unable to taste the solution.

The fit check: A further step, a fit check, is performed and is described in Figure 14.6. It is a self-check, assessing for facial seal and any air leaks and uses a positive and negative pressure test.[52] The fit check should be performed every time a healthcare worker applies a P2 respirator.[9] It requires the healthcare worker to fit the respirator over the mouth and nose. The lower tapes are tied or fitted behind the neck, with the upper tapes tied or fitted above the ears to

the crown of the head. The respirator is then pressed around the bridge of the nose, the cheeks and face.

Once applied, the positive pressure seal is checked by gently exhaling. Adjust the respirator if air escapes. The negative pressure check requires the healthcare worker to gently inhale. The respirator should be drawn in towards the face. If this does not occur, check for air leaks around the face, adjust the tapes, and check for any defects of the respirator.[9]

Other masks/respirators: *Elastomeric masks* are available as half or full fitting face pieces and may provide an alternative to the P2 respirator. They are made from synthetic or rubber materials and provide a tight seal around the face when fit tested. They can be cleaned, disinfected and reused.[53] Although reuse may be an attractive option, the elastomeric mask requires ongoing maintenance. This includes cleaning and disinfection of all the face mask parts including

PRINCIPLES OF FIT CHECKING
HOW TO DON AND FIT CHECK **P2** AND **N95** MASKS
A P2 and N95 mask offers protection from diseases spread by airborne transmission: February 2020

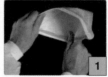

1 SEPARATE THE EDGES OF THE MASK TO FULLY OPEN IT

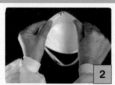

2 BEND THE NOSE WIRE TO FORM A GENTLE CURVE. THE NOSE WIRE REPRESENTS THE TOP OF THE MASK

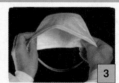

3 HOLD THE MASK UPSIDE DOWN TO EXPOSE THE TWO HEADBANDS

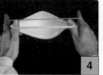

4 USING YOUR INDEX FINGERS AND THUMBS, SEPARATE THE TWO HEADBANDS

5 WHILE HOLDING THE HEADBANDS CUP THE MASK UNDER YOUR CHIN

6 PULL HEADBANDS UP AND OVER YOUR HEAD

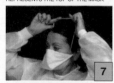

7 PLACE AND POSITION THE LOWER HEADBAND AT THE BASE OF YOUR NECK (UNDER YOUR EARS)

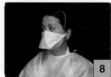

8 PLACE THE UPPER HEADBAND ON THE CROWN OF YOUR HEAD. THE BAND SHOULD RUN JUST ABOVE THE TOP OF YOUR EARS

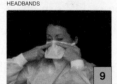

9 GENTLY CONFORM/PRESS THE NOSEPIECE ACROSS THE BRIDGE OF YOUR NOSE BY PRESSING DOWN WITH FINGERS UNTIL THE FIT IS SNUG

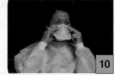

10 CONTINUE TO ADJUST THE MASK UNTIL YOU FEEL YOU HAVE ACHIEVED A GOOD AND COMFORTABLE FACIAL FIT.

A 'fit check' must be performed each time a P2 / N95 mask is worn

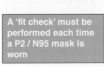

1 GENTLY INHALE. WHEN YOU BREATHE IN THE MASK SHOULD DRAW IN SLIGHTLY TOWARD THE FACE AND COLLAPSE.

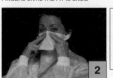

2 WHEN EXHALING THE MASK SHOULD FILL UP WITH AIR. IT IS IMPORTANT AT THIS STAGE TO CHECK THERE IS NO AIR LEAKAGE AROUND THE EDGES OF THE MASK.
CONTINUE ADJUSTING THE SEAL OF THE MASK IF NEEDED.

If you have not achieved a successful fit as instructed above it is important that you seek advice or have someone assist you with fitting and checking your mask.
An incorrectly fitted mask will not provide you with the intended level of protection from airborne infectious diseases.

Brands of P2 / N95 masks may have slight variation. Always refer to the manufacturer's instructions.

Adapted from the NSW Infection Control Resource Centre.

NSW GOVERNMENT | CLINICAL EXCELLENCE COMMISSION

FIGURE 14.6 The fit check

Source: Adapted with permission © NSW Clinical Excellence Commission 2020.

the straps, valves and valve covers. Follow the cleaning instructions provided by the manufacturer and consider advice on how to decontaminate with disinfectants before purchasing an elastomeric mask. It is also recommended that filter components be replaced when they become soiled, clogged or damaged.[53]

Powered air purifying respirators (PAPR) come as a tight-fitting respirator, or as a loose-fitting hood or helmet.[54] These respirators are battery powered and designed to purify the air breathed by using a positive airflow to push air through high-efficiency particulate air (HEPA) filter cartridges or cannisters into the wearer's breathing zone.[54,55] They have a higher assigned protection factor than the P2/N95 respirators and are recommended for use with aerosol-generating procedures.[54] When being used, there are some challenges with communication and mobility, and without proper maintenance there is the risk of battery failure;[54] however, the loose-fitting hood can be worn with facial hair.[56] Consider advice about cleaning and decontamination from the manufacturer before purchasing PAPRs.

Fabric masks should not be considered equal to surgical masks and are not worn by healthcare workers in the healthcare context. Fabric masks are usually made of three layers of fabric material, with recommendations that the outer layer use a water-resistant fabric, such as polyester/polypropylene.[57] Some fabric masks are commercially produced; however, many are homemade and therefore it is not possible to identify the efficiency of the mask to protect a person from respiratory transmission of infection. What is known suggests they provide some protection,[58] especially in confined spaces where social distancing is more difficult.[59] Examples include hotels, public transport and places of worship.

Similar to other masks, after being worn, the fabric mask is contaminated. Therefore, it is important to educate the public to take care to remove the mask using the tapes or elastic and place the soiled mask into a plastic bag until laundering. As well, it is important to emphasise the need for hand hygiene after touching the mask and removal for laundering.[59]

14.6 A shifting paradigm

14.6.1 Droplet or airborne precautions?

At first glance, the principles behind how we designate droplet and airborne precautions appear to be straightforward. We have discussed the size of the particle or droplet that is transmitted as the guide to how we designate the type of precaution required. But what if this can change, depending on what we are doing? For instance, will droplet precautions be sufficient protection when we are suctioning an airway or administering nebulised medications? These are examples of aerosol-generating procedures (AGPs), along with others listed in Box 14.4. An AGP or behaviour is something that generates aerosols that could be smaller in size and/or remain suspended in the air for longer periods. For some people this could include shouting, singing, coughing or sneezing and, as such, increases the risk of transmission of pathogens to healthcare workers.[60] There is much debate about what constitutes an aerosol-generating procedure or behaviour. Note that the examples of potential aerosol-generating procedures provided in Box 14.4 should not be considered exhaustive. There are other human activities and procedures that generate aerosols. The dichotomous way of defining transmission as 'droplet' or 'airborne' is becoming outdated. A more contemporary approach would be to consider using the term 'aerosols', which can be large or very small. The implications of the size of aerosols helps govern the precautions required.

There is evidence that some AGPs and/or behaviours are linked to airborne transmission of pathogens. Consequently, the approach is to be cautious and based on a risk assessment, which considers individual (patient) factors as well as context. Context includes considering important issues such as ventilation, crowding, proximity and time of exposure.

BOX 14.4 Potential aerosol-generating procedures (AGPs)

- Intubation/extubation
- Cardiopulmonary resuscitation
- Tracheostomy
- Ventilation, including non-invasive and manual ventilation
- Bronchoscopy
- Airway suctioning
- Oxygen administration
- Nebulised medication

14.6.2 Does one size fit all with multidrug-resistant organisms?

Contact precautions are routine practice when managing a patient with methicillin-resistant *Staphylococcus aureus* (MRSA) or vancomycin-resistant enterococci (VRE). But are they really necessary? Consider the following scenario.

CASE STUDY 2

Applying contact precautions for multidrug-resistant organisms

In one room you have a patient, Mr Kirby, who has an infected surgical wound. A wound swab revealed that it is *Staphylococcus aureus* and is sensitive to antibiotics. Normal standard precautions are applied. In the single room across the corridor, another patient, Mr Jones, has an infected surgical wound. The wound swab had revealed it was *S. aureus*, but resistant to a range of antibiotics, that is, MRSA. Therefore, contact precautions were initiated. Both patients have *S. aureus*, and the route of transmission will be the same.

1. Why, then, are we instituting contact precautions for only one of the patients, Mr Jones?

2. Is it ethically justifiable to isolate only one patient if the route of transmission remains the same?

Some would argue that it is more difficult to treat MRSA, therefore extra precautions are required. However, evidence suggests that the use of contact precautions does not reduce the incidence of MRSA or VRE.[61,62] Furthermore, it has been suggested that inappropriate use of gloves and other PPE increases the potential for transmission of infection.[63,64] Similarly, an Australian study found that good hand hygiene, using alcohol-based hand rub, was sufficient to effectively remove MRSA from contaminated hands,[65] and increase hand hygiene compliance.[66]

Consider, if the evidence is weak for the use of contact precautions for MRSA and VRE, there is minimal justification for removing a patient's liberty and confining them to a single room.[67] The use of PPE is documented as time consuming[68,69] and impersonal.[68] The patient experience includes stigma leading to mental health symptoms, particularly in the healthcare setting.[70,71] As well, patients under contact precautions experience more adverse events than other patients.[72]

This evidence seems at odds with current guidelines and practice for the management of MROs. Therefore, does that mean we ignore the guidelines? It does suggest we base our practice on evidence. As well, it supports a broader approach to infection prevention and control, where a reduction in MRSA and VRE has been linked to a horizontal approach that incorporates all patients and is hospital-wide. It includes a bundle approach to medical and nursing procedures, a bare below the elbows approach, automatic discontinuation of urinary catheters and other devices after a specified period, bathing with chlorhexidine gluconate and hospital-wide improvements to infection prevention and control.[62] Including guidelines on when to stop contact precautions is also recommended.[73]

14.7 Other considerations

14.7.1 Influence of leadership and culture

The leadership and culture of an organisation can be influential in creating and sustaining a safe environment.[74] Adherence to TBPs is influenced by provision of the necessary resources, including sufficient human resources and time to practise the necessary precautions and follow correct donning and doffing procedures.[74-76] As well, it requires communication that is built on trust, mutual support for each other and collaboration. Strong clinical leadership and positive role modelling will result in a proactive approach, where healthcare workers own the solutions that prevent transmission of infection,[74,77,78] rather than accepting any lapses as normal and acceptable.[79] Concepts of professional obligation and accountability should also be fostered as part of the culture of the organisation and individual healthcare professions.[78]

Therefore, strong leadership and a culture of safety will provide a good foundation for adherence to TBPs and PPE. When it becomes encultured as a 'norm' in the clinical setting or workplace, fellow healthcare workers will support each other to achieve adherence.[79]

14.7.2 Healthcare worker education

Coupled with leadership is education. Though not a new concept, it is widely recognised that knowledge leads to empowerment,[80] a good foundation for proactive healthcare workers to own transmission-based precaution processes.[74]

Education of healthcare workers should include details explaining why processes are followed.[18,28] Providing justifications has the potential to improve recognition of risk associated with transmission of infection and, therefore, the level of protection required.[33] As well, learning how to appropriately don and doff PPE, by developing skills with hands-on training, is recommended as an approach to reduce donning and doffing errors.[18,28,33,34] This could be included in clinical skills assessment tests,[28] adding validity to the process and promoting confidence with the PPE, so enabling optimal use.[77]

As well, educating healthcare workers on healthcare-acquired infections can better inform them of appropriate precautions to adopt. In turn, this supports healthcare workers to provide adequate and accurate information to patients, as well as reducing their own anxieties around potential contamination.[81]

14.7.3 Patient and family perspectives

Any type of TBPs is an uncomfortable experience for patients. It is probable that the patient will be placed in a single room. Single room accommodation has been linked to poorer health outcomes, including adverse events such as patient falls and medication errors, though not consistently.[76,82] Other reports suggest delays in healthcare workers' response to care needs such as toileting, and delays in addressing pain experienced by the patient and any care that required a timely response.[83,84] As well, patients with dementia or other cognitive impairment can create challenges with understanding the need for TBPs or cooperating with it.[76]

Furthermore, patients placed in some form of isolation experienced increased negative feelings about themselves including depression and some reports of anxiety.[76,85] Stigmatisation and fears of contaminating others, associated with healthcare-associated infections such as MRSA and CDI, have also been reported.[81]

Another aspect to consider is the patient's family or visitors when TBPs apply. Signage alone may not be sufficient to inform and educate visitors.[86] Visitors are more likely to use the required PPE when healthcare workers advise them on what to do.

Therefore, healthcare workers should regularly check on the clinical condition of patients on TBPs and be responsive to requests for help. A positive and supportive attitude to patients, using effective therapeutic communication, will create an environment that supports their mental wellbeing, an aspect of care not to be overlooked. Finally, educating family and visitors to wear correct PPE, and providing correct information about appropriate behaviours, is important to ensure the risk of contamination is addressed.

14.7.4 Ethics of transmission-based precautions

Transmission-based precautions pose some ethical issues. The precautions remove a patient's liberty to move around and their autonomy to make certain choices.[76] The removal of autonomy, which is a bioethical principle, is supported by another ethical stance, referred to as 'The doctrine of double effect'. In essence, it is justifying harm to certain individuals, providing there is an overall benefit to others.[87] The harm has been identified as the lack of attention to clinical needs[76,82,83] and is counter to the ethical principles of beneficence and non-maleficence,[67] or as the Hippocratic Oath suggests, 'to do the patient no harm'. However, the harm is counter-balanced by the reduction in transmission of infection, thus protecting an extended group of people from an infectious disease.

Another consideration is the ethical principle of justice. It refers to treating people equally and without prejudice, being fair, and ensuring benefits and burdens are equitably distributed.[88] The acquisition of an infection is in itself unfair, without the additional imposition of TBPs.[67] As well, there are those who might have, but are yet to be diagnosed with, an infectious disease and they are not managed with TBPs.[67,76] A further consideration, in terms of justice, relates to the allocation of single rooms when there are insufficient rooms and, therefore, who should be allocated a single room and who should cohort together.[76] Linked to this are those situations where it is impossible to provide any form of segregation, thus potentially exposing others to the risk of transmission of an infectious agent and failing to meet the ethical principles of beneficence and non-maleficence.

14.7.5 The ethics of finite resources

As a consequence of outbreaks, the resources required to manage a situation may not match the available resources. A hospital will have a finite number of single rooms and even less with specialised air handling. Thus, there are situations where advice from the infection prevention and control staff may require one patient to be removed from isolation for another patient who is considered a higher priority due to the increased risk of transmission of a pathogen. There may also be a shortage of equipment and consumables, resulting in frustration and compromise.[40]

The goal of infection prevention and control is always to prevent and control infectious disease. Thus, thinking of the doctrine of double effect, inevitably some will experience inconvenience and potentially harm, to ensure that a greater number of people remain safe and free of an infectious disease. That is the basis of TBPs.

Conclusion

This chapter commenced by considering the historical practices that have led to transmission-based precautions. With a safety-risk approach, the principles of transmission-based precautions were outlined, with particular emphasis on key attributes, such as P2 respirators for airborne precautions. A detailed explanation of the types of PPE and practices for donning and doffing PPE were provided, again taking a safety-risk approach to prevent contamination. Finally, other considerations appropriate to the implementation and practice of transmission-based precautions were explored.

At all times, a critical and informed approach that identifies the risks involved will support safer practice. In turn, this will reduce the risk of transmission of infection and provide safer healthcare.

Useful websites/resources

- Australasian College for Infection Prevention and Control. https://www.acipc.org.au/
- Centers for Disease Control and Prevention. https://www.cdc.gov/infectioncontrol/guidelines/isolation/index.html
- Clinical Excellence Commission. https://www.cec.health.nsw.gov.au/keep-patients-safe/infection-prevention-and-control/healthcare-associated-infections/policies,-guidelines-and-handbook
- My Health learning videos (CEC). https://www.cec.health.nsw.gov.au/keep-patients-safe/COVID-19/personal-protective-equipment/ppe-training-videos
- National Health & Medical Research Council. https://www.nhmrc.gov.au/about-us/publications/australian-guidelines-prevention-and-control-infection-healthcare-2019
- New Zealand Ministry of Health. https://www.health.govt.nz/our-work/diseases-and-conditions/covid-19-novel-coronavirus/covid-19-information-specific-audiences/covid-19-personal-protective-equipment-workers/personal-protective-equipment-use-health-and-disability-care-settings
- Queensland Health. https://www.health.qld.gov.au/clinical-practice/guidelines-procedures/diseases-infection/infection-prevention
- SA Health. https://www.sahealth.sa.gov.au/wps/wcm/connect/public+content/sa+health+internet/clinical+resources/clinical+programs+and+practice+guidelines/infectious+disease+control
- Tasmanian Department of Health PPE videos. https://www.dhhs.tas.gov.au/publichealth/tasmanian_infection_prevention_and_control_unit/healthcare_worker_education/proper_use_of_personal_protective_equipment
- Victoria (VICNISS). https://www.vicniss.org.au/media/2159/covid-19_how-to-put-on-and-take-off-your-ppe.pdf
- WA Health. https://ww2.health.wa.gov.au/-/media/Files/Corporate/general-documents/Infectious-diseases/PDF/Coronavirus/COVID19-PPE-Poster.pdf

References

1. Risse GB. Mending bodies, saving souls: a history of hospitals. New York: Oxford University Press, 1999.
2. McNeill WH. Plagues and peoples. New York: Penguin Books, 1976.
3. Centers for Disease Control and Prevention. Principles of epidemiology in public health practice, lesson 1: introduction to epidemiology. 3rd ed. Atlanta, Georgia: CDC, 2012. Available from: https://www.cdc.gov/csels/dsepd/ss1978/lesson1/section10.html.
4. Reddy SC, Valderrama AL, Kuhar DT. Improving the use of personal protective equipment: applying lessons learned. Clin Infect Dis. 2019;69(Supplement_3):S165-S170.
5. Clack L, Passerini S, Manser T, Sax H. Likelihood of infectious outcomes following infectious risk moments during patient care—an international expert consensus study and quantitative risk index. Infect Control Hosp Epidemiol. 2018;39(3):280-289.
6. Gregory L, Weston LE, Harrod M, Meddings J, Krein SL. Understanding nurses' workflow: batching care and potential

opportunities for transmission of infectious organisms, a pilot study. Am J Infect Control. 2019;47(10):1213-1218.

7. Chang N-CN, Reisinger HS, Schweizer ML, Jones I, Chrischilles E, Chorazy M, et al. Hand hygiene compliance at critical points of care. Clin Infect Dis. 2020;72(5).811 820.

8. Chang N-C, Jones M, Reisinger HS, Schweizer ML, Chrischilles E, Chorazy M, et al. Hand hygiene and the sequence of patient care. Infect Control Hosp Epidemiol. 2021:1-6.

9. National Health & Medical Research Council. Australian guidelines for the prevention and control of infection in healthcare. NHMRC, 2019.

10. Zimmerman P-A, Browne M, Rowland D. Instilling a culture of cleaning: effectiveness of decontamination practices on non-disposable sphygmomanometer cuffs. J Infect Prev. 2018;19(6):294-299.

11. Knecht VR, McGinniss JE, Shankar HM, Clarke EL, Kelly BJ, Imai I, et al. Molecular analysis of bacterial contamination on stethoscopes in an intensive care unit. Infect Control Hosp Epidemiol. 2019;40(2):171-177.

12. Siegel JD, Rhinehart E, Jackson M, Chiarello L. The healthcare infection control practices advisory committee. 2007 guideline for isolation precautions: preventing transmission of infectious agents in healthcare settings. In: Prevention CfDCa, ed. Atlanta, Georgia: CDC, 2007.

13. John A, Alhmidi H, Cadnum JL, Jencson AL, Donskey CJ. Contaminated portable equipment is a potential vector for dissemination of pathogens in the intensive care unit. Infect Control Hosp Epidemiol. 2017;38(10):1247-9.

14. Telford B, Healy R, Flynn E, Moore E, Ravi A, Geary U. Survey of isolation room equipment and resources in an academic hospital. Int J Health Care Qual Assur. 2019; 32(6):991-1003.

15. Katanami Y, Hayakawa K, Shimazaki T, Sugiki Y, Takaya S, Yamamoto K, et al. Adherence to contact precautions by different types of healthcare workers through video monitoring in a tertiary hospital. J Hosp Infect. 2018; 100(1):70-75.

16. Barker AK, Cowley ES, McKinley L, Wright M-O, Safdar N. An in-room observation study of hand hygiene and contact precaution compliance for Clostridioides difficile patients. Am J Infect Control. 2019;47(10):1273-1276.

17. Harrod M, Petersen L, Weston LE, Gregory L, Mayer J, Samore MH, et al. Understanding workflow and personal protective equipment challenges across different healthcare personnel roles. Clin Infect Dis. 2019;69(Supplement_3): S185-S191.

18. Krein SL, Mayer J, Harrod M, Weston LE, Gregory L, Petersen L, et al. Identification and characterization of failures in infectious agent transmission precaution practices in hospitals: a qualitative study. JAMA Int Med. 2018; 178(8):1016-1022.

19. Hor SY, Hooker C, Iedema R, Wyer M, Gilbert GL, Jorm C, et al. Beyond hand hygiene: a qualitative study of the everyday work of preventing cross-contamination on hospital wards. BMJ Qual Saf. 2017;26(7):552-558.

20. Arriero GD, Taminato M, Kusahara DM, Fram D. Compliance to empirical contact precautions for multidrug-resistant microorganisms. Am J Infect Control. 2020;48(7):840-842.

21. Wilson N, Corbett S, Tovey E. Airborne transmission of COVID-19. BMJ. 2020;370:m3206.

22. Radonovich LJ, Jr, Simberkoff MS, Bessesen MT, Brown AC, Cummings DAT, Gaydos CA, et al. N95 respirators vs medical masks for preventing influenza among health care personnel: a randomized clinical trial. JAMA. 2019;322(9): 824-833.

23. Choi JS, Kim KM. Predictors of respiratory hygiene/cough etiquette in a large community in Korea: a descriptive study. Am J Infect Control. 2016;44(11):e271-e273.

24. Australasian Health Infrastructure Alliance. Australasian health facility guidelines, part D infection prevention and control. North Sydney: Australasian Health Infrastructure Alliance, 2015.

25. Victorian Advisory Committee on Infection Control. Guidelines for the classification and design of isolation rooms in health care facilties. In: Department of Human Services, ed. Melbourne: State Government of Victoria, 2007.

26. Abad CL, Barker AK, Safdar N. A systematic review of the effectiveness of cohorting to reduce transmission of healthcare-associated C. difficile and multidrug-resistant organisms. Infect Control Hosp Epidemiol. 2020;41(6):691-709.

27. Mitchell BG, Williams A, Wong Z. Assessing the functionality of temporary isolation rooms. Am J Infect Control. 2017; 45(11):1231-1237.

28. Phan LT, Maita D, Mortiz DC, Weber R, Fritzen-Pedicini C, Bleasdale SC, et al. Personal protective equipment doffing practices of healthcare workers. J Occup Environ Hyg. 2019; 16(8):575-581.

29. SafeWork Australia. Identify, assess and control hazards. Safe Work Australia, 2020. Available from: https://www.safeworkaustralia.gov.au/risk.

30. Mitchell R, Roth V, Gravel D, Astrakianakis G, Bryce E, Forgie S, et al. Are health care workers protected? An observational study of selection and removal of personal protective equipment in Canadian acute care hospitals. Am J Infect Control. 2013;41(3):240-244.

31. Jones RM, Bleasdale SC, Maita D, Brosseau L. A systematic risk-based strategy to select personal protective equipment for infectious diseases. Am J Infect Control. 2020;48(1):46-51.

32. Hübner N-O, Goerdt A-M, Mannerow A, Pohrt U, Heidecke C-D, Kramer A, et al. The durability of examination gloves used on intensive care units. BMC Infect Dis. 2013;13(1):1.

33. Harrod M, Weston LE, Gregory L, Petersen L, Mayer J, Drews FA, et al. A qualitative study of factors affecting personal protective equipment use among health care personnel. Am J Infect Control. 2020;48(4):410-415.

34. Kwon JH, Burnham C-AD, Reske KA, Liang SY, Hink T, Wallace MA, et al. Assessment of healthcare worker protocol deviations and self-contamination during personal protective equipment donning and doffing. Infect Control Hosp Epidemiol. 2017;38(9):1077-1083.

35. Chughtai AA, Chen X, Macintyre CR. Risk of self-contamination during doffing of personal protective equipment. Am J Infect Control. 2018;46(12):1329-1334.

36. Gurses AP, Dietz AS, Nowakowski E, Andonian J, Schiffhauer M, Billman C, et al. Human factors–based risk analysis to improve the safety of doffing enhanced personal protective equipment. Infect Control Hosp Epidemiol. 2019; 40(2):178.

37. Mumma JM, Durso FT, Casanova LM, Erukunuakpor K, Kraft CS, Ray SM, et al. Common behaviors and faults when doffing personal protective equipment for patients with serious communicable diseases. Clin Infect Dis. 2019; 69:S214-S20.

38. Phan LT, Sweeney D, Maita D, Moritz DC, Bleasdale SC, Jones RM. Respiratory viruses on personal protective equipment and bodies of healthcare workers. Infect Control Hosp Epidemiol. 2019;40(12):1356-60.

39. Phua J, Weng L, Ling L, Egi M, Lim C, Divatia J, et al. Intensive care management of coronavirus disease 2019

(COVID-19): challenges and recommendations. Lancet Respir Med. 2020;8(5):506-517.

40. Rajamani A, Subramaniam A, Shekar K, Haji J, Luo J, Bihari S, et al. Personal protective equipment preparedness in Asia-Pacific intensive care units during the coronavirus disease 2019 pandemic: a multinational survey. Aust Crit Care. 2021;34(2):135-141.

41. Picard C, Edlund M, Keddie C, Asadi L, O'Dochartaigh D, Drew R, et al. The effects of trained observers (dofficers) and audits during a facility-wide COVID-19 outbreak: a mixed-methods quality improvement analysis. Am J Infect Control. 2021;49(9):1136-1141.

42. Al-Amad S, El-Saleh A, Elnagdy S, Al-Nasser F, Alsellemi S. Fingernail length as a predisposing factor for perforations of latex gloves: a simulated clinical experiment. East Mediterr Health J. 2019;25(12):872-877.

43. Wałaszek M, Kołpa M, Różańska A, Wolak Z, Bulanda M, Wójkowska-Mach J. Practice of hand hygiene and use of protective gloves: differences in the perception between patients and medical staff. Am J Infect Control 2018;46(9): 1074-1076.

44. Baloh J, Thom KA, Perencevich E, Rock C, Robinson G, Ward M, et al. Hand hygiene before donning nonsterile gloves: healthcareworkers' beliefs and practices. Am J Infect Control. 2019;47(5):492-497.

45. Jackson SS, Thom KA, Magder LS, Stafford KA, Johnson JK, Miller LG, et al. Patient contact is the main risk factor for vancomycin-resistant Enterococcus contamination of healthcare workers' gloves and gowns in the intensive care unit. Infect Control Hosp Epidemiol. 2018;39(9):1063-1067.

46. Nadimpalli G, O'Hara LM, Pineles L, Lebherz K, Johnson JK, Calfee DP, et al. Patient to healthcare personnel transmission of MRSA in the non–intensive care unit setting. Infect Control Hosp Epidemiol. 2020;41(5):601-603.

47. Baloh J, Reisinger HS, Dukes K, da Silva JP, Salehi HP, Ward M, et al. Healthcare workers' strategies for doffing personal protective equipment. Clin Infect Dis. 2019;69(Supplement_3): S192-S198.

48. Drews FA, Visnovsky LC, Mayer J. Human factors engineering contributions to infection prevention and control. Hum Factors. 2019;61(5):693-701.

49. Roberge RJ. Face shields for infection control: a review. J Occup Environ Hyg. 2016;13(4):235-242.

50. Williams VR, Leis JA, Trbovich P, Agnihotri T, Lee W, Joseph B, et al. Improving healthcare worker adherence to the use of transmission-based precautions through application of human factors design: a prospective multi-centre study. J Hosp Infect. 2019;103(1):101-105.

51. Mitchell BG, Wells A, McGregor A, McKenzie D. Can homemade fit testing solutions be as effective as commercial products? Healthc Infect. 2012;17(4):111-114.

52. Regli A, von Ungern-Sternberg B. Fit-testing of N95/P2-masks to protect health care workers. Med J Aust. 2020; 213(7):293-295.

53. Centers for Disease Control and Prevention. Elastometric respirators: strategies during conventional and surge demand situations: Atlanta, Georgia: CDC, 2020. Available from: https://www.cdc.gov/coronavirus/2019-ncov/hcp/elastomeric-respirators-strategy/index.html.

54. Licina A, Silvers A. Use of powered air-purifying respirator (PAPR) as part of protective equipment against SARS-CoV-2-a narrative review and critical appraisal of evidence. Am J Infect Control. 2021;49(4):492-499.

55. Roberts V. To PAPR or not to PAPR? Can J Respir Ther. 2014;50(3):87-90.

56. Centers for Disease Control and Prevention. Considerations for optimizing the supply of powered air-purifying respirators. Atlanta, Georgia: CDC, 2020. Available from: https://www.cdc.gov/coronavirus/2019-ncov/hcp/ppe-strategy/powered-air-purifying-respirators-strategy.html.

57. Department of Health. How to make a cloth mask. In: Health Do, ed. Canberra: Australian Government, 2020.

58. Ho KF, Lin LY, Weng SP, Chuang KJ. Medical mask versus cotton mask for preventing respiratory droplet transmission in micro environments. Sci Total Environ. 2020;735:139510.

59. Department of Health. Face masks: how they protect you and when to use them. In: Health Do, ed. Canberra: Australian Government, 2020.

60. O'Mahony HR, Martin DS. An anaesthetic and intensive care perspective on infection control measures for the prevention of airborne transmission of SARS-CoV-2. Br J Hosp Med. 2020;81(9):1-9.

61. Furuya EY, Cohen B, Jia H, Larson EL. Long-term impact of universal contact precautions on rates of multidrug-resistant organisms in ICUs: a comparative effectiveness study. Infect Control Hosp Epidemiol. 2018;39(5):534-540.

62. Bearman G, Abbas S, Masroor N, Sanogo K, Vanhoozer G, Cooper K, et al. Impact of discontinuing contact precautions for methicillin-resistant staphylococcus aureus and vancomycin-resistant enterococcus: an interrupted time series analysis. Infect Control Hosp Epidemiol. 2018;39(6):676-682.

63. Burdsall DP, Gardner SE, Cox T, Schweizer M, Culp KR, Steelman VM, et al. Exploring inappropriate certified nursing assistant glove use in long-term care. Am J Infect Control. 2017;45(9):940-945.

64. Loveday HP, Lynam S, Singleton J, Wilson J. Clinical glove use: healthcare workers' actions and perceptions. J Hosp Infect. 2014;86(2):110-116.

65. Jain S, Clezy K, McLaws M-L. Safe removal of gloves from contact precautions: the role of hand hygiene. Am J Infect Control. 2018;46(7):764-767.

66. Cusini A, Nydegger D, Kaspar T, Schweiger A, Kuhn R, Marschall J. Improved hand hygiene compliance after eliminating mandatory glove use from contact precautions—is less more? Am J Infect Control. 2015;43(9):922-927.

67. Harris J, Walsh K, Dodds S. Are contact precautions ethically justifiable in contemporary hospital care? Nurs Ethics. 2019; 26(2):611-624.

68. Godsell MR, Shaban RZ, Gamble J. "Recognizing rapport": health professionals' lived experience of caring for patients under transmission-based precautions in an Australian health care setting. Am J Infect Control. 2013;41(11):971-975.

69. Martin EM, Russell D, Rubin Z, Humphries R, Grogan TR, Elashoff D, et al. Elimination of routine contact precautions for endemic methicillin-resistant staphylococcus aureus and vancomycin-resistant enterococcus: a retrospective quasi-experimental study. Infect Control Hosp Epidemiol. 2016; 37(11):1323-1330.

70. Rump B, De Boer M, Reis R, Wassenberg M, Van Steenbergen J. Signs of stigma and poor mental health among carriers of MRSA. J Hosp Infect. 2017;95(3): 268-274.

71. Day HR, Perencevich EN, Harris AD, Gruber-Baldini AL, Himelhoch SS, Brown CH, et al. Depression, anxiety, and moods of hospitalized patients under contact precautions. Infect Control Hosp Epidemiol. 2013;34(3):251-258.

72. Martin EM, Bryant B, Grogan TR, Rubin ZA, Russell DL, Elashoff D, et al. Noninfectious hospital adverse events decline after elimination of contact precautions for MRSA and VRE. Infect Control Hosp Epidemiol. 2018;39(7):788-796.

73. Banach DB, Bearman G, Barnden M, Hanrahan JA, Leekha S, Morgan DJ, et al. Duration of contact precautions for acute-care settings. Infect Control Hosp Epidemiol. 2018;39(2):127-144.

74. Dubé E, Lorcy A, Audy N, Desmarais N, Savard P, Soucy C, et al. Adoption of infection prevention and control practices by healthcare workers in Québec: a qualitative study. Infect Control Hosp Epidemiol. 2019;40(12):1361-1366.

75. Kim H, Hwang YH. Factors contributing to clinical nurse compliance with infection prevention and control practices: a cross-sectional study. Nurs Health Sci. 2020;22(1):126-133.

76. Gould DJ, Drey NS, Chudleigh J, King MF, Wigglesworth N, Purssell E. Isolating infectious patients: organizational, clinical, and ethical issues. Am J Infect Control. 2018;46(8):e65-e9.

77. Barratt R, Gilbert GL, Shaban RZ, Wyer M, Hor SY. Enablers of, and barriers to, optimal glove and mask use for routine care in the emergency department: an ethnographic study of Australian clinicians. Australas Emerg Care. 2020; 23(2):105-113.

78. Gilbert GL, Kerridge I. The politics and ethics of hospital infection prevention and control: a qualitative case study of senior clinicians' perceptions of professional and cultural factors that influence doctors' attitudes and practices in a large Australian hospital. BMC Health Serv Res. 2019; 19(1):212.

79. Fix GM, Reisinger HS, Etchin A, McDannold S, Eagan A, Findley K, et al. Health care workers' perceptions and reported use of respiratory protective equipment: a qualitative analysis. Am J Infect Control. 2019;47(10):1162-1166.

80. Bradbury-Jones C, Sambrook S, Irvine F. Power and empowerment in nursing: a fourth theoretical approach. J Adv Nurs. 2008;62(2):258-266.

81. Currie K, Melone L, Stewart S, King C, Holopainen A, Clark AM, et al. Understanding the patient experience of health care-associated infection: a qualitative systematic review. Am J Infect Control. 2018;46(8):936-942.

82. Simon M, Maben J, Murrells T, Griffiths P. Is single room hospital accommodation associated with differences in healthcare-associated infection, falls, pressure ulcers or medication errors? A natural experiment with non-equivalent controls. J Health Serv Res Policy. 2016;21(3): 147-155.

83. Siddiqui ZK, Conway SJ, Abusamaan M, Bertram A, Berry SA, Allen L, et al. Patient isolation for infection control and patient experience. Infect Control Hosp Epidemiol. 2019; 40(2):194-199.

84. Chittick P, Koppisetty S, Lombardo L, Vadhavana A, Solanki A, Cumming K, et al. Assessing patient and caregiver understanding of and satisfaction with the use of contact isolation. Am J Infect Control. 2016;44(6):657-660.

85. Hereng O, Dinh A, Salomon J, Davido B. Evaluation in general practice of the patient's feelings about a recent hospitalization and isolation for a multidrug-resistant infection. Am J Infect Control. 2019;47(9):1077-1082.

86. Seibert G, Ewers T, Barker AK, Slavick A, Wright MO, Stevens L, et al. What do visitors know and how do they feel about contact precautions? Am J Infect Control. 2018; 46(1):115-117.

87. Bryan CS, Call TJ, Elliott KC. The ethics of infection control: philosophical frameworks. Infect Control Hosp Epidemiol. 2007;28(9):1077-1084.

88. Butts JB, Rich KL. Nursing ethics across the curriculum and into practice. 4th ed. Burlington MA: Jones & Bartlett, 2016.

CHAPTER 15

Environmental cleaning

MARTIN KIERNAN[i]

Chapter highlights

- A contaminated healthcare environment increases the risk of pathogen transmission to vulnerable patients and clients
- Cleaning and in some cases disinfection processes mitigate this risk
- A cleaning and decontamination bundle approach reduces infections and is cost-effective
- It is critical that processes are monitored for effectiveness and fed back to staff undertaking cleaning in a non-punitive manner

i   Richard Wells Research Centre, University of West London, London, UK

Introduction

It is now accepted that microorganisms found in the healthcare environment are implicated in transmission of healthcare-associated infections (HAIs).[1] Multiple studies have demonstrated this relationship, and large-scale multicentre randomised trials have demonstrated the effectiveness of cleaning and environmental decontamination in terms of actual reductions in HAIs in addition to being a cost-effective intervention.[2,3]

In a relatively short period of time there has been a change in attitudes towards the role of the environment in transmission of pathogens. In 2004, a systematic review[4] concluded that the evidence base for the role of the environment was poor. A further review ten years later came to the opposite conclusion due to a huge increase in the volume of published literature in high quality, peer-reviewed journals.[5] A growing body of evidence of increasingly higher quality, including randomised controlled trials (RCTs), now supports an intuitive view that the environment in which healthcare interventions are undertaken plays a role in the transmission of nosocomial pathogens.[6] Interrupting the chain of transmission, where pathogenic organisms move from a source or reservoir to a vulnerable recipient, is key to any infection prevention and control (IPC) program. Critical components of an IPC strategy aimed at preventing transmission by breaking this chain include hand and environmental hygiene. Patients acquire organisms from the hands of staff and from the environment in which they are being cared for.[6] Once a patient becomes colonised with a pathogen, these organisms can gain access to vulnerable sites such as intravenous lines, urinary catheters and surgical wounds.[7] Reducing contamination of hands and the environment interrupts the chain of transmission and reduces the risk of transmission of organisms from one patient to another.[8-10]

The natural reservoir for many disease-causing pathogens is the human body itself and millions of organisms are shed from the skin and bodily orifices each day. In the absence of cleaning or other forms of decontamination, pathogens can persist in the hospital environment for up to 30 months.[11] Even after these processes take place, healthcare environments are repeatedly recontaminated by microorganisms dispersed from infected/colonised patients, staff and visitors, many of whom are not known to be colonised/infected. The number and range of potential pathogens present in the environment is determined by a range of factors, including the number of people in the environment, the type and volume of activity, whether the surfaces are vertical or horizontal, and whether the surface or item is directly in contact with a source of microorganisms. Other important factors relate to the surfaces on which microorganisms may be deposited, such as whether the surface is rough or smooth—the latter making it easier to clean.

A number of organisms that remain viable in the environment are now recognised as clinically significant. An increasing body of scientific evidence suggests that a contaminated environment plays an important role in the spread of microorganisms and if not cleaned/disinfected on a regular basis, may act as a reservoir for potential pathogens. Potential pathogens carried by humans shed extensively into the environment during medical procedures and patient care activities[12] and these organisms transfer to patients and the hands of staff following contact with environmental surfaces.[10] Further work has demonstrated a risk to subsequent occupants of a room if adequate cleaning and decontamination does not occur.[13]

15.1 Evidence that the environment poses a risk of transmission

Routes of transmission of pathogenic organisms between patients may involve contact with contaminated surfaces,[14] either directly or via contact with healthcare workers who themselves are in contact with the environment.[15,16] A systematic review examining risk of cross-infection to a subsequent occupant of a room previously occupied by a patient known to be colonised with a specific pathogen demonstrated up to a five-fold risk of transmission.[17] Analysis of the papers included in this review demonstrates that suboptimal or ineffective cleaning was likely implicated in this increased risk.[18]

As scientific methods of microorganism identification have developed, so does the evidence base, and whole genome sequencing studies have demonstrated a clear link between healthcare-associated infection (HAI) and contaminated environments,[19] building on former work that demonstrates that organisms responsible for HAI, including MRSA, *C. difficile*, norovirus and VRE, survive and persist on hospital surfaces in numbers sufficient to be transferred to patients either through direct contact or via the hands of healthcare workers.[20,21]

Transmission and infection are therefore a significant risk, and given that the infectious dose for many potential pathogenic organisms appears to be low,[22] it is reasonable to attempt to reduce contamination levels to the minimum possible. For example, for *Staphylococcus aureus* less than 15 cells were required for infection in experimental lesions, less than seven *C. difficile* spores were sufficient to cause CDI[23] and a single norovirus particle is considered able to cause infection—impressive when one considers the volume of particles released when symptom episodes occur.[24] These organisms can persist on surfaces for long periods of time, even years,[11] hence the importance of cleaning and disinfection to minimise the risk of transmission and infection in vulnerable patients.[21,25-29] The survival of microorganisms in the clinical environment is outlined in Table 15.1.[11]

15.1.1 The importance of environmental biofilms

Microorganisms do not live as dispersed individual cells, they accumulate and attach to surfaces forming communities known as biofilms.[30] This is particularly true for bacteria and fungi. Biofilms are ubiquitous in the general environment and may be viewed as slime in wet environments; however, their presence in the healthcare environment is now also considered an area of interest. Both dry and wet biofilms have been implicated in transmission of pathogens.[31,32] Biofilm formation is also not limited to clinically relevant bacteria, and emerging pathogenic fungi such as *Candida auris* have also been shown to form biofilm in the environment.[33] Biofilms can be decontaminated by some disinfectants, including some chlorine-releasing formulations and peracetic acid; however, mechanical action is always required to remove dry biofilm, as biofilm removal from the environment is not straightforward. Studies have demonstrated persistence of multidrug-resistant organisms (MROs) for a year in dry biofilm invisible to the naked eye, even after multiple attempts at terminal cleaning with chlorine.[34,35]

15.2 Key considerations for a cleaning program

When determining what a local cleaning program for a healthcare provider facility should look like, it has been suggested that there are a number of key components.[36] These include the following aspects:

1. A facility-wide risk assessment, including the risk to patients/residents and how susceptible they may be to infection. Secondly, a surface risk profile (the probability of the environment becoming contaminated with pathogens and potential for exposure and/or indirect transmission, and frequency of hand contacts). Thirdly, a pathogen risk profile of the predominant organisms of concern and their likely transmission routes.

2. Disinfectants and equipment selection will be based on the risk assessment. Consider how the identified risks could be mitigated through the use of appropriate agents. Consider cost-effectiveness when doing this also, especially when deciding whether automated room decontamination is necessary. At this point, also consider human factors and whether the methods selected are practically implementable in the facility.

3. The cleaning process and training are critical to success, including adequate staffing ratio, remuneration, equipment, training, supervision and team interactions.

4. Communication between cleaning, clinical and managerial staff has been demonstrated to significantly enhance standards of cleanliness and is critical to the success in building and fostering a team approach. Effective cleaning comes from a team approach rather than the actions of an individual.[3]

5. Assessment of cleanliness should be continuous and used to drive improvement and detect systemic failures in systems or processes that may then be remedied. These assessments should examine not only household-type items but also include clinical equipment that is shared between

TABLE 15.1 Survival of pathogens in healthcare environments

Pathogen	Survival time
S. aureus (including MRSA)	7 days to >12 months
Enterococcus spp. (including VRE)	5 days to >48 months
Acinetobacter spp.	3 days to 11 months
Clostridium difficile (spore form)	>5 months
Norovirus	8 hours to 28 days (temperature-dependent)
Pseudomonas aeruginosa	6 hours to 16 months
Klebsiella spp.	2 hours to >30 months

patients. The results of all cleaning audits should be shared in a non-punitive way with the staff undertaking the cleaning. For further information see the section 'Assessing the effectiveness of environmental cleaning' in this chapter.

15.3 Assessment of level of risk for cleaning and decontamination

The physical environment and equipment within it should be in a good state of repair and non-porous to ensure that cleaning and decontamination procedures are effective. Damaged equipment is impossible to effectively decontaminate.

Assessment of the level of risk is dependent on a number of factors, including the type of procedures to be undertaken in the area, the characteristics of the patient group, the degree of vulnerability of the group and the intelligence from surveillance data that indicates the likely prevalent pathogens.

All equipment should be cleaned and if necessary disinfected in line with the manufacturer's instructions in order to ensure that materials used are compatible with the equipment so as to prevent damage occurring. All equipment that has a requirement for cleaning or decontamination should be supplied with comprehensive instructions on decontamination methods and with a list of compatible agents. If a manufacturer cannot supply adequate information, the item should not be purchased. Equipment must be cleaned by a suitably trained person in a standardised manner after each patient use. Equipment must always be cleaned prior to maintenance in order to protect staff undertaking service or repairs and should be tagged with a decontamination certificate specifying this.

15.3.1 Risk assessment

When considering what procedures need to be undertaken, what equipment and supplies are required, a risk assessment is required. Risk assessment in the context of cleaning means a consideration of the following aspects:

1. What is the known/suspected pathogen? (recognising that not all infections yield a positive microbiology result)

2. What are the potential reservoirs/sources of this organism? (e.g. human, environmental)

3. How may this organism be transmitted, and does it survive well in the environment?

4. What are the physical characteristics of the area to be cleaned? (e.g. single room, multi-occupancy area, toilet or bathing facilities, where high-risk invasive procedures are performed)

5. Is there enough time to adequately decontaminate the area to make it safe for the next occupant?

6. What is the level of risk to patients/persons within this area? (e.g. high risk, such as an intensive care unit, or lower risk, such as a care setting in which invasive medical devices are not used)

7. What agents within the local policy are effective for this organism?

8. Are the agents to be used compatible with the surfaces that require decontamination?

9. Are there any staff health considerations for the use of the selected agents?

10. Are there considerations for the use of the selected method? (e.g. if using an automated system like UV-C or hydrogen peroxide vapour, the area must be completely vacated)

In many cases, a healthcare provider organisation will use local or national guidance to construct a risk assessment that a local guidance for cleaning is based on. Should a situation arise that is not covered by the local policy/procedures, a multidisciplinary team including infection prevention specialists, cleaning specialists and management should undertake a risk assessment for this novel situation.

15.4 Cleaning/decontamination principles and procedures

To make the healthcare environment safe for care of patients, and for the performance of medical and nursing procedures that increase risk because of their invasive nature, cleaning and, in some cases, disinfection should take place. Cleaning means the removal of contamination from an item to a level required either for the intended ensuing use or for its further processing, for example disinfection or sterilisation. Cleaning normally involves a combination of physical and chemical actions and results in a reduction of physical soil. Soil in the context of cleaning and environmental cleaning means contamination of any type, from invisible microorganisms to visible 'dirt' or grime. It does not mean that a surface is free from microorganisms however, and so in some cases a further step, known as disinfection, may be required. Disinfection is an interim stage on from cleaning before sterilisation (complete absence of all microorganisms), and is a process that results in a reduction of microorganisms to a level not thought to be harmful.

15.4.1 The action of detergents

To remove soil from a surface or item, a detergent (or soap) is often applied in the presence of water or another solvent. A surfactant is a compound that lowers the surface tension (or interfacial tension) between two liquids, between a gas and a liquid, or between a liquid and a solid. Surfactants may act as detergents, wetting agents, emulsifiers, foaming agents, or dispersants and the term comes from a combination of the words 'surface', 'active' and 'agent'. Surfactants may be cationic (positively charged), anionic (negatively charged) or non-ionic. Anionic surfactants used in the manufacturing of liquid soaps and detergents may also exhibit antibacterial efficiency because of a dual functionality. The hydrophobic side of these surfactants can dissolve the outer layer of viruses and bacteria, while the hydrophilic side dissolves in water.[37] These agents act as emulsifiers to remove contamination.

A commercially available detergent is a formulation of surfactants which, when mixed in a dilute form, facilitates the removal of soil adherent to a surface. It does this through a variety of mechanisms, but primarily by the formulation acting on surfaces to reduce surface tension to mix the soil into an emulsion that then can either be rinsed or wiped away. A range of components of formulations used in cleaning can be seen in Table 15.2.

Similarly, a soap is also a formulation of surfactants that is less water-soluble than a detergent. Soaps are a mixture of agents with an oil base, whereas detergents are formulated by combining chemical compounds in a mixer.

15.4.2 The action of disinfectants

Biocide literally means 'kills life' and in the context of environmental decontamination means a substance that causes cellular destruction through chemical, mechanical or biological action. Disinfectants are biocides used on surfaces that have an ability to inhibit or inactivate microorganisms. These biocides are classified according to their general chemical types, including alcohols, aldehydes, oxidising agents and halogens. Their general features are described in Table 15.3.

15.4.3 The action of common disinfectant groups

Oxidising agents: Biocides that possess oxidising ability are widely used and include the halogens (chlorine, hypochlorites, bromine and iodine) and peroxygens (chlorine dioxide, peracetic acid, hydrogen peroxide and ozone). In a process called oxidation they remove electrons from a substance, themselves gaining electrons. The result of this on whole cells includes bacterial kill through loss of structure and cellular integrity, cytoplasmic leaks (bactericidal) and inhibition of multiplication (bacteriostasis).[38] In addition to effectiveness against vegetative microorganisms, oxidising agents may also have

TABLE 15.2 Components of a detergent formulation

Component	Action	Examples
Solvent	A liquid used to dissolve soil that is also capable of dissolving other agents for incorporation into a formulation	Water, alcohol, ether
Surfactants	Surfactants (**Surf**ace-**act**ing-ag**ent**s) reduce surface tension at interfaces such as between solid and a gas (air), act as wetting agents, loosen contaminants and reduce foam production. They may be anionic, cationic or non-ionic and are widely used in industry	Sodium laureth sulphate, benzalkonium chloride, cetylpyridinium chloride, dialkyldimethylammonium chloride
Emulsifiers	Substances that stabilise emulsion by increasing kinetic stability. Surfactants may be used as emulsifiers	Sodium stearoyl lactylate
Corrosion inhibitors	Decreases the corrosion rate of a material, typically a metal, that comes into contact with a fluid	Sodium benzoate, calcium gluconate
Chelating agents	Prevents the deposition of mineral salts on a surface	Ethylenediaminetetraacetic acid (EDTA), phosphates

TABLE 15.3 Features of disinfectants

Feature	Description
Range of action	Broadly effective against vegetative (actively metabolising) and spore forms (including viruses); dependent on the specific biocide and exposure conditions (including contact time)
Toxicity to other life forms	Normally toxic to mammals, plants and other life forms; level of toxicity often dependent on concentration
Mode of action	Differs from antibiotics (which normally have only one target) by having multiple targets that can include lipids, proteins, nucleic acids and carbohydrates. Actions are classified as oxidising agents, cross-linking agents, and agents that specifically bind to and disrupt the structure of macromolecules
Stability when 'in-use'	Often degrade rapidly, particularly in the presence of soil and other organic contamination
Type of use	Directly onto a surface or into a liquid; may also be aerosolised to settle on surfaces inaccessible by direct application
Factors that affect activity level	Sensitive to a range of factors including concentration and dilution effects, pH, temperature, humidity, formulation, age of the biocide, and presence of interfering substances
Potential to develop resistance	Limited due to multiple modes of action, particularly in formulations of multiple disinfectants

sporicidal activity. Hydrogen peroxide and peracetic acid activity depends on infiltration into the spore coat and an associated reaction with the spore coat DNA.

Cross-linking agents: Agents such as aldehydes, phenolics, alkylating agents (ethylene oxide) and alcohols cause interactions between macromolecules, particularly proteins and nucleic acids, that lead to loss of structure and function. Alcohols are uncomplicated complexes that possess a hydroxyl (-OH) group attached to a hydrocarbon chain. Short-chained alcohols, including agents commonly used in healthcare such as isopropanol, n–propanol and ethanol, are used as antiseptics and disinfectants. Since alcohols are water and lipid soluble, they also have a rapid effect on surface and membrane-associated proteins.[38]

Other structure-disrupting agents: Biocides that act by disrupting the structures and functions of specific macromolecules include surfactants, quaternary ammonium compounds (QACs) and biguanides (such as chlorhexidine). Surfactants may have hydrophobic (water-repelling, non-polar or lipophilic) and hydrophilic (water-attracting, polar or lipophilic) portions. There are a large number of QACs, each with different activity, and they are extensively used as household, industrial, food preparation and general

healthcare surface disinfectants as they have a dual action of cleaning and disinfection. The full chemical name often describes the structure of the specific agent. QACs are not sporicidal.

Advantages and disadvantages of commonly used disinfectants in healthcare: There is a wide range of disinfectants available from which to select a product appropriate for an intended use; however, each has advantages and disadvantages in terms of mode of action, efficacy against some classes of microorganism and degree of compatibility with a range of surfaces. These are tabulated in Table 15.4, adapted from Rulata and Weber (2019).[39]

15.4.4 Susceptibility of microorganisms to disinfectants

Some organisms are more difficult to destroy than others and there is an accepted hierarchy of susceptibility[40] (Fig 15.1).

15.4.5 Product selection considerations

When choosing a product, the optimal choice will depend on a number of factors. These include:

- What is the target organism? If the target is vegetative bacteria, a number of disinfectants may be suitable; however, spores are difficult to penetrate and destroy and so a sporicidal

TABLE 15.4 Advantages and disadvantages of disinfectants

Disinfectant	Advantages	Disadvantages
Alcohol	Bactericidal, tuberculocidal, fungicidal, virucidal Fast acting Non-corrosive No staining Used to disinfect small surfaces such as rubber stoppers on medication vials No toxic residue	Not sporicidal Microbicidal activity affected by organic matter Slow acting against non-enveloped viruses (e.g. norovirus) unless high % No detergent or cleaning properties Damage some instruments (e.g. harden rubber, deteriorate glue) Flammable (large amounts require special storage) Evaporates rapidly making contact time compliance difficult Not recommended for use on large surfaces Outbreaks ascribed to contaminated alcohol
Chlorine	Bactericidal, tuberculocidal, fungicidal, virucidal Sporicidal (in high concentrations) Fast acting Inexpensive (in dilutable form) Non-flammable Unaffected by water hardness Reduces biofilms on surfaces Relatively stable (e.g. 50% reduction in chlorine concentration in 30 days) Used as a disinfectant in water treatment	Reaction hazard with acids and ammonias (cannot be used for urine spills) Leaves salt residue Corrosive to metals (some ready-to-use products may be formulated with corrosion inhibitors) Unstable active (some ready-to-use products may be formulated with stabilisers to achieve longer shelf life) Microbicidal activity affected by organic matter Discolours/stains fabrics May cause respiratory, skin and eye irritation Odour Irritating at high concentrations
Improved (or accelerated) hydrogen peroxide	Bactericidal, tuberculocidal, fungicidal, virucidal Fast efficacy Easy compliance with wet-treatment times Safe for workers (lowest EPA toxicity category, IV) Benign for the environment No staining EPA-registered Non-flammable	More expensive than most other disinfecting actives Not sporicidal at low concentrations Some materials compatibility issues
Iodophors	Bactericidal, mycobactericidal, virucidal Non-flammable Used for disinfecting blood culture bottles	Not sporicidal Shown to degrade silicone catheters Requires prolonged contact to kill fungi Stains surfaces Used mainly as an antiseptic rather than disinfectant
Phenolics	Bactericidal, tuberculocidal, fungicidal, virucidal Inexpensive (in dilutable form) No staining Non-flammable EPA-registered	Not sporicidal Absorbed by porous materials and irritate tissue Depigmentation of skin caused by certain phenolics Hyperbilirubinemia in infants when phenolic not prepared as recommended
Quaternary ammonium compounds (e.g. benzalkonium chloride, didecyl dimethyl ammonium bromide, dioctyl dimethyl ammonium bromide)	Bactericidal, fungicidal, virucidal against enveloped viruses (e.g. HIV) Good cleaning agents Surface compatibility good No staining Persistent antimicrobial activity when undisturbed Inexpensive	Not sporicidal In general, not tuberculocidal and virucidal against non-enveloped viruses High water hardness and cotton/gauze can make less microbicidal A few reports document asthma as result of exposure to benzalkonium chloride Microbicidal activity affected by organic matter Absorption by cotton, some wipes may diminish microbicidal activity

TABLE 15.4 Advantages and disadvantages of disinfectants—cont'd

Disinfectant	Advantages	Disadvantages
Peracetic acid/ hydrogen peroxide	Bactericidal, fungicidal, virucidal and sporicidal at 3500 ppm (e.g. *Clostridium difficile*) Active in the presence of organic material. Environmentally friendly by-products (acetic acid, O_2, H_2O) Surface compatibility good	Lack of stability in liquid form Potential for material incompatibility (e.g. brass, copper) More expensive than most other disinfecting actives Odour may be irritating Can cause mucous membrane and respiratory health effects

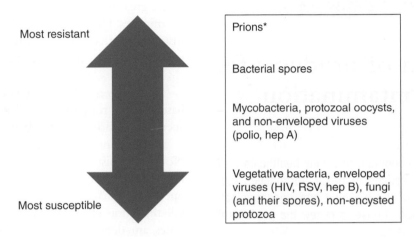

Most resistant

Most susceptible

Prions*

Bacterial spores

Mycobacteria, protozoal oocysts, and non-enveloped viruses (polio, hep A)

Vegetative bacteria, enveloped viruses (HIV, RSV, hep B), fungi (and their spores), non-encysted protozoa

FIGURE 15.1 Hierarchy of organism susceptibility

* Prions are abnormal, pathogenic agents that are transmissible and are able to induce abnormal folding of specific normal cellular proteins called prion proteins that are found most abundantly in the brain. Being proteins and not living cells in the normal sense of the word, they are very difficult to destroy and physical removal is therefore the only way of reducing contamination.

disinfectant may be required. Always check test data against the target organism. You may not find the exact organism; however, test organisms that are selected for standard testing are used by international standards organisations to be a proxy for that class of organism.

- Do you need a virucidal product? Enveloped viruses are easier to destroy than non-enveloped viruses. Some fungi, *Candida auris* for example, are also more difficult to eradicate and manufacturers should be able to supply test data demonstrating efficacy.
- What is the range of compatibility with surfaces? Some disinfectants can damage surfaces, depending on a number of factors including concentration. Always check disinfectant compatibility with the manufacturer of a product that requires

decontamination to ensure that suitable products will be available.

- Is the product likely to be effective when used in the setting? Products are tested for efficacy in laboratories using standard international test methods. Always check that the product has been tested under simulated 'dirty' conditions, as that is more likely to replicate real life. Also, look at the quoted 'contact time' (see the following section for more detailed information) to check that it will be possible for the disinfectant to remain in contact with the surface or item to be decontaminated for enough time.
- Has the product been tested in accredited or respected university laboratories for efficacy? Disinfectant testing is complex and so should always be carried out in laboratories with

accredited and accepted expertise in this specific field.

- Are there any potential staff health issues? Some disinfectants, like chlorine, have been known to cause respiratory issues in some staff members, depending on the degree of exposure and concentrations used. Always check the safety data sheets to look for any potential hazards to staff, for example whether specific PPE is also required.

CASE STUDY 1

Selection of products for decontamination

Situation:

You have just been appointed to a new healthcare facility. The environmental services manager approaches you to undertake a review of the cleaning and decontamination products and you also choose to review the products that the clinical staff are using.

Questions:

1   What factors will you consider when making your selection?

2   Who will you discuss the options with?

3   The predominant organisms responsible for healthcare-associated infections are MRSA and multiresistant *Acinetobacter baumanii*. How does this affect your selection?

4   You have an outbreak of *Clostridium difficile*. Do you change products or continue with your original selection?

15.4.6 The importance of contact time for disinfection

What is contact time? The contact time is how long a surface needs to have wet contact with a disinfectant to result in a meaningful reduction (called a 3-log reduction) in microorganisms. This may sound technical, but a 3-log reduction would reduce the number of microorganisms by 99.9%. This means, for example, that 1,000,000 bacteria would be reduced to 1000, and for some (but not all) organisms this would be a low enough amount to reduce the risk of transmission. The higher the log reduction the more effective the product is at reducing microorganisms. Often, the log reduction is dependent on how long the disinfectant remains in contact with the target surface and the organisms on it. This means by observing the contact time or the 'wet time' you are efficiently and effectively disinfecting the surface you are applying your disinfectant product to. Contact times to achieve a meaningful kill for disinfectants range greatly from anything from 10 seconds to 10 minutes. Disinfectant products should include instructions that direct you to ensure that the surface is visibly wet for the recommended contact time.

Recommended contact time for a disinfectant is based on the results of microbiological testing using an accredited laboratory standard testing method.

Disinfectant labels often state several contact times. Not all organisms are killed at the same rate, as they may have different physical characteristics, for example, enveloped viruses have a lipid layer that makes them easier to kill than non-enveloped viruses. The different contact times are dependent on the microorganisms that the product has demonstrated efficacy against, and the length of time to required kill these microorganisms at the concentration in the specific test conditions (which may be clean or simulated 'dirty'). For example, a disinfectant may have a contact time for norovirus of 30 seconds, but the contact time for hepatitis B virus might be 60 seconds. Unless the target microorganism is known, the longest contact time is the one that should be followed since there could be many different microorganisms present on surfaces. Many disinfectants will kill a wide range of microorganisms with a short contact time. This is important as it may be difficult to maintain a wet surface for the contact time that a manufacturer recommends.

Many things affect contact times, including temperatures/humidity/airflow as it can be difficult even for disinfectants with contact times as short as three minutes to remain wet and therefore active, and it is particularly challenging for disinfectants with high alcohol content, which evaporate quickly. If the disinfectant does dry on the surface before the contact time is reached, label instructions usually require reapplication to ensure that the contact or wet time is met. Another critical component of disinfection is prior cleaning, which is necessary to remove material and biofilms to allow the disinfectant to work as intended.

15.5 Single use equipment

The Therapeutic Goods Administration (TGA) advises that a device designated as only for single use must not be reused. It should be used only on an individual patient during a single procedure and then discarded. The 'single use only' (Fig 15.2) sign is present on the packaging of medical devices and equipment. A medical device that is intended for single patient use, for example nebuliser tubing, means that the device may be used for more than one episode of use on one patient only, and may also have a sign indicating this (Fig 15.3). The device should be reprocessed between each use as per the manufacturer's instructions.

Should an establishment decide to reprocess a single use item, the facility should obtain a licence from the TGA and then will be considered a manufacturer under section 41BG(2) of the *Therapeutic Goods Act 1989*.

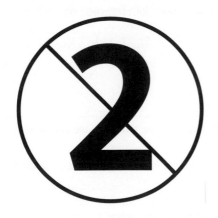

FIGURE 15.2 Single use item symbol

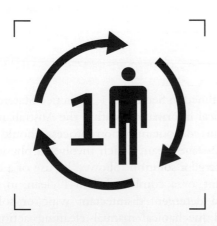

FIGURE 15.3 Single patient use symbol (ISO 15223-2)

15.6 Supporting a safer environment through cleaning and decontamination

The key to providing a safe environment in which to care for patients is to ensure that potentially pathogenic organisms are removed as effectively as possible. In this way, the environment does not become a reservoir of potential pathogens, especially when the environment is inhabited by multiple patients. It is particularly important to make the healthcare environment safe for occupancy by a new patient following the discharge of the previous patient.

The cleaning level required depends on the surfaces and items involved and the risk of contamination. Any surface that is likely to be contaminated with potential pathogens—for example clinical equipment, like vital-signs measuring devices such as blood pressure cuffs—requires cleaning between patient uses, which is more often than general surfaces and fittings.[41] (See Box 15.1.)

15.6.1 The process of cleaning

Although on the face of it cleaning may seem to be quite a simple and straightforward task, a number of important principles should be followed that are infrequently detailed in national decontamination guidelines.

When about to perform any cleaning or decontamination process a systematic approach should be adopted. It has been suggested that a 'Look, Plan, Clean and Dry' approach is a practical method of doing this.[42] (See Table 15.5, modified from Dancer and Kramer (2019).)

15.6.2 Dealing with MROs

Multiresistant organisms (MROs) may be resistant to multiple classes of antimicrobial agents. Increasing levels of antimicrobial resistance amplifies morbidity and mortality associated with infections, meaning prolonged hospital stays and increased costs of healthcare. Although resistant to antibiotics, MROs essentially behave in the same way as fully sensitive organisms when faced with effective cleaning and disinfection processes. An MRO is resistant to antibiotics which each target a single specific mechanism, whereas cleaning and disinfection processes incorporate a number of destructive mechanisms. Although disinfectant resistance has been noted in laboratory studies, in-use concentrations (if correctly prepared) are normally greatly in excess of minimum inhibitory concentrations (MICs).

BOX 15.1 Practical principles of cleaning/decontamination

Some general principles underpin the processes of cleaning and decontamination, many of which are designed to prevent recontamination:

- Clean from top to bottom as the lower areas are likely to be more contaminated
- Clean from inside to out
- Clean from 'clean' to 'dirty'
- Clean using an 'S' shape to ensure that all surfaces are covered and not gone over again using a 'one wipe, one surface, one direction' principle[43]
- Do not transfer organisms from dirty to clean surfaces by reusing wipes and cloths on multiple surfaces
- Never put a soiled cloth back into a disinfectant solution as this means that the disinfectant solution will become both contaminated and possibly ineffective, as chlorine can become deactivated in the presence of organic matter

- Use freshly prepared cleaning fluids according to the manufacturer's instructions and change frequently to avoid cross-contamination
- If using a disinfectant, ensure that surfaces remain wet with the disinfectant to allow time for the organisms to be killed
- Start with high-touch sites and work in a methodical and consistent manner to ensure all surfaces have been cleaned. It may be useful to produce a local checklist with a list of high-touch items, objects, furniture and surfaces that require cleaning in order to assist with this. The list may also indicate the responsibility for each item and could be used for training and auditing
- Clean bathrooms after cleaning the patient room: start with the sink, continue with the shower/bath, and clean the toilet last
- Always use a new cloth between sink, shower/bath and toilet

---

TABLE 15.5 The process of cleaning

LOOK	Visually assess the area or object: general impression, including temperature, smell, visible debris, clutter, space, lighting, patient status, and presence of clinical staff and visitors
PLAN	Organise and prepare for cleaning: wash hands; realign furniture, equipment and patient's belongings for access; removal of litter, food, spillages, debris, etc. Decide what agents will be required
CLEAN	i) Cleaning: remove dirt, smears, stains, grease, dust, etc. according to local policy ii) Disinfection (if required): apply according to manufacturer's recommendation
DRY	Allow time for physical drying (water and cleaning fluids). If detergent and water has been used, the process ends with physical drying of the area (this is equivalent to the rinse and dry stage of hand hygiene, as detergent merely loosens soil for removal). If using a disinfectant or a combined detergent and disinfectant, allow the surfaces to air dry to ensure that the contact time of the disinfectant is achieved. Replace items if moved for cleaning. Assess area, remove equipment and wash hands

Source: Adapted from Dancer and Kramer (2019)[42]

Australian Guidelines recommend that when MROs are encountered, increased environmental cleaning is required.[41] In particular, high-touch surfaces such as bed rails, bedside commodes, door opening and closing handles and tap handles, should be cleaned with a detergent and disinfected with a TGA-listed hospital-grade disinfectant that is listed in the Australian Register of Therapeutic Goods. (See Useful websites/resources at the end of this chapter.)

As outlined in Section 3.1.3 Practice Statement 9 of the practical information within the Australian Guidelines,[41] this decontamination process should involve either a 2-stage clean, which involves a physical clean using detergent solution followed by use of a chemical disinfectant, or a combined 2-in-1 clean, in which a combined detergent/disinfectant wipe or solution is used and mechanical/manual cleaning action is involved. In both cases, the disinfectant should remain on the surface for the contact time required to have effect and this information should be supplied by the manufacturer in the form of test data for the selected disinfectant. Although both methods are effective, a combined cleaning and disinfection process has been demonstrated to be more time-efficient and to simplify the training requirement for staff who have to undertake it.[44]

The most important aspect of dealing with an environment contaminated with MROs is to ensure that all cleaning and decontamination processes are effectively implemented. If this is not done, there is a significant increased risk of transmission to the subsequent occupant of a space.[17]

15.6.3 Cleaning and decontamination during an outbreak

Many outbreaks involve pathogens which are known to contaminate the environment and remain viable and transmissible, thus increasing the risk of prolonging the outbreak. MRSA, *Acinetobacter baumanii*, *Clostridioides difficile* and norovirus are examples of such organisms.[45-48] Australian Guidelines recommend that cleaning frequencies should be increased above the normal standard for the area to ensure any contaminants are removed and that consideration should be given to disinfection of wider areas during outbreaks.[41] What needs to be considered in an outbreak setting is the specific pathogen of interest and whether the range or concentration of disinfectants in routine use is effective against the target organism. *Clostridioides difficile*, for example, is not affected significantly at practical in-use concentrations by chlorine at 1000 parts per million (ppm), requiring 5000 ppm to be effective.[49] Caution has to be taken when considering concentrations of disinfectants in use as they may be corrosive and damage surfaces. Manufacturers' validated cleaning and decontamination guidance should always be consulted to check that a product is approved and is compatible with the product that is being considered.

The challenge of decontaminating the environment is exacerbated by the presence of environmental biofilm. Many studies have demonstrated that viable organisms can be present on surfaces after significant time periods have elapsed.[34,35] Biofilm formation also seems to enhance the virulence and persistence of existing and emerging pathogens.[33,50]

15.6.4 Decontamination of multiple patient use equipment

Studies have shown that equipment that is used by multiple patients is not always effectively decontaminated. One US study demonstrated that a large number of items on a hospital ward had no staff group designated responsible for cleaning them. This study found that 89% of the equipment used by a number of patients—including vital signs monitoring—and cleaned by clinical staff, failed the hygiene benchmark.[51]

A US study demonstrated that multiple significant pathogens could be found on the handles that had been contaminated with harmless fragments of vegetable RNA to allow tracking and demonstrate the potential for transmission. The study also found that 75% of the other vital signs monitoring equipment in the area that had not been marked became positive. The researchers tested whether any cleaning was taking place by the placement of invisible ultraviolet marks and these all remained in place for 14 days, demonstrating that no cleaning was taking place.

Other studies have also demonstrated that benign surrogate markers used to mimic the spread of microorganisms in an intensive care unit, and inoculated onto shared portable equipment, disseminated widely to surfaces in patient rooms and common work areas and to other types of portable equipment.[53] Invisible markers placed on these items to examine whether cleaning was happening showed that items may not be cleaned for up to six days.

It is of course quite possible to effectively render an item safe for multiple patient uses, as reported by researchers in Australia who demonstrated that a disinfectant wipe adequately decontaminated a blood pressure cuff, making it safe to be used on the next person.[54]

Education for staff and feedback of cleaning performance has been shown to improve standards of cleaning for mobile patient equipment and reduce risk to patients.[55]

15.6.5 Non-touch technologies for environmental disinfection

Despite cleaning being accepted as an important factor in reducing transmission, there is evidence that it is frequently inadequate for a number of reasons, including human factors.[45,56,57] This has led to an interest and rise in the use of novel non-touch technologies as an adjunct to traditional cleaning methods.[58] Ultraviolet light (UV-C) and hydrogen peroxide or peracetic acid in gaseous or vapour form are examples of such technologies that may have a useful part to play. A growing body of evidence supports the use of UV-C in enhancing decontamination procedures. Although the log reductions (generally in the region of 3 log_{10}) are not as high as for hydrogen peroxide vapour (6 log_{10}), short cycle times make it an option when time is short and room unavailability must be minimised. The advantages of UV technologies as opposed to gaseous decontamination include the mobility of the equipment, fast cycle times[59] and not having to seal rooms, ventilation systems, fire detection systems and so on, as for hydrogen peroxide vapour systems.

Some examples of non-touch technologies are discussed in more detail below, noting this is an evolving area.

Hydrogen peroxide: The advantage of using gaseous forms of decontamination is that the active agent will be able to reach all parts and surfaces within an area, including parts of the area that are normally difficult or impossible to access by cleaning workers.[60] Hydrogen peroxide non-touch decontamination systems normally come in one of two types— hydrogen peroxide vapour (HPV) and aerosolised hydrogen peroxide (aHP). With many generators, the gas is exhausted from the generator at a velocity great enough to create turbulence within the room which assists with mixing the gas in the room. Studies using an HPV generator with a high exhaust velocity have an acceptable killing around the test room, while dry mist hydrogen peroxide (DMHP), which uses diffusion around the room, only showed efficacy near the generator.[61] Hydrogen peroxide in gaseous form works in the same way as the liquid disinfectant and is a powerful oxidising agent, effective against spores and vegetative bacteria. Clinical studies have demonstrated efficacy in reducing environmental contamination and HAIs.[62-64]

An HPV cycle will normally take around 90–120 min and as the treatment is gaseous, the area has to be sealed for the entirety of this period to prevent egress of toxic agents. This may mean that the use of gaseous decontamination is not possible when, for example, suspended ceilings are used. Other issues include the need to seal off any fire and smoke detectors, as they may be affected or triggered by the process. This may be time-consuming. In one study, when using HPV within a healthcare setting the mean cycle length for decontamination, including the equipment setup, was 139 minutes. In practicality however, this time increased to 206 minutes if the time from the room being vacated by a patient was added to the termination of the decontamination cycle, and this was further extended to 270 minutes from when the room was first vacated to the end of the secondary cleaning following the gaseous decontamination process.[65]

Ultraviolet light (UV-C): The wavelength of UV radiation ranges from 328 nm to 210 nm (3280 A to 2100 A). The maximum bactericidal effect occurs at 240–280 nm.

Mercury vapor lamps emit more than 90% of their radiation at 253.7 nm, which is close to the maximum microbicidal activity.[66,67] The use of UV-C light is a recognised and reliable method of microorganism inactivation that involves exposing air, water or contaminated surfaces to UV-C light. UV technology has been used in germicidal air and water treatment applications since the early 1900s, and in healthcare settings since the 1930s,[68] but has only recently been adopted for surface treatment in hospitals. UV light penetrates the deoxyribonucleic acid (DNA) or ribonucleic acid (RNA) of microorganisms, disrupts the cell's genetic material and renders it unable to replicate due to the damaged genetic material. Bacteria and viruses are more easily killed by UV light than are bacterial spores,[67] and UV-C has been shown to be effective for Carbapenemase-producing *Enterobacteriaceae*,[59] noroviruses[69] and respiratory viruses such as MERS-CoV.[70]

A number of clinical studies demonstrate the effectiveness of this form of automated room disinfection.[71] Research has shown that UV light can effectively reduce environmental contamination and potentially mitigate infection risks,[72] and is effective in reducing microbial burden due to MRSA, VRE and even *C. difficile*, especially when manual cleaning is suboptimal.[73] Spores are generally accepted as being harder to eradicate; however, simply extending the cycle has been shown to be effective against *C. difficile* spores[74] and studies have shown reductions in *C. difficile* infections following introduction.[75] In a more recent paper,[76] 15 minutes of UV-C exposure was added to the standard cleaning and disinfection process for terminal cleaning, demonstrating increased efficacy and a significantly reduced microbial burden. Interestingly, manual cleaning was also shown to be as effective as the UV-C process; however, only when all cleaning processes were undertaken under direct observation, with the cleaning staff being aware that they were being observed and thus likely to be performing optimally.

A large multi-centre cluster-randomised crossover trial has been undertaken.[77] In this study, rooms from which a patient with infection or colonisation with one of a group of target organisms (methicillin-resistant *Staphylococcus aureus*, vancomycin-resistant *enterococci*, *C. difficile* and multidrug-resistant *Acinetobacter*) was discharged were terminally disinfected with one of four strategies:

1. the reference (quaternary ammonium disinfectant, except for *C. difficile*, for which bleach was used) is a standard method widely used in the USA

2. UV (quaternary ammonium disinfectant and disinfecting ultraviolet [UV-C] light except for *C. difficile*, for which bleach and UV-C were used)

3. chlorine; and

4. chlorine and UV-C.

The next patient admitted to that room was considered to be 'exposed'. Primary outcomes were the incidence of infection or colonisation with all target organisms among exposed patients and the incidence of *C difficile* infection among exposed patients in the intention-to-treat population. The results showed the incidence of target organisms among 'exposed' patients to be significantly lower after adding UV to standard cleaning strategies (n=76; 33.9 cases per 10,000 exposure days; relative risk [RR] 0.70, 95% CI 0.50-0.98; p=0.036). The authors concluded that the addition of UV-C to the standard form of room cleaning and disinfection enhanced the effectiveness of room preparation.

When using UV-C devices, questions may arise regarding safe exposure time and the potential risk of accidental exposure. According to NIOSH (National Institute for Occupational Safety and Health) at the Centers for Disease Control and Prevention (CDC), the recommended exposure limit for UV-C is 6000 microwatt-seconds per square centimetre (6 mJ/cm$_2$) for a daily eight-hour work shift. Additionally, manufacturer's guidelines should always be followed and UV-C treatment should be performed in unoccupied rooms with a warning sign placed on or outside the door as an added precaution when the device is in use. Although excessive UV-C exposure has the potential to superficially make skin red and eyes feel painful and gritty, these symptoms typically subside within 24 to 48 hours.[68] Well-designed UV-C devices have safety controls and procedures to minimise the risk of UV-C exposure. For example, a device may be fitted with passive infrared (PIR) safety sensors that are triggered by motion and changes in the infrared radiation above a predefined value (this is different from a motion sensor that detects only motion; this type of sensor could be triggered by insignificant movements). When a door is opened and a person enters the room, the safety sensors detect the person's body heat and shut the device down within seconds.

Limitations of UV-C include the presence of organic matter preventing light penetration, light not reaching shadowed areas and UV intensity, which can be dependent on distance from the surfaces that are being decontaminated and the cleanliness of tubes. Shadow and intensity can be mitigated by using the machine in a minimum of two or three positions (depending on the type of room and where there is an ensuite toilet facility) within the room.[78]

Non-touch automated room decontamination technology continues to develop and the evidence base that these technologies have a part to play in ensuring that rooms are effectively decontaminated by rapid processes that do not interfere with patient flows is steadily increasing.[58,71]

15.6.6 Dealing with body fluid spills

Body fluid spills are a common occurrence in healthcare settings and care needs to be taken when dealing with them. The first thing to do is communicate the hazard and attempt to isolate it to protect others. The next step is to determine what the substance is (blood, urine, faeces or vomitus for example) and then undertake a risk assessment to guide the level of PPE required to deal with the task. Local policy should dictate the procedure to be followed. If there is no risk of a splash to the face or mucous membranes, then gloves will be required as a minimum. Gloves will protect from contamination from any infectious agents potentially present in the spill and from any chemical agents used. Consideration should also be given to clothing protection by use of an apron, depending on the manual process that is required and the agents to be used. If, however, there is a risk of a splash through the intensity of any manual cleaning process or for any other reason, then PPE in the form of face and eye protection should be worn in line with local policy or guidance.

From a procedural point of view, first the spill must be controlled to prevent further spread. If the spill does not contain blood, soak as much of the liquid element up as possible with disposable paper towels. If the spill does contain blood, an attempt to decontaminate should be made prior to the manual removal of the spill. A solution of 1% chlorine (diluted to the correct concentration if necessary), absorbent chlorine-releasing granules or peracetic acid-based absorbent pads may be used for this. The area is then left for two minutes, after which the liquid may be soaked up into disposable paper towels or pads and removed carefully into the appropriate waste stream in line with local guidance. The area is then cleaned with hot water and detergent, dried and the PPE is disposed of according to local guidance, with hand hygiene performed to remove contamination that could have occurred through glove penetration or when removing the PPE. If the spill contains urine, chlorine should not be used, as excess chlorine fumes will be released.

For spills on clothing, sponge off with hot, soapy water and wash as soon as possible in the hottest cycles the garments will stand.

For spills on upholstery or carpets, mop up excess liquid with kitchen roll, sponge with cold water, and clean with hot water and general-purpose detergent.

15.7 Assessing the effectiveness of environmental cleaning

Several different methods of assessing the effectiveness of environmental cleaning and disinfection exist, including visual, use of invisible UV markers, adenosine triphosphate (ATP) measurement and microbiological methods. Some are qualitative and subjective, and others are quantitative. All have their advantages and disadvantages and are not suitable for all settings. The choice of method may depend on a number of things including the risk of transmission from the environment; the risk to the inhabitants of that environment; the physical makeup of the environment; and the resources available. For example, quantitative methods may be used in a high-risk environment, where risk to patients is high because of the use of multiple invasive devices. There are generally hard surfaces that are relatively easy to clean and therefore to measure the effectiveness of cleaning; and there may be some resource in terms of budgets. This is markedly different to a long-term residential care setting in the community where invasive device use is low, surfaces are soft, the environment is not suitable for some monitoring methods, and resources in terms of technology and access to laboratories will not be available. In these situations, qualitative assessments are likely to be adequate in the absence of evidence of ongoing transmission or outbreaks.

15.7.1 Visual assessment

Visual assessment is the generally used measure of cleanliness, despite being an unreliable indicator of microbial contamination. It is an impression of cleanliness and although a surface may be visibly free of soil, this may not reflect that the surface is free of microbial load.[79-82]

To reduce the risk of cross-infection, microbial load on the surface must be below the level required for transmission, recognising that this level is unknown for the majority of pathogens implicated in HAIs. Visual assessments are cheap in terms of consumables and a rapid means of assessing cleanliness, providing a subjective indication of performance and cleaning efficiency. However, this method has been reported to be a poor indicator of quantitative cleanliness in comparison to fluorescent markers and ATP assays.[83-88]

In some settings, where risks are low and other methods unsuitable, impractical and costly, visual inspections are a valid method of assessing whether standards are being met. An example of an assessment tool that could be used in long-term care is provided in Table 15.6.

TABLE 15.6 Example of a cleaning and decontamination audit for long-term care

Ref	Standard	Yes	No	N/A	Notes
1. The environment must be maintained appropriately to reduce and minimise the risk of cross-infection					
1.1	Communal and residents' rooms are free from unpleasant smells/malodours				
1.2	The general environment is clean and free from dust				
1.3	Curtains and blinds are free from stains, dust and cobwebs				
1.4	There is a cleaning program in place for regular decontamination for all curtains and blinds (evidence of signing sheet)				
1.5	Carpeted areas are clean and in a good state of repair				
1.6	There is a robust cleaning program in place for the systematic cleaning of carpets in both communal and residents' rooms (evidence of frequency documented)				
2. Furniture					
2.1	The furniture is in a good state of repair and is free from rips and tears				
1.8	Furniture in residents' areas, e.g. chairs and settees, is made of impermeable and washable materials				

TABLE 15.6 Example of a cleaning and decontamination audit for long-term care—cont'd

Ref	Standard	Yes	No	N/A	Notes
1.9	There is a cleaning program in place for regular decontamination of furniture (evidence of frequency documented)				
3. Bathrooms					
3.1	Bathrooms/washrooms are clean				
3.2	Anti-slip bath/shower mats are clean and hung over the bath/rail to dry between use				
3.3	Lifting aids are waterproof, easy to clean and appropriately maintained, e.g. check underneath bath seats/slings				
3.4	Slings are single resident use or cleaned between each resident				
3.5	Slings contaminated with bodily fluid should be laundered immediately				
3.6	The mechanical hoist is clean and in a good state of repair				
3.7	Baths, sinks and accessories are clean				
3.8	Appropriate cleaning materials are available to clean the bath after use				
3.9	Wall tiles and wall fixtures (including soap dispensers and towel holders) are clean, free from mould and intact				
3.10	Shower curtains are subject to a cleaning program and are clean and free from mould				
3.11	All toilets are visibly clean with no body fluid contamination, lime scale stains, etc				
3.12	Floors including edges and corners are free from dust and grit				
3.13	Flooring is impervious and sealed including edges and corners, and is free of dust and grit				
4. Sluice/dirty utility					
4.1	A dirty utility area is available				
4.2	A separate sink is available for decontamination of patient equipment				
4.3	A sluice hopper is available for disposal of body fluids				
4.4	Separate handwashing facilities are available including liquid soap and paper towels				
4.5	The room is clean and free from inappropriate items				
4.6	The floor is clean and free from spillages				
4.7	Floors including edges and corners are free of dust and grit				
4.8	Cleaning equipment is colour coded as per local policy				
4.9	Wash bowls are stored clean, dry and inverted on a rack, or stored clean and dry in the resident's room (for their use only)				
4.10	Bed pans, commode buckets, urinals and jugs are stored on inverted racks				
4.11	Commodes are visibly clean and cleaned after each use				
4.12	Appropriate facilities are available and are clean and in working order to ensure correct disposal or disinfection of bed pans and urinals (macerator and/or washer disinfector)				

Continued

TABLE 15.6 Example of a cleaning and decontamination audit for long-term care—cont'd

Ref	Standard	Yes	No	N/A	Notes
4.13	Shelves and cupboards are clean inside and out and free of dust, litter or stains				
5. Housekeeping room					
5.1	There is a robust cleaning program schedule in place for regular decontamination throughout the establishment (documented evidence)				
5.2	Equipment used by the cleaning staff is clean, well maintained and stored in a locked area in accordance with local regulations				
5.3	Information on the colour coding system in use is available				
5.4	PPE is available and appropriately used by cleaning staff (gloves and aprons)				
5.5	Products used for cleaning and disinfection comply with policy and are used at the correct dilution				
5.6	Cleaning agents are stored in clearly marked containers				
5.7	Disposable cloths are colour coded				
5.8	Colour-coded buckets and mops are stored dry and inverted				
6. Equipment decontamination					
6.1	There is a comprehensive and up-to-date decontamination policy available				
6.2	The roles and responsibilities for cleaning patient equipment are clearly defined, e.g. bedframes, mattresses, commodes—and documented evidence is available				
6.3	Staff can state the procedure for the decontamination of commonly used patient care equipment, e.g. commodes, mattresses (ask three members of staff)				
6.4	Mattress covers are clean and intact				
6.5	Dressing trolleys are clean and free of rust				
6.6	Bed rails and cot sides (where used) are clean and included in the cleaning program				
6.7	Pillows are clean and intact				
6.8	Wheelchairs and cushions are clean and intact				

15.7.2 Fluorescent markers

Fluorescent gels, powders and lotions have been used to determine whether high-touch surfaces have been cleaned. The marker is easily removed with light pressure with a moist cloth or pre-wetted wipe and is only visible under a UV lamp of the correct wavelength.

The marker is applied to the surface, which is subsequently examined after cleaning has taken place. These methods have been used both as educational tools, including as part of a quality improvement process[56,89-91] and as an audit tool[57,72,92,93] for assessing the thoroughness of cleaning, particularly of high-touch surfaces.[89] It has been shown that fluorescent markers are a useful tool in determining how thoroughly a surface is wiped and mimics microbiological data better than ATP (<500 RLU).[94]

Fluorescent powders have been used for assessing environmental cleanliness.[95] In addition to highlighting surfaces which have not been cleaned, fluorescent powders also demonstrate the potential for transference of microorganisms to clean surfaces and also to highlight deficiencies in techniques when removing PPE[96] and hand hygiene.[97]

15.7.3 Adenosine triphosphate (ATP)

Adenosine triphosphate is the molecule used for energy storage by all types of living cells (animal, plant, bacterial, yeast and mould). ATP transfers energy within living cells to power the enzymes needed for cellular functions. After cell death, ATP is broken down by autolysis within a few minutes.

The ATP collected from a surface reacts with luciferin/luciferase compounds present in the sample swab to create bioluminescence light. The amount of bioluminescence is measured by the Luminometer and is expressed in relative light units (RLU). RLU numbers are directly proportional to the amount of ATP, and therefore the amount of organic/food residue or microbial biomass on the sampled surface. ATP bioluminescence is an indirect measurement of the amount of organic/food residue on a surface that has the potential to support microbial growth and also microbial biomass. In simple terms, it measures the dirt on a surface, indicating the need for cleaning and disinfection.

ATP bioluminescence has been widely used in the food industry and is increasingly being used in healthcare settings; however, as the system is not able to differentiate between the proportion of microbial and non-microbial ATP in the sample, it cannot be used to correlate bacterial numbers.[94]

It is a rapid (20 seconds), easy-to-use method of evaluating cleaning that provides instant feedback. Although studies have recommended that a 500 RLU is an achievable measure of cleanliness,[98] defining a cut-off level will depend on the type of system used.[84,85] When establishing benchmarks it is important to assess the location of the surface (high-touch surface).[99] Using this system, surfaces cleaned by cleaning staff were more likely to pass the cleanliness benchmark than those cleaned by clinical staff (89% of surfaces cleaned by clinical staff failed the benchmark).[51] ATP bioluminescence is increasingly being used as an effective tool for the monitoring and promotion of hospital cleaning.[83,86,87,100-108] It should not, however, be used as the sole indicator for infection risk.

15.7.4 Microbiological sampling

Current Australian guidelines do not advise routine sampling of floors, walls, surfaces and air. Despite the time and resources required for microbial culturing, it represents the most accurate indication of the potential infection risk, although feedback is not instantaneous and many clinical laboratories are not accredited for environmental work.

The presence of indicator organisms, such as *S. aureus*, *C. difficile*, VRE or *Acinetobacter* spp., is indicative of a requirement for increased cleaning.[109] Aerobic colony counts on hand-touch sites should not exceed 5 CFU/cm.^{2}[2,79,109] It should be noted the choice of sampling method (swabs, dipslides, sampling sponges and settling plates) will affect the end result.[110-116] Limitations of microbiological sampling in isolation include how to interpret results. A negative swab from a 2.5cm^2 area in a room does not necessarily mean the room is clean.

CASE STUDY 2

Assessing the effectiveness of cleaning and decontamination

Situation:

You are responsible for assessing the effectiveness of the cleaning program in your facility, which is a 250-bed regional hospital which has a four-bed ICU, three operating theatres and a small burns unit. Resources are limited and so your choice will need to be justified to obtain any funding.

Questions:

1. What methods would you consider and why?
2. How frequently would you perform the monitoring?
3. Would any situation change this?
4. How would you disseminate the results of the monitoring and to whom would you deliver them?

15.8 Feedback of the results of environmental monitoring

There are two groups of staff who will be primarily interested in the results of monitoring of cleaning: the managers or contract monitoring teams, who may be looking for evidence of work completed; and the cleaning staff themselves, who may either be fearful of the consequences of poor performance or looking for opportunities to perform better. There is good evidence from high-quality studies that feedback results in improved performance.[3,56,117,118] There is also evidence that if the feedback is presented well, it is effective. However, for this to happen it must be timely, individualised to a level that an individual recognises the effect of their own practice, and non-punitive.[119] The way the feedback is presented does impact on how it is received, and also on whether it will result in change rather than the recipient simply seeking to defend a position.

Conclusion

Environmental cleaning and, where necessary, decontamination, is highly relevant for healthcare settings. An abundance of evidence exists to show that contamination of the environment with pathogenic organisms occurs, that the organisms persist in the environment;

and that transmission occurs. Although this is now accepted in acute care settings, the SARS-CoV-2 pandemic has demonstrated that the principles, if not identical practices, apply equally in community and long-term care settings. In each area, a proportionate response is required, with risk assessments of individual settings underpinning policy and procedure. Done well, cleaning plays a vital part in patient and resident safety. The staff undertaking these vital roles should have their contribution to patient safety respected and acknowledged, and language should reflect this. Instead of asking 'Is that room clean?' we should ask, 'Is that room safe?'

Useful websites/resources

- Australian Register of Therapeutic Goods. https://www.tga.gov.au/australian-register-therapeutic-goods.
- Australasian College of Infection Prevention and Control. www.acipc.org.au.
- Australian Guidelines for the Prevention and Control of Infection in Healthcare. https://www.nhmrc.gov.au/about-us/publications/australian-guidelines-prevention-and-control-infection-healthcare-2019.
- Australian Commission on Safety and Quality in Healthcare Environmental cleaning section. https://www.safetyandquality.gov.au/our-work/infection-prevention-and-control/environmental-cleaning-and-infection-prevention-and-control-resources.

References

1. Rutala WA, Weber DJ. Disinfection, sterilization, and antisepsis: principles, practices, current issues, new research, and new technologies. Am J Infect Control. 2019;47S:A1-A2.
2. White NM, Barnett AG, Hall L et al. Cost-effectiveness of an environmental cleaning bundle for reducing healthcare-associated infections. Clin Infect Dis. 2020;70:2461-2468.
3. Mitchell BG, Hall L, White N et al. An environmental cleaning bundle and health-care-associated infections in hospitals (REACH): a multicentre, randomised trial. Lancet Infect Dis. 2019;19:410-418.
4. Dettenkofer M, Wenzler S, Amthor S, Antes G, Motschall E, Daschner FD. Does disinfection of environmental surfaces influence nosocomial infection rates? A systematic review. Am J Infect Control. 2004;32:84-89.
5. Donskey CJ. Does improving surface cleaning and disinfection reduce health care-associated infections? Am J Infect Control. 2013;41:S12-19.
6. Weber DJ, Rutala WA, Miller MB, Huslage K, Sickbert-Bennett E. Role of hospital surfaces in the transmission of emerging health care-associated pathogens:norovirus, Clostridium difficile, and Acinetobacter species. Am J Infect Control. 2010;38:S25-33.
7. Lesens O, Mihaila L, Robin F, et al. Outbreak of colonization and infection with vancomycin-resistant Enterococcus faecium in a French university hospital. Infect Control Hosp Epidemiol. 2006;27:984-986.
8. Kundrapu S, Sunkesula V, Jury LA, Sitzlar BM, Donskey CJ. Daily disinfection of high-touch surfaces in isolation rooms to reduce contamination of healthcare workers' hands. Infect Control Hosp Epidemiol. 2012;33:1039-1042.
9. Guerrero DM, Nerandzic MM, Jury LA, Jinno S, Chang S, Donskey CJ. Acquisition of spores on gloved hands after contact with the skin of patients with Clostridium difficile infection and with environmental surfaces in their rooms. Am J Infect Control. 2012;40:556-558.
10. Stiefel U, Cadnum JL, Eckstein BC, Guerrero DM, Tima MA, Donskey CJ. Contamination of hands with methicillin-resistant Staphylococcus aureus after contact with environmental surfaces and after contact with the skin of colonized patients. Infect Control Hosp Epidemiol. 2011;32:185-187.
11. Kramer A, Schwebke I, Kampf G. How long do nosocomial pathogens persist on inanimate surfaces? A systematic review. BMC Infect Dis. 2006;6:130.
12. Alhmidi H, Cadnum JL, Koganti S, et al. Shedding of methicillin-resistant Staphylococcus aureus by colonized patients during procedures and patient care activities. Infect Control Hosp Epidemiol. 2019;40:328-332.
13. Mitchell BG, Wilson F, Wells A. Evaluating environment cleanliness using two approaches:a multi-centred Australian study. Healthcare Infection. 2015;20:95-100.
14. Otter JA, Yezli S, French GL. The role played by contaminated surfaces in the transmission of nosocomial pathogens. Infect Control Hosp Epidemiol. 2011;32:687-699.
15. Chacko L, Jose S, Isac A, Bhat KG. Survival of nosocomial bacteria on hospital fabrics. Indian J Med Microbiol. 2003; 21:291.
16. Bhalla A, Pultz NJ, Gries DM, et al. Acquisition of nosocomial pathogens on hands after contact with environmental surfaces near hospitalized patients. Infect Control Hosp Epidemiol. 2004;25:164-167.

17. Mitchell BG, Dancer SJ, Anderson M, Dehn E. Risk of organism acquisition from prior room occupants: a systematic review and meta-analysis. J Hosp Infect. 2015;91:211-217.

18. Nseir S, Blazejewski C, Lubret R, Wallet F, Courcol R, Durocher A. Risk of acquiring multidrug-resistant Gram-negative bacilli from prior room occupants in the intensive care unit. Clin Microbiol Infect 2011;17:1201-1208.

19. Halachev MR, Chan J, Constantinidou CI, Cumley N, Bradley C, Banks MS, et al. Genomic epidemiology of a protracted hospital outbreak caused by multidrug-resistant Acinetobacter baumannii in Birmingham, England. Genome Med. 2014;6.

20. Dancer SJ. Control of transmission of infection in hospitals requires more than clean hands. Infect Control Hosp Epidemiol. 2010;31:958-960.

21. Tajeddin E, Rashidan M, Razaghi M, et al. The role of the intensive care unit environment and health-care workers in the transmission of bacteria associated with hospital acquired infections. J Infect Pub Health. 2016;9:13-23.

22. Yezli S, Otter JA. Minimum infective dose of the major human respiratory and enteric viruses transmitted through food and the environment. Food Environ Virol. 2011;3:1-30.

23. Lawley TD, Clare S, Deakin LJ, et al. Use of purified Clostridium difficile spores to facilitate evaluation of health care disinfection regimens. Appl Environ Microbiol. 2010;76:6895-6900.

24. Teunis PF, Moe CL, Liu P, et al. Norwalk virus: how infectious is it? J Med Virol. 2008;80:1468-1476.

25. Ling ML, Apisarnthanarak A, Thu le TA, Villanueva V, Pandjaitan C, Yusof MY. APSIC Guidelines for environmental cleaning and decontamination. Antimicrob Resist Infect Control. 2015;4:58.

26. Beggs C, Knibbs LD, Johnson GR, Morawska L. Environmental contamination and hospital-acquired infection: factors that are easily overlooked. Indoor Air. 2015;25:462-474.

27. Weber DJ, Rutala WA. Assessing the risk of disease transmission to patients when there is a failure to follow recommended disinfection and sterilization guidelines. Am J Infect Control. 2013;41:S67-71.

28. Munoz-Price LS, Namias N, Cleary T, et al. Acinetobacter baumannii:association between environmental contamination of patient rooms and occupant status. Infect Control Hosp Epidemiol. 2013;34:517-520.

29. Munoz-Price LS, Lubarsky DA, Arheart KL, et al. Interactions between anesthesiologists and the environment while providing anesthesia care in the operating room. Am J Infect Control. 2013;41:922-924.

30. Donlan RM. Biofilms: microbial life on surfaces. Emerg Infect Dis. 2002;8:881-90.

31. Ledwoch K, Robertson A, Lauran J, Norville P, Maillard JY. It's a trap! The development of a versatile drain biofilm model and its susceptibility to disinfection. J Hosp Infect. 2020;106:757-764.

32. Lemarie C, Legeay C, Kouatchet A, et al. High prevalence of contamination of sink drains with carbapenemase-producing Enterobacteriaccae in 4 intensive care units apart from any epidemic context. Am J Infect Control. 2020;48:230-232.

33. Short B, Brown J, Delaney C, et al. Candida auris exhibits resilient biofilm characteristics in vitro: implications for environmental persistence. J Hosp Infect. 2019;103:92-96.

34. Parvin F, Hu H, Whiteley GS, Glasbey T, Vickery K. Difficulty in removing biofilm from dry surfaces. J Hosp Infect. 2019;103:465-467.

35. Vickery K, Deva A, Jacombs A, Allan J, Valente P, Gosbell IB. Presence of biofilm containing viable multiresistant organisms despite terminal cleaning on clinical surfaces in an intensive care unit. J Hosp Infect. 2012;80:52-55.

36. Assadian O, Harbarth S, Vos M, Knobloch JK, Asensio A, Widmer AF. Practical recommendations for routine cleaning and disinfection procedures in healthcare institutions:a narrative review. J Hosp Infect. 2021;113:104-114.

37. Asker D, Weiss J, McClements DJ. Formation and stabilization of antimicrobial delivery systems based on electrostatic complexes of cationic-non-ionic mixed micelles and anionic polysaccharides. J Agric Food Chem. 2011;59:1041-1049.

38. McDonnell GE. Antisepsis, disinfection, and sterilization: types, action and resistance, 2nd ed. Washington DC: ASM Press, 2017.

39. Rutala WA, Weber DJ. Best practices for disinfection of noncritical environmental surfaces and equipment in health care facilities: a bundle approach. Am J Infect Control. 2019;47S:A96-A105.

40. Walker JT. The importance of decontamination in hospitals and healthcare. In: Walker JT, ed. Decontamination in hospitals and healthcare, 2nd ed. Woodhead Publishing, 2020.

41. National Health and Medical Research Council. Australian guidelines for the prevention and control of infection in healthcare. Canberra: Commonwealth of Australia, 2019.

42. Dancer SJ, Kramer A. Four steps to clean hospitals: look, plan, clean and dry. J Hosp Infect. 2019;103:e1-e8.

43. Williams GJ, Denyer SP, Hosein IK, Hill DW, Maillard JY. Limitations of the efficacy of surface disinfection in the healthcare setting. Infect Control Hosp Epidemiol. 2009;30:570-573.

44. Shepherd E, Leitch A, Curran E, Infection Prevention and Control Team NHS Lanarkshire. A quality improvement project to standardise decontamination procedures in a single NHS board in Scotland. J Infect Prev. 2020;21:241-246.

45. French GL, Otter JA, Shannon KP, Adams NM, Watling D, Parks MJ. Tackling contamination of the hospital environment by methicillin-resistant Staphylococcus aureus (MRSA): a comparison between conventional terminal cleaning and hydrogen peroxide vapour decontamination. J Hosp Infect. 2004;57:31-37.

46. Lerner AO, Abu-Hanna J, Carmeli Y, Schechner V. Environmental contamination by carbapenem-resistant Acinetobacter baumannii: the effects of room type and cleaning methods. Infect Control Hosp Epidemiol. 2020;41:166-171.

47. Endres BT, Dotson KM, Poblete K, et al. Environmental transmission of Clostridioides difficile ribotype 027 at a long-term care facility; an outbreak investigation guided by whole genome sequencing. Infect Control Hosp Epidemiol. 2018;39:1322-1329.

48. Saez-Lopez E, Marques R, Rodrigues N, et al. Lessons learned from a prolonged norovirus GII.P16-GII.4 Sydney 2012 variant outbreak in a long-term care facility in Portugal, 2017. Infect Control Hosp Epidemiol. 2019;40:1164-1169.

49. Barbut F. How to eradicate Clostridium difficile from the environment. J Hosp Infect. 2015;89:287-295.

50. Zeighami H, Valadkhani F, Shapouri R, Samadi E, Haghi F. Virulence characteristics of multidrug resistant biofilm forming Acinetobacter baumannii isolated from intensive care unit patients. BMC Infect Dis. 2019;19:629.

51. Anderson RE, Young V, Stewart M, Robertson C, Dancer SJ. Cleanliness audit of clinical surfaces and equipment: who cleans what? J Hosp Infect. 2011;78:178-181.

52. John AR, Alhmidi H, Cadnum JL, Jencson AL, Gestrich S, Donskey CJ. Evaluation of the potential for electronic thermometers to contribute to spread of healthcare-associated pathogens. Am J Infect Control. 2018;46:708-710.

53. John A, Alhmidi H, Cadnum J, Jencson A, Donskey C. Contaminated portable equipment is a potential vector for dissemination of pathogens in the intensive care unit. Infect Control Hosp Epidemiol. 2017;38:1247-1249.

54. Zimmerman PA, Browne M, Rowland D. Instilling a culture of cleaning: effectiveness of decontamination practices on non-disposable sphygmomanometer cuffs. J Infect Prev. 2018;19.

55. Reese SM, Knepper BC, Kurtz J, et al. Implementation of cleaning and evaluation process for mobile patient equipment using adenosine triphosphate. Infect Control Hosp Epidemiol. 2019;40:798-800.

56. Carling PC, Briggs J, Hylander D, Perkins J. An evaluation of patient area cleaning in 3 hospitals using a novel targeting methodology. Am J Infect Control. 2006;34:513-519.

57. Rupp ME, Adler A, Schellen M, et al. The time spent cleaning a hospital room does not correlate with the thoroughness of cleaning. Infect Control Hosp Epidemiol. 2013;34:101-102.

58. Boyce JM. Modern technologies for improving cleaning and disinfection of environmental surfaces in hospitals. Antimicrob Resist Infect Control. 2016;5:10.

59. Rock C, Curless MS, Nowakowski E, et al. UV-C Light disinfection of carbapenem-resistant enterobacteriaceae from high-touch surfaces in a patient room and bathroom. Infect Control Hosp Epidemiol. 2016;37:996-997.

60. Andersen BM, Rasch M, Hochlin K, Jensen FH, Wismar P, Fredriksen JE. Decontamination of rooms, medical equipment and ambulances using an aerosol of hydrogen peroxide disinfectant. J Hosp Infect. 2006;62:149-55.

61. Fu TY, Gent P, Kumar V. Efficacy, efficiency and safety aspects of hydrogen peroxide vapour and aerosolized hydrogen peroxide room disinfection systems. J Hosp Infect. 2012;80:199-205.

62. Melgar M, Ramirez M, Chang A, Antillon F. Impact of dry hydrogen peroxide on hospital-acquired infection at a pediatric oncology hospital. Am J Infect Control. 2021. doi 10.1016/j.ajic.2021.12.010.

63. Ramirez M, Matheu L, Gomez M, et al. Effectiveness of dry hydrogen peroxide on reducing environmental microbial bioburden risk in a pediatric oncology intensive care unit. Am J Infect Control. 2020;doi 10.1016/j.ajic.2020.08.026.

64. Doll M, Morgan DJ, Anderson D, Bearman G. Touchless technologies for decontamination in the hospital: a review of hydrogen peroxide and UV devices. Curr Infect Dis Rep. 2015;17:498.

65. Otter JA, Puchowicz M, Ryan D, et al. Feasibility of routinely using hydrogen peroxide vapor to decontaminate rooms in a busy United States hospital. Infect Control Hosp Epidemiol. 2009;30:574-577.

66. Rutala WA, Weber DJ. Healthcare infection control practices advisory committee guideline for disinfection and sterilization in healthcare facilities, 2008. Atlanta, GA: Centers for Disease Control, 2008.

67. Russell AD. Ultraviolet radiation. In: Russell AD, Hugo WB, Ayliffe GAJ, eds. Principles and practices of disinfection, preservation and sterilization. Oxford: Blackwell Science, 1999.

68. Kowalski W. Ultraviolet germicidal irradiation handbook: UVGI for air and surface disinfection. Cincinatti, OH: Springer, 2009.

69. Park SY, Kim AN, Lee KH, Ha SD. Ultraviolet-C efficacy against a norovirus surrogate and hepatitis A virus on a stainless steel surface. Int J Food Microbiol. 2015;211:73-78.

70. Bedell K, Buchaklian AH, Perlman S. Efficacy of an automated multiple emitter whole-room ultraviolet-c disinfection system against coronaviruses MHV and MERS-CoV. Infect Control Hosp Epidemiol. 2016;37:598-599.

71. Weber DJ, Rutala WA, Anderson DJ, Chen LF, Sickbert-Bennett EE, Boyce JM. Effectiveness of ultraviolet devices and hydrogen peroxide systems for terminal room decontamination: focus on clinical trials. Am J Infect Control. 2016;44:e77-84.

72. Sitzlar B, Deshpande A, Fertelli D, Kundrapu S, Sethi AK, Donskey CJ. An environmental disinfection odyssey: evaluation of sequential interventions to improve disinfection of Clostridium difficile isolation rooms. Infect Control Hosp Epidemiol. 2013;34:459-465.

73. Wong T, Woznow T, Petrie M, et al. Postdischarge decontamination of MRSA, VRE, and Clostridium difficile isolation rooms using 2 commercially available automated ultraviolet-C-emitting devices. Am J Infect Control. 2016;44:416-420.

74. Cadnum JL, Tomas ME, Sankar T, et al. Effect of variation in test methods on performance of ultraviolet-c radiation room decontamination. Infect Control Hosp Epidemiol. 2016,37:555-560.

75. Pegues D, Gilmar C, Denno M, Gaynes S. CDC Prevention epicenters program. reducing Clostridium difficile infection among hematology-oncology patients using ultraviolet germicidal irradiation for terminal room disinfection. ID Week, San Diego: CDC, 2015.

76. Penno K, Jandarov RA, Sopirala MM. Effect of automated ultraviolet C-emitting device on decontamination of hospital rooms with and without real-time observation of terminal room disinfection. Am J Infect Control. 2017;45:1208-1213.

77. Anderson DJ, Chen LF, Weber DJ, et al. Enhanced terminal room disinfection and acquisition and infection caused by multidrug-resistant organisms and Clostridium difficile (the benefits of enhanced terminal room disinfection study): a cluster-randomised, multicentre, crossover study. Lancet. 2017;389:805-814.

78. Kanamori H, Rutala WA, Gergen MF, Weber DJ. Patient room decontamination against carbapenem-resistant enterobacteriaceae and methicillin-resistant staphylococcus aureus using a fixed cycle-time ultraviolet-c device and two different radiation designs. Infect Control Hosp Epidemiol. 2016;37:994-996.

79. Mulvey D, Redding P, Robertson C, et al. Finding a benchmark for monitoring hospital cleanliness. J Hosp Infect. 2011;77:25-30.

80. Sherlock O, O'Connell N, Creamer E, Humphreys H. Is it really clean? An evaluation of the efficacy of four methods for determining hospital cleanliness. J Hosp Infect. 2009;72:140-146.

81. Boyce JM, Havill NL, Dumigan DG, Golebiewski M, Balogun O, Rizvani R. Monitoring the effectiveness of hospital cleaning practices by use of an adenosine triphosphate bioluminescence assay. Infect Control Hosp Epidemiol. 2009;30:678-684.

82. Cooper RA, Griffith CJ, Malik RE, Obee P, Looker N. Monitoring the effectiveness of cleaning in four British hospitals. Am J Infect Control. 2007;35:338-341.

83. Huang YS, Chen YC, Chen ML, et al. Comparing visual inspection, aerobic colony counts, and adenosine triphosphate bioluminescence assay for evaluating surface cleanliness at a medical center. Am J Infect Control. 2015. doi 10.1016/j.ajic.2015.03.027.

84. Whiteley GS, Derry C, Glasbey T, Fahey P. The perennial problem of variability in adenosine triphosphate (ATP) tests for hygiene monitoring within healthcare settings. Infect Control Hosp Epidemiol. 2015. doi 10.1017/ice.2015.32:1-6.

85. Whiteley GS, Derry C, Glasbey T. Sampling plans for use of rapid adenosine triphosphate (ATP) monitoring must overcome variability or suffer statistical invalidity. Infect Control Hosp Epidemiol. 2015;36:236-237.

86. Gibbs SG, Sayles H, Chaika O, Hewlett A, Colbert EM, Smith PW. Evaluation of the relationship between ATP bioluminescence assay and the presence of organisms

associated with healthcare-associated infections. Healthcare Infect. 2014;19:101.

87. Zambrano AA, Jones A, Otero P, Ajenjo MC, Labarca JA. Assessment of hospital daily cleaning practices using ATP bioluminescence in a developing country. Braz J Infect Dis. 2014;18:675-677.

88. Luick DS, Thompson PA, Loock MH, Vetter SL, Cook J, Guerrero DM. Diagnostic assessment of different environmental cleaning monitoring methods. Am J Infect Control. 2013;41:751-752.

89. Boyce JM, Havill NL, Havill HL, Mangione E, Dumigan DG, Moore BA. Comparison of fluorescent marker systems with 2 quantitative methods of assessing terminal cleaning practices. Infect Control Hosp Epidemiol. 2011;32:1187-1193.

90. Carling PC, Parry MM, Rupp ME, et al. Improving cleaning of the environment surrounding patients in 36 acute care hospitals. Infect Control Hosp Epidemiol. 2008;29:1035-1041.

91. Griffith CJ, Obee P, Cooper RA, Burton NF, Lewis M. Evaluating the thoroughness of environmental cleaning in hospitals. J Hosp Infect. 2007;67:390.

92. Gillespie E, Othman N, Irwin L. Using ultraviolet visible markers in sterilizing departments. Am J Infect Control. 2014;42:1343.

93. Shaughnessy RJ, Cole EC, Moschandreas D, Haverinen-Shaughnessy U. ATP as a marker for surface contamination of biological origin in schools and as a potential approach to the measurement of cleaning effectiveness. J Occup Environ Hyg. 2013;10:336-346.

94. Rutala WA, Gergen MF, Sickbert-Bennett E, Huslage K, Weber DJ. Comparison of four methods to assess cleanliness. APIC, Fort Lauderdale, 2013.

95. Munoz-Price LS, Fajardo-Aquino Y, Arheart KL. Ultraviolet powder versus ultraviolet gel for assessing environmental cleaning. Infect Control Hosp Epidemiol. 2012;33:192-195.

96. Guo YP, Li Y, Wong PL. Environment and body contamination: a comparison of two different removal methods in three types of personal protective clothing. Am J Infect Control. 2014;42:e39-45.

97. Pan SC, Chen E, Tien KL, et al. Assessing the thoroughness of hand hygiene: "seeing is believing". Am J Infect Control. 2014;42:799-801.

98. Griffith CJ, Cooper RA, Gilmore J, Davies C, Lewis M. An evaluation of hospital cleaning regimes and standards. J Hosp Infect. 2000;45:19-28.

99. Dancer SJ. Hospital cleaning in the 21st century. Eur J Clin Microbiol Infect Dis. 2011;30:1473-1481.

100. Whiteley GS, Knight JL, Derry CW, Jensen SO, Vickery K, Gosbell IB. A pilot study into locating the bad bugs in a busy intensive care unit. Am J Infect Control. 2015;43:1270-1275.

101. Roady L. The role of ATP luminometers in infection control. Infect Control Hosp Epidemiol. 2015; doi 10.1017/ice.2015.209:1.

102. Colbert EM, Sayles H, Lowe JJ, Chaika O, Smith PW, Gibbs SG. Time series evaluation of the 3M™ Clean-Trace™ ATP detection device to confirm swab effectiveness. Healthcare Infect. 2015;20:108-114.

103. Colbert EM, Gibbs SG, Schmid KK, et al. Evaluation of adenosine triphosphate (ATP) bioluminescence assay to confirm surface disinfection of biological indicators with vaporised hydrogen peroxide (VHP). Healthcare Infect. 2015; 20:16-22.

104. Chan MC, Lin TY, Chiu YH, et al. Applying ATP bioluminescence to design and evaluate a successful new intensive care unit cleaning programme. J Hosp Infect. 2015; 90:344-346.

105. Smith PW, Beam E, Sayles H, et al. Impact of adenosine triphosphate detection and feedback on hospital room cleaning. Infect Control Hosp Epidemiol. 2014;35:564-569.

106. Branch-Elliman W, Robillard E, McCarthy G, Jr., Gupta K. Direct feedback with the ATP luminometer as a process improvement tool for terminal cleaning of patient rooms. Am J Infect Control. 2014;42:195-197.

107. Malik DJ. Assessment of infection risk from environmental contamination using rapid ATP surface measurements. Am J Infect Control. 2013;41:477-478.

108. Alfa MJ, Fatima I, Olson N. The adenosine triphosphate test is a rapid and reliable audit tool to assess manual cleaning adequacy of flexible endoscope channels. Am J Infect Control. 2013;41:249-253.

109. Dancer SJ. How do we assess hospital cleaning? A proposal for microbiological standards for surface hygiene in hospitals. J Hosp Infect. 2004;56:10-15.

110. Claro T, Galvin S, Cahill O, Fitzgerald-Hughes D, Daniels S, Humphreys H. What is the best method? Recovery of methicillin-resistant Staphylococcus aureus and extended-spectrum beta-lactamase-producing Escherichia coli from inanimate hospital surfaces. Infect Control Hosp Epidemiol. 2014;35:869-871.

111. Galvin S, Dolan A, Cahill O, Daniels S, Humphreys H. Microbial monitoring of the hospital environment: why and how? J Hosp Infect. 2012;82:143-151.

112. Dolan A, Bartlett M, McEntee B, Creamer E, Humphreys H. Evaluation of different methods to recover meticillin-resistant Staphylococcus aureus from hospital environmental surfaces. J Hosp Infect. 2011;79:227-230.

113. Aksoy E, Boag A, Brodbelt D, Grierson J. Evaluation of surface contamination with staphylococci in a veterinary hospital using a quantitative microbiological method. J Small Anim Pract. 2010;51:574-580.

114. Hedin G, Rynback J, Lore B. New technique to take samples from environmental surfaces using flocked nylon swabs. J Hosp Infect. 2010;75:314-317.

115. Otter JA, Havill NL, Adams NM, Cooper T, Tauman A, Boyce JM. Environmental sampling for Clostridium difficile: swabs or sponges? Am J Infect Control. 2009;37:517-518.

116. Weese JS. Environmental surveillance for MRSA. Methods Mol Biol. 2007;391:201-8.

117. Carling PC, Von Beheren S, Kim P, Woods C. Intensive care unit environmental cleaning: an evaluation in sixteen hospitals using a novel assessment tool. J Hosp Infect. 2008;68:39-44.

118. Carling PC, Parry MF, Von Beheren SM. Identifying opportunities to enhance environmental cleaning in 23 acute care hospitals. Infect Control Hosp Epidemiol. 2008;29:1-7.

119. Hysong SJ, Best RG, Pugh JA. Audit and feedback and clinical practice guideline adherence: making feedback actionable. Implement Sci. 2006;1:9.

CHAPTER 16

Disinfection and sterilisation

TERRY McAULEY[i]

Dr GERALD McDONNELL[ii]

Chapter highlights

- An overview of the regulatory framework and a brief history of the applicable standards relating to medical device processing in Australia
- Discussion of the Spaulding Classification and its application to processing of medical devices
- An outline of the key steps in the medical device processing cycle with reference to AS/NZS 418
- Practical guidance on assessing the quality of medical device processing at a healthcare facility

[i] STEAM Consulting Pty Ltd, Greenvale, VIC
[ii] Microbiological Quality and Sterility Assurance, Johnson & Johnson, Raritan, NJ, USA

Introduction

Processing (or reprocessing) is defined as an activity to prepare a new or used healthcare product for its intended use. This can include various steps of cleaning, disinfection and sterilisation of medical devices. Processing is therefore a cornerstone in the prevention of transmission of infectious agents to and between patients undergoing medical and surgical procedures.

In the early 1990s, Standards Australia was tasked with developing an Australian Standard to guide processing of reusable medical devices (RMDs), largely in response to transmission of human immunodeficiency virus (HIV) between four patients that had undergone minor surgical procedures in a doctor's consulting room in 1989. The result was the first edition of AS 4187 in 1994 and a second edition in 1998. Prior to this, both Western Australia (WA) and New South Wales (NSW) had created their own sterilisation and disinfection guidelines although these were only applicable to processing in the hospital setting, thus the publication of a national standard for cleaning, disinfection and sterilisation of devices across all practice settings was a game changer in Australian medical device processing. Soon there were calls for a more practical and achievable standard for office-based practices, particularly in general practice and dentistry settings, resulting in the publication of separate yet related Australian and New Zealand standards for device processing in office-based practices (AS/NZS 4815:2001).

As technologies and devices evolved, AS 4187 was again revised in 2003 and published as a combined Australian and New Zealand standard, with the current edition being AS/NZS 4187:2014.[1] A second edition of AS/NZS 4815 was published in 2006 and remains a current standard.[2] Currently, a new draft standard, AS5369, is in preparation and once published, will replace both AS/NZS 4187 and AS/NZS 4815, recognising that the underpinning principles of cleaning, disinfection and sterilisation are universal despite contextual differences and risks in each practice setting.

Typically, compliance with an Australian Standard (or joint AS/NZ Standard) is voluntary unless the standard has been called into legislation when compliance becomes mandatory. While NSW, South Australia (SA) and Tasmania reference AS/NZS 4187 (and in some cases AS/NZS 4815) in their legislation or regulations, other jurisdictions currently do not. Nonetheless, the Australian Commission for Safety and Quality in Health Care (ACSQHC) requires compliance with AS/NZS 4187 in accordance with National Safety and Quality Health Service Standards (NSQHS) Standard 3 and Advisory AS 18/07,[3] and this is applicable to all Australian health facilities.

Effective processing of RMDs relies upon having appropriately trained, competent personnel that operate validated, monitored and maintained processing equipment. Implementation of the requirements in AS/NZS 4187:2014 hinges on a health facility having robust quality management systems in place.[1] Ensuring a quality systems approach to the processing of RMDs is essential, as breaches in correct processing procedures are frequently reported. Examples include lack of documented policies and procedures, no planned preventative maintenance programs, and poorly trained staff that fail to adhere to manufacturers' instructions for use (IFU) and facility procedures.[4]

16.1 The Australian regulatory framework for medical devices, sterilants and disinfectants

The role of the Therapeutic Goods Administration (TGA) is to ensure that therapeutic goods available in Australia are fit for purpose and are safe to use.[5] The TGA regulates the supply of pharmaceutical products, vaccines, biologics and tissue-based products, blood products, complementary medicines, including vitamins and other supplements, products used to test for or diagnose various diseases or conditions, and medical devices, disinfectants and sterilants, including the manufacturing and advertising of these products.[5] The TGA regulates medical devices under the *Therapeutic Goods Act 1989* and the Therapeutic Goods (Medical Devices) Regulations 2002. The legislation requires medical devices to be included on the Australian Register of Therapeutic Goods (ARTG) unless exempt before they can be legally supplied or sold in Australia or exported from Australia.[6]

Medical devices range from blood pressure monitors to surgical instruments, including equipment and consumable products that are used to prepare medical devices for use or reuse. Medical devices are categorised according to risks and, for regulatory requirements, must meet the 15 Essential Principles.[7,8] Essential Principle 13.4 requires the manufacturer or sponsor of the medical device to provide IFUs. When a medical device is intended to be cleaned, disinfected, packaged or sterilised before use or reuse, these instructions must include appropriate processes to be followed to ensure that the risk of infection from the use of the medical device is minimised, and must also include the number of times a medical device may be safely reused. Note that devices labelled as sterile and single use are not intended to be processed. They are previously sterilised in their primary (sterile maintenance) packaging by the manufacturer using methods such as radiation, gaseous or heat-based sterilisation processes.[9] As these devices are designed for direct use with a patient and not subjected to processing, they are not further considered in this chapter.

Disinfectants are regulated under the *Therapeutic Goods Act 1989*, the Therapeutic Goods Regulations 1990, and the Therapeutic Goods (Standard for Disinfectants and Sanitary Products) Order 2019, usually referred to as TGO 104. It is important to note that TGO 104 does not apply to sterilants as these agents are regulated as medical devices.[10] Hard surface disinfectants—those used for disinfection of general environmental surfaces—are regulated as Other Therapeutic Goods.[11] Hospital- or household-grade disinfectant liquids, sprays, wipes and aerosols that do not make a claim of efficacy against a specific microorganism are exempt from entry on the ARTG; however, if a specific claim of efficacy against microorganisms is made for these products, entry on the ARTG is required.[12]

Skin antiseptic agents are regulated as 'Over the Counter' medicines and must be entered on the ARTG. These products have been assessed by the TGA to ensure that they are appropriate for use on the skin and have been tested by the manufacturer.[11]

Disinfectants and sterilants that are used on medical devices are regulated as Class IIb medical devices and must be entered on the ARTG. In addition, cleaning agents intended for use on medical devices, which do not claim to have disinfectant or sterilant activity, are regulated as Class I medical devices and must also be included in the ARTG.[11] Disinfectants and sterilants intended for use on medical devices must be labelled as 'Instrument Grade' and there are three recognised spectrums of efficacy: low-level, intermediate-level and high-level disinfectants. Semi-critical medical devices that cannot withstand sterilisation or thermal disinfection processes must be cleaned and undergo high-level disinfection using an instrument-grade, high-level disinfectant.[1] A sterilant is a chemical agent, typically other than a gas, that can kill all microorganisms including bacterial endospores to result in a sterility assurance level (SAL) of $\leq 10^{-6}$.[13] This is essentially the same expectation as a sterilisation process used to render the product free from viable microorganisms. Instrument-grade high-level disinfectants are typically chemical sterilants that are used at a shorter exposure time than is required for achievement of sterilisation (or a defined SAL). A high-level disinfectant is expected to kill all microbial pathogens with the exception of large numbers of bacterial endospores when used in accordance with the manufacturer's instructions for use.[14]

An instrument-grade intermediate-level disinfectant is intended for use on non-critical medical devices or patient care items and is expected to be bactericidal, tuberculocidal, virucidal and fungicidal against asexual spores but not necessarily dried sexual or chlamydospores. Instrument-grade intermediate-level disinfectants cannot kill bacterial endospores.[13] An instrument-grade low-level disinfectant may also be used on non-critical medical devices and patient care items but can only reliably kill vegetative bacteria and large or medium-sized lipid (enveloped) viruses. Instrument-grade low-level disinfectants are not able to reliably kill bacterial endospores, mycobacteria, fungi or small non-lipid (non-enveloped) viruses.[13]

The TGA is also responsible for managing the collection of data regarding the safety and efficacy of medicines and medical devices. The medical device incident reporting and investigation scheme (IRIS) provides a framework for manufacturers, sponsors, users or consumers to report adverse events and near adverse events associated with the use of medical devices.[15] Adverse events or near adverse events can be related to mechanical or material failure of the devices, design or manufacturing issues, problems with packaging and labelling, software deficiencies, adverse interactions with other devices, or user or systemic errors. When an adverse (or near adverse) event occurs, the problem should be reported to health facility quality or risk management reporting pathways, where both the supplier of the device and the TGA should be promptly notified. Completed IRIS reports are investigated and risk assessed by the TGA and, where appropriate, information added to the Database of Adverse Events (DAEN) for future reference. During the investigation, the TGA will work with the sponsor or supplier of the device to resolve the issues. In certain circumstances, the outcome of the investigation may be the release of an alert or publication of an article on the TGA website; this may require the supplier to improve labelling or instructions, add warnings, or in some cases to withdraw the product from the market or issue a recall.

- Before purchasing medical devices, sterilants, antiseptic agents and disinfectants, check to ensure that the products have been entered on the ARTG and that instructions for use, including instructions for processing of medical devices, can be effectively followed at the facility.
- Ensure that healthcare workers know how to report problems experienced with medical devices, sterilants, antiseptic agents and disinfectants used within an organisation and that the organisation has the appropriate systems in place to report these problems to the manufacturer/sponsor and the TGA.

16.2 The relationship between Australian and international standards

As discussed in the introduction, processing (or reprocessing) of reusable medical devices (RMDs) in Australia is expected to be undertaken in accordance with either AS/NZS 4187 or AS/NZS 4815. But these standards, particularly AS/NZS 4187, extensively reference European Norm (EN) and International Organisation for Standardisation (ISO) standards. There is some history to this, largely due to Australia being a participant in the Global Harmonization Task Force (GHTF) founded in 1993. The GHTF's goal was to harmonise standards and medical device regulations that affect the safety, quality and performance of medical devices.[16] This was superseded by the International Medical Device Regulators Forum (IMDRF) in 2011, with the same goal. Australia is represented by the TGA.[17]

Standards Australia is a member of ISO. ISO has a Technical Committee (TC-198) that is responsible for a suite of standards under the umbrella title of 'Sterilisation of health care products'. ISO TC-198 was created in 1990 and began working on and publishing cleaning, disinfection and sterilisation-related standards as part of global harmonisation, many of them combining existing EN and ISO standards. ISO has an agreement with the European Committee for Standardization (CEN) that produces EN standards. ISO standards frequently reference applicable EN standards and when EN standards can be applied worldwide they can be published as an ISO standard.[18]

In Australia, Technical Committee HE-023 is responsible for standards relating to processing of medical and surgical instruments. When revising the content of AS/NZS 4187:2003 in preparation for publication of the 2014 edition, the committee took the decision to retire existing Australian standards where a suitable EN or ISO standard existed and to adopt the generic headings for each section within AS/NZS 4187 as used in most of the ISO sterilisation standards. Thus, AS/NZS 4187 frequently cross references the applicable ISO and EN standards, obliging users to have access to copies of the referenced documents and a working knowledge of the contents as they pertain to the Australian context of practice.

- Ensure your organisation has access to copies of the applicable AS, EN and ISO standards.
- Make sure that where applicable, any processing equipment or consumable products such as sterilisers, washer-disinfectors, chemical indicators and sterile barrier systems in use at your facility are provided with, or make a Declaration of Conformity to, the relevant applicable AS, ISO or EN standards.

16.3 The Spaulding Classification

The Spaulding Classification has been used since the 1950s to define RMD processing requirements and continues to be widely used worldwide.[19] To assist in developing a greater understanding of the principles underpinning the Spaulding Classification, the main pathogenic (or disease-causing) forms of microorganisms can be classified based on their resistance to inactivation—ranging from those that are relatively easier to inactivate to those that demonstrate higher resistance, as demonstrated in Figure 16.1. Expected levels of disinfection and sterilisation to inactivate these microorganisms are defined based on this resistance profile.

Essentially the Spaulding Classification is a tool that can be used to categorise devices and patient care equipment into three main types based on risk of transmission of infectious agents to patients: critical, semi-critical and non-critical medical devices, as indicated in Table 16.1.

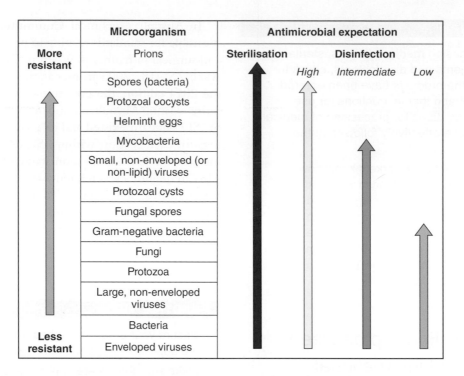

FIGURE 16.1 Microbiological resistance to inactivation and associated level of disinfection and sterilisation
Note that terms such as high, intermediate or low-level disinfection can have scientific and regulatory expectations,
and from a regulatory perspective, can vary regionally
*Note: This resistance list is given as a general guide and the resistance profiles can vary depending on the
specific disinfection or sterilisation method being considered.[9,18] Label claims such as 'bactericidal' or 'virucidal'
can often be misleading, as they imply the ability to be able to kill all bacteria or viruses respectively, although on
closer inspection this may not include certain types of bacteria (e.g. bacterial spores or mycobacteria) or only
certain types of viruses (e.g. enveloped viruses such as HIV or coronaviruses but not necessarily the more resistant
non-enveloped viruses such as polio- or parvo-viruses).
Source: Dr Gerald McDonell*

Critical medical devices are considered the highest risk as they are intended to enter areas of the body that may be considered 'sterile' or typically free from microorganisms. They are recommended to be cleaned, disinfected and sterilised before and between uses to protect the patient from the risk of infection. Terminal sterilisation processes are preferred, referring to the sterilisation of a medical device inside a sterile barrier system that protects the device from contamination after sterilisation and during periods of storage until required for use. In some instances, a medical device may be sterilised without a sterile barrier system for immediate use. In Australia, this practice has been discouraged in most situations (see section 16.13.3 Immediate use sterilisation).

Semi-critical medical devices may only contact mucous membranes that are not considered sterile tissues (e.g. consider the mouth, nasal passages or alimentary tract) or non-intact skin. Consequently, the minimum requirements for processing of these devices is cleaning followed by high-level disinfection.[1] Disinfection can be achieved by using chemical or heat-based processes; however, AS/NZS 4187[1] requires semi-critical devices to undergo sterilisation where they are compatible with a sterilisation process.

Non-critical medical devices are only intended to contact intact skin. In some circumstances, non-critical devices include patient care items that may not come into direct contact with the patient but are touched by the healthcare worker frequently during its use in patient care, for example intravenous infusion pumps. It is important to note that non-critical does not imply 'no risk'. Consider for example that contaminated surfaces can be touched by the hands

TABLE 16.1 The Spaulding Classification of medical devices and patient care equipment and recommended levels of disinfection or sterilisation prior to patient use

Classification	Description	Examples	Processes	Storage
Non-critical	Contact with intact skin	'High-touch' surfaces of patient care equipment e.g. touch screens, keyboards, stethoscopes, blood pressure cuffs, non-invasive ultrasound transducers, intravenous pumps and ventilators	Cleaning followed by disinfection when applicable. It is common for these devices to be cleaned and disinfected in one step using a TGA listed combined detergent and instrument-grade disinfectant product	Clean, dry place to minimise cross-contamination
Semi-critical	Contact with intact mucous membranes or non-intact (or broken) skin	Many types of flexible or rigid endoscopes (depending on their clinical use), intracavity ultrasound transducers, respiratory and anaesthesia equipment, vaginal speculae, anorectal manometry equipment, diaphragm fitting rings	Cleaning and sterilisation preferred where the medical device is compatible. Cleaning followed by high-level disinfection using an instrument-grade disinfectant is acceptable if the device cannot withstand a terminal sterilisation process.	Flexible endoscopes must be stored in an EN 16442 compliant storage cabinet.[20] Other semi-critical medical devices should be stored in a clean, dry, controlled space to prevent cross-contamination.[4] Duration of storage should be consistent with applicable published guidance documents
Critical	Contact with or penetration into sterile body cavities, the bloodstream or other 'sterile' body tissues	Surgical or dental devices or implants, needles, intravenous devices, endoscopes such as laparoscopes, arthroscopes, bronchoscopes	Cleaning, disinfection and steam sterilisation preferred. If the device cannot withstand a terminal steam sterilisation process, a terminal low temperature sterilisation process is acceptable	For devices sterilised in a sterile barrier system, store in a clean, dry and controlled area. Devices sterilised without a sterile barrier system must be used immediately

Source: Terry McAuley, developed from Table 5.1 in AS/NZS 4187:2014[1] and NHMRC[19]

(including sterile-gloved hands) prior to the handling of a device or patient directly and this can be a source of infectious agents. Overall, the focus is on risk reduction to decrease but not eliminate the presence of microorganisms. This, combined with prudent aseptic practices, can be effective and practical. The risks with non-critical devices can be reduced by cleaning and/or low-level disinfection using practical solutions (e.g. widely used disinfection wipes or liquid disinfectants) that both physically remove and/or inactivate common pathogens (vegetative bacteria and certain types of viruses).

Overall, the Spaulding Classification provides a practical guide to safe practices in cleaning, disinfection and sterilisation in healthcare facilities. Scientifically, there remains some debate on the potential to modify these requirements (or indeed, the expectations and limitations of these processes), but they have stood the test of time and experience, even as our knowledge of microbiology has increased. What is clear is that cleaning, disinfection and sterilisation practices are tools that are only as effective as the ways in which they are used in healthcare settings. Effectiveness is dependent on the education and competency of those using these technologies, and also on the maintenance of an appropriate environment in which these processes are undertaken, to minimise the risks of cross-contamination.

PRACTICE TIP 3

- Ensure your organisation has a system of designating medical devices as critical, semi-critical or non-critical, and that a register of these devices is kept that includes the locations where these devices are used and processed, and the approved method of processing.
- Regular audits should be conducted in all areas where medical device processing is occurring to ensure ongoing compliance with organisational policy.

16.4 Processing environments

In Australia, a processing facility is usually referred to as a central sterilising services department (CSSD), although processing can also occur in many different areas within a facility. As contaminated medical devices posing risks to staff are handled in these areas, coupled with the need to safely process devices to ensure patient safety, correct design of these processing areas is important. AS/NZS 4187:2014[1] contains specific requirements for unidirectional workflows, ventilation, surface finishes and fixtures and fittings for processing environments, although this standard does not provide extensive detail to guide the design and construction of a compliant processing facility.

In Australia, most jurisdictions have adopted the requirements in the Australasian Health Facility Guidelines (AusHFG) as the basis for designing and constructing a healthcare facility. The Sterilising Services Unit B.0190 section outlines basic requirements. The guidelines contain various operational models for sterilising services delivery, broad operational policies, and descriptions of each functional area, including requirements for surface finishes, ventilation, lighting, water and steam quality. It also contains reference to requirements in endoscope processing facilities.[21]

In addition to the specifications in the AusHFG, some jurisdictions have other requirements that must be met for health buildings, including specifications directly relating to CSSDs. For example, ventilation specifications in a CSSD are discussed in greater detail in the NSW Health document GL2021_014 Engineering Services Guidelines,[22] despite AS/NZS 4187:2014 referencing the Australian Standard AS 1668.2.[23] Other jurisdictions have comprehensive capital infrastructure guidelines that contain specifications over and above those in the AusHFG. For example, Queensland Health

has published Capital Infrastructure Requirements,[24] Victoria's Health and Human Services Building Authority has published the Engineering Guidelines for Healthcare Facilities,[25] and WA Health has a series of Building Guidelines for Health Facilities.[26] These guidance documents include more detailed requirements for ventilation, lighting, emergency power, surface finishes and other services in health buildings and may also contain requirements specific to CSSDs.

In practice, processing of medical devices usually occurs in three main settings:

1. in a centralised processing facility (CSSD)
2. in a dedicated endoscope processing facility; or
3. at a suitable location at or near to the point of use.

16.4.1 Central sterilising services departments

Critical medical devices and those semi-critical medical devices that are compatible with a sterilisation process should be sent to the CSSD for processing. This ensures that RMDs are cleaned, disinfected and inspected, then where applicable are packaged and sterilised by dedicated, trained and competent personnel.

Both AS/NZS 4187:2014 and the AusHFG Sterilising Services Unit B.0190[21] describe the basic requirements for processing facilities. A well-designed processing facility should be divided into three distinct and physically separated rooms. These rooms are commonly referred to as the:

1. decontamination or cleaning area
2. inspection, assembly and packaging (IAP) area; and
3. sterile storage area.

It is not uncommon to have the sterile storage area located separately to the processing facility, for example some designs require the sterile RMDs to be transported to the operating suite (OS) for storage, rather than the RMDs remaining in a sterile storage room co-located with the processing facility.

These rooms are further supported by other functional spaces and may include, but are not limited to: a dedicated loan set receipt and despatch room; a plant room for water treatment and/or steam generation systems and, if applicable, centralised chemical dosing; storage areas for bulk and clean consumable products used in the preparation of RMDs for use or reuse; waste disposal rooms and staff change rooms; and a break room. Figure 16.2 provides an example of processing facility design and the interrelationships of the associated areas.

RMDs typically move from the decontamination or cleaning room via pass-through processing equipment

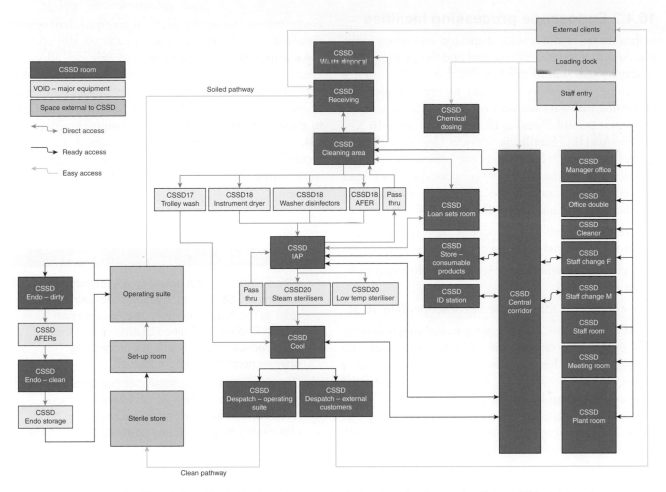

FIGURE 16.2 Processing facility design and detailed internal functional relationships
Source: Terry McAuley and Simon Coupe, Opunake Pty Ltd

such as washer-disinfectors (WDs) or automated flexible endoscope reprocessors (AFERs) to ensure that a soiled RMD cannot bypass a cleaning and associated thermal or chemical disinfection process before moving to the IAP area. An AFER should be provided to clean and disinfect flexible endoscopes (e.g. bronchoscopes, cystoscopes and rhino-laryngoscopes) that are then subjected to terminal low temperature sterilisation. These medical devices, just like the RMDs made of metals, must be cleaned and disinfected prior to sterilisation using an automated cleaning and disinfection process where compatible.

For RMDs that are not compatible with an automated cleaning and disinfection process, a manual cleaning pathway can be created that enables an RMD to be manually cleaned, rinsed with high-quality water and then placed into a pass-through drying cabinet without risk of cross-contamination.

Once cleaned, disinfected and packaged, controls should be in place to ensure that the RMDs cannot bypass a suitable sterilisation process before entering the sterile storage room. This is readily achieved by using pass-through steam and/or low temperature sterilising equipment.

Figure 16.2 also shows pass-through boxes between the IAP and the cleaning area, and the IAP and the cooling area. This is to facilitate the return of loading racks used to hold RMDs in the WDs and sterilisers back to the applicable area, to facilitate throughput without having to use the equipment to pass back the loading racks once emptied.

Ideally, there should be no means of personnel moving directly between each room—rather, personnel should move between each area through a common or central corridor. The described workflow minimises the risks of cross-contamination of RMDs and avoids the inadvertent release of an RMD that has not undergone a validated cleaning, disinfection and sterilisation process.

16.4.2 Endoscope processing facilities

In healthcare facilities with dedicated endoscopy units, it is common to have a dedicated endoscope processing facility located within this functional area, although it is becoming increasingly common to create endoscope processing pathways within a modern CSSD where co-location is possible[21] and as illustrated in Figure 16.3.

The AusHFG Sterilising Services Unit B.0190[21] describes the basic requirements for endoscope processing facilities, similar to the design concepts in a CSSD. A well-designed endoscope processing environment will be separated into three distinct zones:

1. a dirty zone where endoscopes are received and undergo manual cleaning

2. a clean zone where endoscopes are processed in an AFER; and

3. a storage area for processed endoscopes (Fig 16.3).

AFERs are now available with pass-through designs. This enables the creation of an endoscope processing environment that has two physically separate and distinct rooms, one for receiving and manually pre-cleaning the endoscope prior to loading it into the 'dirty' side of the AFER and the second, clean room in which cleaned and disinfected endoscopes are unloaded from the AFER and placed directly into EN 16442 compliant controlled environment storage cabinets, or an equivalent system. Controlled environment storage cabinets also come in a pass-through configuration, and this can allow for creation of a design where the users do not need to enter the processing area to retrieve processed endoscopes for patient use. The use of pass-through AFERs in endoscope processing facility design eliminates the risks of cross-contamination of cleaned and disinfected endoscopes as they are no longer being handled in the same space where soiled endoscopes are being cleaned.

PRACTICE TIP 4

- When planning for a new—or refurbishing an existing—CSSD or endoscope processing facility, refer to the requirements in the Australasian Health Facility Guidelines to ensure that the fundamental requirements for processing environments are being achieved.

- Consider engaging specialist consultants to provide advice on design, workflows, surface finishes, fixtures, ventilation, water quality, and processing equipment and capacity requirements.

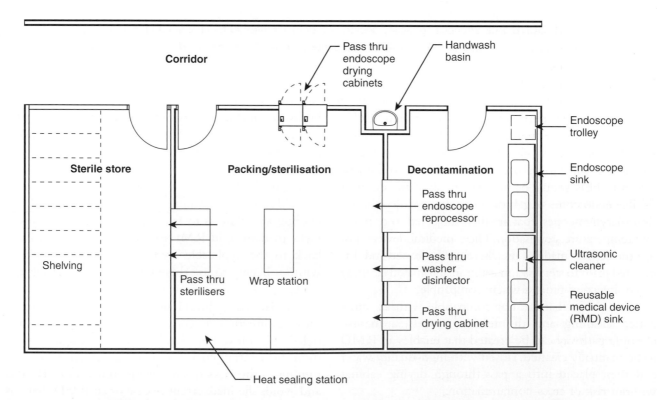

FIGURE 16.3 Best practice layout of a combined RMD and endoscope processing facility

Source: Baade Harbour Australia Pty Ltd and Terry McAuley

16.5 Point of care processing

Point of care processing usually occurs for all non-critical devices and patient care items, but also with some semi-critical devices that are not compatible with a sterilisation process. It is not uncommon to find that point of care processing occurs throughout a health facility, typically in outpatient departments (OPD), such as ENT clinics, speech pathology, respiratory therapy, sleep studies, urology, gynaecology and anorectal clinics, and in inpatient wards and departments, such as emergency department (ED), intensive care unit (ICU), diagnostic imaging (DI) and in the operating suite (OS).

Cleaning and, where required, low or intermediate-level disinfection at the point of care for non-critical devices and patient care items is often a straightforward process, usually using a commercially available detergent or a detergent and disinfectant (2-in-1) wipe system. It is essential that the personnel undertaking the cleaning and disinfection process follow a standardised procedure to ensure that the process is effective, as patient-ready devices have been found to be highly contaminated in numerous studies.[27,28]

Cleaning and high-level disinfection of a semi-critical medical device at the point of care is more challenging, as the microbiological quality of the cleaned and disinfected device can be compromised if there is not an appropriate environment in which the device can be processed and designated personnel competent in undertaking the processing procedures.[4] Ultrasound transducers that are in contact with blood, or have blood contamination occur during use, must undergo cleaning and high-level disinfection.[4,29] Procedures where ultrasound transducers are at risk for contamination with blood include areas such as ED, ICU, DI and in the OS.

AS/NZS 4187:2014[1] states that sheaths/sleeves/protective barriers for RMDs must not be used as a substitute for cleaning, disinfection or sterilisation. RMDs that come into contact with sterile body cavities or that are used on the critical aseptic field should be treated as critical medical devices. Cleaning and high-level disinfection of these RMDs prior to the application of a probe cover is intended to protect the patient from the risk of transmission of infectious agents, should there be a breach in the protective barrier during the procedure. Cleaning and high-level disinfection after use is intended to protect the next patient from the risk of contact with the previous patient's microorganisms.[4]

Often underestimated in the past, semi-critical medical devices are now considered to represent the greatest risk of infection agent transmission, as far more healthcare-associated infections (HAIs) have been reported using these devices when compared with those caused by critical or non-critical devices.[30] Therefore, ensuring that there is an appropriate environment for point of care processing of non-critical RMDs—and in particular for semi-critical RMDs that need to undergo cleaning and high-level disinfection at the point of care—is essential for patient safety and to minimise the risks of cross-contamination.[4] For example, processing a semi-critical device in a dirty utility room that is also used for the disposal or cleaning of human waste containers and disposal of contaminated waste and soiled linen is not an appropriate environment. This is because there is no clear demarcation between soiled and clean activities, workflows may not be unidirectional, and the disinfected device is exposed to the risks of cross-contamination through contact with contaminated environmental surfaces or aerosols generated during disposal procedures.[4]

Wherever practicable, a dedicated processing environment should be created in wards and departments where point of care processing is occurring, when sending these devices to a CSSD is not feasible.[4] The dedicated processing environment should ensure that unidirectional workflows can be achieved and there is clear demarcation between soiled and clean areas to ensure cross-contamination is avoided.[4] Ventilation, surfaces and other finishes must be consistent with AS/NZS 4187:2014 requirements.[1] Personnel undertaking the processing procedures must be trained to follow the RMD manufacturer's IFU, taking into account the cleaning agent and disinfecting agent manufacturer's IFU and ensure their practices in terms of personal protective equipment (PPE) use and disposal is such that soiled PPE is removed prior to handling a cleaned or disinfected device.[4]

PRACTICE TIP 5

Find out whether your organisation is effectively managing point of care processing of non-critical and semi-critical RMDs being used in wards and departments by visiting units such as speech pathology, respiratory therapy, ENT and ENT oncology, urology, gynaecology, obstetrics, sleep studies, ED, ICU and the OS. Ask them to show you what medical devices are being processed at the point of care and then investigate where and how these RMDs are being processed and stored.

16.6 Water quality

Water is used in many stages of RMD processing. The quality of the water required in each stage varies as both the chemical purity and the microbiological quality of the water used can compromise the outcomes of cleaning, disinfection or sterilisation processes.[30] AS/NZS 4187:2014 Amendment Number 2[1] specifies water quality requirements for:

1. cleaning processes

2. final rinse water in manual and automated cleaning and thermal disinfection processes

3. final rinse water in automated cleaning and chemical disinfection processes; and steam generation.

Currently work is in progress to create an International Standard or Guidance document on the quality of water used for processing medical devices and this may change these specifications in future.

16.6.1 Chemical purity of water

Water is a universal solvent and contains many chemicals in an ionic state (ions). The type and number of ions carried in the water will influence its chemical purity and acceptability for processing. For processing, the ionic contaminates of frequent concern are those causing water hardness and chlorides that contribute to the presence of residuals and metal corrosion (Table 16.2). For example, hard water conditions (the presence of a high concentration of calcium or magnesium) can impact on cleaning efficacy as they can make the cleaning

TABLE 16.2 Summary of the possible effects and risks of sources of ionic and other contaminants in water used in processing of medical devices

Contaminant	Observed effect	Risk assessment
pH high or low	Pitting, corrosion	Device damage Potential compromise to cleaning and/or disinfection efficacy
Hardness	Scaling Lime deposits Corrosion potential Potential for generation of non-condensable gases in boiler feedwater	Soil accumulation and deposits Device damage or usability Equipment damage (requiring frequent descaling) Potential compromise to cleaning and/or disinfection efficacy Increased corrosion Compromised sterilisation
Chlorides, chlorine	Pitting, corrosion, rusting Filter damage	Risk to patient and user safety Difficulty cleaning or achievement of sterilisation due to damaged surfaces Device stress and crevice corrosion and instrument breakages Reduced device lifetime Damage to filters, rubber components, RO membranes
Silicates	White-grey/yellowish-brown/bluish-purple deposits; scaling Promotes corrosive effect of chlorides	Risk to patient safety Reduced device lifetime Can make visual inspection more difficult
Heavy and non-ferrous metals	Brown-red deposits Secondary rust	Risk to patient safety Reduced device lifetime Can make visual inspection more difficult
Iron	Corrosive to stainless steel Can form magnetite in steriliser pipework	Risk to patient safety Reduced device lifetime
Phosphates	Promotes corrosive effect of chlorides	Risk to patient safety Reduced device lifetime
Evaporative residue and particulates	Spotting and scaling	Risk to patient safety Can make visual inspection more difficult

Source: Terry McAuley, developed from sources[32–35]

agents less effective, and cause components to precipitate and deposit onto RMD surfaces, resulting in staining. Increasing the temperature (or boiling) of hard water can also cause deposition of these ions onto surfaces, leading to visible 'scale' particulates. Chlorides in water are known to lead to corrosion of metals, and the impact of chlorides increases as the temperature of the water is elevated.[31] AS/NZS 4187:2014[1] requires monthly monitoring and recording of water hardness and chloride levels in water used for cleaning processes.

After cleaning, RMDs undergo rinsing and often thermal disinfection where the temperature of the water in WDs is usually much higher than that used in the cleaning stage of the process. Consequently, the specifications for the chemical purity of final rinse water or for steam generation are more stringent (see AS/NZS 4187:2014, Amendment 2, Tables 7.2 and Table 7.4[1]). For the final rinse water in a WD, the conductivity of the water (as a general indication of the levels of ions present) must be ≤30μS/cm and for steam generation ≤5μS/cm.[1] Once per annum a full laboratory chemical analysis should be undertaken on the final rinse water and water used for steam generation. For WDs, AS/NZS 4187:2014[1] recommends monthly monitoring and recording of conductivity as a method to demonstrate the water treatment system is maintaining conformance within specifications.

Thermolabile endoscopes undergo rinsing at much lower temperatures and the endoscope materials of construction are considered less susceptible to the effects of ions. Therefore, there is no current requirement to test the chemical purity of the final rinse water in an AFER unless it is a requirement of the AFER manufacturer.[1,35]

Steam purity refers to the chemical composition of the steam being used for sterilisation and must be in accordance with AS/NZS 4187:2014, Amendment 2 Table 7.4.[1] At this time, the specifications for water purity used for steam generation in small steam sterilisers are different.[36] Overall, the purity of the water used for steam generation can also influence the 'quality' of the steam. Steam quality refers to the physical properties of steam necessary for effective sterilisation, including variables such as the absence of air or other non-condensable gases (NCGs); excess moisture or wet steam; or the presence of superheat, where the steam is too dry.[1]

Achievement of the chemical purity specifications for water used in the final rinse after cleaning, thermal disinfection and steam generation requires installation of water treatment systems to remove the ionic and other contaminants that can include carbon filters, water softening units, deionising units or reverse osmosis (RO) water treatment systems. As water treatment systems will remove chlorine compounds or similar antimicrobial agents from the water, the risk of microbial contamination and growth can be higher, and this is discussed in the next section.

16.6.2 Microbiological quality of water

At the completion of either cleaning, disinfection or sterilisation, RMDs are required to be of a suitable microbiological quality that will not impact on patient safety. Therefore, processing procedures should not add to the bioburden (population of microorganisms) on the device. As water is often used for final stages of processing (e.g., rinsing following cleaning or chemical disinfection, or for heat disinfection/sterilisation), it is important to control the microbial quality of the water used.[1,32] Treating water to remove chemical contaminates, including sources of chlorine or similar preservatives, will further increase the risks of microbial contamination in water. Gram-negative bacteria and non-tuberculous mycobacteria readily proliferate, even in the purest water.[32] The outer cell wall of Gram-negative bacteria includes lipopolysaccharide complexes known as endotoxins that are released from the bacterial cells when damaged or inactivated. Endotoxins can cause fever and other adverse effects in patients and are potential contaminants on medical devices.[32,33] Endotoxins are heat stable and are not reliably inactivated by heat disinfection or steam sterilisation processes used in healthcare.[37]

Microorganisms are commonly removed from the water supply using filters in combination with water treatment systems intended to remove chemical contaminates.[34] RO water treatment systems are widely used as they can remove both organic and inorganic contaminants.[34] However, with any water treatment system there is still a risk that if not properly designed and controlled, the water distribution network can become contaminated, often with microbial biofilms resulting in unacceptably high levels of microbial contamination and endotoxins.[34] Biofilms are persistent communities of microorganisms that are often associated with water-handling systems. Controls will include system design and routine maintenance.

To ensure that the microbiological quality of the water used in processing will not adversely impact patient safety, Table 7.2 in AS/NZS 4187:2014 Amendment No. 2[1] specifies that final rinse water used in manual cleaning or for the final rinse in a WD has a total viable count (TVC) of ≤100 cfu/100mL and endotoxins must be ≤0.25EU/mL. For AFERs, Table 7.3

requires the TVC is ≤10 cfu/100mL with no detection of *P. aeruginosa* or atypical *Mycobacterium* species, and endotoxins ≤30 EU/mL. Monthly monitoring of the microbiological quality (via TVC) of the final rinse water in WDs and AFERs is required, while endotoxin testing is only required annually.[1]

16.6.3 Design, maintenance and testing of water treatment systems

Well designed and maintained water treatment systems are essential to ensure that water will continue to be produced at the specified quality.[1] For example, filters must be changed on a regular basis to ensure that they continue to function correctly. Records should be kept of filter changes, and these must occur at the frequency specified by the manufacturer. Filter changes may be time based or may be triggered by pressure variations across two consecutive filters in the system indicating particulate accumulation.

It is important to note that carbon filters, water softeners and deionising units can become contaminated with microorganisms if not changed and/or disinfected (also referred to as sanitised) on a regular basis to reduce microbial contamination. With water softening systems, there may be a requirement to regularly top up the salt in the systems, and with deionising units there may be a requirement to regenerate the resin deionising beads. Reference must be made to the water treatment system manufacturer's IFU to identify the frequency of disinfection of the filtration, softening and/or deionising systems and, where applicable, regeneration of the deionising resins.

Filtration is the most common method for treatment of the rinse water supplied to an AFER and management of the water filters must be in accordance with the manufacturer's IFU. Most AFERs require self-disinfection and waterline disinfection cycles to be completed on a regular basis and completion of these tasks must be documented.

RO water systems should be designed with a ring main loop to ensure a continual flow of water at >1m/s to avoid stagnation. Common problems seen in practice are RO systems that have terminal points into a WD or steam generator without a return loop, use of corrugated or other flexible plastic hoses running off the ring main to the equipment that may be coiled on top of the machine, coupled with no regular automated or manual disinfection schedules, or checks of pre-filter pressures and regular pre-filter changes as part of a planned preventative maintenance agreements. With RO water treatment systems, continuous disinfection by heating and circulating the water at >60°C is very effective;[34] however, there are other, possibly lower cost, options for disinfection such as chlorine dioxide, ozone or regular hyper-chlorination. Most RO systems also include UV light disinfection and often endotoxin filters on the exit loop of the ring main to reduce the risk of system contamination.

Most RO water systems also include a water storage system to ensure there is sufficient water to meet or exceed peak demand. It is important to ensure that any water storage tanks do not contaminate the rest of the system through having the tank properly vented with bacterial filters and having a zero-water retention design.

It is important to have sampling ports located at key points throughout the system. The sampling ports must be a sanitary type to protect the system from contamination. Sampling ports are typically located on the exit and return loop on the ring main, often near the water storage tank in addition to having other sampling ports fitted closer to the point of entry into the steam generator and, where applicable, near to the point of entry into WDs.[1,38] If a WD has a rinse water storage/heating tank, the sample must be taken from inside the machine.[38] For AFERs, final rinse water samples are usually taken from the endoscope basin in accordance with the manufacturer's IFU, as most have a 0.2μ filter inside the machine.

PRACTICE TIP 6

Investigate the water quality monitoring systems that are in place in your organisation and ensure that:

- the cleaning process water is monitored for hardness and chlorides monthly

- the final rinse water quality in your washer-disinfectors is being monitored on a monthly basis by recording conductivity; and

- total viable count (TVC) testing is being performed on a regular basis, once the requirement for monthly testing for a 12-month period has demonstrated consistency in results.

Investigate the water quality monitoring for the AFERs in use in your organisation and ensure that:

- TVCs are being performed monthly; and

- the testing includes tests for *Pseudomonas aeruginosa* and non-tubercular mycobacteria (NTM).

16.7 Steps in processing of reusable medical devices

The earlier discussion on the Spaulding Classification (Table 16.1) defined the minimum requirements of processing depending on the risk associated with the use of the reusable device. A summary of these steps is given in Figure 16.4.

Non-critical devices must undergo cleaning, and this may be followed by low or intermediate-level disinfection, semi-critical devices must undergo cleaning and high-level disinfection although if the device is compatible, sterilisation is required, and critical devices must undergo cleaning and sterilisation.[1] It should be noted that many critical medical devices will undergo cleaning in an automated washer-disinfector (or AFER) system that includes a thermal or chemical disinfection step and is then subjected to packaging and terminal sterilisation. Highlighted in this cycle of processing are other important steps such as inspection and, when applicable, storage and transportation.

There are two important standards that define the processing requirements that must be included in instructions for use, ISO 17664-1[39] for critical and semi-critical devices, and ISO 17664-2[40] for non-critical devices. It is the RMD manufacturers' responsibility to provide validated, detailed instructions for use that describe the requirements for processing of a medical device in compliance with the international standards, as well as considering applicable national standards in force in countries in which the device is sold.

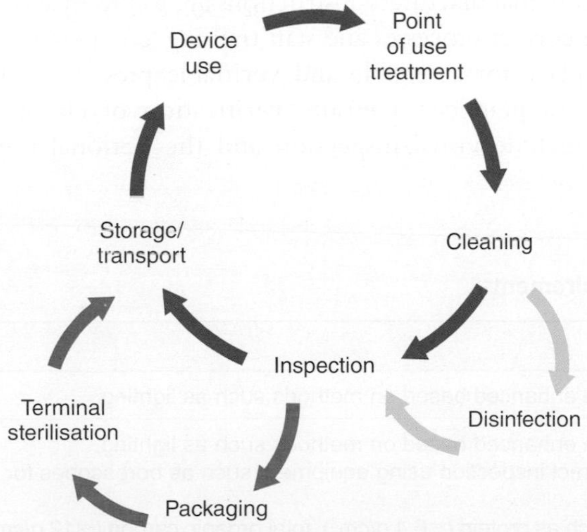

FIGURE 16.4 RMD processing steps
Source: Dr Gerald McDonnell

The instructions should include steps for any point of use treatment and any limitations or restrictions on processing (including the usable life of the device). The manufacturer must also provide instructions for a validated automated method for cleaning and disinfection of the device, unless the device is unable to withstand an automated cleaning and disinfection process. In these circumstances, the manufacturer is obliged to provide a statement alerting the user to this issue.[39] For critical devices, further instructions on packaging, terminal sterilisation, and handling post-sterilisation should be included.

It is the healthcare facility's responsibility to integrate these processing requirements into their quality management system and ensure they are correctly applied. For example, review of new RMDs IFU prior to purchase will help to ensure that the correct water quality, cleaning agents, cleaning brushes, disinfectants (where applicable), washer-disinfector equipment, inspection equipment, packaging materials, sterilising equipment and trained personnel are available.

16.8 Point of use pre-treatment

Point of use pre-treatment is the first step in the processing cycle and is undertaken by the user of the device. This can involve wiping or rinsing gross debris off all surfaces of the device and minimising the drying of soils in and on the device prior to cleaning.[39] This may be achieved by transporting soiled medical devices immediately to the processing facility, or when transportation is delayed, keeping the devices moist until cleaning can occur.[39] Smith et al.[41] described commonly used options to keep devices moist, including spraying them with a pre-cleaning solution, gel or wetting agent; using commercially produced plastic bags with absorbent material that is moistened with water prior to placing the RMDs inside and sealing the bag; or placing RMDs inside readily available plastic bags to which sterile wound pads that have been moistened with sterile water are added and sealing the bag. In this study on the effectiveness of methods to keep neurosurgical RMDs moist between use and subsequent cleaning, the authors concluded that using tap water to wet the tray liner inside the surgical tray before sealing it in a plastic bag could be equally as effective at keeping RMDs moist, in addition to being more cost effective.[41]

According to Bundgaard et al.[42] various international standards or guidelines have recommended that cleaning of RMDs should commence within 6 hours after use, noting that the delay in processing of flexible endoscopes after use should be no more than 60 minutes.[43] However, they also challenged this assumption for surgical RMDs, saying that there was limited scientific data upon which this recommendation had been made. Their study demonstrated that there was no difference in residual protein levels and corrosion occurring on RMDs that had processing delayed for >6 hours, although there was an acknowledgement that extended delays in processing could allow microbial replication to occur as reported in other studies. It was not investigated if the presence of an increased number of microorganisms on RMDs prior to cleaning impacted on the cleanliness of the RMDs after processing. In short, best practice is to minimise the delay between use of RMDs and commencement of cleaning, and where there is an anticipated delay in processing, methods should be implemented to keep the devices moist until cleaning can be undertaken. It is also best practice to only use cleaning or pre-cleaning products labelled for that use. Manufacturers often recommend against the use of other chemicals commonly found in clinical/surgical practice such as antiseptics (e.g. iodine) or saline, as these can damage devices.

PRACTICE TIP 7

Investigate the methods being used for point of use pre-treatment of RMDs at your facility and identify whether the practices are consistent with your local policy and requirements in AS/NZS 4187:2014.

16.9 Cleaning

Cleaning is an essential requisite to ensure device safety, irrespective of how the device is being used. It is defined as the removal of contaminants to the extent necessary for further processing or for intended use.[44]

For non-critical devices, cleaning alone may be appropriate for the physical removal of visible soil and associated microorganisms; for these types of devices or patient care equipment it is often sufficient to perform a one-step cleaning and disinfection process by a pour (or spray)-and-wipe process in accordance with manufacturer's instructions. But as the criticality of the device increases, so do the requirements for cleaning. This is because residuals from the cleaning process itself can lead to negative patient impacts (e.g. toxicity) and particularly if these residuals may not be removed by a subsequent process (as in the case with steam sterilisation, which may even change the residual chemicals to make them toxic to patients). Further, residuals that can remain due to inadequate cleaning can also interfere with the subsequent disinfection and/or sterilisation process, increasing the risk of microorganisms surviving these processes. There are many reports in the literature of this impact that have been implicated as the source of patient infections, even following steam sterilisation.[45-49] The lack of adequate cleaning is therefore the greatest risk in processing of RMDs.

The main criterion for cleaning is to ensure the lack of visible soiling, but recent standardisation in this area has led to more defined criteria for the requirements of cleaning and associated cleaning validation testing for critical and semi-critical devices as summarised in Table 16.3.[38,50,51] These test requirements are performed by the device manufacturer to international and/or regional requirements and provide the basis for cleaning instructions for use by the manufacturer.[39] It is not necessary for healthcare facilities to validate individual device cleaning requirements, but to ensure manufacturers' instructions are followed and that the correct processes and staff training/competency are in place for a reliable and verifiable process.[1] But it is best practice to ensure verification of cleanliness to include visual inspection and the optional use of

---

TABLE 16.3 Recommended end points for RMD cleaning requirements

RMD Spaulding Classification	Cleaning end points
Non-critical	Visual inspection, which can be enhanced based on methods such as lighting
Semi-critical	Visual inspection, which can be enhanced based on methods such as lighting, magnification or the use of indirect inspection using equipment such as borescopes for endoscopic lumen inspection. Detectable levels of analytes such as protein ($\leq$6.4 g/cm^2), total organic carbon ($\leq$12 g/cm^2), or haemoglobin ($\leq$2.2 g/cm^2)

Source: Dr Gerald McDonnell, developed from ISO 15883-1,[38] FDA[50] and ISO 15883-5[51]

cleaning indicator systems that may detect the presence of protein or other soil components. Worst-case devices or device features (that represent product families) may be chosen for this purpose. For cleaning this will typically include device features that may have limited access to the cleaning process, such as restrictive surfaces, moving parts and lumens.

Once received in a processing facility, RMDs are sorted according to the appropriate cleaning pathways. While most RMDs can undergo cleaning in a WD or AFER, many RMDs require pre-cleaning steps prior to being subjected to these processes. For example, multi-component devices may need to be disassembled and jointed instruments opened prior to loading into the WD. Cannulated RMDs require brushing and flushing of the lumens prior to these being connected to the fluid pathway in a WD, and some RMDs may require exposure to an ultrasonic cleaning process prior to being processed in a WD. In all circumstances, review of the manufacturer's IFU is required, as some manufacturers require full manual cleaning of the RMD prior to exposure to an automated cleaning and disinfection process.

Flexible endoscope manufacturers currently require manual pre-cleaning of the endoscope prior to these being loaded into an AFER. This usually involves a leak test being performed, followed by manual cleaning by the passage of a brush or equivalent device down internal channels as specified by the manufacturer. Manufacturers may also require that certain internal channels that cannot be brushed are also adequately flushed prior to further processing in an automated cleaning and disinfection process. These steps are not only important to remove gross soil but also to verify that the internal lumens are not blocked. Some modern types of AFERs have the capability to detect lumens are free flowing, but it is important to ensure that such equipment is used in accordance with the manufacturer's instructions (including manual cleaning steps). Note that attention is not only required to the device but also any accessories used with devices, such as complex valves that can be difficult to clean. A common source of HAIs associated with devices is linked to the inadequate cleaning of internal device structures such as lumens and complex or moving parts.[45-49]

Some RMDs may not be compatible with automated cleaning and disinfection processes and are subject only to manual cleaning. In this case, best practice is to have a dedicated pathway for manually cleaned RMDs, separate to other RMD processing pathways to minimise the risks for cross-contamination.

16.9.1 Manual cleaning processes

ISO 17664-1[39] clearly requires manufacturers of medical devices to warn users if their device cannot undergo an automated cleaning and disinfection process. Health facilities should carefully evaluate device IFUs prior to purchase to ensure that, wherever practicable, RMDs can withstand automated cleaning and disinfection processes, and/or that equipment for cleaning is available.

For effective manual cleaning of an RMD a unidirectional workflow must be followed to avoid risks for cross-contamination. Personnel must be trained to differentiate between soiled and cleaned RMDs and change their PPE according to the stage of the process, so PPE does not become a source for cross-contamination.[4]

Appropriate controls need to be implemented to ensure that the temperature and the quality of the water used in each stage of the cleaning and rinsing processes is controlled where required, that the cleaning agent dosage is correct, that the brushes used for cleaning do not contribute to the bioburden on the RMDs being cleaned and are of the correct size and type, and that the volumes for flushing and rinsing lumens are delivered in accordance with the manufacturer's IFUs.

Training and competency assessment of personnel undertaking manual cleaning processes is essential to minimise risks for patient safety.[4] While AS/NZS 4187:2014 only requires visual inspection of RMDs after cleaning, implementation of routine monitoring of the effectiveness of manual cleaning using a protein or ATP residual test is beneficial.

16.9.2 Ultrasonic cleaning

Some RMD manufacturers' IFUs require subjecting the device to an ultrasonic cleaning process prior to processing in an automated cleaning and disinfection process or as part of a manual cleaning procedure.

There is an Australian Standard for ultrasonic cleaners, AS 2773:2019,[52] although it should be recognised that ultrasonic cleaners may be manufactured in countries outside Australia. This does not preclude their purchase; however, checks should be made to ensure that the ultrasonic cleaners manufactured outside Australia broadly meet the essential principles contained in AS 2773.

Ultrasonic cleaners remove soil from the surfaces of an RMD through a process called cavitation in combination with an applicable cleaning agent. In simple terms, cavitation is the formation and implosion of microscopic bubbles created by high frequency sound waves creating alternating waves of high and low pressure in a solution.[53] This creates a physical cleaning action at the surface of the RMD, effectively dislodging adherent soils.[53] As the bubbles can form in locations on and within an RMD that are difficult to reach with standard cleaning methods, ultrasonic cleaning can be an effective tool in cleaning RMDs with complex geometry.

Typically, an ultrasonic cleaning process is applied to an RMD prior to further processing in a WD or prior to manual cleaning. Where ultrasonic cleaning is required according to the RMD manufacturer's instructions for use, multi-component RMDs should be disassembled, jointed RMDs should be opened, and lumened RMDs should be either connected to a fluid pathway in the machine if available or immersed in a manner that expels all the air from the device lumens and ensures the presence of the cleaning chemistry in the lumen. RMDs should be placed in the manufacturer's loading basket in a single layer and exposed to the process at the recommended energy frequency for the correct exposure time.

However, it is important to note that not all RMDs are compatible with exposure to an ultrasonic cleaning process. For example, RMDs with soft surfaces such as rubber, silicone or plastic absorb the ultrasonic energy, reducing cleaning effectiveness. RMDs with cements or adhesive components such as laparoscopes and arthroscopes can be damaged, as ultrasonic energy can erode the materials holding the fibreoptic bundles and lenses in place.

It is currently controversial if the water and cleaning agent solution used in ultrasonic cleaning systems may only be changed at a minimum of once per day and whenever visibly soiled.[1] Over a period of time, the ultrasonic cleaner can become a source of contamination for other RMDs.[54] This was clearly demonstrated in a study by Vassey et al.,[54] where RMDs that had been exposed to manual cleaning followed by ultrasonic cleaning had significantly more protein residues after the process than RMDs that had not undergone cleaning at all. Therefore, best practice when using an ultrasonic cleaner as part of any cleaning process, either manual or automated, is to use the ultrasonic as a pre-cleaning step after gross soil has been removed from the RMD and follow exposure to the ultrasonic cleaner with a full manual or automated cleaning process. Other options include the use of fresh water and cleaning agent solution in every cycle.

AS/NZS 4187:2104[1] and the applicable standards for ultrasonic cleaning equipment require daily testing and annual qualification of the performance of the equipment to deliver an effective process.

16.9.3 Automated cleaning and disinfection processes

With some limited exceptions, most RMDs are compatible with automated cleaning processes delivered by washer-disinfectors compliant with ISO 15883-1,[38] along with the requirements of other parts of the standard series such as ISO 15883-2[55] for RMDs, or ISO 15883-4[56] for thermolabile endoscopes (AFERs). AS/NZS 4187:2014[1] requires that equipment delivering automated cleaning and disinfection processes undergo performance qualification on an annual basis and be routinely monitored on a cycle-by-cycle basis.

Routine monitoring includes verification that all process parameters have been met during a process cycle and that other tests and checks have been successfully performed, for example monitoring of cleaning agent dosage, water quality and cleaning of the processing equipment in accordance with the manufacturer's IFU.

While there is no current recommended requirement for the routine use of cleaning indicators (or artificial soil tests) on a daily or more frequent basis for monitoring of WDs, it is common practice in most CSSDs to use these tests. It is important to note that AS/NZS 4187 Table 10.1 (Amendment Number 2)[1] requires quarterly testing with artificially soiled loads in the WD in accordance with requirements specified in ISO 15883-1.[38]

All RMDs released from an automated cleaning and disinfection process must be visually inspected prior to release for use if cleaning and disinfection is the terminal process, or if further assembly and packaging is required in preparation for terminal sterilisation. Visual inspection is an essential step in ensuring the safety and quality of processed RMDs, as the human factor can impact on the efficacy of achievement of cleaning and disinfection, despite the use of automated cleaning and disinfection equipment.[4] Therefore, it is essential that personnel are trained and competent at the disassembly and loading of RMDs into WDs and AFERs. Examples include that all device lumens are connected to a fluid flow pathway in the machine, that the manner of RMD presentation does not create the potential for shadowing, and the devices are allowed to drain to allow for drying.[4] Ideally, standardised methods for loading the RMDs in the WDs and AFERs should be instituted and compliance with loading patterns audited on a regular basis.

Automated cleaning and disinfection equipment may or may not include a drying stage as part of the process cycle. If the process cycle includes an effective drying stage, both ISO 15883-1[38] and ISO 15883-4[56] require RMDs and endoscopes to be free from residual water at the completion of the process cycle. Where a drying stage is not included in a process cycle or the drying time has been deliberately reduced by the health facility in order to facilitate throughput, RMDs will need to be dried in an AS 5330 compliant drying cabinet for reusable medical devices[57] and endoscopes may be dried in an EN 16442 compliant controlled environment storage cabinet or equivalent system for processed thermolabile endoscopes.[58] Device lumens are particularly difficult to dry, where the presence of water is not just a concern for the growth of microorganisms over time but can also compromise the safety of terminal sterilisation processes.

It is essential to have an overall quality process in place at the healthcare facility that will include training, monitoring of parametric indicators during any automated process (e.g. chemistry dosing, temperatures and times) as well as visual inspection. Product families that represent the worst-case features and washer-disinfector loads for cleaning may be chosen for this purpose.

16.9.4 Thermal disinfection

In Australia, thermal disinfection processes are commonly applied to RMDs following cleaning in a WD intended for processing of thermally stable RMDs.

Thermal, moist heat (such as hot water or steam) is a traditional and reliable disinfectant or sterilant depending on its use and both are dependent on exposure to defined temperatures over time. For moist heat disinfection, this is practically employed by heating of water to temperatures in excess of 70°C, and exposures at defined time and temperature combinations to reduce the microbial load on or in RMDs. These combinations equate to the requirements for low, intermediate or high levels of chemical disinfection,[59] as indicated in Table 16.4.

Calculation of the required time at temperature combinations utilises a mathematical equation to calculate the A_0 value as described in ISO 15883-1[38] and this is based on a similar equation used for sterilisation to calculate the F_0 value used for steam sterilisation.[59] This is due to the predicable nature of microbial inactivation at these temperatures, and essentially that as the temperature increases above the threshold of 70°C so does the antimicrobial activity. The higher the temperature, the less time it takes to demonstrate the same level of antimicrobial activity. In practical use, it is not uncommon to see all RMDs undergoing thermal disinfection to be processed at an A_0 of up to 3000 although an A_0 of 600 is considered more than acceptable for a high-level disinfection process, particularly for critical devices that will be subjected to a terminal sterilisation process.[60] For non-critical RMDs, AS/NZS 4187:2014[1] suggests an A_0 of 600 may be suitable

TABLE 16.4 Levels of thermal disinfection and time/ temperature requirements

Level of disinfection	Spaulding Classification	Recommended A_0*	Common Australian exposure time and temperature combinations
High level	Interim disinfection of critical device prior to packaging and terminal sterilisation. Semi-critical RMDs that cannot tolerate sterilisation e.g. certain laryngoscope designs	≥600, although 3000 is traditionally common in many countries	**3000** 93°C for 2.5 minutes 90°C for 5 minutes **600** 90°C for 1 minute 83°C for 5 minutes
Intermediate level	Semi-critical RMDs that may or may not undergo sterilisation prior to use, e.g. vaginal speculae, laryngoscope blades	≥600	**600** 90°C for 1 minute 83°C for 5 minutes
Low level	Non-critical RMDs or patient care items that can withstand exposure to thermal disinfection processes, e.g. bed pans, carts or walking frames	≥60	**600** 90°C for 1 minute 83°C for 5 minutes **60** 80°C for 1 minute 70°C for 10 minutes

Source: Terry McAuley, developed from Block[59]
*As defined in the ISO 15883 series of washer-disinfector standards

for items exposed to a thermal disinfection process, even though the minimum requirement in the ISO 15883 series of standards is an A_o of 60.

Release of any load or device following a thermal disinfection process to these requirements can be determined parametrically by verification of the achieved time/temperature requirements in maintained/calibrated automated equipment under the facility's quality requirements.

16.9.5 Chemical disinfection

Chemical disinfection is widely used for processing of non-critical devices and patient care items, and some types of thermolabile semi-critical devices. For non-critical devices and patient care items, disinfection is commonly achieved through using disinfectant-impregnated wipes or solutions. Chemical disinfection of semi-critical devices can be achieved by manual or automated methods. Manual disinfection methods for semi-critical RMDs include application using a wipe system, or through immersion of the device in a disinfectant solution; however, it is preferable that where an RMD is compatible, it is processed in a washer-disinfector for thermolabile medical devices (AFER) that achieves high-level chemical disinfection as part of an automated process.

Examples of the types of antimicrobials used for disinfection of semi-critical RMDs include aldehydes (OPA, glutaraldehyde) and oxidising agents (hydrogen peroxide, peracetic acid, chlorine dioxide), due to their broad-spectrum antimicrobial activity. Some are labelled for use only when used as part of specific equipment (such as AFERs), while others can be used for manual or automated disinfection processes. Disinfectants used on RMDs should be labelled instrument grade and be listed on the ARTG.[12] Each disinfection product is a unique formulation with individual IFU that includes specific instructions regarding the preparation of the disinfectant (e.g. requiring dilution or activation), contact time and temperature (if applicable) requirements for disinfection, shelf-life and safety requirements. Safety information is detailed in safety data sheets which are required to be provided with chemicals.[1]

Product-specific IFU can include requirements for temperature controls to achieve the desired disinfection level and recommended contact times. For manual disinfection methods it is essential that the disinfectant is thoroughly rinsed at the conclusion of the contact time, to avoid hazards to patients from process residuals, noting there may be detailed requirements for water quality—that is, sterile or filtered, volumes of rinse water used, and/or the duration of rinsing—as there are

multiple reports in the literature of the damage to patient tissues from high levels of chemical residuals on semi-critical devices.[61,62]

High-level disinfectants and sterilants can be labelled for single or multiple use. Most are provided with process (or chemical) indicators that are used to verify the presence of the disinfectant at adequate concentration for effectiveness. Close adherence to the chemical indicator IFU is important, as these frequently require the user to perform positive and negative control tests upon opening each new bottle of indicators, along with the need to record the date of opening of the bottle, as the shelf life of the indicators is shortened upon opening, usually to a 3 or 6-month time period.

As chemical disinfectants can be toxic, hazards to the user and the environment must be effectively managed during storage, use or disposal, and they require strict adherence to the manufacturer's IFU.[1]

Automated cleaning and disinfection systems provide many advantages as the process is effectively monitored and controlled, provides evidence of disinfection parameters being achieved on the process record, and the process is reproducible. However, there are some automated or partially automated disinfection systems that use hydrogen peroxide or chlorine dioxide as the disinfectant, although these systems do not include an automated cleaning stage. These types of systems may be useful at the point of care for high-level disinfection of non-critical and semi-critical RMDs that cannot readily withstand processing in an AFER due to non-immersible components, for example ultrasound transducers and trans-oesophageal echocardiogram (TOE) probes. Whilst not a chemical disinfection process, there are also automated systems that use ultraviolet (UV-C) radiation to achieve high-level disinfection of semi-critical RMDs after they have been manually cleaned.

PRACTICE TIP 8

- Investigate the products used for cleaning of non-critical medical devices and identify whether the products being used are intended for use on medical devices.

- Meet with your CSSD manager and discuss the process for obtaining and evaluating the RMD manufacturer's instructions for use. Identify whether this evaluation occurs before or after purchasing of RMDs and what systems are in place if it is identified that all the steps in the cleaning process cannot be effectively followed.

- Identify what RMDs are being manually cleaned and not processed through a washer-disinfector. Evaluate whether the decision to manually clean these RMDs is based on the requirements stated in the manufacturer's instructions for use or is a locally developed practice. If the practice is locally developed, establish why these RMDs are not being exposed to an automated cleaning and disinfection process.
- Visit your CSSD and endoscope processing facility and observe the processes in place for loading the washer-disinfectors. Identify the systems in place to ensure all parts of the RMDs are effectively exposed to the cleaning and disinfection process and whether these loading systems ensure that RMDs with lumens are connected to the fluid pathway, avoid shadowing and facilitate drainage.
- Ask the CSSD and endoscopy staff to show you what process parameters are checked on the cycle record at the completion of the cycle. Identify what happens if the RMDs or the process cycle do not meet acceptance criteria, for example if process parameters are not met or if an RMD or cleaning process indicator is not clean at the end of the process.

16.10 Drying RMDs and endoscopes

After cleaning and rinsing, manually cleaned RMDs should be dried manually using low linting cloths or using an RMD drying cabinet. In Australia, the applicable standard for RMD drying cabinets is AS 5330:2019,[57] although it should be recognised that this type of equipment may be manufactured in countries outside Australia. This does not preclude their purchase, but checks should be made to ensure that they broadly meet the essential principles contained in AS 5330:2019.[57] AS 5330:2019[57] requires RMD drying cabinets to operate in the range of 50–90°C although in practical use most cabinets are operated at the range of 65–75°C for RMDs that are not heat sensitive. Drying may need to be assisted by manual steps prior to placing in the cabinet, such as to ensure the removal of water from lumens or other areas where water can be retained. Drying cabinets must have daily checks of the temperature recorded.[1] Drying cabinets are also required to be cleaned on a regular basis in accordance with the manufacturer's IFU and this may include

washing of reusable filters or replacement of disposable filters.[1,57]

RMDs should not be left to dry in ambient air due to the risks for contamination and being an ineffective process. Other methods may be used to dry RMDs where a drying cabinet is not available, for example by using low linting cloths or medical-grade compressed air.[1] When using medical-grade compressed air, care must be taken to ensure that the air is oil and particulate free and that the use of the air does not pose a hazard to the operator in terms of air embolism, hearing impairment or dispersion of contamination. Figure 16.5 shows an example of a vented cabinet that can be used to mitigate the risks of dispersion of aerosols generated during the use of an air gun to aid in the drying of RMDs.

Endoscopes that have been processed in an AFER should be placed in an EN 16442 compliant storage cabinet or equivalent drying and storage system as soon as possible after the completion of the process cycle. EN 16442 compliant cabinets are required to achieve drying of an endoscope within 3 hours, including lumens.[50] Staff should be trained in the correct use of this equipment to ensure all lumens and device features are adequately dried over time. In the absence or breakdown of a storage cabinet, processed endoscopes will need to be dried before being stored, following the endoscope manufacturer's IFU for manual drying.

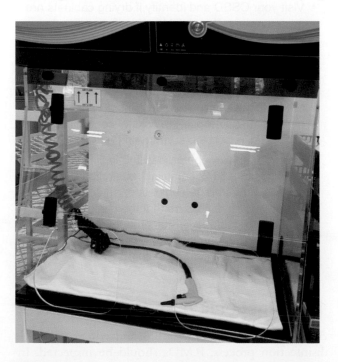

FIGURE 16.5 Vented cabinet and compressed air gun for drying

Source: Terry McAuley

Typically, this involves using 70% alcohol and forced air to dry the internal channels of the endoscope and low linting cloths for drying the exterior surfaces. A study has shown that manual alcohol flushing and rapid forced air drying may not be effective methods for drying endoscope channels and in some cases, reduced the efficiency of channel drying.[63] Drying takes time and is influenced by the air temperature and diameter of each lumen; therefore, this method of drying should only be used in exceptional circumstances.

AS/NZS 4187:2014[1] and the applicable standards for drying equipment require annual qualification of the performance of the equipment to deliver effective drying processes. In the case of EN 16442,[58] there is also a requirement to demonstrate that the storage system can maintain the microbiological quality of the processed endoscope over time during the annual qualification procedures. This includes methods to demonstrate that the quality of the air introduced into the cabinet and the procedures used to clean the cabinet, including decontamination of the attachments at the frequency specified by the manufacturer, do not contribute to endoscope contamination.

requirements defined by the manufacturer (e.g. moving parts). Ideally, the IAP will have good natural lighting and the inspection and packaging workstation should have magnifiers and task lighting to improve inspection capabilities.

For flexible endoscopes, clean gloves should be worn when removing the endoscope from the AFER and visual checks made to ensure it is clean, dry and free from obvious damage (in particular at moving parts and at the distal tips). Surgical RMDs can be handled with clean hands after removal from the WD.

All RMDs must be visually inspected to verify that they are clean, dry, free from soil, cracks, pitting, staining or other damage, and all components are complete and intact. Fine and delicate RMDs may need enhanced visual inspection under a stereo microscope (Fig 16.6) and cannulated RMDs may need inspection using an accessory such as a clean borescope.

In the absence of a borescope, some facilities may pass a brush or pipe-cleaner through device lumens to check for cleanliness. Other RMDs may need to be checked to ensure functionality such as forceps tips align, joints move freely, ratchets hold tension or that

---

PRACTICE TIP 9

- Visit your CSSD and identify if drying cabinets are being used for drying RMDs. Verify that the drying cabinet for heat stable RMDs is being operated between 65–75°C and that the temperature is being checked and recorded daily.

- Identify if air guns are ever used to dry RMDs or to check cleanliness of lumens. Ensure the methods used reduce the risks of contamination of the RMDs and the surrounding environment.

- Visit your endoscope processing facility and identify if EN16442 compliant controlled environment storage cabinets or an equivalent system is in use. Ensure that the cabinets and, where applicable, any attachments are being cleaned at the frequency and using the methods specified in the instructions for use.

16.11 Inspection and maintenance

After completion of the cleaning and, where applicable, disinfection process, RMDs should be inspected. Inspection requirements will include visible cleanliness, dryness, lack of significant damage, and any functional

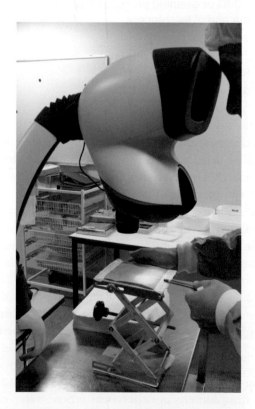

FIGURE 16.6 Enhanced visual inspection using a stereo microscope
Source: Terry McAuley

the blades are sharp. Fibreoptic RMDs may need to be checked to ensure that the light fibres are not broken and insulated RMDs may need to undergo insulation integrity testing between uses.

Multi-component devices may need to be reassembled to ensure all parts are still functional prior to disassembly for sterilisation. ISO 17664:2017[39] requires manufacturers to specify whether an RMD is not to be reassembled or only partially reassembled prior to sterilisation. It is common practice for jointed instruments to be open and unlocked[1] in preparation for sterilisation; however, some manufacturers' IFU allow jointed RMDs to be closed on the first ratchet. A study[64] showed that most common multi-component RMD designs—such as taps on rigid cystoscopes and hysteroscopes, instruments with threads and mated surfaces such as artery clamps—were reliably sterilised in a steam steriliser operating between 132–134°C for a four-minute holding time.

Powered devices such as saws and drills may need to be operated to test their function and, in some cases, to apply lubrication. Lubricants may be required for use on RMDs after exposure to the WD cycle to maintain optimal function. Lubricants, or any other chemicals added to such devices, should be compatible with the sterilisation process and non-toxic if at risk of patient contact. The type and dose of lubricant should be specified. Some RMDs, including some powered tools, may need to be sent to the manufacturer at a specified frequency for maintenance and calibration.

Any damaged or incomplete RMD should be removed from circulation and/or sent for repair. Records should be kept of those RMDs sent for repair. After the return from repair, the RMD must undergo cleaning and disinfection and, if applicable, sterilisation[1] prior to being returned to the tray or set it originated from. Flexible endoscopes that have been returned from repair must undergo full processing prior to being used on a patient and have microbiological testing completed within 72 hours of receipt at the facility.[43]

PRACTICE TIP 10

- Visit your CSSD and observe the processes in place for inspection, maintenance and testing of RMDs as part of the process for preparation for sterilisation. Identify whether visual inspection processes could be enhanced through better lighting, access to magnification systems for

inspection of delicate RMDs, or borescopes for inspecting lumened RMDs.
- Where insulated and electrosurgical RMDs are being processed regularly, ensure there is a system in place for testing the RMDs to ensure there are no breaks in the insulation or integrity of the RMD and that records of this testing are being kept.

16.12 Packaging

Prior to sterilisation, RMDs are packaged in a sterile barrier system (SBS) to preserve the sterile state following the process. SBS should only be used in accordance with their labelled claims and instructions of use. They come in several forms, such as sterilisation wraps, preformed reusable or disposable containers, and pouches, bags or reels collectively referred to as PSBS. Sterilisation wraps and preformed pouches, bags and reels can be made from cellulosic materials, synthetic materials, or blends of both. Reusable containers are typically manufactured from aluminium, whereas disposable containers are made of plastic. Containers frequently use filters made of similar materials to sterilisation wraps to allow for air removal and penetration of the sterilant into and out of the container and to provide microbial barrier properties to protect the container contents during storage. Requirements for packaging of terminally sterilised medical devices are described in ISO 11607-1,[65] recognising that there are nine EN standards specific to different packaging material types, and ISO 11607-2[66] covers requirements for validation of packaging processes.

When assembled in trays as instrument sets, the trays must be large enough to accommodate all RMDs in a single layer without overcrowding and the mass of the tray must be evenly distributed. Care should be taken not to exceed weight requirements in accordance with manufacturers' instructions (for the devices, containers and sterilisers). Tray or container weights in excess of 10 kg can present ergonomic concerns for staff.[67] Tray liners may be used if necessary, to aid in drying and must be intended for this purpose, but not an impediment to air removal and/or sterilant penetration.[67] Note that the two most common causes of the presence of wetness (or lack of drying) following steam sterilisation are overcrowding (or inefficient loading of devices in the steriliser load) and poor steam quality, both of which should be investigated if frequently identified. Sharp and/or delicate RMDs should be protected from damage. Tip protectors, if used, must be intended for this purpose.[65]

The size of the packaging must be appropriate to the size of the RMDs being packaged. For pouches, bags and reels, an allowance of 2 cm around every edge of the RMD is necessary. Where double pouching is used, both pouches must be from the same manufacturer. The inner pouch must not be folded over and must occupy less than 75% of the space in the outer pouch.[67] Handles of RMDs must be placed towards the end of the pouch to be opened and hollowware must have the opening facing the paper side of the pouch.[1] Preformed sterile barrier systems should be heat sealed wherever practicable. Where self-sealing pouches are used, care must be taken to ensure that the seal is completed correctly.

Sterilisation wraps must be large enough to completely cover the RMD on the first pass in order to create a tortuous path.[67] Wrapping may be in the form of an envelope, square, parcel or Pasteur/roll method and if the manufacturer requires more than one sheet to create the sterile barrier, this may be applied simultaneously or sequentially. The grade of the sterilisation wrap should be suitable for the weight, size and shape of the RMD requiring wrapping.

Any tape used to seal RMDs wrapped in a sterilisation wrap must be intended for this purpose[65] and usually includes a Type 1 chemical indicator to facilitate identification of processed from unprocessed products. Sufficient tape should be used to seal the package, but too much tape can compromise the expansion of the pack during the air removal phases of the sterilisation process and create an impediment to air removal and sterilant penetration.[67]

Where reusable sterilisation containers are in use, the containers must be processed through a washer-disinfector after each use. Prior to use, the container must be checked to ensure that the container itself and the gasket is free from damage, the filter is intact or has been changed in accordance with the manufacturer's IFU, and that the lid creates a good seal.[67]

16.12.1 Labelling

All packaged RMDs must be labelled with the name of the RMD or set.[1] Stickers or other labelling systems must be intended for use for labelling of packaged RMDs, and pens used for labelling should be non-toxic, soft-tipped and water resistant.[1] For pouches and reels, the label should be placed on the film without concealing the device; or if writing the label on the package, this should be outside the sterile window area. Labelling on wrapped packages should be on the closure tape, not directly on wrappers. Labelling should remain securely adhered to the sterile barrier system through the sterilisation process and storage until the point of use.

PRACTICE TIP 11

- Obtain several examples of packaged, sterile RMDs and examine the packaging. Ensure that the package label is present and the method of labelling the package is correct. If examining a wrapped RMD, check that there are no holes or other evidence of defects in the wrapper and that when opened, the wrapper is large enough to adequately contain the contents. If examining a pouched item, check that the handles of the RMD are oriented to the end of the pouch to be opened, that the contents of the pouch occupy no more than 75% of the usable space, if double pouched, that the inner pouch has not been folded over and that there is no evidence of breaches to the seal or damage to the paper or the laminate side of the pouch.

- Identify if reusable sterilisation containers are being used at your facility. Ensure that these containers are being processed through a washer-disinfector after each use and that any containers that have dents or damage to the gaskets are being routinely removed from circulation and repaired or replaced.

16.13 Sterilisation

16.13.1 Sterility assurance levels

AS/NZS 4187:2014[1] defines sterilisation to be a validated process that renders a product free from viable microorganisms. The definition recognises that in practical terms there is no method by which the state of being free from microorganisms can be directly proven by classical microbiological techniques. Microbial inactivation kinetics and development of food, industrial and device sterilisation processes use the concept of a sterility assurance level (SAL) of 10^{-6}. A SAL is a probability of a single viable microorganism occurring on an item after a sterilisation process is determined based on known antimicrobial expectations from experimentation combined with mathematical extrapolations into probability.[59]

For the development of any sterilisation process, the first step is to demonstrate that the process has broad-spectrum antimicrobial activity (Fig 16.1). This also allows for the identification of what might be considered as the most resistant microorganism to the process, and in most cases, these are bacterial spores,[59] noting that prions are the most resistant to reprocessing procedures.[68] The second is to study the rate at which the process can kill microbes by incremental exposure of a defined population of microorganisms to the process under various conditions to optimise antimicrobial activity (e.g. investigating the impacts of exposure time, temperature, chemical concentration and humidity). By calculating the survivors, the data can be plotted as the number of survivors over time (or dose) on a linear or logarithmic scale.[59] These studies, initially undertaken in the food industry with heat-based processes, enabled calculation of the average D-value or decimal reduction time. The D-value is defined as the time or dose required to reduce a population of microorganisms by 90% or 1 $\log_{10}$ under specified conditions.[59]

Calculation of D-values using bacterial spores known to be the most resistant to the sterilisation processes under consideration facilitated selection of process parameters and exposure times that achieve an overkill process commonly defined as a 12-log reduction (12D). This assumes that if there were theoretically 10^6 microorganisms of the highest resistance on a device, then exposure to the overkill process would give an initial 6 $\log_{10}$ reduction (where the devices could now be practically considered sterile) and then a further 6 $\log_{10}$ reduction to provide a probability of sterility (SAL) of 10^{-6} (hence an 'overkill' process). This generally accepted SAL for medical devices was incorporated in national and international standards and pharmacopoeias.[59]

Recognising that most sterilisation processes are not able to maintain consistent or homogenous conditions and that other phases in the sterilisation cycle may also contribute to lethality, further mathematical concepts were developed, such as the z-value that describes the change in temperature necessary to achieve a 1 log change in the D-value and the F-value (e.g. F_0) that allows calculation of equivalent lethality over a range of temperatures that can then be correlated to an overall $\log_{10}$ reduction for the process.[59] For heat disinfection processes, with a known D-value and z-valve the total lethality can be predicted, where the higher the temperature and exposure time the greater the antimicrobial efficacy. These are essentially the basics for steam sterilisation processes used in healthcare device processing, and similar concepts apply to chemical sterilisation processes.[59] These process conditions are required to be validated by steriliser manufacturers in accordance with various international standards.

16.13.2 Thermal sterilisation

Thermal sterilisation methods include moist and dry heat. Dry heat sterilisation is not commonly used in healthcare applications in Australia as the process is considerably longer than a moist heat sterilisation process, and thus will not be discussed in this chapter.

Moist heat sterilisation can occur using a variety of process cycles, but Australian health facilities use steam sterilisers that deliver dynamic or active air removal processes compliant with EN 285[75] and EN 13060.[36] These machines use pressure changes (e.g. drawing a vacuum) to remove air out of the chamber and load in the initial stages of the cycle, and again at the end of the cycle, to facilitate drying of the sterilised load. In the initial stages, air is removed to aid in the rapid and even penetration of steam into lumens and crevices of RMDs and porous items. Residual air retained within the load due to inadequate air removal, if introduced through leakage during the cycle, or in the steam as a NCG, can compromise the ability of the steam to condense on the surface and transfer its energy to the load, which is the basis of the antimicrobial activity.

Once air removal has been achieved and steam has filled the chamber, the chamber is pressurised (steam under pressure) to elevate the temperature to the desired parameters for sterilisation. In Australia, the two most common time and temperature relationships are 121°C for 15 minutes and 134°C for 3 minutes, although in practice holding times are typically set for 4 minutes at 134°C, although there are other recognised time/temperature combinations.[1] Any of these time/temperature combinations can be effective, if supported by validation to the appropriate standards.[69]

In the final stage of the process cycle, a vacuum is drawn to remove steam from the chamber and load and to draw sterile filtered air through the chamber. Drawing a vacuum to a certain point reduces the pressure inside the chamber, thereby reducing the boiling point of water, so residual condensate can flash back into steam and be removed. At the completion of the cycle, there should be no detectable moisture on or within the load, as wet packaging materials have the capacity to allow penetration of microbes through the sterile barrier over time, thus compromising sterility. Excessive water in the load can be difficult to get consistently dry, and frequent detection of moisture should be investigated and remediated; the two most common causes of excessive moisture are due to load configuration (including weight) and 'wet' steam.

After removal from the steriliser chamber, the load should be left in a controlled environment to cool to room temperature before handling to minimise the risks for contamination.[87] Infrequently used packaged RMDs may be placed in protective packaging.[65] Protective packaging is usually in the form of a 'dust cover'. Dust covers are plastic packaging that can be hermetically sealed or sealed using an adhesive tape. This protective packaging must be clearly labelled as a dust cover only and must be applied as soon as the packaged RMD is cool and dry, post-sterilisation.[1]

Modern steam sterilisers are designed to allow parametric release of the sterilised loads following the process by verification of the achievement of the process times and temperatures for sterilisation through checking of the cycle record and ensuring that the load items are dry, intact and the external chemical indicators show the correct colour change. Facilities may also choose to use various types of indicators to verify the success of sterilisation processes as outlined in Table 16.5. However, it is important to note that the success of the process is also based on ensuring the overall quality requirements have been met, for example ensuring staff have been trained on correct loading of the machine and undertaking routine monitoring, maintenance and annual performance qualification.

16.13.3 Immediate use sterilisation

According to AS/NZS 4187:2014[1] immediate use sterilisation has also been known as 'flash', 'emergency' and 'fast-track' sterilisation. In decades past, it was not uncommon for health facilities to have insufficient RMD inventory to meet workload demands, leading to the practice of abbreviated processing cycles. The practice often meant RMDs would be manually cleaned (sometimes in the OS itself) and put into the steriliser unwrapped for exposure to a rapid gravity steam cycle with no drying. After completion of the cycle the instruments came out of the steriliser hot and wet; therefore, maintenance of sterility during transfer to the operative field was problematic.

But AS/NZS 4187:2014[1] now clearly states that immediate use sterilisation must not be used routinely as a convenience or as a cost-saving mechanism due to insufficient RMD inventory. Since the implementation of the first edition of AS 4187, this practice has been strongly discouraged as it introduced a different standard of care for patients and compromised patient safety. Consequently, the practice has been addressed in most facilities and is only used for unique emergency situations, such as in the case of a single dropped RMD required during a surgical procedure.

Immediate use sterilisation was a new term introduced in AS/NZS 4187:2014.[1] This term was developed in the USA in 2009 and has been defined as a process in which sterilised RMDs are transferred aseptically to the sterile field in the shortest practicable time after removal from the steriliser.[88] As the RMDs will not be dry at completion of the sterilisation cycle it is essential that they are transferred to the critical aseptic field immediately after sterilisation is complete and in a manner that protects the RMDs from contamination from any source, for example air and environmental contaminants.[1] In some facilities, RMDs are placed in a rigid reusable sterilisation container in order to facilitate aseptic transfer to the critical aseptic field whereas in others the RMD is packaged in a preformed sterile barrier system (paper/laminate pouch) and the drying stage is sufficient to dry this type of sterile barrier system.

The term 'fast-tracking' often refers to needing to prioritise the processing of RMDs so they can be used again within an operative list. This sometimes involves manual cleaning of instruments (that are compatible with and should be processed through an automated cleaning and disinfection process) to save time, and may involve manual drying of instruments, abbreviated inspection procedures prior to packaging, and the use of a sterilisation cycle with an abbreviated drying stage. Frequently, items are not quarantined for the recommended 30-minute cooling period post-sterilisation and thus a risk of compromise to achievement of sterility and sterility maintenance can occur.[87] As with the practice of immediate use sterilisation, fast-tracking of an RMD bypassing routine processing procedures can be a risk for patient safety and thus should be avoided. When planning surgical services, the bare minimum turn-around time for an RMD undergoing steam sterilisation should be calculated at 3–5 hours from use to the point where the RMDs are ready for use again.

16.13.4 Chemical sterilisation

Chemicals are used as an alternative for sterilisation of critical devices at lower temperatures for devices that are heat or high-pressure sensitive. Chemical sterilants are also required to demonstrate broad-spectrum antimicrobial activity (Fig 16.1), but also achieve predictable levels of activity over time when delivered as part

TABLE 16.5 Summary of performance testing and routine monitoring of moist heat and low temperature sterilisers

Performance or routine monitoring tests	Purpose of test	Applicable standards	Small steam steriliser	Large steam steriliser	Low temperature steriliser
Bowie and Dick-type test	Demonstrates achievement of adequate air removal sufficient to enable steam penetration into the test pack	ISO11140-3 ISO11140-4 ISO11140-5[72–74]	Each day of use	Each day of use	Not applicable, but similar types of tests can pose a penetration challenge to the gas (e.g. a PCD test)
Leak rate/ vacuum test	Demonstrates the resistance of the steriliser chamber, pipework and seals to air entry during periods of vacuum	EN 285 EN 13060 AAMI ST8[36,75,76]	As per IFU although typically daily or weekly if air detector fitted	Daily or weekly if air detector fitted	As per IFU
Air detector test (where fitted)	Demonstrates the air detector will fail a process cycle when sufficient air to compromise sterilisation has entered the chamber, usually through a leak or maybe NCGs	EN 285 EN 13060[36,74]	Weekly	Weekly	Not applicable
Process record, as applicable (e.g. time, temperature, pressure, humidity)	Provides a record of the process cycle that can be checked to ensure the equipment is functioning in accordance with the specification and the process parameters have been met for the cycle	EN 285 EN 13060 ISO 14937[36,69,74]	Every cycle	Every cycle	Every cycle
Chemical indicators – external	Allows visual assessment that a product has been exposed to a process cycle	ISO 1 1140-1[77]	Every packaged RMD	Every packaged RMD	Every packaged RMD
Chemical indicators – internal	Allows the user to verify that the product has been exposed to a process cycle	ISO 11140-1[77]	Optional	Optional	Optional
Biological indicators	Demonstrates a cycle has delivered a process that kills resistant spore population	ISO 11138 series[78–84]	Optional	Optional	Optional and often used for routine maintenance
Process challenge devices	Demonstrates a defined resistance to assess process performance (e.g. a steam cycle has achieved sufficient air removal to facilitate steam penetration into a hollow device and that NCGs were not present in the steam to impair the process)	ISO 11140-6 (for steam) [in draft] EN 867-5[85,86]	Optional but recommended for every cycle if no air detector fitted according to AS/NZS 4187	Optional but recommended for every cycle if no air detector fitted according to AS/NZS 4187	Optional or when recommended by the manufacturer
Diagnostic cycle	Varies according to machine – refer to IFU	AS/NZS 4187[1]	N/A	N/A	As per IFU
Product package integrity	Visual quality check completed prior to release of a processed RMD for patient use	AS/NZS 4187[1]	Every packaged RMD	Every packaged RMD	Every packaged RMD

Source: Terry McAuley, developed from AS/NZS 4187:2014

of a validated sterilisation process as required in ISO 14937 or equivalent.[70]

Most terminal chemical sterilisation processes for packaged devices are based on gaseous chemicals such as ethylene oxide (EO), formaldehyde and hydrogen peroxide. Peracetic acid can be used as liquid chemical sterilisation processes for processing RMDs for immediate use, located as close to the point of use as possible; however, aseptic transfer to the critical aseptic field must be able to be achieved.[1]

Gaseous processes typically have three phases during a sterilisation cycle, being conditioning (air removal or humidification), sterilisation (or antimicrobial phase) and aeration (to remove residuals to safe levels). Chemical sterilisation processes can only be claimed to be effective when used under controlled conditions. For example, ethylene oxide requires defined pressure conditions, chemical concentrations, exposure time, temperature and humidity levels. Hydrogen peroxide requires defined pressures (vacuum), sterilant concentrations, exposure times and temperature conditions. Some hydrogen peroxide gas/vapor processes also include the use of a plasma phase (essentially an activated or energised gas) during cycle conditions for various reasons (e.g. for breakdown of peroxide residuals). Liquid chemical processes are similar with conditioning, sterilisation, and rinsing (with water) phases.

These processes will have defined limitations to the maximum sterilisation load (e.g. number of devices of a particular type) and packaging materials (it is common not to include paper-based materials). It is important to understand any IFU specified by the steriliser manufacturer as well as the RMD manufacturer regarding the applicability and preparation of devices for sterilisation. This will include any limitations on packaging materials and the use of process indicators (including BIs, CIs and PCDs). Other requirements will include device/material compatibility and safety requirements (including chemical residuals). During routine healthcare use, verification of controls, including personnel training, load conditions, sterilisation process conditions, maintenance and process indicator verifications such as the use of CIs and BIs, is essential to ensure sterilisation quality.[1]

16.13.5 Performance testing and routine monitoring of sterilisation processes

AS/NZS 4187:2014[1] outlines the performance testing and routine monitoring requirements for sterilisation processes in Table 8.2. For steam sterilisers using a vacuum stage for air removal, there is an expectation that performance tests will be completed before processing loads of RMDs each day the steriliser is used. Performance testing for low temperature testing should be in accordance with the manufacturer's IFU, as machine specification can vary.

The performance and routine monitoring tests to be completed on steam sterilisers are briefly described in Table 16.5. Similar tests are typically performed for low temperature sterilisers, as defined by the manufacturer. Test cycles, and where applicable any products used for the performance testing or routine monitoring of sterilisers, should comply with applicable ISO and EN standards and the manufacturer's IFU.

To ensure that compromised RMDs are not released for patient use it is essential that personnel are appropriately trained and competent at completing performance tests and interpreting the results. Personnel must be trained to check on a cycle-by-cycle basis that the steriliser is delivering the required process, typically established through checking of the process records to ensure correct process parameters were met and through examination of the packages to ensure that they are intact, free from visible moisture, and that the external chemical indicator shows the correct colour change.[1]

PRACTICE TIP 12

- Identify the methods of sterilisation in use at your facility. Ensure that the correct daily and, where applicable, weekly monitoring tests are being completed in accordance with the steriliser manufacturer's instructions for use and with reference to the requirements in Table 8.2 in AS/NZS 4187:2014.

- Ask the CSSD staff to show you what process parameters are checked on the cycle record at the completion of the cycle. Identify what happens if the RMDs or the process cycle do not meet acceptance criteria, for example if process parameters are not met, if the external chemical indicators have not changed colour, or a packaged RMD is not dry at the end of the process.

16.14 Storage and transportation of processed RMDs

After sterilisation, RMDs must be released for patient use and transported to the designated storage locations. Sterile storage locations can be directly adjacent and an integral part of the CSSD, within the OS or maybe in a ward or department.

AS/NZS 4187:2014[1] requires sterile RMDs to be transported and stored in a manner that protects the items from contamination from any source. The principles of sterile storage should also be applied to commercially sterilised medical devices.

The ideal storage environment should be dedicated for that purpose, have smooth, non-porous and easily cleaned surfaces and have temperature and humidity controlled typically between 18–25°C and 35–70% relative humidity.[1] It is good practice to ensure that sterile items are located at least 250 mm above floor level and 440 mm below ceiling level and at least 50 mm away from walls.[87] Sterile packages should not be compressed, bent or punctured during storage and must not be stored on the floor, on window ledges or in uncontrolled environments.[87] Access to the sterile store should be restricted to authorised personnel and the workforce trained in correct storage and handling of sterile products, whether these be produced by CSSD or obtained from a commercial supplier.

Transportation of processed RMDs outside of the controlled CSSD and OS environment usually includes placement of the sterile products into suitable clean plastic containers with lids, case carts or covered trolleys.[87] Where trolleys are used to transport sterile items, these should be enclosed or covered, and the bottom shelf should be solid.[87] Equipment used to transport sterile products should be cleaned before each use. Where processed RMDs are to be transported off-site, the transport vehicle should provide for complete separation of contaminated items from clean and sterile items, with a completely enclosed storage compartment that can protect the sterile items from damage during transport and exposure to extremes in temperature and humidity.[87]

The duration of sterility for a sterile medical device is said to be 'event-related' and this concept applies to both CSSD and commercially produced medical devices.[87] Adverse events can include:

- tears, punctures or other damage to packaging
- compression of packaging by stacking, bundling together with rubber bands, tapes or other methods
- soiling by being in contact with a dirty surface, for example the floor
- exposure to dampness/wetness by contact with wet/damp surfaces or hands
- exposure to excessive humidity or extreme temperatures
- exposure to sunlight/UV sources
- writing on packaging
- multiple episodes of handling; and
- storage for prolonged periods.

Most commercially sterilised products will have an expiry date indicated on the packaging; however, if the product has been subject to an adverse event prior to the expiration date, it must be considered compromised and not used for patient care. For sterile RMDs, the duration of sterility or shelf-life must be determined through an assessment of the quality of the sterile barrier system and the manufacturer's instructions for use in tandem with an assessment of the storage and handling conditions the items will be exposed to. Most sterile barrier system manufacturers will provide guidance on the shelf life recommended for their products.

PRACTICE TIP 13

Evaluate the storage conditions for commercially sterilised products and CSSD produced sterile RMDs. Typical areas for improvement in storage conditions to note in your assessment include whether:
- items are stored on the floor or too close to it
- shelving or storage containers are not being kept clean
- products are still contained in cardboard shipper cartons
- cardboard boxes have been reused as containers or dividers between items
- rubber bands or bulldog clips have been used to bundle items together; and
- sterile items are at risk from contamination from non-sterile products, fluids or items of equipment.

16.15 Quality assurance and quality control in medical device processing

A quality management systems approach to reusable medical device processing should include written policies and procedures, staff training, process validation, monitoring of processes, and routine maintenance of processing equipment. It is not the intention of this chapter to cover all aspects of such a system, but this section considers some central aspects of quality assurance and control.

16.15.1 Validation of processes

AS/NZS 4187:2014[1] requires all cleaning, disinfection, packaging and sterilisation processes to be validated in accordance with the relevant applicable Australian, European or ISO standards. Validation is a term that encompasses activities such as installation qualification (IQ), operational qualification (OQ) and performance qualification (PQ). IQ and OQ are typically undertaken by the manufacturer upon the design and installation of the equipment to verify that the equipment has been installed in a suitable location, that the services meet specification, and that the equipment operates as intended.

PQ of the process is usually undertaken by the healthcare facility, often in conjunction with the manufacturer, and demonstrates that the equipment can deliver an expected, effective process to the range of RMDs being processed by the healthcare facility. Aspects of the PQ must be repeated on an annual basis and/or in situations when a significant change occurs. A significant change may include, but not be limited to, modification of a service or utility, change in process chemicals, sterile barrier systems or introduction of a completely new type of RMD that has no common attributes with other RMDs being processed.

Product families: The concept of product families has been used in commercial sterilisation to maximise the efficiency of industrial sterilisation processes by grouping products with similar characteristics together and exposing them to the same process. The concept has been further extended to device manufacturers when undertaking validation of cleaning, disinfection and sterilising processes applied to medical devices for the purpose of developing reprocessing instructions for devices that share common, worst-case characteristics.[39]

Allocation of RMDs to product families in healthcare assists in the development of processing pathways for RMDs throughout each step in the processing cycle. Product family allocation considers various features of a device that may make it challenging to clean, disinfect or sterilise.

For product family allocation, the methods for product family allocation for RMDs to be steam sterilised are described in Part 3 of the ISO 17665 series; however, this is currently being updated and in future will be included as an appendix to ISO 17665-1.[69]

Allocation of endoscopes into product families is also described in EN16442.[58]

Features of RMD design including lumens or complex moving parts, physical attributes such as mass or surface area, materials of construction such as metals or polymers, and even the method of packaging may influence the success of the cleaning, disinfection, packaging and sterilisation processes. RMD features that may be difficult to clean may be easier to sterilise and vice versa.

Product family allocation is essentially the first stage in identifying RMDs that may be representative of 'worst-case'—the most difficult to clean, disinfect or sterilise RMDs in use at the healthcare facility. These worst-case RMDs and, where applicable, the instrument sets in which they may be contained are then used as the basis for preparing reference loads for PQ of cleaning, disinfection and sterilisation processes.

The sections that follow briefly outline the main requirements for PQ of washer-disinfectors and sterilisers, noting that requirements for PQ of drying, packaging and other processes are not discussed in this chapter.

Washer-disinfector process performance qualification: PQ of the processes delivered by (thermal) washer-disinfectors complying with ISO 15883-1 and ISO 15883-2 involves verifying the efficacy of the cleaning process and achievement of disinfection.

Thermometric tests are completed on the disinfection stage of the process cycle, one test commencing from a cold start and the other three from a hot start. Thermometric tests require a minimum of 12 temperature sensors to be located on chamber walls and throughout the loading space in the chamber. To be completed correctly, only the disinfection stage of the process cycle should be run, as the heat from the wash stages should not have any influence on achievement of the disinfection temperature. Acceptance criteria are met when all temperature sensors are +5°/-0°C of the stated value for disinfection and temperature fluctuation during the disinfection stage is no more than +/- 2°C.

Cleaning efficacy test 1 in ISO 15883-1[38] for washer-disinfectors requires a test soil complying with ISO 15883-5[51] to be applied to a load of representative RMDs, the loading cart and chamber walls and the cleaning stage of the cycle to be disconnected from the rinsing and disinfection stages of the process cycle. At completion of the cleaning stage, all parts of the WD and the load must be free from visible soil and other residues from the test soil.

Cleaning efficacy test 2 is performed after the thermometric tests and cleaning efficacy test 1 has been completed. This test requires three separate loads of patient-soiled RMDs to be processed through a full process cycle intended to be used for those types of RMDs. At the completion of the process cycle the RMDs must be visually clean with no residual protein to be detected using a test method as described in this standard. At the time of writing, ISO 15883-1 was under revision and the cleaning requirements have now been defined in both parts 1 and 5 of the standard (with ISO 15883-5 now upgraded to a standard). In a significant revision, the cleaning, testing and end-point requirements have been updated and these are expected to have an impact on clinical testing over time.

Process residuals and load dryness tests must also be included in the PQ.

PQ of the processes delivered by a (chemical) washer-disinfector complying with ISO 15883-1 and ISO 15883-4 also involves verifying the efficacy of the cleaning process and achievement of disinfection.

Where temperature influences the effectiveness of the disinfection process, thermometric tests must be performed. A minimum of eight temperature sensors must be used in the chamber with at least one probe located in one of the endoscope channels. Temperatures must be 0°C to +5°C of the washing and disinfection temperatures specified by the manufacturer.

Cleaning efficacy tests usually involve the use of a surrogate endoscope that is contaminated with a test soil and may also have test soil coupons located inside the channels. Verification of cleanliness occurs through visual inspection and, in Australia, protein residues.

Disinfection efficacy testing is usually performed by undertaking microbiological sampling of patient-soiled endoscopes after exposure to the process before the endoscopes are dried when completed in accordance with specifications in ISO 15883-4. However, in Australia, there is a longstanding practice of routine microbiological sampling from endoscopes after they have been stored for 12 hours post processing.[43]

Sterilisation process performance qualification: PQ of sterilisation processes involves physical performance qualification (PPQ) using temperature and pressure sensors and microbiological qualification (MPQ) using biological indicators.[1]

This means that the physical process parameters necessary for sterilisation to be achieved, for example

the attainment of time, temperature, and presence of moisture, must be independently confirmed to have been achieved within the RMDs and the worst-case reference load. Temperature sensors should be located within RMDs considered to have the most resistance to steam penetration, for example inside lumened RMDs. The number of temperature sensors used is influenced by the size of the steriliser chamber. For sterilisers with a volume of <60 litres, a minimum of three temperature sensors should be used[36] and for larger sterilisers, a minimum of at least seven temperature sensors should be used.[75]

Process lethality can be further confirmed through the use of biological indicators (BIs) co-located with temperature sensors (in the case of steam sterilisers) throughout the reference load(s).[1] BIs are test systems containing viable microorganisms providing a defined resistance to a specified sterilisation process.[44] They contain high concentrations (typically 10^6) of bacterial spores, due to their resistance profile to inactivation. This validation approach is a combination and modification of parametric measurements combined with a full-cycle overkill method.[69] This assumes a greater than expected level of microbial contamination prior to sterilisation and that the types of microorganisms normally present on the device demonstrate a lower level of resistance to inactivation.

As an alternative, often used for low temperature sterilisation processes, validation could use BIs with 10^6 bacterial spores placed at various locations within a representative, worst-case steriliser load and then showing them to be inactivate at ≤1/2 sterilisation cycle.[70] This would practically confirm at least a worst-case 12 log reduction of test microorganisms over a full sterilisation cycle with the most resistant form of microorganism, well in excess of antimicrobial activity needed for a typical critical RMD.[71] Examples of bacterial spores used for this purpose include those of *Geobacillus stearothermophilus* for steam, hydrogen peroxide gas, vapor or plasma processes, and *Bacillus atrophaeus* for EO or dry heat sterilisers.

PRACTICE TIP 14

- Visit the CSSD at your facility and ask the CSSD manager to explain the methods used to allocate RMDs into product families. Identify the master products that are representative for each product family.

- Ask to see the validation report for a (thermal) washer-disinfector and identify whether the methodology for thermometric tests was consistent with requirements in ISO 15883-1 with respect to the number and location of temperature sensors and whether the disinfection stage was run in isolation from the other process stages; and for cleaning efficacy test 1, whether the cleaning stage was run in isolation from the other process stages. If non-conformances are identified, discussion with the validation services provider may be required.

- Ask to see the validation report for a steam steriliser and establish whether the reference load contained a load representative of the most difficult to sterilise RMDs from each product family as applicable for the process cycle undergoing PQ. Identify whether the number of temperature sensors used meets the minimum number requirement, whether any temperature sensors were located inside lumened RMDs and if biological indicators were included within the packs with temperature sensors. If non-conformances are identified, discussion with the validation services provider may be required.

16.16 Criteria for release of processed RMDs

In Australia, release of processed RMDs predominantly follows the concept of parametric release, where products are released from a sterilisation process on the basis that the process records demonstrated that the sterilisation process variables had been delivered within defined tolerances.[44] The concept of parametric release can also be applied to other processes used for cleaning, disinfection and packaging of RMDs. At the completion of every process cycle, process parameters should be checked and an assessment of the processed RMDs undertaken prior to release of the RMDs to the next step in the processing cycle.[1] Release criteria for each process are described in Table 9.1 in AS/NZS 4187:2014.

For manual cleaning processes, the RMD must be free from visible soil. For automated cleaning and disinfection processes, the RMD must be visibly clean, and the process record must be checked to verify that the correct process parameters have been achieved, for example volume of cleaning agent or chemical disinfectant dosage and the correct temperatures in each process stage being reached.

For terminal sterilisation processes the packs must be dry, intact, the chemical indicator shows the correct colour changes, and the process record shows that the correct process parameters have been achieved, for example, correct exposure time, temperature, pressure and, if applicable, chemical dosage or concentration.

Some low temperature sterilisation processes require the use of both parametric and non-parametric release criteria for the release of a load. For example, ethylene oxide sterilisation processes require the use of biological indicators in every process cycle and verification of sufficient aeration time for the removal of residuals.[1] In these cases, processed RMDs are not released for use in patient care until the results from the incubation of the biological indicators are known.

16.17 Traceability

AS/NZS 4187:2014 requires critical and semi-critical RMDs to be tracked through the processing cycle and to patient use; however, the minimum requirement for traceability is to enable a non-conforming product to be able to be tracked to the patient(s) it had been used on, in the event of a recall being necessary.[1]

Other traceability documentation is required to meet requirements in AS/NZS 4187:2014, for example details of the person responsible for loading and unloading the equipment and authorising load release, results of process monitoring and, where applicable, details of chemical batch numbers and expiry dates for low temperature and high-level disinfection processes.

It is also important to note that the Australian Commission for Safety and Quality in Health Care Advisory AS 18/07[3] requires health facilities to have a traceability system that enables semi-critical and critical equipment, instruments and devices to be tracked to the patient and the procedure. In practical terms, this equates to being able to identify the disinfection or sterilisation process cycle that an RMD or a set of RMDs has been exposed to.

For disinfection processes, this is achieved through documentation of the serial number of the semi-critical RMD and linking this to the record of the manual or automated cleaning and disinfection process that the item has been exposed to. The tracking documentation may be kept as a local record or may be included in the patient's medical record in accordance with local policy.

For critical RMDs, traceability is achieved through attaching a tracking label to the packaged item that provides the date of sterilisation, the identification of the steriliser and the number of the cycle the RMD was processed in. This type of labelling is often referred to as batch labelling and typically only identifies the RMDs as a set or single packaged item that was processed on a particular day in that sterilisation cycle.

To meet the traceability requirements in Advisory AS 18/07, sets of RMDs would need to be managed as a single unit, with the instruments remaining on their designated trays and the set able to be uniquely identified, for example General Set Number 1. Tracking of individually packaged RMDs is more challenging, although there are systems available that can be used for this purpose.

The Australian Government Department of Health requires that RMDs used on tissues that have a higher infectivity risk for Creutzfeldt-Jakob Disease (CJD) are tracked to an individual instrument level to an individual patient.[68] This means that each individual RMD, whether it is contained within a set or packaged as a single instrument, must be labelled in a manner that allows it to be uniquely identified and to be linked to the use on individual patients, in the case of a look-back investigation being required. Achievement of this level of traceability almost obligates the use of electronic traceability systems that enable these unique codes to be scanned into the system. This ensures that instruments do not migrate between sets and are not used in another low CJD risk specialty and enables the retrieval of data that identifies every patient on whom that RMD or set of RMDs had been used.

AS/NZS 4187:2014 recognises that health facilities should be working towards the implementation of electronic traceability systems, as these systems:

- enable RMDs to be tracked throughout each stage of the processing cycle
- include safety features such as warnings if an item has not passed through the correct steps in the processing cycle
- facilitate education of personnel through the use of photographs and guided instructions on disassembly, assembly, inspection and packaging; and
- enable the capture of important business data such as purchase, maintenance and repair records, turn-around times, locations during transport and storage and non-conformances.

PRACTICE TIP 15

- Review the systems in place for traceability of RMDs at your facility. Identify whether it is possible to track the use of individual RMDs used on higher-infectivity tissues to individual patients. This includes RMDs used for neurosurgery, surgery involving the spinal cord or olfactory epithelium, and procedures on the posterior chamber of the eye and optic nerve. It is also good practice to be able to track RMDs used on the anterior chamber of the eye to individual patients.
- If procedures on higher-infectivity tissues are not performed at your facility, ensure that systems are in place that enable a particular RMD or set of RMDs to be tracked from use on a patient to the washer-disinfector and steriliser cycles in which they were processed.

Conclusion

This chapter has focused on the importance of:
- internationally harmonised instructions for processing from all suppliers and that are available electronically
- standard requirements for cleaning chemistries/ detergents
- limits and requirements for establishing device lifetime
- validation and safety requirements for cleaning effectiveness
- recognised tertiary level qualifications for managers
- consistency in training and competency demonstration for technicians
- capacity calculation tools for equipment and staffing
- the implementation of quality management systems
- environmental controls for storage and transportation of sterile RMDS
- safety requirements in handling devices known or suspected to be contaminated with transmissible spongiform encephalopathy disease agents (e.g. CJD); and
- environmental impact considerations (e.g. water and chemical waste management).

Useful websites/resources

- Therapeutic Goods Administration: Information for health professionals. https://www.tga.gov.au/health-professionals; https://www.tga.gov.au/medical-devices; https://www.tga.gov.au/behind-news/regulation-medical-devices; https://www.tga.gov.au/disinfectants-sterilants-and-sanitary-products; https://www.tga.gov.au/reporting-problems

- Australasian Legal Information Institute: Free access to Australasian legal materials. http://www.austlii.edu.au

- Standards Australia: Information on Australian standards. http://www.standards.org.au

- International Organisation for Standardisation: Information on international standards. https://www.iso.org/standards.html

- Australasian Health Facility Guidelines: Resources for good health facility design. https://www.healthfacilityguidelines.com.au/

- Instrument Reprocessing Working Group: Resources for RMD reprocessing. https://en.a-k-i.org/rote-broschuere

References

1. Standards Australia. (AS/NZS 4187:2014/Amdt 2: 2019) Reprocessing of reusable medical devices in health service organizations. Sydney: SAI Global, 2019.
2. Standards Australia. (AS/NZS 4815:2006) Office-based health care facilities—reprocessing of reusable medical and surgical instruments and equipment, and maintenance of the associated environment. Sydney: SAI Global, 2006.
3. Australian Commission for Safety and Quality in Health Care. (AS 18/07) Reprocessing of reusable medical devices in health service organisations. Sydney: National Safety and Quality Health Service (NSQHS), 2021.
4. Bradley CR, et al. Guidance for the decontamination of intracavity medical devices: the report of a working group of the Healthcare Infection Society. J Hosp Infect. 2019; 101(1):1-10.
5. Therapeutic Goods Administration (TGA). TGA basics. Canberra: Australian Government Department of Health. Available from: https://www.tga.gov.au/tga-basics.
6. Therapeutic Goods Administration (TGA). How to tell if a medical device is legally supplied for use in Australia. Canberra: Australian Government Department of Health. Available from: https://www.tga.gov.au/node/3980.
7. Therapeutic Goods Administration (TGA). Australian regulatory guidelines for medical devices (ARGMD) [26 November 2020]. Canberra: Australian Government Department of Health. Available from: https://www.tga.gov.au/node/5308.
8. Therapeutic Goods Administration (TGA). Manufacture of medical devices: quality management [29 April 2013]. Canberra: Australian Government Department of Health. Available from: https://www.tga.gov.au/node/4430.
9. McDonnell GE. Antisepsis, disinfection, and sterilization: types, action, and resistance. 2nd ed. John Wiley & Sons, 2020.
10. Therapeutic Goods Administration (TGA). Changes to labelling and regulation of hard surface disinfectants (commencing 1 April 2019) [23 December 2019]. Canberra: Australian Government Department of Health. Available from: https://www.tga.gov.au/node/874734.
11. Therapeutic Goods Administration (TGA). Disinfectants, sterilants and sanitary products. [21 December 2020]. Canberra: Australian Government Department of Health. Available from: https://www.tga.gov.au/node/4395.

12. Therapeutic Goods Administration (TGA). Disinfectant Claim Guide - specific claims and non-specific claims [15 March 2021]. Canberra: Australian Government Department of Health. Available from: https://www.tga.gov.au/node/874788.
13. Therapeutic Goods Administration (TGA). Guidelines for the evaluation of sterilants and disinfectants [1 February 1998]. Canberra: Australian Government Department of Health. Available from: https://www.tga.gov.au/node/5327.
14. Therapeutic Goods Regulations 1990, Statutory Rules No. 394, 1990. (Commonwealth).
15. Therapeutic Goods Administration (TGA). Medical device incident reporting & investigation scheme (IRIS) [30 October 2019]. Canberra: Australian Government Department of Health. Available from: https://www.tga.gov.au/node/4580.
16. World Health Organization (WHO). Global harmonization task force (GHTF). Geneva: WHO. Available from: https://www.who.int/medical_devices/collaborations/force/en/.
17. International Medical Device Regulators Forum (IMDRF). About International Medical Device Regulators Forum. Available from: https://www.imdrf.org/about
18. The European Committee for Standardization (CEN) the European Committee for Electrotechnical Standardization (CENELEC). Making standards for Europe: about us. Available from: https://www.cencenelec.eu/ABOUTUS/Pages/default.aspx.
19. National Health and Medical Research Council (NHMRC) and Australian Commission on Safety and Quality in Health Care (ACSQHC). Australian guidelines for the prevention and control of infection in healthcare. Canberra: NHMRC, ACSQHC, 2019.
20. Devereaux BM, et al. Australian infection control in endoscopy consensus statements on carbapenemase-producing Enterobacteriaceae. J Gastroenterol Hepatol. 2019;34(4): 650-658.
21. Australasian Health Infrastructure Alliance (AHIA). Australasian Health Facility Guidelines. Available from: https://www.healthfacilityguidelines.com.au/.
22. NSW Ministry of Health. Engineering Services Guidelines (GL2021_014). 2021; File No. 03/7793-2. Available from: https://www1.health.nsw.gov.au/pds/ActivePDSDocuments/GL2021_014.pdf.

23. Standards Australia Committee. ME–062, (AS 1668.2-2012) The use of ventilation and airconditioning in buildings. Part 2: Mechanical ventilation in buildings. Sydney: SAI Global, 2021.

24. Queensland Health. Capital infrastructure requirements, volume 4 engineering and infrastructure, section 2: manual. Brisbane: Queensland Government, 2020.

25. Victorian Health and Human Services Building Authority. Engineering guidelines for healthcare facilities. Melbourne: State Government of Victoria, 2020. Available from: https://www.vhhsba.vic.gov.au/engineering-guidelines-healthcare-facilities.

26. Western Australia Department of Health. Building guidelines: Western Australian health facilities guidelines for architectural requirements. Perth: WA Government, 2018. Available from: https://ww2.health.wa.gov.au/-/media/Files/Corporate/general-documents/Licensing/PDF/standards/building-guidelines-architectural-requirements.pdf.

27. Whiteley GS, et al. A new sampling algorithm demonstrates that ultrasound equipment cleanliness can be improved. Am J Infect Control. 2018;46(8):887-892.

28. Keys M, et al. Efforts to attenuate the spread of infection (EASI): a prospective, observational multicentre survey of ultrasound equipment in Australian emergency departments and intensive care units. Crit Care Resusc. 2015;17(1):43-46.

29. Australasian Society for Ultrasound in Medicine (ASUM) and the Australasian College for Infection Prevention and Control (ACIPC). Guidelines for reprocessing ultrasound transducers. Australas J Ultrasound Med. 2017;20(1):30-40.

30. Rutala WA, DJ Weber. New developments in reprocessing semicritical items. Am J Infect Control. 2013;41(5):S60-S66.

31. The Instrument Reprocessing Working Group (AKI). Instrument reprocessing – reprocessing of instruments to retain value. Tenth anniversary ed. Darmstadt, Germany: Arbeitskreis Instrumenten-Aufbereitung [Instrument Preprocessing Working Group], 2016. Available from: https://www.mmmgroup.com/sites/default/files/brochures/instrument_reprocessing_-_publication_en_0.pdf.

32. Association for the Advancement of Medical Instrumentation (AAMI). Technical Information Report (AAMI TIR34: 2014): Water for the reprocessing of medical devices. Arlington, VA: AAMI, 2014. Available from: https://www.aami.org/.

33. UK Department of Health and Social Care. Health technical memorandum 01-01: management and decontamination of surgical instruments (medical devices) used in acute care. Part C: steam sterilization. London: UK Government, 2016. Available from: https://www.england.nhs.uk.

34. UK Department of Health and Social Care. Health technical memorandum 01-01: management and decontamination of surgical instruments (medical devices) used in acute care. Part D: washer-disinfectors. London: UK Government, 2016. Available from: https://www.england.nhs.uk.

35. UK Department of Health and Social Care. Health technical memorandum 01-06: decontamination of flexible endoscopes. Part B: design and installation. London: UK Government, 2016. Available from: https://www.england.nhs.uk.

36. Comité Européen de Normalisation (CEN). European Standard (EN 13060:2014+A1: 2018) Small steam sterilizers. Brussels: CEN–CENELEC Management Centre, 2018.

37. Australian Government. Medical device standards order (endotoxin requirements for medical devices) 2018. Canberra: Australian Government, 2018.

38. International Organization for Standardization (ISO). (ISO 15883-1:2006) Washer-disinfectors. Part 1: general requirements, terms and definitions and tests. Geneva: ISO, 2006.

39. International Organization for Standardization (ISO). (ISO 17664-1:2017) Processing of health care products — information to be provided by the medical device manufacturer for the processing of medical devices. Part 1: critical and semi-critical medical devices. Geneva: ISO, 2017.

40. International Organization for Standardization (ISO). (ISO 17664-2:2021) Processing of health care products — information to be provided by the medical device manufacturer for the processing of medical devices. Part 2: non-critical medical devices. Geneva: ISO, 2021.

41. Smith A, et al. Reducing the risk of iatrogenic Creutzfeldt-Jakob disease by improving the cleaning of neurosurgical instruments. J Hosp Infect. 2018;100(3):e70-e76.

42. Bundgaard K, et al. Challenging the six-hour recommendation for reprocessing sterilizable medical equipment. J Hosp Infect. 2019;101(1):13-19.

43. Devereaux BM, Jones D, Wardle E, on behalf of the Infection Control in Endoscopy Committee. Infection prevention and control in endoscopy 2021. Melbourne: Gastroenterological Society of Australia, 2021.

44. International Organization for Standardization (ISO). (ISO 11139:2018) Sterilization of health care products — Vocabulary of terms used in sterilization and related equipment and process standards. Geneva: ISO, 2021.

45. Kovaleva J, et al. Transmission of infection by flexible gastrointestinal endoscopy and bronchoscopy. Clin Microbiol Rev. 2013;26(2):231-254.

46. Alfa MJ. Medical instrument reprocessing: current issues with cleaning and cleaning monitoring. Am J Infect Control. 2019;47s:a10-a16.

47. Tosh PK, et al. Outbreak of Pseudomonas aeruginosa surgical site infections after arthroscopic procedures: Texas, 2009. Infect Control Hosp Epidemiol. 2011; 32(12):1179-1186.

48. Wendelboe AM, et al. Outbreak of cystoscopy related infections with Pseudomonas aeruginosa: New Mexico, 2007. J Urol. 2008;180(2):588-592; discussion 592.

49. Southworth PM. Infections and exposures: reported incidents associated with unsuccessful decontamination of reusable surgical instruments. J Hosp Infect. 2014; 88(3):127-131.

50. US Food and Drug Administration (FDA). Reprocessing medical devices in health care settings: validation methods and labeling. Maryland, USA: FDA, 2015. Available from: https://www.fda.gov/media/80265/download.

51. International Organization for Standardization (ISO). (ISO 15883-5) Washer-disinfectors — Part 5: Performance requirements and test method criteria for demonstrating cleaning efficacy. Geneva: ISO, 2021.

52. Standards Australia. (AS 2773:2019) Ultrasonic cleaners for health service organisations. Sydney: SAI Global, 2019.

53. Kovach SM. Research: ensuring cavitation in a medical device ultrasonic cleaner. Biomed Instrum Technol. 2019;53(4):280-285.

54. Vassey M, et al. A quantitative assessment of residual protein levels on dental instruments reprocessed by manual, ultrasonic and automated cleaning methods. Br Dent J. 2011;210(9):E14-E14.

55. International Organization for Standardization (ISO). (ISO 15883-2:2006) Washer-disinfectors. Part 2: requirements and tests for washer-disinfectors employing thermal disinfection for surgical instruments, anaesthetic equipment, bowls, dishes, receivers, utensils, glassware, etc. Geneva: ISO, 2006.

56. International Organization for Standardization (ISO). (ISO 15883-4:2018) Washer-disinfectors. Part 4: requirements and tests for washer-disinfectors employing chemical disinfection for thermolabile endoscopes. Geneva: ISO, 2018.

57. Standards Australia, (AS 5330:2019) Drying cabinets for reusable medical devices. Sydney: SAI Global; 2019.

58. Comite Europeen de Normalisation (CEN). European Standard (EN 16442:2015) - Controlled environment storage cabinet for processed thermolabile endoscopes. Brussels: CEN-CENELEC Management Centre, 2015.

59. McDonnell G. Microorganisms and resistance. In: McDonnell G and Hansen J, eds. Block's disinfection, sterilization, and preservation. Philadelphia: Wolters Kluwer, 2020.

60. McCormick PJ, et al. Moist heat disinfection and revisiting the A0 concept. Biomed Instrum Technol. 2016;50(Suppl 3): 19-26.

61. Baiomi A, et al. Chemical colitis caused by hydrogen peroxide vaginal douche: a case report. World J Gastrointest Endosc. 2019;11(9):486-490.

62. Shih HY, et al. Glutaraldehyde-induced colitis: case reports and literature review. Kaohsiung J Med Sci. 2011;27(12):577-580.

63. Nerandzic M, et al. Efficacy of flexible endoscope drying using novel endoscope test articles that allow direct visualization of the internal channel systems. Am J Infect Control. 2021;49(5):614-621.

64. Haas I, et al. Steam sterilisation of reusable surgical instruments effectiveness limits. Central Service (Zentral Sterilisation). 2009;17(4):257-267.

65. International Organization for Standardization (ISO). (ISO 11607-1:2019) Packaging for terminally sterilized medical devices. Part 1: requirements for materials, sterile barrier systems and packaging systems. Geneva: ISO, 2019.

66. International Organization for Standardization (ISO). (ISO 11607-2:2019) Packaging for terminally sterilized medical devices. Part 2: validation requirements for forming, sealing and assembly processes. Geneva: ISO, 2019.

67. International Organization for Standardization (ISO). (ISO/TS 16775:2014) Packaging for terminally sterilized medical devices. Guidance on the application of ISO 11607-1 and ISO 11607-2. Geneva: ISO, 2019.

68. Australian Government Department of Health. Infection Control Guidelines - Creutzfeldt-Jakob disease. 2013. 15 April 2013 [This document provides recommendations for infection prevention and control procedures to minimise the risk of transmission of Creutzfeldt-Jakob disease (CJD) in healthcare settings.] Available from: https://www1.health.gov.au/internet/main/publishing.nsf/Content/icg-guidelines-index.htm.

69. International Organization for Standardization (ISO). (ISO 17665-1:2006) Sterilization of health care products — Moist heat. Part 1: requirements for the development, validation and routine control of a sterilization process for medical devices. Geneva: ISO, 2006.

70. International Organization for Standardization (ISO). (ISO 14937:2009) Sterilization of health care products. General requirements for characterization of a sterilizing agent and the development, validation and routine control of a sterilization process for medical devices. Geneva: ISO, 2009.

71. Cloutman-Green E, et al. Biochemical and microbial contamination of surgical devices: a quantitative analysis. Am J Infect Control. 2015;43(6):659-61.

72. International Organization for Standardization (ISO). (ISO 11140-3:2007) Sterilization of health care products — chemical indicators. Part 3: class 2 indicator systems for use in the Bowie and Dick-type steam penetration test. Geneva: ISO, 2007.

73. International Organization for Standardization (ISO). (ISO 11140-4:2007) Sterilization of health care products — chemical indicators. Part 4: class 2 indicators as an alternative to the Bowie and Dick-type test for detection of steam penetration. Geneva: ISO, 2007.

74. International Organization for Standardization (ISO). (ISO 11140-5:2007) Sterilization of health care products — chemical indicators. Part 5: class 2 indicators for Bowie and Dick-type air removal tests. Geneva: ISO, 2007.

75. Comite Europeen de Normalisation (CEN). European Standard (EN 285:2015) - Sterilization - steam sterilizers - large sterilizers. Brussels: CEN-CENELEC Management Centre, 2015.

76. Association for the Advancement of Medical Instrumentation (AAMI). (ANSI/AAMI ST8:2013) Hospital steam sterilizers. Geneva: ISO, 2013.

77. International Organization for Standardization (ISO). (ISO 11140-1:2014) Sterilization of health care products — chemical indicators. Part 1: general requirements. Geneva: ISO, 2014.

78. International Organization for Standardization (ISO). (ISO 11138-1:2017) Sterilization of health care products — biological indicators. Part 1: general requirements. Geneva: ISO, 2017.

79. International Organization for Standardization (ISO). (ISO 11138-2:2017) Sterilization of health care products — biological indicators. Part 2: biological indicators for ethylene oxide sterilization processes. Geneva: ISO, 2017.

80. International Organization for Standardization (ISO). (ISO 11138-3:2017) Sterilization of health care products — biological indicators. Part 3: biological indicators for moist heat sterilization processes. Geneva: ISO, 2017.

81. International Organization for Standardization (ISO). (ISO 11138-4:2017) Sterilization of health care products — biological indicators — Part 4: biological indicators for dry heat sterilization processes. Geneva: ISO, 2017.

82. International Organization for Standardization (ISO). (ISO 11138-5:2017) Sterilization of health care products — Biological indicators. Part 5: biological indicators for low-temperature steam and formaldehyde sterilization processes. Geneva: ISO, 2017.

83. International Organization for Standardization (ISO). (ISO 11138-7:2019) Sterilization of health care products — biological indicators. Part 7: guidance for the selection, use and interpretation of results. Geneva: ISO, 2019.

84. International Organization for Standardization (ISO). (ISO/DIS 11138-8) Sterilization of health care products — biological indicators. Part 8: method for validation of a reduced incubation time for a biological indicator.

85. International Organization for Standardization (ISO). (ISO/CD 11140-6.2) Sterilization of health care products — chemical indicators. Part 6: class 2 indicators and process challenge devices for use in performance testing of steam sterilizers [under development].

86. Comité Européen de Normalisation de Normalisation (CEN). European Standard (EN 867-5:2001) – non-biological systems for use in sterilizers. Part 5: specification for indicator systems and process challenge devices for use in performance testing for small sterilizers Type B and Type S. Brussels: CEN-CENELEC Management Centre, 2001.

87. Association for the Advancement of Medical Instrumentation (AAMI). (ANSI/AAMI ST79:2017) Comprehensive guide to steam sterilization and sterility assurance in health care facilities. Arlington, VA: AAMI, 2017. Available from: https://www.aami.org/.

88. The Joint Commission. Instrument reprocessing - immediate use steam sterilization (IUSS). Washington DC: The Joint Commission, 2021. Available from: https://www.jointcommission.org/standards/standard-faqs/ambulatory/infection-prevention-and-control-ic/000002122/.

CHAPTER 17

Urinary tract infections

PROFESSOR BRETT G. MITCHELL[i-iii]

Chapter highlights

- Urinary tract infections are common and many are associated with the use of an indwelling urinary catheter
- In the era of antimicrobial resistance (AMR), prevention of catheter-associated urinary tract infections (CAUTI) is paramount
- Prevention of CAUTI includes reducing unnecessary catheter insertion, correct insertion and maintenance, and prompt removal

i   School of Nursing, Avondale University, Lake Macquarie, NSW

ii School of Nursing and Midwifery, Monash University, VIC

iii Central Coast Local Health District, Gosford Hospital, NSW

Acknowledgements: The author wishes to acknowledge contributions from Grace Prael and Dr Cassie Curryer in preparing this chapter.

Introduction

Urinary tract infection (UTI) constitutes one of the most frequent infections and highest burdens of non-communicable infectious disease globally, with an estimated worldwide incidence of 2–3%, or around 150 million persons/year.[1] The prevalence of UTI varies across demographic groups but is greater in some populations, such as women, persons over 65 years of age, persons who use urinary catheterisation for urine voiding, and the immunocompromised.[1-6] This chapter provides:

- an overview of UTI prevalence, diagnosis and treatment
- a discussion about the importance of UTI prevention in the context of increasing antimicrobial resistance
- strategies for the prevention of catheter-associated UTIs.

A note on terminology: A variety of terms are used to describe UTI in community and hospital settings and for UTI arising from the use of catheterisation. In this chapter, the term CAUTI refers to *catheter-associated* urinary tract infection. The focus of this chapter is on CAUTI.

17.1 Epidemiology of urinary tract infections

The prevalence of UTI varies across geographical contexts and among population groups but has been found to be associated with gender, both older and younger age, sexual activity, obesity, chronic diseases such as diabetes, genetic susceptibility, being a hospitalised patient or long-term care resident requiring catheterisation, and having a spinal cord injury.[1,3,6-10] Urinary tract infection and bacteriuria are prevalent among older adults.[8] In the community, the prevalence of UTI is estimated to be 0.7%,[11] and accounts for 1.2% of Australian general practice consultations.[12] The burden of UTI is additionally associated with a significant economic burden tied to clinician consultations, antibiotic costs, laboratory investigation costs and hospital admissions. In Australia, acute UTI accounts for 75,617 potentially preventable hospitalisations, with an estimated cost of over $367 million.[13] In the hospital settings, UTIs are one of the most common healthcare-associated infections.[14] There are an estimated 70,000 UTIs acquired in Australian public hospitals each year.[15] Further information about the epidemiology of UTIs in Australian hospitals has been published.[16]

Previous history of UTI increases the risk of having UTIs, for example, having ≥5 UTIs over the lifetime is a strong predictor of new UTI among postmenopausal women aged ≤75 years (OR:6.9, CI:3.5–13.6).[11] Females of all ages are susceptible to UTI, whereas in men, older age and prostate enlargement are associated with an increased risk of UTI.[1,7,17] Fifty to sixty percent of adult women will experience at least one UTI in their lifetime, and as many as 20–30% of those may go on to experience recurrent UTIs.[10,18] The gender disparity in UTI prevalence is such that women have up to 50 times greater UTI risk than men.[19] For Australian women, UTIs are also the most frequent driver of potentially preventable hospitalisations.[20] The higher incidence of UTI among women is often attributed to women having a shorter distance between the anus and urethral opening than men. Vaginal and perineal microenvironments may also facilitate colonisation of uropathogens. Among women, pregnancy and post-menopause are also common risk factors.[3,7]

For children and infants, a higher risk of UTI is associated with being an infant under one year of age, being born prematurely, having congenital abnormalities of the urinary tract, prior history of UTI, and bladder or bowel dysfunction (constipation).[2,21,22] Under 6 months of age, UTI incidence is much higher in uncircumcised boys than girls.[7,23] The incidence rate for boys decreases from 5.3% (≤6 months old) to around 2% (ages 1–6 years). In comparison, the incidence of UTI among girls is reversed (2% ≤6 months), rising to 11% at ages 1–6 years.[2] Thereafter, incidence rates of UTI continue to be higher for girls than boys.

Persons with spinal cord injuries or multiple sclerosis (MS) are also at higher risk of developing a UTI, in part due to the higher percentage requiring intermittent (self) catheterisation for voiding urine.[3,4,6] In one study, almost two-thirds of persons with MS who presented to emergency departments, or were admitted for UTI, were using a urinary catheter.[4] Urinary tract infection associated with catheterisation (CAUTI) is discussed in more detail later in this chapter.

17.2 What are urinary tract infections?

Urinary tract infection involves bacterial or fungal infiltration, often by endogenous bodily organisms (e.g. native to the gastrointestinal tract), of traditional non-host areas for such bacteria or fungi. There is often confusion between UTI and bacteriuria, which can lead to misdiagnosis and inappropriate antimicrobial use. Urinary tract infection is defined when there are signs or symptoms of infection, often alongside microbiological results. Bacteriuria is the presence of bacteria in the urine, often defined as the presence of $\geq 10^5$ CFU/mL bacteria in urine. Around 40% of men and women living in long-term residential care present with asymptomatic bacteriuria (ASB), and as many as one-third experience long-term colonisation.[24] Recurrent UTIs are defined as having two or more symptomatic UTI episodes within a 6-month period, or three or more episodes within a 12-month period.[25,26] Infection of the urinary tract may be caused by a number of species of bacteria, most frequently *E. coli.* and less commonly other organisms (Fig 17.1).[1,17,27]

17.2.1 Mechanisms underlying urinary tract infection

Normally, the urinary tract resists infection using a variety of protective physiological mechanisms.[7,27] These include:

- low pH of urine that makes the tract inhospitable to harmful microorganisms, thus preventing uropathogenic colonisation
- flushing action of urine flow
- mucosal lining that makes bacterial penetration (uroepithelial adhesion) challenging.

The pathogenesis of UTI typically involves the contamination of tissues surrounding the urethra with bacteria or fungi.[7,27] The pathogen then colonises the urethra, before travelling to the bladder. Physiological structures of bacteria that promote adhesion to the host (pili and adhesins) facilitate this. Urinary tract infections can involve the upper (ureters and kidney) and lower (bladder, urethra) urinary tract, but are frequently limited to the lower urinary tract.[27] Differentiation of these types of UTI is relevant when selecting for which patient populations require long-term follow-up and extended antibiotic treatment.

17.2.2 Symptoms of UTI

The definition of what constitutes a UTI includes clinical signs and symptoms, as well as the results of urine cultures. Common symptoms include:

- painful urination (often described as a burning sensation)
- urinary frequency/urgency (dysuria)

- flank pain or costovertebral angle tenderness
- fever.[8,26,28]

17.3 Diagnostic methods for UTI

Diagnosis of UTI is clinically challenging.[29] Signs and symptoms can vary according to the age and sex of the patient and be non-specific or, alternatively, associated with catheterisation. Bacteriuria is common, can be asymptomatic, and may be misdiagnosed as UTI.[29,30] For patients who are not catheterised, diagnosis of UTI generally involves obtaining a clean-catch urine sample from a patient with suspected infection.[30] The sample should be collected from midstream urine, to avoid contamination with organisms dwelling on the entrance to the urethra, which could otherwise confound the results. Perineal cleansing before collecting the sample is recommended for women, but might not necessarily confer lower contamination rates.[29] Urinary samples collected from indwelling urinary catheters should be collected from the sampling port (and not the collection bag) to reduce likelihood of contamination.[29] Urine samples should be submitted in a sterile, leak-proof container or collection tube with boric acid preservative, and kept refrigerated at 4–10°C for up to 24 hours. Unpreserved urine culture specimens should be received in the laboratory within 2 hours of collection.[29]

17.3.1 Dipstick urinalysis

Nitrate-detecting dipstick tests that function via ammonia sensitivity are available as an alternative to laboratory-based tests such as urine cultures, including for home use. Urine dipsticks are able to detect nitrites in the presence of bacteria $>10^5$ CFU/mL, leukocyte esterase (white blood cells) and very low levels of blood in the urine, which may increase probability of UTI. Dipstick urinalysis can, however, lack sensitivity and specificity, hence a negative dipstick may not rule out the possibility of UTI, and dipstick urinalysis may also fail to distinguish between symptomatic and asymptomatic UTI.[28,31]

Where other symptoms are suggestive of UTI, a urine culture should always be performed. A study that examined differences in dipstick testing for symptomatic and asymptomatic UTI among patients up to 65 years of age found similar specificity (76.7% vs 70.4%) between groups, and higher sensitivity among symptomatic (73.7%) than asymptomatic (64.3%) patients. Moreover, almost two-thirds of patients who had positive dipstick results returned negative urine cultures, risking over-diagnosis.[28]

17.3.2 Microscopic urinalysis

Microscopic urinalysis is performed using either manual or automated light microscopy to identify the presence of leukocytes (pyuria) or bacteria, and is useful for ruling out and diagnosing UTI when used in conjunction with results of clinical presentation.[28] In older adults, microscopic urinalysis should be interpreted with care, due to the presence of both bacteriuria and pyuria without symptomatic infection. The absence of bacteriuria does not rule out UTI.[28] During pregnancy, microscopic urinalysis has low to moderate sensitivity for asymptomatic bacteriuria (ASB), hence urine dipstick testing may provide more accurate results.[28]

17.3.3 Urine culture

Urine culture analysis is considered the gold standard for diagnosis of UTI.[28,29] Once collected, the urine sample is cultured and the colony-forming units per millilitre of urine calculated. Antimicrobial susceptibility testing is also typically performed.[29] Urine cultures that show significant growth of a single uropathogen are considered positive, while cultures with mixed flora may indicate contamination.[28,29] The presence of significant bacterial growth may not reflect an active infection, for example, approximately 5% of premenopausal women, 30–50% of older women living in residential aged care, and between 2–10% of pregnant women have asymptomatic bacteriuria.[28] In the presence of symptoms, culture results can confirm the type of causative bacteria and antimicrobial sensitivity, thus helping to inform treatment decisions and potentially reduce risk of antimicrobial resistance.

17.3.4 Diagnosis in infants and children under 16 years

Diagnosis of UTI in infants and children (≤16 years) can be challenging due to non-specific symptoms such as lethargy and irritability, and difficulty in obtaining urine specimens. A systematic approach to diagnosing UTI is therefore needed. For infants and toddlers, bladder catheterisation and suprapubic aspiration are the recommended methods of urine collection and are considered to be 'gold standard' for UTI diagnostic purposes due to lower rates of contamination than compared to clean-catch methods.[32] Where a urine collection bag is used, it should only be attached for 15–30 minutes. Post voiding, the bag should be removed and the urine analysed without delay. To aid quick voiding of urine in infants, an innovative approach (Quick-Wee method) has been successfully used.[33]

Urine collection in infants and very young children should be performed or supervised by an experienced healthcare professional, due to risks of infection and the difficulty of catheterising young males.[32] A Swiss consensus on diagnosing UTI in children strongly recommends that diagnosis of UTI by urine dipstick (leukocyte esterase and nitrate) or microscopy alone is not sufficient to definitively confirm the presence of UTI. Other contexts such as previous history, risk factors and urine culture results should be considered in making a diagnosis.[32]

17.4 UTI treatment, prevention and antimicrobial resistance (AMR)

17.4.1 Treatment of UTI

Treatment of UTI should be guided by national and local guidelines, which will take into account local epidemiology and antimicrobial resistance. It is generally not recommended to treat asymptomatic bacteriuria in infants, children or healthy non-pregnant women.[34]

17.4.2 Prevention of UTI

A number of approaches have been and continue to be explored to prevent community-acquired UTI or UTIs not associated with urinary catheters. These approaches include using complementary medicines and probiotics, increasing fluid intake, and behavioural modifications such as improving bowel habits (avoiding constipation) and relaxed urine voiding techniques.[35-37] In a systematic review exploring increased fluid intake for the prevention of UTIs, the authors concluded that there was a lack of enough robust randomised control studies to draw conclusions about the effectiveness of this intervention for UTI prevention.[38] A Cochrane review published in 2015, investigating the effect of probiotics in the prevention of UTI in adults and children, concluded that from the available literature, there was no evidence that probiotics reduced UTIs,[35] while another Cochrane review found no benefit from cranberry juice in reducing UTIs.[39]

Although not necessarily supported by clinical research, prevention strategies recommended by government bodies and expert groups include:

- drinking sufficient water and other fluids to flush the urinary system
- after going to the toilet, wiping from front to back (urethra to anus)

- treating vaginal infections in a timely manner
- avoiding spermicide-containing products
- using a water-based lubricant during sex
- passing urine as soon as the urge to urinate is felt
- emptying the bladder after sex
- avoiding potentially irritating feminine products
- avoiding constipation.[40-43]

17.4.3 Antimicrobial resistance

Antimicrobial resistance is a growing concern in medicine and infectious diseases research, with real consequences for everyday clinical practice.[44-49] The efficacy of first-line antibiotics that have commonly been used to treat UTI is declining.[45] Chapter 3 contains more information about AMR. There are a number of broad antimicrobial stewardship principles that are directly relevant to UTIs. It is important to refer to your local and national guidelines for appropriate and specific advice.

17.5 Classifications and definitions of UTIs by geographical location

There are various types or classifications of UTI. These are outlined in Table 17.1. Urinary tract infections are sometimes defined by their place of acquisition, for example community-acquired or hospital-acquired. In this section, these concepts are explored in more detail.

17.5.1 Community-acquired UTI

Typically, community-acquired UTIs could be considered to be those occurring in community-dwelling individuals, occurring less than 48 hours after hospital admission, or more than 48 hours after hospital discharge. However, there are many caveats to this broad approach and professional organisations and government bodies have guidelines on what may constitute a healthcare-associated UTI—meaning that others could be assumed to be community-acquired.

17.5.2 Community-acquired or healthcare-associated UTI

Some UTIs could fall into both categories: community-acquired and healthcare-associated. One example is intermittent catheterisation. A significant number of people in the community undertake intermittent self-catheterisation to empty their bladders due to a chronic condition or disability, such as a spinal cord injury. The proportion of people undertaking intermittent catheterisation and experiencing ≥1 UTIs per year is estimated to be around 45%.[52] Urinary tract infection may also occur in long-term residential care settings where indwelling or intermittent catheterisation (IC) is performed. For example, between 5–10% of long-term care residents requiring chronic indwelling catheterisation will develop a UTI.[11]

17.5.3 Healthcare-associated (or hospital-acquired) UTI (HAUTI)

A broad example of a healthcare-associated UTI is one that was not present on admission to hospital and occurs more than 48 hours after admission to hospital.[53] These infections (HAUTIs) have been associated with increases in length of stay in hospital, morbidity and mortality.[54] The incidence of HAUTIs from one study in Australia, which observed 162,503 patient admissions, was 1.73%.[54] They represent one of the most common

TABLE 17.1 Classification of urinary tract infections adopted by the European Association of Urology[51]

Classification of UTIs	
Uncomplicated UTIs	Acute, sporadic or recurrent lower (uncomplicated cystitis) and/or upper (uncomplicated pyelonephritis) UTI, limited to non-pregnant women with no known relevant anatomical and functional abnormalities within the urinary tract or comorbidities
Complicated UTIs	All UTIs which are not defined as uncomplicated
Recurrent UTIs	Recurrent episodes of uncomplicated and/or complicated UTIs. The frequency of episodes is at least three UTIs per year or two UTIs in the last 6 months
Catheter-associated UTIs	Catheter-associated urinary tract infection (CAUTI) refers to UTIs occurring in a person whose urinary tract is currently catheterised or has had a catheter in place within the past 48 hours
Urosepsis	Urosepsis is defined as life-threatening organ dysfunction caused by a dysregulated host response to infection originating from the urinary tract and/or male genital organs[50]

Source: Bonkat, G., Pickard, R., Bartoletti, R., Bruyère, F., Geerlings, S., Wagenlehner, F., ... & Veeratterapillay, R. (2021). Urological infections. Arnhem: European Association of Urology.

types of infections acquired in hospitals,[14] with an estimated 70,000 HAUTIs occurring each year in Australian public hospitals.[15] Catheter-associated UTIs are one of the most frequent examples of UTIs in hospital.

17.6 Catheter-associated UTI (CAUTI)

Around 16–25% of hospital inpatients will have an indwelling urinary catheter inserted at some point during care.[55,56] The risk of acquiring a CAUTI rises by 3–7% daily while ever the catheter remains in place.[34] An estimated 80% of UTIs acquired in hospitals are catheter-associated.[1] In Australia, a 2014 point prevalence study found that the prevalence of hospital-acquired UTI in Australian hospitals was 1.2%, with CAUTI being the vast majority at 0.9%.[55] CAUTI can lead to complications including cystitis, prostatitis, endocarditis, septic arthritis, meningitis, increased hospital stay and mortality.[53,54] Even short-term catheterisation may increase the risk of complications, due to persistent inflammation, impaired host defence mechanisms, microbial colonisation, and biofilm formations on urinary catheter devices.[7,57] A large proportion of CAUTIs are considered preventable.[7,58]

17.6.1 Definitions of CAUTI

An example of a definition for CAUTI is provided in Table 17.2. This definition was developed by the Centers for Disease Control and Prevention (CDC) and National Healthcare Safety Network.[53] There are other definitions for CAUTIs in patients one year of age or less. A healthcare-associated CAUTI must meet the definition of a CAUTI (Table 17.2), in addition to meeting the definition of being healthcare-associated. More detail regarding epidemiology and surveillance definitions for healthcare-associated infections is provided in Chapter 10.

17.6.2 Strategies to prevent CAUTI

Strategies for preventing CAUTI could be broadly summarised into five approaches:

1. appropriate urinary catheter use

2. correct techniques and approaches for urinary catheter insertion

3. correct techniques and approaches for urinary catheter maintenance

4. prompt removal of urinary catheters

5. quality improvement programs, which could include audit, surveillance and administrative infrastructure[59-61] (Fig 17.1).

17.6.3 Appropriate use

Reducing inappropriate urinary catheter use is one of the simplest strategies for preventing CAUTI. Each day of urinary catheterisation increases the risk of both bacteriuria and CAUTI.[62,63] For this reason, minimising

TABLE 17.2 Example of a catheter-associated urinary tract infection (CAUTI) definition[53]

CAUTI definition (all ages)	Additional considerations
1. Patient had an indwelling urinary catheter that had been in place for more than 2 consecutive days[a] in an inpatient location on the date of event *AND* was either: • present for any portion of the calendar day on the date of event, *OR* • removed the day before the date of event *AND* 2. Patient has at least one of the following symptoms: • fever (>38.0°C)[b] • suprapubic tenderness, costovertebral angle pain or tenderness[c] • urinary urgency or frequency, dysuria[d] • *(for patients ≤1 year of age)* fever (>38.0°C)[b] or hypothermia (36.0°C), lethargy, apnoea, bradycardia or vomiting[e] *AND* 3. Patient has a urine culture with no more than two species of organisms identified, at least one of which is a bacterium at concentrations of ≥10⁵ CFU/mL	(a) UTI occurring within the 2-day period is not classified as CAUTI, but may meet criteria for a healthcare-associated infection[53] (b) Fever is a non-specific symptom of infection and cannot be excluded from UTI[53] (c) Having no other recognised cause, and excluding generalised 'abdominal pain' or 'low back pain' (symptoms are too general)[53] (d) Symptoms of urinary urgency, frequency or dysuria can be indicative of catheterisation (rather than UTI) and so cannot be used when/if the catheter is in place[53] (e) *(for patients ≤1 year of age)* lethargy, apnoea, bradycardia, and/or vomiting which has no other recognised cause

Source: Adapted from The CDC NHSN Urinary Tract Infection (Catheter-Associated Urinary Tract Infection [CAUTI] and Non-Catheter-Associated Urinary Tract Infection [UTI]) Events guideline.

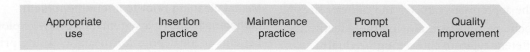

FIGURE 17.1 Overview of strategies to prevent CAUTI

catheter use, both insertion and duration, is one of the most important ways to prevent CAUTIs. The CDC recommends using catheters only where indicated and to minimise duration, particularly among those at higher risk of CAUTI.[60] The Practice tip box provides an overview of indicators for appropriate and inappropriate use of catheterisation.

PRACTICE TIP 1

INDICATORS FOR INDWELLING URINARY CATHETERISATION

- Acute urinary retention or bladder obstruction
- Direct measurement of urinary output in patients with critical illness
- Perioperative use for selected surgical procedures, e.g.:
  - urologic or other surgery on contiguous structures of the genitourinary tract
  - anticipated prolonged surgery duration (remove catheter in post-anaesthesia care unit)
  - patients receiving large-volume infusions or diuretics during surgery
  - for monitoring of intraoperative urinary output.
- Where operative patients have an indication for indwelling catheter, this should be removed as soon as possible post-operatively, and preferably ≤24 hours, unless otherwise appropriate
- Removal of urine from patients who require long-term immobilisation (such as for pelvic fracture, traumatic injury)
- In patients who have an open sacral or perineal wound
- To improve comfort in end-of-life (palliative) care

Source: Adapted from the Centers for Disease Control and Prevention[60]

There are a number of situations that constitute inappropriate use of indwelling urinary catheters. These include:

- using urinary catheters in patients and residential care (aged care) residents for management of incontinence

- routine use of indwelling catheterisation in operative patients (use only as necessary)
- prolonged postoperative duration without appropriate indications (e.g. prolonged effect of epidural anaesthesia)
- obtaining urine for cultures or other diagnostic tests when the patient can voluntarily void.[60,64]

Alternatives to indwelling catheter use may be considered, and include: intermittent catheterisation, use of a bedside urine receptable or bottle, absorbent garments designed for incontinent patients, and/or external condom catheter (male patients only).[59] A portable ultrasound bladder scanner may be used to assess the need for catheterisation before a catheter is placed intermittently, preventing unnecessary catheterisations and thus reducing the rate of CAUTI.[59,65]

17.6.4 Insertion practice: techniques and approaches for urinary catheter insertion

Using the correct, aseptic technique for inserting urinary catheters is important for reducing risk of microscopic trauma to the urinary tract and CAUTI. Correct insertion technique can be difficult to achieve, however, due to a variety of factors such as differences in genitourinary anatomy, physical patient factors, time and/or privacy pressures, apprehension among nursing staff about vocalising and reporting insertion errors, and being unable to maintain current knowledge about urinary catheter insertion practices.[66] It is important, therefore, that practices are regularly reviewed with a view to quality improvement and patient safety.

Insertion of urinary catheters should be undertaken by a person trained and deemed competent to undertake this procedure. There are a number of principles of indwelling urinary catheter insertion.[60,67] These include:

- only insert a urinary catheter if clinically indicated (see previous section)[67]
- follow relevant policies or procedures, and ensure that staff members performing the procedure are trained[67]

- choose the appropriate catheter and catheter size[67,68]
  - A Cochrane review exploring the effectiveness of different types of indwelling urethral catheters in reducing the risk of UTI in adults who require short-term urethral catheterisation in hospitals was published in 2014.[68] The authors concluded that silver alloy-coated catheters were not associated with a statistically significant reduction in symptomatic CAUTI. Nitrofurazone-impregnated catheters reduced the risk of symptomatic CAUTI and bacteriuria, although the magnitude of reduction was low and hence may not be clinically important.[68]
- use an aseptic technique and sterile equipment (including a sterile drape) when inserting and connect the catheter or a sterile system[67]
- clean the urethral meatus before insertion of the catheter[67]
  - consider the emerging evidence available for suitable cleaning solutions.[67] There is emerging evidence that using chlorhexidine for cleaning the urethral meatus prior to insertion reduces the risk of CAUTI and is cost-effective.[58,69,70]
- use a sterile, single use lubricant when inserting the catheter[67]
  - male patients may require the application of anaesthetic gel prior to the insertion of the catheter
- following insertion, attach the urinary catheter to the drainage device and secure the catheter and the drainage device to the patient[67]
- document insertion of the device in the patient medical record, including the date, time, product and clinical indication.[67]

Meatal cleaning prior to indwelling urinary catheter insertion: There is some evidence that using antiseptics, compared to non-antiseptics, for meatal cleaning prior to using indwelling urinary catheters may help to prevent bacteriuria and/or CAUTI (OR 0.84, 95% CI 0.69–1.02).[70] Antiseptics such as chlorhexidine or povidone-iodine for meatal cleaning are showing some value at reducing the incidence of CAUTI, compared to alternatives such as saline (OR=0.65, 95% CI 0.42–0.99).[70] A multi-centred randomised control trial, the largest undertaken to date, found that chlorhexidine 0.1% reduces the incidence of CAUTI by 94% at 7 days post insertion, compared to saline.[58] This approach was also found to be cost saving for health services.[69]

Meatal cleaning prior to intermittent (self) catheterisation: In a systematic review exploring the benefits of antiseptics for meatal cleaning prior to intermittent catheterisation, there was a suggestion of some potential benefits of using chlorhexidine to reduce the risk of UTI.[52] However, only two studies were identified that explored this topic and both had significant limitations, making interpretation difficult.[52]

17.6.5 Maintenance practice: techniques and approaches for urinary catheter maintenance

There are a number of measures that can be undertaken to reduce the risk of CAUTI once a catheter is inserted.[60,71,72] These include:

- connecting the catheter to a sterile closed system (bag) and maintaining a closed drainage system, unless clinically indicated
- changing urinary catheters only when clinically needed or as per manufacturer's instructions
- ensuring appropriate hand hygiene when handling catheters
- using a sampling port to obtain urine samples
- ensuring that the catheter tubing is kept kink-free
- keeping the collection bag below the level of the bladder.

There is no need to:

- routinely instil antiseptic or antimicrobial solutions into urinary drainage bags
- clean the periurethral area with antiseptics to prevent CAUTI while the catheter is in place.

17.6.6 Prompt removal

The period of time that a catheter remains in place is the principal determining factor of rates of bacteriuria and CAUTI, and with each day of catheterisation, the risk of CAUTI rises.[34] Removing catheters as early as possible is therefore one of the most important strategies for CAUTI prevention.[60,71] Barriers,[73] such as catheters going 'unnoticed', a lack of accurate and up-to-date patient catheter documentation, and unclear role responsibilities for assessing catheter removal can impede the timely removal of catheters.[73] To counter these barriers, a number of different approaches to support prompt removal of catheters have been used, including rounding checklists; written, verbal or visual reminders; and automatic stop orders.[59,74-80]

Many organisations use criteria-initiated urinary catheter removal protocols to enable healthcare workers, such as nurses, to remove urinary catheters that are no longer necessary.[81,82] There are also several global campaigns, with associated resource material, to support the early removal of catheters. These include 'CatheterOut' in the United States[83] and Choosing Wisely Canada's campaign 'Lose the Tube'.[84]

An integrative review undertaken by Meddings and colleagues found evidence that reminders and stop orders appear to reduce the incidence of CAUTI. As such these should be used to improve patient safety.[65] In a meta-analysis of 11 studies, the rate of CAUTI (episodes per 1000 catheter-days) was reduced by 53% (rate ratio 0.47; 95% CI 0.30–0.64) with the use of a reminder or stop order.[65]

17.7 Quality improvement programs

The prevention of CAUTI through quality improvement can include audits, surveillance and administrative infrastructure. Quality improvement processes are intertwined with other prevention strategies, such as appropriate use, and appropriate insertion and maintenance, as well as those to promote the removal of catheters.

17.7.1 Surveillance

Surveillance of CAUTI—or surrogate measures for CAUTI—are important as the cornerstone for any infection prevention and control program. Further details on broad surveillance approaches are provided in Chapter 10. CAUTI surveillance should be undertaken following an organisational risk assessment because, depending on the surveillance approach used, it can be resource intensive. Where CAUTI surveillance is undertaken, standardised methodologies and definitions should be used to enable benchmarking.[60] Feedback to clinical staff of any surveillance undertaken is vitally important.

17.7.2 Audit

As ongoing surveillance of CAUTIs can be resource intensive, depending on the infrastructure of the organisation, another approach to support quality improvement is audits. Auditing in the context of CAUTI prevention could include, but is not limited to:

- the use of point prevalence studies[14,55,85]
- compliance with policies or procedures, such as the need for catheterisation
- monitoring of the duration of catheterisation
- the appropriate use of antimicrobials.

17.7.3 Administrative

There are a number of administrative approaches that can be used, in conjunction with other approaches, that may help reduce the risk of CAUTI. Ensuring that staff are trained and competent in the appropriate use, selection, insertion, maintenance and removal of short-term indwelling urethral catheters is one such recommendation.[71] This extends not only to healthcare organisations, but also to those responsible for undergraduate education. Where a patient with a urinary catheter is discharged or transferred, there should be a clearly documented plan for the reasons for catheterisation and a date for removal or review.[71] Other systems to aid best practice include having clear policies and/or procedures for catheter insertion, maintenance and removal; availability and use of bladder scanners; and the continuing education of professional staff.[71]

17.7.4 Other strategies for preventing CAUTI

Prophylactic antibiotic treatments: While the routine use of systemic antibiotics for prophylaxis against CAUTI has been used in the past, this practice is not currently recommended.[7,86]

Conclusion

Urinary tract infections are common, and in healthcare many are associated with indwelling urinary catheter use. The current gold standard for preventing CAUTI includes limiting insertion to those who meet defined criteria; following correct insertion and maintenance practices; and ensuring the prompt removal of urinary catheters. Approaches to each of these have been detailed in this chapter. Quality improvement and administrative measures can help support these approaches.

Useful websites/resources

- Agency for Healthcare Research and Quality. https://www.ahrq.gov/hai/tools/cauti-hospitals/index.html
- The Centers for Disease Control and Prevention. https://www.cdc.gov/hai/ca_uti/uti.html
- Clinical Excellence Commission. https://www.cec.health.nsw.gov.au/keep-patients-safe/infection-prevention-and-control/cauti-prevention
- Clinical Excellence, Queensland Health. https://clinicalexcellence.qld.gov.au/sites/default/files/docs/clinical-networks/cauti-prevention-position-statement.pdf
- The Australian Commission on Safety and Quality in Health Care (ACSQHC). https://www.safetyandquality.gov.au/standards/nsqhs-standards/preventing-and-controlling-infections-standard

References

1. Öztürk R, Murt A. Epidemiology of urological infections: a global burden. World J Urol. 2020; 38(11):2669-2679.
2. 't Hoen LA, Bogaert G, Radmayr C, Dogan HS, Nijman RJM, Quaedackers J, et al. Update of the EAU/ESPU guidelines on urinary tract infections in children. J Pediatr Urol. 2021;17(2):200-207.
3. Storme O, Tirán Saucedo J, Garcia-Mora A, Dehesa-Dávila M, Naber KG. Risk factors and predisposing conditions for urinary tract infection. Ther Adv Urol. 2019;11: 1756287218814382.
4. Li V, Barker N, Curtis C, Porter B, Panicker JN, Chataway J, et al. The prevention and management of hospital admissions for urinary tract infection in patients with multiple sclerosis. Mult Scler Relat Disord. 2020;45:102432.
5. Gao Y, Danforth T, Ginsberg DA. Urologic management and complications in spinal cord injury patients: a 40- to 50-year follow-up study. Urology. 2017;104:52-58.
6. Kim Y, Cho MH, Do K, Kang HJ, Mok JJ, Kim MK, et al. Incidence and risk factors of urinary tract infections in hospitalised patients with spinal cord injury. J Clin Nurs. 2021;30(13-14):2068-2078.
7. Flores-Mireles A, Hreha TN, Hunstad DA. Pathophysiology, treatment, and prevention of catheter-associated urinary tract infection. Top Spinal Cord Inj Rehabil. 2019;25(3):228-240.
8. Zeng G, Zhu W, Lam W, Bayramgil A. Treatment of urinary tract infections in the old and fragile. World J Urol. 2020; 38(11):2709-2720.
9. Carrondo MC, Moita JJ. Potentially preventable urinary tract infection in patients with type 2 diabetes – a hospital-based study. Obes Med. 2020;17:100190.
10. Pigrau C, Escolà-Vergé L. Recurrent urinary tract infections: from pathogenesis to prevention. Med Clín (Barc) (English edition). 2020;155(4):171-177.
11. Tandogdu Z, Wagenlehner FME. Global epidemiology of urinary tract infections. Curr Opin Infect Dis. 2016;29(1):73-79.
12. Australian Commission on Safety and Quality in Health Care. The second Australian atlas of healthcare variation. Canberra: Australian Commission on Safety and Quality in Health Care, 2017.
13. Australian Institute of Health and Welfare. Australia's health, 2020. Data insights. Australia's health series no. 17. Cat. no. AUS 231. Canberra: AIHW, 2020.
14. Russo PL, Stewardson AJ, Cheng AC, Bucknall T, Mitchell BG. The prevalence of healthcare associated infections among adult inpatients at nineteen large Australian acute-care public hospitals: a point prevalence survey. Antimicrob Resist Infect Control. 2019;8(1):114.
15. Mitchell BG, Shaban RZ, MacBeth D, Wood C-J, Russo PL. The burden of healthcare-associated infection in Australian hospitals: a systematic review of the literature. Infect Dis Health. 2017;22(3):117-128.
16. Shaban RZ, Mitchell BG, Russo PL, MacBeth D. Epidemiology of healthcare-associated infections in Australia. Sydney: Elsevier, 2021.
17. Flores-Mireles AL, Walker JN, Caparon M, Hultgren SJ. Urinary tract infections: epidemiology, mechanisms of infection and treatment options. Nat Rev Microbiol. 2015;13(5):269-284.
18. Medina M, Castillo-Pino E. An introduction to the epidemiology and burden of urinary tract infections. Ther Adv Urol. 2019;11:1756287219832172.
19. Zalmanovici Trestioreanu A, Green H, Paul M, Yaphe J, Leibovici L. Antimicrobial agents for treating uncomplicated urinary tract infection in women. Cochrane Database Syst Rev. 2010;(10):Cd007182.
20. Australian Institute of Health and Welfare. Disparities in potentially preventable hospitalisations across Australia: exploring the data. Cat. no. HPF 51. Canberra: AIHW, 2020.
21. Zaffanello M, Banzato C, Piacentini G. Management of constipation in preventing urinary tract infections in children: a concise review. The European Research Journal. 2019; 5(2):236-243.
22. Khan A, Jhaveri R, Seed PC, Arshad M. Update on associated risk factors, diagnosis, and management of recurrent urinary tract infections in children. J Pediatric Infect Dis Soc. 2018; 8(2):152-159.
23. Leung AKC, Wong AHC, Leung AAM, Hon KL. Urinary tract infection in children. Recent Pat Inflamm Allergy Drug Discov. 2019;13(1):2-18.
24. Biggel M, Heytens S, Latour K, Bruyndonckx R, Goossens H, Moons P. Asymptomatic bacteriuria in older adults: the most fragile women are prone to long-term colonization. BMC Geriatr. 2019;19(1):170.
25. Harding C, Rantell A, Cardozo L, Jacobson SK, Anding R, Kirschner-Hermanns R, et al. How can we improve investigation, prevention and treatment for recurrent urinary tract infections – ICI-RS 2018. Neurourol Urodyn. 2019; 38(S5): S90-S7.
26. Kranz J, Schmidt S, Lebert C, Schneidewind L, Mandraka F, Kunze M et al. The 2017 update of the German clinical guideline on epidemiology, diagnostics, therapy, prevention, and management of uncomplicated urinary tract infections in adult patients: part 1. Urol Int. 2018;100(3):263-270.

27. Klein RD, Hultgren SJ. Urinary tract infections: microbial pathogenesis, host–pathogen interactions and new treatment strategies. Nat Rev Microbiol. 2020;18(4):211-226.

28. Chu CM, Lowder JL. Diagnosis and treatment of urinary tract infections across age groups. Am J Obstet Gynecol. 2018;219(1):40-51.

29. Claeys KC, Blanco N, Morgan DJ, Leekha S, Sullivan KV. Advances and challenges in the diagnosis and treatment of urinary tract infections: the need for diagnostic stewardship. Curr Infect Dis Rep. 2019;21(4):11.

30. Godbole GP, Cerruto N, Chavada R. Principles of assessment and management of urinary tract infections in older adults. JPPR. 2020; 50(3):276-283.

31. Ohly N, Teece S. Accuracy of negative dipstick urine analysis in ruling out urinary tract infection in adults. Emerg Med J. 2003;20(4):362-363.

32. Buettcher M, Trueck J, Niederer-Loher A, Heininger U, Agyeman P, Asner S, et al. Swiss consensus recommendations on urinary tract infections in children. Eur J Pediatr. 2021; 180(3):663-674.

33. Kaufman J, Fitzpatrick P, Tosif S, Hopper SM, Donath SM, Bryant PA, et al. Faster clean catch urine collection (Quick-Wee method) from infants: randomised controlled trial. BMJ. 2017; 357: j1341.

34. Nicolle LE, Gupta K, Bradley SF, Colgan R, DeMuri GP, Drekonja D, et al. Clinical practice guideline for the management of asymptomatic bacteriuria: 2019 update by the Infectious Diseases Society of America. Clin Infect Dis. 2019;68(10):e83-e110.

35. Schwenger EM, Tejani AM, Loewen PS. Probiotics for preventing urinary tract infections in adults and children. Cochrane Database Syst Rev. 2015;(12):Cd008772.

36. Ortega Martell JA, Naber KG, Milhem Haddad J, Tirán Saucedo J, Domínguez Burgos JA. Prevention of recurrent urinary tract infections: bridging the gap between clinical practice and guidelines in Latin America. Ther Adv Urol. 2019;11:1756287218824089.

37. Zhu M, Wang S, Zhu Y, Wang Z, Zhao M, Chen D, et al. Behavioral and dietary risk factors of recurrent urinary tract infection in Chinese postmenopausal women: a case–control study. J Int Med Res. 2019; 48(3):0300060519889448.

38. Fasugba O, Mitchell BG, McInnes E, Koerner J, Cheng AC, Cheng H, et al. Increased fluid intake for the prevention of urinary tract infection in adults and children in all settings: a systematic review. J Hosp Infect. 2020;104(1):68-77.

39. Jepson RG, Mihaljevic L, Craig J. Cranberries for preventing urinary tract infections. Cochrane Database Syst Rev. 2004; (1):Cd001321.

40. Department of Health Victoria. Urinary tract infections (UTI). In: Health Do, ed.:Victorian Government, 2021.

41. Mayo Clinic. Urinary tract infection (UTI) i. 2021. [cited 6 Jul 2021] Available from: https://www.mayoclinic.org/diseases-conditions/urinary-tract-infection/symptoms-causes/syc-20353447.

42. Cleveland Clinic. Urinary tract infections 2021. [cited 6 Jul 2021] Available from: https://my.clevelandclinic.org/health/diseases/9135-urinary-tract-infections.

43. National Health Service. Urinary tract infections. 2020. [cited 6 Jul 2021] Available from: https://www.nhs.uk/conditions/urinary-tract-infections-utis/.

44. Bader MS, Loeb M, Leto D, Brooks AA. Treatment of urinary tract infections in the era of antimicrobial resistance and new antimicrobial agents. Postgrad Med. 2020;132(3):234-250.

45. Fasugba O, Mitchell BG, Mnatzaganian G, Das A, Collignon P, Gardner A. Five-year antimicrobial resistance patterns of urinary Escherichia coli at an Australian tertiary hospital: time series analyses of prevalence data. PLoS One. 2016; 11(10):e0164306.

46. Ny S, Edquist P, Dumpis U, Gröndahl-Yli-Hannuksela K, Hermes J, Kling A-M, et al. Antimicrobial resistance of Escherichia coli isolates from outpatient urinary tract infections in women in six European countries including Russia. J Glob Antimicrob Resist. 2019;17:25-34.

47. Sugianli AK, Ginting F, Parwati I, de Jong MD, van Leth F, Schultsz C. Antimicrobial resistance among uropathogens in the Asia-Pacific region: a systematic review. JAC-Antimicrob Resist. 2021; 3(1).

48. Naziri Z, Derakhshandeh A, Soltani Borchaloee A, Poormalekenia M, Azimzadeh N. Treatment failure in urinary tract infections: a warning witness for virulent multi-drug resistant ESBL-producing Escherichia coli. Infect Drug Resist. 2020;13:1839-1850.

49. Fasugba O, Gardner A, Mitchell BG, Mnatzaganian G. Ciprofloxacin resistance in community- and hospital-acquired Escherichia coli urinary tract infections: a systematic review and meta-analysis of observational studies. BMC Infect Dis. 2015;15(1):545.

50. Singer M, Deutschman CS, Seymour CW, Shankar-Hari M, Annane D, Bauer M, et al. The third international consensus definitions for sepsis and septic shock (Sepsis-3). JAMA. 2016; 315(8): 801-810.

51. Bonkat G, Bartoletti R, Bruyère F, Cai T, Geerlings SE, Köves B, et al. European Association of Urology guidelines: urological infections. Arnhem: EAU Guidelines Office; 2021.

52. Mitchell BG, Prael G, Curryer C, Russo PL, Fasugba O, Lowthian J, et al. The frequency of urinary tract infections and the value of antiseptics in community-dwelling people who undertake intermittent urinary catheterization: a systematic review. Am J Infect Control. 2021;49(8):1058-1065.

53. Centers for Disease Control and Prevention, National Healthcare Safety Network. Urinary tract infection (catheter-associated urinary tract infection [CAUTI] and non-catheter-associated urinary tract infection [UTI]) events. Atlanta: CDC, 2021.

54. Mitchell BG, Ferguson JK, Anderson M, Sear J, Barnett A. Length of stay and mortality associated with healthcare-associated urinary tract infections: a multi-state model. J Hosp Infect. 2016; 93(1): 92-99.

55. Gardner A, Mitchell B, Beckingham W, Fasugba O. A point prevalence cross-sectional study of healthcare-associated urinary tract infections in six Australian hospitals. BMJ Open. 2014; 4(7): e005099.

56. Shackley DC, Whytock C, Parry G, Clarke L, Vincent C, Harrison A, et al. Variation in the prevalence of urinary catheters: a profile of National Health Service patients in England. BMJ Open. 2017;7(6):e013842.

57. Ricardo SIC, Anjos IIL, Monge N, Faustino CMC, Ribeiro IAC. A glance at antimicrobial strategies to prevent catheter-associated medical infections. ACS Infect Dis. 2020;6(12):3109-30.

58. Fasugba O, Cheng AC, Gregory V, Graves N, Koerner J, Collignon P, et al. Chlorhexidine for meatal cleaning in reducing catheter-associated urinary tract infections: a multicentre stepped-wedge randomised controlled trial. Lancet Infect Dis. 2019;19(6): 611-619.

59. Agency for Healthcare Research and Quality. AHRQ safety program for reducing CAUTI in hospitals. Implementation guide. Rockville, MD: AHRQ, 2015.

60. Centers for Disease Control and Prevention. Guideline for prevention of catheter-associated urinary tract infections, 2009. Updated 6 Jun 2019. Atlanta: CDC, 2009.

61. Mitchell BG. Meatal cleansing with chlorhexidine reduces catheter-associated infection. Nursing Times. 2019;115(9):21-22.

62. Letica-Kriegel AS, Salmasian H, Vawdrey DK, Youngerman BE, Green RA, Furuya EY, et al. Identifying the risk factors for catheter-associated urinary tract infections: a large cross-sectional study of six hospitals. BMJ Open. 2019;9(2):e022137.

63. Fukuoka K, Furuichi M, Ito K, Morikawa Y, Watanabe I, Shimizu N, et al. Longer duration of urinary catheterization increases catheter-associated urinary tract infection in PICU. Pediatr Crit Care Med. 2018;19(10).

64. Mitchell B, Ware C, McGregor A, Brown S, Wells A, Stuart RL, et al. ASID (HICSIG)/AICA position statement: preventing catheter-associated urinary tract infections in patients. Healthcare Infection. 2011;16(2):45-52.

65. Meddings J, Rogers MAM, Krein SL, Fakih MG, Olmsted RN, Saint S. Reducing unnecessary urinary catheter use and other strategies to prevent catheter-associated urinary tract infection: an integrative review. BMJ Qual Saf. 2014;23(4):277-289.

66. Lough ME, Eller S, Mayer B. Registered nurses' experiences with urinary catheter insertion: a qualitative focus group study. Appl Nurs Res. 2020;55:151293.

67. National Health and Medical Research Council. Australian guidelines for the prevention and control of infection in healthcare (2019). Canberra: NHMRC, 2021.

68. Lam TB, Omar MI, Fisher E, Gillies K, MacLennan S. Types of indwelling urethral catheters for short-term catheterisation in hospitalised adults. Cochrane Database Syst Rev. 2014;(9): Cd004013.

69. Mitchell BG, Fasugba O, Cheng AC, Gregory V, Koerner J, Collignon P, et al. Chlorhexidine versus saline in reducing the risk of catheter associated urinary tract infection: a cost-effectiveness analysis. Intl J Nurs Stud. 2019;97:1-6.

70. Mitchell B, Curryer C, Holliday E, Rickard CM, Fasugba O. Effectiveness of meatal cleaning in the prevention of catheter-associated urinary tract infections and bacteriuria: an updated systematic review and meta-analysis. BMJ Open. 2021;11(6):e046817.

71. Loveday HP, Wilson JA, Pratt RJ, Golsorkhi M, Tingle A, Bak A, et al. Epic3: national evidence-based guidelines for preventing healthcare-associated infections in NHS hospitals in England. J Hosp Infect. 2014;86 Suppl 1:S1-70.

72. National Health and Medical Research Council (NHMRC). Australian guidelines for the prevention and control of infection in healthcare (2019). Canberra: NHMRC, 2019.

73. Quinn M, Ameling JM, Forman J, Krein SL, Manojlovich M, Fowler KE, et al. Persistent barriers to timely catheter removal identified from clinical observations and interviews. Jt Comm J Qual Patient Saf. 2020;46(2):99-108.

74. Nassikas NJ, Monteiro JFG, Pashnik B, Lynch J, Carino G, Levinson AT. Intensive care unit rounding checklists to reduce catheter-associated urinary tract infections. Infect Control Hosp Epidemiol. 2020;41(6):680-683.

75. Siegel BI, Figueroa J, Stockwell JA. Impact of a daily PICU rounding checklist on urinary catheter utilization and infection. Pediatr Qual Saf. 2018;3(3):e078.

76. Mitchell BG, Northcote M, Cheng AC, Fasugba O, Russo PL, Rosebrock H. Reducing urinary catheter use using an electronic reminder system in hospitalized patients: a randomized stepped-wedge trial. Infect Control Hosp Epidemiol. 2019;40(4):427-31.

77. Shadle HN, Sabol V, Smith A, Stafford H, Thompson JA, Bowers M. A bundle-based approach to prevent catheter-associated urinary tract infections in the intensive care unit. Crit Care Nurse. 2021;41(2):62-71.

78. Gazarin M, Ingram-Crooks J, Hafizi F, Hall L, Weekes K, Casselman C, et al. Improving urinary catheterisation practices in a rural hospital in Ontario. BMJ Open Qual. 2020;9(1).

79. Menegueti MG, Ciol MA, Bellissimo-Rodrigues F, Auxiliadora-Martins M, Gaspar GG, Canini S, et al. Long-term prevention of catheter-associated urinary tract infections among critically ill patients through the implementation of an educational program and a daily checklist for maintenance of indwelling urinary catheters: a quasi-experimental study. Medicine (Baltimore). 2019; 98(8):e14417.

80. Elkbuli A, Miller A, Boneva D, Puyana S, Bernal E, Hai S, McKenney M. Targeting catheter-associated urinary tract infections in a trauma population: a 5-s bundle preventive approach. J Trauma Nurs. 2018;25(6): 366-373.

81. Clinical Excellence Commission. Reducing catheter-associated urinary tract infections: quick guide on criteria-initiated urinary catheter removal. NSW Ministry of Health, 2016.

82. Schiessler MM, Darwin LM, Phipps AR, Hegemann LR, Heybrock BS, Macfadyen AJ. Don't have a doubt, get the catheter out: a nurse-driven CAUTI prevention protocol. Pediatr Qual Saf. 2019;4(4):e183.

83. Catheter Out. Catheter out. 2022. [cited 17 Feb 2022] Available from: https://www.catheterout.org/about.html.

84. Canadian Society of Internal Medicine. Lose the tube: a toolkit for appropriate use of urinary catheters in hospitals. 2019.

85. Mitchell BG, Fasugba O, Beckingham W, Bennett N, Gardner A. A point prevalence study of healthcare associated urinary tract infections in Australian acute and aged care facilities. Infect Dis Health. 2016;21(1):26-31.

86. Taich L, Zhao H, Cordero C, Anger JT. New paradigms in the management of recurrent urinary tract infections. Curr Opin Urol. 2020;30(6):833-837.

CHAPTER 18

Surgical site infections

PROFESSOR RAMON Z. SHABAN[i-iv]

Dr DEBOROUGH MACBETH[v]

PAUL SIMPSON[vi]

Dr CATHERINE VIENGKHAM[i]

Dr CHRISTINE RODER[vii]

Chapter highlights

- The prevailing national and international definitions of surgical site infections (SSIs) based on wound type and depth
- Current epidemiology and burden of SSIs, both internationally and in Australia
- Common causes of SSIs, and the pathophysiology and presentation of infection
- Endogenous and exogenous factors that increase the risk of acquiring an SSI
- A summary of the current infection prevention and control (IPC) interventions recommended within Australian and international guidelines

i Susan Wakil School of Nursing and Midwifery, Faculty of Medicine and Health, University of Sydney, Sydney, NSW

ii Public Health Unit, Centre for Population Health, Western Sydney Local Health District, North Parramatta, NSW

iii Sydney Infectious Diseases Institute, Faculty of Medicine and Health, University of Sydney, Sydney, NSW

iv New South Wales Biocontainment Centre, Western Sydney Local Health District, Westead, NSW

v Gold Coast Hospital and Health Service, Southport, QLD

vi Infection Prevention and Control Service, Redcliffe Hospital, Metro North Health, Brisbane, QLD

vii Barwon South West Public Health Unit, Barwon Health, Geelong, VIC

Introduction

Modern history has seen substantial advances in the management of surgical incisions and wounds, as well as developments in techniques used before, during and after surgical procedures to ensure healthy wound healing and prevent infection. In general, the introduction of antimicrobials, aseptic technique and general advances in medical care have made significant contributions to lowering both the risk and dangers of surgical site infections (SSIs) since the beginning of the 20th century.[1] Despite this, SSIs remain a serious and frequent hospital-acquired complication that can occur after surgical procedures, and one which often leads to longer hospital stays, greater healthcare costs and increased patient morbidity and mortality.[2,3] It comprises one of the nine healthcare-associated infection (HAI) complications defined by the Australian Commission on Safety and Quality in Health Care (ACSQHC),[4] and is exacerbated by the increasing use of surgical procedures and the emergence of multidrug-resistant organisms (MROs).[5] This chapter provides an overview of the current surveillance definitions

and epidemiology of SSIs in Australia and worldwide. It then summarises the current infection prevention and control (IPC) interventions recommended by the literature and current guidelines.

18.1 Definitions of surgical site infections

Broadly speaking, SSIs are infections that are acquired as a direct result of a surgical procedure. More specific definitions have also been developed for the purposes of surveillance by the United States' Centers for Disease Control and Prevention (CDC) via the National Healthcare Safety Network (NHSN), as well as the European Centre of Disease Prevention and Control (ECDC). These definitions are summarised in Table 18.1. They are relatively well established and are widely adopted, both internationally and, to some degree, in state-based SSI surveillance systems in Australia. For more detailed explanations about them and their applications, refer to the source documents referenced at the end of this chapter.

TABLE 18.1 Definitions of 'surgical site infections' as provided by the CDC National Healthcare Safety Network and the ECDC

United States CDC/NHSN[10]		
Superficial incisional SSI	**Deep incisional SSI**	**Organ/space SSI**
Date of event occurs within 30 days of operative procedure AND involves skin and subcutaneous tissue of the incision AND patient has at least <u>one</u> of the following: a) purulent drainage from the superficial incision b) organism(s) identified from an aseptically obtained specimen from the superficial incision or subcutaneous tissue by a culture or non-culture based microbiologic testing method which is performed for purposes of clinical diagnosis or treatment c) a superficial incision that is deliberately opened by a surgeon or attending physician* and culture or non-culture based testing of the superficial incision or subcutaneous tissue is not performed AND patient has at least <u>one</u> of the following signs or symptoms: localised pain or tenderness; localised swelling; erythema; or heat d) diagnosis of a superficial incisional SSI by surgeon or attending physician	Date of event occurs within the NHSN specified period after the operative procedure AND involves deep soft tissues of the incision (e.g. fascia and muscle layers) AND patient has at least <u>one</u> of the following: a) purulent drainage from the deep incision b) a deep incision that spontaneously dehisces, or is deliberately opened or aspirated by a surgeon or attending physician AND organism(s) identified from the deep soft tissues of the incision by a culture or non-culture based microbiologic testing method which is performed for purposes of clinical diagnosis or treatment or culture or non-culture based microbiologic testing method is not performed AND patient has at least <u>one</u> of the following signs or symptoms: fever (>38°C); localised pain or tenderness c) an abscess or other evidence of infection involving deep incision that is detected on gross anatomical or histopathologic exam, or imaging test	Date of event occurs within the NHSN specified period after the operative procedure AND involves any part of the body deeper than the fascial muscle layers that is opened or manipulated during the operative procedure AND meets at least <u>one</u> criterion for a listed NHSN organ/space infection site AND patient has at least <u>one</u> of the following: a) purulent drainage from a drain that is placed into the organ/space (e.g. closed suction drainage system, open drain, T-tube drain, CT-guided drainage) b) organism(s) identified from fluid or tissue in the organ/space by a culture or non-culture based microbiologic testing method which is performed for purposes of clinical diagnosis or treatment c) an abscess or other evidence of infection involving the organ/space that is detected on gross anatomical or histopathologic exam, or imaging test evidence suggestive of infection

TABLE 18.1 Definitions of 'surgical site infections' as provided by the CDC National Healthcare Safety Network and the ECDC—cont'd

Europe (ECDC)[9]

Superficial incisional SSI	Deep incisional SSI	Organ/space SSI
Infection occurs within 30 days after the operation AND involves only skin and subcutaneous tissue of the incision AND at least <u>one</u> of the following: a) purulent drainage with or without laboratory confirmation, from the superficial incision b) organisms isolated from an aseptically obtained culture of fluid or tissue from the superficial incision c) at least one of the following signs or symptoms of infection: pain or tenderness, localised swelling, redness or heat and superficial incision is deliberately opened by surgeon, unless incision is culture-negative d) diagnosis of superficial incisional SSI made by surgeon or attending physician	Infection occurs within 30 days after the operation if no implant[†] is left in place or within 90 days if implant is in place AND the infection appears to be related to the operation and infection involves deep soft tissue (e.g. fascia, muscle) of the incision AND at least <u>one</u> of the following: a) purulent drainage from the deep incision but not from the organ/space component of the surgical site b) a deep incision spontaneously dehisces or is deliberately opened by a surgeon when the patient has at least one of the following signs or symptoms: fever (>38°C), localised pain or tenderness, unless incision is culture-negative c) an abscess or other evidence of infection involving the deep incision is found on direct examination, during reoperation, or by histopathologic or radiologic examination d) diagnosis of deep incisional SSI made by a surgeon or attending physician	Infection occurs within 30 days after the operation if no implant[†] is left in place or within 90 days if implant is in place AND the infection appears to be related to the operation and infection involves any part of the anatomy (e.g. organs and spaces) other than the incision that was opened or manipulated during an operation AND at least <u>one</u> of the following: a) purulent discharge from a drain that is placed through a stab wound into the organ/space b) organisms isolated from an aseptically obtained culture of fluid or tissue in the organ/space c) an abscess or other evidence of infection involving the organ/space that is found on direct examination, during reoperation, or by histopathologic or radiologic examination d) diagnosis of organ/space SSI made by a surgeon or attending physician

Source: Adapted from Control ECfDPa, 2017;[9] and Network NHS[10]
*The term physician for the purpose of application of the NHSN SSI criteria may be interpreted to mean a surgeon, infectious disease physician, emergency physician, other physician on the case, or physician's designee (nurse practitioner or physician's assistant).
†The US National Healthcare and Safety Network definition: a non-human-derived implantable foreign body (e.g. prosthetic heart valve, non-human vascular graft, mechanical heart or hip prosthesis) that is permanently placed in a patient during surgery.[10]

The CDC/NHSN and ECDC distinguish three types of SSIs based on the depth of the infection (Fig 18.1):

1. *Superficial incisional SSIs* are infections that involve the skin and subcutaneous tissue.

2. *Deep incisional SSIs* are infections that involve deep soft tissue, including the muscle and tissue that surround the muscle.

3. *Organ or space SSIs* are infections that involve any areas deeper than the skin and muscle layers, including body organs or space between the organs.

Currently, there is no nationally agreed upon definition for SSIs in Australia. However, most healthcare guidelines available at national (i.e. the ACSQHC) and state and territory levels either directly adopt or reference the CDC/NHSN criteria for SSIs.[6,7] In recognition of the absence of a formal definition in Australia, the ACQSHC published Approaches to Surgical Site Infection Surveillance for Acute Care Settings in Australia[6] in 2017. In this document, the Commission provided an overview of the components necessary for SSI surveillance and presented several recommendations for defining SSIs, such as the need to consider patient risk factors, the type of surgical procedure, the inclusion period, the wound type and the acceptable markers of infection. Additionally, as with all HAIs, SSIs may be identified using codes derived from the International Statistical Classification of Diseases and Related Health Problems, Tenth Revision, Australian Modification (ICD–10–AM), which currently distinguishes three diagnoses for SSIs:

1. wound infection following a procedure, not elsewhere classified

2. infection of amputation stump; and

3. infection of obstetric surgical wound.[8]

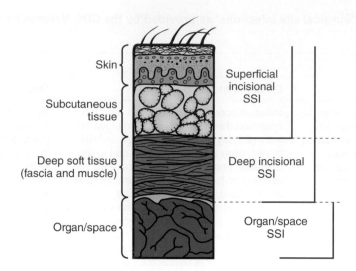

FIGURE 18.1 The three categories of surgical site infections defined by the CDC National Healthcare Safety Network and the ECDC[9,10]

Sources: Control ECfDPa. Surveillance of surgical site infections and prevention indicators in European hospitals – HAISSI protocol. Solna: European Centre for Disease Prevention and Control 2017; Network NHS. Surveillance for Surgical Site Infection (SSI) Events. Atlanta: CDC, 2020

While these codes are useful for the broader classification of healthcare-acquired complications, they are not nuanced enough to provide the clinically validated SSI data to be used and evaluated by IPC professionals to inform practice.

18.2 Epidemiology and burden of surgical site infections

18.2.1 Epidemiology of SSIs in Australia

Accurate national incidence rates of SSIs in Australia are difficult to ascertain because of the current absence of a nationally established definition and surveillance system. Nevertheless, there remain several sources from which these rates may be estimated. State-based SSI surveillance systems do exist as part of broader HAI programs within individual jurisdictions and are overseen at state, territory and local levels.[6,11] Surveillance definitions vary across jurisdictions and are generally limited to the mandatory reporting of a select number of surgical procedures, such as hip arthroplasty, knee arthroplasty, coronary artery bypass grafts (CABGs) and caesarean sections. Victoria is unique in its inclusion of a greater number of surgical procedures, such as breast and colorectal surgeries and spinal fusion. An overview of publicly available SSI surveillance data for Victoria, South Australia and Western Australia is presented in Table 18.2.

TABLE 18.2. The most recently reported, publicly available jurisdictional SSI surveillance data reported for Victoria, South Australia and Western Australia*

Procedure	VIC[12]	SA[7]	WA[13]
CBGB	RI 1: 2.1 (n = 1,489) RI 2: 6.2 (n = 503)	–	–
CBGC	RI 1: 0.8 (n = 129) RI 2: 5.6 (n = 36)	–	–
Other cardiac surgery	RI 1: 0.8 (n = 257) RI 2: 0.6 (n = 171)	–	–
Breast surgery	RI 0: 0 (n = 30) RI 1: 0 (n = 140)	–	–

TABLE 18.2. The most recently reported, publicly available jurisdictional SSI surveillance data reported for Victoria, South Australia and Western Australia*—cont'd

Procedure	VIC[12]	SA[7]	WA[13]
Caesarean sections	RI 0: 0.5 (n = 6,303) RI 1: 0.7 (n = 5,930) RI 2: 1.6 (n = 757)	RI 0: 0.4 RI 1: 0.1 RI 2: 0 (n = 4,397)	Risk all: 1.32 (n = 1,436) RI 0: 0.4 (n = 4,800) RI 1: 0.59 (n = 3,038) RI 2: 1.76 (n = 626) RI 3: 2.0 (n = 50)
Hip replacement/arthroplasty	RI 0: 0.5 (n = 2,292) RI 1: 0.8 (n = 3,441) RI 2: 1.4 (n = 902)	RI 0: 0.1 RI 1: 1.2 RI 2: 0.6 (n = 2,097)	Risk all: 0.63 (n = 315) RI 0: 0.54 (n = 2,600) RI 1: 0.89 (n = 1,682) RI 2: 2.74 (n = 219) RI 3: 0 (n = 17)
Knee replacement/arthroplasty	RI 0: 0.3 (n = 2,415) RI 1: 0.5 (n = 3,374) RI 2: 0.8 (n = 1,429)	RI 0: 0.1 RI 1: 0.5 RI 2: 0.3 (n = 2,148)	Risk all: 0.8 (n = 377) RI 0: 0.43 (n = 3,708) RI 1: 0.64 (n = 2,671) RI 2: 1.77 (n = 451) RI 3: 10.0 (n = 20)
Colorectal surgery	RI -1: 2.4 (n = 533) RI 0: 3.6 (n = 700) RI 1: 1.4 (n = 144) RI 2: 9.0 (n = 434)	–	–
Spinal fusion	RI 0: 0 (n = 64) RI 1: 3.4 (n = 119) RI 2: 5.9 (n = 68)	–	–
Hernia repair	RI 0: 0.3 (n = 303) RI 1: 0 (n = 382) RI 2: 1.6 (n = 124)	–	–
RI definitions	Risk stratification is based on the CDC/NHSN risk index	Risk stratification is based on the CDC/NHSN risk index	Risk stratification is based on the CDC/NHSN risk index. Risk 'All' applies to HISWA hospitals that perform less than 100 procedures annually and are not required to assign a risk index score

* Reported as number of infections per 100 procedures, separated by the risk index (RI) of patients
Source: Adapted from Epidemiology of healthcare associated infections[11]

Furthermore, peer-reviewed publications from both Australian and international literature offer geographically diverse insights into the rates of SSIs over both short and long periods of observation. Table 18.3 provides an overview of Australian peer-reviewed literature reporting on the incidence of surgical site or wound infections per 100 procedures. All states and territories, except for the Northern Territory, are reported on across these studies. The definitions used for SSIs vary widely in these studies, ranging from having no stated definition, to using those established by the CDC/NHSN, ECDC or the ICD-10-AM. These variations, in addition to differences in the types of surgical procedures or populations monitored, prevent the collation of averaged data. However, infection rates broadly range between 0.37% to 9.64% and are highly dependent on the types of surgical procedures performed and the assessed risk. Procedures like colorectal surgery have consistently been associated with a higher incidence of SSIs compared to other surgeries which is likely due to the nature of the surgical site. In general, both these values and their range correspond closely to those reported by both peer-reviewed literature and formal surveillance systems in other countries. A recent review and meta-analysis of 488,594 patients that examined the worldwide incidence of SSIs found

TABLE 18.3. Data on surgical site infections identified from literature research

Author	Year	State (# hospitals)	Year(s) monitored	Population	HAI monitored	SSI definition used	Key findings
Austin[15]	2017	NSW (1)	2011-2014	98 ECMO patients	Wound	Wound infection (WI): CDC/NHSN criteria for superficial incisional SSI or skin/soft tissue infection; Sternal WI: CDC/NHSN criteria for deep incisional or organ/space SSI.	20 per 1000 ECMO days
Bagheri[16]	2017	NSW (?)	2002-2013	58,096 surgical patients	SSIs (colorectal)	'Infection following a surgical procedure' code (ICD-10-AM T81.4) associated with colorectal surgeries was used for the study	9.64%
Betts[17]	2019	QLD (?)	2009-2015	All inpatient live births in QLD in study period	Surgical wound infection	Obstetric surgical wound infection (ICD-10-AM O86)	0.37%
Chandrananth[18]	2016	VIC (3)	2011-2014	1,019 patients undergoing hip or knee arthroplasty	SSI (adherence vs. non-adherence to antibiotic guidelines)	CDC/NHSN definition of SSIs	Total: 2.7% Adherent: 1.7% Non-adherent: 5.0%
Furuya-Kanamori[19]	2017	NSW (?)	2002-2013	237,187 patients who underwent colorectal, joint replacement, spinal or cardiac procedures	SSIs (joint replacement, colorectal, spinal, and cardiac operations)	'Infection following a surgical procedure' (ICD-10-AM T81.4) and 'Infection due to prosthetic device, implants and grafts' (ICD-10-AM T82.6-T82.7, T83.5-T83.6, T84.5-T84.7, T85.7)	Colorectal: 9.64% Joint replacement: 3.33% Spinal: 2.33% Cardiac: 5.66%

Author	Year	State (# hospitals)	Year(s) monitored	Population	HAI monitored	SSI definition used	Key findings
Jarratt[20]	2013	SA (1)	2003-2011	All hospital	SSI	CDC/NHSN definition of SSIs	MRO: 55.3%; Non-MRO: 65.9%
Kelly[21]	2017	WA (1)	2000-2002, 2010-2012	184 patients who underwent major lower limb amputation	WIs	None	2000-2002: 26.4%. 2010-2012: 12.4%
Lavers[22]	2018	WA (1)	2015-2017	250 patients who underwent breast procedures	SSIs	None	5.2%
Russo[23]	2019	All except NT (19)	2018	2767 acute adult inpatients	SSIs	ECDC definition of SSIs	3.6%
Tao[24]	2015	VIC (1)	2012	88 orthopaedic patients	SSIs	CDC/NHSN definition of SSIs	7%
Worth[25]	2015	VIC (81)	2002-2013	164,721 surgical patients	SSIs	CDC/NHSN definition of SSIs	2.8%

Source: Adapted from Shaban RZ, et al, 2021[11]
* ECMO = extracorporeal membrane oxygenation

an incidence rate of 11% in general surgery patients within 30 days of their procedure.[14]

18.2.2 Burden of SSIs

Surgical site infections comprise a large subset of HAIs and are a source of substantial clinical and economic burden on patients and the healthcare systems. In Australia, data obtained from two public hospitals over a two-year period found that patients who acquired an SSI spent an average of 14.2 days longer in hospital compared to patients who did not.[26] Longer length of stay (LOS) directly contributed to greater healthcare costs, with the need for additional bed days, medical staff, use of antibiotics, administration of other treatments for infection (e.g. reoperations, debridement), possible readmission and excess mortality. There are also notable productivity costs, with both patients and their carers requiring longer absences from work or being unable to perform their work to their usual capacity for an extended period of time.[27-29]

Estimates of the economic burden of SSIs in Australia vary between procedures. One study approximated a base cost of $1005 for every additional hospital day resulting from an HAI.[29] This value is broadly consistent with the estimated additional cost of $12,419 per patient that developed an SSI following coronary artery bypass graft.[28] These costs increase exponentially with complex procedures, such as hip and knee replacement surgeries.[30] The 2017–2018 Australian and New Zealand Audit of Surgical Mortality reported that between 2012 and 2018, 34.1% of the 24,375 audited surgical patients that died had a clinically significant infection.[31] Of these patients, 57.9% acquired these infections at some point during their admission. Approximately 8% were SSIs and an additional 67.4% were infections acquired postoperatively. In conjunction with organ failure, respiratory failure and cardiac events, septicaemia accounted for the greatest proportion of deaths following surgery.

Similar outcomes have been observed worldwide. A systematic review of the healthcare burden of SSIs across six European countries found that patients with SSIs unanimously reported increased length of hospital stays across multiple types of surgical procedures, as well as consistently higher rates of mortality.[32] Notably, the discrete increase in length of stay varied widely depending on the type of surgical procedure performed, ranging from an average of 2.1 days in a study of unspecified surgeries to as high as 54 days in a study observing orthopaedic and trauma surgery.[33, 34] In general, length of stay and mortality for patients who developed an SSI were 2–3 times greater compared to those who did not.[32,35] The increase in healthcare costs closely corresponded to greater LOS, although the exact costs varied considerably from country to country, based on differences in the estimated cost of bed days and additional resources. In the US, SSIs are quoted as one of the costliest HAIs, approaching US$20,785 per case and over US$3 billion in total annual healthcare costs across adult inpatients in US acute care hospitals.[36,37]

18.3 Aetiology of surgical site infections

18.3.1 Microbiological causes of SSIs

The site of the surgical wound must be contaminated in order for an SSI to occur. The risk of SSI after microbial contamination can be broadly calculated using the following equation:

$$Risk\ of\ SSI = \frac{Dose\ of\ bacterial\ contamination \times virulence}{Resistance\ of\ patient}$$

Surgical sites that are contaminated with over 10^5 microorganisms per gram of tissue have an elevated risk of infection.[38] There are multiple sources from which microbial contamination of the surgical site may occur. The most accepted cause of an SSI occurring after elective surgery under standard methods of antisepsis is an intraoperative contamination event. The predominant source of microbes involved in SSIs originate from either the natural flora from the patient's skin or the surrounding tissues of the incision (e.g. *Staphylococcus aureus*), or from deeper structures involved in the operative procedure (e.g. *Escherichia coli*, enterococci and anaerobes when the incision is close to gastrointestinal organs).

However, studies of microbial cultures taken from surgical wounds at the end of surgery appear to refute the intraoperative contamination theory. An alternative explanation is the inoculation of the surgical site with endogenous microorganisms from other sites on the patient. It has been postulated that the so-called Trojan horse mechanism may play a significant role. Although currently unproven, this mechanism suggests infection caused by pathogens far from the surgical site, such as the patient's gums or intestinal tract.[39] This may also occur from sites where patients have had a prosthesis or implant.[40,41] Exogenous sources of microorganisms are also possible but have been reported less frequently, typically resulting from contamination of surgical personnel, equipment or the environment. Carriage of both *S. aureus* and group A streptococci by surgical staff has been implicated in previous SSI outbreaks.[42-44]

Table 18.4 and Table 18.5 summarise the most common microorganisms isolated in SSIs from different types of surgical procedures reported in Australia and internationally. In general, *S. aureus* is the most frequently reported microorganism isolated from SSIs involving clean procedures which do not enter the gastrointestinal, gynaecologic or respiratory tracts. It is typically followed in frequency by Coagulase-negative Staphylococci (CoNS) and other Gram-positive bacteria like Streptococcus spp. Infections caused by Gram-negative bacteria like *E. coli* and *Pseudomonas aeruginosa*, as well as anaerobes, also become more common when specific organs are entered.

TABLE 18.4 Distribution of common microorganisms isolated from SSIs following state-reported surgeries

Surgery	Common organisms	Victoria (2018–2020)[12]	South Australia (2015–2020)[7]	Western Australia (2017–2018)[13]
Caesarean section	*Staphylococcus aureus*	69%	45%	41%
	Streptococcus spp.	0%	6.4%	2.3%*
	E. coli	10%	5.0%	–
	Coagulase-negative Staphylococcus	4%	3.5%	7.6%
	Enterobacter spp.	1%	3.2%	0%
	Other Gram-negative bacteria	8%	13.5%	23% (includes E. coli)
Hip replacement/ arthroplasty	*Staphylococcus aureus*	–	30%	44%
	Coagulase-negative Staphylococcus	–	14%	31%
	Pseudomonas aeruginosa	–	9.3%	–
	Streptococcus spp.	–	8.3%	14%*
	Enterococcus spp.	–	8.3%	2.8%
	Other Gram-negative bacteria	–	23%	1.1% (includes P. aeruginosa)
Knee replacement/ arthroplasty	*Staphylococcus aureus*	–	40%	29%
	Coagulase-negative Staphylococcus	–	19%	16%
	Enterococcus spp.	–	8.7%	8.2%
	Pseudomonas aeruginosa	–	6.8%	–
	Streptococcus spp.	–	5.8%	12%*
	Other Gram-negative bacteria	–	15%	33% (includes P. aeruginosa)
Cardiac bypass surgery	*Staphylococcus aureus*	23%	–	–
	Coagulase-negative Staphylococcus	22%	–	–
	Pseudomonas aeruginosa	11%	–	–
	E. coli	8%	–	–
	Other Gram-negative bacteria	15%	–	–
	Candida albicans	5%	–	–

Continued

TABLE 18.4 Distribution of common microorganisms isolated from SSIs following state-reported surgeries—cont'd

Surgery	Common organisms	Victoria (2018–2020)[12]	South Australia (2015–2020)[7]	Western Australia (2017–2018)[13]
Colorectal surgery	*E. coli*	25%	–	–
	Pseudomonas aeruginosa	21%	–	–
	Enterococcus spp.	16%	–	–
	Staphylococcus aureus	11%	–	–
	Coagulase-negative Staphylococcus	6%	–	–
	Candida albicans	5%	–	–

Source: Adapted from Mangram AJ, et al. 1999[41]
* Statistic includes case numbers for Streptococcus spp. and 'other Gram-positive species'

TABLE 18.5 Organisms commonly isolated from different surgical procedures

Surgery type	Common organisms	Surgery type	Common organisms
Placement of graft, prosthesis or implant	*S. aureus*, CoNS*	Appendectomy	Gram-negative bacilli, anaerobes
Cardiac	*S. aureus*, CoNS	Biliary tract	Gram-negative bacilli, anaerobes
Neurosurgery	*S. aureus*, CoNS	Colorectal	Gram-negative bacilli, anaerobes
Breast	*S. aureus*, CoNS	Gastroduodenal	Gram-negative bacilli, streptococci, oropharyngeal anaerobes
Ophthalmic	*S. aureus*, CoNS, streptococci, Gram-negative bacilli	Head and neck	*S. aureus*, streptococci, oropharyngeal anaerobes
Orthopaedic	*S. aureus*, CoNS, Gram-negative bacilli	Obstetric and gynaecological	Gram-negative bacilli, enterococci, Group B streptococci, anaerobes
Non-cardiothoracic	*S. aureus*, CoNS, *Streptococcus pneumoniae*, Gram-negative bacilli	Urological	Gram-negative bacilli
Vascular	*S. aureus*, CoNS		

Source: Adapted from Mangram AJ, et al.1999[41]
* CoNs = Coagulase-negative Staphylococcus

18.3.2 Presentation of surgical site infections

If microbial contamination at the surgical site is minimal, the infection may be effectively neutralised by the patient's innate immune response, which then facilitates the process for wound healing. However, if the microorganisms overwhelm the initial immune reaction, the body then engages a greater systemic inflammatory response, involving the upregulation of neutrophil activity and the release of Interleukin (IL)-1, IL-6, and other proinflammatory signals by the activated monocyte and serve as endocrine signals responsible for fever.[45]

As the infection progresses, the surgical wound releases pus, resulting from the accumulation of necrotic tissue, neutrophils, bacteria and proteinaceous fluid. The site will also exhibit the classic signs of inflammation: redness, swelling, increase in heat, pain or tenderness and inhibition of function. While these symptoms are typical of acute wound infections, chronic wound infection has been defined by a different set of symptoms, including friable granulation tissue, wound breakdown, increasing pain and foul odour. Wound infection significantly inhibits the healing process and can be potentially life threatening.

18.4 Risk factors for surgical site infections

The risk of developing an SSI is likely to be multifactorial and influenced by both *endogenous* and *exogenous* factors and processes (Table 18.6).[3] Endogenous factors encompass those relating to the patient, and are further classified into non-modifiable and modifiable factors. Non-modifiable endogenous factors include patient age, sex, history of infection and preexisting comorbid conditions or illnesses that cannot be feasibly treated. Modifiable factors include the use of substances such as alcohol, tobacco and other drugs, nutrition, activity level and those preexisting conditions which can feasibly be treated or improved prior to the surgical procedure if given enough time (e.g. glycaemic control and diabetic status, immunosuppression).

Exogeneous risk factors encompass all non-patient factors. This typically includes features relating to the physical environment and facility, the operative personnel, and the surgical procedure itself. Features in the physical environment include sufficient ventilation in the operating theatre, the presence of transient staff during surgery, and the adequacy of environmental cleaning and equipment sterilisation. Personnel-related risk factors include surgeon experience and the number of staff within the operating theatre. Lastly, surgical procedure risk factors are the most extensive and can

be further categorised into risks during the following surgical phases:

1. The *preoperative* phase is the period between the decision for the need for surgery and when everything is ready for the operation to start—i.e., the patient is on the operating table (including the preparation of operative staff). Preoperative risk factors include:
   - the duration of hospital stay prior to the procedure
   - the adequacy of skin preparation and hair removal; and
   - the appropriate administration of antibiotic prophylaxis.

2. The *intraoperative* phase is the period from when the patient is on the operating table to when the operation has finished, and the wound is closed. Intraoperative risk factors include:
   - the duration and complexity of the surgery
   - blood transfusion
   - adherence to aseptic technique; and
   - maintenance of patient glucose, oxygenation and body temperature.

3. The *postoperative* phase encompasses the end of the intraoperative phase to the resolution of the surgical procedure, including the administration of dressings, wound drains and negative-pressure wound therapy. Postoperative risk factors include:
   - the safe and appropriate application of dressing
   - wound management; and
   - antibiotic prophylaxis.

TABLE 18.6 Examples of endogenous and exogenous SSI risk factors

Endogenous factors		Exogenous factors
Non-modifiable	Modifiable	Operative personnel and environment
• age • sex • previous skin or soft tissue infection • existing chronic comorbidities • immune status	• diabetic status[47] • obesity • substance use—tobacco, alcohol, illicit drugs • nutrition • activity/exercise status • medications	• duration of surgery • emergency surgery • length of preoperative hospital stay • wound class (see Table 18.7) • presence of visitors during surgery • suboptimal prophylaxis or prophylaxis redosing • contaminated personnel, equipment and/or instruments • postoperative wound management • maintenance of homeostasis (blood glucose, oxygenation, body temperature)

Source: Adapted from Uçkay I et al[46]

Most surgical procedures will involve different combinations of exogenous and endogenous risk factors, which must be carefully considered by both physicians and patients prior to undergoing the surgery. Furthermore, the deliberate categorisation of patients into similar groups on the basis of risk is also important for the surveillance of infection rates and the assessment of the effectiveness of IPC measures. The basic SSI risk index is used to assign surgical patients into categories based on the presence of three major risk factors: wound contamination class, physical status of patient and procedure duration.[9,10] While it has its limitations, the basic SSI risk index is currently the most commonly used risk adjustment method in Australia. More complex risk adjustment methods, such as the NHSN Standardised Infection Ratio (SIR), have evolved from logistic regression modelling using large data sets.[48,49] The SIR is a summary measure that adjusts for facility and patient factors, and is well suited to electronically available data and national data sets.

Wound contamination can be classified into four classes which describe the cleanliness and condition of wounds (Table 18.7). The classification system was developed by the National Academy of Sciences and the National Research Council Cooperative Research study in 1964 and was later modified and used by the

TABLE 18.7 Wound contamination classification as presented by the CDC/NHSN and ECDC, and examples of common procedures associated with each wound type

Class	Type	Description	Common procedures
W1	Clean	An uninfected operative wound in which no inflammation is encountered and the respiratory, alimentary, genital or uninfected urinary tract is not entered. In addition, clean wounds are primarily closed and, if necessary, drained with closed drainage. Operative incisional wounds that follow non-penetrating (blunt) trauma should be included in this category if they meet the criteria	• reducible inguinal hernia • thromboendarterectomy • repair of initial incisional or ventral hernia • excision of breast lesion • excision of cyst, fibroadenoma, or other benign or malignant tumour
W2	Clean-contaminated	An operative wound in which the respiratory, alimentary, genital or urinary tracts are entered under controlled conditions and without unusual contamination. Specifically, operations involving the biliary tract, appendix, vagina and oropharynx are included in this category, provided no evidence of infection or major break in technique is encountered	• laparoscopy, surgical; cholecystectomy • laparoscopy, surgical, gastric restrictive procedure • laparoscopy, surgical; cholecystectomy with cholangiography • laparoscopy, surgical, appendectomy • colectomy, partial; with anastomosis
W3	Contaminated	Open, fresh, accidental wounds. In addition, operations with major breaks in sterile technique (e.g. open cardiac massage) or gross spillage from the gastrointestinal tract, and incisions in which acute, non-purulent inflammation is encountered are included in this category	• laparoscopy, surgical, appendectomy • laparoscopy, surgical; cholecystectomy • appendectomy • laparoscopy, surgical; cholecystectomy with cholangiography • enterectomy, resection of small intestine; single resection and anastomosis
W4	Dirty-infected	Old traumatic wounds with retained devitalised tissue and those that involve existing clinical infection or perforated viscera. This definition suggests that the organisms causing postoperative infection were present in the operative field before the operation	• laparoscopy, surgical, appendectomy • appendectomy; for ruptured appendix with abscess or generalised peritonitis • colectomy, partial; with end colostomy and closure of distal segment • incision and drainage of ischiorectal and/or perirectal abscess (separate procedure) • enterectomy, resection of small intestine; single resection and anastomosis

Source: CDC/NHSN and ECDC,[9,10] classification based on Altemeier et al (1984).[51] Procedures based on findings from Ortega et al.[52]

TABLE 18.8 **The American Society of Anaesthesiologists (ASA) physical status classification**

ASA Score	Definition	Examples
A1	A normal healthy patient	Healthy, non-smoking, no or minimal alcohol use
A2	A patient with mild systemic disease or condition	Mild diseases or conditions only without substantive functional limitations examples include (but not limited to): current smoker, social alcohol drinker, pregnancy, obesity (30 < BMI* < 40), well-controlled diabetes mellitus or hypertension, mild lung disease
A3	A patient with severe systemic disease	Substantive functional limitations; one or more moderate to severe diseases Examples include (but not limited to): poorly controlled diabetes mellitus or hypertension, chronic obstructive pulmonary disease, morbid obesity (BMI ≥ 40), active hepatitis, alcohol dependence or abuse, implanted pacemaker, moderate reduction of ejection fraction, end stage renal disease undergoing regularly scheduled dialysis, premature infant postconceptional age <60 weeks
A4	A patient with an incapacitating systemic disease that is a constant threat to life	Examples include (but not limited to): ongoing cardiac ischemia or severe valve dysfunction, severe reduction of ejection fraction, sepsis, disseminated intravascular coagulation or end stage renal disease not undergoing regularly scheduled dialysis
A5	A moribund patient who is not expected to survive without the operation	Examples include (but not limited to): ruptured abdominal/thoracic aneurysm, massive trauma, intracranial bleed with mass effect, ischaemic bowel in the face of significant cardiac pathology or multiple organ/system dysfunction

Source: Adapted from ASA physical status classification system, ASA House of Delegates, 2014[9]; and ECDC 2017.[53]
* BMI: body mass index

CDC/NHSN for risk stratification.[50] For the basic risk index, wounds that are classified as either 'clean' or 'clean-contaminated' are given a risk score of 0, and those classified as 'contaminated' or 'dirty-infected' are given a risk score of 1.

The physical status of the patient is determined by the American Society of Anaesthesiologists' (ASA) physical status classification (Table 18.8), which was first developed in the 1940s and then adopted in its modern five-class format from the 1960s.[53] The suffix 'E' can also be added to each category to signify emergency surgery. For basic risk assessment, patients with an ASA classification of A1 or A2 are given a risk score of 0, and patients with a classification of A3, A4 or A5 are given a risk score of 1.

The final component of the risk index is the procedure duration. Operations with a longer duration inherently carry a larger risk; however, length associated with greater risk is not equal across all procedure types. Risk score is determined by whether the operation falls under or exceeds a threshold or 'cut-off' approximate to the 75th percentile of the duration of the surgery for the operative procedure (rounded to the nearest whole hour). These thresholds vary between procedures and are summarised in Table 18.9. If the duration of the operation is below or equal to the 75th percentile cut-off, it is given a risk score of 0. If it is over, it is given a risk score of 1. The basic SSI risk index is the sum of the scores from each of the major risk categories listed above, with the lowest possible value of 0 to the highest possible value of 3. The data presented in Table 18.2 are an example of where epidemiological data on SSIs are collected and stratified based on this basic risk index.

18.5 Infection prevention and control interventions

Efforts to reduce the risk of SSI have employed a range of evidence-based strategies.[3,54,55] Many of these strategies have undergone extensive systematic review to inform the recommendations of international guidelines released by organisations such as the WHO[3] and the Joint Commission International.[56] Different interventions may be performed at different phases during the operation. Ultimately, the effectiveness of any strategy, alone, or in tandem, can only be determined through robust and systematic data collection. Table 18.10 provides a summary of

TABLE 18.9 75th percentile cut-off values for duration of operative procedure categories

Abbreviation	Description	75th percentile cut-off value (hours)
CARD	cardiac surgery	5
CABG	coronary artery bypass graft, unspecified	5
CBGB	coronary artery bypass graft with both chest and donor site incisions	5
CBGC	coronary artery bypass graft with chest incision only	4
CHOL	cholecystectomy	2
COLO	colon surgery	3
CSEC	caesarean section	1
HPRO	hip arthroplasty	2
KPRO	knee arthroplasty	2
LAM	laminectomy	2
REC	rectum surgery	4

TABLE 18.10 Commonly proposed IPC interventions to be performed at preoperative, intraoperative and postoperative phases

Preoperative	Intraoperative	Postoperative
• preoperative bathing • hair removal • antimicrobial prophylaxis • blood glucose	• surgical hand hygiene • surgical attire • skin antisepsis • aseptic technique • surgical procedure • antimicrobial sutures • maintaining homeostasis: oxygenation normothermia blood glucose	• wound management • continue maintaining homeostasis: oxygenation normothermia blood glucose

Source: World Health Organization, 2018[3]; and Soule B, 2018[56]

common interventions that have been examined in reducing rates of SSIs across each operative phase.

18.5.1 Preoperative

Hair removal: Historically, removing hair from the planned site of surgical incision was part of routine preoperative care. The rationale was in part based on the idea that hair represents a potential source of bacteria and therefore a potential increased risk of SSI.[3] However, a Cochrane systematic review has found no statistically significant difference in SSI rates between hair removal and no hair removal interventions.[57] Hair removal may be necessary in some circumstances to provide acceptable exposure and preoperative skin marking. It may also aid suturing and the application of wound dressings. However, razors should not be used for hair removal because they increase the risk of SSI, possibly due to micro-abrasions. If hair is required to be removed, the use of electric clippers with a single use head is recommended on the day of surgery.[3]

Preoperative bathing: Preoperative bathing or showering of the whole body has been considered good practice prior to surgery due to the likely reduction in skin bacterial load, particularly at the incision site. In general, either plain or antimicrobial soap containing 2%-4% chlorhexidine gluconate (CHG) is recommended for this purpose.[3] A 2012 Cochrane systematic review concluded that there is no strong evidence of the benefit of preoperative showering or bathing with CHG over the use of soap in reducing SSI.[57] Consideration should be given to the potential for induced CHG resistance.[3] It is also not uncommon for patients to demonstrate hypersensitivity, and in some rare cases, an allergic reaction to CHG.[57,58]

Antimicrobial prophylaxis: Antimicrobial prophylaxis is the preoperative administration of antimicrobial agents to reduce SSI rates.[59-61] Antimicrobial prophylaxis may be indicated in procedures that carry a high risk of infection (e.g. colorectal surgery); procedures where consequences of infection are severe (e.g. prosthetic implants); or for any procedure if the patient has underlying medical conditions that increase the risk of SSI (e.g. is immunosuppressed).[59-61] The use of antimicrobials to treat established infections or preoperative decolonisation is not considered antimicrobial prophylaxis.[59,61] The main groups of organisms covered by antimicrobial prophylaxis include skin-dwelling Gram positive organisms such as Staphylococci and Streptococci, coliforms such as *E. coli*, and gut-related anaerobes.[60]

Appropriate prescribing of antimicrobial prophylaxis should be in accordance with local and therapeutic guidelines and consider indication, antimicrobial agent, route and timing of administration, dose and duration.[59-61] Choice of antimicrobial agent is influenced by the surgical procedure, associated risk factors, patient factors such as β-lactam allergy, and the expected microbiological flora at the incision site.[59-61] Effective prophylaxis requires the serum and tissue concentrations of the antimicrobial agent to be greater than the minimum inhibitory concentration (MIC) at the time of incision.[59-61] For most procedures, achieving this requires a single dose to be administered intravenously within 60 minutes of incision.[59-61] Dosing may be influenced by patient factors including age (e.g. paediatric patients), weight and renal function.[59-61] Agents with prolonged infusion times (e.g. vancomycin and fluoroquinolones) should be given 120 minutes before incision.[59] There is little evidence that post-procedure dosing reduces the risk of SSI, and most guidelines recommend providing antimicrobial prophylaxes for less than 24 hours.[59,61]

The risks associated with antimicrobial prophylaxis include allergic reaction, antibiotic-associated diarrhoea, *Clostridioides difficile* colitis, drug interactions, phlebitis associated with intravenous administration, and drug toxicity.[59-61]

18.5.2 Intraoperative

Blood glucose control: A rise in blood glucose is commonly observed in the operative and postoperative periods due to a surgical stress response. This response results in increased secretion of catabolic hormones, inhibition of insulin secretion and insulin resistance.[62] Several observational studies showed that hyperglycaemia is associated with an increased risk of SSI.[63-65] Overall, there is low-quality evidence that a protocol with a more stringent blood glucose level target has a significant benefit in reducing SSI rates when compared to a conventional protocol. However, the WHO suggests the use of protocols for intensive perioperative blood glucose control for both diabetic and non-diabetic adult patients undergoing surgical procedures to reduce the risk of SSI.[3]

Maintaining patient homeostasis: Maintaining patient homeostasis perioperatively and postoperatively reduces the risk of SSI and this can be achieved by avoiding hypothermia, hypoxia and decreased perfusion.[66] Hypothermia, defined as a core body temperature below 36°C, may occur perioperatively and postoperatively in major surgical procedures.[3] Maintaining perioperative normothermia is considered an important component of perioperative care.[67,68] Some well-designed studies support normothermia in reducing the risk of SSI. However, it remains unclear exactly how maintaining normothermia reduces the risk of SSI.[3]

Once a surgical incision has been made, wound perfusion and oxygenation are critical for acute inflammation and optimal surgical wound healing.[69] National and international guidelines recommend that adult patients undergoing general anaesthesia with endotracheal intubation should receive 80% fraction of inspired oxygen (FiO2) perioperatively and, where possible, in the immediate postoperative period (2–6 hours) to reduce the risk of SSI.[3,54,55] This traditional view has been challenged with a recent meta-analysis showing no statistically significant difference in postoperative SSI when comparing patients receiving an FiO2 of 80% to those receiving an FiO2 of 30%.[70] However, it has been suggested that hyperoxygenation may be beneficial when normovolemia (expected circulating body fluid) and normothermia are also maintained.[3]

Sutures: There is a lack of high-quality evidence supporting the use of sutures over staples in terms of wound infection, readmission rate, adverse events and postoperative pain, although low-quality evidence suggests sutures reduce postoperative pain and improve grade of satisfaction with the cosmetic outcome.[71] There is strong evidence supporting tricolon-coated sutures to reduce the risk of SSIs, particularly in clean and contaminated surgical procedures.[72]

18.5.3 Postoperative

Wound management: A surgical incision or surgical wound, when not infected, heals by primary intention once the wound edges are brought together by either sutures, staples or clips.[73] Routinely, surgical wounds are covered with a sterile dressing. Such dressings act as a protective barrier against external contamination until the wound is healed and impermeable to pathogenic organisms. These dressings can also aid healing by absorbing wound exudate and keeping the wound dry.[3]

Since the 1800s, advances in surgical wound management have been driven largely by military conflict. Evolution in the aseptic treatment of wounds by pioneers such as Lister drew attention to the use of clean dressings. In the second half of the 19th century a surgeon called Gamgee developed an absorbent antiseptic dressing. In the 1960s the principles around moist wound healing were established and resulted in the development of dressings such as films and hydrocolloids.[74]

Despite many differing types of dressings for surgical wounds, according to a 2016 Cochrane systematic review, it remains unclear if one type of dressing is superior to another for preventing SSI. In fact, the Cochrane review found no strong evidence that covering the wound at all reduces the risk of SSI. Furthermore, there is no clear evidence that any dressing type improves scarring, pain control, patient suitability or ease of removal.[73] The WHO has also conducted a systematic review and found low-quality evidence that advanced dressings significantly reduce SSI rates compared to standard dressings. In particular, when comparing standard dressings to more advanced dressings, such as hydrocolloid dressings, low-quality evidence showed neither benefit nor harm.[3] Decisions about types of dressing remain largely based on clinical preference with the cost of dressing an element of consideration.[75] Table 18.11 lists some commonly used types of dressings and the rationale for their use.

Recent innovations have included the use of negative pressure wound therapy (NPWT) for surgical wounds. NPWT has become popular, in particular with sternal wound management following cardiac surgery for high-risk patients. A 2011 systematic review did not find evidence to support NPWT having a positive effect on wound healing or proof of superiority over conventional wound dressings.[78] However, a 2015 Australian-based study found significant reductions in sternal wound infections. This study recommends use on patients considered at high risk due to one or more of the following issues: increased body mass index, diabetes and/or previous chest radiation.[79]

18.5.4 Care bundles

A care bundle is a set of evidence-based interventions that, when used together, significantly improve patient outcomes.[80] Bundles are structured practices which simplify decisions and aim to reduce errors.[81] Care bundles were first used by intensive care practitioners aiming to improve ventilated patients' outcomes. A large multi-centre conducted in 2004 introduced an

TABLE 18.11 Commonly used dressings for various wound types

Dressing type	Rationale
Protective dressings	
Gauze	inexpensive easily accessible easy to apply
Impregnated gauze	non-adherent preserves moisture
Antimicrobial dressings	
Antibacterial ointments	can be applied to areas where dressings are difficult to apply
Iodine-based	absorbent not to be used in thyroid disorders
Silver-based	broad spectrum with low resistance
Absorbent dressings	
Foam	absorbs moderate exudate
Hydrogels	can absorb minimal wound exudate or rehydrate wound absorption function predominant
Hydro-fibres and alginates	absorbs heavy exudate
Autolytic debridement	
Films	occlusive allows exchange of gases
Hydrogels	can absorb minimal wound exudate or rehydrate wound absorption function predominant
Hydrocolloids	occlusive not for exudative or infected wounds

Sources: Yao K, et al, 2013[75]; Murphy PS, et al, 2012[76]; and Walter C, et al, 2012[77]

evidenced-based bundle that resulted in an average of 44.5% reduction in ventilator-associated pneumonia.[82] This bundle approach within intensive care units (ICUs) was extended to include prevention of central line–associated bloodstream infection (CLABSI). It proved successful in reducing CLABSI rates and demonstrated that the improvement could be sustained over time.[83,84]

Bundled approaches such as the WHO surgical safety checklist are widely used within the surgical environment.[85,86] More recently care bundles have been used within the perioperative environment to reduce the risk of SSI. An example of a care bundle targeting the prevention of SSIs after hip and knee replacement surgeries is presented in Table 18.12. Although these bundles have consistently demonstrated success internationally,

TABLE 18.12 Example of an evidence-based surgical care bundle developed by Project JOINTS (Joining Organisations IN Tackling SSIs), an initiative funded by the US Federal Government, targeting the prevention of SSIs after hip and knee replacement surgeries

Project JOINTS Care Bundles
SSI prevention bundle
1. Use an alcohol-containing antiseptic agent for preoperative skin preparation
2. Instruct patients to bathe or shower with chlorhexidine gluconate (CHG) soap for at least 3 days before surgery
3. Screen patients for *S. aureus* and decolonise *S. aureus* carriers with 5 days of intranasal mupirocin, and bathing or showering with CHG soap for at least 3 days before surgery
Surgical Care Improvement Project (SCIP) bundle
1. Appropriate use of prophylactic antibiotics:
• prophylactic antibiotic received within 1 hour prior to surgical incision
• prophylactic antibiotic selection for surgical patients consistent with national guidelines
• prophylactic antibiotics discontinued within 24 hours after surgery end time.
2. Appropriate hair removal
3. Hair removal must not be performed with a razor, but instead a clean clipper should be used outside of the procedure room

Source: How-to guide: prevent surgical site infection for hip and knee arthroplasty. Cambridge, MA: Institute for Healthcare Improvement, 2012[87]

they remain a relatively new initiative in Australia and are currently not consistently or uniformly implemented within Australian healthcare.[72,81]

Conclusion

Despite considerable advances in the measures used to prevent infections following surgical procedures over the past century, SSIs continue to impart a heavy burden on both patients and the healthcare system. International and national epidemiological data indicate that SSIs are one of the most frequent and expensive HAIs and one that is highly vulnerable to the modern emergence of multidrug-resistant organisms, such as MRSA.

Yet it is notable that in Australia, our current knowledge of the incidence of SSIs remains a broad estimate due to the absence of any comprehensive, formal surveillance system or a nationally consistent surveillance definition.

This chapter has explored the current international frameworks released by the CDC/NHSN and ECDC with regard to defining and classifying SSIs, and determining the patient and procedural risk factors for acquiring an SSI. We also highlighted the extensive and ongoing research examining the effectiveness of numerous infection prevention and control interventions, as well as the considerable efforts to synthesise this research to offer evidence-based recommendations.

Useful websites/resources

- Global guidelines for the prevention of surgical site infection, second edition. Geneva: World Health Organization, 2018. Available from: https://www.who.int/publications/i/item/global-guidelines-for-the-prevention-of-surgical-site-infection-2nd-ed
- Australian Commission on Safety and Quality in Health Care. Approaches to Surgical Site Infection Surveillance. Sydney: ACSQHC, 2017. Available from: https://www.safetyandquality.gov.au/sites/default/files/migrated/Approaches-to-Surgical-Site-Infection-Surveillance.pdf

References

1. Young PY, Khadaroo RG. Surgical site infections. Surgical Clinics. 2014;94(6):1245-64.
2. Bull A, McGechie D, Richards M, Russo P, Worth I. Surgical site infection. In: Cruickshank M, Ferguson J, eds. Reducing harm to patients from health care associated infection: the role of surveillance. Canberra: ACSQHC, 2008.
3. World Health Organization. Global guidelines for the prevention of surgical site infection. 2nd ed. Geneva: WHO, 2018.
4. Care ACoSaQiH. Hospital-acquired complications (HACs) list – specifications – Version 3.1 (12th ed). Sydney: ACSQHC, 2019.
5. Australian Institute of Health and Welfare. Hospitals at a glance 2017–18: surgery in Australia's hospitals. Canberra: AIHW, 2019.
6. Care ACoSaQiH. Approaches to surgical site infection surveillance. Sydney: ACSQHC, 2017.
7. Government of South Australia. South Australian healthcare-associated infection surveillance program: surgical site infection annual report 2020. Adelaide: Communicable Diseases Control Branch, 2021.

8. Authority IHP. Classifications 2019. Darlinghurst: Independent Hospital Pricing Authority, 2019.
9. Control ECfDPa. Surveillance of surgical site infections and prevention indicators in European hospitals – HAISSI protocol. Solna: European Centre for Disease Prevention and Control, 2017.
10. Network NHS. Surveillance for surgical site infection (SSI) events. Atlanta: Centers for Disease Control, 2020.
11. Shaban RZ, Mitchell B, Russo P, Macbeth D. Epidemiology of healthcare-associated infections in Australia. Elsevier Health Sciences, 2021.
12. Doherty Institute. Healthcare-associated infection in Victoria: surveillance report 2019-20. Melbourne: Doherty Institute, 2021.
13. Communicable Disease Control Directorate. Healthcare infection surveillance Western Australia: annual report 2017-18. Perth, Australia: Communicable Disease Control Directorate, 2018.
14. Gillespie BM, Harbeck E, Rattray M, Liang R, Walker R, Latimer S, et al. Worldwide incidence of surgical site infections in general surgical patients: a systematic review and meta-analysis of 488,594 patients. Int J Surg. 2021;95:106136.
15. Austin DE, Kerr SJ, Al-Soufi S, Connellan M, Spratt P, Goeman E, et al. Nosocomial infections acquired by patients treated with extracorporeal membrane oxygenation. Crit Care Resusc. 2017;19(Suppl 1):68-75.
16. Bagheri N, Furuya-Kanamori L, Doi SAR, Clements ACA, Sedrakyan A. Geographical outcome disparities in infection occurrence after colorectal surgery: an analysis of 58,096 colorectal surgical procedures. Int J Surg. 2017;44:117-21.
17. Betts KS, Kisely S, Alati R. Predicting common maternal postpartum complications: leveraging health administrative data and machine learning. BJOG. 2019;126(6):702-709.
18. Chandrananth J, Rabinovich A, Karahalios A, Guy S, Tran P. Impact of adherence to local antibiotic prophylaxis guidelines on infection outcome after total hip or knee arthroplasty. J Hosp Infect. 2016;93(4):423-427.
19. Furuya-Kanamori L, Doi SAR, Smith PN, Bagheri N, Clements ACA, Sedrakyan A. Hospital effect on infections after four major surgical procedures: outlier and volume-outcome analysis using all-inclusive state data. J Hosp Infect. 2017;97(2):115-121.
20. Jarratt LS, Miller ER. The relationship between patient characteristics and the development of a multi-resistant healthcare-associated infection in a private South Australian hospital. Healthcare Infection. 2013;18:94-101.
21. Kelly DA, Pedersen S, Tosenovsky P, Sieunarine K. Major lower limb amputation: outcomes are improving. Ann Vasc Surg. 2017;45:29-34.
22. Lavers A, Yip WS, Sunderland B, Mackenzie S, Seet J, Czarniak P. Surgical antibiotic prophylaxis use and infection prevalence in non-cosmetic breast surgery procedures at a tertiary hospital in Western Australia – a retrospective study. Peer J. 2018;6:e5724.
23. Russo PL, Stewardson AJ, Cheng AC, Bucknall T, Mitchell BG. The prevalence of healthcare associated infections among adult inpatients at nineteen large Australian acute-care public hospitals: a point prevalence survey. Antimicrob Resist Infect Control. 2019;8:114.
24. Tao F, Jiang R, Chen Y, Chen R. Risk factors for early onset of catheter-related bloodstream infection in an intensive care unit in China: a retrospective study. Med Sci Monit. 2015;21:550-556.
25. Worth LJ, Bull AL, Spelman T, Brett J, Richards MJ. Diminishing surgical site infections in Australia: time trends in infection rates, pathogens and antimicrobial resistance using a comprehensive Victorian surveillance program, 2002–2013. Infect Control Hosp Epidemiol. 2015;36(4):409-416.
26. KPMG. Report commissioned by the Australian Commission on Safety and Quality in Health Care. 2013.
27. Graves N, Halton K, Doidge S, Clements A, Lairson D, Whitby M. Who bears the cost of healthcare-acquired surgical site infection? J Hosp Infect. 2008;69(3):274-282.
28. Jenney AW, Harrington GA, Russo PL, Spelman DW. Cost of surgical site infections following coronary artery bypass surgery. ANZ J Surg. 2001;71(11):662-664.
29. Graves N, Halton K, Paterson D, Whitby M. Economic rationale for infection control in Australian hospitals. Healthcare Infection. 2009;14(3):81-88.
30. Cruickshank M, Ferguson J, Bull A. Reducing harm to patients from health care associated infection: the role of surveillance. Chapter 3: Surgical site infection–an abridged version. Healthcare Infection. 2009;14(3):109-114.
31. Royal Australasian College of Surgeons. Australian and New Zealand audit of surgical mortality national report 2017-2018. Kent Town: RACS, 2018.
32. Badia J, Casey A, Petrosillo N, Hudson P, Mitchell S, Crosby C. Impact of surgical site infection on healthcare costs and patient outcomes: a systematic review in six European countries. J Hosp Infect. 2017;96(1):1-15.
33. Edwards C, Counsell A, Boulton C, Moran C. Early infection after hip fracture surgery: risk factors, costs and outcome. J Bone Joint Surg Br. 2008;90(6):770-777.
34. Arroyo AA, Casanova PL, Soriano JV, Torra i Bou J-E. Open-label clinical trial comparing the clinical and economic effectiveness of using a polyurethane film surgical dressing with gauze surgical dressings in the care of post-operative surgical wounds. International Wound Journal. 2015;12(3):285-292.
35. Cossin S, Malavaud S, Jarno P, Giard M, L'Hériteau F, Simon L, et al. Surgical site infection after valvular or coronary artery bypass surgery: 2008–2011 French SSI national ISO-RAISIN surveillance. J Hosp Infect. 2015;91(3):225-230.
36. Anderson DJ, Pyatt DG, Weber DJ, Rutala WA, Group NCDoPHHA. Statewide costs of health care-associated infections: estimates for acute care hospitals in North Carolina. Am J Infect Control. 2013;41(9):764-768.
37. Zimlichman E, Henderson D, Tamir O, Franz C, Song P, Yamin CK, et al. Health care–associated infections: a meta-analysis of costs and financial impact on the US health care system. JAMA Intern Med. 2013;173(22):2039-2046.
38. Raahave D. Wound contamination and postoperative infection. A review. Dan Med Bull. 1991;38(6):481-485.
39. Alverdy JC, Hyman N, Gilbert J. Re-examining causes of surgical site infections following elective surgery in the era of asepsis. Lancet Infect Dis. 2020;20(3):e38-e43.
40. Owens C, Stoessel K. Surgical site infections: epidemiology, microbiology and prevention. J Hosp Infect. 2008;70:3-10.
41. Mangram AJ, Horan TC, Pearson ML, Silver LC, Jarvis WR, Committee HICPA. Guideline for prevention of surgical site infection, 1999. Infect Control Hosp Epidemiol. 1999;20(4):247-80.
42. Berkelman RL, Martin D, Graham DR, Mowry J, Freisem R, Weber JA, et al. Streptococcal wound infections caused by a vaginal carrier. JAMA. 1982;247(19):2680-2682.
43. McIntyre DM. An epidemic of Streptococcus pyogenes puerperal and postoperative sepsis with an unusual carrier site—the anus. Am J Obstet Gynecol. 1968;101(3):308-314.
44. Weber S, Herwaldt LA, McNutt L-A, Rhomberg P, Vaudaux P, Pfaller MA, et al. An outbreak of Staphylococcus aureus in a pediatric cardiothoracic surgery unit. Infect Control Hosp Epidemiol. 2002;23(2):77-81.
45. Rasa K, Pagani L, Coimbra R, Sartelli M. Infections in surgery: prevention and management. Springer, 2021.
46. Uçkay I, Harbarth S, Peter R, Lew D, Hoffmeyer P, Pittet D. Preventing surgical site infections. Exp Rev Anti Infect Ther. 2010;8(6):657-670.

47. Martin ET, Kaye KS, Knott C, Nguyen H, Santarossa M, Evans R, et al. Diabetes and risk of surgical site infection: a systematic review and meta-analysis. Infect Control Hosp Epidemiol. 2016;37(1):88-99.

48. Mu Y, Edwards JR, Horan TC, Berrios-Torres SI, Fridkin SK. Improving risk-adjusted measures of surgical site infection for the National Healthcare Safety Network. Infect Control Hosp Epidemiol. 2011;32(10):970-86.

49. National Healthcare Safety Network. The NHSN Standardized Infection Ratio (SIR). USA: NHSN, 2022.

50. Onyekwelu I, Yakkanti R, Protzer L, Pinkston CM, Tucker C, Seligson D. Surgical wound classification and surgical site infections in the orthopaedic patient. J Am Acad Orthop Surg Glob Res Rev. 2017;1(3):e022.

51. Altemeier WA, et al. Manual on control of infection in surgical patients. 2nd ed. Philadelphia, PA: JB Lippincott, 1984.

52. Ortega G, Rhee DS, Papandria DJ, Yang J, Ibrahim AM, Shore AD, et al. An evaluation of surgical site infections by wound classification system using the ACS-NSQIP. J Surg Res. 2012;174(1):33-38.

53. American Society of Anesthesiologists. ASA physical status classification system. ASA House of Delegates, 2014.

54. Berrios-Torres SI, Umscheid CA, Bratzler DW, Leas B, Stone EC, Kelz RR, et al. Centers for Disease Control and Prevention guideline for the prevention of surgical site infection, 2017. JAMA Surg. 2017;152(8):784-791.

55. National Institute for Health and Care Excellence. NICE guideline [NG125] surgical site infections: prevention and treatment. London: NIfHaC, 2019.

56. Soule B. Evidence-based principles and practices for preventing surgical site infections toolkit. Joint Commission International, 2018.

57. Webster J, Osborne S. Preoperative bathing or showering with skin antiseptics to prevent surgical site infection. Cochrane Database Syst Rev. 2012(9).

58. Krautheim A, Jermann T, Bircher A. Chlorhexidine anaphylaxis: case report and review of the literature. Contact Dermatitis. 2004;50(3):113-116.

59. Bratzler DW, Dellinger EP, Olsen KM, Perl TM, Auwaerter PG, Bolon MK, et al. Clinical practice guidelines for antimicrobial prophylaxis in surgery. Surg Infect (Larchmt). 2013;14(1):73-156.

60. Dryden M. Surgical antibiotic prophylaxis. Surgery (Oxford). 2019;37(1):19-25.

61. Ierano C, Nankervis J-AM, James R, Rajkhowa A, Peel T, Thursky K. Surgical antimicrobial prophylaxis. Australian Prescriber. 2017;40(6):225.

62. Kao LS, Phatak UR. Glycemic control and prevention of surgical site infection. Surg Infect (Larchmt). 2013;14(5):437-444.

63. Ata A, Lee J, Bestle SL, Desemone J, Stain SC. Postoperative hyperglycemia and surgical site infection in general surgery patients. Arch Surg. 2010;145(9):858-864.

64. Ma T, Lu K, Song L, Wang D, Ning S, Chen Z, et al. Modifiable factors as current smoking, hypoalbumin, and elevated fasting blood glucose level increased the SSI risk following elderly hip fracture surgery. J Invest Surg. 2019; 33(8):750-758.

65. Okabayashi T, Shima Y, Sumiyoshi T, Kozuki A, Tokumaru T, Iiyama T, et al. Intensive versus intermediate glucose control in surgical intensive care unit patients. Diabetes Care. 2014; 37(6):1516-1524.

66. Kurz A, Fleischmann E, Sessler D, Buggy D, Apfel C, Akça O, et al. Effects of supplemental oxygen and dexamethasone on surgical site infection: a factorial randomized trial. Br J Anaesth. 2015;115(3):434-443.

67. Lehtinen SJ, Onicescu G, Kuhn KM, Cole DJ, Esnaola NF. Normothermia to prevent surgical site infections after gastrointestinal surgery: holy grail or false idol? Annals of Surgery. 2010;252(4):696.

68. Yamada K, Nakajima K, Nakamoto H, Kohata K, Shinozaki T, Oka H, et al. Association between normothermia at the end of surgery and postoperative complication following orthopedic surgery. Clin Infect Dis. 2020;70(3):474-482.

69. Chambers A, Leaper D. Role of oxygen in wound healing: a review of evidence. J Wound Care. 2011;20(4):160-164.

70. Smith BK, Roberts RH, Frizelle FA. O2 no longer the Go2: a systematic review and meta-analysis comparing the effects of giving perioperative oxygen therapy of 30% FiO2 to 80% FiO2 on surgical site infection and mortality. World J Surg. 2020;44(1):69-77.

71. Cochetti G, Abraha I, Randolph J, Montedori A, Boni A, Arezzo A, et al. Surgical wound closure by staples or sutures?: systematic review. Medicine. 2020;99(25).

72. Bull A, Wilson J, Worth L, Stuart R, Gillespie E, Waxman B, et al. A bundle of care to reduce colorectal surgical infections: an Australian experience. J Hosp Infect. 2011;78(4):297-301.

73. Dumville JC, Gray TA, Walter CJ, Sharp CA, Page T, Macefield R, et al. Dressings for the prevention of surgical site infection. Cochrane Database Syst Rev. 2016(12).

74. Watret L, White R. Surgical wound management: the role of dressings. Nursing Standard (through 2013). 2001; 15(44):59.

75. Yao K, Bae L, Yew WP. Post-operative wound management. Australian Fam Physician. 2013;42(12):867-870.

76. Murphy PS, Evans GR. Advances in wound healing: a review of current wound healing products. Plastic Surg Int. 2012;2012:190436.

77. Walter C, Dumville J, Sharp C, Page T. Systematic review and meta-analysis of wound dressings in the prevention of surgical-site infections in surgical wounds healing by primary intention. J Br Surg. 2012;99(9):1185-1194.

78. Peinemann F, Sauerland S. Negative-pressure wound therapy: systematic review of randomized controlled trials. Deutsches Ärzteblatt International. 2011;108(22):381.

79. Jennings S, Vahaviolos J, Chan J, Worthington MG, Stuklis RG. Prevention of sternal wound infections by use of a surgical incision management system: first reported Australian case series. Heart Lung Circ. 2016;25(1):89-93.

80. McCarron K. Understanding care bundles. Nursing made incredibly easy. 2011;9(2):30-33.

81. Proops EM. Implementing a surgical site infection care bundle: implications for perioperative practice. J Periop Nurs. 2019;32(2):25-28.

82. Resar R, Pronovost P, Haraden C, Simmonds T, Rainey T, Nolan T. Using a bundle approach to improve ventilator care processes and reduce ventilator-associated pneumonia. Jt Comm J Qual Patient Saf. 2005;31(5):243-248.

83. DePalo VA, McNicoll L, Cornell M, Rocha JM, Adams L, Pronovost PJ. The Rhode Island ICU collaborative: a model for reducing central line–associated bloodstream infection and ventilator-associated pneumonia statewide. Qual Saf Health Care. 2010;19(6):555-561.

84. Pronovost PJ, Watson SR, Goeschel CA, Hyzy RC, Berenholtz SM. Sustaining reductions in central line–associated bloodstream infections in Michigan intensive care units: a 10-year analysis. Am J Med Qual. 2016;31(3):197-202.

85. WHO Patient Safety & WHO. WHO guidelines for safe surgery 2009: safe surgery saves lives: World Health Organization, 2009.

86. Gawande A. Checklist manifesto, the (HB). Penguin Books India, 2010.

87. How-to guide: prevent surgical site infection for hip and knee arthroplasty. Cambridge, MA: Institute for Healthcare Improvement, 2012.

CHAPTER 19

Pneumonia and other respiratory infections

Dr OYEBOLA FASUGBA[i-ii]

ASSOCIATE PROFESSOR ANDREW STEWARDSON[iii]

Chapter highlights

- The majority of hospital-acquired pneumonia (HAP) occurs in non-ventilated patients
- Non-ventilator-associated pneumonia (NV-HAP) is an underappreciated major patient safety issue associated with prolonged hospital stay and increased healthcare costs, patient morbidity and mortality
- Diagnosing NV-HAP may pose a challenge as the clinical and radiological features are non-specific
- Oral hygiene plays a significant role in reducing the occurrence of NV-HAP and consistent implementation of a comprehensive oral care protocol is essential
- Prevention and control of influenza and respiratory syncytial viruses requires the use of a multifaceted intervention strategy

i   Nursing Research Institute, St Vincent's Health Network Sydney, St Vincent's Hospital, Melbourne, VIC
ii School of Nursing, Midwifery and Paramedicine, Australian Catholic University, Australia
iii Department of Infectious Diseases, The Alfred Hospital and Central Clinical School, Monash University, VIC

Introduction

Hospital-acquired pneumonia (HAP) is one of the most common hospital-acquired infections and can be either ventilator-associated (VAP) or non-ventilator-associated (NV-HAP). The proportion of patients at risk for NV-HAP is substantially larger than those at risk for VAP as the vast majority of patients in hospital do not require mechanical ventilation.[1,2] Hence, NV-HAP occurs more frequently than VAP and is associated with higher overall costs and more deaths.[1,2] Other commonly encountered hospital-acquired respiratory tract infections include influenza and respiratory syncytial viruses (RSV).[3,4] These infections can be spread by direct contact with infected healthcare staff, visitors and family, and other infected patients. Transmission can also occur indirectly from patient to patient due to poor hand hygiene practices among healthcare staff. Hospital-acquired respiratory tract infections can sometimes be fatal as hospitalised patients are often vulnerable and may suffer more severe disease or complications;[5] therefore, it is important to develop a good understanding of these infections.

This chapter focuses on NV-HAP. A brief discussion on influenza and respiratory syncytial viruses is also provided. VAP is discussed in more detail in Chapter 28.

19.1 Epidemiology

NV-HAP is a major patient safety concern that is associated with significant health and economic burden for patients and the healthcare system worldwide.[1] It is a leading cause of death in critically ill patients.[6]

19.1.1 Prevalence and incidence

In Australia, the prevalence of HAP among adult patients in a sample of large public hospitals was 2.4% in 2018, the second most prevalent healthcare-associated infection (HAI) after surgical site infection.[7] Point prevalence surveys in Europe (2011–2012) and the United States (2010) have estimated the prevalence of HAP in acute hospitals to be 1.3% and 1.0%, respectively.[8,9] Estimates of incidence are more challenging and tend to be extrapolated from prevalence data or based on administrative data sets, i.e. ICD codes. An estimated 17,854 episodes of HAP occurred in Australian public hospitals in 2015–2016.[10] However, the proportion of hospital-acquired pneumonia that were NV-HAP was not reported. The population-based incidence of HAP in Europe was modelled at 138 cases per 100,000 population annually, using ECDC point prevalence data.[11] Based on administrative data sets, the proportion of patients diagnosed with NV-HAP in US acute care hospitals in 2012 was 1.3–1.6%, equivalent to a rate of 3.63 per 1000 patient days.[12] In 2014, the incidence rate in 21 US hospitals was estimated to be 0.12–2.28 cases per 1000 patient days.[13]

19.1.2 Morbidity and mortality

Among Australian patients, the length of hospital stay has been shown to be 19 days longer for those with HAP compared to those without HAP.[14] This raw difference, however, cannot be entirely attributed to HAP, as patients with longer hospital stay are at greater risk of HAP. A high-quality estimate of the health impact comes from Europe, where it is estimated that HAP results in 26,972 deaths and a burden of 169 disability-adjusted life years (DALYs) per 100,000 population each year.[11] In the US, mortality attributed to NV-HAP has been found to range between 13.1% to 30%,[12,15,16] with additional inpatient hospital stay of 9198–11,826 days and hospital readmission rate of 19.3% for patients with NV-HAP.[13] NV-HAP also directly impacts ICU utilisation, with one in five patients with NV-HAP requiring intensive care unit admission.[17] Patients with NV-HAP transferred to the ICU have a longer length of hospital stay with consequent increase in mortality and hospital costs.[13]

19.1.3 Economic impact

NV-HAP is associated with increased total hospital costs. Data from Australia suggest that each hospitalisation involving an HAP may be associated with $39,406 in extra costs.[14] Estimated NV-HAP acute care treatment costs in the United States range from US$28,008 to $40,000 per patient.[12,15]

19.1.4 Aetiology and risk factors

A wide variety of organisms can cause NV-HAP (Table 19.1). While bacterial organisms, especially aerobic Gram-negative bacilli, have traditionally been considered the main aetiological agents, respiratory viruses are also likely to play an important role.[3,18,19] Pathogens that cause NV-HAP are similar to those that cause VAP (see Chapter 28).[18] Fungi are an important cause NV-HAP in immunocompromised and critically ill patients.[3,19,20] Many infections are polymicrobial and in recent years, multidrug-resistant organisms have also been identified as important causative organisms in NV-HAP.[21] *Legionella pneumophila* is a rare but important cause of severe HAP associated with inhalation of contaminated water in the healthcare environment.

TABLE 19.1 Causative organisms for NV-HAP

Type of organism	Examples
Bacteria (Gram-negative bacilli)	*Klebsiella pneumoniae, Escherichia coli, Pseudomonas aeruginosa, Acinetobacter species, Enterobacter species, Legionella pneumophila*
Bacteria (Gram-positive cocci)	*Staphylococcus aureus*
Viruses	Rhinovirus, influenza, parainfluenza, metapneumovirus, SARS-CoV-2
Fungi	*Aspergillus* species

Since 2020, SARS-CoV-2 has been widely reported as a cause of HAP, following transmission from staff, visitors or other patients.[22-26]

Several risk factors have been shown to influence the development of NV-HAP and knowledge of these risk factors is important for its prevention and control.[27] Some risk factors include increasing age, male sex, comorbidities, patients undergoing surgery, prolonged hospital stay, underlying chronic lung disease (e.g. chronic obstructive pulmonary disease, chronic bronchitis), smoking, malnutrition, immunosuppression, diabetes, admission to an intensive care unit, limited mobility, poor oral hygiene associated with dental plaque build-up, and aspiration of organisms from the oral microbiome.[1,6,14,27-29] Patients with multiple risk factors, such as older adults and young children with comorbidities, are particularly vulnerable.[27] In some cases, patients may also present with few to no risk factors, including patients on maternity wards and healthy young adults.[2,12]

19.1.5 Pathogenesis/pathophysiology

NV-HAP develops following an imbalance between a patient's normal host defence mechanism and the ability of organisms to colonise and invade the lower respiratory tract, thereby overwhelming the host's defences with subsequent inflammation of the lung parenchyma.[19,30,31] Micro-aspiration of the causative organism, either from the oropharynx or gastrointestinal tract, into the lower respiratory tract is a key step for bacterial NV-HAP. This is more likely to occur among patients with oral, pharyngeal or gastric colonisation by relevant causative agents, and those with decreased conscious state and impaired cough reflex.[17,19] Contamination of the oral cavity can result from poor oral hygiene

and the formation of dental plaque.[15] Contamination of gastric contents is more likely among patients with reduced acidity of gastric contents.[32] Inhalation of the causative agent, an alternative mode of acquisition, is more relevant for viruses, fungi and *Legionella pneumophila*.

19.1.6 Definitions: how NV-HAP is diagnosed

Similar to all hospital-acquired infections, NV-HAP are infections that are not present on admission and have symptoms of infection occurring ≥ 48 hours after admission to the hospital.[33] Various definitions have been used to identify patients with NV-HAP. While there is no gold standard definition for the diagnosis of NV-HAP,[34] commonly applied criteria include those published by widely recognised international organisations and professional associations or societies.

According to the definitions published in the United States by the Centers for Disease Control and Prevention (CDC), the diagnosis of NV-HAP is based on the presence of a combination of radiographic evidence (e.g. a new or progressive and persistent pulmonary infiltrate on chest radiograph), clinical signs and symptoms (e.g. fever >38°C or >100.4°F, abnormal white blood cell count, purulent sputum or secretions, oxygenation impairment) and laboratory evidence of infection (e.g. positive culture).[33]

The 2016 clinical practice guidelines provided by the Infectious Diseases Society of America and the American Thoracic Society define NV-HAP as an episode of pneumonia that occurs 48 hours or more after admission, is not incubating at the time of admission and not associated with mechanical ventilation.[34] The diagnosis of NV-HAP is suspected if the patient has a new or progressive radiographic lung infiltrate, along with clinical findings such as the new onset of fever, purulent sputum, leucocytosis and decline in oxygenation which suggest that the infiltrate is of an infectious origin.[32,34]

The Association of Medical Microbiology and Infectious Disease Canada and the Canadian Thoracic Society's clinical practice guidelines for HAP and VAP in adults states that diagnosis of a pneumonia in hospitalised patients is based on abnormal clinical manifestations (e.g. fever >38°C or <36°C, leukopenia or leucocytosis, purulent tracheal secretions and decreased oxygen saturation) combined with abnormal radiological findings (e.g. presence of new or progressive radiographic infiltrates).[30]

Other methods that have been used to diagnose NV-HAP include criteria applied by the European

Centre for Disease Prevention and Control (ECDC) in their point prevalence survey of healthcare-associated infections (HAIs) and antimicrobial use. The standardised criteria are based on a combination of clinical symptoms and signs, radiological evidence and microbiology tests and are subdivided into five categories.[35] This allows reasonable comparisons by IPC professionals between data from hospitals, against national data as well as within and between country comparisons.[1,35] Biomarkers (e.g. procalcitonin), the clinical pulmonary infection score and administratively coded data[36] have also been considered for the diagnosis of NV-HAP.[34]

PRACTICE TIP 1

It is important to note that diagnosing NV-HAP may pose a challenge as the clinical features are non-specific and may be mimicked by other infectious and non-infectious clinical conditions such as acute respiratory distress syndrome, congestive heart failure and pulmonary embolism. Chest radiography and laboratory investigations may also not provide definitive confirmation for NV-HAP. Hence, newer criterion (e.g. lung ultrasound) must be evaluated and the use of sputum must be encouraged in patients with NV-HAP, to demonstrate its lower respiratory tract origin and quality.[37] While invasive diagnostic techniques such as bronchoscopy may be required, particularly in immunocompromised patients,[30,34] it is not clear whether they are associated with improvements in patient outcomes.[37]

To apply the definitions for NV-HAP described above into practice, see Case study 1.

CASE STUDY 1

Diagnosing NV-HAP

Situation:

A 56-year-old male patient on the fourth day of hospital admission develops a low-grade fever and mild cough. He is not on mechanical ventilation. Three hours later, his temperature increases to 39.5°C with frequent coughing that is productive of purulent sputum. He also appears to have difficulty with breathing. Think about the definitions above.

What diagnostic tests will help in clarifying the diagnosis of NV-HAP in this patient?

Solution:

In this situation, early identification of the possibility of NV-HAP is necessary and could include the following tests:

1. monitor vital signs: temperature, respiratory rate, heart rate, blood pressure
2. white cell count
3. arterial oxygenation saturation
4. arterial blood gases if indicated
5. chest x-ray (posteroanterior and lateral views)
6. respiratory tract cultures

19.2 Surveillance of NV-HAP

An accurate surveillance system may assist with the prevention of healthcare-associated infections (HAIs). However, while NV-HAP is one of the most common HAIs most hospitals do not routinely conduct prospective surveillance for NV-HAP. A major reason for this is the complexity, non-specificity and subjectivity of the definitions for NV-HAP which result in the lack of a gold standard definition as discussed in the previous section.[38,39] Surveillance based on microbiological diagnosis of NV-HAP is likely to be ineffective because high-quality lower respiratory microbiological samples are difficult to obtain.[40] Another difficulty in undertaking surveillance for NV-HAP is the time-consuming and resource-intensive nature of manual surveillance.[41] Data are difficult to abstract because they are inconsistently documented in patients' records and typically require reading free-text medical notes rather than analysing structured data.[39] In addition, almost every hospitalised patient must be tracked for NV-HAP surveillance in contrast to surveillance for VAP, where a relatively small number of patients receive mechanical ventilation.[39]

Suggested strategies for surveillance include:

- combining pharmacy records of antibiotic prescriptions for respiratory infection with electronic patient records
- mandating clinicians to report NV-HAP based on specific diagnostic criteria. This approach will be supported by pharmacy or IPC teams
- using a combination of clinical and microbiological surveillance techniques.[40]

The use of administrative data for surveillance of NV-HAP has been suggested by some researchers. An Australian study found that administrative coding data accurately identified HAP in 86% of cases.[42] However, administrative coding data, which is not designed for detection of HAIs, is more frequently found to perform poorly when compared to clinical or surveillance criteria.[38]

19.3 Prevention and control of NV-HAP

19.3.1 A multifaceted oral healthcare protocol in the hospital setting

Good oral or dental care plays a significant role in reducing the occurrence of NV-HAP and has been identified as the most common preventive strategy.[1,15,43] During a patient's first 48 hours in hospital changes occur in the oral microbiome, especially in the absence of regular oral care, that are associated with virulent HAP-causing organisms.[44] Consistent implementation of a comprehensive oral care protocol is therefore essential to prevent NV-HAP and there is substantial evidence in support of this.[45-47] Oral care interventions have also been found to be cost-effective.[2,47]

Examples of oral care interventions shown to be beneficial include: oral care kits containing an antiseptic (cetylpyridinium chloride and 1.5% hydrogen peroxide); oral care by swabbing with an antiseptic (chlorhexidine gluconate vs metronidazole); oral care kits and using a toothbrush containing sodium bicarbonate and an antiseptic; and moisturiser, toothbrushes and oral swabs impregnated with sodium bicarbonate and an antiseptic rinse (1.5% hydrogen peroxide).[1] While a number of antiseptic agents such as chlorhexidine gluconate, sodium bicarbonate, hydrogen peroxide, povidone–iodine and cetylpyridinium chloride have been explored in studies, current evidence remains unclear about the most effective antiseptic for oral care in the prevention of NV-HAP.[1]

Given the role of dental plaque build-up leading to microbial colonisation in the oral cavity of non-mechanically ventilated patients, a comprehensive oral care NV-HAP prevention program should include brushing the teeth and tongue with toothpaste to remove oral biofilm.[15,44] While optimal tooth brushing frequency for oral care in non-ventilated patients remains unknown, brushing the teeth twice a day is considered routine practice and generally recommended.[48,49] Increasing toothbrushing frequency by once per day

may reduce the odds of developing NV-HAP by 40% in non-ICU acute care patients.[48] Decreasing bacterial colonisation and plaque formation with adequate oral care products, toothbrushing frequency and appropriate healthcare staff could potentially decrease the development or severity of NV-HAP.[49] Healthcare staff should refer to their hospital's oral care protocols for recommendations and implement accordingly.

In ICU patients with NV-HAP, oral care also involves the use of toothbrushing to prevent NV-HAP.[50] A suction or soft-bristled toothbrush, toothpaste, gel, antiseptic oral rinse and/or non-petroleum-based moisturiser are recommended depending on whether the patient is independent and/or has dentures.[49] Poor documentation of oral hygiene in non-ventilated ICU patients has also been identified[50] which may impact the implementation of prevention strategies. Hence, ICUs should not only develop a standardised evidence-based oral care protocol but should also audit oral care documentation to ensure compliance with protocol recommendations.[51]

It is important to consider the challenges that may be encountered when implementing an oral care prevention program in the acute care setting. These include: nurse-to-patient staffing ratios, patient refusals and care resistant behaviours, particularly in patients with dementia. In the ICU setting, patients often depend on nurses for care. ICU nurses typically care for one or two patients and can therefore routinely and more readily provide oral care as part of their NV-HAP prevention protocol. In comparison, the patient-to-nurse ratio in the non-ICU acute care setting may be significantly higher, making provision of oral care more difficult.[48]

19.3.2 Residential aged care facilities (RACF) and long-term care facilities

Pneumonia is associated with substantial morbidity and mortality among residents of residential aged care facilities (RACF) and long-term care facilities.[52] Proper oral care is an important component of strategies to prevent pneumonia in residential aged care facilities.[29,52] Aged care residents are prone to poor oral health because they have reduced access to professional dental care and are unable to maintain the practice of good personal oral hygiene.[52] In addition, they have an increased rate of dental plaque colonisation which acts as a potential reservoir for pathogens associated with pneumonia.[52] Periodontal disease increases an aged care resident's risk for developing pneumonia that could potentially become fatal if not properly prevented and treated.

There is evidence to show that one in every ten pneumonia-related aged care deaths could be prevented by improving the resident's oral health status.[53] Hence, oral disease prevention could potentially be the standard of care in RACF to reduce and prevent elderly patients from contracting pneumonia.[29] There is low-quality evidence to suggest that professional oral care (a combination of brushing teeth and mucosa, cleaning dentures, using mouth rinse, and making check-up visits to a dentist) could reduce mortality due to pneumonia in RACF residents when compared to usual oral care (generally less intensive, self-administered, or provided by nursing home staff without special training in oral hygiene).[52] Although the professional oral care model may not be feasible in the acute care setting due to high patient-to-nurse ratios, it should be considered as a standard of care in a RACF.[48]

Establishing a multifaceted oral healthcare protocol which includes preventive strategies targeted at plaque removal, periodontal disease and dental caries prevention, as well as care of dentures, should be considered in this setting. It is important to also note that nurses, physicians and dental hygienists have a role to play in the detection, education and implementation of prevention strategies for residents at risk in RACF.[29] A collaborative approach between these groups of clinicians is vital to the implementation of an effective oral care protocol.

19.3.3 Other strategies

Other preventive strategies should also be aimed at targeting potential modifiable risk factors. These strategies involve basic nursing care procedures and are relatively inexpensive but require time, prioritisation, vigilance and integration into routine care. Key preventive strategies include:[1,15,43]

- *protecting the patient from aspiration*—to reduce the risk of NV-HAP in hospitalised non-ventilated patients, it is important to identify the risk for aspiration and implement strategies to reduce this risk. In addition to a normal physiology that includes micro-aspiration, other factors that increase aspiration risk in this group of patients are reduced mobility and supine positioning, medications that reduce the level of consciousness, and presence of nasogastric and orogastric tubes.[44] Recognised preventive strategies for aspiration include elevation of the head of the bed, teaching the patient techniques for optimising cough and airway clearance, and daily assessment for continued use of orogastric and nasogastric tubes. Use of these devices should be discontinued as soon as they are no longer clinically indicated.[44]

- *prompt diagnosis and treatment of dysphagia*— dysphagia screening has the potential to reduce the occurrence of NV-HAP.[54,55] Patients with dysphagia have an increased risk of aspiration, hence it is recommended to manage dysphagia promptly in these patients to prevent development of HAP.[48] A validated swallow screen tool should be used prior to commencing oral food and fluid intake. Patients who pass the procedure can advance to normal feeding while those who fail are referred to a speech pathologist for further evaluation.[44]

- *increased physical activity or mobilisation*—lack of physical activity in hospitalised patients with subsequent decreased clearance of secretions may contribute to the development of NV-HAP.[56] Hence, physiotherapeutic interventions focusing on increasing an inpatient's mobility have been investigated. For example, an early mobility bundle intervention consisting of extra targeted physiotherapy and collaboration with ward staff to encourage and promote physical activity has been shown to reduce the incidence of NV-HAP in medical patients.[56] Rotation therapy (turning) has also been recommended. Implementation of a manual turning and passive mobilisation program (the 'turn-mob' program) could reduce the incidence of NV-HAP in hospitalised patients with acute ischaemic stroke during their stay at the hospital and up to 14 days after discharge.[57]

Other important strategies include improved hand hygiene, prevention of viral infections, strengthening host defences to infection and multi-modal programs for the prevention of nosocomial influenza cross-infection. Prevention bundles have also been shown to be effective. A recent study conducted in a tertiary care center in Switzerland found that implementation of a five-measure NV-HAP prevention bundle consisting of oral care, dysphagia screening and management, mobilisation, discontinuation of non-indicated proton-pump inhibitors and respiratory therapy led to a reduction in NV-HAP.[58]

In Australia, selected best practices for the prevention of NV-HAP include maintaining good oral hygiene, use of allied health interventions such as chest physiotherapy and swallowing assessment and management, and appropriate vaccination of staff and patients where indicated.[14] Figure 19.1 provides some examples of interventions to prevent NV-HAP.[15]

It is important to also adhere to standard and transmission-based IPC precautions to minimise

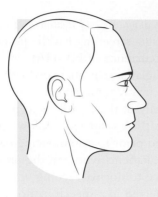

Selected interventions to prevent colonisation:
- Provide information about optimal pulmonary state.
- Optimise functional reserve capacity.
- Strengthen patient's resistance to atelectasis.
- Maintain patient's resistance to infection:
  — Perform hand hygiene.
  — Institute a routine oral hygiene regimen.
  — Eliminate oral bacterial reservoirs.
  — Consult with a dental professional.
  — Protect oral epithelial cells and nasal passages by providing moisture and avoiding large-bore nasogastric tubes.
  — Avoid unnecessary antibiotics.
  — Avoid unnecessary stress ulcer prophylaxis (if necessary, consider a cytoprotective agent).
  — Consider chlorhexidine oral rinse or chlorhexidine bath for select patient populations.

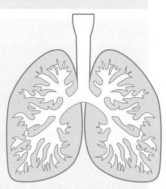

Selected interventions to prevent aspiration:
- Teach techniques for optimising cough and airway clearance.
- Avoid unnecessary medications that reduce level of consciousness.
- Maintain head of the bed at 30 degrees or greater unless contraindicated.
- Encourage ambulation.
- Provide subglottic suctioning.
- Consult with speech and/or swallowing professionals when appropriate.

Holistic prevention strategies:
- Administer vaccines and immunisations.
- Provide smoking cessation counselling.
- Institute environmental infection control measures.
- Encourage personal hygiene, including hand hygiene.
- Evaluate the patient's risk for aspiration.
- Provide dementia screening.
- Assess the patient's nutritional status.
- Encourage routine professional dental care.

FIGURE 19.1 Selected interventions to prevent NV-HAP

Source: Davis, J., & Finley, E. (2018). A second breadth: Hospital-acquired pneumonia in Pennsylvania, nonventilated versus ventilated patients. PA Patient Saf. Advis, 15, 48–59. http://patientsafety.pa.gov/ADVISORIES/Pages/201809_NVHAP.aspx#

transmission of respiratory organisms that cause NV-HAP. Respiratory precautions to consider include:[5,59]

- placing patients with NV-HAP in a single room where a transmissible pathogen is confirmed or suspected (or cohort where appropriate)
- respiratory hygiene and cough etiquette, e.g. practising hand hygiene after coughing, sneezing or using tissues
- correct use of personal protective equipment (PPE), e.g. face mask, eye protection, gloves.

To apply the prevention and control strategies for NV-HAP described above into practice, see Case studies 2 and 3.

CASE STUDY 2

Preventing NV-HAP

Situation:

You have been assigned to care for a post surgical elderly male who has been on admission for six weeks following a diagnosis of diabetic foot ulcer. He also has a history of smoking and chronic obstructive pulmonary disease. He currently has limited mobility due to his ulcer. How could you assist in preventing NV-HAP?

Solution:

Given your knowledge of the risk factors for NV-HAP, you undertake the following NV-HAP preventive strategies for your patient:

- adhere to standard IPC precautions such as hand hygiene
- institute the hospital's oral hygiene protocol
- encourage ambulation
- provide counselling on smoking cessation
- evaluate the patient's risk for aspiration.

CASE STUDY 3

Preventing NV-HAP

Situation:

A patient on your ward develops a stroke while on admission. She remains conscious but has an impaired cough reflex. How could you assist in preventing NV-HAP?

Solution:

To prevent micro-aspiration of pharyngeal and gastric bacteria due to accumulation of secretions:

- teach the patient techniques for optimising cough and airway clearance
- avoid unnecessary medications that reduce her level of consciousness
- maintain head of the bed at 30° or greater unless contraindicated
- institute the hospital's oral hygiene protocol.

PRACTICE TIP 2[15]

- All healthcare staff should receive training in oral care.
- Use of a comprehensive oral care protocol is highly recommended.
- Always use PPE when assisting patients with oral care, including gloves, mask and face shield.
- To be successful, preventive interventions should be performed at appropriate intervals.

19.4 Influenza

Influenza is a common respiratory hospital–acquired infection in adult and paediatric populations. Infection with hospital-acquired influenza virus has been associated with increased morbidity, mortality and healthcare costs.[60] The prevalence of hospital-acquired influenza is highly variable among hospitalised patients in Australia, but has been reported to be as high as 9.6% during a period of high influenza activity in the community.[61]

Transmission of influenza virus is primarily by inhalation of particles which are produced when infected people cough or sneeze in close contact to susceptible individuals.[67] Indirect transmission via contact with virus-contaminated surfaces may also occur.[63] Infected patients, visitors and healthcare staff can introduce influenza virus into the hospital setting where it can be transmitted from patient to healthcare staff or vice versa. Patient-to-patient transmission may also occur due to breakdown in infection control practices.[62]

A number of strategies have been shown to be effective in the prevention and control of hospital-acquired influenza virus infection. These include vaccination of healthcare staff and patients at high risk of infection.[64,65] Compliance with hand hygiene and use of personal protective equipment (e.g. gloves, masks, gowns) by staff, particularly when managing patients with suspected influenza virus infection, should be undertaken. Implementation of respiratory hygiene and cough etiquette practices, including isolation of patients with confirmed infection, has also been recommended.[63] Rapid diagnostic testing for influenza in suspected patients also supports infection prevention efforts to reduce hospital transmission through patient isolation or cohorting.[66,67] Prompt and accurate diagnosis has the potential to prevent serious, complicated, or even fatal outcomes in patients.[67] In addition, sick healthcare staff should be excluded from the hospital setting and remain at home until their symptoms have resolved.[59]

19.5 Respiratory syncytial virus (RSV)

Respiratory syncytial virus is another important cause of hospital-acquired respiratory infection, especially in infants and children.[62] Older adults, particularly those who are immunocompromised, can also be infected by RSV.[68] Transmission of RSV is similar to influenza virus, spreading via respiratory particles, contaminated hands of infected people and fomites.[62,69] Compared to community-acquired RSV infection, children with hospital-acquired infection have longer paediatric intensive care unit stay (median (interquartile range) 7.5 (5–12) vs 5 (3–9)) and higher mortality (29% vs 4%).[70]

Prevention and control of hospital-acquired RSV requires the use of a multifaceted intervention strategy. Interventions shown to be effective in reducing hospital transmission of RSV include strict hand hygiene compliance; single room isolation for infected symptomatic patients or cohort nursing if no individual isolation rooms are available; and use of personal protective equipment (e.g. gowns, gloves, masks and eye protection goggles) by staff.[71] Another measure is limiting visitor contact with infected patients.[62] The use of rapid tests is also potentially beneficial as an infection control measure for RSV by improving outbreak prevention.[66]

19.6 Coronavirus (COVID-19)

COVID-19 is an infectious disease caused by the SARS-CoV-2 virus with the potential to cause severe pneumonia and death.[72] Given that this is a new respiratory virus, the evidence base is rapidly changing and regularly being updated. For the latest information on the prevention, control and management of COVID-19, visit the websites listed in Useful websites/resources below.

Conclusion

Hospital-acquired pneumonia in non-ventilated patients is a preventable condition with significant health and economic impacts for patients and health systems worldwide. More research into the prevention of this hospital-acquired infection is needed. Healthcare staff should be trained to identify those at risk of NV-HAP and institute evidence-based oral care protocols which are currently recognised as the most common preventive strategy for NV-HAP.

Useful websites/resources

- Australian Guidelines for the Prevention and Control of Infection in Health Care—chapter 3. https://www.nhmrc.gov.au/sites/default/files/documents/infection-control-guidelines-feb2020.pdf
- Mouth Care Matters—Improving Oral Health. https://mouthcarematters.hee.nhs.uk/
- This Health Education England (HEE) initiative provides access to training materials, posters, and resources to assist healthcare workers in improving the oral health of patients in hospital.
- Centers for Disease Control and Prevention (CDC). https://www.cdc.gov/coronavirus/2019-ncov/hcp/infection-control-recommendations.html
- World Health Organization (WHO). https://www.who.int/health-topics/coronavirus#tab=tab_1
- National COVID-19 Clinical Evidence Taskforce. https://covid19evidence.net.au/
- Commonwealth of Australia Department of Health. https://www.health.gov.au/committees-and-groups/infection-prevention-and-control-expert-group-iceg

References

1. Mitchell BG, Russo PL, Cheng AC, Stewardson AJ, Rosebrock H, Curtis SJ, et al. Strategies to reduce non-ventilator-associated hospital-acquired pneumonia: a systematic review. Infect Dis Health. 2019;24(4):229-239.
2. Quinn B, Baker DL, Cohen S, Stewart JL, Lima CA, Parise C. Basic nursing care to prevent nonventilator hospital-acquired pneumonia. J Nurs Scholarsh. 2014;46(1):11-19.
3. Shorr AF, Zilberberg MD, Micek ST, Kollef MH. Viruses are prevalent in non-ventilated hospital-acquired pneumonia. Respir Med. 2017;122:76-80.
4. Manchal N, Mohamed MRS, Ting M, Luetchford H, Francis F, Carrucan J, et al. Hospital acquired viral respiratory tract infections: an underrecognized nosocomial infection. Infect Dis Health. 2020;25(3):175-180.
5. Public Health England. Infection control precautions to minimise transmission of acute respiratory tract infections in healthcare settings. London: Public Health England; 2016.
6. Torres A, Niederman MS, Chastre J, Ewig S, Fernandez-Vandellos P, Hanberger H, et al. International ERS/ESICM/ESCMID/ALAT guidelines for the management of hospital-acquired pneumonia and ventilator-associated pneumonia: guidelines for the management of hospital-acquired pneumonia (HAP)/ventilator-associated pneumonia (VAP) of the European Respiratory Society (ERS), European Society of Intensive Care Medicine (ESICM), European Society of Clinical Microbiology and Infectious Diseases (ESCMID) and Asociación Latinoamericana del Tórax (ALAT). Eur Respir J. 2017;50(3).
7. Russo PL, Stewardson AJ, Cheng AC, Bucknall T, Mitchell BG. The prevalence of healthcare associated infections among adult inpatients at nineteen large Australian acute-care public hospitals: a point prevalence survey. Antimicrob Resist Infect Control. 2019;8(1):1-8.
8. Magill SS, Edwards JR, Bamberg W, Beldavs ZG, Dumyati G, Kainer MA, et al. Multistate point-prevalence survey of health

care–associated infections. N Eng J Med. 2014;370(13): 1198-1208.

9. European Centre for Disease Prevention and Control. Point prevalence survey of healthcare-associated infections and antimicrobial use in European acute care hospitals. Stockholm: ECDC; 2013.

10. Independent Hospital Pricing Authority. Activity based funding admitted patient care 2015-16, acute admitted episodes, excluding same day.

11. Cassini A, Plachouras D, Eckmanns T, Abu Sin M, Blank H-P, Ducomble T, et al. Burden of six healthcare-associated infections on European population health: estimating incidence-based disability-adjusted life years through a population prevalence-based modelling study. PLoS Medicine. 2016;13(10):e1002150.

12. Giuliano KK, Baker D, Quinn B. The epidemiology of nonventilator hospital-acquired pneumonia in the United States. Am J Infect Control. 2018;46(3):322-327.

13. Baker D, Quinn B. Hospital acquired pneumonia prevention initiative-2: incidence of nonventilator hospital-acquired pneumonia in the United States. Am J Infect Control. 2018;46(1):2-7.

14. Australian Commission on Safety and Quality in Health Care. Healthcare-associated infections. ACSQHC; 2018.

15. Davis J, Finley E. A second breath: hospital-acquired pneumonia in Pennsylvania, nonventilated versus ventilated patients. Pennsylvania Patient Safety Authority. 2018;15(3):1-12.

16. Micek ST, Chew B, Hampton N, Kollef MH. A case-control study assessing the impact of nonventilated hospital-acquired pneumonia on patient outcomes. Chest. 2016;150(5): 1008-1014.

17. Saied WI, Martin-Loeches I, Timsit J-F. What is new in non-ventilated ICU-acquired pneumonia? Intensive Care Med. 2020;46(3):488-491.

18. Feng D-Y, Zhou Y-Q, Zou X-L, Zhou M, Zhu J-X, Wang Y-H, et al. Differences in microbial etiology between hospital-acquired pneumonia and ventilator-associated pneumonia: a single-center retrospective study in Guang Zhou. Infect Drug Resist. 2019;12:993.

19. Jain V, Vashisht R, Yilmaz G, Bhardwaj A. Pneumonia pathology: StatPearls Publishing, Treasure Island (FL), 2020.

20. Shamim S, Agarwal A, Ghosh BK, Mitra M. Fungal pneumonia in intensive care unit: when to suspect and decision to treatment: a critical review. J Assoc Chest Physicians. 2015;3(2):41.

21. Djordjevic ZM, Folic MM, Jankovic SM. Distribution and antibiotic susceptibility of pathogens isolated from adults with hospital-acquired and ventilator-associated pneumonia in intensive care unit. J Infect Public Health. 2017;10(6):740-744.

22. Papamanoli A, Nakamura J, Fung J, Abata J, Karkala N, Tsui ST, et al. Incidence of hospital-acquired and ventilator-associated pneumonia in patients with severe COVID 19 on high flow oxygen. Open Forum Infectious Diseases. 2020; 7(Supplement_1):S260-S1.

23. Wang D, Hu B, Hu C, Zhu F, Liu X, Zhang J, et al. Clinical characteristics of 138 hospitalized patients with 2019 novel coronavirus–infected pneumonia in Wuhan, China. JAMA. 2020;323(11):1061-1069.

24. Søgaard KK, Baettig V, Osthoff M, Marsch S, Leuzinger K, Schweitzer M, et al. Community-acquired and hospital-acquired respiratory tract infection and bloodstream infection in patients hospitalized with COVID-19 pneumonia. J Intensive Care. 2021;9(1):10.

25. Carter B, Collins J, Barlow-Pay F, Rickard F, Bruce E, Verduri A, et al. Nosocomial COVID-19 infection: examining the risk of mortality. The COPE-Nosocomial Study (COVID in Older PEople). J Hosp Infect. 2020;106(2):376-384.

26. Rickman HM, Rampling T, Shaw K, Martinez-Garcia G, Hail L, Coen P, et al. Nosocomial transmission of coronavirus disease 2019: a retrospective study of 66 hospital-acquired cases in a London teaching hospital. Clin Infect Dis. 2020; 72(4):690-593.

27. Vignari M. Non-ventilator health care-associated pneumonia (NV-HAP): NV-HAP risk factors. Am J Infect Control. 2020; 48(5):A10-A3.

28. Strassle PD, Sickbert-Bennett EE, Klompas M, Lund JL, Stewart PW, Marx AH, et al. Incidence and risk factors of non–device-associated pneumonia in an acute-care hospital. Infect Control Hosp Epidemiol. 2020;41(1):73-79.

29. Kanzigg LA, Hunt L. Oral health and hospital-acquired pneumonia in elderly patients: a review of the literature. American Dental Hygienists' Association. 2016;90(suppl 1): 15-21.

30. Rotstein C, Evans G, Born A, Grossman R, Light RB, Magder S, et al. Clinical practice guidelines for hospital-acquired pneumonia and ventilator-associated pneumonia in adults. Can J Infect Dis Med Microbiol. 2008;19(1):19-53.

31. Vallecoccia MS, Dominedò C, Cutuli SL, Martin-Loeches I, Torres A, De Pascale G. Is ventilated hospital-acquired pneumonia a worse entity than ventilator-associated pneumonia? Eur Respir Rev. 2020;29(157).

32. Society AT, America IDSo. Guidelines for the management of adults with hospital-acquired, ventilator-associated, and healthcare-associated pneumonia. Am J Respir Crit Care Med. 2005;171(4):388.

33. Centers for Disease Control and Prevention. CDC/NHSN Surveillance definition of healthcare-associated infection and criteria for specific types of infections in the acute care setting. CDC, 2013.

34. Kalil AC, Metersky ML, Klompas M, Muscedere J, Sweeney DA, Palmer LB, et al. Management of adults with hospital-acquired and ventilator-associated pneumonia: 2016 clinical practice guidelines by the Infectious Diseases Society of America and the American Thoracic Society. Clin Infect Dis. 2016;63(5):e61-e111.

35. European Centre for Disease Prevention and Control. Point prevalence survey of healthcare-associated infections and antimicrobial use in European acute care hospitals – protocol version 5.3. Stockholm: European Centre for Disease Prevention and Control, 2016.

36. Redondo-González O, Tenías JM, Arias Á, Lucendo AJ. Validity and reliability of administrative coded data for the identification of hospital-acquired infections: an updated systematic review with meta-analysis and meta-regression analysis. Health Serv Res. 2018;53(3):1919-1956.

37. Ranzani OT, De Pascale G, Park M. Diagnosis of nonventilated hospital-acquired pneumonia: how much do we know? Curr Opin Crit Care. 2018;24(5):339-346.

38. Batlle HR, Klompas M, Program CPE. Accuracy and reliability of electronic versus CDC surveillance criteria for non-ventilator hospital-acquired pneumonia. Infect Control Hosp Epidemiol. 2020;41(2):219-221.

39. Ji W, McKenna C, Ochoa A, Batlle HR, Young J, Zhang Z, et al. Development and assessment of objective surveillance definitions for nonventilator hospital-acquired pneumonia. JAMA Netw Open. 2019;2(10):e1913674.

40. Ewan VC, Witham MD, Kiernan MA, Simpson AJ. Hospital-acquired pneumonia surveillance-an unmet need. Lancet Respir Med. 2017;5(10):771-772.

41. Wolfensberger A, Jakob W, Hesse MF, Kuster S, Meier A, Schreiber P, et al. Development and validation of a semi-automated surveillance system—lowering the fruit for non-ventilator-associated hospital-acquired pneumonia (nvHAP) prevention. Clin Microbiol Infect. 2019;25(11):1428.e7-e13.

42. Bartley D, Panchasarp R, Bowen S, Deane J, Ferguson J. How accurately is hospital acquired pneumonia documented for the correct assignment of a hospital acquired complication (HAC)? Infect Dis Health. 2021;26(1):67-71.

43. Pássaro L, Harbarth S, Landelle C. Prevention of hospital-acquired pneumonia in non-ventilated adult patients: a narrative review. Antimicrob Resist Infect Control. 2016; 5(1):1-11.

44. Quinn B, Giuliano KK, Baker D. Non-ventilator health care-associated pneumonia (NV-HAP): best practices for prevention of NV-HAP. Am J Infect Control. 2020;48(5, Supplement): A23-A7.

45. Munro S, Baker D. Reducing missed oral care opportunities to prevent non-ventilator associated hospital acquired pneumonia at the Department of Veterans Affairs. Applied Nurs Res. 2018;44:48-53.

46. Pedersen PU, Larsen P, Håkonsen SJ. The effectiveness of systematic perioperative oral hygiene in reduction of postoperative respiratory tract infections after elective thoracic surgery in adults: a systematic review. JBI Database System Rev Implement Rep. 2016;14(1):140-173.

47. Talley L, Lamb J, Harl J, Lorenz H, Green L. HAP prevention for nonventilated adults in acute care: can a structured oral care program reduce infection incidence? Nursing Management. 2016;47(12):42-48.

48. McNally E, Krisciunas GP, Langmore SE, Crimlisk JT, Pisegna JM, Massaro J. Oral care clinical trial to reduce non–intensive care unit, hospital-acquired pneumonia: lessons for future research. J Healthc Qual. 2019;41(1):1-9.

49. Vollman K, Sole ML, Quinn B. Endotracheal tube care and oral care practices for ventilated and non-ventilated patients. AACN Procedure Manual for High Acuity, Progressive and Critical Care, 7th ed. St Louis, MO: Elsevier, 2017, p. 32-9.

50. Emery KP, Guido-Sanz F. Oral care practices in non-mechanically ventilated intensive care unit patients: an integrative review. J Clin Nursi. 2019;28(13-14):2462-2471.

51. American Association of Critical Care Nurses. AACN practice alert: oral care for acutely and critically ill patients 2017 [cited 26 February 2021]. Available from: https://www.aacn.org/clinical-resources/practice-alerts/oral-care-for-acutely-and-critically-ill-patients.

52. Liu C, Cao Y, Lin J, Ng L, Needleman I, Walsh T, et al. Oral care measures for preventing nursing home-acquired pneumonia. Cochrane Database System Rev. 2018; 9(9):CD012416.

53. Sjögren P, Nilsson E, Forsell M, Johansson O, Hoogstraate J. A systematic review of the preventive effect of oral hygiene on pneumonia and respiratory tract infection in elderly people in hospitals and nursing homes: effect estimates and methodological quality of randomized controlled trials. J Am Geriatr Soc. 2008;56(11):2124-2130.

54. Schrock JW, Lou L, Ball BA, Van Etten J. The use of an emergency department dysphagia screen is associated with decreased pneumonia in acute strokes. Am J Emerg Med. 2018;36(12):2152-2154.

55. Titsworth WL, Abram J, Fullerton A, Hester J, Guin P, Waters MF, et al. Prospective quality initiative to maximize dysphagia screening reduces hospital-acquired pneumonia prevalence in patients with stroke. Stroke. 2013;44(11): 3154-3160.

56. Stolbrink M, McGowan L, Saman H, Nguyen T, Knightly R, Sharpe J, et al. The Early Mobility Bundle: a simple enhancement of therapy which may reduce incidence of hospital-acquired pneumonia and length of hospital stay. J Hosp Infect. 2014;88(1):34-39.

57. Grajales Cuesy P, Lavielle Sotomayor P, Talavera Piña JO. Reduction in the incidence of poststroke nosocomial pneumonia by using the "turn-mob" program. Journal of Stroke and Cerebrovascular Diseases. 2010;19(1): 23-28.

58. Wolfensberger A, Clack L, von Felten S, Hesse MF, Saleschus D, Meier M, et al. Prevention of non-ventilator-associated hospital-acquired pneumonia in Switzerland: a type 2 hybrid effectiveness–implementation trial. Lancet Infect Dis. 2023;/ S1473-3099(22)00812-X.

59. National Health and Medical Research Council. Australian Guidelines for the Prevention and Control of Infection in Healthcare. Canberra: NHMRC, 2019.

60. Vanhems P, Bénet T, Munier-Marion E. Nosocomial influenza: encouraging insights and future challenges. Curr Opin Infect Dis. 2016;29(4):366-372.

61. Parkash N, Beckingham W, Andersson P, Kelly P, Senanayake S, Coatsworth N. Hospital-acquired influenza in an Australian tertiary centre 2017: a surveillance based study. BMC Pulmonary Med. 2019;19(1):1-9.

62. Bonvehí PE, Temporiti ER. Transmission and control of respiratory viral infections in the healthcare setting. Curr Treat Options Infect Dis. 2018;10(2):182-196.

63. Centers for Disease Control and Prevention, National Center for Immunization and Respiratory Diseases. Prevention strategies for seasonal influenza in healthcare settings-guidelines and recommendations. United States: Centers for Disease Control and Prevention, 2018.

64. Godoy P, Torner N, Soldevila N, Rius C, Jane M, Martínez A, et al. Hospital-acquired influenza infections detected by a surveillance system over six seasons, from 2010/2011 to 2015/2016. BMC Infect Dis. 2020;20(1):80.

65. O'Reilly F, Dolan GP, Nguyen-Van-Tam J, Noone P. Practical prevention of nosocomial influenza transmission, 'a hierarchical control' issue. Occup Med (Lond). 2015;65(9): 696-700.

66. Wabe N, Li L, Lindeman R, Yimsung R, Dahm MR, Clezy K, et al. The impact of rapid molecular diagnostic testing for respiratory viruses on outcomes for emergency department patients. Med J Aust. 2019;210(7):316-320.

67. Green DA, StGeorge K. Rapid antigen tests for influenza: rationale and significance of the FDA reclassification. J Clin Microbiol. 2018;56(10):e00711-00718.

68. Frange P, Toubiana J, Parize P, Moulin F, Scemla A, Leruez-Ville M. Preventing respiratory syncytial virus infections in hospitalized children and adults: should we do better? Infect Prev Pract. 2020;2(2):100041.

69. Barr R, Green CA, Sande CJ, Drysdale SB. Respiratory syncytial virus: diagnosis, prevention and management. Therap Adv Infect Dis. 2019;6:2049936119865798.

70. Thorburn K, Eisenhut M, Riordan A. Mortality and morbidity of nosocomial respiratory syncytial virus (RSV) infection in ventilated children—a ten year perspective. Minerva Anestesiologica. 2012;78(7):782.

71. French CE, McKenzie BC, Coope C, Rajanaidu S, Paranthaman K, Pebody R, et al. Risk of nosocomial respiratory syncytial virus infection and effectiveness of control measures to prevent transmission events: a systematic review. Influenza Other Respir Viruses. 2016;10(4):268-290.

72. Attaway AH, Scheraga RG, Bhimraj A, Biehl M, Hatipoğlu U. Severe Covid-19 pneumonia: pathogenesis and clinical management. BMJ. 2021;372.

CHAPTER 20

Bloodstream infections

Dr PATRICIA E. FERGUSON[i-iii]

KATHY DEMPSEY[iv]

Chapter highlights

- Bloodstream infections (BSIs) are healthcare-associated if they develop as a consequence of healthcare, or are associated with the infection caused by a prosthetic or invasive device
- Healthcare-associated BSIs were identified in 14% of all healthcare-associated infections (HAIs) in a large Australian study, and were associated with 46% of all HAI deaths, an estimated 3200 deaths per year[28]
- Many healthcare-associated BSIs can be prevented with infection prevention measures, including surveillance and governance
- Healthcare-associated *Staphylococcus aureus* BSI rates are used as a marker of the quality and safety of healthcare delivery. These rates are required to be reported by facilities within Australia to national and state governing bodies

i   Centre for Infectious Diseases and Microbiology, The University of Sydney, Sydney, NSW
ii Clinical Senior Lecturer, The University of Sydney
iii Westmead Hospital, Westmead, NSW
iv Healthcare-associated Infection and Infection Prevention and Control Program, Clinical Excellence Commission, Sydney, NSW

Acknowledgement: The authors wish to thank Dr Rebecca Sparks, Microbiology Registrar, Centre for Infectious Diseases and Microbiology, Westmead, NSW.

Introduction

Bloodstream infections by definition require a positive result from blood that has been placed into a culture bottle, and incubated at 35°C for 5–7 days. Blood culture bottles contain enriched non-selective broth that assists growth of aerobes, anaerobes and yeasts.[3,17,18] A set of bottles, specific for aerobic and anaerobic growth, is used to maximise results in adults, although a single bottle is used in paediatric patients.

Incubation occurs in a designated incubator in a microbiology laboratory. While most bacteria are identified in 2–3 days, bottles are routinely incubated for 5–7 days, and this can be extended out to 21 days for fastidious organisms including *Brucella* spp. or yeasts.[3,18] *Mycobacteria* spp. usually require both specific broth and a prolonged incubation for detection. If fastidious organisms are being considered, discussion with the laboratory is essential to ensure correct bottles and incubation periods are used.

Growth of organisms within blood culture bottles produces turbidity or haemolysis of the broth that can be detected by the naked eye, and a change in the pH or redox potential that can be detected by an automated incubator.[3,18]

Preliminary information on the likely bacteria is then determined manually using Gram stain and microscopy to determine the shape and configuration of organisms.[3] The culture broth is also inoculated onto solid media plates, incubated and then assessed further for growth, appearance of colonies on the plate, results of specific biochemical or antigen tests,[3] or mass spectroscopy[18] to achieve a final identification. This can take 1–2 more days until a final result is available.

An initial antibiotic susceptibility profile can be inferred from the Gram stain and microscopy results, which determine the likely class of bacteria. This can guide initial antibiotic prescribing when combined with local susceptibility knowledge. Antibiotic susceptibility testing takes a further 12–24 hours to achieve a result, depending on the methods used.

Some laboratories may employ molecular based methods (including PCR) which can assist in rapid identification of organisms in addition to a limited number of resistance genes, which can provide results within as little as 1–2 hours. This is performed on simple specialised machinery; however, the technology remains costly at present.[18]

The earliest a blood culture 'flags positive' is approximately 12 hours. This time to culture positivity may reflect the burden of bacteria within the bloodstream, with shorter time indicating a greater burden of organisms.[3]

It is essential that blood cultures are taken prior to onset of antibiotics, or as close as possible to antibiotics being administered, to maximise the likelihood of a positive result in the setting of a true bloodstream infection. Two or more sets of blood cultures should be collected for increased yield and to determine pathogenicity of low pathogenic organisms[18] (see 20.1.3 BSI with low pathogenic organisms).

20.1 Definitions

Standardised definitions for bloodstream infection (BSI) have been developed and are used for the purpose of healthcare surveillance and research. The most thorough definitions are published by the Centers for Disease and Prevention National Healthcare Safety Network,[19] an online resource used for surveillance of infections in USA. This is updated regularly. (See Useful websites/resources at the end of this chapter.)

20.1.1 Primary bloodstream infection

Primary BSI is a laboratory-confirmed BSI that is not a result of an infection at another body site.[20] This requires clinical examination and investigation to exclude the presence of an underlying infection as the source of the BSI, and is a diagnosis of exclusion.

20.1.2 Secondary bloodstream infection

Secondary BSI is one that has resulted from infection at another site, for example a urinary tract infection, pneumonia or cellulitis.[20] This requires a consistent clinical picture (symptoms, signs and laboratory or imaging findings) and onset of clinical features within a window period of 3 days either prior to, or following, blood culture collection.[20]

20.1.3 BSI with low pathogenic organisms

There are a number of organisms termed 'commensals' that are frequently found within the oral mucosa or on the skin surface. These organisms can be identified if the aseptic technique for collection of blood cultures has been compromised and the specimen contaminated with organisms in oral droplets or colonising skin. This can occur if the venepuncture site is not adequately cleaned, or if the site becomes contaminated after cleaning, such as with further palpation or both inadequate hand hygiene or inadequate skin preparation. Commensals are low pathogenic organisms that

TABLE 20.1 Frequently identified commensals*

Oral organisms	Viridans group streptococci
	Aerococcus spp.
	Rhodococcus spp.
Skin organisms	Coagulase-negative staphylococci (including *S. epidermidis, S. capitis*)
	Corynebacterium spp. (not *C. diphtheria*)
	Micrococcus spp.
	Bacillus spp. (not *B. anthracis*)
	Propionibacterium acnes

**Complete lists of commensals are available online, e.g. from NHSN Organism list (see Useful websites/resources)*

infrequently cause infection in healthy individuals; however, they can cause significant infection in patients with immunosuppression, intravascular access or prosthetic devices. Frequently identified commensals are listed in Table 20.1.

Confirmation of a BSI with low pathogenic organisms requires two positive blood culture collections with the identical organisms from separate blood draws taken within 2 consecutive calendar days.[20] Clinical evidence of infection is also required. In all ages this is one of fever >38.0°C, chills or hypotension. In children under 1 year of age, this is one of fever >38.0°C, hypothermia <36.0°C, chills, hypotension, apnoea or bradycardia.[20]

A contamination rate of 5.6% was found in an Australian study of blood cultures collected in an emergency department with a culture of frequently taking cultures through the intravenous cannulae,[21] compared to the maximum acceptable contamination rate of <3% in microbiology laboratories.

It is imperative that aseptic technique is followed when collecting blood for culture to reduce the likelihood of culturing non-pathogenic organisms. Steps to guide an aseptic technique for blood culture collection are included in Box 20.1.

20.1.4 Mucosal barrier injury BSI

This is a subgroup of primary BSI with low pathogenic organisms from the gastrointestinal tract. It specifically refers to the translocation of gastrointestinal organisms in immunosuppressed patients with neutropenia or allogeneic haematopoietic stem cell recipients with gastrointestinal graft versus host disease or severe diarrhoea.[20] This will be discussed further in the chapter on infections in cancer.

BOX 20.1 Steps to sterile blood culture collection

1. Prepare sterile field with chlorhexidine
2. Apply tourniquet proximal to the sterile field
3. Follow hand hygiene procedure and don gloves (sterile gloves if vein may need to be palpated again)
4. Collect blood using minimal equipment, e.g. safety butterfly inserted into blood culture bottle
5. Remove cap from blood culture bottle immediately before connecting to the tubing from butterfly
6. Use a vacuum connector with needle (single use, sterile) if required
7. Do not collect through a vascular access device, unless investigating a possible catheter-related BSI, in which case paired samples should be taken simultaneously through the device and a peripheral vein for comparison
8. Ensure adequate blood is collected in the bottles—20 mL is the recommended amount in adults, and 0.5–3 mL for infants or children. The volume of blood collected is directly associated with the likelihood of a positive result in a patient that is bacteraemic.[3]

Source: Royal College of Pathologists of Australasia. RCPA Manual - Pathology tests - Blood culture, 2022. Available from: https://www.rcpa.edu.au/Manuals/RCPA-Manual/Pathology-Tests/B/Blood-culture.

20.1.5 Healthcare-associated BSI (HA-BSIs)

BSIs are deemed to be healthcare-associated if they develop as a consequence of healthcare, or are associated with the infection of a prosthetic or invasive device. BSIs were identified in 10% of healthcare-associated infections (HAIs) in an Australian point prevalence study,[22] similar to proportions of 8.7–13% from international point prevalence studies.[23-26] Primary, secondary and mucosal barrier injury BSIs can all be healthcare-associated.

HA-BSIs cause significant impact on patients' morbidity, mortality and length of hospital stay. The European CDC has reported that 3.5% of patients in European intensive care units (ICU) over a 4-year period developed HA-BSIs, with an attributed mortality of

5% and an additional 14 days stay in ICU.[27] In Australia, it is estimated that HA-BSIs contribute to 3200 deaths per year.[28] While HA-BSIs were present in only 14% of all HAIs in a large Australian study, they were associated with 46% of all HAI deaths.[28]

While many bacteria can be implicated in HA-BSIs, *Staphylococcus aureus* is a frequent and important pathogen, and internationally has become a marker for safe healthcare delivery and infection prevention measures within a healthcare facility[29] and is a key performance indicator for acute care hospitals in Australia.[30]

20.2 *Staphylococcus aureus* bloodstream infections (SABSIs)

Staphylococcus aureus is a Gram-positive cocci that colonises the nares in 20–40% of the population[31] and can colonise other parts of the body, including the throat, axilla, groin and rectum.[32] *S. aureus* is readily transmitted from person to person with direct contact, and can spread within families and sports teams.[33] Within the healthcare setting, *S. aureus* can be transmitted on healthcare worker hands and shared equipment.

S. aureus infections develop when the cutaneous and mucosal barriers of the skin become disrupted due to chronic skin conditions, intravascular devices or surgical procedures.[31]

S. aureus can enter the bloodstream following localised infection, or direct intravenous inoculation, as occurs with non-sterile intravenous injection or from a contaminated intravascular catheter.[31]

S. aureus is a virulent organism, and SABSIs are associated with high morbidity and mortality. Metastatic infection complicates 8% of *S. aureus* bloodstream infections,[34] with preference for bones, joints and heart valves, causing osteomyelitis, septic arthritis and endocarditis respectively. Sites with prosthetic material are at increased risk of seeding, resulting in complicated infections involving pacemakers, heart valves, joints and internal fixation devices and the surrounding native tissue.[4]

20.2.1 Microbiology—MSSA and MRSA

Historically, *S. aureus* was treated with methicillin, a beta-lactam antibiotic. In 1961, *S. aureus* that was resistant to methicillin was described and was termed methicillin-resistant *Staphylococcus aureus* (MRSA). Although methicillin is no longer used for treatment due to toxicity, and has been replaced by other beta-lactams for first-line treatment (flucloxacillin or first generation cephalosporins, cefazolin or cephalothin), the terms MRSA and MSSA for methicillin-susceptible *S. aureus* remain.

MRSA was initially described with hospital outbreaks and termed healthcare-associated MRSA (HA-MRSA).[31] Community acquisition of MRSA (CA-MRSA) also occurs. Indigenous Australians in Western Australia and the Northern Territory have high prevalence of CA-MRSA; it is identified in up to 60% of skin and soft tissue infections requiring treatment in these populations.[35-37]

MRSA infections require treatment with alternate classes of antibiotics—with vancomycin, a glycopeptide, primarily used. Treatment with vancomycin has inherent difficulties. Prescribing is based on patient weight, age and renal function, and requires drug monitoring to ensure effective dosing without toxicity.[38] More recently, resistance to vancomycin has been detected with increasing frequency, from 2% before 2006 to 7% of all *S. aureus* isolates in 2015–20 worldwide, with the highest proportions in Africa (16%) and Asia (5%).[39] Treatment options for these organisms are limited and problematic.

The Australian Group on Antimicrobial Resistance (AGAR) monitors national SABSI isolates for resistance and molecular epidemiology. The latest report describes 2734 unique episodes of SABSI analysed in 2020 with the following features:

- 66.7% male
- median age 61 years, mean 56 years, range 0–102
- 79.7% were community onset
- MSSA 82.4%
- MRSA 17.6%
- all-cause mortality at 30 days—13.5%
- all-cause mortality in MSSA—13.3%
- all-cause mortality in MRSA—14.2%[1]

A recent Australian study identified ten factors associated with developing community and healthcare-associated SABSIs, with six of these reflecting healthcare exposure. The proportions of these factors in the SABSIs studied are:

- animal exposure (41%)
- recent hospitalisation (39%)
- presence of a medical device (37%)
- prior antibiotic therapy (35%)
- recent healthcare attendance (32%)
- recent surgical procedure (21%)
- receipt of immunosuppression (20%)
- injecting drug use (9%)
- chronic skin disease (9%)
- residence in long-term care facility (4%).[34]

20.2.2 Community and healthcare-associated SABSI

Effective surveillance requires strict definitions for data classification, with standardised definitions being reviewed and updated. The current Australian definitions are provided by the Australian Commission on Safety and Quality in Health Care (ACSQHC)[4] (Box 20.2) and are discussed further below. For further discussion on different definitions used internationally, see the companion volume to this text, *HAI Epidemiology*.

Community-onset SABSI refers to the collection of an initial positive blood culture prior to or within 48 hours of a hospital presentation, and is associated with skin and soft tissue infections and intravenous drug use.

BOX 20.2 Healthcare-associated *S. aureus* bloodstream infection definitions

Hospital-onset SABSI requires:

• collection of the initial positive blood culture >48 hours after presentation to hospital

AND

• no evidence the infection was present on admission or <48 hours following discharge.

Healthcare-associated SABSI with community onset requires:

• initial positive blood culture collected prior to admission or <48 hours of admission; a recent healthcare intervention

AND one of the following:

• complication or the presence of an indwelling medical device:
  - <30 days of a surgical procedure where SABSI is related to the surgical procedure OR
  - <90 days of a surgical procedure where SABSI is related to a deep incisional/organ space infection related to a surgically implanted device OR
  - <48 hours of a related instrumentation or incision OR
  - is associated with neutropenia contributed to by cytotoxic therapy and is unrelated to the presence of an indwelling device.[4]

Source: Reproduced with permission from Implementation Guide for the Surveillance of Staphylococcus aureus bloodstream infection, Australian Commission on Safety and Quality in Health Care – License Agreement – Elsevier Australia – 05/06/2023 – Page 5 developed by the Australian Commission on Safety and Quality in Health Care (ACSQHC). ACSQHC: Sydney 2021.

Hospital-onset SABSI refers to the collection of an initial positive blood culture >48 hours after admission/presentation to hospital, or <48 hours following discharge.

SABSI can also be healthcare-associated with community onset, if the initial positive blood culture was collected prior to or within 48 hours of admission, and with recent healthcare interventions:

• presence or complication of an indwelling medical device

• within 30 days of a surgical procedure where SABSI is related to the surgical procedure

• within 90 days of a surgical procedure where SABSI is related to a deep incisional/organ space infection associated with a surgically implanted device

• within 48 hours of a related instrumentation or incision

• associated with neutropenia contributed to by cytotoxic therapy and is unrelated to the presence of an indwelling device[4]—this is discussed further in Chapter 30.

HA-SABSIs are recognised as a marker of the quality and safety of healthcare delivery. There are many governance measures and infection prevention and control strategies to prevent HA-SABSIs. HA-SABSI rates are now used universally as a surveillance indicator for healthcare delivery.

Within Australia, SABSIs associated with hospital care are reported nationally to the Australian Institute of Health and Welfare (AIHW), and also to state health bodies. These can be accessed online at the AIHW website[40] and individual facilities' data at MyHospital[41] (see Useful websites/resources).

20.2.3 Healthcare-associated SABSI—epidemiology

The true burden of HA-SABSI within Australia is difficult to determine, as data are captured and published in different formats and with different definitions. While all public hospitals are required to submit data to AIHW, private hospitals are not, with only 28% of private hospitals providing data in 2019–2020.[2]

The Australian *Staphylococcus aureus* Sepsis Outcome Programme (ASSOP) within AGAR reported that 20% of the total SABSIs monitored by their group annually between 2018–2020 had hospital onset. This refers to approximately 550 hospital-onset SABSIs per year.[1,42,43]

In contrast, AIHW data from July 2019 to June 2020 reports 1630 episodes from 183 private and >700 public hospitals, covering 26.7 million occupied bed days (OBD).[2] The rate of infection was 0.71/10,000

TABLE 20.2 Rates of healthcare-associated *S. aureus* bloodstream infections reported in Australia using ASSOP[1] and AIHW[2]

Group	Year	Group	Number of HA-SABSIs	Denominator	Rate
ASSOPP	2020	All BSI reported to AGAR	555	Total cases	20.3%
AIHW	2019–2020	Public hospitals (n>700)	1428	20.1M OBD	0.71/10,000 OBD
		Private hospitals (n=183)	202	6.6M OBD	0.30/10,000 OBD

OBD: occupied bed days
Sources: Adapted from ASSOP[1] and AIHW[2]

OBD in public and 0.30/10,000 OBD in private hospitals.[2] Within private hospitals, 63 hospitals (34.4%) reported HA-SABSIs, with a rate that ranged from 0.09 to 1.80 per 10,000 OBD at these facilities.[2] See Table 20.2 for further detail.

HA-SABSIs are reported from all types of public hospitals, with the greatest proportion from major hospitals (55%), as shown in Table 20.3.[2] The higher rates and proportion of cases seen in major, large and children's hospitals may reflect that these facilities treat a greater proportion of patients at risk of SABSI compared to the small and medium hospitals.[2] Across states and territories within Australia the rates range from 0.34/10,000 OBD in the Northern Territory to 0.81/10,000 OBD in Tasmania and the Australian Capital Territory.[2]

It is important to recognise that the incidence rates of HA-SABSIs have reduced substantially in recent years. A study of 132 hospitals in four Australian states or territories (24% of all hospitals) showed a 63% reduction in the annual rate of hospital-onset SABSI from 1.72/10,000 OBD in 2002 to 0.64/10,000 OBD in 2013[44] with further reductions seen since. This improvement followed the introduction of surveillance and reporting, as discussed above. Furthermore, processes to detect, monitor and prevent SABSIs have been incorporated into the Australian Commission on Safety and Quality in Health Care (ACSQHC) Accreditation Standards for health facilities.[11] These are discussed in 20.4 Prevention methods—HA SABSIs and 20.6 Investigation, surveillance and governance.

20.2.4 Clinical outcomes

The clinical outcomes following HA-SABSIs are substantial. Within Australia, patients who develop a HA-SABSI will have their hospital stay prolonged by 5.3 days, or 7.9 days if this is an MRSA BSI.[45] There is also a threefold greater increased risk of in-hospital death, and additional hospital costs estimated in 2020 at $A14,507 per episode, and $A21,720 if this is with MRSA.[45]

HA-SABSIs also have risks for metastatic seeding and localised infections, including osteomyelitis, septic arthritis and endocarditis, with further increased morbidity and mortality.[46,47]

20.3 Device-related infections

Medical devices are a frequent source for HA-BSIs and can also be associated with infections caused by other bacteria and fungi.

A medical device was associated with 37% of all SABSIs in an Australian study, including those with community acquisition. Intravascular access devices were present in 54% of these, with peripheral intravenous cannulae (PIVCs) most frequent in 33%, haemodialysis access devices in 12%, and peripherally inserted central venous catheters (PICC) in 9%; the remaining 46% of devices were not further described.[34]

Non-intravascular medical devices that are associated with HA-BSI include orthopaedic devices (prosthetic

TABLE 20.3 Rates of healthcare-associated *S. aureus* bloodstream infections reported from different sized hospitals to AIHW, Australia, 2019–2020[2]

	Rate/ 10,000 OBD	Proportion of total cases
Major hospital	0.96	55%
Large hospital	0.91	33%
Medium hospital	0.46	6%
Small hospital	0.32	3%
Children's hospital	0.91	4%

Source: Australian Institute of Health and Welfare. Bloodstream infections associated with hospital care 2019–2020. AIHW, 2022

joints, internal and external fixation devices), cardiac devices (pacemakers, defibrillators, prosthetic valves), ventricular shunts and peritoneal dialysis catheters—although any prosthetic material placed in situ can be associated with infection.

20.3.1 Intravascular catheter-associated BSIs

Intravascular catheters are devices placed within a vessel for treatment delivery, blood withdrawal or haemodynamic monitoring. Their presence was documented in 70% of acute adult inpatients in a large Australian point prevalence study, with peripheral intravenous devices in 55% and central venous devices in 15%.[22] Intravenous catheters cause more than 3500 cases of BSIs annually in Australia, with a large proportion of these deemed potentially preventable.[6]

Peripheral intravenous catheters (PIVC): Peripheral intravenous catheters are short, plastic devices inserted in a vein in a peripheral limb for short-term treatment. PIVCs are an important risk for *S. aureus* bloodstream infections.[46]

Central venous access devices (CVADs): Central venous access devices are intravascular catheters where the tip is located close to, or at, the heart or one of the great vessels. These are inserted either centrally or peripherally, as outlined below and shown in Fig 20.1:

- *non-tunnelled central venous catheters (CVCs).* These central lines are placed in the subclavian or internal jugular or femoral vein, with the distal tip lying in the superior vena cava.[48] These are frequently used in intensive care units for intravenous treatments and haemodynamic monitoring.

- *tunnelled CVCs.* These central lines are tunnelled in the subcutaneous tissue between an insertion point and where the catheter enters the blood vessel. Some have a cuff that sits in the subcutaneous tunnel (cuffed catheters).[48] These are frequently used to provide short- and long-term haemodialysis, and are present in 1/7 patients receiving haemodialysis in Australia.[47]

- *peripherally inserted central catheters (PICCs).* These central lines are inserted into peripheral veins (usually brachiocephalic vein in the upper limb)

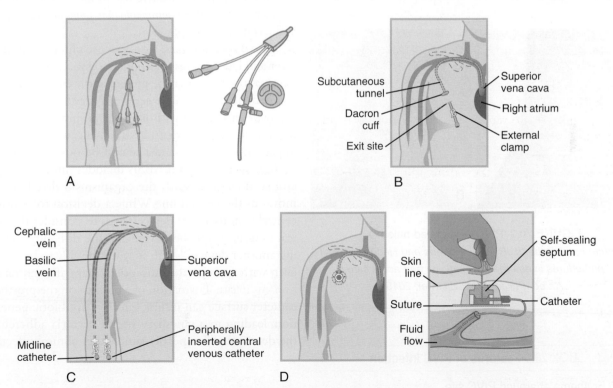

FIGURE 20.1 Central venous access devices. A, Non-tunnelled central venous catheter placed in the subclavian vein. B, Tunnelled central venous catheter C, Peripherally inserted central venous catheter (PICC). D, Implanted venous access device or port

Source: Malarvizhi S. Black's Medical-surgical nursing: Clinical management for positive outcomes,
First South Asia Edition. Elsevier India, 2019.

with the distal tip lying in the superior vena cava.[48] These are frequently used for prolonged intravenous antibiotics.

- *implanted ports.* These are surgically inserted devices that sit under the skin and are accessed with specific port needles.[48] These are frequently associated with prolonged haematology and oncology treatments.

20.3.2 PIVC-associated SABSIs

PIVC-associated SABSIs that have clinical evidence of phlebitis, skin or soft tissue infection at a current or previously used cannulation site meet the definition for a secondary BSI related to this clinical infection (Fig 20.2 and Box 20.3). Other SABSIs may be related to direct inoculation of a catheter hub or injection using non-sterile technique; no clinical findings may be present when this has occurred. This can help to explain how the presence of a PIVC is identified as the main risk factor associated with developing HA-SABSI, whether or not infection of the insertion site is present.[50]

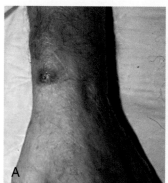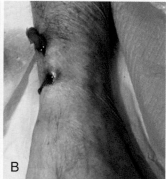

FIGURE 20.2 PIVC-associated phlebitis
Source: From Roberts JR, et al. Roberts and Hedges' clinical procedures in emergency medicine and acute care. 7th ed. Philadelphia: Elsevier, 2019.

BOX 20.3 Features of PIVC infection

- Erythema at/around PIVC site
- Presence of purulent exudate
- Pain
- Tenderness
- Thickening of vein
- Fever

20.3.3 Central-line associated bloodstream infections (CLABSIs)

It is estimated that 15% of patients with a CVC will have a catheter-related complication, including infection.[51] Central-line associated bloodstream infections (CLABSIs) are most frequent in intensive care units (ICUs), where the majority of patients have CVCs in situ. ICU-associated CLABSIs are discussed further in Chapter 28.

CLABSIs also occur outside of the ICU setting in the patient populations outlined above. Estimates of CLABSIs in Australian dialysis patients range from 3.5–5.89 per 1000 catheter days, with 30% associated with *S. aureus* bloodstream infection.[47] Specific risks that relate to dialysis patients include prolonged duration in situ and variations in aseptic technique compliance when accessing for dialysis in a variety of settings, including home haemodialysis.

The ACSQHC has standardised definitions for CLABSIs, based on international definitions (Box 20.4).

The common causative microorganisms of CLABSIs include *S. aureus*, coagulase negative Staphylococci, Enterococci, Gram-negative bacilli including *Pseudomonas aeruginosa* and *Stenotrophomonas maltophilia*, Candida and polymicrobial infections.[46,47,51]

CLABSIs often have non-specific clinical features of fever and leucocytosis without an identifiable source. Inflammation or pus may be present at the catheter exit site, and patients may develop signs of systemic infection (fever, hypotension, tachycardia) after flushing of the line.[51] It is essential to consider CLABSI as a cause for infection in patients with fever and a central venous access device.

Management of CLABSIs includes directed antimicrobial therapy towards the organisms isolated and removal of the central line. While a decision to remove a central venous access device needs to consider the clinical indication for the device and the difficulty in placing another device,[51] BSIs may not be able to be cleared even with appropriate antibiotic therapy if a central line remains in situ. Formation of a biofilm on the prosthetic catheter surface can inhibit effective antibiotic penetration, leading to a sanctuary site of bacteria adherent to the device that can perpetuate further clinical infection.

20.4 Prevention methods— HA-SABSIs

2.4.1 Hand hygiene

An association between hand hygiene and prevention of HA-SABSI was shown in a large study of 132 Australian hospitals over six years. This used linkage data of facility

BOX 20.4 Central line-associated bloodstream infection definition

CLABSI requires:

Laboratory-confirmed BSI in a patient where the central line was in place for >48 hours on the date of the event

AND

The central line was in place on the date of the event or the day before. If the central line was in place for >48 hours and then removed, the following criteria must be fully met on the day of removal or the next day.

Criterion 1:

A patient at any age has a recognised bacterial or fungal pathogen cultured from one or more blood cultures

AND

The organism cultured from blood is **not** related to an infection at another site.

Criterion 2:

A patient of any age has at least one of the following signs/symptoms: fever (>38ºC), chills or hypotension

OR

A patient <1 year of age has at least one of the following signs/symptoms: fever (>38ºC core), hypothermia (<36ºC core), apnoea or bradycardia

AND

The organism cultured from blood is **not** related to an infection at another site

AND

The same (matching) potential contaminant (low pathogenic organism as outlined above) is cultured from **two** or more sets of blood cultures drawn on separate occasions within 24 hours.[5]

Source: Reproduced with permission from Implementation Guide: Surveillance of Central-Line Associated Bloodstream Infection (2019), developed by the Australian Commission on Safety and Quality in Health Care (ACSQHC). ACSQHC: Sydney 2019.

hand hygiene results following implementation of the National Hand Hygiene Initiative (NHHI) and the corresponding HA-SABSIs data reported to AIHW between 2010–11 and 2016–17.[52] For every 10% increase in hand hygiene compliance as measured by the 'Your 5 Moments for Hand Hygiene', there was a corresponding relative reduction in the incidence of HA-SABSI of 15%.[52] This was seen across all hospitals submitting data (principal referral hospitals and Group A and B hospitals).[52]

It is important to recognise that this refers not only to healthcare workers washing their hands, but to the implementation of a hand hygiene system that includes education, auditing, reporting, governance and inclusion in hospital accreditation programs.[53] The NHHI website provides a comprehensive description of this Australian program (see Useful websites/resources below).

While environmental cleaning is a key component to reducing many HAIs, including infection with VRE, it has not been shown to reduce SABSI rates.[54]

20.4.2 Clearance of MRSA

Eliminating *S. aureus* colonisation can reduce the risk of subsequent infections, and is a strategy used in a variety of settings including recurrent folliculitis and prior to elective surgery. Decolonisation consists of a 5–10 day regimen of daily chlorhexidine body washes accompanied by fresh sheets, towels and clothes with thrice-daily intranasal mupiricin.[31] To be cleared of MRSA, patients that are not on MRSA-targeted therapy and do not have an open wound or invasive device require evidence from repeated swabs that MRSA has not been identified. While studies have shown mixed impact on surgical site infections following MRSA decolonisation, subsequent colonisation can occur with MSSA, or recolonisation with MRSA, and no evidence for an effect on SABSI rates has been shown.[31]

20.4.3 Medical device management

The key principles of aseptic technique and device management have been instrumental in reducing both PIVC and CVC-related BSIs. These are now referred to as 'bundles' of care that occur at insertion and when accessing intravenous devices. See Box 20.5 for an outline of the principles discussed below.

Peripherally inserted Intravascular catheters (PIVC) management: It is essential to consider the need for a PIVC before insertion, including if oral treatment alternatives (fluids and medications) may be possible. A recent point prevalence study has shown that 34% of peripheral cannulae inserted in emergency departments were not used, and that this was the case in half of patients with a triage category of 4 or 5, indicating less severe illness acuity.[55]

Introducing PIVC bundles that include components of intravenous device management has been associated with a reduction in PIVC-associated SABSIs both

---

**BOX 20.5 Key principles of intravenous
device management**

1. Only place and use intravascular devices that are required—consider alternative options before inserting
2. Choose appropriate device and placement site
3. Use aseptic technique for insertion
4. Use aseptic technique when accessing intravenous devices
5. Ensure early removal when no longer required
6. Frequently review and consult documentation to guide appropriate removal
7. Consider alternative access based on clinical progress, e.g. for prolonged intravenous treatment

---

nationally and internationally, with components outlined below.[50,56-58]

Measures to improve aseptic technique compliance at PIVC insertion have included review of current insertion technique within a facility or jurisdiction, followed by education, aseptic technique training and competency, and introduction of PIVC equipment packs with consistent equipment including skin disinfectant[12,50,56] with 70% alcohol + 2% chlorhexidine (consider povidone-iodine and alcohol or aqueous chlorhexidine if allergy is present).[8]

Documentation of date and time of insertion has been enhanced, with stickers included with key PIVC equipment that are to be placed both at the PIVC site and in medical records.[8] Healthcare workers inserting PIVCs are encouraged to document their names in the medical record.[50] Frequent clinical review of the PIVC site and documentation within the medical record[50,56] should occur every shift or every eight hours, and removed if there are signs of inflammation, the PIVC is unable to be used, or is no longer required.[10,12,50,56]

While studies have shown that the risk for SABSI increases if a PIVC remains in situ >72 hours,[58] it is unclear if automatic removal at 72 hours is necessary. Options include reviewing the PIVC, assessing for signs of inflammation, and reviewing the indication and expected duration that IV access is required. Some states or facilities have chosen to include automatic removal at 72 hours in their bundles if they do not think this clinical review process will occur.[50]

These bundles have been associated with a pronounced reduction in the rate of PIVC-associated SABSI.[50,56] An Australian study showed a 63% decrease in PIVC-associated SABSIs from 0.39/10,000 OBD to 0.14/10,000 OBD in the 15 months following stepwise bundle introduction compared with the 12 months prior to intervention.[50] While this also showed an increase in compliance with bundle components, these remained suboptimal in the PIVCs audited, with less than 50% of all components being met.[50]

The Australian Guidelines for the Prevention and Control of Infection in Healthcare (2019) have developed a table based on current evidence to reduce the infection risk to patients from intravascular access devices by device type. These steps are provided in Box 20.6.

**BOX 20.6 Minimising the infection risk to patients from intravascular access
devices by device type**

	Peripheral Intravenous Catheter (PIVC)	Peripheral Inserted Central Catheter (PICC)	Central Venous Catheter (CVC)
Need for intravascular catheterisation	All types of intravascular access devices should be used only when clinically indicated and deemed necessary, and when all other alternatives have been considered (such as oral medication). Select the most appropriate device and site for the patient after assessing the need for the device and duration of therapy.[9]		
		The risk factors associated with inserting central lines should be considered prior to insertion, and all risks should be minimised, where possible.	

BOX 20.6 Minimising the infection risk to patients from intravascular access devices by device type—cont'd

	Peripheral Intravenous Catheter (PIVC)	Peripheral Inserted Central Catheter (PICC)	Central Venous Catheter (CVC)
Skin preparation	Healthcare workers should allow sufficient contact time for site preparation, ensuring the following: • remove hair, if necessary, using clippers (not shavers)[14] • clean a site large enough for insertion before applying antisepsis and allowing to dry completely • decontaminate the site using a single use application of alcohol-based chlorhexidine gluconate solution (2% chlorhexidine gluconate in 70% isopropyl alcohol)[9] • if insertion through or close to mucous membranes is necessary, use aqueous solution supplemented with 2% chlorhexidine • for patients with a history of chlorhexidine sensitivity, use 5% alcohol-based povidone-iodine solution or 10% aqueous povidone-iodine if insertion is close to or through mucous membranes (see *Recommendation 39* for further information).		
Device selection	Choose the shortest and smallest gauge suitable for the prescribed therapy as this can reduce the risk of phlebitis. This must be well secured to prevent dislodgement.	Use a central catheter with the least number of lumens, connectors and ports possible[8] Consider the length of time that the catheter is likely to be in situ. If total parenteral nutrition is being administered, a single lumen should be reserved for that use. There is evidence to suggest that antimicrobial coated or impregnated catheters can reduce the risk of BSI. However, the magnitude of the benefits differs according to the healthcare setting, and significant benefits have primarily been reported in ICUs.[59]	
Site selection	In selecting the best insertion site, consider: • using the patient's non-dominant forearm, where possible • using the basilic or brachial veins on the posterior (dorsal) forearm, where possible • that the metacarpal veins on the dorsum of the hand are easiest to visualise but more liable to clot and are prone to vessel damage. Where possible avoid using: • areas of flexion (i.e. wrist and antecubital fossa), as this may predispose to phlebitis • areas below previous cannulation, bruised or phlebitic areas • an infected limb, or a limb with a PICC or implanted venous access device • the arm on the side of the body where lymph node clearance/ fistulas may be located • lower limbs, due to the risk of deep vein thrombosis • the anterior (ventral) forearm veins, especially the cephalic vein, in patients with chronic renal failure.	In selecting the best insertion site, consider using the non-dominant arm where possible.	Use a subclavian site, rather than a jugular or a femoral site, in adult patients for CVC placement.

Continued

BOX 20.6 Minimising the infection risk to patients from intravascular access devices by device type—cont'd

	Peripheral Intravenous Catheter (PIVC)	Peripheral Inserted Central Catheter (PICC)	Central Venous Catheter (CVC)
Insertion	All healthcare workers who insert intravascular access devices should be appropriately trained or under the supervision of a trained clinician. Required competencies and accreditation are determined according to healthcare facility policy. Perform hand hygiene immediately prior to the insertion of all catheters, either by washing with antimicrobial handwash solution and water or using an alcohol-based hand rub. Multiple insertion attempts increase risk of infection. To avoid this, each healthcare facility should have a documented inserter escalation pathway, and a process for identifying difficult vascular access patients early so that they are referred to the appropriately skilled inserter.		
	Use aseptic technique for the insertion of PIVCs.	Use maximum sterile barrier precautions for insertion of central venous catheters; there is evidence that they can reduce immediate post-insertion skin colonisation.	
		When PICC insertion is done at the bedside (i.e. the patient's room), establish a suitable aseptic field and maintain this throughout the procedure.	Using a two-dimensional ultrasound can offer benefits in safety and quality when compared with an anatomical landmark technique. If using ultrasound guidance, healthcare workers should be appropriately trained in this technique and the principles of asepsis applied throughout the procedure, including the use of sterile ultrasound gel. See ultrasound care guidelines for further information. Consideration may be given to the use of CVC insertion bundles.
Dressing and securement	Use either sterile gauze or sterile, transparent, semi-permeable dressing to cover the catheter site. There is insufficient evidence to suggest the use of one dressing type over the other. Patient preference and clinician preference are currently acceptable factors to consider when choosing a dressing type. If a patient is diaphoretic or if the site is bleeding or oozing, use gauze dressing until this is resolved. Inspect dressing (device and site) at each shift. If there is any moisture or leaking, or the dressing becomes damp, loose, soiled or lifting then it should be replaced. Replacement of dressings: • gauze dressings should be replaced at least every 24 hours • CVAD/PICC transparent dressings should be replaced every 7 days • PIVCs are a short-term device and change may not be required until the device is removed.		

BOX 20.6 Minimising the infection risk to patients from intravascular access devices by device type—cont'd

	Peripheral Intravenous Catheter (PIVC)	Peripheral Inserted Central Catheter (PICC)	Central Venous Catheter (CVC)
Maintenance	Use hand antisepsis and aseptic technique for catheter site care and for accessing the system. The safe maintenance of an intravascular access device includes: good practice in caring for the patient's catheter hub and connection port to avoid contamination by staff hands, the use of an appropriate site dressing regimen, and using flush solutions to maintain the patency of the line. Examine the dressing, device and site at each shift and promptly remove a catheter that is no longer required. Replace the catheter site dressing if it becomes damp, loosened or soiled–do not reinforce a suboptimal dressing with tape. Using chlorhexidine-impregnated dressings at the catheter insertion site has been shown to reduce intravascular access device-related BSI and device colonisation rates. The safety of these dressings has not been established in low birth-weight neonates who may be at risk of skin or systemic toxicity. Patients should be educated to alert healthcare staff if they experience any discomfort at the insertion site including pain, burning, swelling or bleeding. When using a needleless connector, the hub should be scrubbed (70% alcohol wipe is the application of choice) before each access to minimise the risk of microbial contamination.		
Device replacement	All catheters should be checked at each shift and removed when no longer required or if infection is suspected. All catheters inserted in an emergency situation (e.g. by emergency ambulance services or during cardiac arrest) should be removed and replaced when the patient is stable and within 24 hours of insertion.		
	Do not routinely replace PIVCs in neonates and children. There are two options for the replacement of PIVCs in adults. See text for more detailed information.		Do not routinely replace CVCs.
Replacement of administration sets	All administration sets should be replaced when disconnected from the hub or if the catheter is changed. Leave administration sets that do not contain lipids, blood or blood products in place for intervals of up to 96 hours. Change administration sets used for intermittent infusion of blood, blood products or lipid emulsions (including 3–1 parenteral nutrition solutions) when the infusion is complete or at least every 24 hours. Change administration sets used to infuse propofol every 12 hours or as per manufacturer's guidelines. Change administration sets used to infuse heparin every 24 hours.		

Sources: Queensland Health Guidelines[37]; NSW Clinical Excellence Committee Guidelines[57]; epic Guidelines[52]; CDC Guidelines[54] ACQSHC guidelines[33,51,53] and Australian and New Zealand Intensive Care Society Guidelines[58]

Central venous access device (CVAD) management: The required duration and use for a CVAD (haemodialysis, haemodynamic monitoring, chemotherapy, prolonged antibiotics or total parenteral nutrition [TPN]) will determine the most appropriate device to be placed, location of insertion and number of lumens. As a greater number of lumens increases risk for CLABSI when adjusted for the degree of underlying illness,[8] inserting the lowest number of lumens required is prudent. Patients receiving TPN have increased risk for CLABSI,[8] and this is further increased if TPN is given in lumens with other treatments, making a dedicated lumen for TPN necessary.[8]

The site of CVAD placement can impact on CLABSI as a result of the density of skin flora and the risk of thrombophlebitis. Insertion at the subclavian or internal jugular vein are preferred due to a lower infection rate than is seen using the femoral vein.[8]

Antimicrobial or antiseptic agents, including chlorhexidine and silver sulfadiazine, may be incorporated into the physical structure of CVCs or their cuffs, and have been shown in a meta-analysis to reduce the onset of CLABSI, but not sepsis, all-cause mortality or catheter-related local infection.[59] A reduction in colonisation of the CVC was also found in patients within ICU settings, but not patients in haematology-oncology units, or requiring TPN.[59] Decisions regarding the use of these products should be made if the CLABSI rates within a specific patient population (ICU, haematology, renal) remain elevated despite maximising all other measures.

The importance of aseptic technique while inserting CVCs with maximal sterile barrier precautions (sterile gloves and gown, cap, mask and full size sterile drape) was first noted in 1994 to be associated with a six-fold lower rate of CLABSI than when the inserter used only sterile gloves and small sterile drape.[60] These findings have subsequently been developed into bundles to maximise asepsis during insertion.

The Australian and New Zealand Intensive Care Society has resources available to guide insertion and post-insertion care of CVCs to reduce CLABSIs,[13,61] which can be used in both the ICU and non-ICU setting, including education modules (see Useful websites/resources).

An insertion checklist,[61] to be completed by an observer at the bedside during the procedure, is used to calculate compliance with the guidelines. There is signed agreement on this form that the observer can interrupt the proceduralist during insertion if asepsis is breached. The checklist is an important surveillance tool, with compliance rates included in the ACSQHC requirements for accreditation, and for investigation if CLABSI rates increase within a unit. For further discussion regarding CVC prevention in ICU see Chapter 28.

Additional components of the management of CVCs include documentation and frequent review, with attention to length of the catheter, integrity of the securement method, dressing, attached lines[62] and presence of inflammation. CVCs should be replaced when clinically indicated and removed when no longer required. Routine replacement of CVCs and use of guidewire exchange have been associated with increased rates of infection[8] and should not occur. Patient education is vital to ensure the lines are not accessed, damaged or soiled, and for patients to alert their clinical team if signs of infection develop.

Ongoing intravascular device management during use: It is essential to provide meticulous care to peripheral and central intravenous lines when accessing these for treatments. Hand hygiene, aseptic technique, and compliance with standard and transmission-based precautions are necessary, and are guided by the infection or organisms involved.

When accessing ports, these should be thoroughly cleaned ('scrub the hub') for at least 15 seconds, generating friction by scrubbing in a twisting motion with a single use 70% (v/v) alcohol-impregnated swab.[7] If alcoholic chlorhexidine or 10% povidone-iodine is used, the drying time may vary (20 seconds or more) depending on the product and it should be allowed to air dry prior to accessing.[63] Intravenous giving sets should not be disconnected, except for transient controlled disconnections, such as changing IV infusions. If this occurs, the entire IV tubing should be replaced.[7]

When preparing and administering intravenous medications and fluids, hand hygiene is required before and after preparation of medications or solutions, as well as before and after administration. It is essential to disinfect the medication access diaphragm on a vial, intravenous access port, or needleless connector and allow this to dry, as outlined above, before accessing.[7]

Clinical review of intravenous devices: Ongoing review of intravenous devices is required to determine:

* the ongoing need for the device
* patency; and
* presence at the insertion site of erythema, exudate, swelling, tenderness or pain.[62]

Peripheral intravenous site assessment scores (PIVAS) are tools that have been developed to assist with detection of inflammation or phlebitis at PIVC sites. While a number of clinical aids have been developed, robust evidence is lacking on their ability to determine the presence of phlebitis, and on the impact such a tool has on preventing subsequent SABSIs.[64] An example is shown in Figure 20.3,[16] with a monitoring tool for ongoing review of a patient's PIVC. One Australian PI-VAS has recently been shown to have high content validity among international vascular access nurses and clinicians, and high inter-rater reliability on medical-surgical wards in three hospitals.[65] This is both an assessment and decision-making tool that includes steps for infection control measures and documentation.[65] There is no current evidence on its uptake outside of a study setting or its impact on SABSIs (see Fig 20.4).

20.5 Prevention of other healthcare-associated infections

Secondary bloodstream infections can complicate any HAI, including pneumonia and catheter-associated urinary tract infections. Surgical site infections are frequently associated with SABSI. Prevention methods for these conditions are discussed in the appropriate chapters.

Peripheral Intravenous Assessment Score (PIVAS)

Sample PIVAS Tool:

0	PIVC SITE APPEARS HEALTHY No signs of adverse reaction	No signs of phlebitis Routine observation of PIVC
1	**One** of the following is observed Slight pain near PIVC site or slight redness near PIVC site	Possible first signs of phlebitis Observe PIVC (early removal if no longer required)
2	**Two** of the following is observed Pain near PIVC site Erythema Swelling	Early signs of phlebitis **RESITE** cannula
3	**All of** the following is observed Pain along path of cannula Erythema Induration	Medium signs of phlebitis **RESITE** cannula Consider treatment
4	**The following** are present and extensive Pain along path of cannula Erythema Swelling Palpable venous cord	Advanced stage of phlebitis (or start of thrombophlebitis) **RESITE** cannula Consider treatment
5	**All** are present and extensive Pain along path of cannula Erythema Swelling Palpable venous cord Pyrexia	Advanced stage of thrombophlebitis Initiate treatment **RESITE** cannula

A

FIGURE 20.3 PIVAS+ sample monitoring tool

Source: Jackson A. Infection control—a battle in vein: infusion phlebitis.
Nursing Times. 1998;94(4):68–71. Reproduced with permission.

Continued

FIGURE 20.3—cont'd

Sample monitoring tool

	Day 1 __/__/__			Day 2 __/__/__			Day 3 __/__/__			Day 4 __/__/__			Day 5 __/__/__			Day 6 __/__/__			Day 7 __/__/__		
	AM	PM	ND	AM	PM	ND	AM	PM	ND	AM	PM	ND	AM	PM	ND	AM	PM	ND	AM	PM	ND
PIVC observed	✓																				
PIVAS score																					
Dressing – appearance and integrity																					
Dressing – replacement																					
Replacement of infusion system																					
Flushing PIVC																					
Other																					
Signature of observer																					

Reason for removal: ❏ Treatment completed/ceased   ❏ Other _____

❏ PIVAS at removal (circle): 1 2 3 4 5   ❏ Occlusion   ❏ PIVC dislodgement   ❏ Patient request

Comments

B

PIVAS: peripheral intravenous assessment score

20.6 Investigation, surveillance and governance

Investigating and reporting of all HA-SABSIs and CLABSIs is an important component of prevention bundles to ensure oversight of case numbers, potentially preventable factors, and impact of interventions to improve process issues contributing to infections.[12]

This may be conducted by a multidisciplinary team including infection control, infectious diseases and patient safety officers.

For healthcare-associated intravascular device-related SABSIs, the ACSQHC recommends the following steps:

1. Ensure the SABSI meets the criteria for investigation
2. Investigate the BSI episode using an investigation checklist to identify potentially contributing factors (refer to Fig 20.5 and the investigation checklist from Queensland Health)[66]
3. Undertake an event analysis

4. Develop an action plan and report outcomes in accordance with local governance processes.[12]

Several investigation tools are included at the end of this chapter, with three case studies that illustrate how the tools can be used.

Oversight of SABSI rates, clinical outcomes and contributing factors should occur at multiple governance levels, including at:

- the clinical level for individual cases (admitting medical officer and nurse unit manager)[56,57]
- department morbidity and mortality meetings
- facility infection control meetings; and
- an executive level, such as patient safety or accreditation meetings.

Governance structures to review these key health safety measures are a requirement in the ACQSHC Standards for Accreditation.[11]Accountability and transparency in rates is also encouraged, with HA-SABSI rates available publicly on MyHealth website,[41] and facilities encouraged to display their rates for patients and visitors to see.

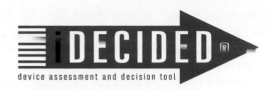

I

IDENTIFY if a device is present

D

DOES the patient need the device?
If no longer in active use, consider device removal.

E

EFFECTIVE function?
Is the device functioning as intended?
If not, troubleshoot as per policy or remove device.

C

COMPLICATION-FREE?
If complications are noted, troubleshoot or remove device.

I

INFECTION prevention
Hand hygiene before and after patient and device care.
Careful handling and disinfection of device access points.

D

DRESSING & securement
Ensure dressings are clean, dry and intact.
Secure devices to prevent tugging or patient injury.

E

EVALUATE & EDUCATE
Discuss device plan with patient & family. Educate as needed.

D

DOCUMENT your decision
Continue, troubleshoot, change dressing, or remove device.

*Always consider local policy,
and consult with team & patient as required.*

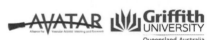
#IDECIDEDassessment

FIGURE 20.4 I-DECIDED peripheral intravenous catheter assessment and decision tool
Source: © Griffith University 2022. Reproduced with permission

PRACTICE TIP 1

ESSENTIAL KNOWLEDGE FOR INFECTION CONTROL PROFESSIONALS

1. A bloodstream infection (BSI) requires a positive blood culture to be defined as a BSI

2. The earliest a blood culture 'flags positive' is 12 hours. Time to culture may indicate burden of bacteria

3. Blood cultures are taken prior to onset of antibiotics

4. Aseptic technique must be followed when collecting blood cultures to reduce contamination

5. Healthcare-associated bloodstream infection (HA-BSI) is defined where the BSI is a consequence of healthcare, or is associated with infection of a prosthetic or invasive device

6. *Staphylococcus aureus* is an important and frequent pathogen. As many IPC measures can reduce the risk for SABSIs, rates of SABSI are used as a marker for healthcare delivery.

7. Surveillance requires clear definitions

8. Community-onset SABSI refers to collection of the initial positive blood culture prior to or within 48 hours of a hospital presentation and is associated with skin and soft tissue infections and intravenous drug use

9. Hospital-onset SABSI refers to collection of the initial positive blood culture >48 hours after admission/presentation to hospital, or <48 hours following discharge

10. SABSI can also be healthcare-associated, with community onset, if the initial positive blood culture was collected prior to or within 48 hours of admission, and with recent healthcare interventions

11. Medical devices are a frequent source of HA-BSIs

12. Non-intravascular medical devices that are associated with HA-BSIs include orthopaedic devices (prosthetic joints, internal and external fixation devices), cardiac devices (pacemakers, defibrillators, prosthetic valves), ventricular shunts and peritoneal dialysis catheters, although any prosthetic material placed in situ can be associated with infection

13. Intravascular catheter-associated BSIs can be associated with peripheral intravenous catheters (PIVC); central venous access devices (CVAD) or peripherally inserted central venous catheter (PICC)

14. Features of PIVC infection include: erythema at or around the PIVC site; presence of purulent exudate; pain; tenderness; thickening of vein; or fever

15. CLABSI is a central line-associated BSI

16. Prevention of HA-SABSI includes:
    - hand hygiene
    - clearance of MRSA colonisation
    - medical device management—optimal insertion, management and removal of intravascular devices
    - prevention of other HAIs
    - investigation, surveillance and governance.

Conclusion

Healthcare-associated bloodstream infections are frequent, important complications of care, with potentially devastating complications, and are responsible for almost half of all deaths from HAI. *S. aureus* bloodstream infections can be prevented when there is high compliance with many infection control programs, including hand hygiene, aseptic technique, intravascular device care, surveillance, and governance of patient safety outcomes. As such, it is recognised as a key indicator for the provision of safe healthcare delivery, and is used as a surrogate marker to compare facilities or show improvements over time.

This chapter has focused on the prevention methods that are necessary components for safe care, and to prevent HA-BSIs. It is essential to detect and report HA-BSIs, and to carry out investigations of individual cases. This will enable fine-tuning and tailoring of processes to individual facilities, teams and patient groups.

Useful websites/resources

- Management of Peripheral Intravenous Catheters Clinical Care Standard. Australian Commission on Safety and Quality in Health Care. https://www.safetyandquality.gov.au/standards/clinical-care-standards/management-peripheral-intravenous-catheters-clinical-care-standard

- Centers for Disease Control and Prevention, National Healthcare Safety Network, https://www.cdc.gov/nhsn/pdfs/pscmanual/pcsmanual_current.pdf

- Australian Institute of Health and Welfare, www.aihw.gov.au

- AIHW MyHospital (To search for individual hospitals), www.aihw.gov.au/reports-data/myhospitals/my-local-area

- Australian and New Zealand Intensive Care Society – CLABSI project, www.anzics.com.au/clabsi/

- National Hand Hygiene Initiative, https://www.safetyandquality.gov.au/our-work/infection-prevention-and-control/national-hand-hygiene-initiative

References

1. Coombs GW, Daley DA, Yee NWT, Shoby P, Mowlaboccus S. Australian group on antimicrobial resistance (AGAR). Australian Staphylococcus aureus Sepsis Outcome Programme (ASSOP) Annual Report 2020. Commun Dis Intell (2020). 2022;46.

2. Australian Institute of Health and Welfare. Bloodstream infections associated with hospital care 2019–2020. AIHW, 2022 [updated 18/02/2022].

3. Royal College of Pathologists of Australasia. RCPA manual - pathology tests - blood culture. RCPA, 2022. Available from: https://www.rcpa.edu.au/Manuals/RCPA-Manual/Pathology-Tests/B/Blood-culture.

4. Australian Commission on Safety and Quality in Health Care. Implementation guide for the surveillance of Staphylococcus aureus bloodstream infection. Sydney: ACSQHC, 2021.

5. Australian Commission on Safety and Quality in Health Care. Implementation guide: sureveillance of central line-associated bloodstream infection. Sydney: ACSQHC, 2019.

6. Queensland Health. Intravascular device management 2019. Queensland Government, 2019. [updated 24 Dec 2019] Available from: https://www.health.qld.gov.au/clinical-practice/guidelines-procedures/diseases-infection/infection-prevention/intravascular-device-management.

7. Clinical Excellence Commission. Infection prevention and control practice handbook. Sydney: CEC, 2020.

8. Loveday HP, Wilson JA, Pratt RJ, Golsorkhi M, Tingle A, Bak A, et al. Epic3: National evidence-based guidelines for preventing healthcare-associated infections in NHS hospitals in England. J Hosp Infect. 2014;86 Suppl 1:S1-70.

9. Centers for Disease Control and Prevention. Guidelines for the prevention of intravascular catheter-related infections 2011. CDC, 2011. Available from: https://www.cdc.gov/infectioncontrol/guidelines/bsi/recommendations.html.

10. Australian Commission on Safety and Quality in Health Care. Management of peripheral intravenous catheters clinical care standard. Sydney: ACSQHC, 2021.

11. Australian Commission on Safety and Quality in Health Care. National Safety and Quality Health Service (NSQHS) Standards: Preventing and controlling infections standard. Sydney: ACSQHC, 2021.

12. National Health and Medical Research Council, Australian Commission on Safety and Quality in Health Care. Australian guidelines for the prevention and control of infection in healthcare (2019). [cited 31 Aug 2021] Canberra: NHMRC/ACSQHC, 2019.

13. Australian and New Zealand Intensive Care Society. Central line insertion and maintenance guideline 2012. Available from: https://www.anzics.com.au/wp-content/uploads/2018/08/ANZICS_Insertionmaintenance_guideline2012_04.pdf.

14. World Health Organization. Global guidelines for the prevention of surgical site infection 2018. Geneva: WHO, 2009. Available from: https://www.who.int/publications/i/item/global-guidelines-for-the-prevention-of-surgical-site-infection-2nd-ed.

15. Bonsall L. NursingCenter [Internet]. Lippincott, 2015. Available from: https://www.nursingcenter.com/ncblog/february-2015-%281%29/complications-of-peripheral-i-v-therapy.

16. Jackson A. Infection control—a battle in vein: infusion phlebitis. Nursing Times. 1998;94(4):68-71.

17. Leber AL, ed. Clinical microbiology procedures handbook. 4th ed. American Society for Microbiology, 2016.

18. American Society for Microbiology, Manual of clinical microbiology. 12th ed. Washington, DC: ASM Press, 2019.

19. Centers for Disease and Prevention National Healthcare Safety Network, Patient safety component manual, CDC, 2022. Available at https://www.cdc.gov/nhsn/pdfs/pscmanual/pcsmanual_current.pdf.

20. Centers for Disease Control and Prevention. National Healthcare Safety Network (NHSN) Patient safety component manual. Chapter 4: Bloodstream infection event (central line-associated bloodstream infection and non-central line associated bloodstream infection) January 2022. CDC, 2022. Available from: https://www.cdc.gov/nhsn/pdfs/pscmanual/pcsmanual_current.pdf.

21. Brown JD, Chapman S, Ferguson PE. Blood cultures and bacteraemia in an Australian emergency department: evaluating a predictive rule to guide collection and their clinical impact. Emerg Med Australas. 2017;29(1):56-62.

22. Russo PL, Stewardson AJ, Cheng AC, Bucknall T, Mitchell BG. The prevalence of healthcare associated infections among adult inpatients at nineteen large Australian acute-care public hospitals: a point prevalence survey. Antimicrob Resist Infect Control. 2019;8:114.

23. Zarb P, Coignard B, Griskeviciene J, Muller A, Vankerckhoven V, Weist K, et al. The European Centre for Disease Prevention and Control (ECDC) pilot point prevalence survey of healthcare-associated infections and antimicrobial use. Euro Surveill. 2012;17(46).

24. Cai Y, Venkatachalam I, Tee NW, Tan TY, Kurup A, Wong SY, et al. Prevalence of healthcare-associated infections and antimicrobial use among adult inpatients in Singapore acute-care hospitals: results from the first national point prevalence survey. Clin Infect Dis. 2017;64(suppl_2):S61-s7.

25. Cairns S, Gibbons C, Milne A, King H, Llano M, MacDonald L, et al. Results from the third Scottish National Prevalence Survey: is a population health approach now needed to prevent healthcare-associated infections? J Hosp Infect. 2018;99(3):312-317.

26. Magill SS, O'Leary E, Janelle SJ, Thompson DL, Dumyati G, Nadle J, et al. Changes in prevalence of health care-associated infections in U.S. hospitals. N Engl J Med. 2018;379(18): 1732-1744.

27. European Centre for Disease Prevention and Control. Incidence and attributable mortality of healthcare-associated infections in intensive care units in Europe, 2008-2012. Surveillance Report. Stockholm: ECDC, 2018.

28. Lydeamore MJ, Mitchell BG, Bucknall T, Cheng AC, Russo PL, Stewardson AJ. Burden of five healthcare associated infections in Australia. Antimicrob Resist Infect Control. 2022;11(1):69.

29. Dendle C, Martin RD, Cameron DR, Grabsch EA, Mayall BC, Grayson ML, et al. Staphylococcus aureus bacteraemia as a quality indicator for hospital infection control. Med J Aust. 2009;191(7):389-392.

30. Australian Commission on Safety and Quality in Health Care. Surveillance for Staphylococcus aureus bloodstream infection (BSI) 2022. Sydney: ACSQHC, 2020. Available from: www.safetyandquality.gov.au/our-work/infection-prevention-and-control/hai-surveillance/surveillance-staphylococcus-aureus-bloodstream-infection-sabsi.

31. Lee AS, de Lencastre H, Garau J, Kluytmans J, Malhotra-Kumar S, Peschel A, et al. Methicillin-resistant Staphylococcus aureus. Nat Rev Dis Primers. 2018;4:18033.

32. Marshall C, McBryde E. The role of Staphylococcus aureus carriage in the pathogenesis of bloodstream infection. BMC Res Notes. 2014;7:428.

33. Shaban RZ, Li C, O'Sullivan MVN, Kok J, Dempsey K, Ramsperger M, et al. Outbreak of community-acquired Staphylococcus aureus skin infections in an Australian professional football team. J Sci Med Sport. 2021;24(6): 520-525.

34. Holmes NE, Robinson JO, van Hal SJ, Munckhof WJ, Athan E, Korman TM, et al. Morbidity from in-hospital complications is greater than treatment failure in patients with Staphylococcus aureus bacteraemia. BMC Infect Dis. 2018;18(1):107.

35. Davey RX, Tong SYC. The epidemiology of Staphylococcus aureus skin and soft tissue infection in the southern Barkly region of Australia's Northern Territory in 2017. Pathology. 2019;51(3):308-312.

36. Cameron JK, Hall L, Tong SYC, Paterson DL, Halton K. Incidence of community onset MRSA in Australia: least reported where it is most prevalent. Antimicrob Resist Infect Control. 2019;8:33.

37. Macmorran E, Harch S, Athan E, Lane S, Tong S, Crawford L, et al. The rise of methicillin resistant Staphylococcus aureus: now the dominant cause of skin and soft tissue infection in Central Australia. Epidemiol Infect. 2017;145(13):2817-2826.

38. Therapeutic Guidelines: Antibiotic. Melbourne: Therapeutic Guidelines Ltd, 2021.

39. Wu Q, Sabokroo N, Wang Y, Hashemian M, Karamollahi S, Kouhsari E. Systematic review and meta-analysis of the epidemiology of vancomycin-resistance Staphylococcus aureus isolates. Antimicrob. 2021;10(1):101.

40. Australian Institute of Health and Welfare. AIHW, 2022. Available from: www.aihw.gov.au.

41. Australian Institute of Health and Welfare. MyHospitals [Internet]. AIHW, 2020. Available from: https://www.aihw.gov.au/reports-data/myhospitals/my-local-area.

42. Coombs GW, Daley DA, Mowlaboccus S, Lee YT, Pang S. Australian Group on Antimicrobial Resistance (AGAR) Australian Staphylococcus aureus Sepsis Outcome Programme (ASSOP) Annual Report 2018. Commun Dis Intell (2018). 2020;44.

43. Coombs GW, Daley DA, Mowlaboccus S, Pang S. Australian Group on Antimicrobial Resistance (AGAR) Australian Staphylococcus aureus Sepsis Outcome Programme (ASSOP) Annual Report 2019. Commun Dis Intell (2018). 2020;44.

44. Mitchell BG, Collignon PJ, McCann R, Wilkinson IJ, Wells A. A major reduction in hospital-onset Staphylococcus aureus bacteremia in Australia-12 years of progress: an observational study. Clin Infect Dis. 2014;59(7):969-975.

45. Lee XJ, Stewardson AJ, Worth LJ, Graves N, Wozniak TM. Attributable length of stay, mortality risk, and costs of bacterial health care-associated infections in Australia: a retrospective case-cohort study. Clin Infect Dis. 2021; 72(10):e506-e514.

46. Pujol M, Hornero A, Saballs M, Argerich MJ, Verdaguer R, Cisnal M, et al. Clinical epidemiology and outcomes of peripheral venous catheter-related bloodstream infections at a university-affiliated hospital. J Hosp Infect. 2007;67(1):22-29.

47. Krishnan A, Irani K, Swaminathan R, Boan P. A retrospective study of tunnelled haemodialysis central line-associated bloodstream infections. J Chemother. 2019;31(3):132-136.

48. Clinical Excellence Commission. Healthcare associated infection (HAI) Clinical indicator manual - Version 3.3 - September 2021. Sydney: CEC, 2021.

49. American College of Surgeons. Understanding your central line (CVAD) 2022. [Internet] Available from: https://www.facs.org/media/2tcnbb4f/understanding_your_central_line.pdf.

50. Rhodes D, Cheng AC, McLellan S, Guerra P, Karanfilovska D, Aitchison S, et al. Reducing Staphylococcus aureus bloodstream infections associated with peripheral intravenous cannulae: successful implementation of a care bundle at a large Australian health service. J Hosp Infect. 2016;94(1):86-91.

51. Smith RN, Nolan JP. Central venous catheters. BMJ. 2013; 347:f6570.

52. Grayson ML, Stewardson AJ, Russo PL, Ryan KE, Olsen KL, Havers SM, et al. Effects of the Australian National Hand Hygiene Initiative after 8 years on infection control practices, health-care worker education, and clinical outcomes: a longitudinal study. Lancet Infect Dis. 2018; 18(11):1269-1277.

53. Australian Commission on Safety and Quality in Health Care. National Hand Hygiene Initiative 2022. Sydney; ACSQHC, 2022. Available from: https://www.safetyandquality.gov.au/our-work/infection-prevention-and-control/national-hand-hygiene-initiative.

54. Mitchell BG, Hall L, White N, Barnett AG, Halton K, Paterson DL, et al. An environmental cleaning bundle and health-care-associated infections in hospitals (REACH): a multicentre, randomised trial. Lancet Infect Dis. 2019;19(4):410-418.

55. Thomas C, Cabilan CJ, Johnston ANB. Peripheral intravenous cannula insertion and use in a tertiary hospital emergency department: a cross-sectional study. Australas Emerg Care. 2020;23(3):166-172.

56. Bruno M, Brennan D, Redpath MB, Bowens G, Murphy J, Love B, et al. Peripheral-venous-catheter-related Staphylococcus aureus bacteraemia: a multi-factorial approach to reducing incidence. J Hosp Infect. 2011;79(2):173-174.

57. Kok J, O'Sullivan MV, Gilbert GL. Feedback to clinicians on preventable factors can reduce hospital onset Staphylococcus aureus bacteraemia rates. J Hosp Infect. 2011;79(2):108-114.

58. Freixas N, Bella F, Limón E, Pujol M, Almirante B, Gudiol F. Impact of a multimodal intervention to reduce bloodstream infections related to vascular catheters in non-ICU wards: a multicentre study. Clin Microbiol Infect. 2013;19(9): 838-844.

59. Lai NM, Chaiyakunapruk N, Lai NA, O'Riordan E, Pau WS, Saint S. Catheter impregnation, coating or bonding for reducing central venous catheter-related infections in adults. Cochrane Database Syst Rev. 2016;3(3):Cd007878.

60. Raad, II, Hohn DC, Gilbreath BJ, Suleiman N, Hill LA, Bruso PA, et al. Prevention of central venous catheter-related infections by using maximal sterile barrier precautions during insertion. Infect Control Hosp Epidemiol. 1994;15(4 Pt 1): 231-238.

61. Australian and New Zealand Intensive Care Society. Central line insertion checklist 2018. Sydney: ACSQHC, 2018. Available from: https://www.anzics.com.au/wp-content/uploads/2018/08/ANZICS-Central-Line-Insertion-Checklist.pdf.

62. Queensland Health. Recommendations for the prevention of infection in intra-vascular devices. [cited December 2019] Brisbane: Queensland Government, 2019.

63. Slater K, Fullerton F, Cooke M, Snell S, Rickard CM. Needleless connector drying time-how long does it take? Am J Infect Control. 2018;46(9):1080-1081.

64. Ray-Barruel G, Polit DF, Murfield JE, Rickard CM. Infusion phlebitis assessment measures: a systematic review. J Eval Clin Pract. 2014;20(2):191-202.

65. Ray-Barruel G, Cooke M, Chopra V, Mitchell M, Rickard CM. The I-DECIDED clinical decision-making tool for peripheral intravenous catheter assessment and safe removal: a clinimetric evaluation. BMJ Open. 2020; 10(1):e035239.

66. Queensland Health. Appendix 7 - Staphylococcus aureus bloodstream investigation checklist. Recommendations for the prevention of infection in intra-vascular devices 2019. Brisbane: Queensland Government, 2019.

CHAPTER 21

Gastrointestinal infections

Dr CHONG WEI ONG[i,ii]

Chapter highlights

- *Clostridioides difficile* is the most common infectious cause of healthcare-associated diarrhoea, followed by noroviruses. Both can occur sporadically or as part of outbreaks
- Although *C. difficile* infection (CDI) has traditionally been considered healthcare-associated, there is increasing recognition of community-associated CDI, some of which is imported into healthcare facilities
- Prevention and control of CDI in healthcare facilities involves antimicrobial stewardship, timely diagnosis, implementation of contact precautions and rigorous environmental cleaning and disinfection with sporicidal agents
- Noroviruses are a leading cause of gastroenteritis outbreaks in healthcare facilities, have a low infectious dose, can persist in the environment for long periods and are relatively resistant to many disinfectants
- Prevention and control of norovirus in healthcare facilities involves timely diagnosis, implementation of contact precautions (with droplet precautions added if indicated) and rigorous environmental cleaning and disinfection
- Rotavirus infection incidence in the community and healthcare settings has diminished markedly since the implementation of national vaccination programs

i   Canberra Health Services, Canberra, ACT
ii Calvary Public Hospital Bruce, Canberra, ACT

Introduction

Healthcare-associated diarrhoea (HCAD) is a common complication in hospitalised patients. Unlike community and outbreak-associated diarrhoea, non-infectious causes predominate. The cause is often multifactorial, including medications, enteral nutrition and underlying disease processes (e.g. inflammatory bowel disease, diverticular disease, graft-versus-host disease).[1] Although clinicians focus on *Clostridioides difficile* infection (CDI), clinical studies indicate that 12–32% of hospitalised patients develop diarrhoea but ≤20% of cases are attributable to CDI.[2]

Amongst infectious causes of HCAD, CDI is by far the most common cause, but only accounts for 4–25% of HCAD cases.[1] Norovirus is the most common infectious cause of non-*C. difficile* hospital onset diarrhoea.[3] Other infectious causes of hospital onset diarrhoea include rotavirus (and other viruses), and very rarely community-acquired pathogens such as enterotoxigenic *Escherichia coli* and *Salmonella* spp.[1] Although toxigenic strains of *Klebsiella oxytoca*, *Clostridium perfringens* and *Staphylococcus aureus* have been implicated in antibiotic-associated diarrhoea,[4] data are limited, diagnostic testing is generally not readily available, and their risk of nosocomial transmission causing outbreaks is not well defined. The contribution of these to the total healthcare-associated infection (HAI) burden within Australia is uncertain. Healthcare-associated outbreaks of parasitic infection have been reported,[5] but mainly from developing countries, and their significance in the Australian context is also uncertain.

Each year, patients in Australia experience a large number of hospital-acquired gastrointestinal (GI) infections, with 2863 occurring in public hospitals in 2015–16 (rate 6.42 per 10,000 hospitalisations).[6] These cause significant morbidity and prolong hospital length of stay. The Australian Guidelines for the Prevention and Control of Infection in Healthcare summarise the necessary actions required for managing patients in healthcare facilities who have various GI infections.[7]

This chapter primarily focuses on the two most common infectious causes of healthcare-associated diarrhoea—*C. difficile* and noroviruses, with a brief section on rotaviruses. Although healthcare-associated cases of infection with *Salmonella* spp.,[8] *Shigella* spp.,[9] *Campylobacter* spp.,[10] *Listeria* spp.[11] and hepatitis A[12] have been documented, these are now infrequent causes of HAI in developed countries and generally represent community-associated or foodborne infections imported into healthcare facilities, with very limited transmission in healthcare settings. Therefore, they are not covered in this text.

21.1 Clostridioides difficile

21.1.1 Background

Clostridioides (formerly *Clostridium*) *difficile* is a leading cause of healthcare-associated infections (HAIs) and an important public health threat, having been associated with substantial morbidity and mortality worldwide. Increasingly, cases are recognised among individuals of all ages beyond the traditionally recognised at-risk groups (e.g. elderly, hospitalised patients, or those having antimicrobial therapy).[13] In 2017, nearly 223,900 people in the United States (US) alone required hospital care for *C. difficile* and at least 12,800 people died.[14] Though the global healthcare costs associated with CDI are not known, these are likely to be substantial, with 2016 estimates suggesting attributable costs in the US alone of US$6.3 billion per year and total US annual hospital management requiring nearly 2.4 million inpatient days.[15] A recent systematic review and meta-analysis suggested that CDI accounts for increased hospital length of stay ranging from 3.0 to 21.6 days.[16] Key highlights related to CDI are shown in Box 21.1.

21.1.2 Epidemiology

In 1978, *C. difficile* was identified as the causative pathogen in the majority of cases of antibiotic-associated diarrhoea and the nearly exclusive cause of pseudomembranous

---

BOX 21.1 CDI

- *Clostridiodes difficile* is acquired through ingestion of spores transmitted from other patients through the hands of healthcare personnel or the environment
- *C. difficile* infection (CDI) is defined as the presence of symptoms plus positive stool microbiological test results—either one alone is insufficient for diagnosis
- Antibiotic use is the most widely recognised risk factor for CDI, but many others exist
- Apart from antibiotic cessation, the mainstay of CDI treatment comprises specific antibiotics targeting the organism
- Prevention and control of CDI in healthcare facilities involves antimicrobial stewardship, timely diagnosis, implementation of contact precautions and rigorous environmental cleaning and disinfection with sporicidal agents

colitis (PMC), with clindamycin implicated in many early cases.[17] From 2001 onwards, CDI was observed in North America and Europe to be more frequent, severe, refractory to standard therapy, and more likely to relapse than previously described.[17,18] This was attributed to a marked increase in a previously uncommon strain of *C. difficile* with variations in toxin genes,[18] variously designated North American pulsed-field type 1 (NAP1), restriction endonuclease analysis group BI, and PCR ribotype 027 (sometimes also referred to as BI/NAP1/027).[19] Prior to the year 2000, strains with this typing profile had accounted for fewer than 1% of US *C. difficile* isolates.[18] This strain appeared hypervirulent, causing higher rates of severe disease and more deaths.[20] In one study, the attributable mortality from nosocomial CDI was 16.7%.[21] CDI caused by ribotype 027 infection was also more likely to relapse.[22] It caused many outbreaks, especially in older persons and in healthcare facilities.[19] Cases have been documented in Australia since 2009.[23]

Another ribotype considered hypervirulent is 078.[24] Since 2005, an increase in the prevalence of CDI due to PCR ribotype 078 has been noticed in The Netherlands.[25] This strain, the predominant strain in pigs and calves, causes disease of similar severity to ribotype 027. However, compared to disease caused by ribotype 027, CDI due to ribotype 078 affects a younger population and is more frequently community-associated. More recently, ribotype 023 has been noted to be emerging as another hypervirulent organism, with severe infections akin to 027 and 078.[26] In Australia, severe CDI has been associated with the previously uncommon ribotype 244, with an outbreak occurring from 2010–2012.[27] Cases were mainly of community-onset.[28]

The total burden of CDI in Australia is uncertain since it is not a public health notifiable disease nationally. The Australian Commission on Safety and Quality in Health Care (ACSQHC) annually monitors the prevalence of CDI diagnoses in Australian public hospitals.[29] Between 2011 and 2016, the average was 4.0 per 10,000 patient days, with average length of stay being 17.7 days and 2.2% of all hospital cases classed as severe.[30]

CDI acquisition was directly attributable to hospital care in 24.9% of separations assigned a CDI diagnosis. More recently, ACSQHC data showed that hospital-diagnosed CDI did not show a clear increasing or decreasing trend overall from 2012–18.[31]

Apart from CDI, asymptomatic colonisation can occur. Healthy adult studies have shown various asymptomatic carriage rates, ranging from 0–17.5%.[32] In hospitalised adults, up to 18% may have asymptomatic *C. difficile* carriage; these patients shed *C. difficile* in stool but do not have diarrhoea or other clinical symptoms.[33] In long-term care facilities, the rate of asymptomatic colonisation may be as high as 51%.[34] These persons serve as a reservoir for environmental contamination. After symptomatic recovery from an episode of CDI, carriage often persists for several weeks.[19] In neonates and infants less than 1 year of age, asymptomatic colonisation is common (up to 90% and 35–40%, respectively) and yet they rarely develop symptomatic CDI.[35,36] By approximately 2–3 years of age, asymptomatic colonisation rates decrease to <5%, similar to rates in non-hospitalised adults. An Australian study which tested 1380 randomly selected asymptomatic hospital patients found that 76 (5.5%) and 28 (2.0%) patients were colonised with toxigenic and non-toxigenic *C. difficile*, respectively.[37]

21.1.3 Risk factors

Antibiotic use is the most widely recognised and modifiable risk factor for CDI.[38–41] It increases the risk for developing CDI by 7- to 10-fold during and up to 1 month after treatment and by approximately 3-fold for 2 months subsequently.[42] CDI usually occurs 5–10 days after commencing antibiotic therapy, although symptoms have been described as early as 2 days and as late as 10 weeks after antibiotic treatment.[43] Antibiotics disrupt the barrier function of the normal colonic microbiota, providing a niche for *C. difficile* to multiply and elaborate toxins.[44] Although any antibiotic can predispose to colonisation by *C. difficile*, the most frequently implicated include fluoroquinolones, clindamycin and broad-spectrum beta-lactams.[45] Use of broad-spectrum antimicrobials, multiple antibiotic agents and increased treatment duration all contribute to the incidence of CDI.[46,47]

Advanced age is associated with CDI frequency and severity. In a 2002 Quebec outbreak, the frequency of CDI among persons ≥65 years was 10-fold higher than that observed in younger adults.[21]

Other established risk factors for CDI include hospitalisation and severe comorbid illness.[41,48] Additional risk factors include enteral tube feeding, gastrointestinal surgery, cancer chemotherapy, hematopoietic stem cell or solid organ transplantation, inflammatory bowel disease, cirrhosis, chronic kidney disease and gastric acid suppression therapy.[17,41,49,50]

21.1.4 Healthcare-associated infection (HA-CDI)

In 1986, the first prospective case control study of CDI was published and showed 87% of 149 cases to be healthcare-associated (and hospital-acquired).[51]

However, about 20% of control patients were also identified as asymptomatic carriers. Transmission of *C. difficile* occurs in hospital, as evidenced by a study showing that admission of asymptomatic patients carrying *C. difficile* in their stool preceded the acquisition of that specific strain by other patients on the same ward in 84% of instances.[52] Prior hospitalisation in the preceding 30 days was also shown to be a risk factor for *C. difficile* carriage detected at admission, suggesting acquisition from hospital is likely. In 2007, the US Centers for Disease Control and Prevention (CDC) proposed a surveillance definition for hospital-acquired *C. difficile*-associated disease (CDAD), where symptom onset occurred >48 hours after hospital admission in a patient with diarrhoea or toxic megacolon combined with a positive laboratory assay result and/or endoscopic or histopathologic evidence of PMC.[53]

21.1.5 Community-associated infection (CA-CDI)

Community-acquired CDI was first described in the 1980s in patients who received antibiotics in the outpatient setting.[54] In 2007, the CDC proposed a surveillance definition for community-acquired CDAD, where symptom onset occurred in the community or ≤48 hours after admission to a healthcare institution (provided that symptom onset was more than 12 weeks after the last discharge from a healthcare institution).[53] Similar to HA-CDI, the patient had to have symptoms of diarrhoea or toxic megacolon combined with a positive laboratory assay result and/or endoscopic or histopathologic evidence of PMC. Although previously thought to be uncommon, CA-CDI cases have been increasing in the last two decades, particularly in patient populations previously thought to be at lower risk, including younger patients and those without prior antibiotic exposure.[55] In the US, approximately half of all CDI cases originate in the community.[56] Of the community-associated cases, over 80% are estimated to be associated with outpatient health care exposure.[57] A recent review of 39 studies found that the incidence of community-acquired CDI has almost doubled in the past decade.[58] Approximately half of all CDI cases were attributed to community origin. Individuals who were younger, female, in the presence of infants, frequently used proton pump inhibitors or specific classes of antibiotics, or lived near farms and livestock were at higher risk for community-acquired CDI. Additionally, approximately 40% of all community-acquired cases required

hospitalisation, where severity was linked to hyper-virulent ribotypes 027 and 078 with poor outcomes. Although CDI is most commonly associated with antibiotic exposure, a US study of almost 1000 CA-CDI cases found that found that 36% of cases had no documented prior use of antibiotics.[59] Further, 18% of cases had no outpatient healthcare exposure, and 41% only had low-level outpatient exposure. The importation of CA-CDI cases into the hospital has been implicated in potentially maintaining HA-CDI transmission.[60] However, more recently, a US study of 40 CA-CDI cases (defined as testing positive for stool toxin either with no previous hospital admission or greater than 12 weeks following discharge) found that 100% had some history of hospitalisation if the timeframe considered was the prior 12 months rather than 12 weeks, and this was supported by genomic analysis, suggesting that even CA-CDI may possibly have nosocomial origins.[61]

21.1.6 Microbiology and pathogenesis

C. difficile is an anaerobic Gram-positive, spore-forming bacillus first described in 1935.[62] It was named 'difficult clostridium' because of difficulty related to its isolation and growth on conventional media.

C. difficile strains have the potential to release two exotoxins that mediate colitis and diarrhoea: toxin A and toxin B. Toxin B is a major factor for the virulence of *C. difficile* and is over 10 times more potent than toxin A for causing colonic mucosal damage.[63] *C. difficile* diarrhoea is mediated by genes for toxin A (tcdA) and toxin B (tcdB), which inactivate members of the Rho family of guanosine triphosphatases, leading to colonocyte death, loss of intestinal barrier function, and neutrophilic colitis.[64] A minority of *C. difficile* clinical isolates are non-toxigenic and considered non-pathogenic.[65] The new epidemic strain, ribotype 027, was resistant to fluroquinolones, produced a binary toxin and increased quantities of toxins A and B.[17]

C. difficile can exist in spore (in the environment) and vegetative (in the intestine) forms. Spores are resistant to heat, acid, many disinfectants and antibiotics. After ingestion, spores survive the acid environment of the stomach, germinate on exposure to bile in the small intestine and proliferate in, and colonise or infect, the colon.[66] These vegetative, toxin-producing forms cause the illness CDI, but also become susceptible to antimicrobial agents. However, toxigenic *C. difficile* can sometimes colonise the gut without causing CDI.

21.1.7 Clostridioides difficile transmission

C. difficile is a ubiquitous organism, able to survive for long periods in the environment through spore formation. *C. difficile* is present in diverse environmental sites such as surface water, drinking water, swimming pools and soil, and in a wide variety of animals, including dogs, cats, horses, sheep and pigs.[67] Humans probably ingest *C. difficile* spores frequently, but remain asymptomatic and uncolonised as a result of the colonisation resistance of an intact gut microbiota.[39]

C. difficile is acquired through ingestion of spores usually transmitted from other patients through the hands of healthcare personnel or the environment.[41,68] Spores can persist on environmental surfaces or equipment for months and place patients at risk.[69] The hospital environment, healthcare worker hands and patients' home environment have all been shown to be contaminated by *C. difficile* spores.[70] The organism can be cultured readily from items and inert surfaces in patient rooms as well as the hands, clothing and stethoscopes of healthcare workers[70,71] and is transmitted readily between patients.[72] CDI patients are a reservoir for environmental contamination and transmission of infection to others, regardless of whether toxin is detected by enzyme immunoassay in stool.[73] Asymptomatic carriers of toxigenic *C. difficile* are also capable of transmitting *C. difficile*, resulting in CDI in others.[74] However, a whole genome sequencing study found that transmission is more likely to occur from patients with CDI than from patients with asymptomatic colonisation.[75]

In the past, it has been thought that CDI is transmitted predominantly within healthcare settings from symptomatic patients. However, genetically diverse sources, in addition to symptomatic patients, play a major part in *C. difficile* transmission.[76] A review of 24 studies specifically reporting on sources of CDI and specific transmission pathways within and/or beyond healthcare facilities found that contact with symptomatic carriers (53%), the hospital environment (40%) and asymptomatic carriers (20%) were the most commonly reported transmission pathways within healthcare settings (total 15 studies), while the leading sources for acquisition of *C. difficile* in the community (total 11 studies) included direct contact with symptomatic and asymptomatic carriers in the community, including infants (30%) and residents of long-term non–acute care facilities (30%), followed by contact with contaminated environments in outpatient care settings (20%) and exposure to livestock or farms (20%).[68]

21.1.8 Clinical features and complications

The clinical spectrum of *C. difficile* ranges from asymptomatic colonisation, mild and self-limiting disease, to a severe, life-threatening PMC, toxic megacolon, sepsis syndrome and death.[32]

As opposed to asymptomatic carriage, CDI can be defined as the presence of typical clinical features of bowel inflammation (e.g. diarrhoea, ileus, toxic megacolon) plus either evidence of the presence of toxin-producing *C. difficile* in faecal samples or PMC on colonoscopy.[40] The period between initial colonisation with *C. difficile* and the occurrence of CDI (i.e., incubation period) is not well-defined. Earlier studies estimated it to be a median of 2–3 days[77] but a more recent study suggests that it is greater than 1 week, ranging between 8–28 days.[78] In patients who develop CDI due to antibiotics, symptoms can occur concurrently with antibiotic initiation or even several weeks after antibiotic discontinuation.[39]

Watery diarrhoea ($\geq$3 loose stools in 24 hours) is the cardinal symptom of CDI,[40,79] but may occasionally be bloody.[80] Other manifestations include lower abdominal pain, fever, nausea, anorexia and tenesmus.[39,41] CDI may also present with unexplained peripheral blood leucocytosis $> 15 \times 10^9$/L in hospitalised patients (even in the absence of diarrhoea at the time of leucocytosis).[81] Diarrhoea subsequently develops in most cases. Lower GI endoscopy, if performed, may demonstrate colonic abnormalities, ranging from oedema, erythema, friability and ulceration to PMC, which is a hallmark of CDI.[39,41,82] In some cases, CDI presents with ileus, where the bowel motility is diminished and radiological signs of bowel distension are seen. Ileus is often associated with more severe disease or even fulminant colitis.[39,41,82] Such patients may have little or no diarrhoea, and should not be mistaken for someone with mild CDI or resolving CDI. In rare instances, CDI may present with protein-losing enteropathy (in the absence of fulminant colitis),[83] appendicitis,[84] small bowel enteritis[85] or other extra-intestinal manifestations such as cellulitis, soft tissue infection, bacteraemia, and reactive arthritis.[86–88]

Complications of the most severe forms of CDI include hypotension or shock, the development of toxic megacolon, intestinal perforation and acute peritonitis.[39] ICU admission may be required for multi-organ failure. Surgery may also be required, including colectomy.

In practice, it is important to distinguish between non-severe and severe CDI since this influences treatment decisions. Within the Australian context, for clinical purposes, severe CDI is defined as an episode of CDI with one or more features listed in Box 21.2.[40,82] There is no consensus definition of disease severity for CDI for children.[40]

Defining recurrent and refractory CDI is also important for making decisions regarding treatment. Recurrent CDI is defined as CDI re-occurring within 8 weeks of the onset of a previous episode which had resolution of symptoms.[40] It has also been defined as complete abatement of CDI symptoms while on appropriate therapy, followed by reappearance of symptoms within 2–8 weeks after treatment has been stopped.[41] Recurrent CDI results from the same or a different *C. difficile* strain but in clinical practice it is impossible to distinguish relapse from new infection.[89] Diagnosis and management do not differ between these.[41] Refractory CDI is defined as failure to demonstrate clinical improvement following 3–4 days of recommended therapy.[40]

21.1.9 Diagnosis

CDI cannot be distinguished clinically from other causes of acute diarrhoea without laboratory testing to identify the presence of toxin or toxin-producing organisms in the faeces.[40] Conversely, laboratory testing cannot distinguish between asymptomatic colonisation and symptomatic infection with *C. difficile*.[90] Therefore, the diagnosis of CDI usually requires a combination of clinical assessment and laboratory testing.

CDI should be suspected in any hospitalised patient who develops acute diarrhoea or any person in the community who develops acute diarrhoea after a course of antibiotics or in association with immunosuppressive therapy, where there is no alternative explanation (e.g. laxative use).[41,43]

Testing should only be performed on unformed stools, because a positive result from formed stool only signifies colonisation rather than CDI.[41,43,91] Suitable faecal samples are those that are liquid or soft (i.e. take the shape of the container).[41] When ileus is present, rectal swabs are suitable specimens.[43,92,93]

In addition to clinician-initiated testing, Australian laboratories are advised to initiate *C. difficile* testing on stool specimens from all hospitalised patients over the age of 2 with diarrhoea occurring ≥48 hours or >72 hours after admission, irrespective of the physician's request.[40,91,94,95] A Dutch study showed that this increased the number of patients diagnosed with CDI by 33%.[96]

In patients with negative results, repeat testing of faecal specimens (by enzyme immunoassay [EIA] for toxin A and B or nucleic acid amplification for toxin genes) within 7 days should not be performed as it does not increase the diagnostic yield significantly.[41,97]

There has been considerable debate over the best laboratory methods for testing for CDI. At present, there is still no definite international consensus on which is the single best gold standard test nor which is the optimal method for CDI diagnosis.[39,41,98,99]

Broadly speaking, there are five test types, as summarised in Table 21.1.

Cell cytotoxicity neutralisation assay (CCNA) [also known as cell cytotoxicity assay (CCTA) or cell culture cytotoxicity neutralisation assay (CCCNA)]: CCNA, historically considered the gold standard test, is now considered to lack sufficient sensitivity to be the gold standard for assay comparison studies. Compared to toxigenic culture, it has sensitivity of approximately 75–85%.[100] *C. difficile* toxin is detected when stool filtrate applied to a cell monolayer causes a cytopathic effect which can be neutralised with specific

TABLE 21.1 Summary of available tests for *Clostridioides difficile* infection

Test	Sensitivity	Specificity	Substance detected	Comments
Toxigenic culture	Very high	Low [Moderate if coupled with a toxin production test]	Toxigenic *C. difficile* vegetative cells or spores	The more sensitive of two gold standards compared with cell cytotoxicity; positive result does not prove toxin production *in vivo*
Nucleic acid amplification tests	Very high	Low to moderate	*C. difficile* nucleic acid (toxin genes)	Positive result does not prove toxin production *in vivo*
Glutamate dehydrogenase enzyme immunoassay	High	Low	*C. difficile* common antigen	Positive result requires another test to distinguish between toxigenic and non-toxigenic *C. difficile*; not adequate as stand-alone test for CDI due to low specificity
Cell cytotoxicity neutralisation assay	Moderate to high	Very high	Free toxins	The less sensitive of two gold standards compared with toxigenic culture
Toxin A and B enzyme immunoassays	Low to high [Variable sensitivity – generally considered low]	High	Free toxins	Not adequate as stand-alone test for CDI due to variable sensitivity

anti-toxin.[101] CCNA has fallen out of favour as a routine diagnostic test due to inadequate sensitivity, relatively prolonged turnaround time, and the requirement for expertise in maintenance of cell cultures and interpretation of results.[98]

Toxigenic culture (TC): Toxigenic culture (TC) is considered a newer gold standard test.[39,77,100] It involves isolating the organism from faecal specimens and then determining if the cultured isolate is a strain capable of producing toxin by using other methods (e.g. CCNA, immunoassay or NAAT), since non-toxigenic strains exist.[91,98] Detection in a stool sample, however, does not necessarily imply toxin production *in vivo* (i.e. in the patient) at the time of sample collection.[98] TC has a long turnaround time and requires specific technical expertise. However, culture enables typing of isolates and antibiotic susceptibility testing.[100]

Toxin enzyme immunoassays (EIA): Enzyme immunoassays for *C. difficile* toxin use antibodies to detect toxin A and/or B presence in stool samples. These assays are less expensive, less labour intensive, have a much quicker turn-around time than CCNA or TC[98] and have relatively high specificity, but have been considered to have variable[98] or low sensitivity compared to CCNA or TC.[102,103] Thus toxin EIAs

should not be considered adequate stand–alone tests for the diagnosis of CDI.[43,74,98,104] However, when combined with a sensitive screening test such as a GDH assay, and/or a NAAT, they provide evidence of *C. difficile toxin* production *in vivo* (when testing faecal specimens) or *in vitro* (when testing isolates).[91]

Glutamate dehydrogenase (GDH) immunoassays: Glutamate dehydrogenase (GDH) is a metabolic enzyme produced at high levels in all isolates of *C. difficile* both toxigenic and non–toxigenic strains.[98] There are many different EIAs for GDH detection. They are generally considered very sensitive for presence of *C. difficile*. However, positive faecal specimens must always be followed up with a confirmatory test, such as a toxin EIA or a molecular test for toxin genes, in order to detect toxigenicity. GDH EIAs are not specific for *C. difficile*[39] and can cross-react with *C. sordellii*.[98]

Nucleic acid amplification tests (NAAT): These molecular assays detect conserved gene targets within the pathogenicity locus of *C. difficile*, including the gene(s) responsible for toxin production, often *tcdB*, but also *tcdA,* or both.[91,98] The methodology used for NAAT is generally polymerase chain reaction (PCR) or loop-mediated isothermal amplification (LAMP).[39] These tests appear to be very sensitive and specific for toxigenic *C. difficile* presence in stool.[39,41,91] NAAT is considered to be the most sensitive, rapid single test, but can be considered costly relative to EIA.[39] Like TC, they detect toxigenic *C. difficile* in stool but not necessarily *in vivo* toxin production.[39,91,98]

Multi-step testing

Many laboratories do not utilise CCNA and TC in routine diagnostics due to the expense, expertise and logistics required, as well as the slow turn-around time.

The GDH EIA and toxin EIA tests are unsuitable to be used alone due to issues with specificity and sensitivity, respectively. Therefore, various multi-step test algorithms have been recommended and are in use.[40,92,94,98] These often combine a screening test with high sensitivity (e.g. GDH EIA, NAAT) with a subsequent test of high specificity for CDI (e.g. toxin-EIA, CCNA, NAAT).[92,98]

Although NAAT has been used as a single test for CDI, the increased rate of CDI diagnosis by NAAT has led some investigators to question whether NAAT is too sensitive as a stand-alone test.[105] Studies have shown that patients diagnosed by NAAT alone had less CDI-related morbidity and mortality than those using a multi-step algorithm that included toxin-detection.[106,107] The critical question is whether patients diagnosed by NAAT alone (without toxin detected) require treatment. They either have mild CDI (that may or may not require treatment) or are carriers with diarrhoea due to another cause (who require no treatment but should be isolated nonetheless because they may transmit *C. difficile*).

Interpretation of test results: Treating clinicians and infection control practitioners (ICPs) should be familiar with interpreting *C. difficile* laboratory reports, so that relevant actions can be taken. The three key points to remember are:

1. patients who are toxin EIA positive are likely to have CDI

2. patients who are NAAT (i.e. toxin gene) positive but toxin EIA negative may or may not have CDI

3. patients who are only GDH EIA positive alone are very unlikely to have CDI.

These are summarised in Table 21.2.

Non-microbiological diagnostic investigations: Findings of PMC on endoscopic or histologic examination are highly suggestive of CDI, even though colonoscopy is not routinely requested in

suspected CDI.[39] Suggestive radiographic features include dilatation of the large bowel without involvement of the small bowel and thickening of the bowel wall (including the 'accordion' sign and 'double-halo' sign associated with submucosal oedema).[108]

21.1.10 Treatment

General measures: General treatment measures include:[82]

- discontinuation of unnecessary antimicrobial therapy
  - before effective treatment for CDI was known, stopping the offending antibiotic resulted in symptom resolution in 20–25% of patients[39]
- adequate replacement of fluid and electrolytes
- potential avoidance of anti-motility medications
  - antimotility agents (e.g. loperamide, opiates) have traditionally been avoided due to potential for worsening CDI,[109] especially in the absence of specific therapy, but the evidence that they cause harm is equivocal, so the addition of an antimotility agent as an adjunct to specific antibacterial therapy for CDI may be safe, although no prospective or randomised studies are available[110]
- reviewing proton pump inhibitor use and ceasing if possible. [40,104,111]

Specific therapy: The mainstay of specific treatment comprises antibiotics active against *C. difficile*, with selection dependent on CDI severity and whether the episode is classified as initial, recurrent or refractory. For details, readers are referred to specific recommendations published by the Australasian Society of Infectious Diseases[40] or jointly by the Infectious Diseases Society of America (IDSA) and Society for Healthcare Epidemiology of America (SHEA).[41] Therapeutic success should not be based on repeat stool testing, as asymptomatic carriage of *C. difficile* at 30 days post-treatment has been estimated at 25–30%.[40]

Faecal microbiota transplantation (FMT) and other microbial replacement therapies: Since CDI results from antibiotic-induced disruption of the normal gut microbiome enabling *C. difficile* colonisation and infection, it has been thought that microbial replacement therapies may help combat CDI. FMT has been the primary method for providing microbial

TABLE 21.2 Interpretation of *C. difficile* test results in patients with compatible clinical symptoms

GDH EIA	TOXIN EIA [or CCNA]	NAAT [or TC]	Interpretation	Clinical management	Infection control management
POS or not performed	NEG	NEG	No toxigenic *C. difficile* present; CDI highly unlikely	No clear indication for treatment	Transmission-based precautions not required
Not performed	Not performed	NEG	No toxigenic *C. difficile* present; CDI highly unlikely	No clear indication for treatment	Transmission-based precautions not required
POS	POS	POS or not performed	Toxigenic *C. difficile* present and toxin being produced; CDI very likely	Treat for CDI	Transmission-based precautions required
Not performed	POS	POS or not performed	Toxigenic *C. difficile* present and toxin being produced; CDI very likely	Treat for CDI	Transmission-based precautions required
POS or not performed	NEG	POS	Toxigenic *C. difficile* present but no evidence of toxin being produced; CDI is possible but not confirmed, patient could be merely colonised	Assess for other causes of diarrhoea in a patient with toxigenic *C. difficile* colonisation; consider treating for CDI if clinical situation warrants or if toxin EIA result is suspected to be false negative	Transmission-based precautions advisable since patient is colonised with toxigenic *C. difficile* and could be a reservoir for spread

NEG = negative and POS = positive

replacement therapy for treating recurrent CDI.[112] It involves the transfer of microbiota from a healthy donor to an unwell patient, usually involving donor faeces. FMT from a healthy donor counteracts the infection susceptibility by recovering the natural microbiota in the recipient. Sometimes more than one FMT treatment is required. In general, FMT protocols utilise donor stool suspended in normal saline prior to administration (via colonoscopy, enema, or nasoduodenal/nasojejunal tube). Careful donor screening and selection as well as recipient health evaluation are necessary.[113,114]

In a meta-analysis of trials (both randomised and non-randomised) comparing FMT with placebo or antibiotics for recurrent CDI, the weighted pooled cure rate from randomised controlled trials (RCTs) was 68% for FMT versus 43% for the comparator.[115] However, it was noted that FMT had lower cure rates in RCTs than in open-label and observational studies. FMT cure rates for all included studies ranged from 43–97%.

Although FMT is known to be effective therapy in recurrent CDI, there is limited evidence which

suggests that it is also effective for treating primary CDI.[116,117] Australian consensus statements recommend FMT for patients with recurrent CDI and consideration of FMT in patients with primary, refractory or severe CDI.[113]

Other methods of microbial replacement include capsule-based therapies (containing spores or full-spectrum stool microbiota) and microbial enemas derived from donor stool.[112]

Novel therapies: A host of other novel therapies and preventative strategies for primary and recurrent *C. difficile* infections have been published.[118,119] Readers can refer to the referenced reviews.

21.1.11 Prevention and control

Screening and surveillance: Continuous surveillance of CDI in hospitals is an important quality improvement activity that contributes to safer care for patients and informs strategies to minimise preventable CDI. Surveillance enables monitoring of the occurrence and spread of *C. difficile* in healthcare and the timely detection of outbreaks. Surveillance at jurisdictional and national levels enables detection of changes in epidemiology, identification of populations at risk and characterisation of the molecular epidemiology of CDI strains.

In Australia, national surveillance of hospital-identified CDI captures both community and healthcare-associated events, with cases sub-classified (in some jurisdictions) based on exposure into:[79]

- healthcare-associated, community-onset
- healthcare-associated, healthcare facility-onset
- community-onset
- indeterminate
- unknown.

Transmission-based precautions: Ideally, patients with three or more loose stools within a 24-hour period should be placed under contact precautions in a single room with dedicated toilet facilities but, if unavailable, an alternative is implementing contact precautions within the bed space and allocating a dedicated toilet/bathroom or commode to the patient, with daily cleaning and disinfection using a sporicidal agent.[69] Patient isolation to control *C. difficile* in healthcare facilities is not supported by very strong evidence, with the limited studies suggesting the impact may possibly be greater during outbreaks than with endemic *C. difficile*.[120–122] Australian NHMRC guidelines recommend that patients in healthcare facilities with CDI should be managed under standard plus contact precautions for the duration of their illness.[7] However, the ASID-ACIPC position statement states that contact precautions and isolation must remain in place for a further 48 hours after the last episode of diarrhoea.[69] US guidelines also favour continuation of contact precautions for at least 48 hours after resolution of diarrhoea, although the quality of evidence for this recommendation is low.[41] Continuation of contact precautions beyond resolution of diarrhoea is reasonable since persistent stool shedding of *C. difficile* spores is common and also patients' skin and their environment have been shown to remain contaminated even after diarrhoea cessation.[123] Onset of ileus or toxic megacolon in CDI may be associated with an unexpected reduction in bowel motions. Such patients would still require contact precautions.[69]

Cleaning and disinfection: Consistent environmental cleaning and disinfection should be ensured, since the environment plays a role in *C. difficile* transmission.[124] Spores are resistant to cleaning and disinfection with many currently used agents,[69] especially quaternary ammonium compounds.[125] *C. difficile* contaminated surfaces or fomites should be cleaned and disinfected with a sporicidal agent.[69] Hypochlorite solutions or other chorine-based disinfectants are often recommended.[7,69] High levels of chlorine (5000 mg/L free chlorine) have been shown to have consistent efficacy against *C. difficile* spores, but lower levels (e.g. 1000 and 3000 mg/L free chlorine) have variable efficacy.[126] Newer products such as peracetic acid and accelerated hydrogen peroxide-containing agents also have sporicidal activity, but chlorine dioxide appears to be less active.[127,128]

Ideally, patient care equipment, such as thermometers, blood pressure cuffs, wheelchairs and stethoscopes, should be dedicated to each patient with *C. difficile* and any shared patient care equipment should be cleaned and disinfected after being used by each patient.[69]

No-touch disinfection technologies such as UV light (UVL) and hydrogen peroxide vapour (HPV) may be used as adjuncts to routine cleaning and disinfection.[129] However, their exact role needs to be better defined. UVL has been shown in a systematic review to decrease CDI.[130] A cluster randomised trial showed that adding UVL to standard cleaning strategies did reduce CDI, but adding UVL to bleach cleaning did not reduce CDI incidence.[131] A more recent study showed CDI rates did not decrease when UVL was implemented in hospitals with low baseline rates and high manual cleaning compliance.[132] HPV has been associated with greater reduction in spore forming organisms than UVL.[133] However, the above systematic review did not show that HPV decreases CDI rates.[130] The ASID-ACIPC position statement advises users to choose only devices with demonstrated bactericidal and sporicidal capabilities and preferably one that has been shown to reduce hospital-associated infections.[69]

Improving cleaning alone, without other measures, may not be sufficient to control HA-CDI. One multi-centre randomised trial, which compared standard cleaning to enhanced cleaning (that included monitoring of environmental services personnel performance by fluorescent marker and environmental cultures) demonstrated that an enhanced cleaning program improved the thoroughness and effectiveness of cleaning but did not reduce the incidence of HA-CDI.[134] A separate systematic review also found that implementation of environmental cleaning bundles was able to increase removal of surface markers and decrease the percentage of positive *C. difficile* cultures, but had no effect on CDI incidence rates.[135]

Hand hygiene: Although evidence exists that alcohol-based handrub (ABHR) is not very active against *C. difficile* spores,[136] and that soap and water are more effective,[137] studies have not shown an increase in CDI with the use of ABHR during outbreaks.[137,138] Also, ABHR is very active against the vegetative forms of CDI,[136] which predominate over spore forms in stool.[139] The ASID-ACIPC Position statement recommends the primary use of ABHR for hand hygiene when caring for patients with CDI.[69] Australian guidelines recommend that ABHR should be used following glove removal.[7] If gloves have been worn, a lower density of contamination of the hands would be expected and ABHR remains the agent of choice for hand hygiene. However, hands should be washed with soap and water if gloves were not worn or were breached and hands visibly soiled. This facilitates the mechanical removal of spores.

Antimicrobial stewardship (AMS): Modelling studies suggest that CDI incidence would be reduced by effective AMS, both in the in-patient (e.g. acute hospital) and outpatient setting, including long-term care facilities.[140,141] This has also been demonstrated in interventional studies involving restrictions on antimicrobial use.[120,142] AMS has been shown to reduce CDI rates both in healthcare and community settings, even in the absence of implementation of key infection control measures.[143,144] Prevention and control of CDI should include an AMS program that is aimed at minimising the frequency and duration of antibiotic use and promoting a narrow-spectrum antibiotic policy.[69] Since both PPIs and antibiotics are independently associated with CDI, reducing the co-administration of these drugs could be considered as part of AMS programs, and can be effectively achieved by an automated alert system when electronic prescribing is used.[145]

Outbreak control measures: An increase in institutional CDI incidence or unusual clustering of cases on a ward should prompt investigation to determine if an outbreak is occurring. Various steps in an epidemiological investigation of a suspected or proven outbreak are outlined in Box 21.3.[69,146]

Probiotics: A revised Cochrane review of 31 RCTs including 8672 patients found that moderate certainty evidence suggests that probiotics are effective for preventing CDI.[147] However, post hoc subgroup analyses indicated that probiotics are effective among

> **BOX 21.3 Steps in a CDI outbreak investigation and management[69,146]**
>
> 1. Verify diagnosis of all CDI cases by ensuring laboratory confirmation
> 2. Establish the outbreak. Identify that additional cases constitute an outbreak by comparing the number against previous case numbers
> 3. Construct a working case definition. For the purpose of control in the early stages of the outbreak until laboratory confirmation is available for all cases, a case definition may be based on clinical presentation, such as episodes of diarrhoea, and an epidemiological risk factor (e.g. contact of a CDI laboratory-confirmed patient)
> 4. Communicate the outbreak to healthcare facility staff and encourage early reporting of suspected cases
> 5. Search for additional cases, passively through the laboratory and actively with the help of healthcare staff
> 6. Implement control and prevention measures
> 7. Develop and test a hypothesis for the outbreak
> 8. Re-evaluate hypothesis and if found necessary based on data, reconsider/refine and re-evaluate the hypothesis
> 9. Re-evaluate the implementation of control and prevention measures
> 10. Communicate final findings

trials with a CDAD baseline risk >5% but not those with a baseline risk ≤5%. The difficulty in translating this into clinical practice is that 'probiotics' are not a single entity, and it is unclear which probiotic agent has reproducible efficacy in CDI prevention. Moreover, there is also the potential for organisms in probiotic formulations to cause infections in vulnerable patients, including those with bowel inflammation.[148]

While probiotics may be beneficial in some studies, Australian and US guidelines do not recommend probiotic therapy in prevention or adjunctive treatment of CDI due to no definite evidence of benefit and concerns regarding reports of harm.[40,41] In a large RCT of lactobacilli and bifidobacteria as probiotic therapy, there was no demonstrable benefit of this probiotic mixture preventing CDI.[149]

Prevention bundles: Although bundled interventions targeting catheter-associated urinary tract infections (CAUTI) and central line-associated bloodstream infections (CLABSI) have had success in reducing the rates of those device-associated HAIs, the evidence for efficacy of bundled interventions in reducing CDI incidence in the inpatient setting is relatively lacking, given the lack of RCTs of intervention bundles.[150] There are, however, reports of successful use of intervention bundles outside of controlled studies, especially in outbreak settings.[151–153]

CASE STUDY 1

Clostridioides difficile infection

Situation:

Mrs Jackson, aged 67, is hospitalised for community-acquired pneumonia. On day 16 of intravenous ceftriaxone therapy, she develops fever and six episodes of non-bloody diarrhoea. What are your considerations in managing this situation if CDI is suspected?

Answer:

- A stool sample should be sent for *C. difficile* testing
- She should be managed under contact precautions, ideally in a single room with dedicated toilet facilities
- Contact precautions should continue for at least the duration of the illness, although continuing these for at least 48 hours after the last diarrhoeal episode has also been guideline-recommended
- At minimum, daily cleaning and disinfection with a sporicidal agent should be instituted
- Staff and visitors should be reminded to adhere to hand hygiene
- Her medical treating team should be alerted to:
  - consider commencing *C. difficile* specific treatment
  - review her need for ongoing IV antibiotics: given that 16 days is a very long course for pneumonia, input from the hospital AMS service is recommended.

21.2 Noroviruses

21.2.1 Epidemiology

Noroviruses are a leading cause of acute gastroenteritis across all age groups, being associated with 18% of all cases.[154] Worldwide, the World Health Organization (WHO) has estimated that noroviruses annually cause 685 million cases of diarrhoea and 212,489 deaths.[155] Noroviruses are the leading cause of foodborne disease worldwide, but contaminated food is estimated to account for <20% of all norovirus cases, suggesting other modes of transmission are important.[156] Cases may be sporadic or part of outbreaks. Outbreaks occur in closed settings, such as hospitals, hotels, cruise ships, day-care centres and residential aged care institutions as well as retail food and institutional foodservice settings.[157] Norovirus is a leading cause of outbreaks in healthcare institutions. A study of three hospital systems in England from 2002–03 identified 227 outbreaks, with norovirus implicated in 63% of those.[158]

One meta-analysis showed that norovirus prevalence tended to be higher in cases of acute gastroenteritis in community (24%) and outpatient (20%) settings compared with inpatient (17%, p=0·066) settings.[154] The high prevalence of norovirus in the community makes it difficult to prevent introduction into healthcare settings, including long-term and acute care facilities, where infection can spread and result in severe illness.[159] Surveillance data from high-income countries indicate that most outbreaks occur in healthcare facilities.[158] These outbreaks result in significant healthcare costs, disruption of operations and morbidity. In Queensland from May–August 2008, norovirus was the confirmed aetiological agent in 39 (68%) of 60 viral gastroenteritis outbreaks in residential aged care facilities.[160] Norovirus was detected in 52% of gastroenteritis outbreaks surveyed in Victoria in 2016, with 77% of the norovirus outbreaks occurring in healthcare settings.[161] In 2017, NSW Health reported that norovirus accounted for 22 of 29 hospital outbreaks of gastroenteritis with stool collected, and also 140 of 259 aged care outbreaks of gastroenteritis with stool collected, making it the leading pathogen for outbreaks where the aetiologic agent was identified.[162] Key highlights related to norovirus infection are shown in Box 21.4.

21.2.2 Virus

The syndrome of sudden-onset, self-limiting vomiting and diarrhoea, peaking in the colder season in temperate regions, was first described in 1929 and named 'Hyperemesis hemis' or 'winter-vomiting disease'.[163]

BOX 21.4 Norovirus infection

- Norovirus infection results from ingestion of virus particles and causes vomiting and diarrhoea, with virus shedding into these body fluids, which can then contaminate the environment

- Transmission may be foodborne or person to person (due to direct or indirect contact with infected persons or contaminated fomites as well as droplets)

- Although norovirus infection is generally self-limiting, immunocompromised persons can experience chronic infection with prolonged symptoms and virus shedding

- Diagnosis is best established by nucleic acid testing of stool samples

- Prevention and control of norovirus in healthcare facilities involves timely diagnosis, implementation of contact precautions (with droplet precautions added if indicated) and rigorous environmental cleaning and disinfection

In 1972, the causative agent, Norwalk virus, was identified and characterised.[164] Norwalk virus subsequently became the prototypic agent of the genus *Norovirus*, one of five genera within the family Caliciviridae.[165]

Noroviruses are single-stranded, non-enveloped, positive sense RNA viruses ranging from 26 to 34 nm in diameter.[157,165] The genus *Norovirus* consists of a genetically diverse group of viruses associated with acute gastroenteritis in a wide range of mammalian host species that include humans, dogs, cats, pigs, mice, sheep and cattle.[166] Phylogenetically, they can be segregated into different genogroups and further into genotypes based on amino acid sequences of the complete VP1 (major capsid protein) gene. Currently, noroviruses are classified into at least 10 genogroups (GI–GX), which are subdivided into a total of at least 48 genotypes.[166] Human infections are mainly caused by GI, GII and GIV viruses.[165] Point mutations and frequent recombination between strains result in significant genetic diversity, which has implications for laboratory diagnostic tests, natural immunity following infection and vaccine development.[167] Since the mid-1990s, GII.4 viruses have been the predominant circulating strains worldwide. Older variants are replaced by new GII.4 variants every 2–4 years, possibly due to herd immunity.[168,169]

Since 2012 GII.4 Sydney is the most contemporary GII.4 variant.[170] GII.17 emerged and became predominant in many areas in Asia from 2014–16 and was detected in other countries, but its prevalence has declined since then.[171]

Noroviruses may survive freezing, heating to 72 °C, low concentration chlorine disinfection and can persist on surfaces for up to 7 days, enhanced by the presence of organic residue.[172–176]

Human challenge studies have found a low infectious dose for this virus, implying that it is highly infectious.[177,178] However, the precise dose is not certain due to differences in estimated infectivity by different mathematical dose-response models.[179] In addition, infectivity and pathogenicity depend on host and pathogen factors. For example, histo-blood group antigen secretor-negative status in humans appears protective for infection. Also, the estimated infection risk is higher for GI than GII.[179]

21.2.3 Transmission

The faecal-oral route is the main mode of transmission.[180] Human challenge study subjects develop symptoms of disease after oral ingestion of virus and then shed virus in both faeces and vomitus.[181] Persons can become infected by ingestion of contaminated food or water, contact with contaminated environmental surfaces or contact with infected persons (i.e. person-to-person transmission).[182] Contaminated water includes both drinking water as well as recreational water (e.g. lakes, swimming pools).[157] Contaminated food includes uncooked or undercooked foods (e.g. shellfish, cake frosting, salads, meats) as well as previously cooked food subsequently contaminated by an infected food handler's hands. Environmental contact and person-to-person transmission occur in closed or semi-closed settings and result from direct or indirect exposure to faeces or vomitus of infected persons. Unlike stool shedding, vomiting is more likely to result in significant environmental contamination, leading to transmission by fomites and, potentially, airborne droplets.[181]

Although aerosolisation and droplets (usually from the infected person vomiting) have been implicated in transmission, the final common pathway is ultimately ingestion of virus particles (virions) arriving in the mouth or upper aerodigestive tract.[157] Air samples collected in patients' rooms, nurses stations and hallways during healthcare norovirus outbreaks have been shown to contain detectable viral RNA.[183] An outbreak study showed viral RNA detection on environmental surfaces (e.g. overbed tables, washbasins, lockers and air vents) and in environmental dust in rooms, suggesting dispersion in the air.[184] There have been a few outbreak reports where air was considered the most likely pathway for virus transfer.[185–187] One study found that detection of airborne norovirus RNA was strongly associated with a shorter time period since the infected person's last vomiting episode (but not the last diarrhoea episode) and was more likely to occur in outbreak settings rather than sporadic cases.[188] RNA could be detected in patient rooms, toilets and corridors. Particles as small as <1 μm had detectable RNA, suggesting that airborne transmission is a possibility,[188] since aerosol particles smaller than 10 μm can be suspended in air for several hours, be transported long distances in air currents, and easily be inhaled.[189] In general, while evidence exists for the potential for airborne transmission, the role of droplet and airborne transmission has not been well-characterised, and the risk to staff and patients not clearly quantified.

The environment clearly plays a role in the transmission of norovirus. In experimental studies, fingertips coming into contact once with faecally contaminated toilet tissue could transfer norovirus sequentially for up to seven clean surfaces.[190] Subsequently, clean hands touching the contaminated surfaces were able to transfer norovirus to other objects, such as door handles, taps and telephones. The environmental persistence of norovirus has been implicated in outbreaks within and outside healthcare facilities. In one incident, two carpet fitters were infected after working on a carpet in a hospital ward where an outbreak had ended 13 days earlier.[191] In a GI.6 outbreak involving 27 flight attendants across 8 different flight sectors over 6 days, aircraft contamination (following a passenger vomiting on the plane) was implicated.[192] Another outbreak involved over 300 cases of gastroenteritis among 1229 school children who had attended a lunchtime school concert the day after a concert attendee had vomited in the auditorium and adjacent toilet the preceding evening.[193]

Within healthcare facilities, it appears that the majority of outbreaks occur due to person-to-person transmission (directly or indirectly) after introduction by a single index case.[194] However, foodborne outbreaks have also been described.[194,195]

21.2.4 Clinical features and complications

Asymptomatic infection is possible, being common especially in children, with asymptomatic shedding rates ranging from 1–49%, depending on the cohort studied.[180] A recent meta-analysis of 81 studies calculated that the pooled prevalence of asymptomatic norovirus infection is about 7% and varies depending on different countries, settings and objects of study, but the pooled prevalence in the context of outbreak exposures is as high as 18%.[196]

Symptomatic disease ranges from mild to severe. After an incubation period of 12–48 hours, illness begins with acute onset of nausea, vomiting, abdominal cramps and myalgias.[57] Fever occurs in less than 50% of cases.[197] Non-bloody diarrhoea and/or vomiting are the commonest symptoms.[180] Resolution of symptoms generally occurs in 1–3 days, but symptoms can last for longer in hospitalised patients, the elderly and children.[157,180,198,199] Viral shedding is generally considered to persist in stool up to about 3–4 weeks.[200,201]

Several complications of norovirus diarrhoea are recognised. Dehydration and renal failure may occur.[202,203] Post-infectious irritable bowel syndrome may occur.[204] Other post-infectious sequelae may include dyspepsia, constipation and/or reflux.[205]

Amongst the elderly in healthcare facility outbreak settings, norovirus has been associated with increased morbidity, need for healthcare and mortality.[206–208] A study involving 407 outbreaks reported by 308 nursing homes showed that norovirus outbreaks were associated with significant concurrent increases in all-cause hospitalisation and mortality, concentrated in the first two weeks and the first week of the outbreak, respectively.[209]

In preterm neonates admitted to neonatal intensive care units, necrotising enterocolitis (NEC) has been associated with norovirus infection.[210] One Australian case-control study showed that 40% (4/10) of NEC infants had norovirus RNA detected compared with 9% (4/45) of non-NEC infants (OR: 6.83, 95% CI: 1.3–34.9,P = 0.021).[211] In infants, norovirus infection has also been associated with benign infantile convulsions with gastroenteritis (BICG).[203]

Immunocompromised patients are significantly impacted by norovirus infection, with diarrhoea sometimes having a chronic rather than acute course and viral shedding being prolonged.[212] In some haematology and oncology patients, virus shedding continues for weeks after symptom resolution, with some patients remaining symptomatic or shedding for months and even over one year.[213] Chronic infection can occur in recipients of solid organ[214] and haemopoietic stem cell transplants,[215] as well as patients with primary immunodeficiencies, including combined variable immunodeficiency.[216]

21.2.5 Diagnosis

In the past, a major challenge in outbreak control involved the difficulty in identifying norovirus early in the time course of an outbreak. Traditionally, the epidemiologic diagnosis had been made using Kaplan's criteria,[217] as outlined in Box 21.5. However, the usefulness in real-time is limited by the delay in excluding bacterial pathogens and the need for accumulation of sufficient numbers of cases to make it meaningful, enabling an outbreak to become established. Furthermore, the criteria are highly specific (99–100%) but not very sensitive (63–68%).[218,219] More recently, a classification and regression tree (CART) modelling profile has been proposed as an alternative, as shown in Box 21.6.[219] CART-derived characteristics for norovirus were assessed to be 85.7% sensitive and 92.4% specific (i.e. much more sensitive than Kaplan's criteria while maintaining high specificity) and were more effective in distinguishing confirmed norovirus outbreaks from confirmed non-viral outbreaks within the US National Outbreak Reporting System database.[219]

BOX 21.5 Kaplan's criteria for diagnosing an outbreak of gastroenteritis caused by norovirus[217]

All of the following should be present:

- vomiting in more than half of affected persons
- average incubation period of 24 to 48 hours
- average illness duration of 12 to 60 hours
- absence of bacterial pathogen in stool culture

Source: Data from Kaplan JE, Feldman R, Campbell DS, Lookabaugh C, Gary GW. The frequency of a Norwalk-like pattern of illness in outbreaks of acute gastroenteritis. Am J Public Health. 1982;72(12):1329–1332. doi:10.2105/ajph.72.12.1329

BOX 21.6 CART-derived characteristics for diagnosing an outbreak of gastroenteritis caused by norovirus[219]

All of the following should be present:

- fever-to-vomiting ratio <1
- proportion with bloody stools <0.1
- proportion with vomiting ≥0.26

Laboratory testing is required for aetiologic diagnosis of outbreaks and sporadic cases. In Australia, the Public Health Laboratory Network has published a laboratory case definition, with definitive criteria for norovirus met by a positive result on either an antigen detection test or nucleic acid amplification test (NAAT), and suggestive criteria met by detection of norovirus-like viral particles by electron microscopy (EM).[220]

Stool samples are the most suitable specimens. Although noroviruses can be detected in vomitus, this should only be collected after consultation with nominated laboratories. Viral loads appear to be higher in faeces than vomitus.[181] Also, some laboratories may not have assays validated for testing vomitus.

Since noroviruses could not be cultivated in cell lines until very recently, viral culture is not used in routine diagnosis.[180,221] EM, the original method of norovirus diagnosis, is unavailable in most laboratories. Estimated sensitivity is poor (17%),[222] but may be improved (58%) by using post-infectious sera (i.e. immune EM).[223] Serum specimens are not recommended for routine laboratory diagnosis of norovirus illness.[224] Over 90% of adults have norovirus IgG antibodies but remain at risk of re-infection.[180]

Antigen detection tests performed on stool comprise enzyme immunoassays (EIAs) and rapid immunochromatographic (ICT) assays. These are relatively simpler and more rapid than NAAT. Since some antibodies are genotype-specific (or even strain-specific), broadly cross-reactive antibody pools are needed to ensure that infections from a diverse range of strains are not missed. Antigen assay performance varies with differing norovirus genotypes, as shown in overseas[225] and Australian[226] studies. Depending on the assay used, EIA specificity ranges from 65–100% and sensitivity from 31–92%, compared with reverse-transcription polymerase chain reaction (RT–PCR).[180] Rapid ICT specificity ranges from 88–100% and sensitivity from 17–90%, compared with RT–PCR.[180] Given their moderate to high specificity but limited sensitivity, antigen tests are more useful in identifying norovirus as the cause of an outbreak (where multiple stool samples are tested) rather than diagnosing a sporadic case.[157,220] In order to reach a 90% probability of detecting a norovirus outbreak, at least 6 patients should be tested if an ELISA is used.[227]

NAATs detect targets within the RNA genome of noroviruses. RT-PCR is the gold standard for the detection and typing of norovirus, and numerous conventional and real-time norovirus RT-PCR assays have been developed.[180] Multiplex PCR assays can detect noroviruses as well as other pathogens in one test.[180] Other NAAT methods are nucleic acid sequence-based amplification (NASBA) and RT–loop-mediated iso-thermal amplification (RT-LAMP).[180] Although RT–PCR is more sensitive than direct antigen detection and electron microscopy, false negative results are possible due to norovirus genetic diversity (i.e. the PCR primers may not detect all variants), low virus concentration in faeces, improper specimen storage, inefficient RNA extraction and faecal reverse transcriptase inhibitors.[228] Detection of norovirus RNA in a patient's stool does not always imply it is the cause of symptoms, since a proportion of healthy individuals in the community may have detectable norovirus in stools despite absence of recent symptoms.[229] Stool viral loads are lower in asymptomatic than symptomatic GII strain infection. Therefore, patients with diarrhoea and detectable GII norovirus but low viral loads may have another cause for their symptoms and merely incidental norovirus co-infection. Viral load testing is not routinely available.

21.2.6 Treatment

Since no specific antiviral therapy has proven to be effective, norovirus treatment consists of supportive measures such as fluid plus electrolyte replacement and symptomatic management of headaches, myalgias and nausea. Analgesics and antiemetics may be prescribed. The effect of antimotility agents has not been rigorously studied. In immunocompromised patients, reduction in immunosuppression, if feasible, is advisable.[180,216,230]

Potential treatment options which have been previously reported in limited numbers of very small studies include nitazoxanide,[231] oral immunoglobulin[232] and ribavirin.[233] However, no conclusive recommendations can be made. More recently, many new drugs and compounds have been investigated, some showing favourable *in vitro* results. At present, no drugs have yet been clinically approved, and the majority of candidates are still in the early stages of preclinical development.[234]

21.2.7 Prevention and control

Screening and surveillance: Since sporadic norovirus cases are not notifiable diseases in many jurisdictions, there is no national surveillance program for all individual norovirus cases. However, outbreaks are notifiable and OzFoodNet focuses on Australian foodborne disease surveillance, including gathering data on norovirus outbreaks.[235]

Transmission-based precautions: Within healthcare institutions, measures need to be taken to interrupt person-to-person transmission of norovirus, thereby preventing or limiting outbreaks.

Symptomatic patients should be separated from uninfected persons,[235] usually in a single room in order to minimise transmission. They should not leave their room or use common areas until 48 hours after resolution of symptoms. Ideally, separate toilet facilities should be allocated for infected patients. In outbreak settings, several guidelines recommend cohorting patients into groups on the basis of 'symptomatic', 'exposed asymptomatic' and 'unexposed asymptomatic' status.[157,235–237] In the past, whole ward or unit closure was considered as a central control measure for managing norovirus outbreaks in healthcare facilities. However, efficient control may be achieved by the early closure of bays (within 3 days of the first case becoming ill), before extensive transmission has occurred within a clinical area.[238–240] This may lead to cost savings and less overall disruption to ward functioning.

Current Australian guidelines recommend that patients with suspected or confirmed norovirus infection be managed with standard plus contact precautions, with droplet precautions added if indicated, based on a risk assessment.[7] Transmission-based precautions should be maintained for a minimum of 48 hours after the resolution of symptoms. This may be extended if patients are incontinent or if an outbreak is present.

There have been some differences in guidelines from various authorities and changes over time, which are summarised in Table 21.3 below.[7,236,237,241,242] In particular, the instructions on mask use are not uniform, due to ongoing debate over the relative contribution of droplets and aerosols in transmission.

In terms of healthcare worker PPE, in addition to gowns and gloves, Australian guidelines recommend using a surgical mask while a patient is symptomatic. Persons who clean areas heavily contaminated with faeces or vomitus may also benefit from wearing masks since virus can be aerosolised from these body substances.[7]

Hand hygiene: Controversies surround the optimal method of hand hygiene, with a key issue being whether alcohol-based hand rub (ABHR) or soap plus water is superior.

In general, laboratory studies to evaluate the ability of a hand disinfection product to reduce virus infectivity use virus culture in the presence and absence of exposure to the product. However, human noroviruses could not be cultured until recently, so prior evaluations used one of two methods. The first involved measuring human norovirus using quantitative RT–PCR

TABLE 21.3 Differences in basic guidance for norovirus infection control management[7,236,237,241,242]

Organisation/ country	CDC USA	NHMRC Australia	CDC USA [current]	Norovirus Working Party UK [current]	NHMRC Australia [current]
Year	2007	2010	2011	2012	2019
Infection control precautions	Standard Contact (faecally incontinent cases)	Contact + Droplet (faecally incontinent cases)	Standard (sporadic case) Contact (outbreak)	'Contact'	Standard + Contact (+ Droplet based on risk assessment)
Remarks	Mask use if cleaning heavily soiled area	Mask use if patient symptomatic	Mask use if anticipated facial splash especially from vomiting patient	Mask only if there is a risk of droplets or aerosols	Mask use if patient symptomatic

in the presence and absence of exposure to hand sanitiser. However, the detection of RNA does not necessarily correlate with infectivity. Sanitisers may damage the viral capsid, removing the ability to bind receptors and cause infection, without necessarily rendering RNA undetectable.[243] Thus, 'false positive' results may be obtained after effective use of a hand sanitiser. Specialised binding RT–PCR studies show that a proportion of norovirus detectable by RT–PCR is actually representative of non-binding (i.e. non-infectious) virus.[244] The second method involved extrapolating results from culture of surrogate viruses with similar properties, such as Feline calicivirus (FCV) or Murine norovirus (MNV), in the presence and absence of exposure to hand sanitiser. But correlation between results obtained with FCV and MNV is variable and correlation of both to RT–PCR studies is poor.[245,246] Thus, prior to reliably culturing human noroviruses, there appears to have been no optimal method to determine which hand disinfection product is most active against them. As a result, studies have had conflicting results. Some RT-PCR-based laboratory studies indicate that ABHR is much less active against norovirus, which is non-enveloped, than soap and the physical rinse with water.[243,247] However, some surrogate virus culture-based studies indicate that ABHR is effective against MNV[248] and even superior to soaps.[249] Today, MNV, a gastrointestinal tract virus, is widely used to determine the activity against noroviruses rather than the respiratory tract pathogen FCV. Ethanol at concentrations between 62.4–85.8% (w/w) is usually effective against MNV in 30 seconds or 1 minute.[250] WHO handrub formulations containing ethanol are active against MNV as a surrogate of human norovirus,

whereas the formulations containing isopropanol have rather poor virucidal activity against MNV.[251] To aid in resolving the issue, a new technique has been developed to evaluate norovirus inactivation by various chemicals using recombinant norovirus virus-like particles (VLPs) as a surrogate for human norovirus.[252] In recent times and progressing into the future, studies involving human norovirus cultured in human intestinal enteroids derived from small intestinal tissue may also help resolve ongoing uncertainty regarding the best chemicals for disinfecting not only hands but also environmental surfaces.[221]

In a cross-sectional survey of US long-term care facilities where 29 of 73 outbreaks had norovirus confirmed, facilities self-reporting that staff were equally or more likely to use ABHR than soap and water for routine hand hygiene had higher odds of a confirmed norovirus outbreak than facilities with staff less likely to use ABHR.[253] It was concluded that preferential use of ABHR over soap and water for routine hand hygiene might be associated with increased risk of norovirus outbreaks. However, others disputed this conclusion, pointing out that association did not imply causation and that the multivariate analysis had failed to take into account actual hand hygiene compliance.[254] The critics suggested that an alternate hypothesis for the association should have been considered, that is, better infection control practices (of which ABHR use was an indicator) led to better outbreak detection and confirmation, as supported by the original study's finding on univariate analysis that having an infection control practitioner in the facility was associated with a greater likelihood of a confirmed norovirus outbreak.[254]

Successful hospital norovirus outbreak control where ethanol ABHRs were used for hand hygiene has been reported,[255] including directly observed hand hygiene practice using the ABHR,[256] although the extent of contribution of the ABHR product is unclear, amidst a host of other interventions.

At present, the jury is still out. WHO experts 'recommend the use of alcohol-based handrubs during outbreaks of noroviral gastroenteritis.'[257] On the other hand, the US CDC states that '… hand washing with soap and running water … reduce norovirus contamination … whereas hand sanitisers might serve as an effective adjunct … but should not be considered a substitute …'.[157] For known or suspected norovirus, current Australian guidelines[7] recommend that hand hygiene is performed as follows:

- if gloves have not been worn, have been breached, or there is visible contamination of the hands despite glove use, use soap and water to facilitate the mechanical removal of spores. After washing, hands should be dried thoroughly with a single-use towel
- if gloves have been worn, a lower density of contamination of the hands would be expected and ABHR remains the agent of choice for hand hygiene.

Decisions on which hand hygiene product to advocate in healthcare settings should take into account the impact of product choice and compliance on transmission of other pathogens (e.g. MRSA).

Cleaning and disinfection: The surfaces of a high-contact objects (i.e. doorknobs, toilet seats and faucets) can be contaminated with up to 10^4 virions per object, which strongly suggests that reductions in levels of 3–4 log_{10} are required to eliminate norovirus contamination on high-contact surfaces.[258]

A range of chemicals and techniques/technologies can potentially be applied.

It has been shown that accelerated hydrogen peroxide and quaternary ammonium compounds (QAC) are less effective than sodium hypochlorite for the inactivation of MNV and FCV on stainless steel surfaces.[259] A study of seven disinfectant preparations showed that sodium hypochlorite alone, peracetic acid plus hydrogen peroxide and a mixture containing glutaraldehyde plus QAC plus isopropanol were most active against both MNV and FCV, whereas ethanol alone and chlorhexidine plus isopropanol had significant activity against MNV but not FCV.[260] Another study showed that QAC were largely inactive against human norovirus and FCV

and MNV. Ethanol appeared to be largely inactive against human norovirus and FCV but showed activity against MNV. Human norovirus strains were more resistant to sodium hypochlorite than were either of the animal surrogates, with the human strains requiring at least 500 ppm of hypochlorite to achieve statistically significant reduction (≥ 3.0 log) in virus concentration.[261]

One key difficulty in determining the optimal chemicals for disinfection is that various studies have used different concentrations, contact times, surfaces, test formats and target measures or surrogates to evaluate disinfectant efficacy.

Several guidelines recommend the use of sodium hypochlorite at a concentration of at least 1000ppm.[157,235,237] Up to 5000ppm may be used.[157]

In an experimental study,[190] single-step wiping with a cloth soaked in detergent, as well as after single-step wiping with a cloth soaked in detergent following surface application of hypochlorite (5000 ppm available chlorine) for 1 min, both failed to remove all traces of norovirus from a faecally contaminated surface. Norovirus was only undetectable after a two-step process involving using a cloth soaked in detergent to wipe away all organic matter prior to application of hypochlorite for ≥ 1 min and then re-wiping. Where a surface was not norovirus-free after wiping, virus was shown to be transferred to cleaners' hands as well as to a second surface wiped with the same cloth. Wiping the same surface twice with a cloth rinsed in detergent and wrung out in between the two wiping attempts also failed to remove all traces of virus. Inadequate environmental cleaning and disinfection procedures not only allow norovirus to persist but can facilitate its spread.

If bleach cannot be used due to the risk of damage to material surfaces, a Therapeutic Goods Administration-listed hospital-grade disinfectant with specific norovirus claims should be used, in addition to standard cleaning practices.[7] Further detail on environmental cleaning is provided in Chapter 16. Further detail on Therapeutic Goods Administration and the Australian regulatory framework for medical devices, sterilants and disinfectants is provided in Chapters 15 and 16.

Enhanced cleaning and disinfection protocols may control and prevent the spread of noroviruses.[262] The cleaning frequency may need to be increased, with greater attention paid to high-traffic areas and frequently touched surfaces (e.g. curtains, door handles, flush handles, toilet seats, taps, hand rails, light switches and telephones.)[157,236,237,263] Cleaning and disinfection should proceed from low-contamination areas to high-contamination areas.[237] Steam cleaning can be considered for soft furnishings (e.g. rugs, carpets, chairs and other fabrics) that are adversely affected by chemicals.[236,237]

The role of newer disinfection technologies in controlling norovirus outbreaks is not well defined. Neutral electrolysed water (NEW) is a novel chlorine-based disinfectant that can be used at reduced concentrations, making it more environmentally friendly and less corrosive than bleach. Experiments showed that 250 ppm NEW effectively eliminated (defined as a 5-$\log_{10}$ reduction) human norovirus GII.4 Sydney on clean stainless steel surfaces after a 30 minute exposure.[264] Supporting studies showed that, like bleach, NEW causes inactivation by disrupting the virus capsid. Hydrogen peroxide vapor (HPV) has been shown to be able to inactivate MNV and FCV both in a laboratory setting[265] and when placed in various positions in a non-occupied patient room,[266] possibly implying this may be effective for human norovirus also. In a separate study, hydrogen peroxide delivered by fog showed promising virucidal activity against FCV by meeting the United States EPA 4-$\log_{10}$ reduction criteria for an anti-noroviral disinfectant; however, a fogged chlorine dioxide-surfactant-based product did not achieve a 4-$\log_{10}$ inactivation. Ultraviolet C (UVC) light has been shown to inactivate MNV on stainless steel surfaces[267] and the human norovirus surrogate MS2 on glass or plastic coupons.[268] In a study involving vinyl and granite floors contaminated with human faeces containing norovirus GII, cleaning followed by disinfection using 1% sodium hypochlorite was shown to be superior to cleaning followed by disinfection using a manual UVC device.[269] Ozone gas from a portable commercial generator has been shown to inactivate norovirus in settings such as hotel rooms, cruise ship cabins and healthcare facilities.[270] Recently, the new biguanide olanexidine gluconate hand rub has demonstrated strong virucidal efficacy against human norovirus.[271]

Outbreak control measures: The main approaches to preventing and containing norovirus outbreaks have been detailed in several guidelines and are summarised in Box 21.7.[7,157,159,236,258]

BOX 21.7 Key infection control recommendations for the control of norovirus outbreaks in healthcare settings[7,157,159,236,258]

Outbreak identification

- Define start of outbreak to enable the initiation of enhanced norovirus infection control measures (e.g. two or more associated patients with gastroenteritis onsets within 24–48 hours of each other)

Patient isolation/cohorting and transmission-based precautions

- Place patients with norovirus gastroenteritis on contact precautions for a minimum of 48 hours after the resolution of symptoms. Patients should have separate/dedicated toilet facilities if possible
- When symptomatic patients cannot be accommodated in single occupancy rooms, efforts should be made to cohort patients into separate groups (e.g. grouped among those who are symptomatic, exposed but asymptomatic, and unexposed), with dedicated nursing staff providing care
- Minimise patient movements within a ward or unit during norovirus outbreaks
- Symptomatic and recovering patients should not leave the patient care area unless it is for essential care or treatment. (Ideally, patients should not be transferred to other wards or facilities until a minimum of 48 hours after the resolution of symptoms.)
- Consider suspending group activities
- Healthcare personnel who have recovered from recent suspected norovirus infection associated with this outbreak may be best suited to care for exposed or symptomatic patients

Personal protective equipment (PPE)

- If norovirus infection is suspected, individuals entering the patient care area should wear PPE according to contact and standard precautions (i.e. gowns and gloves, and among vomiting patients, face masks)

Hand hygiene

- Actively promote adherence to hand hygiene among healthcare personnel, patients and visitors in patient care areas affected by outbreaks of norovirus gastroenteritis

Environmental cleaning

- Perform routine cleaning and disinfection of frequently touched environmental surfaces

Continued

BOX 21.7 Key infection control recommendations for the control of norovirus outbreaks in healthcare settings—cont'd

- Increase the frequency of cleaning and disinfection of patient care areas and frequently touched surfaces during outbreaks of norovirus gastroenteritis
- Clean and disinfect surfaces, starting from the areas with a lower likelihood of norovirus contamination, then to areas with greater likelihood
- Use standard precautions for handling soiled patient-service items or linens, which includes the appropriate use of PPE
- Consider changing privacy curtains routinely and upon patient discharge or transfer

Patient transfer and ward closure

- Closure of wards to new admissions or transfers may be a measure to attenuate the magnitude of a norovirus outbreak
- Early bay closure (within 3 days of the first case becoming ill) may be effective for controlling norovirus outbreaks, particularly when this is combined with other infection control measures, thereby avoiding the need for ward closures
- Consider patient transfers only if receiving facilities are able to maintain contact precautions
- During outbreaks, medically suitable individuals recovering from norovirus gastroenteritis can be discharged to their place of residence

Staff management

- Exclude ill staff from work for a minimum of 48 hours after the resolution of symptoms. Once staff return to work, strict adherence to hand hygiene must be maintained

- Establish protocols for staff cohorting in the event of a norovirus outbreak
- Exclude non-essential healthcare providers, students and volunteers from working in areas experiencing outbreaks of norovirus

Visitors

- Restrict non-essential visitors from affected areas during outbreaks
- For those facilities where it is necessary to have continued visitation privileges, screen and exclude visitors with symptoms consistent with norovirus infection

Diagnostics

- Submit stool specimens as early as possible during a suspected norovirus gastroenteritis outbreak and ideally from individuals during the acute phase of illness
- In the absence of clinical laboratory diagnostics for norovirus, or in the case of delay in obtaining laboratory results, use Kaplan's clinical and epidemiologic criteria to identify a norovirus gastroenteritis outbreak

Food safety

- Determine whether food is the cause of the outbreak and withdraw implicated food
- Discard exposed food
- Exclude ill food-handling staff for at least 48 hours after symptom resolution
- Close communal dining areas
- Ensure proper food preparation, storage and serving
- Eliminate bare-handed contact with ready-to-eat foods

Although multiple recommendations for outbreak control have been made, the evidence base is very limited, with most recommendations based on low-quality evidence or expert opinion.[7,236,263] A systematic review of 72 outbreaks in semi-enclosed settings found no evidence that implementing infection control measures affected the duration of outbreaks, or the attack rates either overall (all settings combined) or within particular settings.[272] Nevertheless, the authors concluded that: 'Sound infection control procedures are key to controlling norovirus outbreaks but unfortunately, the present body of the published literature does not provide an evidence-base for the value of specific measures.'[272]

Vaccination: In 2016, the WHO stated that the development of a norovirus vaccine should be considered a priority.[273] Unfortunately, the development of an effective norovirus vaccine has been extremely difficult, due to the inability to culture the virus until recently, the significant genetic diversity of strains, the lack of long-lasting immunity following natural infection, and the lack of a reliable immune marker to indicate whether an individual is protected from an infection and related disease.[274] Although there are several vaccines in pre-clinical and clinical development, there are currently no vaccines in routine clinical use and available to the wider global population.

CASE STUDY 2

Norovirus infection

Situation:

Mr Jones, aged 80, has been admitted to hospital from a nursing home for cellulitis. The day after admission, he develops frequent vomiting and diarrhoea but you are not notified until three days later. By then, Mr Smith, in the next bed within the same four-bed bay, has developed diarrhoea. Mr Smith has been using the ward kitchenette to make toast each morning. The other two patients in that bay are asymptomatic. A nurse who cared for Mr Jones has called in sick with nausea and diarrhoea. What are your considerations in managing this situation if norovirus infection is suspected?

Answer:

- Stool samples from both Mr Jones and Mr Smith (and the unwell nurse, if possible) should be sent for norovirus testing
- Both Mr Jones and Mr Smith should be managed with contact precautions, with additional droplet precautions for Mr Jones due to vomiting. If available, they can each be moved into a single room with ensuite, or cohorted with a shared toilet. These should remain in place for at least 48 hours after symptom resolution
- The two asymptomatic persons may have been exposed and are incubating the virus. Managing them under contact precautions pre-emptively could be considered
- The four-bed bay and, especially, any shared toilet, should be thoroughly cleaned and disinfected more frequently. Bay closure should be considered
- The ward kitchenette should be closed and thoroughly cleaned and disinfected
- Staff, patients and visitors should be reminded to adhere to hand hygiene
- All ward staff and patients should be checked for symptoms, in case there are undiscovered cases. Ongoing surveillance should be implemented

- The unwell nurse should remain away from work for at least 48 hours after symptom resolution
- Depending on when her symptoms began, any other patients who have been cared for by that nurse may have already been exposed and are incubating the virus
- If the sick individuals have norovirus confirmed, an outbreak has occurred and it may be necessary to notify public health authorities. There may also be cases in Mr Jones' nursing home
- Depending on the outbreak extent, broader measures may be required (e.g. visitor restrictions, ward closures, limitations on staff movements)

21.3 Rotavirus

21.3.1 Background and epidemiology

Rotaviruses are non-enveloped RNA viruses, classified according two surface proteins they contain—the 'G' glycoprotein and the protease-cleaved 'P' protein.[275] Rotavirus strains are most commonly referred to by their G serotype.

Rotavirus infection was previously the commonest cause of severe gastroenteritis in infants and young children,[275] but both rotavirus-specific and all-cause hospital presentations for gastroenteritis markedly decreased following nationwide vaccination introduced in Australia in 2007, [276,277] with over 70% reduction in rotavirus-specific cases.[276] Compared with their non-Indigenous peers, Aboriginal and Torres Strait Islander infants and children are hospitalised with rotavirus gastroenteritis about 3–5 times more often, are younger at hospitalisation and have a longer average duration of hospital stay (5 vs 2 days).[275]

Rotavirus is an important cause of nosocomial gastroenteritis, particularly in children.[278–281] Following vaccine introduction however, various countries have reported a marked and sustained decrease in incidence of nosocomial rotavirus gastroenteritis.[282–284] Rotavirus is also capable of infecting adults, including travellers and people caring for children, and can also cause outbreaks amongst older adults in residential facilities.[285]

There are limited data on nosocomial rotavirus infections in Australia. Prior to the vaccination era, it was recognised as a significant problem in paediatric wards and hospitals, with at least 14–19% of all rotavirus infections being hospital acquired.[279,281] From 1997–2000, rotavirus was implicated in 13% of

53 gastroenteritis outbreaks in aged care facilities in Victoria.[286]

Rotaviruses are shed in the stool of infected persons. Transmission occurs by the faecal–oral route, through close person-to-person contact and fomites. Transmission via droplets has also been hypothesised but not proven.[287] Rotavirus transmission through contaminated food and water appears to be uncommon.[288] In temperate Australia, rotavirus infections follow a seasonal pattern. The peak incidence is in mid to late winter. The northern tropical and arid regions do not show a consistent seasonal pattern.[275] Rotavirus is highly communicable, as evidenced by the nearly universal infection of children by age 5 years in the pre-vaccine era. Infected persons shed large quantities of virus in their stool, beginning 2 days before the onset of diarrhoea and for up to 10 days after onset of symptoms,[288] but viral shedding can range from 4–57 days.[289] Spread within healthcare facilities, households[290] and childcare settings[291] is common.

21.3.2 Clinical features and diagnosis

The incubation period is 1–3 days.[275] Infection may be asymptomatic, may cause self-limited watery diarrhoea, or may result in severe diarrhoea with fever and vomiting. In children, the classic presentation of rotaviral infection is fever and vomiting for 2–3 days, followed by non-bloody diarrhoea. Symptoms generally resolve in 3–7 days.[288] Infected adults can be asymptomatic or may have mild illness.[285] Both adults and children with underlying immunodeficiency are at risk of chronic and more severe symptoms and prolonged viral shedding.[285]

Diagnosis requires stool samples submitted for either antigen testing or nucleic acid amplification testing by RT-PCR. PCR may detect vaccine-strain virus in recently vaccinated infants, leading to overdiagnosis, so typing is required.[292]

21.3.3 Management, prevention and control

Rotavirus disease is usually self-limited. Management consists of fluid and electrolyte replacement. Dietary management is an important factor in the care of children with acute diarrhoea. Breastfeeding should be encouraged and, for older children, the maintenance of adequate protein–calorie intake during the diarrhoea episode using age-appropriate foods should be encouraged.[287]

Within healthcare institutions, patients with rotavirus infections should be managed with standard and contact precautions for the duration of their illness.[7,241] Australian guidelines state that alcohol-based hand hygiene products are less effective than hand washing with soap and water for this infectious agent.[7] Consistent environmental cleaning and disinfection and frequent removal of soiled diapers should be practised. Prolonged shedding may occur in both immunocompetent and immunocompromised children and the elderly.

The National Rotavirus Reference Centre undertakes surveillance and characterisation of rotavirus strains causing annual epidemics of severe diarrhoea in young children throughout Australia.[293] In Australia, live-attenuated oral rotavirus vaccines are recommended for all infants before they are 6 months old, if there are no contraindications. A course of vaccination prevents rotavirus gastroenteritis of any severity in approximately 70% of recipients and prevents severe rotavirus gastroenteritis and rotavirus hospitalisation for 85–100% of recipients for up to 3 years.[275]

Conclusion

C. difficile and noroviruses are the two most common agents implicated in healthcare-associated diarrhoea of infectious aetiology. They remain significant causes of morbidity and their management consumes healthcare resources. Vaccination has reduced the overall impact of rotaviruses.

Useful websites/resources

- Australian Guidelines for the Prevention and Control of Infection in Healthcare. https://www.nhmrc.gov.au/about-us/publications/australian-guidelines-prevention-and-control-infection-healthcare-2019
- *C. diff (Clostridioides difficile)*. US Centers for Disease Control and Prevention (CDC). https://www.cdc.gov/cdiff/index.html
- *Clostridioides difficile*: guidance, data and analysis. Public Health England. https://www.gov.uk/government/collections/clostridium-difficile-guidance-data-and-analysis
- Norovirus. US Centers for Disease Control and Prevention (CDC). https://www.cdc.gov/norovirus/index.html

- Rotavirus. US Centers for Disease Control and Prevention (CDC). https://www.cdc.gov/rotavirus/index.html
- Surveillance for Clostridioides difficile infection - Implementation Guide. https://www.safetyandquality. gov.au/our-work/healthcare-associated-infection/consultation-on-clostridium-difficile

References

1. Turner NA, Saullo JL, Polage CR. Healthcare associated diarrhea, not Clostridioides difficile. Curr Opin Infect Dis. 2020;33(4):319-326. doi:10.1097/QCO.0000000000000653.
2. Polage CR, Solnick JV, Cohen SH. Nosocomial diarrhea: evaluation and treatment of causes other than Clostridium difficile. Clin Infect Dis. 2012;55(7):982-989. doi:10.1093/cid/cis551.
3. Hitchcock MM, Gomez CA, Banaei N. Low yield of film array GI Panel in hospitalized patients with diarrhea: an opportunity for diagnostic stewardship intervention. J Clin Microbiol. 2018;56(3). doi:10.1128/JCM.01558-17.
4. Larcombe S, Hutton ML, Lyras D. Involvement of bacteria other than Clostridium difficile in antibiotic-associated diarrhoea. Trends Microbiol. 2016;24(6):463-476. doi:10.1016/j.tim.2016.02.001.
5. Jarrin C, Bearman G. Parasites. Guide to infection control in the healthcare setting. 2018. [cited 4 Dec 2020]. Available from: https://isid.org/guide/pathogens/parasites/.
6. Australian Commission on Safety and Quality in Health Care. Hospital-acquired complication - 3. Healthcare-associated infection fact sheet. 2018. [cited 4 Dec 2020]. Available from: https://www.safetyandquality.gov.au/publications-and-resources/resource-library/hospital-acquired-complication-3-healthcare-associated-infection-fact-sheet.
7. NHMRC. Australian guidelines for the prevention and control of infection in healthcare. National Health and Medical Research Council, 2019. Available from: http://www.legislationreview.nhmrc.gov.au/_files_nhmrc/publications/attachments/cd33_infection_control_healthcare.pdf.
8. Lee MB, Greig JD. A review of nosocomial Salmonella outbreaks: infection control interventions found effective. Public Health. 2012;127(3):199-206. doi:10.1016/j.puhe.2012.12.013.
9. Mccall B, Stafford R, Cherian S, et al. An outbreak of multi-resistant Shigella sonnei in a long-stay geriatric nursing centre. Commun Dis Intell. 2000;24(9):272-275.
10. Jelovcan S, Schmid D, Lederer I, et al. Cluster of nosocomial campylobacteriosis, Austria 2006. J Hosp Infect. 2008;69(1):97-98. doi:10.1016/j.jhin.2008.01.010.
11. Graham JC, Lanser S, Bignardi G, Pedler S, Hollyoak V. Hospital-acquired listeriosis. J Hosp Infect. 2002;51(2):136-139. doi:10.1053/jhin.2002.1234.
12. Burkholder BT, Coronado VG, Brown J, et al. Nosocomial transmission of hepatitis A in a pediatric hospital traced to an anti-hepatitis A virus-negative patient with immunodeficiency. Pediatr Infect Dis J. 1995;14(4):261-266. doi:10.1097/00006454-199504000-00003.
13. Lessa FC, Gould CV, McDonald LC. Current status of Clostridium difficile infection epidemiology. Clin Infect Dis. 2012;55(suppl_2):S65-S70. doi:10.1093/cid/cis319.
14. Centers for Disease Control and Prevention. Antibiotic resistance threats in the United States, 2019. US Department of Health and Human Services, CDC, 2019. doi:http://dx.doi.org/10.15620/cdc:82532.
15. Zhang S, Palazuelos-Munoz S, Balsells EM, Nair H, Chit A, Kyaw MH. Cost of hospital management of Clostridium difficile infection in United States—a meta-analysis and modelling study. BMC Infect Dis. 2016;16(1):447. doi:10.1186/s12879-016-1786-6.
16. Marra AR, Perencevich EN, Nelson RE, et al. Incidence and outcomes associated with Clostridium difficile infections: a systematic review and meta-analysis. JAMA Netw Open. 2020;3(1):e1917597-e1917597. doi:10.1001/jamanetworkopen.2019.17597
17. Bartlett JG. Narrative review: the new epidemic of Clostridium difficile-associated enteric disease. Ann Intern Med. 2006;145(10):758-764. doi:10.7326/0003-4819-145-10-200611210-00008
18. McDonald LC, Killgore GE, Thompson A, et al. An epidemic, toxin gene–variant strain of Clostridium difficile. N Engl J Med. 2005;353(23):2433-2441. doi:10.1056/NEJMoa051590
19. Freeman J, Bauer MP, Baines SD, et al. The changing epidemiology of Clostridium difficile infections. Clin Microbiol Rev. 2010;23(3):529-549. doi:10.1128/CMR.00082-09
20. Miller M, Gravel D, Mulvey M, et al. Health care-associated Clostridium difficile infection in Canada: patient age and infecting strain type are highly predictive of severe outcome and mortality. Clin Infect Dis. 2010;50(2):194-201. doi:10.1086/649213
21. Pépin J, Valiquette L, Cossette B. Mortality attributable to nosocomial Clostridium difficile-associated disease during an epidemic caused by a hypervirulent strain in Quebec. Can Med Assoc J. 2005;173(9):1037-1042. doi:10.1503/cmaj.050978
22. Pepin J, Alary M-E, Valiquette L, et al. Increasing risk of relapse after treatment of Clostridium difficile colitis in Quebec, Canada. Clin Infect Dis. 2005;40(11):1591-1597. doi:10.1086/430315
23. Riley TV, Thean S, Hool G, Golledge CL. First Australian isolation of epidemic Clostridium difficile PCR ribotype 027. Med J Aust. 2009;190(12):706-708.
24. Kamuju V, Kumar S, Khan WH, Vivekanandan P. Hypervirulent Clostridium difficile ribotypes are CpG depleted. Virulence. 2018;9(1):1422-1425. doi:10.1080/21505594.2018.1509669
25. Goorhuis A, Bakker D, Corver J, et al. Emergence of Clostridium difficile infection due to a new hypervirulent strain, polymerase chain reaction ribotype 078. Clin Infect Dis. 2008;47(9):1162-1170. doi:10.1086/592257
26. Shaw HA, Preston MD, Vendrik KEW, et al. The recent emergence of a highly related virulent Clostridium difficile clade with unique characteristics. Clin Microbiol Infect. 2020;26(4):492-498. doi:10.1016/j.cmi.2019.09.004
27. Lim SK, Stuart RL, Mackin KE, et al. Emergence of a ribotype 244 strain of Clostridium difficile associated with severe disease and related to the epidemic ribotype 027 strain. Clin Infect Dis. 2014;58(12):1723-1730. doi:10.1093/cid/ciu203
28. Eyre DW, Tracey L, Elliott B, et al. Emergence and spread of predominantly community-onset Clostridium difficile PCR ribotype 244 infection in Australia, 2010 to 2012. Euro Surveill. 2015;20(10):21059. doi:10.2807/1560-7917.es2015.20.10.21059
29. Australian Commission on Safety and Quality in Health Care. Clostridium difficile infection - 2017 data snapshot.

ACSQHC, 2019. Available from: https://www.safetyandquality.gov.au/publications-and-resources/resource-library/clostridium-difficile-infection-2017-data-snapshot-1.

30. Australian Commission on Safety and Quality in Health Care. Clostridium difficile infection. Monitoring the national burden of Clostridium difficile. ACSQHC, 2018. Available from: https://www.safetyandquality.gov.au/publications-and-resources/resource-library/clostridium-difficile-infection-monitoring-national-burden-clostridium-difficile-0.

31. Australian Commission on Safety and Quality in Health Care. Clostridioides difficile infection - 2018 data snapshot. ACSQHC, 2020. Available from: https://www.safetyandquality.gov.au/sites/default/files/2020-10/attachment_1_clostridium_difficile_infection_2018_data_snapshot_report.pdf.

32. Schäffler H, Breitrück A. Clostridium difficile – from colonization to infection. Front Microbiol. 2018;9:646. doi:10.3389/fmicb.2018.00646

33. Donskey CJ, Kundrapu S, Deshpande A. Colonization versus carriage of Clostridium difficile. Infect Dis Clin North Am. 2015;29(1):13-28. doi:10.1016/j.idc.2014.11.001

34. Riggs MM, Sethi AK, Zabarsky TF, Eckstein EC, Jump RLP, Donskey CJ. Asymptomatic carriers are a potential source for transmission of epidemic and nonepidemic Clostridium difficile strains among long-term care facility residents. Clin Infect Dis. 2007;45(8):992-998. doi:10.1086/521854

35. Enoch DA, Butler MJ, Pai S, Aliyu SH, Karas JA. Clostridium difficile in children: colonisation and disease. J Infect. 2011;63(2):105-113. doi:10.1016/j.jinf.2011.05.016

36. Lees EA, Miyajima F, Pirmohamed M, Carrol ED. The role of Clostridium difficile in the paediatric and neonatal gut - a narrative review. Eur J Clin Microbiol Infect Dis. 2016; 35(7):1047-1057. doi:10.1007/s10096-016-2639-3

37. Furuya-Kanamori L, Clements ACA, Foster NF, et al. Asymptomatic Clostridium difficile colonization in two Australian tertiary hospitals, 2012-2014: prospective, repeated cross-sectional study. Clin Microbiol Infect. 2017;23(1):48.e1-48.e7. doi:10.1016/j.cmi.2016.08.030

38. Guh AY, Adkins SH, Li Q, et al. Risk factors for community-associated Clostridium difficile infection in adults: a case-control study. Open Forum Infect Dis. 2017;4(4):ofx171. doi:10.1093/ofid/ofx171

39. Gerding DN, Young VB, Donskey CJ. Clostridioides difficile (formerly Clostridium difficile) infection. In: Bennett JE, Dolin R, Blaser MJ, eds. Mandell, Douglas, and Bennett's principles and practice of infectious diseases. 9th ed. Elsevier, 2020, p. 2933-2947.

40. Trubiano JA, Cheng AC, Korman TM, et al. Australasian Society of Infectious Diseases updated guidelines for the management of Clostridium difficile infection in adults and children in Australia and New Zealand. Intern Med J. 2016; 46(4):479-493. doi:10.1111/imj.13027

41. McDonald LC, Gerding DN, Johnson S, et al. Clinical practice guidelines for Clostridium difficile infection in adults and children: 2017 Update by the Infectious Diseases Society of America (IDSA) and Society for Healthcare Epidemiology of America (SHEA). Clin Infect Dis. 2018;66(7):e1-e48. doi:10.1093/cid/cix1085

42. Hensgens MPM, Goorhuis A, Dekkers OM, Kuijper EJ. Time interval of increased risk for Clostridium difficile infection after exposure to antibiotics. J Antimicrob Chemother. 2012;67(3):742-748. doi:10.1093/jac/dkr508

43. Cheng AC, Ferguson JK, Richards MJ, et al. Australasian Society for Infectious Diseases guidelines for the diagnosis and treatment of Clostridium difficile infection. Med J Aust. 2011;194(7):353-358.

44. Britton RA, Young VB. Role of the intestinal microbiota in resistance to colonization by Clostridium difficile.

Gastroenterology. 2014;146(6):1547-1553. doi:10.1053/j.gastro.2014.01.059

45. Brown KA, Khanafer N, Daneman N, Fisman DN. Meta-analysis of antibiotics and the risk of community-associated Clostridium difficile infection. Antimicrob Agents Chemother. 2013;57(5):2326-2332. doi:10.1128/AAC.02176-12

46. Stevens V, Dumyati G, Fine LS, Fisher SG, van Wijngaarden E. Cumulative antibiotic exposures over time and the risk of Clostridium difficile infection. Clin Infect Dis. 2011;53(1):42-48. doi:10.1093/cid/cir301

47. Tabak YP, Srinivasan A, Yu KC, et al. Hospital-level high-risk antibiotic use in relation to hospital-associated Clostridioides difficile infections: retrospective analysis of 2016-2017 data from US hospitals. Infect Control Hosp Epidemiol. 2019; 40(11):1229-1235. doi:10.1017/ice.2019.236

48. Loo VG, Bourgault A-M, Poirier L, et al. Host and pathogen factors for Clostridium difficile infection and colonization. N Engl J Med. 2011;365(18):1693-1703. doi:10.1056/NEJMoa1012413

49. Yan D, Chen Y, Lv T, et al. Clostridium difficile colonization and infection in patients with hepatic cirrhosis. J Med Microbiol. 2017;66(10):1483-1488. doi:10.1099/jmm.0.000596

50. Kwok CS, Arthur AK, Anibueze CI, Singh S, Cavallazzi R, Loke YK. Risk of Clostridium difficile infection with acid suppressing drugs and antibiotics: meta-analysis. Am J Gastroenterol. 2012;107(7):1011-1019. doi:10.1038/ajg.2012.108

51. Gerding DN, Olson MM, Peterson LR, et al. Clostridium difficile-associated diarrhea and colitis in adults. A prospective case-controlled epidemiologic study. Arch Intern Med. 1986; 146(1):95-100.

52. Clabots CR, Johnson S, Olson MM, Peterson LR, Gerding DN. Acquisition of Clostridium difficile by hospitalized patients: evidence for colonized new admissions as a source of infection. J Infect Dis. 1992;166(3):561-567. doi:10.1093/infdis/166.3.561

53. McDonald LC, Coignard B, Dubberke E, Song X, Horan T, Kutty PK. Recommendations for surveillance of Clostridium difficile-associated disease. Infect Control Hosp Epidemiol. 2007;28(2):140-145. doi:10.1086/511798

54. Stergachis A, Perera DR, Schnell MM, Jick H. Antibiotic-associated colitis. West J Med. 1984;140(2):217-219. https://pubmed.ncbi.nlm.nih.gov/6730468

55. Khanna S, Pardi DS. The growing incidence and severity of Clostridium difficile infection in inpatient and outpatient settings. Expert Rev Gastroenterol Hepatol. 2010;4(4): 409-416. doi:10.1586/egh.10.48

56. Kwon JH, Olsen MA, Dubberke ER. The morbidity, mortality, and costs associated with Clostridium difficile infection. Infect Dis Clin North Am. 2015;29(1):123-134. doi:10.1016/j.idc.2014.11.003

57. Lessa FC, Mu Y, Bamberg WM, et al. Burden of Clostridium difficile infection in the United States. N Engl J Med. 2015; 372(9):825-834. doi:10.1056/NEJMoa1408913

58. Ofori E, Ramai D, Dhawan M, Mustafa F, Gasperino J, Reddy M. Community-acquired Clostridium difficile: epidemiology, ribotype, risk factors, hospital and intensive care unit outcomes, and current and emerging therapies. J Hosp Infect. 2018;99(4):436-442. doi:10.1016/j.jhin.2018.01.015

59. Chitnis AS, Holzbauer SM, Belflower RM, et al. Epidemiology of community-associated Clostridium difficile infection, 2009 through 2011. JAMA Intern Med. 2013;173(14):1359-1367. doi:10.1001/jamainternmed.2013.7056

60. Walker AS, Eyre DW, Wyllie DH, et al. Characterisation of Clostridium difficile hospital ward–based transmission using extensive epidemiological data and molecular typing. PLOS

Med. 2012;9(2):e1001172. https://doi.org/10.1371/journal.pmed.1001172

61. Thornton CS, Rubin JE, Greninger AL, Peirano G, Chiu CY, Pillai DR. Epidemiological and genomic characterization of community-acquired Clostridium difficile infections. BMC Infect Dis. 2018;18(1):443. doi:10.1186/s12879-018-3337-9

62. Hall IC, O'Toole E. Intestinal flora in newborn infants with a description of a new pathogenic anaerobe Bacillus difficilis. Am J Dis Child. 1935;49:390.

63. Riegler M, Sedivy R, Pothoulakis C, et al. Clostridium difficile toxin B is more potent than toxin A in damaging human colonic epithelium in vitro. J Clin Invest. 1995; 95(5):2004-2011. doi:10.1172/JCI117885

64. Leffler DA, Lamont JT. Clostridium difficile infection. N Engl J Med. 2015;372(16):1539-1548. doi:10.1056/NEJMra1403772

65. Natarajan M, Walk ST, Young VB, Aronoff DM. A clinical and epidemiological review of non-toxigenic Clostridium difficile. Anaerobe. 2013;22:1-5. doi:10.1016/j.anaerobe.2013.05.005

66. Peniche AG, Savidge TC, Dann SM. Recent insights into Clostridium difficile pathogenesis. Curr Opin Infect Dis. 2013;26(5):447-453. doi:10.1097/01.qco.0000433318.82618.c6

67. al Saif N, Brazier JS. The distribution of Clostridium difficile in the environment of South Wales. J Med Microbiol. 1996; 45(2):133-137. doi:10.1099/00222615-45-2-133

68. Durovic A, Widmer AF, Tschudin-Sutter S. New insights into transmission of Clostridium difficile infection—narrative review. Clin Microbiol Infect. 2018;24(5):483-492. doi:10.1016/j.cmi.2018.01.027

69. Stuart RL, Marshall C, Harrington G, Sasko L, McLaws M-L, Ferguson J. ASID/ACIPC position statement - infection control for patients with Clostridium difficile infection in healthcare facilities. Infect Dis Heal. 2019;24(1):32-43. doi:10.1016/j.idh.2018.10.001

70. Kim KH, Fekety R, Batts DH, et al. Isolation of Clostridium difficile from the environment and contacts of patients with antibiotic-associated colitis. J Infect Dis. 1981; 143(1):42-50. doi:10.1093/infdis/143.1.42

71. Gerding DN, Johnson S, Peterson LR, Mulligan ME, Silva JJ. Clostridium difficile-associated diarrhea and colitis. Infect Control Hosp Epidemiol. 1995;16(8):459-477. doi:10.1086/648363

72. Samore MH, Venkataraman L, DeGirolami PC, Arbeit RD, Karchmer AW. Clinical and molecular epidemiology of sporadic and clustered cases of nosocomial Clostridium difficile diarrhea. Am J Med. 1996;100(1):32-40. doi:10.1016/s0002-9343(96)90008-x

73. Mawer DPC, Eyre DW, Griffiths D, et al. Contribution to Clostridium difficile transmission of symptomatic patients with toxigenic strains who are fecal toxin negative. Clin Infect Dis. 2017;64(9):1163-1170. doi:10.1093/cid/cix079

74. Donskey CJ, Sunkesula VCK, Stone ND, et al. Transmission of Clostridium difficile from asymptomatically colonized or infected long-term care facility residents. Infect Control Hosp Epidemiol. 2018;39(8):909-916. doi:10.1017/ice.2018.106

75. Kong LY, Eyre DW, Corbeil J, et al. Clostridium difficile: investigating transmission patterns between infected and colonized patients using whole genome sequencing. Clin Infect Dis. 2019;68(2):204-209. doi:10.1093/cid/ciy457

76. Eyre DW, Cule ML, Wilson DJ, et al. Diverse sources of C. difficile infection identified on whole-genome sequencing. N Engl J Med. 2013;369(13):1195-1205. doi:10.1056/NEJMoa1216064

77. Cohen SH, Gerding DN, Johnson S, et al. Clinical practice guidelines for Clostridium difficile infection in adults: 2010 update by the Society for Healthcare Epidemiology of America (SHEA) and the Infectious Diseases Society of America (IDSA). 2010;31(5). doi:10.1086/651706

78. Curry SR, Muto CA, Schlackman JL, et al. Use of multilocus variable number of tandem repeats analysis genotyping to determine the role of asymptomatic carriers in Clostridium difficile transmission. Clin Infect Dis. 2013;57(8):1094-1102. doi:10.1093/cid/cit475

79. Australian Commission on Safety and Quality in Health Care. Implementation guide for the surveillance of Clostridioides difficile infection. ACSQHC, 2020. Available from: https://www.safetyandquality.gov.au/sites/default/files/2020-07/surveillance_guide_cdi_july_2020_indesign_final.pdf.

80. Knoop FC, Owens M, Crocker IC. Clostridium difficile: clinical disease and diagnosis. Clin Microbiol Rev. 1993;6(3):251-265. doi:10.1128/cmr.6.3.251

81. Wanahita A, Goldsmith EA, Marino BJ, Musher DM. Clostridium difficile infection in patients with unexplained leukocytosis. Am J Med. 2003;115(7):543-546. doi:10.1016/s0002-9343(03)00420-0

82. Debast SB, Bauer MP, Kuijper EJ. European Society of Clinical Microbiology and Infectious Diseases: update of the treatment guidance document for Clostridium difficile infection. Clin Microbiol Infect. 2014;20 Suppl 2:1-26. doi:10.1111/1469-0691.12418

83. Dansinger ML, Johnson S, Jansen PC, Opstad NL, Bettin KM, Gerding DN. Protein-losing enteropathy is associated with Clostridium difficile diarrhea but not with asymptomatic colonization: a prospective, case-control study. Clin Infect Dis. 1996;22(6):932-937. doi:10.1093/clinids/22.6.932

84. Brown TA, Rajappannair L, Dalton AB, Bandi R, Myers JP, Kefalas CH. Acute appendicitis in the setting of Clostridium difficile colitis: case report and review of the literature. Clin Gastroenterol Hepatol Off Clin Pract J Am Gastroenterol Assoc. 2007;5(8):969-971. doi:10.1016/j.cgh.2007.04.016

85. Hayetian FD, Read TE, Brozovich M, Garvin RP, Caushaj PF. Ileal perforation secondary to Clostridium difficile enteritis: report of 2 cases. Arch Surg. 2006;141(1):97-99. doi:10.1001/archsurg.141.1.97

86. Jacobs A, Barnard K, Fishel R, Gradon JD. Extracolonic manifestations of Clostridium difficile infections. Presentation of 2 cases and review of the literature. Medicine (Baltimore). 2001;80(2):88-101. doi:10.1097/00005792-200103000-00002

87. Shmerling RH, Caliendo AM. Case records of the Massachusetts General Hospital. Weekly clinicopathological exercises. Case 19-1998. A 70-year-old man with diarrhea, polyarthritis, and a history of Reiter's syndrome. N Engl J Med. 1998;338(25):1830-1836. doi:10.1056/NEJM199806183382508

88. Gupta A, Patel R, Baddour LM, Pardi DS, Khanna S. Extraintestinal Clostridium difficile infections: a single-center experience. Mayo Clin Proc. 2014;89(11):1525-1536. doi:10.1016/j.mayocp.2014.07.012

89. Barbut F, Richard A, Hamadi K, Chomette V, Burghoffer B, Petit JC. Epidemiology of recurrences or reinfections of Clostridium difficile-associated diarrhea. J Clin Microbiol. 2000;38(6):2386-2388. doi:10.1128/.38.6.2386-2388.2000

90. Bagdasarian N, Rao K, Malani PN. Diagnosis and treatment of Clostridium difficile in adults: a systematic review. JAMA. 2015;313(4):398-408. doi:10.1001/jama.2014.17103

91. Public Health Laboratory Network. Clostridium difficile infection (CDI) laboratory case definition. 2016. [cited 11 Aug 2020]. Available from: https://www1.health.gov.au/internet/main/publishing.nsf/Content/cda-phlncd-clostridium-difficile-infection-(CDI).htm

92. Crobach MJT, Planche T, Eckert C, et al. European Society of Clinical Microbiology and Infectious Diseases: update of the diagnostic guidance document for Clostridium difficile infection. Clin Microbiol Infect. 2016;22 Suppl 4:S63-81. doi:10.1016/j.cmi.2016.03.010

93. Kundrapu S, Sunkesula VCK, Jury LA, Sethi AK, Donskey CJ. Utility of perirectal swab specimens for diagnosis of Clostridium difficile infection. Clin Infect Dis. 2012; 55(11):1527-1530. doi:10.1093/cid/cis707

94. Ferguson JK, Cheng AC, Gilbert GL, et al. Clostridium difficile laboratory testing in Australia and New Zealand: national survey results and Australasian Society for Infectious Diseases recommendations for best practice. Pathology. 2011;43(5):482-487. doi:10.1097/PAT.0b013e328348c9b4

95. Wilcox MH. Preface: Clostridium difficile Infection. Infect Dis Clin North Am. 2015;29(1):xiii-xiv. doi:10.1016/j.idc.2014.12.001

96. van den Berg RJ, Vaessen N, Endtz HP, Schülin T, van der Vorm ER, Kuijper EJ. Evaluation of real-time PCR and conventional diagnostic methods for the detection of Clostridium difficile-associated diarrhoea in a prospective multicentre study. J Med Microbiol. 2007;56(Pt 1):36-42. doi:10.1099/jmm.0.46680-0

97. Aichinger E, Schleck CD, Harmsen WS, Nyre LM, Patel R. Nonutility of repeat laboratory testing for detection of Clostridium difficile by use of PCR or enzyme immunoassay. J Clin Microbiol. 2008;46(11):3795-3797. doi:10.1128/JCM.00684-08

98. Burnham C-AD, Carroll KC. Diagnosis of Clostridium difficile infection: an ongoing conundrum for clinicians and for clinical laboratories. Clin Microbiol Rev. 2013;26(3):604-630. doi:10.1128/CMR.00016-13

99. Kraft CS, Parrott JS, Cornish NE, et al. A laboratory medicine best practices systematic review and meta-analysis of nucleic acid amplification tests (NAATs) and algorithms including NAATs for the diagnosis of Clostridioides (Clostridium) difficile in adults. Clin Microbiol Rev. 2019;32(3). doi:10.1128/CMR.00032-18

100. Planche T, Wilcox M. Reference assays for Clostridium difficile infection: one or two gold standards? J Clin Pathol. 2011;64(1):1-5. doi:10.1136/jcp.2010.080135

101. Chang TW, Bartlett JG, Gorbach SL, Onderdonk AB. Clindamycin-induced enterocolitis in hamsters as a model of pseudomembranous colitis in patients. Infect Immun. 1978;20(2):526-529. doi:10.1128/IAI.20.2.526-529.1978

102. O'Connor D, Hynes P, Cormican M, Collins E, Corbett-Feeney G, Cassidy M. Evaluation of methods for detection of toxins in specimens of feces submitted for diagnosis of Clostridium difficile-associated diarrhea. J Clin Microbiol. 2001;39(8):2846-2849. doi:10.1128/JCM.39.8.2846-2849.2001

103. Eastwood K, Else P, Charlett A, Wilcox M. Comparison of nine commercially available Clostridium difficile toxin detection assays, a real-time PCR assay for C. difficile tcdB, and a glutamate dehydrogenase detection assay to cytotoxin testing and cytotoxigenic culture methods. J Clin Microbiol. 2009;47(10):3211-3217. doi:10.1128/JCM.01082-09

104. Crobach MJT, Dekkers OM, Wilcox MH, Kuijper EJ. European Society of Clinical Microbiology and Infectious Diseases (ESCMID): data review and recommendations for diagnosing Clostridium difficile-infection (CDI). Clin Microbiol Infect. 2009;15(12):1053-1066. doi:10.1111/j.1469-0691.2009.03098.x

105. Wilcox MH. Overcoming barriers to effective recognition and diagnosis of Clostridium difficile infection. Clin Microbiol Infect. 2012;18 Suppl 6:13-20. doi:10.1111/1469-0691.12057

106. Longtin Y, Trottier S, Brochu G, et al. Impact of the type of diagnostic assay on Clostridium difficile infection and complication rates in a mandatory reporting program. Clin Infect Dis. 2013;56(1):67-73. doi:10.1093/cid/cis840

107. Polage CR, Gyorke CE, Kennedy MA, et al. Overdiagnosis of Clostridium difficile infection in the molecular test era. JAMA Intern Med. 2015;175(11):1792-1801. doi:10.1001/jamainternmed.2015.4114

108. Kawamoto S, Horton KM, Fishman EK. Pseudomembranous colitis: spectrum of imaging findings with clinical and pathologic correlation. Radiographics. 1999;19(4):887-897. doi:10.1148/radiographics.19.4.g99jl07887

109. Kato H, Kato H, Iwashima Y, Nakamura M, Nakamura A, Ueda R. Inappropriate use of loperamide worsens Clostridium difficile-associated diarrhoea. J Hosp Infect. 2008;70(2):194-195. doi:10.1016/j.jhin.2008.06.010

110. Koo HL, Koo DC, Musher DM, DuPont HL. Antimotility agents for the treatment of Clostridium difficile diarrhea and colitis. Clin Infect Dis. 2009;48(5):598-605. doi:10.1086/596711

111. Janarthanan S, Ditah I, Adler DG, Ehrinpreis MN. Clostridium difficile-associated diarrhea and proton pump inhibitor therapy: a meta-analysis. Am J Gastroenterol. 2012;107(7):1001-1010. doi:10.1038/ajg.2012.179

112. Cho JM, Pardi DS, Khanna S. Update on treatment of Clostridioides difficile infection. Mayo Clin Proc. 2020; 95(4):758-769. doi:10.1016/j.mayocp.2019.08.006

113. Haifer C, Kelly CR, Paramsothy S, et al. Australian consensus statements for the regulation, production and use of faecal microbiota transplantation in clinical practice. Gut. 2020; 69(5):801-810. doi:10.1136/gutjnl-2019-320260

114. Cammarota G, Ianiro G, Tilg H, et al. European consensus conference on faecal microbiota transplantation in clinical practice. Gut. 2017;66(4):569-580. doi:10.1136/gutjnl-2016-313017

115. Tariq R, Pardi DS, Bartlett MG, Khanna S. Low cure rates in controlled trials of fecal microbiota transplantation for recurrent Clostridium difficile infection: a systematic review and meta-analysis. Clin Infect Dis. 2019;68(8):1351-1358. doi:10.1093/cid/ciy721

116. Juul FE, Garborg K, Bretthauer M, et al. Fecal microbiota transplantation for primary Clostridium difficile infection. N Engl J Med. 2018;378(26):2535-2536. doi:10.1056/NEJMc1803103

117. Roshan N, Clancy AK, Borody TJ. Faecal microbiota transplantation is effective for the initial treatment of Clostridium difficile infection: a retrospective clinical review. Infect Dis Ther. Published online 2020. doi:10.1007/s40121-020-00339-w

118. Dieterle MG, Rao K, Young VB. Novel therapies and preventative strategies for primary and recurrent Clostridium difficile infections. Ann NY Acad Sci. 2019;1435(1):110-138. doi:10.1111/nyas.13958

119. Ooijevaar RE, van Beurden YH, Terveer EM, et al. Update of treatment algorithms for Clostridium difficile infection. Clin Microbiol Infect. 2018;24(5):452-462. doi:https://doi.org/10.1016/j.cmi.2017.12.022

120. Hsu J, Abad C, Dinh M, Safdar N. Prevention of endemic healthcare-associated Clostridium difficile infection: reviewing the evidence. Am J Gastroenterol. 2010;105(11):2327-2339; quiz 2340. doi:10.1038/ajg.2010.254

121. Ratnayake L, McEwen J, Henderson N, et al. Control of an outbreak of diarrhoea in a vascular surgery unit caused by a high-level clindamycin-resistant Clostridium difficile

PCR ribotype 106. J Hosp Infect. 2011;79(3):242-247. doi:10.1016/j.jhin.2011.06.013

122. Longtin Y, Paquet-Bolduc B, Gilca R, et al. Effect of detecting and isolating Clostridium difficile carriers at hospital admission on the incidence of C difficile infections: a quasi-experimental controlled study. JAMA Intern Med. 2016;176(6):796-804. doi:10.1001/jamainternmed.2016.0177

123. Sethi AK, Al-Nassir WN, Nerandzic MM, Bobulsky GS, Donskey CJ. Persistence of skin contamination and environmental shedding of Clostridium difficile during and after treatment of C. difficile infection. Infect Control Hosp Epidemiol. 2010;31(1):21-27. doi:10.1086/649016

124. Weber DJ, Anderson DJ, Sexton DJ, Rutala WA. Role of the environment in the transmission of Clostridium difficile in health care facilities. Am J Infect Control. 2013;41(5, Supplement):S105-S110. doi:https://doi.org/10.1016/j.ajic.2012.12.009

125. Mayfield JL, Leet T, Miller J, Mundy LM. Environmental control to reduce transmission of Clostridium difficile. Clin Infect Dis. 2000;31(4):995-1000. doi:10.1086/318149

126. Macleod-Glover N, Sadowski C. Efficacy of cleaning products for C. difficile: environmental strategies to reduce the spread of Clostridium difficile-associated diarrhea in geriatric rehabilitation. Can Fam Physician. 2010;56(5):417-423.

127. Doan L, Forrest H, Fakis A, Craig J, Claxton L, Khare M. Clinical and cost effectiveness of eight disinfection methods for terminal disinfection of hospital isolation rooms contaminated with Clostridium difficile 027. J Hosp Infect. 2012;82(2):114-121. doi:https://doi.org/10.1016/j.jhin.2012.06.014

128. Perez J, Springthorpe VS, Sattar SA. Activity of selected oxidizing microbicides against the spores of Clostridium difficile: relevance to environmental control. Am J Infect Control. 2005;33(6):320-325. doi:https://doi.org/10.1016/j.ajic.2005.04.240

129. Weber DJ, Rutala WA, Anderson DJ, Chen LF, Sickbert-Bennett EE, Boyce JM. Effectiveness of ultraviolet devices and hydrogen peroxide systems for terminal room decontamination: focus on clinical trials. Am J Infect Control. 2016;44(5):e77-e84. doi:10.1016/j.ajic.2015.11.015

130. Marra AR, Schweizer ML, Edmond MB. No-touch disinfection methods to decrease multidrug-resistant organism infections: a systematic review and meta-analysis. Infect Control Hosp Epidemiol. 2018;39(1):20-31. doi:DOI: 10.1017/ice.2017.226

131. Anderson DJ, Chen LF, Weber DJ, et al. Enhanced terminal room disinfection and acquisition and infection caused by multidrug-resistant organisms and Clostridium difficile (the benefits of enhanced terminal room disinfection study): a cluster-randomised, multicentre, crossover study. Lancet. 2017;389(10071):805-814. doi:https://doi.org/10.1016/S0140-6736(16)31588-4

132. McMullen K, Guth RM, Wood H, et al. Impact of no-touch ultraviolet light room disinfection systems on Clostridioides difficile infections. Am J Infect Control. Published online 2020. doi:https://doi.org/10.1016/j.ajic.2020.08.030

133. Havill NL, Moore BA, Boyce JM. Comparison of the microbiological efficacy of hydrogen peroxide vapor and ultraviolet light processes for room decontamination. Infect Control Hosp Epidemiol. 2012;33(5):507-512. doi:DOI: 10.1086/665326

134. Ray AJ, Deshpande A, Fertelli D, et al. A multicenter randomized trial to determine the effect of an environmental

disinfection intervention on the incidence of healthcare-associated Clostridium difficile infection. Infect Control Hosp Epidemiol. 2017;38(7):777-783. doi:10.1017/ice.2017.76

135. Chau JPC, Liu X, Lo SHS, Chien WT, Wan X. Effects of environmental cleaning bundles on reducing healthcare-associated Clostridioides difficile infection: a systematic review and meta-analysis. J Hosp Infect. 2020;106(4):734-744. doi:10.1016/j.jhin.2020.08.019

136. Wullt M, Odenholt I, Walder M. Activity of three disinfectants and acidified nitrite against Clostridium difficile spores. Infect Control Hosp Epidemiol. 2003;24(10):765-768. doi:DOI: 10.1086/502129

137. Jabbar U, Leischner J, Kasper D, et al. Effectiveness of alcohol-based hand rubs for removal of Clostridium difficile spores from hands. Infect Control Hosp Epidemiol. 2010;31(6):565-570. doi:DOI: 10.1086/652772

138. Dubberke ER, Carling P, Carrico R, et al. Strategies to prevent Clostridium difficile infections in acute care hospitals: 2014 Update. Infect Control Hosp Epidemiol. 2014;35(6):628-645. doi:10.1086/676023

139. Jump RLP, Pultz MJ, Donskey CJ. Vegetative Clostridium difficile survives in room air on moist surfaces and in gastric contents with reduced acidity: a potential mechanism to explain the association between proton pump inhibitors and C. difficile-associated diarrhea? Antimicrob Agents Chemother. 2007;51(8):2883-2887. doi:10.1128/AAC.01443-06

140. Barker AK, Alagoz O, Safdar N. Interventions to reduce the incidence of hospital-onset Clostridium difficile infection: an agent-based modeling approach to evaluate clinical effectiveness in adult acute care hospitals. Clin Infect Dis. 2018;66(8):1192-1203. doi:10.1093/cid/cix962

141. Rhea S, Jones K, Endres-Dighe S, et al. Modeling inpatient and outpatient antibiotic stewardship interventions to reduce the burden of Clostridioides difficile infection in a regional healthcare network. PLoS One. 2020;15(6):1-16. doi:10.1371/journal.pone.0234031

142. Feazel LM, Malhotra A, Perencevich EN, Kaboli P, Diekema DJ, Schweizer ML. Effect of antibiotic stewardship programmes on Clostridium difficile incidence: a systematic review and meta-analysis. J Antimicrob Chemother. 2014;69(7):1748-1754. doi:10.1093/jac/dku046

143. Graber CJ. Clostridium difficile infection: stewardship's lowest hanging fruit? Lancet Infect Dis. 2017;17(2):123-124. doi:10.1016/S1473-3099(16)30416-9

144. Lawes T, Lopez-Lozano J-M, Nebot CA, et al. Effect of a national 4C antibiotic stewardship intervention on the clinical and molecular epidemiology of Clostridium difficile infections in a region of Scotland: a non-linear time-series analysis. Lancet Infect Dis. 2017;17(2):194-206. doi:https://doi.org/10.1016/S1473-3099(16)30397-8

145. Kandel CE, Gill S, McCready J, Matelski J, Powis JE. Reducing co-administration of proton pump inhibitors and antibiotics using a computerized order entry alert and prospective audit and feedback. BMC Infect Dis. 2016;16(1):355. doi:10.1186/s12879-016-1679-8

146. Centers for Disease Control and Prevention. Principles of epidemiology in public health practice-an introduction to applied epidemiology and biostatistics. 3rd ed. Centers for Disease Control and Prevention, 2006. Available from: https://stacks.cdc.gov/view/cdc/6914/cdc_6914_DS1.pdf.

147. Goldenberg JZ, Yap C, Lytvyn L, et al. Probiotics for the prevention of Clostridium difficile-associated diarrhea in adults and children. Cochrane Database Syst Rev. 2017;12(12):CD006095. doi:10.1002/14651858.CD006095.pub4

148. Kothari D, Patel S, Kim S-K. Probiotic supplements might not be universally-effective and safe: a review. Biomed Pharmacother. 2019;111:537-547. doi:https://doi.org/10.1016/j.biopha.2018.12.104

149. Allen SJ, Wareham K, Wang D, et al. Lactobacilli and bifidobacteria in the prevention of antibiotic-associated diarrhoea and Clostridium difficile diarrhoea in older inpatients (PLACIDE): a randomised, double-blind, placebo-controlled, multicentre trial. Lancet. 2013;382(9900): 1249-1257. doi:10.1016/S0140-6736(13)61218-0

150. Barker AK, Ngam C, Musuuza JS, Vaughn VM, Safdar N. Reducing Clostridium difficile in the inpatient setting: a systematic review of the adherence to and effectiveness of C. difficile prevention bundles. Infect Control Hosp Epidemiol. 2017;38(6):639-650. doi:10.1017/ice.2017.7

151. Muto CA, Blank MK, Marsh JW, et al. Control of an outbreak of infection with the hypervirulent Clostridium difficile BI strain in a university hospital using a comprehensive "bundle" approach. Clin Infect Dis. 2007;45(10):1266-1273. doi:10.1086/522654

152. Weiss K, Boisvert A, Chagnon M, et al. Multipronged intervention strategy to control an outbreak of Clostridium difficile infection (CDI) and its impact on the rates of CDI from 2002 to 2007. Infect Control Hosp Epidemiol. 2009;30(2):156-162. doi:10.1086/593955

153. Koll BS, Ruiz RE, Calfee DP, et al. Prevention of hospital-onset Clostridium difficile infection in the New York metropolitan region using a collaborative intervention model. J Healthc Qual. 2014;36(3):35-45. doi:10.1111/jhq.12002

154. Ahmed SM, Hall AJ, Robinson AE, et al. Global prevalence of norovirus in cases of gastroenteritis: a systematic review and meta-analysis. Lancet Infect Dis. 2014;14(8):725-730. doi:10.1016/S1473-3099(14)70767-4

155. Pires SM, Fischer-Walker CL, Lanata CF, et al. Aetiology-specific estimates of the global and regional incidence and mortality of diarrhoeal diseases commonly transmitted through food. PLoS One. 2015;10(12):e0142927. https://doi.org/10.1371/journal.pone.0142927

156. Kirk MD, Pires SM, Black RE, et al. World Health Organization estimates of the global and regional disease burden of 22 foodborne bacterial, protozoal, and viral diseases, 2010: a data synthesis. PLOS Med. 2015;12(12):e1001921. https://doi.org/10.1371/journal.pmed.1001921

157. Centers for Disease Control and Prevention. Updated norovirus outbreak management and disease prevention guidelines. MMWR Recomm Reports Morb Mortal Wkly Report. 2011;60(RR-3):1-18.

158. Lopman BA, Reacher MH, Vipond IB, et al. Epidemiology and cost of nosocomial gastroenteritis, Avon, England, 2002-2003. Emerg Infect Dis. 2004;10(10):1827-1834. doi:10.3201/eid1010.030941

159. Kambhampati A, Koopmans M, Lopman BA. Burden of norovirus in healthcare facilities and strategies for outbreak control. J Hosp Infect. 2015;89(4):296-301. doi:10.1016/j.jhin.2015.01.011

160. Davis C, Vally H, Bell R, Sheehan F, Beard F. Viral gastrointestinal outbreaks in residential care facilities: an examination of the value of public health unit involvement. Aust N Z J Public Health. 2014;38(2): 177-183. doi:10.1111/1753-6405.12171

161. Bruggink LD, Triantafilou MJ, Marshall JA. The molecular epidemiology of norovirus outbreaks in Victoria, 2016. Commun Dis Intell. 2018;42.

162. Communicable Diseases Branch. NSW OzFoodNet Annual Surveillance Report: 2017. Health Protection NSW, 2018.

163. Zahorsky J. Hyperemesis hemis or the winter vomiting disease. Arch Pediatr. 1929;46:391-395.

164. Kapikian AZ, Wyatt RG, Dolin R, Thornhill TS, Kalica AR, Chanock RM. Visualization by immune electron microscopy of a 27-nm particle associated with acute infectious nonbacterial gastroenteritis. J Virol. 1972;10(5): 1075-1081. doi:10.1128/JVI.10.5.1075-1081.1972

165. Dolin R, Treanor JJ. 176 - Noroviruses and sapoviruses (caliciviruses). 9th ed. Bennett JE, Dolin R, Blaser MJ, eds. Elsevier Inc, 2020. doi:10.1016/B978-0-323-48255-4.00176-4

166. Chhabra P, de Graaf M, Parra GI, et al. Updated classification of norovirus genogroups and genotypes. J Gen Virol. 2019; 100(10):1393-1406. doi:10.1099/jgv.0.001318

167. Glass RI, Parashar UD, Estes MK. Norovirus gastroenteritis. N Engl J Med. 2009;361(18):1776-1785. doi:10.1056/NEJMra0804575

168. Siebenga JJ, Vennema H, Zheng D-P, et al. Norovirus illness is a global problem: emergence and spread of norovirus GII.4 variants, 2001-2007. J Infect Dis. 2009;200(5): 802-812. doi:10.1086/605127

169. Green KY. Caliciviridae: the noroviruses. In: Knipe DM, Howley PM, eds. Fields' virology. 6th ed. Volume 1. 6th ed. Lippincott Williams & Wilkins, 2013.

170. Kroneman A, Vega E, Vennema H, et al. Proposal for a unified norovirus nomenclature and genotyping. Arch Virol. 2013;158(10):2059-2068. doi:10.1007/s00705-013-1708-5

171. Atmar RL, Ramani S, Estes MK. Human noroviruses: recent advances in a 50-year history. Curr Opin Infect Dis. 2018;31(5):422-432. doi:10.1097/QCO.0000000000000476

172. Weber DJ, Rutala WA, Miller MB, Huslage K, Sickbert-Bennett E. Role of hospital surfaces in the transmission of emerging health care-associated pathogens: norovirus, Clostridium difficile, and Acinetobacter species. Am J Infect Control. 2010;38(5 Suppl 1):S25-33. doi:10.1016/j.ajic.2010.04.196

173. Seitz SR, Leon JS, Schwab KJ, et al. Norovirus infectivity in humans and persistence in water. Appl Environ Microbiol. 2011;77(19):6884-6888. doi:10.1128/AEM.05806-11

174. Podewils LJ, Zanardi Blevins L, Hagenbuch M, et al. Outbreak of norovirus illness associated with a swimming pool. Epidemiol Infect. 2007;135(5):827-833. doi:10.1017/S0950268806007370

175. Keswick BH, Satterwhite TK, Johnson PC, et al. Inactivation of Norwalk virus in drinking water by chlorine. Appl Environ Microbiol. 1985;50(2):261-264. doi:10.1128/AEM.50.2.261-264.1985

176. D'Souza DH, Sair A, Williams K, et al. Persistence of caliciviruses on environmental surfaces and their transfer to food. Int J Food Microbiol. 2006;108(1):84-91. doi:10.1016/j.ijfoodmicro.2005.10.024

177. Atmar RL, Opekun AR, Gilger MA, et al. Determination of the 50% human infectious dose for Norwalk virus. J Infect Dis. 2014;209(7):1016-1022. doi:10.1093/infdis/jit620

178. Teunis PFM, Moe CL, Liu P, et al. Norwalk virus: how infectious is it? J Med Virol. 2008;80(8):1468-1476. doi:10.1002/jmv.21237

179. Teunis PFM, Le Guyader FS, Liu P, Ollivier J, Moe CL. Noroviruses are highly infectious but there is strong variation in host susceptibility and virus pathogenicity.

Epidemics. 2020;32:100401. doi:10.1016/j.epidem.2020. 100401

180. Robilotti E, Deresinski S, Pinsky BA. Norovirus. Clin Microbiol Rev. 2015;28(1):134-164. doi:10.1128/ CMR.00075-14

181. Kirby AE, Streby A, Moe CL. Vomiting as a symptom and transmission risk in norovirus illness: evidence from human challenge studies. PLoS One. 2016;11(4):1-10. doi:10. 1371/journal.pone.0143759

182. Matthews JE, Dickey BW, Miller RD, et al. The epidemiology of published norovirus outbreaks: a review of risk factors associated with attack rate and genogroup. Epidemiol Infect. 2012;140(7):1161-1172. doi:DOI: 10.1017/S0950268812000234

183. Bonifait L, Charlebois R, Vimont A, et al. Detection and quantification of airborne norovirus during outbreaks in healthcare facilities. Clin Infect Dis. 2015;61(3):299-304. doi:10.1093/cid/civ321

184. Nenonen NP, Hannoun C, Svensson L, et al. Norovirus GII.4 Detection in environmental samples from patient rooms during nosocomial outbreaks. Tang Y-W, ed. J Clin Microbiol. 2014;52(7):2352 LP - 2358. doi:10.1128/JCM. 00266-14

185. Sawyer LA, Murphy JJ, Kaplan JE, et al. 25- to 30-nm virus particle associated with a hospital outbreak of acute gastroenteritis with evidence for airborne transmission. Am J Epidemiol. 1988;127(6):1261-1271. doi:10.1093/ oxfordjournals.aje.a114918

186. Chadwick PR, Walker M, Rees AE. Airborne transmission of a small round structured virus. Lancet. 1994;343(8890):171. doi:10.1016/s0140-6736(94)90959-8

187. Marks PJ, Vipond IB, Carlisle D, Deakin D, Fey RE, Caul EO. Evidence for airborne transmission of Norwalk-like virus (NLV) in a hotel restaurant. Epidemiol Infect. 2000;124(3):481-487. doi:10.1017/s0950268899003805

188. Alsved M, Fraenkel C-J, Bohgard M, et al. Sources of airborne norovirus in hospital outbreaks. Clin Infect Dis. 2020;70(10):2023-2028. doi:10.1093/cid/ciz584

189. Gralton J, Tovey E, McLaws M-L, Rawlinson WD. The role of particle size in aerosolised pathogen transmission: a review. J Infect. 2011;62(1):1-13. doi:10.1016/j.jinf.2010.11.010

190. Barker J, Vipond IB, Bloomfield SF. Effects of cleaning and disinfection in reducing the spread of Norovirus contamination via environmental surfaces. J Hosp Infect. 2004;58(1):42-49. doi:https://doi.org/10.1016/j.jhin. 2004.04.021

191. Cheesbrough JS, Barkess-Jones L, Brown DW. Possible prolonged environmental survival of small round structured viruses. J Hosp Infect. 1997;35(4):325-326. doi:10.1016/ S0195-6701(97)90230-9

192. Thornley CN, Emslie NA, Sprott TW, Greening GE, Rapana JP. Recurring norovirus transmission on an airplane. Clin Infect Dis. 2011;53(6):515-520. doi:10.1093/cid/cir465

193. Evans MR, Meldrum R, Lane W, et al. An outbreak of viral gastroenteritis following environmental contamination at a concert hall. Epidemiol Infect. 2002;129(2):355-360. doi:DOI: 10.1017/S0950268802007446

194. Petrignani M, van Beek J, Borsboom G, Richardus JH, Koopmans M. Norovirus introduction routes into nursing homes and risk factors for spread: a systematic review and meta-analysis of observational studies. J Hosp Infect. 2015;89(3):163-178. doi:10.1016/j.jhin.2014.11.015

195. Parrón I, Álvarez J, Jané M, et al. A foodborne norovirus outbreak in a nursing home and spread to staff and their

household contacts. Epidemiol Infect. 2019;147:e225-e225. doi:10.1017/S0950268819001146

196. Qi R, Huang Y, Liu J, et al. Global prevalence of asymptomatic norovirus infection: a meta-analysis. EClinicalMedicine. 2018;2:50-58. doi:10.1016/j. eclinm.2018.09.001

197. Arness MK, Feighner BH, Canham ML, et al. Norwalk-like viral gastroenteritis outbreak in U.S. Army trainees. Emerg Infect Dis. 2000;6(2):204-207. doi:10.3201/ eid0602.009918

198. Lopman BA, Reacher MH, Vipond IB, Sarangi J, Brown DWG. Clinical manifestation of norovirus gastroenteritis in health care settings. Clin Infect Dis. 2004;39(3):318-324. doi:10.1086/421948

199. Goller JL, Dimitriadis A, Tan A, Kelly H, Marshall JA. Long-term features of norovirus gastroenteritis in the elderly. J Hosp Infect. 2004;58(4):286-291. doi:10.1016/j. jhin.2004.07.001

200. Rockx B, De Wit M, Vennema H, et al. Natural history of human calicivirus infection: a prospective cohort study. Clin Infect Dis. 2002;35(3):246-253. doi:10.1086/341408

201. Costantini VP, Cooper EM, Hardaker HL, et al. Epidemiologic, virologic, and host genetic factors of norovirus outbreaks in long-term care facilities. Clin Infect Dis. 2016;62(1):1-10. doi:10.1093/cid/civ747

202. Biçer S, Çöl D, Küçük Ö, et al. Is there any difference between the symptomatology and clinical findings of viral agents causing dehydration? Minerva Pediatr. 2018;70(2): 165-174. doi:10.23736/S0026-4946.16.04259-X

203. Petrignani M, Verhoef L, de Graaf M, Richardus JH, Koopmans M. Chronic sequelae and severe complications of norovirus infection: a systematic review of literature. J Clin Virol. 2018;105:1-10. doi:10.1016/j.jcv.2018. 05.004

204. Zanini B, Ricci C, Bandera F, et al. Incidence of post-infectious irritable bowel syndrome and functional intestinal disorders following a water-borne viral gastroenteritis outbreak. Am J Gastroenterol. 2012;107(6):891-899. doi:10. 1038/ajg.2012.102

205. Porter CK, Faix DJ, Shiau D, Espiritu J, Espinosa BJ, Riddle MS. Postinfectious gastrointestinal disorders following norovirus outbreaks. Clin Infect Dis. 2012; 55(7):915-922. doi:10.1093/cid/cis576

206. Van Asten L, Siebenga J, Van Den Wijngaard C, et al. Unspecified gastroenteritis illness and deaths in the elderly associated with norovirus epidemics. Epidemiology. 2011; 22(3):336-343. doi:10.1097/EDE.0b013e31821179af

207. Trivedi TK, Desai R, Hall AJ, Patel M, Parashar UD, Lopman BA. Clinical characteristics of norovirus-associated deaths: a systematic literature review. Am J Infect Control. 2013;41(7):654-657. doi:10.1016/j.ajic.2012.08.002

208. Hall AJ, Curns AT, McDonald LC, Parashar UD, Lopman BA. The roles of Clostridium difficile and norovirus among gastroenteritis-associated deaths in the United States, 1999-2007. Clin Infect Dis. 2012;55(2):216-223. doi:10.1093/ cid/cis386

209. Trivedi TK, DeSalvo T, Lee L, et al. Hospitalizations and mortality associated with norovirus outbreaks in nursing homes, 2009-2010. JAMA. 2012;308(16):1668-1675. doi:10.1001/jama.2012.14023

210. Turcios-Ruiz RM, Axelrod P, St John K, et al. Outbreak of necrotizing enterocolitis caused by norovirus in a neonatal intensive care unit. J Pediatr. 2008;153(3):339-344. doi:10. 1016/j.jpeds.2008.04.015

211. Stuart RL, Tan K, Mahar JE, et al. An outbreak of necrotizing enterocolitis associated with norovirus genotype GII.3. Pediatr Infect Dis J. 2010;29(7):644-647. doi:10.1097/inf.0b013e3181d824e1

212. Bok K, Green KY. Norovirus gastroenteritis in immunocompromised patients. N Engl J Med. 2012;367(22):2126-2132. doi:10.1056/NEJMra1207742

213. Ludwig A, Adams O, Laws H-J, Schroten H, Tenenbaum T. Quantitative detection of norovirus excretion in pediatric patients with cancer and prolonged gastroenteritis and shedding of norovirus. J Med Virol. 2008;80(8):1461-1467. doi:10.1002/jmv.21217

214. van Beek J, van der Eijk AA, Fraaij PLA, et al. Chronic norovirus infection among solid organ recipients in a tertiary care hospital, the Netherlands, 2006-2014. Clin Microbiol Infect. 2017;23(4):265.e9-265.e13. doi:10.1016/j.cmi.2016.12.010

215. Swartling L, Ljungman P, Remberger M, et al. Norovirus causing severe gastrointestinal disease following allogeneic hematopoietic stem cell transplantation: a retrospective analysis. Transpl Infect Dis. 2018;20(2):e12847. doi:10.1111/tid.12847

216. Brown L-AK, Clark I, Brown JR, Breuer J, Lowe DM. Norovirus infection in primary immune deficiency. Rev Med Virol. 2017;27(3):e1926. doi:10.1002/rmv.1926

217. Kaplan JE, Feldman R, Campbell DS, Lookabaugh C, Gary GW. The frequency of a Norwalk-like pattern of illness in outbreaks of acute gastroenteritis. Am J Public Health. 1982;72(12):1329-1332. doi:10.2105/ajph.72.12.1329

218. Turcios RM, Widdowson M-A, Sulka AC, Mead PS, Glass RI. Reevaluation of epidemiological criteria for identifying outbreaks of acute gastroenteritis due to norovirus: United States, 1998–2000. Clin Infect Dis. 2006;42(7):964-969. doi:10.1086/500940

219. Lively JY, Johnson SD, Wikswo M, Gu W, Leon J, Hall AJ. Clinical and epidemiologic profiles for identifying norovirus in acute gastroenteritis outbreak investigations. Open Forum Infect Dis. 2018;5(4):ofy049. doi:10.1093/ofid/ofy049

220. Public Health Laboratory Network - Department of Health. Norovirus laboratory case definition (LCD). 2006. [cited 25 Aug 2020]. Available from: https://www1.health.gov.au/internet/main/publishing.nsf/Content/cda-phlncd-norwalk.htm#,:text=1 Definitive Criteria,Nucleic Acid Amplification (NAA).

221. Estes MK, Ettayebi K, Tenge VR, et al. Human norovirus cultivation in nontransformed stem cell-derived human intestinal enteroid cultures: success and challenges. Viruses. 2019;11(7):9-11. doi:10.3390/v11070638

222. Fisman DN, Greer AL, Brouhanski G, Drews SJ. Of gastro and the gold standard: evaluation and policy implications of norovirus test performance for outbreak detection. J Transl Med. 2009;7(1):23. doi:10.1186/1479-5876-7-23

223. Rabenau HF, Stürmer M, Buxbaum S, Walczok A, Preiser W, Doerr HW. Laboratory diagnosis of norovirus: which method is the best? Intervirology. 2003;46(4):232-238. doi:10.1159/000072433

224. Centers for Disease Control and Prevention. Norovirus - specimen collection. 2018. [cited 27 Dec 2020]. Available from: https://www.cdc.gov/norovirus/lab/specimen-collection.html

225. Ambert-Balay K, Pothier P. Evaluation of 4 immunochromatographic tests for rapid detection of norovirus in faecal samples. J Clin Virol. 2013;56(3):194-198. doi:10.1016/j.jcv.2012.11.001

226. Bruggink LD, Witlox KJ, Sameer R, Catton MG, Marshall JA. Evaluation of the RIDA®QUICK immunochromatographic norovirus detection assay using specimens from Australian gastroenteritis incidents. J Virol Methods. 2011;173(1):121-126. doi:https://doi.org/10.1016/j.jviromet.2011.01.017

227. Duizer E, Pielaat A, Vennema H, Kroneman A, Koopmans M. Probabilities in norovirus outbreak diagnosis. J Clin Virol. 2007;40(1):38-42. doi:https://doi.org/10.1016/j.jcv.2007.05.015

228. Patel MM, Widdowson M-A, Glass RI, Akazawa K, Vinjé J, Parashar UD. Systematic literature review of role of noroviruses in sporadic gastroenteritis. Emerg Infect Dis. 2008;14(8):1224-1231. doi:10.3201/eid1408.071114

229. Phillips G, Lopman B, Tam CC, Iturriza-Gomara M, Brown D, Gray J. Diagnosing norovirus-associated infectious intestinal disease using viral load. BMC Infect Dis. 2009;9(1):63. doi:10.1186/1471-2334-9-63

230. Angarone MP, Sheahan A, Kamboj M. Norovirus in transplantation. Curr Infect Dis Rep. 2016;18(6):17. doi:10.1007/s11908-016-0524-y

231. Rossignol J-F, El-Gohary YM. Nitazoxanide in the treatment of viral gastroenteritis: a randomized double-blind placebo-controlled clinical trial. Aliment Pharmacol Ther. 2006;24(10):1423-1430. doi:10.1111/j.1365-2036.2006.03128.x

232. Gairard-Dory A-C, Dégot T, Hirschi S, et al. Clinical usefulness of oral immunoglobulins in lung transplant recipients with norovirus gastroenteritis: a case series. Transplant Proc. 2014;46(10):3603-3605. doi:10.1016/j.transproceed.2014.09.095

233. Woodward JM, Gkrania-Klotsas E, Cordero-Ng AY, et al. The role of chronic norovirus infection in the enteropathy associated with common variable immunodeficiency. Am J Gastroenterol. 2015;110(2):320-327. doi:10.1038/ajg.2014.432

234. Netzler NE, Enosi Tuipulotu D, White PA. Norovirus antivirals: where are we now? Med Res Rev. 2019;39(3):860-886. doi:10.1002/med.21545

235. Communicable Diseases Network Australia. Guidelines for the public health management of gastroenteritis outbreaks due to norovirus or suspected viral agents in Australia. Australian Government Department of Health and Ageing, 2010. Available from: https://www.health.gov.au/internet/main/publishing.nsf/Content/cda-cdna-norovirus.htm/$File/norovirus-guidelines.pdf

236. MacCannell T, Umscheid CA, Agarwal RK, Lee I, Kuntz G, Stevenson KB. Guideline for the prevention and control of norovirus gastroenteritis outbreaks in healthcare settings. Infect Control Hosp Epidemiol. 2011;32(10):939-969. doi:DOI: 10.1086/662025

237. Norovirus Working Party. Guidelines for the management of norovirus outbreaks in acute and community health and social care settings. United Kingdom Government, 2012. Available from: https://www.gov.uk/government/publications/norovirus-managing-outbreaks-in-acute-and-community-health-and-social-care-settings

238. Haill CF, Newell P, Ford C, et al. Compartmentalization of wards to cohort symptomatic patients at the beginning and end of norovirus outbreaks. J Hosp Infect. 2012;82(1):30-35. doi:10.1016/j.jhin.2012.05.015

239. Illingworth E, Taborn E, Fielding D, Cheesbrough J, Diggle PJ, Orr D. Is closure of entire wards necessary to control norovirus outbreaks in hospital? Comparing the effectiveness of two infection control strategies. J Hosp Infect. 2011;79(1):32-37. doi:10.1016/j.jhin.2011.04.024

240. Harris JP, Adak GK, O'Brien SJ. To close or not to close? Analysis of 4 years' data from national surveillance of norovirus outbreaks in hospitals in England. BMJ Open. 2014;4(1):e003919-e003919. doi:10.1136/bmjopen-2013-003919

241. Siegel JD, Rhinehart E, Jackson M, Chiarello L, Committee HCICPA. 2007 Guideline for isolation precautions: preventing transmission of infectious agents in health care settings. Am J Infect Control. 2007;35(10 Suppl 2):S65-S164. doi:10.1016/j.ajic.2007.10.007

242. NHMRC. Australian guidelines for the prevention and control of infection in healthcare. Commonwealth of Australia, 2010.

243. Liu P, Yuen Y, Hsiao H-M, Jaykus L-A, Moe C. Effectiveness of liquid soap and hand sanitizer against Norwalk virus on contaminated hands. Appl Environ Microbiol. 2010;76(2):394-399. doi:10.1128/AEM.01729-09

244. Li D, Baert L, Van Coillie E, Uyttendaele M. Critical studies on binding-based RT-PCR detection of infectious noroviruses. J Virol Methods. 2011;177(2):153-159. doi:https://doi.org/10.1016/j.jviromet.2011.07.013

245. Sattar SA, Ali M, Tetro JA. In vivo comparison of two human norovirus surrogates for testing ethanol-based handrubs: the mouse chasing the cat! PLoS One. 2011;6(2):e17340. https://doi.org/10.1371/journal.pone.0017340

246. Park GW, Barclay L, Macinga D, Charbonneau D, Pettigrew CA, Vinjé J. Comparative efficacy of seven hand sanitizers against murine norovirus, feline calicivirus, and GII.4 norovirus. J Food Prot. 2010;73(12):2232-2238. doi:10.4315/0362-028x-73.12.2232

247. Tuladhar E, Hazeleger WC, Koopmans M, Zwietering MH, Duizer E, Beumer RR. Reducing viral contamination from finger pads: handwashing is more effective than alcohol-based hand disinfectants. J Hosp Infect. 2015;90(3):226-234. doi:10.1016/j.jhin.2015.02.019

248. Paulmann D, Steinmann J, Becker B, Bischoff B, Steinmann E, Steinmann J. Virucidal activity of different alcohols against murine norovirus, a surrogate of human norovirus. J Hosp Infect. 2011;79(4):378-379. doi:10.1016/j.jhin.2011.04.029

249. Steinmann J, Paulmann D, Becker B, Bischoff B, Steinmann E, Steinmann J. Comparison of virucidal activity of alcohol-based hand sanitizers versus antimicrobial hand soaps in vitro and in vivo. J Hosp Infect. 2012;82(4):277-280. doi:10.1016/j.jhin.2012.08.005

250. Kampf G. Efficacy of ethanol against viruses in hand disinfection. J Hosp Infect. 2018;98(4):331-338. doi:10.1016/j.jhin.2017.08.025

251. Suchomel M, Steinmann J, Kampf G. Efficacies of the original and modified WHO-recommended hand rub formulations. J Hosp Infect. Published online 26 August 2020. doi:10.1016/j.jhin.2020.08.006

252. Sato J, Miki M, Kubota H, et al. Effects of disinfectants against norovirus virus-like particles predict norovirus inactivation. Microbiol Immunol. 2016;60(9):609-616. doi:10.1111/1348-0421.12435

253. Blaney DD, Daly ER, Kirkland KB, Tongren JE, Kelso PT, Talbot EA. Use of alcohol-based hand sanitizers as a risk factor for norovirus outbreaks in long-term care facilities in northern New England: December 2006 to March 2007. Am J Infect Control. 2011;39(4):296-301. doi:10.1016/j.ajic.2010.10.010

254. Longtin Y, Voss A, Allegranzi B, Pittet D. Norovirus outbreaks and alcohol-based handrub solutions: association does not prove causation. Am J Infect Control. 2012;40(2):191; author reply 192. doi:10.1016/j.ajic.2011.05.002

255. Khanna N, Goldenberger D, Graber P, Battegay M, Widmer AF. Gastroenteritis outbreak with norovirus in a Swiss university hospital with a newly identified virus strain. J Hosp Infect. 2003;55(2):131-136. doi:https://doi.org/10.1016/00195-6701(03)00257-0

256. Cheng VCC, Tai JWM, Ho YY, Chan JFW. Successful control of norovirus outbreak in an infirmary with the use of alcohol-based hand rub. J Hosp Infect. 2009;72(4):370-371. doi:10.1016/j.jhin.2009.04.021

257. World Health Organization. System change – changing hand hygiene behaviour at the point of care. [cited 27 Aug 2020]. Available from: https://www.who.int/gpsc/tools/faqs/system_change/en/

258. Barclay L, Park GW, Vega E, et al. Infection control for norovirus. Clin Microbiol Infect. 2014;20(8):731-740. doi:10.1111/1469-0691.12674

259. Chiu S, Skura B, Petric M, McIntyre L, Gamage B, Isaac-Renton J. Efficacy of common disinfectant/cleaning agents in inactivating murine norovirus and feline calicivirus as surrogate viruses for human norovirus. Am J Infect Control. 2015;43(11):1208-1212. doi:10.1016/j.ajic.2015.06.021

260. Zonta W, Mauroy A, Farnir F, Thiry E. Comparative virucidal efficacy of seven disinfectants against murine norovirus and feline calicivirus, surrogates of human norovirus. Food Environ Virol. 2016;8(1):1-12. doi:10.1007/s12560-015-9216-2

261. Tung G, Macinga D, Arbogast J, Jaykus L-A. Efficacy of commonly used disinfectants for inactivation of human noroviruses and their surrogates. J Food Prot. 2013;76(7):1210-1217. doi:10.4315/0362-028X.JFP-12-532

262. Heijne J, Teunis P, Morroy G, et al. Enhanced hygiene measures and norovirus transmission during an outbreak. Emerg Infect Dis. 2009;15:24-30. doi:10.3201/1501.080299

263. University of South Australia. Literature Review Report - In healthcare settings, what is the current epidemiology and latest evidence on transmission pathways and infection prevention and control measures for norovirus gastroenteritis? National Health and Medical Research Council, 2017. Available from: https://www.nhmrc.gov.au/about-us/publications/australian-guidelines-prevention-and-control-infection-healthcare-2019.

264. Moorman E, Montazeri N, Jaykus L-A. Efficacy of neutral electrolyzed water for inactivation of human norovirus. Schaffner DW, ed. Appl Environ Microbiol. 2017;83(16):e00653-17. doi:10.1128/AEM.00653-17

265. Zonta W, Mauroy A, Farnir F, Thiry E. Virucidal efficacy of a hydrogen peroxide nebulization against murine norovirus and feline calicivirus, two surrogates of human norovirus. Food Environ Virol. 2016;8(4):275-282. doi:10.1007/s12560-016-9253-5

266. Holmdahl T, Walder M, Uzcátegui N, et al. Hydrogen peroxide vapor decontamination in a patient room using feline calicivirus and murine norovirus as surrogate markers for human norovirus. Infect Control Hosp Epidemiol. 2016;37(5):561-566. doi:10.1017/ice.2016.15

267. Park SY, Kim A-N, Lee K-H, Ha S-D. Ultraviolet-C efficacy against a norovirus surrogate and hepatitis A virus on a stainless steel surface. Int J Food Microbiol. 2015;211:73-78. doi:10.1016/j.ijfoodmicro.2015.07.006

268. Wallace RL, Ouellette M, Jean J. Effect of UV-C light or hydrogen peroxide wipes on the inactivation of methicillin-resistant Staphylococcus aureus, Clostridium difficile spores and norovirus surrogate. J Appl Microbiol. 2019;127(2):586-597. doi:10.1111/jam.14308

269. Ciofi-Silva CL, Bruna CQM, Carmona RCC, et al. Norovirus recovery from floors and air after various

decontamination protocols. J Hosp Infect. 2019;103(3): 328-334. doi:10.1016/j.jhin.2019.05.015

270. Hudson JB, Sharma M, Petric M. Inactivation of norovirus by ozone gas in conditions relevant to healthcare. J Hosp Infect. 2007;66(1):40-45. doi:10.1016/j.jhin.2006.12.021

271. Imai K, Hagi A, Inoue Y, Amarasiri M, Sano D. Virucidal efficacy of olanexidine gluconate as a hand antiseptic against human norovirus. Food Environ Virol. 2020;12(2):180-190. doi:10.1007/s12560-020-09422-4

272. Harris JP, Lopman BA, O'Brien SJ. Infection control measures for norovirus: a systematic review of outbreaks in semi-enclosed settings. J Hosp Infect. 2010;74(1):1-9. doi:10.1016/j.jhin.2009.07.025

273. Giersing BK, Vekemans J, Nava S, Kaslow DC, Moorthy V. Report from the World Health Organization's third Product Development for Vaccines Advisory Committee (PDVAC) meeting, Geneva, 8-10th June 2016. Vaccine. 2019;37(50):7315-7327. doi:10.1016/j.vaccine.2016.10.090

274. Esposito S, Principi N. Norovirus vaccine: priorities for future research and development. Front Immunol. 2020;11: 1383. Available from: https://www.frontiersin.org/article/10.3389/fimmu.2020.01383.

275. Australian Technical Advisory Group on Immunisation (ATAGI). The Australian Immunisation Handbook 10th Ed (2018 Update). Australian Government Department of Health, 2018. Available from: https://immunisationhandbook.health. gov.au/.

276. Dey A, Wang H, Menzies R, Macartney K. Changes in hospitalisations for acute gastroenteritis in Australia after the national rotavirus vaccination program. Med J Aust. 2012;197(8):453-457. doi:10.5694/mja12.10062

277. Buttery JP, Lambert SB, Grimwood K, et al. Reduction in rotavirus-associated acute gastroenteritis following introduction of rotavirus vaccine into Australia's national childhood vaccine schedule. Pediatr Infect Dis J. 2011; 30(1 Suppl):S25-9. doi:10.1097/INF.0b013e3181fefdee

278. Frühwirth M, Heininger U, Ehlken B, et al. International variation in disease burden of rotavirus gastroenteritis in children with community- and nosocomially acquired infection. Pediatr Infect Dis J. 2001;20(8):784-791. doi:10.1097/00006454-200108000-00013

279. Ringenbergs ML, Davidson GP, Spence J, Morris S. Prospective study of nosocomial rotavirus infection in a paediatric hospital. Aust Paediatr J. 1989;25(3):156-160. doi:10.1111/j.1440-1754.1989.tb01441.x

280. Gleizes O, Desselberger U, Tatochenko V, et al. Nosocomial rotavirus infection in European countries: a review of the epidemiology, severity and economic burden of hospital-acquired rotavirus disease. Pediatr Infect Dis J. 2006; 25(1 Suppl):S12-21. doi:10.1097/01.inf.0000197563.03895.91

281. Snelling T, Cripps T, Macartney K, Dalton D, Kesson A, Isaacs D. Nosocomial rotavirus infection in an Australian children's hospital. J Paediatr Child Health. 2007;43(4):318. doi:10.1111/j.1440-1754.2007.01068.x

282. Standaert B, Strens D, Li X, Schecroun N, Raes M. The sustained rotavirus vaccination impact on nosocomial infection, duration of hospital stay, and age: the RotaBIS study (2005-2012). Infect Dis Ther. 2016;5(4):509-524. doi:10.1007/s40121-016-0131-0

283. Zlamy M, Kofler S, Orth D, et al. The impact of rotavirus mass vaccination on hospitalization rates, nosocomial rotavirus gastroenteritis and secondary blood stream infections. BMC Infect Dis. 2013;13:112. doi:10.1186/1471-2334-13-112

284. Macartney KK, Porwal M, Dalton D, et al. Decline in rotavirus hospitalisations following introduction of Australia's national rotavirus immunisation programme. J Paediatr Child Health. 2011;47(5):266-270. doi:10.1111/j.1440-1754. 2010.01953.x

285. Anderson EJ, Weber SG. Rotavirus infection in adults. Lancet Infect Dis. 2004;4(2):91-99. doi:10.1016/S1473-3099(04)00928-4

286. Marshall J, Botes J, Gorrie G, et al. Rotavirus detection and characterisation in outbreaks of gastroenteritis in aged-care facilities. J Clin Virol. 2003;28(3):331-340. doi:10.1016/s1386-6532(03)00081-7

287. Crawford SE, Ramani S, Tate JE, et al. Rotavirus infection. Nat Rev Dis Prim. 2017;3. doi:10.1038/nrdp.2017.83

288. Centers for Disease Control and Prevention (CDC). Rotavirus. In: Hamborsky J, Kroger A, Wolfe S, eds. Epidemiology and prevention of vaccine-preventable diseases. 13th ed. Public Health Foundation, 2015, p. 263-274. Available from: http://www.cdc.gov/vaccines/pubs/pinkbook/downloads/rota.pdf.

289. Richardson S, Grimwood K, Gorrell R, Palombo E, Barnes G, Bishop R. Extended excretion of rotavirus after severe diarrhoea in young children. Lancet. 1998;351(9119): 1844-1848. doi:10.1016/S0140-6736(97)11257-0

290. Wikswo ME, Parashar UD, Lopman B, et al. Evidence for household transmission of rotavirus in the United States, 2011-2016. J Pediatric Infect Dis Soc. 2020;9(2):181-187. doi:10.1093/jpids/piz004

291. Ferson MJ, Stringfellow S, McPhie K, McIver CJ, Simos A. Longitudinal study of rotavirus infection in child-care centres. J Paediatr Child Health. 1997;33(2):157-160. doi:10.1111/j.1440-1754.1997.tb01020.x

292. Whiley DM, Ye S, Tozer S, et al. Over-diagnosis of rotavirus infection in infants due to detection of vaccine virus. Clin Infect Dis. 2020;71(5):1324-1326. doi:10.1093/cid/ciz1196

293. Australian Government Department of Health. Rotavirus: Australian Rotavirus Surveillance Program annual reports. 1999. [cited 4 April 2022]. Available from: https://www1. health.gov.au/internet/main/publishing.nsf/Content/cda-pubs-annlrpt-rotavar.htm.

CHAPTER 22

Significant and multiresistant organism infections, and antimicrobial resistance

Dr JAMES WOLFE[i]

Dr SANCHIA WARREN[i]

Dr LOUISE COOLEY[i]

Chapter highlights

- Overview of the epidemiology, microbiology, antimicrobial resistance (AMR) and infection prevention and control (IPC) measures for Gram-positive bacteria, including *Staphylococcus aureus* and Enterococcus spp.
- Overview of the epidemiology, microbiology, AMR and IPC measures for Gram-negative bacteria, including Enterobacterales, Acinetobacter spp., *Pseudomonas aeruginosa, Burkholderia cepacia* and *Stenotrophomonas maltophilia*
- Overview of the epidemiology, microbiology, AMR and IPC measures for other bacteria, such as *Mycobacterium tuberculosis*, and fungal species, including *Candida auris*

i   Department of Microbiology and Infectious Diseases, Royal Hobart Hospital, Hobart, TAS

Introduction

Multidrug-resistant infections and antimicrobial resistance (AMR) are major and urgent global public health threats. AMR describes when infectious organisms (including bacteria, fungi, viruses and parasites) render certain antimicrobial agents ineffective. That is, they are no longer killed by those antimicrobial agents. Resistance to antimicrobials can lead to poor outcomes in situations that require suboptimal antimicrobials to be used as an alternative. In rarer and more extreme cases, some infections have no antimicrobial treatment options. Infection control and antimicrobial stewardship (AMS) programs are important elements in the fight against AMR. This chapter discusses clinically relevant organisms that have demonstrated AMR and the recommended infection prevention and control (IPC) measures.

22.1 Staphylococcus aureus

Staphylococcus aureus was first isolated in the 1880s and usually appears on microscopy as clusters of Gram-positive cocci.[1] It is a common organism that typically colonises skin and the nasal passage or upper respiratory tract in humans without causing disease. At the same time, *S. aureus* is a leading cause of both community and hospital-acquired infections. Clinical infections caused by *S. aureus* include bacteraemias, infective endocarditis, skin and soft tissue infections (e.g. cellulitis and abscesses), bone and joint infections (e.g. osteomyelitis and prosthetic joint infections), central nervous system infections and sometimes respiratory disease. Primary urinary tract infections with *S. aureus* are unusual, especially if there has not been any instrumentation to the urinary tract. If *S. aureus* is isolated from a urine sample, it should prompt evaluation for bacteraemia. A focus of infection is not found in up to a quarter of cases of *S. aureus* bacteraemia (SAB).

SABs are generally classified as complicated or uncomplicated, which is relevant for determining antibiotic treatment durations. Complicated infections are those that have prolonged blood culture positivity, relapse of fever, abnormal cardiac valvular morphology, no identifiable source of infection, evidence of metastatic infection or intravascular prosthetic devices. Complicated SABs are generally treated with a longer intravenous course of antibiotics, typically up to 4–6 weeks. Uncomplicated SABs usually require a known source without metastatic complications or underlying risk for this (such as cardiac valvulopathies) and with quickly cleared blood cultures. These are typically treated with two weeks of intravenous antibiotics. It is worth mentioning that there is data emerging to support shorter durations of the intravenous part of a patient's total antibiotic course, including in SABs and infective endocarditis cases, but this is beyond the scope of this chapter.

Mortality associated with invasive SABs is up to 15–50%.[2] Higher mortality has been associated with more resistant *S. aureus* organisms. Treatment of *S. aureus* infections has evolved over the years alongside increasing rates of antibiotic resistance. Early treatments utilised penicillin, but soon required directed semi-synthetic anti-staphylococcal penicillins (ASPs) when resistance began to emerge and methicillin-susceptible *S. aureus* (MSSA) was observed. Subsequently, methicillin-resistant *S. aureus* (MRSA) emerged, which harbours resistance to nearly the entire class of beta-lactam antibiotics.

22.1.1 Epidemiology

More than 30% of the human population is persistently colonised with *S. aureus*, with some estimates of intermittent carriage being up to 60%.[3] In some, this colonisation may be transient, while in others it does persist. Some populations are at higher risk of *S. aureus* colonisation, including healthcare workers and patients with frequent contact with healthcare settings. *S. aureus* can be transmitted by direct or indirect contact between people or on contact with fomites (inanimate objects contaminated with an infectious organism) or contaminated surfaces or equipment.

Globally, *S. aureus* is one of the most frequently isolated organisms in bloodstream infections. Rates of SAB have generally remained stable over recent decades; however, the proportion of MRSA in these bacteraemias has fluctuated over time. From 49 institutions across Australia in 2020, a total of 2734 episodes of SAB were reported, 17.6% of which were methicillin-resistant.[4] The highest rates of SAB occur at the extremes of age and males are generally at higher risk than females. People living with human immunodeficiency virus (HIV) and those who require haemodialysis have also demonstrated significantly higher incidences of SAB.

SABs are generally differentiated into those that are healthcare-acquired (including hospital- or community-onset infections) or community-acquired. The use of intravascular catheters is a frequently implicated risk factor for healthcare-acquired infections. Community-acquired SABs occur in patients who have not had recent contact with the healthcare system. These patients are more likely to present with complicated infection, including metastatic sites of infection, or with clinically inapparent sources of infection, such as vertebral osteomyelitis. Risk factors for community-acquired SABs include the use of injecting drugs or known *S. aureus* colonisation.

22.1.2 Microbiology

S. aureus are Gram-positive cocci that usually occur in clusters, described as 'appearing like a bunch of grapes'. Colonies are often golden or yellow on media. *S. aureus* cultures both aerobically and anaerobically and is coagulase-positive, which differentiates it from coagulase-negative staphylococcus species including, for example, *Staphylococcus epidermidis*, *Staphylococcus haemolyticus* and *Staphylococcus hominis*. Molecular methods (including polymerase chain reaction; PCR) can be used to detect *S. aureus* in the laboratory. Commercial MALDI-TOF MS (matrix-assisted laser desorption/ionisation-time-of-flight mass spectrometry) systems are commonly used on culture isolates to reliably confirm the identity of *S. aureus*. Disc diffusion and automated broth dilution methods (e.g. Vitek) are used for antimicrobial susceptibility testing in the laboratory.

22.1.3 Antimicrobial resistance

S. aureus isolates exist on a spectrum, from those that retain susceptibility to narrow-spectrum antibiotics to those that are broadly antibiotic-resistant. On occasion, some *S. aureus* isolates remain susceptible to narrow-spectrum penicillins, such as penicillin G. These organisms are referred to as penicillin-susceptible *S. aureus* (PSSA). It is not known whether treatment of these isolates with penicillin is more, or less, successful than using an anti-staphylococcal penicillin (ASP) such as flucloxacillin.

More commonly, MSSA isolates are susceptible to semi-synthetic ASPs but resistant to earlier penicillins. In these organisms, resistance to penicillins is mediated by the beta-lactamase gene *blaZ* encoding a penicillinase enzyme. Susceptibility is usually tested in the laboratory using oxacillin, requiring a minimal inhibitory concentration ≤ 2 mg/L. ASPs maintain activity against MSSA isolates. Examples of these antibiotics that are commonly used in clinical practice in Australia include flucloxacillin and dicloxacillin. Cefazolin, a first-generation cephalosporin, also maintains activity against MSSA isolates.

MRSA isolates are resistant to the semi-synthetic ASPs.[5] MRSA was first observed within a year of the first clinical use of the semi-synthetic ASPs. Methicillin resistance is mediated by the *mecA* gene, which encodes penicillin binding protein 2a (PBP2a). PBP2a is a unique transpeptidase that is not inhibited well by β-lactam antibiotics. Hence, while other PBPs with transpeptidase activity might be inhibited, PBP2a is able to continue peptidoglycan crosslinking even in the presence of β-lactam antibiotics. This confers resistance of MRSA to this class of antibiotics, which includes but is not limited to penicillins and cephalosporins. (A notable exception is ceftaroline, a fifth-generation cephalosporin that is active against MRSA.) A *mecC* gene has recently been found in MRSA isolated from livestock, wildlife and companion animals, including domestic cats.[6-8] In Australia, invasive MRSA infections are typically treated using intravenous vancomycin, a bacteriostatic glycopeptide antibiotic. Notably, the coagulase-negative staphylococci sometimes cause clinically relevant infections similar to those of *S. aureus*, including infective endocarditis. These organisms frequently carry the *mecA* gene and will be phenotypically methicillin-resistant isolates that are similarly treated with vancomycin, as above.

S. aureus isolates with reduced vancomycin susceptibility have been reported since the late 1990s. Vancomycin-intermediate and vancomycin-resistant *S. aureus* (VISA and VRSA, respectively) have elevated minimum inhibitory concentrations (MICs) to vancomycin (4–8 and ≥ 16 µg/ml). Mechanisms of resistance in these isolates continue to be investigated. Heterogeneous VISA isolates are susceptible to vancomycin but with minority populations of the organism with a vancomycin MIC >2 µg/ml. High rates of vancomycin use may be a risk factor for development of resistance. Fortunately, VISA and VRSA isolates often maintain susceptibility to non-beta-lactam antibiotics with anti-staphylococcal activity, including trimethoprim/sulfamethoxazole, rifampicin and linezolid.

22.1.4 Infection prevention and control

General preventative measures are important in prevention of resistant staphylococcal infection and spread. This includes hand hygiene and personal hygiene where there are shared facilities. Education programs in hospitals and in the community are important in increasing the uptake and successful use of hygiene measures. Cautious wound care and keeping wounds covered may limit transmission. This includes covering minor wounds, such as boils or abscesses affecting healthcare workers, to limit transmission to patients.

Different regions of Australia have different rates of MRSA for both colonisation and clinically relevant infections. As a result, infection prevention practices may vary between regions and hospitals. For example, hospitals that serve communities where there is a high prevalence of MRSA may not institute contact precautions for patients who have screened positive for MRSA carriage or patients with MRSA infection. Some institutes may isolate patients with MRSA colonisation or infection based on the risk of exposure, such as in orthopaedic wards where prosthetic joint replacements are performed. At institutes where rates of MRSA are low, all patients affected by MRSA may be managed under contact precautions. Staphylococcal decolonisation is an option for patients who have screened positive for MRSA colonisation and are undergoing high-risk surgical procedures. Examples of these include prosthetic cardiac valve replacement or prosthetic joint replacements.

The appropriate use of narrower-spectrum antibiotics is critical and AMS programs play a vital role in this regard.

22.2 Enterococcus

Enterococci are commensal organisms of the gastrointestinal tract that can cause a variety of opportunistic infections in humans. Over time, resistance rates to first-line antimicrobials, such as amoxicillin in the case of *Enterococcus faecium*, have shifted the need to treat this organism with vancomycin. Vancomycin's mechanism of action against enterococci is through the antibiotic binding to the D-alanyl-D-alanine (D-Ala-D-Ala) terminus of cell wall precursors and preventing synthesis of the cell wall. However, the subsequent emergence of vancomycin-resistant Enterococcus (VRE) has meant this organism has become a multidrug-resistant healthcare-associated pathogen of concern. Acquisition of plasmid-mediated vancomycin-resistance genes (e.g. *vanA*, *vanB* and *vanD* gene clusters) alters the vancomycin binding site of the Enterococcus. Hence there is decreased affinity of the antibiotic for the binding site, rendering it resistant. The VRE resistance genes confer varying MICs for vancomycin.

The Clinical and Laboratory Standards Institute (CLSI) defines the vancomycin susceptibility and resistance in enterococci as vancomycin susceptible (MIC ≤4 mcg/mL) and vancomycin resistant (MIC ≥32 mcg/mL), with MICs between these values considered intermediate. However, intermediate isolates are not recommended for vancomycin treatment if therapy is indicated. The European Committee on Antimicrobial Susceptibility (EUCAST) defines vancomycin susceptibility as ≤4 mg/L and resistance as >4 mg/L. Similarly, linezolid resistance can occur in this organism, where linezolid may be a last-line antimicrobial treatment for an already resistant organism.

22.2.1 Epidemiology

First detected in Europe in the 1980s, VRE has spread worldwide. Prior to the advent of VRE, *E. faecalis* was the more common organism, but there has been a shift to *E. faecium* predominance and increasing rates of VRE. Initially, VRE was associated with outbreaks and epidemics, but it is now endemic in many large hospitals internationally. There is evidence of clonal spread within institutions with differing multi-locus sequence types present in various parts of Australia implying local spread.[9]

The vast majority of VRE is in *E. faecium*. Clinical infection with VRE is associated with poorer clinical outcomes as outlined in the AGAR (Australian Group on Antimicrobial Resistance), and Enterococcus spp. is a priority organism for surveillance and antimicrobial resistance strategies with AURA (Antimicrobial Use and Resistance in Australia).[9] The rates of VRE infection appear to be declining in Australia; however, they still remain higher compared to many European countries. Prior to 2018, the predominant VRE genotype in Australia was vanB, which contrasted with the findings worldwide where vanA predominated.[4,10,11] More recently, vanA and vanB VRE now appear to be circulating in equal numbers.

Clinically, *E. faecium* is most commonly associated with urinary tract infections, biliary tract infections, other intraabdominal infections and septicaemia; while *E. faecalis* has a similar clinical manifestation it is also more likely to be implicated in infective endocarditis. They are typically seen in hospitalised patients where their integument has been breached either through devices or surgery with vulnerable populations (e.g. the elderly, immunocompromised or those with multiple comorbidities). Enterococcal bacteraemia is associated with significant mortality with rates of 18.1% in Australia in 2020.[4]

22.2.2 Microbiology

Enterococci are Gram-positive cocci that occur in short chains, pairs or singly. They typically grow easily on blood agar within 24 hours and generally exhibit alpha haemolysis or no haemolysis. Some *E. faecalis* isolates may exhibit beta-haemolysis. Enterococcal species were previously identified using phenotypic methods, but MALDI-TOF MS now provides rapid identification to genus and species.

Chromogenic agar can be utilised for the screening for colonisation with or detection of VRE. These specialised selective agars allow for growth of VRE (*E. faecalis* and *E. faecium*) while inhibiting growth of competing organisms including vancomycin susceptible Enterococci. Colour differentiation in the colonies allows rapid identification for phenotypic VRE from these chromogenic agars. Susceptibility testing using the EUCAST or CLSI breakpoints can detect VRE. The vanA phenotype has inducible high-level resistance to vancomycin and teicoplanin whereas the inducible vanB phenotype has mid to high-level resistance to vancomycin only. The other van phenotypes vary in their level of vancomycin resistance; however, it is vanA and vanB that are the most clinically relevant and transmissible via plasmids. Molecular methods are used to determine the presence of vanA or vanB gene. This can be utilised on clinical or screening isolates. The vanA and vanB genes can be inducible and therefore may be detected by molecular methods but not exhibit vancomycin resistance at the time of susceptibility testing.

22.2.3 Infection prevention and control

The Australian Commission on Safety and Quality in Health Care (ACSQHC) outlines a multimodal approach to the prevention of VRE in healthcare settings.[12] It is clear from the evidence of varying sequence types in different states and territories of Australia that IPC is key to minimising spread and transmission. The core strategies are expanded from the basis in the Australian Infection Prevention and Control Guidelines.

VRE is known to be carried on the hands of healthcare workers acquired during patient care or in contact with the surrounding environment. Hand hygiene should be effective and in line with the ACSQHC's National Hand Hygiene Initiative (NHHI) and the '5 Moments for Hand Hygiene' program. Gowns or aprons should be used on entering the room or patient zone, with the type of gown or apron depending on the degree of risk of contact of clothing with surfaces and the potential for exposure to blood and body fluids. Gloves should be applied when entering the room or patient zone to prevent transmission through environmental contamination. Other personal protective equipment (PPE) can be considered as part of standard precautions to minimise risk of exposure to blood/body fluids (e.g. eyewear). Gloves and gowns/aprons should be removed prior to leaving the patient zone or room and hand hygiene should be performed. High-touch objects and the patient surrounds should be cleaned with a suitable detergent and disinfected twice a day. Disinfection should include the use of a Therapeutic Goods Administration (TGA)-listed hospital-grade product or a chlorine-based product such as sodium hypochlorite. The room should also be cleaned and disinfected on transfer or discharge of the patient from the room. Ideally, single use patient care equipment should be used. Reusable equipment should be cleaned and disinfected between patients.

Monitoring of antimicrobial use and possible associations with VRE colonisation at the healthcare setting should occur, followed by the implementation of strategies to adjust prescribing practice. The incidence of VRE infection and/or colonisation should be monitored by institutions and reported in accordance with the relevant state or territory reporting requirements. High-risk units and places where patients have existing risk factors for VRE acquisition should consider undergoing screening for colonisation with VRE. These include intensive care units (ICUs), nephrology units, haematology and oncology units or wards and solid organ transplant units. Regular screening of patients at considerable risk of carriage may be implemented, for example prolonged ICU admission, renal dialysis units or haematology wards. Where decolonisation or clearance for VRE has no agreed process, local and state policies should be consulted. VRE-colonised patients should have an alert in the medical record allowing easy identification, including on readmission. Alerts, including electronic alerts, should only be modified in consultation with the IPC team. Staff and consumers should receive education and relevant information on VRE colonisation and infection.

22.3 Enterobacterales

The order Enterobacterales (and family Enterobacteriaceae) encompasses a collection of Gram-negative bacteria, some of which are commensal organisms of the human gastrointestinal and hepatobiliary tracts. These taxonomies have notably undergone significant changes over past decades.[13] Common examples seen in clinical practice include *Escherichia coli*, *Klebsiella pneumoniae* and Salmonella spp. Enterobacterales are Gram-negative rod-shaped bacteria (or bacilli) and they represent a significant cause of invasive, clinically relevant infections in humans. These include bacteraemias, which may complicate infections such as cholecystitis, ascending cholangitis, infective colitis, diverticulitis, appendicitis, intraabdominal abscesses and urinary tract infections including pyelonephritis or prostatitis. Infections of the respiratory tract may occur while skin and soft tissue infections are uncommon. Enterobacterales species may be associated with central line-associated bloodstream infections (CLABSIs), especially in high-risk settings such as the ICU.

22.3.1 Epidemiology

Risk factors for invasive Gram-negative bacillary infections include immunosuppressive disorders (including solid organ or haematologic transplants, HIV infection or systemic glucocorticoid treatment), diabetes, haemodialysis, chronic liver failure and underlying respiratory diseases. The elderly are also at higher risk. Increased rates of antimicrobial resistance may explain higher rates of Enterobacterales infections. There may also be some effect of seasonality, where warmer external temperatures are associated with higher rates of invasive Gram-negative bacillary infections. Some Enterobacterales species have been responsible for significant foodborne disease outbreaks. These include Salmonella spp., *E. coli*, *Shigella* and *Yersinia enterocolitica*. They are also important pathogens in healthcare-associated infections, including catheter-associated urinary tract infections (CAUTIs) and surgical site infections and CLABSIs.

As will be discussed below, there are several mechanisms of antimicrobial resistance observed in the Enterobacterales. These confer variable spectra of antimicrobial resistance. There is some epidemiologic risk for more broadly resistant Enterobacterales, where they are typically seen in higher proportions in particular geographic regions. Notably, the rates of these broadly resistant Enterobacterales are being observed increasingly widely across the world.

22.3.2 Microbiology

Enterobacterales are Gram-negative, non-spore forming bacilli. Culture using blood agar typically shows medium to large colonies that are glistening and grey. They may demonstrate beta-haemolysis. A number of PCR targets exist and offer the opportunity for rapid detection of a number of the Enterobacterales.

22.3.3 Antimicrobial resistance

Beta-lactamases: Beta-lactamases are enzymes that open the beta-lactam ring of an antibiotic, rendering the antibiotic inactive. Some beta-lactamases are reasonably narrow in the spectrum of beta-lactam antibiotics that they can hydrolyse. Beta-lactam-beta-lactamase-inhibitor (BLBLI) antibiotics utilise beta-lactamase inhibitors to overcome antimicrobial resistance conferred by beta-lactamases. Examples of BLBLI antibiotics include amoxicillin with clavulanic acid and piperacillin with tazobactam.

Extended-spectrum beta-lactamases (ESBLs): In contrast to the narrower-spectrum beta-lactamases, ESBLs confer resistance to most beta-lactam antibiotics,

including penicillin, cephalosporins and monobactams.[14] ESBL varieties include TEM, SHV, CTX-M, OXA and others like PER, VEB and GES beta-lactamases. Importantly, EBSLs cause a variety of resistance profiles, and there are enzymes within the above ESBL varieties that are in fact not ESBLs and confer resistance only to penicillins and narrow-spectrum cephalosporins (e.g. TEM-1 and TEM-2, which are considered 'inhibitor-resistant'). Some beta-lactamases are both ESBLs and inhibitor-resistant.

Many ESBLs are plasmid-mediated. Genes encoding ESBLs are carried on plasmids, which are small, circular, double-stranded DNA molecules, distinct from chromosomal DNA. Plasmids can replicate independently and can be passed between bacteria, offering a method of disseminating antimicrobial resistance. Some ESBLs occur as the result of amino acid substitution.

Laboratory detection of ESBL-producing organisms is based on demonstrating resistance to oxymino-beta-lactam substrates such as ceftriaxone or cefotaxime, where beta-lactamase inhibitors (such as clavulanic acid) block this resistance. Given the heterogeneity of ESBLs, susceptibility to several oxymino-beta-lactam substrates should be tested. Disc diffusion and broth dilution techniques are used for susceptibility testing. Methods for susceptibility testing include automated systems (such as Vitek), double disc tests and E-test strips. Additionally, antimicrobial resistance mechanisms may be detected by nucleic acid testing genomic sequencing.

Carbapenemase-producing Enterobacteriaceae (CPE): CPE isolates produce carbapenemases, which are enzymes known as beta-lactamases that hydrolyse carbapenems and confer resistance to a broad spectrum of antibiotic classes.[15] Organisms that produce carbapenemases may also be referred to as carbapenem-resistant Enterobacteriaceae (CRE). Carbapenemases are organised into classes A, B, C and D based on amino acid homology in the Ambler molecular classification system. Class A, C and D beta-lactamases share a serine residue in the active site. Class B beta-lactamases are referred to as metallo-beta-lactamases (MBLs) since they require the presence of zinc for activity. A few notable examples of carbapenemases will be briefly described here.

The *K. pneumoniae* carbapenemase (KPC) group is the most clinically important of the Class A carbapenemases.[16] These enzymes are plasmid-mediated and can be transmitted from *Klebsiella* spp. to Enterobacterales of other genera. KPCs are the most common carbapenemases observed in the United States.

The New Delhi metallo-beta-lactamase (NDM-1) was quick to spread throughout the world after it was first described in 2009 in a Swedish patient hospitalised in India.[17] NDM-1-producing isolates have been recorded particularly in association with healthcare contact in high-risk countries, such as India and Pakistan. It has been observed in *K. pneumoniae*, *E. coli* and *Enterobacter cloacae*, as well as some non-Enterobacterales Gram-negative bacilli (e.g. *Acinetobacter*). NDM-1 MBLs were first described in Japan and have spread to other parts of Asia, Europe, North and South America and Australia.

Class D beta-lactamases are known as OXA-type enzymes. OXA group enzymes may be transmitted on plasmids or chromosomally encoded and are the most common CPE detected in Australia.

ESCAPPM organisms: The ESCAPPM acronym describes a collection of organisms that harbour inducible beta-lactamases. That is, chromosomally mediated expression of beta-lactamases can be upregulated, typically on exposure to a beta-lactam agent. AmpC beta-lactamases are an example of these.[18] While these organisms may test susceptible to beta-lactam antibiotics in the laboratory, the risk with initiating treatment with these agents is that organisms develop resistance to them, sometimes within a single treatment course.

The acronym has expanded over time, and is more comprehensively represented by 'KESCHAPPM':

- *Klebsiella aerogenes* (formerly *Enterobacter aerogenes*)
- Enterobacter spp.
- Serratia spp.
- *Citrobacter freundii* (excluding other non-freundii Citrobacter species)
- Hafnia spp.
- Aeromonas spp.
- *Proteus vulgaris* (and some other species, excluding *Proteus mirabilis*)
- Providencia spp.
- *Morganella morganii*.

Importantly, not all ESCAPPM organisms have the same resistance profile. Their inducible beta-lactamases occur at variable levels and variable affinities for different penicillin and cephalosporin antibiotics. Clinical cure rates and risk of phenotypic resistance to different beta-lactam agent varies based on the organism and the site of infection.

22.3.4 Antimicrobial treatment options

The preferred treatment options for invasive infections with ESBL-producing organisms are carbapenems, such as meropenem. Ertapenem is an alternative carbapenem if the individual organism tests susceptible, and has a slightly narrower spectrum compared to meropenem. ESBL phenotype can be influenced by the number of amino acid substitutions, where broader resistance is observed with more substitutions. Lower mortality rates were observed with meropenem in a randomised trial that compared its use with piperacillin-tazobactam in patients with ESBL-producing Enterobacteriaceae bacteraemias.[19] Piperacillin-tazobactam is therefore generally not recommended for invasive ESBL-producing infections. It is sometimes considered as a treatment option for less invasive infections where high drug concentrations can be achieved, such as in uncomplicated acute cystitis.

There are limited antimicrobial treatment options for CPE isolates and treatments should be guided by expert infectious diseases advice. Treatment of choice is influenced by the carbapenemase detected. For organisms that possess a serine carbapenemase, ceftazidime-avibactam (a late third generation cephalosporin with a beta-lactamase) and other novel BLBLI combination drugs are used. For isolates that produce MBLs, aztreonam-based combination regimens might be used, such as aztreonam and ceftazidime-avibactam. Where these drugs cannot be used, polymyxin-based regimens may be an option, such as colistin used with a second agent.

22.3.5 Infection prevention and control

Environmental, animal and food contamination with ESBL-producing Enterobacterales is well reported. A foodborne healthcare-associated outbreak of SHV1 and CTX-M-15-producing *K. pneumoniae* provided evidence of food being a transmission vector for ESBL-producing *K. pneumoniae*.[20] Screening of high-risk patients for broadly resistant Enterobacterales occurs in healthcare settings. Hospitalised patients known to be colonised or infected with broadly resistant Enterobacterales are managed with contact precautions.

22.4 Acinetobacter spp.

Acinetobacter spp. have emerged over the last few decades as an organism of concern particularly in ICUs. They can cause severe healthcare-associated infections. With high levels of intrinsic resistance and increasing resistance to antimicrobials, the mainstay of therapy is often broad-spectrum carbapenems. Increasing resistance to last line antimicrobials is occurring. Due to this ability to acquire resistance to many classes of antimicrobials, the World Health Organization has listed carbapenem-resistant *Acinetobacter baumannii* on the critical-priority pathogens list for effective drug development.[9]

22.4.1 Epidemiology

Acinetobacter spp. are commonly found in the environment, particularly in water and soil in humid environments, as well as in sewage, food and animal specimens. Infection may be seen after environmental exposure and has been particularly associated with times of warfare (e.g. Korean, Vietnam, Iraq wars) and natural disaster (2004 South East Asia Tsunami). *A. baumanii* is also increasingly associated with healthcare-associated outbreaks due to the organism's innate survival ability. Community-acquired infection is more commonly seen in Australia and Asia and frequently in the wet season. In one study 10% of severe community-acquired pneumonia in the northern Australian monsoon season was due to *A. baumannii*.[21]

Colonisation with Acinetobacter (ACB) is more common than infection; however, distinguishing between the two is difficult. Independent risk factors for colonisation with resistant strains of ACB include:

- prior colonisation with MRSA
- prior antimicrobial use (fluoroquinolones and beta-lactams, in particular carbapenems)
- glucocorticoid therapy
- presence of central access lines and/or mechanical ventilation
- current or prior ICU admission
- recent surgery
- malignancy; and
- being bedridden.

Colonisation of the skin or mucosae (predominantly respiratory or urinary) can last for weeks. Most frequently, ACB complex is associated with ventilator-associated pneumonia or bloodstream infections.[22]

Several terms relating to the resistance profile of *A. baumanii* have been used including MDR (multidrug-resistant), XDR (extensive drug-resistant) and PDR (pan drug-resistant). In 2011 the European and United States Centers for Disease Control and Prevention (ECDC and CDC) proposed the following definitions:

- Multidrug-resistant—isolate is non-susceptible to at least one agent in three or more antibiotic classes
- Extensively drug-resistant—isolate is non-susceptible to at least one agent in all but two or fewer antibiotic classes; and

- Pan drug-resistant—isolate is non-susceptible to all agents.

22.4.2 Microbiology

There are over 50 different species in the Acinetobacter genus but the vast majority are not known to cause human disease and have low pathogenicity. *A. baumanii* is the most commonly studied and associated with human disease. *Acinetobacter calcoaceticus* and *A. baumanii* were previously difficult to distinguish and were often grouped into a complex—the *A. calcoaceticus-A. baumannii* complex—comprising of four genospecies. *Acinetobacter lowoffi* is also a commonly reported healthcare-associated pathogen associated with bloodstream and line infection.[22]

The Gram-negative cocci-bacilli is easily isolated in the laboratory on standard media (blood agar, MacConkey agar). They typically grow quickly within 24–48 hours under aerobic conditions. While traditionally it was sometimes difficult to identify further or split the organism based on phenotypic testing, the advent of rapid diagnostic methods (e.g. MALDI-TOF MS) now allows quick and accurate identification.

22.4.3 Susceptibility testing

A. baumanii complex can easily acquire or develop resistance to nearly all antibiotics that may be used for treatment of infection. The EUCAST and CLSI provide breakpoints for the interpretation of susceptibility testing. Of note, testing for colistin susceptibility should ideally occur via broth microdilution due to the poor ability of colistin to diffuse through the agar.

These organisms can acquire a wide range of resistance mechanisms. Acinetobacter spp. all have an intrinsic or inbuilt AmpC beta-lactamase, meaning all will be resistant to cephalosporins. The acquisition of those beta-lactamases inducing carbapenem resistance is of more concern. This is often compounded by the presence of efflux pumps and porins reducing the presence of available carbapenem or access of the antimicrobial to the organism. Fluroquinolones, colistin and sulphonamides can also acquire resistance through genetic mechanisms.[23] It is for this reason that *A. baumanii* is considered a critical priority pathogen by the WHO. Similarly, the ACSQHC, through AURA, includes *A. baumanii* with confirmed carbapenem resistance due to presence of carbapenemase as a National Alert System for Critical Antimicrobial Resistance (CARAlert) organism.[9]

22.4.4 Infection prevention and control

The basic principles of early recognition of colonisation or infection with Acinetobacter spp. with aggressive prevention of spread aims to halt the establishment of strains in the hospital setting. As with most multidrug-resistant Gram-negative organisms, a multimodal approach should be undertaken. In line with the Australian Guidelines for the Prevention and Control of Infection in Healthcare, patients with a multidrug-resistant Acinetobacter spp. should be managed under contact and standard precautions for the duration of their illness. In the absence of resistance, standard precautions suffice; however, there should be vigilance for the spread of this organism, particularly in the intensive care setting.

Acinetobacter spp. are able to survive and persist on fomites. As such, cleaning and disinfection is paramount in the management of this organism. Hand hygiene compliance and cleaning of high-touch surfaces has been shown to reduce the rate of colonisation with multidrug-resistant Acinetobacter in the intensive care setting. Indeed, stringent environmental cleaning regimens have been shown to decrease environmental colonisation with the organism and henceforth decrease the rate of colonisation in patients and intensive care outbreaks. However, the multimodal role is important. In one setting, enhanced cleaning alone was insufficient to curb an outbreak and the rate of colonisation was higher as ventilator use increased. Adherence to hand hygiene in addition to the cleaning strategies is required to prevent healthcare-associated spread.[12]

22.5 Pseudomonas aeruginosa

Pseudomonas aeruginosa is a worldwide pathogen with emerging multi-resistance and is prevalent in a wide spectrum of infections. It can be multidrug-resistant and can also acquire carbapenemases with subsequent severe hospital-acquired infections associated with a high mortality rate, especially in immunocompromised hosts.

22.5.1 Epidemiology

P. aeruginosa is an opportunistic pathogen. It is commonly found in the environment, particularly in areas with water, and is an important plant pathogen. Sources of community infection include contaminated contact lens solution and 'hot-tub folliculitis'.

It is most worrying as a healthcare-associated pathogen due to its ability to survive in the environment (e.g. sinks) and its preference for patients with altered host defence mechanisms (e.g. poor phagocytosis in febrile neutropenia, skin defence in burns, abnormal physiology in cystic fibrosis (CF)). This, coupled with its ability to rapidly develop resistance to many broad-spectrum antimicrobials, raises concern. It is one of the most frequent sources of ventilator-associated pneumonia and is associated with significant morbidity and mortality. Recently, P. aeruginosa has emerged as a common cause of secondary pneumonia in COVID-19 patients.[9] It has also been implicated in catheter-associated urinary tract infection (CAUTI), wound infection and bacteraemia, and its role in CF is well established.

22.5.2 Microbiology

P. aeruginosa is a non-fermentative Gram-negative rod within the large and complex genus of Pseudomonas. The organism grows aerobically on a variety of media as it has very simple nutritional requirements. It has a characteristic grape-like odour and typically green pigmentation. A key feature in its identification is that it is oxidase positive. Colonies may be mucoid or non-mucoid. These varied phenotypes are typically the same clone of Pseudomonas, but the mucoid forms are exhibiting adaptation to the lung environment and the development of biofilms. The biofilm mucoid forms are typically more resistant to antimicrobials, reflecting its tolerant state. Identification by MALDI-TOF MS is now commonplace, replacing the phenotypic identification systems.

Both the EUCAST and CLSI have established breakpoints for P. aeruginosa using both disc diffusion and gradient strip testing for MIC. The exception to this is colistin which requires broth microdilution due to the drug's inability to diffuse adequately through solid agar. The organism exhibits intrinsic resistance to many antimicrobial classes, with inducible AmpC beta-lactamases conferring all P. aeruginosa resistant to ampicillin, amoxicillin, amoxicillin-clavulanate, first and second generation cephalosporins and cefotaxime and ceftriaxone. Intrinsic efflux pumps also contribute to resistance to tetracyclines and sulphonamides. P. aeruginosa has the ability to acquire many resistant mechanisms including beta-lactamases, impermeability mutations, aminoglycoside modifying enzymes, plasmid-mediated quinolone resistance and efflux pumps, which can render it multi-resistant to many antimicrobials.[23]

Of great concern, as with any Gram-negative bacteria, is the acquisition of carbapenemases (metallo-beta-lactamases) via plasmid-mediated means. Typically, these are able to spread between other Gram-negatives and also on the plasmid are accompanied by other resistance mechanisms. Examples include plasmid-mediated IMP and VIM as well as the New-Delhi metallo-beta-lactamase (NDM-1), which has spread from

Enterobacterales and has been identified in *P. aeruginosa*. Due to varying expression of these carbapenemases they can sometimes be difficult to detect, as the MIC to the carbapenem may indeed be within the susceptible range. The ACSQHC through AURA has criteria to capture this circumstance and when carbapenem resistance is confirmed due to presence of carbapenemase, it is reported as a CARAlert organism.[9]

22.5.3 Infection prevention and control

The IPC management of multidrug-resistant or carbapenemase-resistant *P. aeruginosa* requires enhanced precautions, identification of carriage of at-risk patients via isolation in clinical specimens. Overall management of *P. aeruginosa* is multi-pronged and includes:[12]

- adherence to hand hygiene practices with alcohol-based hand rub
- use of PPE with standard and contact precautions; and
- stringent infection control cleaning schedules with disinfectant.

These are integral to the management and prevention of spread of CPEs. Furthermore, AMS assists in preventing the development of multidrug resistance.

22.6 Burkholderia cepacia

Burkholderia cepacia complex (BCC) is an emerging opportunistic pathogen in healthcare settings and vulnerable populations. This is an important organism due to limited effective antimicrobials for treatment and the organism's ability to survive certain disinfectants.[24]

22.6.1 Epidemiology

BCC is ubiquitous in soil, water and plants and is able to adapt to a variety of environments. Previously known as *Pseudomonas cepacia*, it emerged as a significant pathogen for patients with CF in the 1980s and is associated with decline in pulmonary function.[25] It poses little threat to immunocompetent hosts but has been associated with UTIs, bloodstream infections, peritonitis and pneumonia in immunocompromised patients. In particular, patients with CF and chronic granulomatous diseases are particularly susceptible. Healthcare-associated outbreaks have occurred due to environmental or medical device contamination. This has included contaminated medical solutions (ultrasound gels, mouthwash, medications) and contaminated disinfectants.[26-28] Outbreaks have occurred in ICUs associated with ventilators.[29] Pseudo-outbreaks have occurred due to contamination within the medical laboratory.

22.6.2 Microbiology

BCC is one of over 70 named species within the genus Burkholderia. BCC comprises at least 21 closely related species of different genomovars. It is an aerobic non-spore forming, oxidase positive, Gram-negative bacillus which may require at least 3 days to grow on media (e.g. MacConkey). They have a characteristic dirt or soil-like odour. Phenotypically they are very similar within the complex; however, the advent of MALDI-TOF MS within the clinical laboratory permits rapid identification.

22.6.3 Antimicrobial resistance

BCC organisms are resistant to many antimicrobial agents. Combinations of chromosomal beta-lactamases and impermeability can mean resistance to beta-lactam agents. Intrinsic resistance occurs via a variety of mechanisms to aminoglycosides, polymyxins, ciprofloxacin, tetracyclines and chloramphenicol. These resistance combinations mean there are limited antimicrobials suitable to test susceptibility for that can perhaps treat the infection.

The EUCAST does not provide breakpoints for interpretation of susceptibilities due to there being little evidence linking interpretation of susceptibility or MIC and clinical outcome. Furthermore, there are some difficulties undertaking susceptibility testing due to the need for broth microdilution over specific gradient strips (e.g. E-test). The CLSI have established breakpoints for a limited number of antimicrobials using gradient strips for interpretation of MIC.

22.6.4 Infection prevention and control

BCC can adapt to its environment. It can spread via fomites and has also been implicated in person-to-person transmission. Factors proven to be linked with healthcare-associated transmission of BCC include contaminated fomites and equipment, poor hand hygiene and cohorting of CF patients. As such, international CF guidelines recommended single rooms for CF patients, as well as considering having BCC colonised patients separated by wards depending on their biovars.[30]

The Australian Guidelines for the Prevention and Control of Infection in Healthcare recommend standard, contact and droplet precautions for CF patients with BCC colonisation or infection. However, contact and droplet precautions criteria are not established, and should be considered on a case-by-case basis depending on degree of infection, environment and resistance profile.[9] Given its ability to contaminate medical disinfectants and solutions, studies have shown varying biocide susceptibility. High MICs for chlorhexidine (>100 mg/L) and triclosan (>500 mg/L), among others, was exhibited amongst BCC isolates. BCC remained viable in some commercial biocide solutions, and established CF outbreak strains were shown to have elevated chlorhexidine MIC. This highlights the importance of multimodal prevention strategies.

22.7 Stenotrophomonas maltophilia

Stenotrophomonas maltophilia was first isolated in 1943 and has more recently emerged as an important healthcare-associated multidrug-resistant infection.[31] It is a Gram-negative bacillus closely related to *Pseudomonas* and is the only one of its genus known to cause infections in humans. It is commonly isolated in samples from the respiratory tract where it is often considered a commensal organism. When it causes invasive infections, it is usually as an opportunistic pathogen, especially among patients with immunocompromising conditions. *S. maltophilia* most often affects debilitated patients, such as those in the ICU. The most common infections caused by *S. maltophilia* are bacteraemias and pneumonias. Less frequently, *S. maltophilia* can cause skin and soft tissue infections, osteomyelitis, meningitis, endocarditis and infections of the urinary and biliary tracts.

It is important to differentiate between clinical infection and colonisation when considering treating *S. maltophilia*. Treatment should be prompt when it is considered a true pathogen. Growth from a usually sterile site, such as blood and pleural or peritoneal fluid, should be considered pathogenic. Isolation of *S. maltophilia* from upper respiratory tract samples may be pathogenic in the absence of an alternative organism and with clinical evidence of pneumonia, especially in at-risk patients.

22.7.1 Epidemiology

Typically, *S. maltophilia* infections occur in patients with frequent or significant contact with healthcare settings. Risk factors for invasive *S. maltophilia* infection include admission to the ICU, mechanical ventilation, central venous catheters, treatment with broad-spectrum antibiotics, and other immunosuppressing or debilitating conditions like HIV infection, cystic fibrosis, solid organ or haematologic malignancies and neutropenias.[32] Outbreaks of *S. maltophilia* have occurred in some of these at-risk patient populations in hospital wards, including the ICU.

22.7.2 Microbiology

S. maltophilia is a ubiquitous, non-fermentative, Gram-negative bacillus that has a few polar flagella. It has been recovered from environmental sources including soils, plant roots, animals and water systems. *S. maltophilia* is an obligate aerobe and grows well on laboratory culture plates including blood and MacConkey agars. It can be reliably identified in the laboratory using standard biochemical tests and is also accurately identified using automated methods (e.g. MALDI-TOF MS).

22.7.3 Antimicrobial resistance

Intrinsic and acquired resistance mechanisms contribute to the broadly antibiotic-resistant profile of *S. maltophilia*. Two inducible, chromosomally encoded beta-lactamases confer resistance to beta-lactams (namely L1 and L2), including a penicillinase and a clavulanic acid-sensitive cephalosporinase.[31] *S. maltophilia* is also resistant to aminoglycosides due to an aminoglycoside acetyl-transferase. Temperature-dependent changes in the outer membrane lipopolysaccharide (LPS) structure provide added resistance to aminoglycosides, as warmer temperatures alter the chemical composition of the LPS. Efflux pumps confer resistance to other antibiotic classes. Resistance to carbapenems should be presumed for all *S. maltophilia* isolates.

As a result, there are very limited antibiotic options for the treatment of *S. maltophilia*. First-line treatment is limited to trimethoprim-sulfamethoxazole. Rates of susceptibility of *S. maltophilia* to trimethoprim-sulfamethoxazole remain high, although resistance has been increasingly reported among some patient populations. For some patients, use of trimethoprim-sulfamethoxazole is precluded, for example by hypersensitivity reactions, drug toxicities (including myelosuppression, renal impairment and hyperkalaemia). In these cases, fluoroquinolones are a potential alternative antibiotic choice, particularly levofloxacin. There is a risk of selecting out resistant mutant populations of *S. maltophilia* where fluoroquinolones are used. Furthermore, formation of biofilm aids in the evasion of antibiotics.

22.7.4 Infection prevention and control

Surveillance programs have identified *S. maltophilia* as a frequently isolated organism in the ICU, representing 4.3% of a total 74,394 Gram-negative bacillus isolates in a study of ICUs in the United States between 1993 and 2004.[23] Antimicrobial stewardship plays a two-fold preventative role in managing *S. maltophilia* infections. Firstly, it aids in reducing the incidence of *S. maltophilia* infections by limiting the use of broad-spectrum antibiotics. Secondly, it reduces the risk of inducing more broadly resistant strains by limiting their exposure to antibiotics. Hand hygiene and contact isolation have been used in the ICU to reduce spread of *S. maltophilia*.

22.8 Mycobacterium tuberculosis

Tuberculosis refers to infections caused by *Mycobacterium tuberculosis* (TB).[33] This organism is usually spread by inhaling aerosols. The most common manifestation of TB is with pulmonary disease, often with cavitating lung lesions and less frequently with the widespread changes of miliary tuberculosis. Pleural disease also occurs. Of the extra-pulmonary sites of TB infection, peripheral lymphadenitis is the next most common. Infections of any other body system are possible, including the central nervous system (such as TB meningitis), gastrointestinal system (such as TB ileitis) and renal, ocular, genitourinary and cutaneous infections. Treatment of TB infections typically requires multidrug therapy for extended time periods; first-line therapy usually comprises the four drugs of isoniazid, rifampicin, pyrazinamide and ethambutol. Emergence of drug-resistant strains of TB is a challenge for both treatment and for public health. Exposure to TB can also result in latent TB infection, where there is no clinically apparent disease. Courses of treatment for latent TB reduce the lifetime risk of TB reactivation.

A number of non-tuberculous Mycobacteria also cause disease in humans. Examples include Mycobacterium avium complex, *Mycobacterium ulcerans*, *Mycobacterium abscessus*, *Mycobacterium leprae* (leprosy), *Mycobacterium chelonae*, *Mycobacterium fortuitum* and *Mycobacterium marinum*.

22.8.1 Epidemiology

Most people affected by TB are in low- and middle-income countries. Countries with the highest rates of TB include China, India, Bangladesh, Pakistan, Indonesia, the Philippines, Nigeria and South Africa. TB infections in Australia are generally acquired overseas, either in people who have migrated from high incidence countries or by travel to an endemic country, although some Australia-born populations are at higher risk, including Indigenous Australians in remote communities. An estimated one-quarter of the world's population is infected with TB. The majority of these infections are latent disease. Close to 10 million people develop clinical TB disease each year.[34]

22.8.2 Microbiology

TB is an example of an acid-fast bacillus (AFB) and is not seen on microscopy using the conventional Gram stain. Ziehl–Neelsen staining is used to demonstrate TB on microscopy. TB is a slow-growing mycobacterium and requires specific nutrient support and extended times of culture in the laboratory; TB cultures are usually incubated for six weeks. PCR allows the possibility of rapid identification of TB as well as assessing for rifampicin resistance mutations (using the *rpoB* gene). Histology can support the diagnosis where there is clinical suspicion, typically showing the presence of granulomas often with central necrosis or caseation.

22.8.3 Antimicrobial resistance

Drug-resistant TB is resistant to at least one of the four first-line anti-tuberculous drugs listed above. Multidrug-resistant TB (MDR-TB) is resistant to at least isoniazid and rifampicin. Extensively drug-resistant TB (XDR-TB) describes MDR-TB that is also resistant to a fluoroquinolone and at least one other intravenous anti-tuberculous drug. Drug resistance is either primary, where it is present at the time of infection, or acquired, where it has occurred during a treatment course. In Australia, MDR-TB is uncommon (around 2%) and cases of XDR-TB are rare.[35] The vast majority of these cases occur in patients who were born overseas.

22.8.4 Infection prevention and control

Pulmonary TB disease is described as 'smear-positive' when AFBs are demonstrated on sputum sample. Patients with smear-positive disease are considered to have a density of TB infection that poses a much higher risk of transmission, compared to those with smear-negative disease. In general, TB is less infectious than many other (typically viral) organisms that infect the respiratory tract. Hours of close contact is generally necessary for transmission.

In Australia, TB is a notifiable disease to public health authorities. Public health programs are involved in assessing the contacts of patients diagnosed with TB and screening them for TB infection, whether active or latent. Such contacts can then be offered TB therapies if appropriate, thereby reducing the risk of further exposures and further transmission.

22.9 Candida auris

The fungal pathogen *Candida auris* is an emerging, multidrug-resistant yeast implicated in healthcare outbreaks with substantial mortality. It was first isolated in 2009 from a patient in Japan[36] being isolated from an ear discharge swab, hence its name 'auris'. Over the following decade it has spread to all continents, leading to outbreaks in hospitals internationally, including Australia. The first detection was in Perth, Western Australia, in 2015[37] and has subsequently led to outbreaks in other Australian states.[38] Detection of *C. auris* is reportable in some Australian states and has been included in the Australian National Alert System for Critical Antimicrobial Resistances (CARAlert) since 2019. Eight isolates were reported from three states between 2019–20.[9]

22.9.1 Epidemiology

C. auris is a relatively recent pathogen, with the earliest isolate identified retrospectively in 1996 in Korea. There are four major discrete clades based on genetic and genomic data and the location of the first isolates: the Southeast Asian (I), the East Asian (II), the South African (III) and the South American (IV).[36]

22.9.2 Microbiology

C. auris is a newly emerged member of the Candida/ Clavispora clade. It has a typical oval-elongated budding yeast form on Gram stain. Culture-based methodologies are key to detecting *C. auris*. Growth rates are slow, requiring up to 10 days of incubation. As a result, many laboratories utilise an enrichment step to reduce incubation periods. As well as growing on standard *Candida*-specific media (Sabarouds dextrose agar), specialised *Candida*-chromogenic media, on which colonies develop individual species-specific colours, may be used to provide preliminary identification of *C. auris* in potentially mixed cultures. Many commercial laboratory systems can misidentify *C. auris*, however, the commercial MALDI-TOF MS systems available in Australia accurately differentiate *C. auris* from other fungal species.[39]

Susceptibility testing should be performed using standardised laboratory methods or the isolate should be referred to a reference laboratory. MICs should be reported, as susceptibility breakpoints have not been developed by the major susceptibility testing methods. Almost all *C. auris* isolates have increased MIC to fluconazole. In addition, lower-level resistance to Amphotericin B and echinocandins has been reported and appears to be clade dependent.[36] Concerningly, rapid emergence of multidrug-resistance (resistance to more than two antifungal classes) may develop during therapy. Referral of the isolate for whole genome sequencing and phylogenetic analysis is recommended to determine clade, possible source of infection and potential local transmission.[38]

22.9.3 Infection prevention and control

Guidelines and recommendations for the management of *C. auris* in the healthcare setting have been produced in Australia and internationally. A multimodal management strategy is recommended for the control of *C. auris* in the healthcare setting. These include active screening and isolation of at-risk patients, surveillance strategies, environmental cleaning and disinfection. The Australasian Society for Infectious Diseases (ASID) has provided a position statement on the diagnosis, management and prevention of *C. auris* in hospitals.[40] The ASID recommendations for the management of *C. auris* in healthcare settings include pre-emptive isolation and screening for high-risk individuals. This includes patients transferred from a hospital with endemic or an outbreak of *C. auris*, patients admitted following at least an overnight stay in an overseas healthcare institution in the previous 12 months, or close contacts of *C. auris* patients (i.e., current room contacts and past room contacts within the previous month). Cleaning should be performed using both detergent and disinfectant as per the manufacturer's instructions. Products with sporicidal activity should be used for disinfection and patient rooms should be cleaned and disinfected at least daily. A thorough terminal clean should occur once the patient is discharged from a room and shared patient equipment should be cleaned and disinfected between patients. Alcohol-based hand rubs are recommended when hands are not visibly soiled. If hands are visibly soiled, washing with soap and water is recommended.

Screening and surveillance are recommended in hospitals where more than one patient with *C. auris* is identified. Point prevalence surveys of an entire ward or facility may be conducted to assess the extent of transmission and to identify all colonised patients. Repeated screening of currently hospitalised patients (such as weekly screening) should be considered if further cases are identified despite other measures. The sites recommended for screening are at least composite axilla and groin swabs. Additional screening sites are suggested to enhance yield, including specimens collected from vascular line exit sites, wounds, drain tube outputs and urine.

Placement of an alert in the medical record of patients colonised or infected with *C. auris* ensures appropriate isolation measures are taken at readmission. If a patient is to be transferred, the receiving facility must also be notified of the patient's status and required infection control precautions. There must be appropriate management of indwelling devices, implementation of effective local antifungal stewardship programs, and clinical governance systems with authority to mandate effective care-bundles and healthcare worker adherence to multimodal IPC strategies in facilities where *C. auris* is identified.

Conclusion

AMR presents a constantly evolving threat to healthcare and the effective treatment of both common and severe infections. It is one of the most serious issues for the future of healthcare and the health of humans in general. Over the past century, increasing numbers of microorganisms are exhibiting multidrug resistance, with many proving resistant to a broad range of drugs. Containing AMR requires a comprehensive and multi-pronged approach. At the forefront of this is prevention, and adherence to an array of IPC practices to prevent infection in the first place. Additionally, widespread implementation of AMS programs aims to reduce the inappropriate prescription and use of antimicrobials and thereby inhibit rates of resistance from rising.

Useful websites/resources

- Antimicrobial Resistance Australia: https://www.amr.gov.au/
- Australia's National Antimicrobial Resistance Strategy–2020 and beyond: https://www.amr.gov.au/resources/australias-national-antimicrobial-resistance-strategy-2020-and-beyond
- AURA 2021: Fourth Australian report on antimicrobial use and resistance in human health: https://www.safetyandquality.gov.au/publications-and-resources/resource-library/aura-2021-fourth-australian-report-antimicrobial-use-and-resistance-human-health
- ACSQHC National Safety and Quality Health Service Preventing and Controlling Infections Standard: Antimicrobial stewardship: https://www.safetyandquality.gov.au/standards/nsqhs-standards/preventing-and-controlling-infections-standard/antimicrobial-stewardship

References

1. Tong SYC, Davis JS, Eichenberger E, Holland TL, Fowler Jr VG. *Staphylococcus aureus* infections: epidemiology, pathophysiology, clinical manifestations, and management. Clinical Microbiol Rev. 2015;28(3):603-661.
2. van Hal SJ, Jensen SO, Vaska VL, Espedido BA, Paterson DL, Gosbell IB. Predictors of mortality in Staphylococcus aureus bacteremia. Clin Microbiol Rev. 2012;25(2):362-386.
3. Kluytmans J, van Belkum A, Verbrugh H. Nasal carriage of Staphylococcus aureus: epidemiology, underlying mechanisms, and associated risks. Clin Microbiol Rev. 1997;10(3):505-520.
4. Coombs GW, Daley DA, Yee NWT, Shoby P, Mowlaboccus S. Australian Group on Antimicrobial Resistance (AGAR) Australian Staphylococcus aureus Sepsis Outcome Programme (ASSOP) Annual Report 2020. Commun Dis Intell (2018). 2022;46.
5. Turner NA, Sharma-Kuinkel BK, Maskarinec SA, Eichenberger EM, Shah PP, Carugati M, et al. Methicillin-resistant *Staphylococcus aureus*: an overview of basic and clinical research. Nat Rev Microbiol. 2019;17(4):203-218.
6. Aklilu E, Hui Ying C. First mecC and mecA positive livestock-associated methicillin resistant Staphylococcus aureus (mecC MRSA/LA-MRSA) from dairy cattle in Malaysia. Microorganisms. 2020;8(2):147.
7. Paterson GK, Larsen AR, Robb A, Edwards GE, Pennycott TW, Foster G, et al. The newly described mecA homologue, mecALGA251, is present in methicillin-resistant Staphylococcus aureus isolates from a diverse range of host species. J Antimicrob Chemother. 2012;67(12):2809-2813.
8. García-Álvarez L, Holden MT, Lindsay H, Webb CR, Brown DF, Curran MD, et al. Meticillin-resistant Staphylococcus aureus with a novel mecA homologue in human and bovine populations in the UK and Denmark: a descriptive study. Lancet Infect Dis. 2011;11(8):595-603.
9. Australian Commission on Safety and Quality in Health Care. AURA 2021: Fourth Australian report on antimicrobial use and resistance in healthy humans. Sydney: ACSQHC, 2021.
10. Coombs GW, Daley DA, Mowlaboccus S, Lee YT, Pang S. Australian Group on Antimicrobial Resistance (AGAR) Australian Enterococcal Sepsis Outcome Programme (AESOP) Annual Report 2018. Commun Dis Intell (2018). 2020;44.
11. Coombs GW, Daley DA, Mowlaboccus S, Pang S. Australian Group on Antimicrobial Resistance (AGAR) Australian Enterococcal Sepsis Outcome Programme (AESOP) Annual Report 2019. Commun Dis Intell (2018). 2020;44.
12. National Health and Medical Research Council. Australian Guidelines for the Prevention and Control of Infection in Healthcare. Canberra: Commonwealth of Australia, 2019.
13. Janda JM, Abbott SL. The changing face of the family Enterobacteriaceae (Order: "Enterobacterales"): new members, taxonomic issues, geographic expansion, and new diseases and disease syndromes. Clin Microbiol Rev. 2021;34(2).
14. Jacoby GA, Munoz-Price LS. The new beta-lactamases. N Engl J Med. 2005;352(4):380-391.

15. Bonomo RA, Burd EM, Conly J, Limbago BM, Poirel L, Segre JA, et al. Carbapenemase-producing organisms: a global scourge. Clin Infect Dis. 2018;66(8):1290-1297.

16. Walther-Rasmussen J, Høiby N. Class A carbapenemases. J Antimicrob Chemother. 2007;60(3):470-482.

17. Yong D, Toleman MA, Giske CG, Cho HS, Sundman K, Lee K, et al. Characterization of a new metallo-beta-lactamase gene, bla(NDM-1), and a novel erythromycin esterase gene carried on a unique genetic structure in Klebsiella pneumoniae sequence type 14 from India. Antimicrob Agents Chemother. 2009;53(12):5046-5054.

18. Jacoby GA. AmpC beta-lactamases. Clin Microbiol Rev. 2009;22(1):161-182.

19. Harris PNA, Tambyah PA, Lye DC, Mo Y, Lee TH, Yilmaz M, et al. Effect of piperacillin-tazobactam vs meropenem on 30-day mortality for patients with E coli or Klebsiella pneumoniae bloodstream infection and ceftriaxone resistance: a randomized clinical trial. JAMA. 2018; 320(10):984-994.

20. Calbo E, Freixas N, Xercavins M, Riera M, Nicolás C, Monistrol O, et al. Foodborne nosocomial outbreak of SHV1 and CTX-M-15-producing *Klebsiella pneumoniae*: Epidemiology and control. Clin Infect Dis. 2011;52(6): 743–749.

21. Anstey NM, Currie BJ, Hassell M, Palmer D, Dwyer B, Seifert H. Community-acquired bacteremic Acinetobacter pneumonia in tropical Australia is caused by diverse strains of Acinetobacter baumannii, with carriage in the throat in at-risk groups. J Clin Microbiol. 2002;40(2):685-686.

22. Ibrahim S, Al-Saryi N, Al-Kadmy IMS, Aziz SN. Multidrug-resistant Acinetobacter baumannii as an emerging concern in hospitals. Mol Biol Rep. 2021;48(10):6987-6998.

23. Lockhart SR, Abramson MA, Beekmann SE, Gallagher G, Riedel S, Diekema DJ, et al. Antimicrobial resistance among Gram-negative bacilli causing infections in intensive care unit patients in the United States between 1993 and 2004. J Clin Microbiol. 2007;45(10):3352-3359.

24. Kim JM, Ahn Y, LiPuma JJ, Hussong D, Cerniglia CE. Survival and susceptibility of Burkholderia cepacia complex in chlorhexidine gluconate and benzalkonium chloride. J Ind Microbiol Biotechnol. 2015;42(6):905-913.

25. Isles A, Maclusky I, Corey M, Gold R, Prober C, Fleming P, et al. Pseudomonas cepacia infection in cystic fibrosis: an emerging problem. J Pediatr. 1984;104(2):206-210.

26. Dos Santos Saalfeld SM, Shinohara DR, Dos Anjos Szczerepa MM, Martinez HV, Vieira de Campos E, Mitsugui CS, et al. Consecutive outbreaks of Burkholderia cepacia complex caused by intrinsically contaminated chlorhexidine mouthwashes. Am J Infect Control. 2020; 48(11):1348-1353.

27. Bilgin H, Altınkanat Gelmez G, Bayrakdar F, Sayın E, Gül F, Pazar N, et al. An outbreak investigation of Burkholderia cepacia infections related with contaminated chlorhexidine mouthwash solution in a tertiary care center in Turkey. Antimicrob Resist Infect Control. 2021;10(1):143.

28. Hutchinson J, Runge W, Mulvey M, Norris G, Yetman M, Valkova N, et al. Burkholderia cepacia infections associated with intrinsically contaminated ultrasound gel: the role of microbial degradation of parabens. Infect Control Hosp Epidemiol. 2004;25(4):291-296.

29. Peterson AE, Chitnis AS, Xiang N, Scaletta JM, Geist R, Schwartz J, et al. Clonally related Burkholderia contaminans among ventilated patients without cystic fibrosis. Am J Infect Control. 2013;41(12):1298-1300.

30. Saiman L, Siegel JD, LiPuma JJ, Brown RF, Bryson EA, Chambers MJ, et al. Infection prevention and control guideline for cystic fibrosis: 2013 update. Infect Control Hosp Epidemiol. 2014;35 Suppl 1:S1-s67.

31. Brooke JS. Stenotrophomonas maltophilia: an emerging global opportunistic pathogen. Clin Microbiol Rev. 2012;25(1):2-41.

32. Calza L, Manfredi R, Chiodo F. Stenotrophomonas (Xanthomonas) maltophilia as an emerging opportunistic pathogen in association with HIV infection: a 10-year surveillance study. Infection. 2003;31(3):155-161.

33. Natarajan A, Beena PM, Devnikar AV, Mali S. A systemic review on tuberculosis. Indian J Tuberc. 2020;67(3):295-311.

34. Furin J, Cox H, Pai M. Tuberculosis. Lancet. 2019;393(10181): 1642-1656.

35. Bright A, Denholm J, Coulter C, Waring J, Stapledon R. Tuberculosis notifications in Australia, 2015-2018. Commun Dis Intell (2018). 2020;44.

36. Du H, Bing J, Hu T, Ennis CL, Nobile CJ, Huang G. Candida auris: epidemiology, biology, antifungal resistance, and virulence. PLoS Pathog. 2020;16(10):e1008921.

37. Heath CH, Dyer JR, Pang S, Coombs GW, Gardam DJ. Candida auris sternal osteomyelitis in a man from Kenya visiting Australia, 2015. Emerg Infect Dis. 2019;25(1):192-194.

38. Lane CR, Seemann T, Worth LJ, Easton M, Pitchers W, Wong J, et al. Incursions of Candida auris into Australia, 2018. Emerg Infect Dis. 2020;26(6):1326-1328.

39. Ghosh AK, Paul S, Sood P, Rudramurthy SM, Rajbanshi A, Jillwin TJ, et al. Matrix-assisted laser desorption ionization time-of-flight mass spectrometry for the rapid identification of yeasts causing bloodstream infections. Clin Microbiol Infect. 2015;21(4):372-378.

40. Ong CW, Chen SC, Clark JE, Halliday CL, Kidd SE, Marriott DJ, et al. Diagnosis, management and prevention of Candida auris in hospitals: position statement of the Australasian Society for Infectious Diseases. Intern Med J. 2019;49(10):1229-1243.

CHAPTER 23

High consequence infectious diseases and biocontainment for health protection

PROFESSOR RAMON Z. SHABAN[i-iv]

Dr MATTHEW V. N. O'SULLIVAN[iv,v]

Dr CECILIA Z. LI[i]

Dr CATHERINE VIENGKHAM[i]

Chapter highlights

- The nature and relevance of high consequence infectious diseases (HCID) in Australia relative to the international context
- The role and principles of biocontainment for health protection within contemporary Australian health systems
- The current state of preparedness of the Australian healthcare system in view of the ongoing threat of HCIDs

i   Susan Wakil School of Nursing and Midwifery, Faculty of Medicine and Health, University of Sydney, Sydney, NSW
ii Sydney Infectious Diseases Institute, Faculty of Medicine and Health, University of Sydney, Sydney, NSW
iii Public Health Unit, Centre for Population Health, Western Sydney Local Health District, Westmead, NSW
iv New South Wales Biocontainment Centre, Western Sydney Local Health District, Westmead, NSW
v   Centre for Infectious Diseases and Microbiology, New South Wales Health Pathology, ICPMR, Westmead, NSW

Introduction

This chapter provides an overview of high consequence infectious diseases (HCIDs) their impact in Australia, and the current state of biocontainment preparedness and response across the country. HCIDs are broadly defined as acute infectious diseases that have a high case mortality, are highly communicable, and are difficult to prevent, contain and treat. International outbreaks of HCIDs, such as SARS, MERS-CoV and Ebola virus disease (EVD), have been occurring with greater frequency and often result in considerable mortality. For example, the 2014–15 EVD outbreak in West Africa, which subsequently spread across Africa, Europe and the United States, yielded 28,600 cases and more than 11,300 deaths.[1,2] As of February 2023 the global outbreak of COVID-19, which initially was classified as an HCID, has seen over 784,000,000 confirmed cases and 6,800,000 deaths. These outbreaks highlight the need for adequate preparation to contain and manage cases should such diseases reach or emerge in Australia.

Healthcare workers (HCWs) are particularly vulnerable to outbreaks of HCIDs, being in positions where they are more likely to become infected and to spread infection. The impacts of HCID outbreaks on the healthcare system are considerable. Although no longer categorised as an HCID, the global experience of COVID-19 has demonstrated that HCWs are under immense psychological pressure, resulting from an ever-changing environment, increased workload, potentially scarce resources, and the stress caused by constant exposure to potentially deadly disease.

Many countries, including Australia, have established systems and protocols to follow in the event of HCID outbreaks. One of the key strategies in managing HCIDs is through biocontainment and the establishment of dedicated facilities for the purposes of containing infected individuals and preventing the disease from spreading. Furthermore, biocontainment facilities play a key role by allowing for the safe and secure maintenance and study of active samples and materials related to HCIDs. Different standards of biosafety exist worldwide. Biocontainment facilities may exist within formal and established specialist healthcare facilities, such as tertiary or quaternary hospitals, or as stand-alone isolated facilities that operate for the primary purpose of researching highly dangerous diseases and organisms.

23.1 International definitions of HCIDs

There is currently no international consensus regarding which diseases or pathogens are classified as HCIDs. There also are no universally accepted criteria for defining which diseases and pathogens constitute an HCID. In 2019, Cieslak et al[3] reported that there was no consensus about which pathogens or diseases would require high-level containment and clinical care. However, it is generally agreed that the all of the following criteria for a disease should be considered when deciding on HCID categorisation:

- *Infectivity* (ID_{50}): the dose of the pathogen (in their respective units) that is required to infect 50% of people who are exposed
- *Communicability* (R_0): the contagiousness of the disease. This is usually expressed in terms of reproductive number, where R_0 quantifies the number of secondary cases that may result from a single primary case. Diseases with $R_0 > 1$ indicate any disease that has the potential to transmit, with contagiousness increasing with greater R_0 values
- *Hazard:* the dangerousness of the disease. This is usually measured in the associated morbidity and mortality rates (number of fatalities/number of infections)
- *Treatment availability:* the availability of licensed and effective medical countermeasures, such as treatment and preventative vaccines.

Considering these criteria, an HCID would be a disease that has high infectivity, high communicability, high hazard and little to no treatment availability. There are only a few diseases that necessarily meet all four criteria and most diseases will usually meet one or two. For example, diseases like anthrax and botulism, caused by exposures to the bacteria *Bacillus anthracis* and *Clostridium botulinum* respectively, are highly hazardous and associated with a high case fatality when left untreated. However, exposure to the bacteria in both cases is either through contact with animals or the consumption of improperly prepared food, and the risk of transmission is low. Furthermore, vaccines and antibiotics exist to treat anthrax, and antitoxins exist for botulism. So, while both diseases are highly dangerous to an infected individual, the low chance of transmission means that care in a regular healthcare facility, under normal protocols, is sufficient and patients are unlikely to require a high-level containment facility.

On the other hand, diseases like rubella and mumps are highly transmissible from person to person and typically spread through inhalation or oral contact with the respiratory droplets or secretions of an infected individual. However, the prognosis for both diseases is usually excellent, with most individuals remaining asymptomatic over the course of their infection, or recovering with little to no additional complications. Vaccines for rubella and mumps are well established and are part of immunisation programs that administer them to children at specific ages in most developed countries. Indeed, the availability of treatments forms a crucial differentiator in this criteria, as similarly contagious and yet more deadly diseases such as measles and smallpox have both been effectively eradicated with the widespread adoption of vaccinations.

While the above criteria for characterising HCIDs currently remain abstract recommendations, many nations have independently taken steps towards regulating the need for high-level containment and handling of certain organisms. For example, the UK and USA have both established formal lists for organisms and diseases that require high-level containment. Public Health England provides a useful definition for HCIDs that is generally echoed internationally. In the UK, an HCID:

* is an acute infectious disease
* typically has a high case fatality rate
* may not have effective prophylaxis or treatment
* is often difficult to recognise and detect rapidly
* is able to spread in the community and within healthcare settings
* requires an enhanced individual, population and system response to ensure it is managed effectively, efficiently and safely.[4]

Public Health England further classifies HCIDs as being either 'contact HCIDs' or 'airborne HCIDs'.[4] Contact HCIDs are predominantly spread by direct contact with an infected person or fluids, or by indirect contact with contaminated surfaces and fomites. Airborne HCIDs are usually spread by respiratory droplets or transmission. Table 23.1 provides the current list of HCIDs recognised the United Kingdom Health Security Agency (UKHSA) (as of June 2021). While the novel coronavirus disease, COVID-19, was initially classified by Public Health England as an HCID, this status was dropped by 19 March 2020[4] once more information came to light and the lower mortality rate of the disease was more clearly defined.

In the US, the Centers for Disease Control and Prevention (CDC) includes the National Center for Emerging and Zoonotic Infectious Diseases (NCEZID), which oversees the Division of High Consequence Pathogens and Pathology (DHCPP). The DHCPP serves to improve public health and safety by investigating, monitoring and controlling agents responsible for highly lethal diseases. They have compiled a list known as the Diseases of High Consequence Pathogens and Pathology which includes a total of 57 disease-causing agents (Table 23.2). This list differs from that of United Kingdom Health Security Agency (UKHSA) primarily with the inclusion of less transmissible but still highly dangerous diseases caused by bacterial infections and prions.

23.2 Defining HCIDs in Australia

At the time of writing, in 2023, there is no formal national definition or designated list of HCIDs in Australia. However, there are established and legislated lists of agents that require specific management in the case of infected individuals; or increased regulation, containment or security in the case of the handling of active samples. National biosecurity in Australia is governed and administered by two federal departments: the Department of Health and Aged Care and the Department of Agriculture, Water and the Environment. Most relevantly, the Department of Health and Aged Care enacts measures to minimise the risk of diseases caused by viruses, bacteria and other microorganisms entering or emerging in Australia that have the potential to cause

TABLE 23.1 United Kingdom Health Security Agency (UKHSA) classifications of contact and airborne HCIDs

Contact HCIDs	Airborne HCIDs
• Argentine haemorrhagic fever (Argentine mammarenavirus, formerly Junin virus) • Bolivian haemorrhagic fever (Machupo mammarenavirus) • Crimean Congo haemorrhagic fever (CCHF) • Ebola virus disease (EVD) • Lassa fever • Lujo virus disease (Lujo mammarenavirus) • Marburg virus disease (MVD) • Severe fever with thrombocytopaenia syndrome (SFTS)	• Andes virus infection (hantavirus) • Avian influenza A H7N9 and H5N1 • Avian influenza A H5N6 and H7N7 • Middle East respiratory syndrome (MERS) • Mpox (monkeypox) (Clade I only) • Nipah virus infection • Pneumonic plague (*Yersinia pestis*) • Severe acute respiratory syndrome (SARS)

Source: Public Health England. High consequence infectious diseases (HCID) 2018[4]

TABLE 23.2 High consequence infectious diseases: pathogens and pathology

Prions	• Bovine spongiform encephalopathy (BSE) • Sporadic, genetic and iatrogenic Creutzfeldt-Jakob disease (CJD) • Chronic wasting disease • Guillain-Barre syndrome • Gerstmann-Straussler-Schneiker syndrome • Reye syndrome • Fatal familial insomnia • Kawasaki syndrome/disease
Viral	• Ebola virus • Sudan virus • Bundibugyo virus • Tai Forest virus • Reston virus • Marburg virus • Ravn virus • Rift Valley fever virus • Crimean-Congo haemorrhagic fever • Hantavirus pulmonary syndrome (HPS) associated viruses • Haemorrhagic fever with renal syndrome (HFRS) associated viruses • Nipah virus • Hendra virus • Lassa virus • Lujo virus disease (Lujo mammarenavirus) • Tick-borne encephalitis (TBE) complex viruses • Far-eastern TBE virus • Omsk haemorrhagic virus • Kyasanur Forest disease virus
Bacterial	• Actinomycoses and nocardiosis • Anthrax • Brucellosis • Buruli ulcer • Capnocytophaga • Glanders (*Burkholderia mallei*) • Hansen's disease (leprosy) • Leptospirosis • Melioidosis (*Burkholderia pseudomallei*) • Pasteurella sp. infections • Rat-bite fever
Poxvirus and rabies	• Bovine papular stomatitis virus • Cowpox virus • Monkeypox virus • Pseudocowpox virus • Skunkpox virus • Variola virus (Smallpox) • Non-rabies lyssavirus • Molluscum contagiosum virus tan • Orf virus • Raccoonpox virus • Tanapox • Volepox • Rabies virus

harm to the Australian population, food security and economy. Currently, four lists have been established under different legislation.

Two of these are relevant to the detection of diseases in individuals:

• Listed Human Diseases (LHDs), as classified under the *Biosecurity Act 2015*.[5] This list pertains to the management of individuals who have, or are suspected to have, the disease when entering Australian states or territories; and

• the list of *nationally notifiable diseases*, governed by the Australian Government Department of Health and Aged Care and Communicable Diseases Network Australia (CDNA).[6]

The other two are relevant to the handling and storage of disease samples in laboratories:

• *Risk Group 4* microorganisms, classified by Standards Australia and Standards New Zealand, for the specific requirement of high-level containment in PC4 laboratories;[7] and

• *Security Sensitive Biological Agents (SSBA)*, overseen by the *National Health Security Act 2007*.[8] This list contains agents that are additionally regarded as potential security threats in the context of bioterrorism.

23.2.1 Listed Human Diseases

The *Biosecurity Act 2015*[5] includes a list of specific diseases (Listed Human Diseases) which are recognised as contagious and have the potential to cause significant harm to human health. These diseases are determined by the Director of Human Biosecurity, in consultation with the chief health officers for each state and territory and the Director of Biosecurity. Last updated in September 2020, the list is shown in Table 23.3.

TABLE 23.3 Listed Human Diseases under the *Biosecurity Act 2015*

Listed Human Diseases	
• Human influenza with pandemic potential • Severe acute respiratory syndrome (SARS) • Smallpox • Yellow fever	• Plague • Middle East respiratory syndrome (MERS) • Viral haemorrhagic fevers • Human coronavirus with pandemic potential

Source:[5,56]

Chapter 2 of the Biosecurity Act details the biosecurity measures put in place in circumstances where a Listed Human Disease is identified or suspected, to manage the risk of the disease entering, emerging, establishing itself or spreading in Australia. This legislation also details the penalties put in place for failing to comply with biosecurity measures. When entering the country, individuals can be asked to:

• provide a declaration of vaccination status or other prophylaxis

• complete a questionnaire in regard to their health

• provide evidence of where they have been prior to entering Australia

• provide a declaration in relation to the specific LHD; and

• be screened.

Furthermore, operators of passenger aircraft and vessels are also required to provide contact information for the identified or suspected individual and to prevent unloading or disembarking where necessary.

An officer may require any individual to answer questions or provide written information if they are satisfied that the person has one or more signs or symptoms of a listed human disease, or if they have been exposed to a listed human disease. Officers may require individuals to remain in place for a period of time (although no longer than six hours) and to comply with biosecurity measures. Biosecurity measures include managing contacts, decontamination, undergoing examination, providing body samples, receiving a vaccination, treatment or medication, reporting of health status to an officer over a specified period, restricting behaviour, risk minimisation, limiting traveller movement and isolation measures.

23.2.2 National notifiable diseases

The National Notifiable Diseases Surveillance System (NNDSS) was established in 1990 under the Communicable Diseases Network Australia.[9] Communicable disease surveillance also operates at state and local levels. Legislation requires that each detected case is reported to state and territory health departments. These departments collect notifications of communicable diseases under their public health legislation. Computerised, deidentified unit records of notifications are supplied to the Australian Government Department of Health and Aged Care daily, for collation, analysis and publication on the internet (updated daily), and in the quarterly journal *Communicable Diseases Intelligence*. Jurisdictions produce a weekly surveillance report to provide a profile of influenza from a number of perspectives, including laboratory-confirmed notifications and hospitalisations due to influenza.[6]

The notification system in Australia enables public health authorities to detect outbreaks and abnormal rates of infectious diseases. There are 73 Australian nationally notifiable diseases including blood-borne, gastrointestinal, listed human, vaccine-preventable and vectorborne diseases, sexually transmissible infections, zoonoses and other bacterial diseases.[9] Additionally, diseases such as Creutzfeldt-Jakob disease and HIV are under national surveillance performed by surveillance bodies other than the Department of Health and Aged Care.[10]

23.2.3 Risk Group 4 microorganisms

The Australian and New Zealand Standard for laboratory safety (AS/NZS 2243.3-2010 – Safety in Laboratories, Part 3: Microbiological safety and containment) follows on from the WHO guidelines for classifying microorganisms that are infectious to humans and animals.[7] The classification groups organisms into four incremental risk categories based on the pathogenicity of the agent, the mode of transmission, the availability of effective preventative measures and the availability of effective treatment. The risk groups are as follows:

* Risk Group 1 (RG1): low individual and community risk
* Risk Group 2 (RG2): moderate individual risk, limited community risk
* Risk Group 3 (RG3): high individual risk, limited to moderate community risk; and
* Risk Group 4 (RG4): high individual and community risk.

Risk Group 4 microorganisms are defined as those causing potentially life-threatening human or animal disease, representing a significant risk to personnel, that may be readily transmissible from one individual to another, and for which there are limited effective treatments or preventative measures. It is recommended that microorganisms belonging to certain risk groups be contained in facilities with respective PC levels or higher. Some of the microorganisms that are currently classified under RG4 are listed in Table 23.4.

23.2.4 List of Security Sensitive Biological Agents

The Department of Health and Aged Care also administers the List of Security Sensitive Biological Agents

TABLE 23.4 List of Risk Group 4 viruses classified by Australian Standards and New Zealand Standards 2010 Safety in laboratories

List of RG4 viruses	
• Lassa fever virus • Venezuelan haemorrhagic fever (Guanarito mammarenavirus) • Bolivian haemorrhagic fever (Machupo mammarenavirus) • Mopeia viruses • Hazara virus • Marburgvirus • Omsk haemorrhagic fever virus • Herpes virus simiae (B virus) • Nipah virus	• Chapare haemorrhagic fever (Chapare mammarenavirus) • Argentine haemorrhagic fever (Argentine mammarenavirus, formerly Junin virus) • Brazilian haemorrhagic fever (Brazilian mammarenavirus, formerly Sabia virus) • Crimean-Congo haemorrhagic fever virus • Ebola virus disease • Kyasanur Forest disease • Tick-borne encephalitis • Hendra virus

and the SSBA Regulatory Scheme. The SSBA differentiates itself from the Listed Human Diseases in that it specifically regulates the handling of biological agents and toxins as distinct elements, separate from their infection of humans. This list primarily exists to regulate agents that pose security risks and health impacts, specifically with the aim of preventing use in terrorism and criminal activity. The former Council of Australian Governments (COAG) Health Council—now the Health Ministers' Meeting (HMM)—first agreed to a national review of hazardous materials, harmful biological materials, radiological sources and chemicals in 2002. The COAG Biological working group sourced information from existing national, international and research databases to compile a preliminary list of biological agents that would warrant assessment for further regulation. Out of an initial list of 200 candidate agents, 22 were recommended for regulation after individual risk assessments. A review of the 22-item list was conducted in 2016. After public consultation with states and territories, members of the regulated community and other key stakeholders, the removal of two Tier 2 agents (*Salmonella* Typhi and *Vibrio cholerae*) was recommended. This recommendation was subsequently approved by the Minister for Health.

Similar to the United States' Select Agents and Toxins list, the agents in the SSBA are categorised into Tier 1 (highest security concern, with more

TABLE 23.5 List of Security Sensitive Biological Agents under the *National Health Security Act 2007*

Tier 1 SSBAs	Tier 2 SSBAs
• Abrin • *Bacillus anthracis* • Botulinum toxin (0.5 mg) • Ebola virus • Foot-and-mouth disease virus • Highly pathogenic influenza virus, infecting humans • Marburgvirus • Ricin (5 mg) • Rinderpest virus • SARS coronavirus • Variola virus (smallpox) • *Yersinia pestis* (plague)	• African swine fever virus • Capripoxvirus (Sheep pox virus and Goat pox virus) • Classical swine fever virus • *Clostridium botulinum* (Botulism; toxin-producing strains) • *Francisella tularensis* (Tularaemia) • Lumpy skin disease virus • Peste-de-petits-ruminants virus • Yellow fever virus (non-vaccine strains)

Source:[8,11]

stringent requirements for handling and mandatory background checks for personnel) and Tier 2 (high security risk, with proportionally lower handling requirements and non-mandatory personnel background checks). The current 20-item list of SSBAs—as last updated in the February 2016 Review of Biological Agents of Security Concern Report—is shown in Table 23.5.[11] Currently, the Minister for Health and Aged Care has the power to add or remove agents from the list after consultation with Commonwealth agencies of relevant expertise, as well as from state and territory advisors.

The Security Sensitive Biological Agent Regulatory Scheme was established in the *National Health Security Act 2007* with the purpose of managing access to SSBAs to ensure that the agents were secure and did not provide opportunities for bioterrorism, and to allow full access to the agents by those with a legitimate need, such as government laboratories, universities, research facilities, diagnostic laboratories and hospitals. Entities that were allowed to handle SSBAs were required to report specific events to the Department of Health and Aged Care, such as the receipt, transport, disposal and acquisition of agents, as well as any incidents or changes in the handling of the agents. All facilities handling SSBAs must comply with the NHS Act and the National Health Security Regulations 2008 (NHS Regulations), which detail who and what is regulated, reporting requirements, legitimate purposes for handling, exemptions, administration, compliance and monitoring. Furthermore, the SSBA Standards under the *National Health Security Act 2007* also set mandatory requirements relating to the secure handling, transport, storage and disposal of SSBAs, how these requirements may be met and best practices.

A risk assessment algorithm was developed to provide a quantitative assessment for the regulated agents. An end-to-end Matrix Assisted Risk Assessment (MARA) was used to calculate each agent's security threat and health impact. The health impact score, specifically for agents affecting humans and human health, was assessed as an averaged score across three criteria: morbidity/mortality, transmissibility and difficulty to treat.

Morbidity considered the impact on individuals and on the health systems with regard to the cost of care required to manage the illness or injury caused by the agent. Mortality was based on the case fatality rate (CFR)—the proportion of individuals who die from contracting an illness after exposure to the agent. Transmissibility assessed the potential for the agent to spread from person to person. Lastly, difficulty to treat assessed whether treatments, therapies and vaccines were readily available and accessible, and how effective those treatments were both pre- and post-exposure to the agent.

The security threat assessment considered two criteria: interest and feasibility. Interest assessed the level of interest in an agent for use by terrorist, criminal or issue-motivated groups of concern in Australia. Feasibility assessed the availability, ease of production and ease of dissemination of the agent. The overall risk assessment scores were obtained by multiplying the health impact and security threat scores.

23.3 Australian experience of HCIDs

Since settlement, Australia has seen a relatively small number of highly detrimental infectious disease outbreaks compared to other countries. The HCIDs listed in Table 23.1 from the United Kingdom Health Security Agency (UKHSA) are not endemic in Australia, and in comparison with other countries our experience with HCIDs is limited. Australia is geographically vast, with a dispersed population. It is a high-income country with stable systems of government, high living standards and strongly developed public healthcare systems based on universal health care. The Australian federal, state and territory governments share responsibility for funding, operating, managing and regulating the health system, which is established constitutionally.[12] National coordination of response to a national public health crisis, such as an infectious disease outbreak, includes several national-level bodies and agencies. Furthermore, the country's geographical isolation as an island nation with a comparably small and sparsely dispersed population, combined with strict biosecurity and quarantine laws, readily act to inhibit the arrival and subsequent spread of diseases, particularly those already noted internationally.

Nevertheless, Australia has experienced several major outbreaks that have deleteriously affected the population and caused fatalities across multiple states. In the 19th century, multiple smallpox outbreaks occurred across New South Wales and Victoria. Lack of access to records mean that the total number of deaths caused by these outbreaks remains unclear; however, it was known that the disease disproportionately affected First Nations peoples.[13-15] In 1919, the global H1N1 influenza A pandemic reached Australian shores and from there spread to every state across the country. This influenza strain was particularly virulent and was estimated to cause upwards of 12,000 deaths across both the young and the old.[16-19] By this time, federal, state and territory governments boasted more established measures for outbreak control, such as quarantine and border closures. Despite several more outbreaks from different influenza strains occurring in the 1950s, 1960s and 2000s,[20,21] the 1919 outbreak remains the most deadly influenza epidemic Australia has experienced to date.

The first case of COVID-19 in Australia was identified in Victoria on 25 January 2020. Initially classified as an HCID, the pandemic resulted in major changes to Australia's social and economic landscape.[22-24] The first cases of COVID-19 in Australia[25] were quarantined in high-level biocontainment facilities in Victoria, New South Wales, Queensland and South Australia. In addition, during the early phase of the COVID-19 pandemic in Melbourne[26] the Royal Melbourne Hospital included the following key components in its response:

- regular communications between multidisciplinary working groups, including the infectious diseases, infection prevention and control (IPC) and emergency medicine units

- establishment of a sub-waiting area in the emergency department (ED) as well as a separate fever clinic for use during surge response

- enhanced IPC measures, including signage about PPE training and distribution of PPE and hand sanitisers

- creation of clinical assessment pathways for confirmed/suspected patients

- establishment of bilingual signage, screening questionnaires and discharge forms

- regular education and training sessions for staff to ask questions and also provide updates on evolving clinical information and epidemiology.

The declassification of COVID-19 as an HCID has resulted in considerable changes to the clinical management of patients with COVID-19 in hospital and non-hospital health and community-based settings. Whereas during the initial outbreak all cases were managed in hospitals, now most cases (depending on clinical indication) are managed in the home or other community settings.[27] In most instances, cases that are managed at home will have met the following criteria:

- a risk assessment has been conducted regarding the suitability of the accommodation and living arrangements, including who else is in the home and their vulnerability to severe disease

- it can be assured that the home environment permits separation of the case from other household members

- the case and household contacts are counselled about risk, and appropriate infection control measures are in place

- there is a reasonable level of confidence of the compliance of the case.

For example, during the COVID-19 outbreak in Western Sydney (NSW), patients clinically assessed to be at a low to medium risk of developing serious illness were being managed and monitored remotely by community health teams and general practitioners in an effort to reduce the burden on hospitals.[28] This was a joint initiative between Western Sydney Local Health District and Western Sydney Primary Health Network.[29]

23.4 Risk to healthcare workers

Frontline HCWs caring for and managing patients with HCIDs are among those at the highest risk of contracting the infection. The 2003 Severe Acute Respiratory Syndrome (SARS) outbreak saw a total of 8096 cases reported and 774 deaths.[30] Infections acquired by HCWs accounted for 1706 cases, equating to 21% of the total. For some countries, like Canada, Vietnam and Singapore, the total percentage of cases accounted for by HCWs reached over 40%.[31] Similarly, during the 2014–16 EVD outbreak in West Africa, case fatality rates ranged from 28–67% in Sierra Leone, Liberia and Guinea.[2] Levels of EVD infection in HCWs in Guinea were reported to be 42.2 times higher than in non-HCWs.[32]

Neither of the aforementioned outbreaks reached epidemic levels in Australia, which only reported six cases during the SARS pandemic and was not affected at all by the EVD outbreaks.[2,30] However, the 2020 COVID-19 epidemic necessitated rapid responses and severe adaptations by the Australian healthcare systems, which were keenly felt by their workers. Quigley et al[33] estimated the burden of COVID-19 on HCWs during the first six months of the pandemic in Australia. They found that HCWs comprised 6.03% of all reported infections and estimated that they were almost three times more likely to contract the disease compared to the general community.

Furthermore, HCWs are also highly prone to suffering poor psychological outcomes when dealing with HCIDs.[34,35] A 2021 study by Fryk et al[36] reported on the knowledge, attitudes and practices of Australian doctors and nurses from emergency and intensive care, and infectious diseases units in managing HCIDs, notably viral haemorrhagic fevers (VHF). The study indicated that while the majority of participants stated that they were familiar with hospital protocols about VHF and the signs and symptoms of VHF, almost two-thirds felt anxious about managing a patient with suspected/confirmed VHF. Their responses revealed concerns about risk of infection, transmitting disease to family members, dealing with uncertainty and feeling unprepared. Since the beginning of the COVID-19 pandemic, research on healthcare staff in response to the disease has been rapid and abundant, both in Australia and internationally.[37] Studies conducted on the knowledge, preparedness and experiences of Australian HCWs revealed the following concerns about working and managing patients during the 2020 COVID-19 outbreak:[38-47]

- higher workloads and working longer hours than usual
- feeling anxious and more stressed at work
- concern about exposure to COVID-19 and contracting SARS-CoV-2 from patients
- not receiving training in the use of PPE as well as scarcity of PPE
- rapidly changing and overload of information.

Preparedness is key to the management and containment of an HCID outbreak, and to prevent transmission to HCWs and to the community. As such, it is critical to strengthen healthcare systems and surveillance networks and prepare HCWs by providing them with ongoing training and education and provision of adequate PPE. Consistent and ongoing communications during rapidly evolving information is also key to helping HCWs feel prepared to care for and manage patients with HCIDs. Supporting and maintaining an adequately trained healthcare workspace, especially during surge capacity, is also essential in order to avoid psychological distress and burnout. Furthermore, a situation where an outbreak of disease that is as transmissible as COVID-19, but more deadly, remains an alarming possibility. These reasons highlight the necessity for dedicated biocontainment facilities that are capable of treating the infected, as well as reducing the risk of further spread to both the general population and to HCWs.

23.5 Designated biocontainment facilities for HCIDs

23.5.1 A brief history of biocontainment facilities

The concept of containment facilities has been evolving since the late 1960s. In 1969, the US Army's Medical Research Institute of Infectious Diseases (USAMRIID) began constructing its first biocontainment unit. The unit, colloquially referred to as 'the Slammer', was officially opened in 1971.[48,49] In addition to providing a dedicated facility for treating patients infected with dangerous pathogens, the unit was also marked to handle the remote possibility of astronauts, deployed on space missions such as Apollo 11, returning to earth with unrecognised biological agents.[49] At the same time, new viruses were being discovered where accidental exposure during research caused serious illness and fatalities. For example, the Lassa arenavirus which causes a viral haemorrhagic fever known as Lassa haemorrhagic fever (LHF) led to critical illness in its discoverer, Dr Casals, and the death of fellow staff and technicians.[48] Thereafter, the newly built biocontainment unit also offered a protective measure for scientists studying dangerous and potentially deadly diseases.

The Slammer was decommissioned in 2012 owing to its primarily observational role to a total of 21 patients (none of whom became ill or otherwise demonstrated signs of infection) over its 40-year operating period. However, the often-unpredictable re-emergence of HCIDs, like EVD, and the frequently detrimental outcomes of such outbreaks have highlighted the fact that dedicated infrastructure is still crucial. In the early 2000s, two biocontainment facilities were opened and are still in operation—one at the Emory University in Atlanta and the other at the University of Nebraska Medical Center in Omaha. The 2014 EVD outbreak, which reached the US,[50] was particularly critical in catalysing the development of biocontainment facilities for the purposes of housing infected patients. A total of 11 individuals were infected with EVD and were treated under high-level biocontainment conditions across four US hospitals, including the two aforementioned facilities. Of these 11 patients, ten made full recoveries, and only one died. In Europe, biocontainment units in Britain, France, Spain, the Netherlands, Norway, Switzerland and Italy also successfully cared for patients during the EVD outbreak. Overall, the mortality rate among patients treated under HLCC conditions was 18%, comparing favourably to historical mortality rates of 50–90% for the disease.

In addition to the containment and treatment of individuals infected with HCIDs, the extant threat of a bioterrorism event or laboratory accident with a highly infectious and pathogenic agent such as smallpox must be considered. Several biocontainment facilities have now been developed and established around the world, including in Australia. The following section provides an overview of containment facilities in the context of healthcare and in laboratory settings.

23.5.2 Features of biocontainment facilities in healthcare

It should be noted that Australia currently (in 2023) does not have national regulations for biocontainment facilities in healthcare settings. However, we can use the lessons learnt from previous outbreaks of HCIDs in countries with similar health infrastructure, such as the EVD outbreaks that affected the US and UK, to inform our own practices. These outbreaks have crucially elucidated that management of patients with HCIDs must occur within highly specialised facilities to minimise risk of transmission to HCWs. These purpose-built facilities should be designed to ensure high-level containment of the pathogens and to maximise the critical care capabilities for patient care. Table 23.6

TABLE 23.6 Features of a biocontainment facility for patient care

Feature	Description
Transportation to facility	• The decision and method of transporting an infected patient should come after expert clinical risk assessment[60] • Transport of infectious disease patients ranges from standard ambulance practice to specially constructed vehicles with inbuilt filters, isolation pods and purpose-trained teams[58,61] • Standard staff training in the correct use of PPE and infection control practices remains an effective baseline standard for transport,[60] though the level of physical protection used by patients, ambulance staff and the vehicle itself will depend on disease characteristics and patient status[62] • Facilities should have secure entry and exit points for patient transfer • Vehicles used must be thoroughly decontaminated prior to normal use[62]
Separated from regular patient areas	• Ideally, biocontainment facilities should be physically separated from other areas, whether this is by being in an entirely separate building or forming an isolated part of an existing structure
On-site diagnostic laboratory	• On-site laboratories are crucial for providing rapid point-of-care testing to monitor patient health and effectiveness of treatment. Discharging patients typically requires the return of negative serologic tests (or some equivalent) to ensure they no longer carry the infection[63,64] • Laboratories must be accredited and fully equipped to handle active disease specimens safely and securely • Appropriate biosafety and containment measures must be in place and regularly inspected, such as proper ventilation, PPE, biological safety cabinets, staff training, equipment and effluent decontamination[65]
On-site or portable specialist services	• Services such as radiology and ultrasounds, as well as treatments or therapeutic services, such as renal replacement therapy[66-69] • Protocols in place to limit the threat of exposures to specialists performing these services and that all products and equipment used are appropriately handled and decontaminated
Pharmacy services	• Can be provided remotely but with infrastructure to provide urgent medications that are delivered on time and with minimal waste[59]

Continued

TABLE 23.6 Features of a biocontainment facility for patient care—cont'd

Feature	Description
Waste handling	• Large quantities of solid and liquid waste are created during patient care[61] • Solid waste, such as PPE, linens and equipment used in biomedical procedures, must be decontaminated prior to disposal. This is typically performed using autoclaves, which should also be routinely verified to ensure proper sterilisation • Liquid waste, such as blood, bodily fluids and urine, is handled differently depending on municipal regulations and water treatment facilities.[58,70] A risk assessment will typically determine whether it is disposed of directly through the drain or requires physical or chemical sterilisation prior to disposal[60]
Critical care capabilities	• Facilities must be equipped to provide critical care, as well as to determine what procedures can be offered to patients when weighed against risk to staff, e.g. life support interventions, open incision surgery • Critical care physicians are essential members of any healthcare team when treating HCID patients and should be capable of delivering all critical care interventions when necessary
Advanced telecommunication	• Two-way communication systems should be installed and allow communication and monitoring of staff between rooms. Systems should include a camera, microphone and screen which are of high enough quality so that clarity of audio and facial recognition is achieved even under PPE • As visitors are typically not permitted to enter an HCID facility, additional telecommunication systems should also allow family members and visitors to interact with patients and staff remotely[59]
Emergency power generating system	• Either all, or select, critical systems—such as ventilation systems—should be connected to an automatic, emergency back-up power supply in case of a black-out
Ventilation and controlled airflow	• Units are typically completely sealed and airtight to prevent leakage • Ventilation systems exist to protect against the spread of airborne pathogens. Directional airflow, when air moves from less to more contaminated areas, is highly recommended (typically, inwards and away from entries and exits) • Patient rooms are typically maintained at negative air pressure relative to adjacent areas with air changed between 12 to 15 times per hour • Air is funnelled towards the ceiling where it is passed through HEPA filters that capture 99.99% of particles prior to being exhausted • Exhaust air should be completely exhausted to the outside, away from the facility or any other occupied building and must not be recirculated
Dedicated donning and doffing areas	• Each patient room has either a shared, or dedicated, anteroom for donning and doffing. Separate anterooms are favourable to promote unidirectional staff flow and reduce the risk of cross-contamination • Double, interlocking doors on either end of anterooms, separating patient rooms from 'clean' corridors • These areas should be large enough to store all necessary PPE for donning, dunk tanks to contain all disposed PPE • They also include decontamination facilities and products, such as showers, handbasins and disinfectant
Security and surveillance	• On some occasions, security may be required in patient care areas. Protocols should be in place in instances where a patient needs to be restrained to limit patient harm and personnel infection • Operational surveillance systems to monitor, regulate and record non-healthcare personnel (e.g. housekeeping, security, maintenance staff) who enter the unit
Equipment decontamination, cleaning and maintenance	• All equipment used in the facility should be selected to facilitate easy decontamination, or otherwise be replaced with disposable alternatives • All surfaces in the facility e.g. floors, walls, furniture, should be non-porous, seamless and easy to clean[49] • When a room is in use, daily cleaning is performed by medical and nursing staff. Cleaning services are employed when the room is readied to receive a new patient, or at patient discharge or death. This is to mitigate risk of harm to non-clinical staff • All permanent equipment will require regular and thorough maintenance to ensure correct function • Clear procedures must be in place to respond to different incidents e.g. spills, soiled items

Source:[57-60]

TABLE 23.7 Features of biocontainment workforce for patient care

Feature	Description
Coordination of trained multidisciplinary teams	• Active biocontainment services will involve a multidisciplinary team including, but not limited to, infectious disease specialists, emergency and critical care workers, IPC and pathology and laboratory services • The team requires a designated leader, usually a senior clinician who is responsible for team coordination, training, liaison and communication • A nursing lead is also recommended for ward management and training of nursing staff • Clear roles and delegation of responsibilities for members should be established at the beginning of team formation and staff hire[71]
Staff training and preparedness	• All staff need to be trained and prepared in the appropriate processes, procedures and systems that are unique to the biocontainment facility, notably as these may introduce new or additional precautions to their practice in standard healthcare facilities • This includes, but is not limited to, specific PPE donning and doffing protocols, hazard and waste management, patient interaction, equipment operation, reporting, expected responsibilities and work hours, and maintenance of their training over the course of their service
Staff communication	• All teams must establish clear channels for top-down communication, as well as streamlined communication strategies between staff, such as a regularly updated log of patient status that can be easily understood by takeover staff • The electronic communications systems in place must be of high quality and secure, and a dedicated process should be active for incident reporting and management • The time, frequency and purposes of team meetings are established early on, regularly maintained, documented and its information disseminated to all staff
Staff mental health and wellbeing	• Personnel are encouraged to have access to psychological and spiritual support • Some recommend a dedicated psychological team and process for determining 'fitness for duty' • Regular staff meetings should encourage and facilitate staff discussion and allow clear communication and issues to be addressed, e.g. counselling can be administered where appropriate
Pre- and post-exposure prophylaxis	• Prior to working with confirmed or suspected patients, staff should be prepared in their knowledge of the disease, modes of transmission and vaccinations[62] • Ensure post-exposure prophylactic procedures are in place in the event that an HCW becomes exposed to, or is suspected to have become exposed to, a HCID[72]
Correspondence with local public health authorities	• Local health authorities should be kept up to date on cases and fatalities • Correspondence with media is also crucial for case finding, identifying close contacts and other potential community infections, as well as informing the public
Emergency evacuation	• Evacuation plans must be in place and tested when the facility is not in use • Plans should be able to maintain patient containment and be capable for transporting patients to another fully equipped facility or a suitable temporary shelter

Source:[57-59]

contains a comprehensive overview of the structural features required in a biocontainment unit and Table 23.7 highlights the key workforce features.

23.5.3 Features of biocontainment in laboratories

The containment and safety standards for working with microorganisms and potentially dangerous agents are set out by the Joint Standards Australia/Standards New Zealand Committee CH-026, Safety in Laboratories.[7] The Standards exist separately from formal legislation and no requirements set by the Standards are enforced by law unless they are specifically included in an act or regulation in that jurisdiction. At time of writing, they have been incorporated into several formal pieces of legislation, including the Gene Technology Regulations 2001 and the Work Health and Safety Regulations 2011, and remain the defining and globally adopted benchmark for guiding microbiological safety in laboratories. The Standards describe a Physical Containment (PC) level system with four levels (PC1 to PC4) that are assigned for working with microorganisms of increasing risk factors.

Certain basic work practices are enforced across all levels, such as limiting laboratory access to authorised persons, no eating or drinking, and the appropriate use and disposal of PPE. Personnel should also actively aim to minimise the production of aerosols and the dissemination of microbiological material and fungi. Other practices include clearly identifying and dating cultures, ensuring appropriate chemical storage, using exhaust ventilation or a fume cupboard when handling hazardous substances, and regularly decontaminating communal surfaces such as workbenches, door handles, fridges, equipment and phones. The differences between each PC level are summarised in Table 23.8 and the broader relevant types of associated containment measures are illustrated in Figure 23.1.

TABLE 23.8 A non-exhaustive comparison of construction, ventilation, work practices and containment equipment standards across PC1 to PC4 laboratory facilities

	Physical Containment Level			
	PC1	PC2	PC3	PC4
External building construction				
Laboratory isolation	No	No	Yes	Yes
Separation from office spaces	No	Yes	Yes	Yes
Areas and stairs connecting laboratories classification	No	Yes	Yes	Yes
Lift classification	No	No	Yes	Yes
External access to valves and control equipment	No	No	Yes	Yes
Automatic emergency power supply	No	Rec.	Rec.	Yes
Internal facility construction				
Biological hazard signs	No	Yes	Yes	Yes
Sealable room for gaseous decontamination	No	No	Yes	Yes
Number of doors to enter/exit	1	1	2	4
Self-locking doors	No	No	Yes	Yes
Airlock	No	No	Yes	Yes
Airlock with shower	No	No	Rec.	Yes
Decontamination and waste management				
Autoclave/pressure steam steriliser	No	Yes	Yes[a]	Yes[a]
Effluent treatment	No	No	Yes/No	Yes
Pass-through dunk tanks	No	No	Rec.	Yes
Ventilation				
Negative air pressure and inward airflow	No	Rec.	Yes	Yes
HEPA-filtered air exhaust	No	No	Yes	Yes
HEPA-filtered air supply	No	No	Yes/No[b]	Yes
Zero internal air recirculation	No	No	No	Yes
Security, surveillance and alarms				
Video surveillance and monitoring	No	No	Yes	Yes
Transparent panels between areas to observe personnel	No	No	Yes	Yes[c]
Two-way communication systems	No	No	Yes	Yes
Alarm to indicate loss of negative air pressure	No	No	Yes	Yes
Alarm to indicate open doors	No	No	No	Yes
Safety equipment				
Biological safety cabinets	No	Yes (Class I, II)	Yes (Class III)	Yes (Class III)

TABLE 23.8 A non-exhaustive comparison of construction, ventilation, work practices and containment equipment standards across PC1 to PC4 laboratory facilities—cont'd

	Physical Containment Level			
	PC1	PC2	PC3	PC4
Cytotoxic drug safety cabinets	No	Yes	Yes	Yes
Centrifuges	No	Yes	Yes	Yes
Vacuum system with filters and disinfectant traps	No	No	Yes	Yes
Work practices				
Specialised personnel training in microorganism handling	No	Yes	Yes	Yes
Double sealing for transfer of active samples	No	Yes	Yes	Yes
Complete clothing change	No	No	Yes	Yes
Regulated annual inspections	No	No	Yes	Yes
Periodic blood sample testing	No	No	Yes	Yes
Immunisations	No	No	Yes	Yes
Full body shower upon exit	No	No	No	Yes
One-piece positive pressure suit	No	No	No	Yes

Source:Data from Standards Australia SNZ. AS/NZS 2243.3-2010 Safety in laboratories Part 3: Microbiological safety and containment – 6th Edition. Australia: Standards Australia; 2010.
[a] Preferably double-ended
[b] Supply air is filtered but does not necessary require HEPA filters
[c] All glass and transparent material used must be impact resistant and be able to withstand changes in pressure

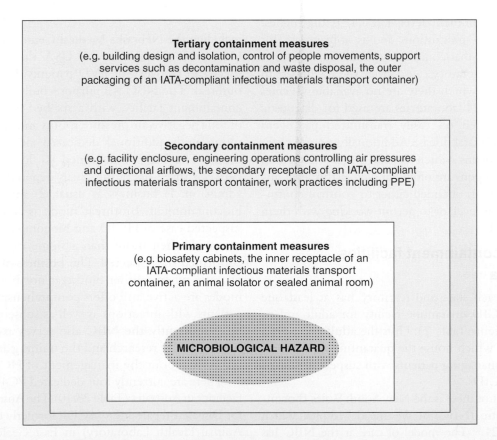

FIGURE 23.1 Primary, secondary and tertiary containment measures
Source: Image courtesy of Standards Australia and Standards New Zealand.

Physical containment level 1 (PC1) is suitable for work with microorganisms where the hazard levels are low. Here, personnel are sufficiently protected by standard laboratory practices. Organisms are classified as Risk Group 1, well-characterised agents which do not cause disease in healthy humans or, alternatively, specimens that have been inactivated and no longer require higher-level containment. Due to the relative ease and safety of maintaining a PC1 laboratory, these are the types of laboratories generally used as teaching spaces for high schools and universities.

Physical containment level 2 (PC2) is suitable for work involving agents of moderate potential hazard to personnel and the environment. This includes microbes that may cause mild disease in humans but which are difficult to contract via aerosol in a laboratory setting. Research, diagnostic laboratories and health services frequently operate at this level.

Physical containment level 3 (PC3) is appropriate for work involving microbes which can cause serious and potentially lethal disease via the inhalation of aerosols. It is commonly used for research and diagnostic work involving various microbes which can be transmitted by aerosols and/or cause severe disease.

Physical containment level 4 (PC4) is the highest level of biosafety precautions and is appropriate for work with agents that could easily be aerosol-transmitted within the laboratory, cause severe to fatal disease in humans, and for which there are no available vaccines or treatments. PC4 laboratories are used for diagnostic work and research on easily transmitted pathogens which can cause fatal disease. Additionally, poorly characterised pathogens which appear closely related to dangerous pathogens are often handled at this level until sufficient data is obtained either to confirm continued work at this level, or to permit working with them at a lower level.

23.5.4 Biocontainment facilities in Australia

In Australia, each state and territory has at least one designated HCID quarantine facility for adult and/or paediatric patients. Table 23.9 lists the adult and paediatric hospitals which house the quarantine facilities responsible for managing patients with suspected and/or confirmed HCIDs.

The newest of these is the New South Wales Biocontainment Centre (NBC) at Westmead Hospital which opened in 2021.[51] The model of care at the NBC has been modelled on international biocontainment units,

TABLE 23.9 Designated quarantine facilities for HCIDs in Australia

State/Territory	Name of HCID quarantine facility
Australian Capital Territory	1. Canberra Hospital
New South Wales	2. Westmead Hospital 3. Children's Hospital at Westmead
Northern Territory	4. Royal Darwin Hospital
Queensland	5. Royal Brisbane and Women's Hospital 6. Queensland Children's Hospital 7. Cairns Hospital
South Australia	8. Royal Adelaide Hospital 9. Women's and Children's Hospital Adelaide
Tasmania	10. Royal Hobart Hospital
Victoria	11. Royal Melbourne Hospital 12. The Royal Children's Hospital
Western Australia	13. Sir Charles Gairdner Hospital
	14. Perth Children's Hospital

including the Nebraska Medical Center and the Emory University Hospital in the USA that facilitated the successful recovery of EVD patients during the 2014 outbreak. The NBC is a purpose-built, state-wide biocontainment facility, with a six-bed base, comprising of four negative air pressure rooms and two quarantine rooms with additional dedicated airlocks and anterooms. The NBC is designed to flex up and down between three operating levels depending on patient admission: 1) business as usual, 2) biothreat, and 3) biocontainment. Biothreat mode is activated with a suspected case of HCID and biocontainment mode is activated when more than a single case of HCID is confirmed or suspected. The business-as-usual mode operates when neither biothreat nor biocontainment modes are active and offers comprehensive services to patients with infections as well as subsequent follow-up. Importantly, the NBC also serves as a state-wide site for HCID research and the training and education of HCWs about the management of HCIDs.

There are currently four dedicated PC4 containment facilities in Australia (Table 23.10). The Australian Centre for Disease Preparedness (ACDP, formerly the Australian Animal Health Laboratory) in East Geelong, Victoria, being the oldest.[52,53] It houses a purpose-built Diagnostic

TABLE 23.10 List of PC4 containment facilities in Australia

Location	Name of facility
Geelong, Victoria	1. Australian Centre for Disease Preparedness (formerly the Australian Animal Health Laboratory)
Melbourne, Victoria	2. Victorian Infectious Diseases Reference Laboratory and Doherty Institute for Infection and Immunity
Westmead, New South Wales	3. Institute of Clinical Pathology and Medical Research
Brisbane, Queensland	4. Queensland Health Forensic and Scientific Services

Emergency Response Laboratory[54] as well as a PC4 Zoonosis Suite and Bioimaging Facility.[55]

Conclusion

While the possibility of an HCID outbreak occurring in Australia remains low, increasing international travel significantly adds to the risk of an HCID being imported into the country. Interdepartmental cooperation between jurisdictions is key to an effective HCID response. As such, it is imperative for our healthcare systems and HCID quarantine facilities to continue to prepare for future large-scale infectious diseases threats by consolidating their emergency response and outbreak management plans.

Useful websites/resources

- United Kingdom Health Security Agency (UKHSA). https://www.gov.uk/guidance/high-consequence-infectious-diseases-hcid
- NSW Health Clinical Excellence Commission: https://www.cec.health.nsw.gov.au/keep-patients-safe/infection-prevention-and-control/high-consequence-infectious-diseases
- Commonwealth Scientific and Industrial Research Organisation (CSIRO). https://www.csiro.au/en/about/facilities-collections/ACDP
- Centers for Disease Control and Prevention. https://www.cdc.gov/ncezid/dhcpp/vspb/diseases.html
- European Centre for Disease Prevention and Control. https://www.ecdc.europa.eu/en/publications-data/health-emergency-preparedness-imported-cases-high-consequence-infectious-diseases

References

1. Centers for Disease Control and Prevention. Ebola virus disease distribution map: cases of ebola virus disease in Africa since 1976. United States of America: CDC, 2021 [cited 17 March 2022]. Available from: https://www.cdc.gov/vhf/ebola/history/distribution-map.html.
2. Organization WH. Ebola virus disease 2021 [updated 23 February 2021]. Available from: https://www.who.int/news-room/fact-sheets/detail/ebola-virus-disease.
3. Cieslak TJ, Herstein JJ, Kortepeter MG, Hewlett AL. A methodology for determining which diseases warrant care in a high-level containment care unit. Viruses. 2019;11(9).
4. Public Health England. High consequence infectious diseases (HCID) 2018 [updated 25 January 2023]. Available from: https://www.gov.uk/guidance/high-consequence-infectious-diseases-hcid.
5. Biosecurity Act 2015 (Commonwealth).
6. Communicable Diseases Network Australia. National Notifiable Diseases Surveillance System – current CDNA fortnightly report. Canberra: Commonwealth of Australia, 2022 [cited 08 March 2022]. Available from: https://www1.health.gov.au/internet/main/publishing.nsf/Content/cdnareport.htm.
7. Standards Australia/SNZ. AS/NZS 2243.3-2010 Safety in laboratories part 3: microbiological safety and containment - 6th Edition. Sydney: Standards Australia, 2010.
8. National Health Security Act 2007 (Commonwealth).
9. Australian Government Department of Health. Australian national notifiable diseases by disease type. Canberra: Commonwealth of Australia, 2021 [cited 08 March 2022]. Available from: https://www1.health.gov.au/internet/main/publishing.nsf/Content/cda-surveil-nndss-casedefs-distype.htm.
10. Australian Government Department of Health. Surveillance systems reported in communicable diseases intelligence, 2016. Canberra: Commonwealth of Australia, 2020 [cited 05 March 2022]. Available from: https://www1.health.gov.au/internet/main/publishing.nsf/Content/cda-surveil-surv_sys.htm.
11. Australia Government Department of Health. Review of biological agents of security concern. In: Department of Health, editor. Canberra: Commonwealth of Australia, 2016.
12. Australian Government Department of Health. The Australian health system. Canberra: Commonwealth of Australia, 2019 [cited 05 March 2022]. Available from: https://www.health.gov.au/about-us/the-australian-health-system.
13. Cousen N. "The smallpox on Ballarat": nineteenth-century public vaccination on the Victorian goldfields. The Journal of Public Record Office Victoria. 2018(16).
14. Mear C. The origin of the smallpox outbreak in Sydney in 1789. Australia: The Free Library, 2008 [cited 09 March 2022]. Available from: https://www.thefreelibrary.com/The+origin+of+the+smallpox+outbreak+in+Sydney+in+1789.-a0180278188.

15. Poulter J. The smallpox holocaust that swept Aboriginal Australia - red hot echidna spikes are burning me. Australia: Can Do Better, 2014 [cited 08 March 2022]. Available from: https://candobetter.net/node/3720.

16. Cumpston JHL. Influenza and maritime quarantine in Australia. Melbourne, Australia: Authority of the Minister for Trade and Customs, 1919.

17. Curson P, McCracken K. An Australian perspective of the 1918–1919 influenza pandemic. New South Wales Public Health Bulletin. 2006;17(8):103-7.

18. Downes C, Mitchell S. Closed borders and broken agreements: Spanish Flu in Australia. Australia: National Archives of Australia, 2021 [cited 08 March 2022]. Available from: https://www.naa.gov.au/blog/closed-borders-and-broken-agreements-spanish-flu-australia#:~:text=On%20 1%20February%2C%20Queensland%20closed,and%20 restrictions%20at%20land%20borders.

19. Paton R. Report on the influenza epidemic in New South Wales in 1919. Sydney: Department of Public Health, 1920.

20. Collignon PJ. Swine flu—lessons learnt in Australia. Med J Aust. 2010;192(7):364-365.

21. Huf B, Mclean H. Epidemics and pandemics in Victoria: historical perspectives. Melbourne: Department of Parliamentary Services, Parliament of Victoria; 2020.

22. Australian Government Department of Health. Coronavirus (COVID-19) case numbers and statistics. Canberra, Department of Health; 2022 [cited 05 March 2022]. Available from: https://www.health.gov.au/health-alerts/ covid-19/case-numbers-and-statistics.

23. Storen R, Corrigan N. COVID-19: a chronology of state and territory government announcements (up until 30 June 2020). In: Parliament of Australia, editor. Canberra: Commonwealth of Australia, 2020.

24. Team C-NIRS. COVID-19 Australia: Epidemiology Report 57: Reporting period ending 16 January 2022. Commun Dis Intell (2018). 2022;46.

25. Shaban RZ, Li C, O'Sullivan MVN, Gerrard J, Stuart RL, Teh J, et al. COVID-19 in Australia: our national response to the first cases of SARS-CoV-2 infection during the early biocontainment phase. Intern Med J. 2021;51(1):42-51.

26. Rojek AM, Dutch M, Camilleri D, Gardiner E, Smith E, Marshall C, et al. Early clinical response to a high consequence infectious disease outbreak: insights from COVID-19. Med J Aust. 2020;212(10):447-50 e1.

27. Communicable Diseases Network Australia. Coronavirus Disease 2019 (COVID-19): CDNA National Guidelines for Public Health Units. Department of Health, 24 June 2021.

28. McDonald K. Western Sydney COVID-19 patients now being remotely monitored at home. Pulse+IT. 15 April 2020.

29. General practices and hospitals delivering as 'one Western Sydney health system' during COVID-19 pandemic [press release], 14 April 2020.

30. World Health Organization. Summary of probable SARS cases with onset of illness from 1 November 2002 to 31 July 2003. Geneva: WHO, 2015.

31. Silverman A, Simor A, Loutfy MR. Toronto emergency medical services and SARS. Emerg Infect Dis. 2004;10(9):1688.

32. Grinnell M, Dixon MG, Patton M, Fitter D, Bilivogui P, Johnson C, et al. Ebola virus disease in health care workers-Guinea, 2014. Morb Mortal Wkly Rep. 2015;64(38): 1083-1087.

33. Quigley AL, Stone H, Nguyen PY, Chughtai AA, MacIntyre CR. Estimating the burden of COVID-19 on the Australian healthcare workers and health system during the first six months of the pandemic. Int J Nurs Stud. 2021;114:103811.

34. Spoorthy MS, Pratapa SK, Mahant S. Mental health problems faced by healthcare workers due to the COVID-19 pandemic–a review. Asian J Psychiatr. 2020;51:102119.

35. Vizheh M, Qorbani M, Arzaghi SM, Muhidin S, Javanmard Z, Esmaeili M. The mental health of healthcare workers in the COVID-19 pandemic: a systematic review. J Diabetes Metab Disord. 2020;19(2):1967-1978.

36. Fryk JJ, Tong S, Marshall C, Rajkhowa A, Buising K, MacIsaac C, et al. Knowledge, attitudes and practices of healthcare workers within an Australian tertiary hospital to managing high-consequence infectious diseases. Infect Dis Health. 2021;26(2):95-103.

37. Williams R, Kaufman KR. Narrative review of the COVID-19, healthcare and healthcarers thematic series. BJPsych Open. 2022;8(2).

38. Halcomb E, McInnes S, Williams A, Ashley C, James S, Fernandez R, et al. The experiences of primary healthcare nurses during the COVID-19 pandemic in Australia. J Nurs Scholarsh. 2020;52(5):553-563.

39. Li C, Sotomayor-Castillo C, Nahidi S, Kuznetsov S, Considine J, Curtis K, et al. Emergency clinicians' knowledge, preparedness and experiences of managing COVID-19 during the 2020 global pandemic in Australian healthcare settings. Australas Emerg Care. 2021.

40. Nahidi S, Sotomayor-Castillo C, Li C, Currey J, Elliott R, Shaban RZ. Australian critical care nurses' knowledge, preparedness and experiences of managing SARS-COV-2 and COVID-19 pandemic. Australian Critical Care. 2021.

41. Sotomayor-Castillo C, Nahidi S, Li C, Hespe C, Burns PL, Shaban RZ. General practitioners' knowledge, preparedness, and experiences of managing COVID-19 in Australia. Infect Dis Health. 2021;26(3):166-172.

42. Sotomayor-Castillo C, Nahidi S, Li C, Macbeth D, Russo P, Mitchell B, et al. Infection control professionals' and infectious diseases physicians' knowledge, preparedness, and experiences of managing COVID-19 in Australian healthcare settings. Infect Dis Health. 2021 Nov;26(4):249-257.

43. Shanahan MC, Akudjedu TN. Australian radiographers' and radiation therapists' experiences during the COVID-19 pandemic. J Med Radiat Sci. 2021;68(2):111-120.

44. Foley DA, Chew R, Raby E, Tong SYC, Davis JS, Australasian Society for Infectious Diseases Clinical Research N. COVID-19 in the pre-pandemic period: a survey of the time commitment and perceptions of infectious diseases physicians in Australia and New Zealand. Intern Med J. 2020;50(8):924-930.

45. Foley DA, Kirk M, Jepp C, Brophy-Williams S, Tong SYC, Davis JS, et al. COVID-19 and paediatric health services: a survey of paediatric physicians in Australia and New Zealand. J Paediatr Child Health. 2020;56(8):1219-1224.

46. Lord H, Loveday C, Moxham L, Fernandez R. Effective communication is key to intensive care nurses' willingness to provide nursing care amidst the COVID-19 pandemic. Intensive Crit Care Nurs. 2021;62:102946.

47. Dobson H, Malpas CB, Burrell AJ, Gurvich C, Chen L, Kulkarni J, et al. Burnout and psychological distress amongst Australian healthcare workers during the COVID-19 pandemic. Australas Psychiatr. 2021;29(1):26-30.

48. Kortepeter MG, Cieslak TJ. Biocontainment units: moving to the next phase of evolution. Health Secur. 2019;17(1):74-76.

49. Cieslak TJ, Kortepeter MG. A brief history of biocontainment. Curr Treat Options Infect Dis. 2016;8(4):251-258.

50. McCarthy M. Surgeon from Sierra Leone treated for Ebola in Nebraska dies. BMJ (Online). 2014;349.

51. Marie Bashir Institute. NSW Biocontainment Centre: NSW Chief Health Officer visits Westmead: The University of

Sydney, 2021 [updated 29 June 2021]. Available from: https://www.sydney.edu.au/marie-bashir-institute/news-and-events/news/2021/06/29/nsw-biocontainment-centre.html.

52. Commonwealth Scientific and Industrial Research Organisation (CSIRO). About the Australian Centre for Disease Preparedness 2021. Available from: https://www.csiro.au/en/about/facilities-collections/ACDP/About-ACDP.

53. Commonwealth Scientific and Industrial Research Organisation (CSIRO). Engineering underpinning the science 2021. Available from: https://www.csiro.au/en/about/facilities-collections/ACDP/Engineering-underpinning-the-science.

54. Commonwealth Scientific and Industrial Research Organisation (CSIRO). Diagnostic emergency response laboratory 2021. Available from: https://www.csiro.au/en/about/facilities-collections/ACDP/Diagnostic-emergency-response-laboratory.

55. Commonwealth Scientific and Industrial Research Organisation (CSIRO). PC4 Zoonosis Suite and Bioimaging Facility 2021 [Available from: https://www.csiro.au/en/about/facilities-collections/ACDP/PC4-Zoonsis-suite-and-bioimaging-facility.

56. Australian Government Department of Health. Listed Human Diseases Canberra: Commonwealth of Australia, 2020 [cited 11 March 2022]. Available from: https://www1.health.gov.au/internet/main/publishing.nsf/Content/ohp-biosec-list-diseases.htm.

57. Fusco FM, Schilling S, Puro V, Brodt HR, Follin P, Jarhall B, et al. EuroNHID checklists for the assessment of high-level isolation units and referral centres for highly infectious diseases: results from the pilot phase of a European survey. Clin Microbiol Infect. 2009;15(8):711-719.

58. Garibaldi BT, Chertow DS. High-containment pathogen preparation in the intensive care unit. Infect Dis Clin North Am. 2017;31(3):561-576.

59. Garibaldi BT, Kelen GD, Brower RG, Bova G, Ernst N, Reimers M, et al. The creation of a biocontainment unit at a tertiary care hospital. the Johns Hopkins Medicine experience. Ann Am Thorac Soc. 2016;13(5):600-608.

60. Bannister B, Puro V, Fusco FM, Heptonstall J, Ippolito G, Group EW. Framework for the design and operation of high-level isolation units: consensus of the European Network of Infectious Diseases. Lancet Infect Dis. 2009;9(1):45-56.

61. Sykes A. An international review of high level isolation units. Winston Churchill Memorial Trust, 2018.

62. Isakov A, Miles W, Gibbs S, Lowe J, Jamison A, Swansiger R. Transport and management of patients with confirmed or suspected Ebola virus disease. Annals Emerg Med. 2015;66(3):297-305.

63. Jelden KC, Gibbs SG, Smith PW, Schwedhelm MM, Iwen PC, Beam EL, et al. Nebraska Biocontainment Unit patient discharge and environmental decontamination after Ebola care. Am J Infect Control. 2015;43(3):203-205.

64. Iwen PC, Smith PW, Hewlett AL, Kratochvil CJ, Lisco SJ, Sullivan JN, et al. Safety considerations in the laboratory testing of specimens suspected or known to contain Ebola virus. Oxford, UK: Oxford University Press, 2015.

65. World Health Organization. Laboratory biosafety manual. 3rd ed. Geneva: WHO, 2004.

66. Bluemke DA, Meltzer CC. Ebola virus disease: radiology preparedness. Radiology. 2015;274(2):527-531.

67. Moreno CC, Kraft CS, Vanairsdale S, Kandiah P, Klopman MA, Ribner BS, et al. Performance of bedside diagnostic ultrasound in an Ebola isolation unit: the Emory University Hospital experience. AJR Am J Roentgenol. 2015;204(6):1157-1159.

68. Auffermann WF, Kraft CS, Vanairsdale S, Lyon GM, Tridandapani S. Radiographic imaging for patients with contagious infectious diseases: how to acquire chest radiographs of patients infected with the Ebola virus. AJR Am J Roentgenol. 2015;204(1):44-48.

69. Connor MJ, Kraft C, Mehta AK, Varkey JB, Lyon GM, Crozier I, et al. Successful delivery of RRT in Ebola virus disease. J Am Soc Nephrol. 2015;26(1):31-37.

70. Lowe JJ, Olinger PL, Gibbs SG, Rengarajan K, Beam EL, Boulter KC, et al. Environmental infection control considerations for Ebola. Am J Infect Control. 2015;43(7):747-749.

71. Smith PW, Boulter KC, Hewlett AL, Kratochvil CJ, Beam EJ, Gibbs SG, et al. Planning and response to Ebola virus disease: an integrated approach. Am J Infect Control. 2015;43(5):441-446.

72. Jacobs M, Aarons E, Bhagani S, Buchanan R, Cropley I, Hopkins S, et al. Post-exposure prophylaxis against Ebola virus disease with experimental antiviral agents: a case-series of health-care workers. Lancet Infect Dis. 2015;15(11):1300-1304.

CHAPTER 24

Construction, redevelopment and the built environment

Dr DEBOROUGH MACBETH[i]

Chapter highlights

- Key elements of the process for planning and designing health facilities
- The role of facility design in infection prevention and control
- Key resources to assist in construction and refurbishment
- The infection control resource requirements for a project

Introduction

The impact of the built environment in relation to infection prevention and control (IPC) is clearly demonstrated in the literature describing outbreaks of infection associated with pathogens such as Legionella, norovirus, *Clostridioides difficile*, *Mycobacterium tuberculosis*, carbapenemase-producing Enterobacteriaceae, and other multidrug-resistant bacteria, and the range of guidelines developed to prevent and control them.[1-8] Control of outbreaks has required changes to the physical environment and often additional cleaning and disinfection of surfaces. The choice of surfaces, fabrics and finishes during facility design is therefore an important consideration in preventing and controlling infections, especially in terms of durability and cleanability.[9]

In addition, the dynamic nature of healthcare necessitates changes to the built environment. Such changes may be related to emerging technologies and treatment modalities, emerging pathogens, or various demographic pressures amongst the Australian population such as ageing and obesity, and the healthcare services required to respond. In many instances modification of existing facilities is undertaken to accommodate these changing needs; however, on occasion, new health facilities will be constructed on greenfield sites. This chapter explores the built environment and its impact on IPC as well as the challenges associated with renovation and refurbishment of existing buildings and the construction of new buildings. It is designed to guide the infection control professional (ICP) in relation to some of the issues to be considered when planning for construction or renovation and some of the resources available to assist. Standard 3 of the National Safety and Quality Health Service Standards requires health service organisations to ensure and maintain a clean, safe and hygienic environment with reference to the maintenance, repair and upgrade of buildings.[10]

24.1 Environmental risks

The role of the environment as both a potential source of infection and a potential mode of infection transmission is well documented in multiple case reports of infection outbreaks in health facilities. Legionella has caused infection due to poorly designed or inadequately maintained air-handling systems and legionella has also been transmitted to vulnerable patients through water via showers and taps over handbasins.[11] Aspergillosis among vulnerable patients has resulted when the patients were exposed to the dust caused through demolition of existing buildings during renovation.[12] More recently, the healthcare environment has been identified as the potential source of exposure to severe acute respiratory syndrome coronavirus (SARS-CoV-2).[13]

Airborne pathogens such as measles, tuberculosis and varicella can be carried on air currents from the source of infection to other patients as well as staff and visitors.[14-17] Alternatively, the environment can be used to contain the pathogenic material and protect others if designed to do so and functioning correctly. Engineering controls can be incorporated into the design of the building to help protect patients and prevent infection.[6,18] One such example is the operating room which is constructed to include special air-handling systems to control temperature and humidity but also to ensure the constant flow of ultra-clean air over the operative site through high-efficiency particulate air (HEPA) filters.[19] Another example of the protective role of the built environment is the inclusion of negative pressure isolation rooms designed to accommodate patients with infections transmitted via the airborne route.[19] These rooms isolate the patient and have special air-handling components that draw air from the adjacent outside corridors into the room rather than allowing contaminated air from within the room out into adjacent areas where patients, staff and visitors may be exposed. Furthermore, the air is not recirculated through the facility but exhausted externally, usually above the facility where it mixes with outside air thereby rendering it innocuous. Standard single rooms with ensuite bathrooms also provide protection to others by accommodating infectious patients in isolation from other patients and visitors and allowing staff to don personal protective equipment (PPE) before entering.

In order to provide protection, the built environment must be easy to clean as well as providing the means of isolating infectious patients; otherwise, once the patient is discharged and another patient is admitted to the same room, the new patient is at risk of acquiring the previous patient's infection from the environment.[20] This is demonstrated by the increased risk of acquiring multidrug-resistant organisms (MROs) such as multi-resistant *Staphylococcus aureus* (MRSA) when the patient is accommodated in a room recently vacated by a patient known to be colonised or infected with MRSA.[21] Although the room was cleaned between the discharge of the first patient and admission of the second patient, the cleaning regimen failed to remove all contaminants. Therefore, the design of facilities including the furniture, fixtures, materials and surfaces are important components of the planning process to ensure appropriate consideration is given to how easy it is to clean the room, how the fabrics and surfaces will stand up to repeated cleaning and the use of chemicals. Other considerations include whether and to what extent regular maintenance will be required and the inclusion of required maintenance on a regular maintenance schedule so that maintenance records can provide some assurance that the work is being done.

24.2 Managing risk: the hierarchy of control

Recognising that the built environment is a potential contributor to the risk of infection transmission within health facilities, it is helpful to consider that risk and how it might be managed by applying the risk management hierarchy of controls.[22] The controls that have the highest benefit include substitution, isolation and engineering controls, and examples of all these are used to manage infection risks associated with the process of building and refurbishment as well as being incorporated into the facility design itself (Fig 24.1).

Substitution to remove risk is applied when considering fabrics and finishes. Use fluid-impervious and easily cleaned materials and scratch-resistant surfaces. Isolation of the infection risk is at work when single rooms and special isolation rooms are considered and included in the facility footprint. In addition, engineering controls such as HEPA filtered air or negative pressure air

handling are incorporated into the plan to limit the risk of contamination onto the sterile field in the operating room and to prevent contaminated air from recirculating outside isolation rooms respectively. The hoarding erected around the work area during refurbishment activities is a mechanism designed to isolate the risk by containing the dust and debris until it can be placed in closed receptacles for removal from the site. Before risks can be controlled, they must be identified and that requires a structured approach to the project.

24.3 A structured approach

All construction projects require a systematic and structured approach. A project team will be appointed, and responsibilities allocated. The ICP needs to find their place in, and define their relationship with, this team. The project commences with planning and progresses through the various phases of consultation, review, construction and commissioning. An overview of some of the considerations within each of these elements follows.

24.3.1 Planning

The first phase of planning commences well before the project team is appointed. The aim of the project will be determined, and various departments asked to submit plans describing the proposed services to be provided in the new facilities. Projected service delivery targets, population increases, new technologies and other information will be incorporated and considered as the basis for deciding the size of the project and the cost versus allocated budget before architectural plans can be prepared.

At the outset of the planning stage the ICP should consider establishing some infection control design principles to guide the decision making across the project. This is an opportunity for the ICP to try and establish a decision-making framework that the architects, engineers and designers must apply throughout the planning process. It is particularly important when the project is large and complex, and it is unlikely the ICP will be able to attend every planning and design meeting. Simple decisions such as what handbasins will be required in common settings and where they will be placed require the expertise of the ICP. The Australasian Health Facility Guidelines (AusHFG) list the different types of handbasin and their intended purpose; however, ICP input will be required. For example, according to the AusHFG, a Type A handbasin is required in procedural areas but the ICP needs to define what constitutes a procedural area for the project team.[19]

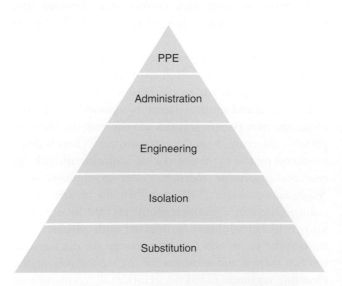

FIGURE 24.1 Hierarchy of controls

Placement of the handbasins is also important. In any project, space is at a premium, so early decisions about the placement of handbasins can help ensure they are not simply added as an afterthought and placed wherever the plan allows. If they are to support good infection control practice, they need to be placed where they are visible and accessible for staff but far enough away from patients to prevent any risk of aerosol drift from the handbasin to the patient. The widespread use of alcohol-based hand rub (ABHR) has led to a mindset that handbasins are either not required or not as many are required. However, healthcare workers (HCWs) need access to handbasins for occasions where hands are visibly soiled, where care is provided to patients with infections caused by spore-forming pathogens, and where surgical scrubbing is required—acknowledging that there is now ABHR approved for surgical hand antisepsis.

Workflow is also an important consideration when planning and designing facilities. Flow should be from clean to dirty. This is most evident in areas such as the Central Sterilising Department (CSD) where dirty instruments come into the department at one entry point and move through cleaning, drying, packaging and sterilisation and then into the clean store and out of the department at a separate point on their way back to where they will next be used (Fig 24.2). This one-way flow prevents contamination of clean areas. Workflow is also important in dirty utility rooms, food services areas, laundries and procedural areas. Designing an area to support appropriate workflow will support appropriate infection control practice.

For the ICP, planning should not just involve considerations around design principles but also how the ICP will manage the additional workload associated with the project. Some accommodation will be required if the ICP is to assist with the project and still meet the requirements of their usual role. This could potentially provide a professional development opportunity for another member of the infection control team who may be supported to take on some of the lead ICP responsibilities. The ICP may need to negotiate additional resources for the department to assist with the workload. It might mean accepting some administrative support and refining some of the usual activities to identify any administrative components that could be handed over in order to make time for the project work.

24.3.2 Consultation

The importance of consultation with all stakeholders cannot be overstated. Background consultation with key stakeholders prior to a meeting with the project team can help ensure the ICP is not blindsided by some previously unrecognised and potentially contentious issue. Taking time to work with the stakeholders and understand their needs and goals can assist in building and strengthening relationships between the ICP and other members of the team which in turn leads to support from stakeholders for the ICP. Very few ICPs will have

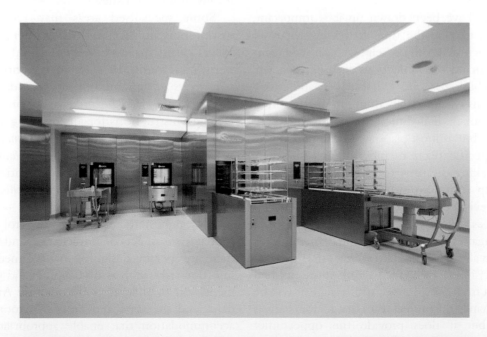

FIGURE 24.2 Clean industrial surfaces appropriate for central sterilising department

the range of experience required to understand every element of each service included in the project, so consultation that provides the ICP with a clear understanding of the nature and aim of the specific service provision allows the ICP to apply the infection control principles to the specific practice context. It also allows the ICP the time to research and prepare for project meetings. In addition, stakeholders will be more amenable and supportive of the ICP's recommendations and advice when the ICP has taken the time to understand the service needs and explain the basis of any recommendations.

Consultation with the infection control team throughout the project can also be beneficial in terms of exposing less experienced members of the team to the planning process and the basis for decision making. More experienced team members can provide additional advice to support the ICP working on the project. Furthermore, inclusion of the rest of the team provides some capacity for others to step in when necessary. It is also worth including the broader team—such as infectious diseases physicians and medical microbiologists—in these meetings. This is particularly the case where there are contentious issues because it is not uncommon for dissatisfied stakeholders or project team members to try and source advice from someone else, especially if they believe there is someone more senior or influential to whom they can appeal.

24.3.3 Review

Once the plans have been drawn up it is important, where possible, to take the time to review them all prior to construction. It can be helpful to gather a team of people that includes the infectious diseases physician, medical microbiologist and other ICPs and work through the plans systematically to ensure that nothing has been overlooked. It is difficult to ensure there are no design flaws but as most plans are developed in isolation, with specific team members reviewing their own section, taking the time to review the plans as a whole can help ensure consistency across the project and allow for review of the intersection points between different services and departments. Involvement of the broader team again serves to expose newer members to the process and allow people who weren't in the meetings where decisions were made to look at the finished product from a fresh perspective. At this stage, it will be difficult to convince the project team that major changes are required but it does provide the opportunity to identify any major design flaws before construction

begins. It also provides reassurance for the ICP to have colleagues review the plans.

24.3.4 Construction

Tempting as it is to think that once construction commences the workload will diminish, that is not the case, especially in large projects. The ICP may need to undertake site visits (wearing appropriate PPE—high-visibility vests, hard hats and steel-capped boots) to look at fit-out. This includes identifying where in each area specific items should be placed such as sharps containers, glove dispensers, paper-towel dispensers, ABHR and so forth. This process is important but also time consuming as it requires the ICP to attend the site, so the time allocated needs to include travel to and from the site.

24.3.5 Commissioning

The AusHFG Part D provides guidance on the areas for review prior to handover of the new facility.[19] Once the project nears completion, the ICP is generally required to review the areas to approve the work and ensure that it meets requirements. This is the time to identify any defects for rectification, check that all the necessary equipment and amenities have been included in the design and fit-out, and that hand hygiene and PPE dispensers have been installed and are available and accessible. Check that surfaces and spaces have been thoroughly cleaned and that surfaces and joints are free of gaps. The use of a checklist acts as a prompt for review of specific issues.[19]

Some specialised areas may require additional work for commissioning such as operating rooms and other 'clean' spaces like stem cell laboratories and sterile storerooms. In these areas, although somewhat controversial, air sampling can provide some reassurance that the HEPA filters are working effectively. Detailed instructions for air sampling are available in *Infection Control Principles for the Management of Construction, Renovation, Repairs and Maintenance within Health Care Facilities*, (second edition), produced by the Loddon Mallee Region Infection Control Resource Centre.[23,24]

Although there are infection control considerations related to all aspects of construction and refurbishment, there are specific design elements aimed at mitigating infection risks, such as air-handling and water management systems that meet the relevant Australian Standards and the type and design of rooms for patient accommodation that enable appropriate isolation of patients with infectious diseases and conditions.[19]

24.4 Infection control by design

Architects and designers want to build something distinctive, a showcase of their talents to use as an example of their skill when pitching for future contracts. They often use their previous projects as the basis for their knowledge and skill when discussing design decisions. The ICP must be prepared with as much evidence as possible to substantiate any recommendations, especially if the recommendations do not coincide with the view of other members of the project team. When faced with the claim that the issue at hand was not a problem during a previous project elsewhere, it is often prudent for the ICP to contact a colleague at the other facility to see whether Infection Prevention and Control had any input into that design element, and, whether there have been any problems associated with the design since occupation. It is not at all uncommon to learn that either the ICP had no input into the design, or raised the same objections but was overruled. Sometimes, problems that arose were not apparent until the new facility was occupied and functioning. By this time the architects have moved onto the next project and remain unaware of any problems.

The built environment can also act as either a barrier to appropriate infection control practice or a means of cueing and supporting appropriate practice.[25] To demonstrate, think about the behaviours that are considered acceptable in one environment compared with another. Behaviours considered appropriate in a sports stadium would not be tolerated in a church, temple or mosque. There are established behavioural norms and they exist in the healthcare environment as well. The relatively uncontrolled and unpredictable nature of the emergency department (ED) environment accommodates a range of behaviours and practices that would not be acceptable in the controlled environment of the operating room (OR). In the ED, HCWs must be prepared to manage any patient presenting with any problem or issue, whereas in the OR, access is regulated, managed and controlled.

The ED is designed for rapid assessment, triage, review, treatment and referral or discharge as appropriate. Multiple patients are managed in the space simultaneously with various members of the extended healthcare team having responsibility for a number of patients at any time.[26] In contrast, the OR is designed to focus the attention of all the team members on one patient at a time. Roles are clearly defined, and responsibilities allocated. Activity within the OR is orchestrated with each player allocated specific space to occupy and specific tasks to perform. The environment in each respective area supports the activities and approaches specific to that area.

While the ED may be divided into different compartments, outside of the resuscitation room, the compartments are largely communal, characterised by open bays containing trolleys, beds or chairs and usually separated only by means of a curtain. Movement of staff from patient to patient is unhindered and undifferentiated. In contrast, movement between patients in the OR is well defined with an entire OR designated for the use of one patient at a time. The team is allocated to that specific patient in the specific OR. Movement from that patient requires the HCW to pass through a door to leave the room which is itself a cue to the end of the patient encounter. Such cues can signal behaviours such as hand hygiene and PPE removal.

The infection risks associated with the OR—where surgical incisions negate the protection offered by intact skin, and invasive devices such as intravascular cannulae and endotracheal tubes bypass normal defence mechanisms—are mitigated by a range of elements in the OR environment that support infection control practice.[27] The fact that access to the OR is restricted, and those entering must pass through the change rooms and change their attire, signals a transition from the environment outside the OR and entry into a special space where different rules apply and those entering must separate themselves from the outside. Some infection control practices have been ritualised in the OR including hand hygiene, or at least the surgical scrub, and gowning and gloving of the scrub team prior to contact with the patient. There is clear delineation of the sterile field through the use of drapes, and those allowed access to the sterile field are identifiable and linked by the colour of their sterile gowns to the drapes that define the sterile field. In this way the scrub team becomes an extension of the sterile field and the patient. Thus, the role of each person, at least in relation to the sterile field, is visibly cued.

Within the OR, teams are specialised and therefore able to focus on the same surgical procedures performed over and over again. The concept of surgical conscience is an accepted principle within the OR where it is expected that all staff will monitor themselves and their colleagues for any potential breaches in asepsis and call them out for rectification, irrespective of professional boundaries that might exist elsewhere in the health facility. The built environment supports these principles through the separate space allocated for scrubbing, and the space inside the OR where gowning and gloving is undertaken and assisted and visible to all. Once the patient is draped and the procedure begins, movement around the sterile field is limited and carefully choreographed and monitored for any breach.

This is a simple illustration of how the built environment can support infection control practice by cueing appropriate behaviour. Similarly, the ICP should consider how the design of the facility could be used to cue appropriate behaviour and support desired practice. Placement of hand hygiene products and handbasins, the number of single rooms versus multi-bed bays, and the design of specific spaces to direct workflows can all be used to support infection control practice. All these issues need to be considered by the ICP during planning and used to support design decisions.

Design decisions do not rest solely with the ICP who is one of a team of people having input into the design process, each with their own priorities and goals. Negotiation and compromise will be required and therefore the ICP needs to determine what is negotiable from an infection control perspective. Compromise is likely to be required more frequently when the project is a renovation or extension of an existing facility.

24.5 New build versus renovation

A new build on a greenfield site is paradoxically both more complex and much easier than renovation of an existing site. A new build is generally a much larger project; however, design decisions are not impacted by the existing structures. A renovation, on the other hand, often occurs while health service provision continues and must align with the existing structures. Thus, the renovation is associated with two additional challenges: first, the ICP must consider mitigation strategies designed to protect vulnerable patients from infection associated with the dust and debris caused by the demolition that is inevitably associated with renovation; and the ICP must ensure that the compromises required to fit the renovation into the existing structure do not impact negatively on infection prevention and control. A simple example of the latter might be the placement of handbasins being determined by where they can be slotted into the plans rather than being installed where they support infection control practice and workflow.

The control of dust and debris is critical, especially if the renovation is taking place adjacent to vulnerable populations such as immunocompromised patients. A thorough risk assessment needs to be conducted, with mitigation strategies identified to control for each risk.

The resulting risk management plan will be detailed and include allocation of responsibilities to specific individuals with associated checklists and documentary evidence of compliance for each stage before the next phase commences. The Loddon and Mallee checklist for refurbishment is a valuable tool that can assist the ICP in developing a risk mitigation plan.[23] Case study 1 below provides a practical example of the planning and consultation required for refurbishment.

CASE STUDY 1

Renovation risk mitigation

In preparation for relocation to a new hospital, the current special care nursery was to be renovated to include two neonatal intensive care beds. The service would be operating at the new facility on a much larger scale; however, it was deemed prudent to establish a scaled down version in the current facility to help establish the service and the lines of communication and partnerships that would be essential to its success prior to the relocation.

The ICP was contacted to provide input into the plans for the new service as well as to advise how the work could be undertaken while the existing nursery continued to function.

Considerations

1. How would contractors and materials move in and out of the construction zone without travelling through the existing facility?

2. How could the air-handling system continue to function without contamination from the construction zone?

3. What strategies, if any, would be needed to ensure the contractors did not become a source of infection for the neonates in the adjacent area?

Actions

The ICP met with the project manager and construction lead. A separate area for entry and egress of personnel and materials was identified and it was agreed that this would be the only route to and from the construction zone except in the event of an emergency.

The air-handling system in the construction zone was isolated from the remainder of the system so that no dust or debris from the construction zone could enter the air-handling system supplying the nursery.

Floor-to-ceiling hoarding was constructed between the construction zone and the nursery and sealed to prevent dust or debris from the zone entering the nursery. An exhaust system was established within the construction zone to remove any airborne contaminants from the zone venting directly outside to the external environment, thereby improving the air quality in the zone and further reducing the risk of contamination of the nursery.

All the actions identified were discussed and agreed and developed into a risk management plan with responsibilities for each element assigned to individuals, including timeframes and deliverables in the form of signed checklists for each phase of the renovation.

A copy of the plan was provided to the nurse unit manager (NUM) of the nursery and the ICP met with the NUM and nursery staff to explain the mitigation strategies and answer any questions.

Once the hoarding was in place and the mitigation strategies had been implemented, the ICP inspected the area to confirm compliance prior to work commencing.

Outcome

The renovation was completed without incident. The ICP established a professional relationship with the contractor and the project lead.

In contrast, the construction of a new facility on a greenfield site does not have the constraints associated with building while continuing to offer health services on the same site, and because there are no existing buildings, there are no requirements to build into and align with existing buildings. However, the size and complexity of the project is potentially significant. Such a project will involve the employment and reassignment of multiple staff. External staff will include architects, designers, engineers and contractors. Internally, the health organisation will reassign existing staff to lead various elements of the project and act as project officers, liaising between external participants and internal stakeholders. It is often the case that the work is divided into sections or specialty groups, each with its own architect, designer and project lead. Thus, multiple planning and design meetings can be held simultaneously.

Ideally, the ICP should attend every planning meeting, at least in the beginning to establish specific infection control design rules; however, if meetings are held concurrently this is unachievable. The ICP may need to prioritise attendance at specific meetings or hold a meeting with all the project leads to establish the infection control design rules. It is prudent for the ICP to set aside time towards the end of the planning phase to review all detailed designs before they are accepted as the final version to try and ensure there are no glaringly obvious design flaws. It is worth remembering that you will live with the things you overlook for many years ahead.

A new build project can consume hours of the ICP's time and energy, and while new staff are employed and others redeployed to concentrate on the planning of the new facility, the ICP is usually expected to participate in the project within the existing resource allocation. This places significant strain on the ICP because the usual work deliverables are still expected in addition to all the meetings that are suddenly added to the schedule. While that time can be accounted, there is no measure of the multiple email requests for advice and information, or the research required to find the evidence upon which to base advice and decisions.

The competing tension between the infection control principles and aesthetics of design can make it appear that these two are in opposition; however, the provision of an aesthetically pleasing work environment can result in the occupants working to ensure it is well maintained. Furthermore, patients presenting to a facility take cues from the built environment as to the level of care they are likely to receive. For example, their confidence is likely to be negatively impacted if they encounter poorly maintained and unhygienic facilities and environments. Conversely, patients entering a clean, well-maintained, modern facility are likely to be confident that the care they receive will be cutting edge, competent and professional (Fig 24.3). The key is to find a balance between aesthetics and practicality. Arguably, any aesthetic element is likely to be lost if it cannot be cleaned and maintained easily. While almost anything can be cleaned, the more difficult it is to clean, or where cleaning requires special equipment or expertise, the less likely the cleaning will occur. An example of one of the design issues that can arise is outlined in Case study 2 below, which also serves to demonstrate some of the issues associated with the negotiation and competing agendas that can impact the decision making.

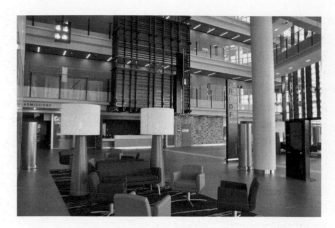

FIGURE 24.3 Well-maintained, modern health facility

CASE STUDY 2

Carpet in a new build

One of the many challenges encountered by the ICP working on the planning of a new facility was the issue of carpet as a floor covering choice in clinical areas. The architects and designers expressed a view that carpet should be the floor covering of choice in patient rooms and corridors in wards. The ICP held a different view due to the difficulty associated with cleaning carpet especially in the context of likely frequent body fluid contamination. One of the project leads convened a meeting of key stakeholders to discuss the issue and asked a carpet manufacturer to present to the group regarding the benefits of carpeting and to address the cleaning requirements.

Unfortunately, the carpet manufacturer was not asked to leave the room once the presentation was complete but allowed to stay and participate in the ensuing discussion. Arguably, this represented a conflict of interest; however, the matter was not addressed at the time. The ICP had to make arguments against the installation of carpet in clinical areas to the group with the carpet manufacturer able to comment on the points offered.

The discussion became quite tense during the meeting with a clear line of demarcation drawn between the carpet manufacturer, architects and designers on one side and the ICP on the other with the remainder of the group left to decide the outcome. The designers pointed to their last project where a new hospital was constructed, and carpet laid in the clinical areas without any objection or problem. The carpet manufacturer outlined the various properties of the carpet that could benefit patients such as reducing the harm from falls. The project lead asked for evidence that carpet posed an infection control risk and of course this was very difficult to find in terms of literature or scientific studies. It seemed the ICP would be defeated on this issue.

However, after the meeting the ICP contacted the hospital mentioned by the designers and spoke with the ICP at that facility. That ICP stated they had not been involved or consulted regarding the decision to lay carpet in clinical areas and since the hospital became operational, the difficulty arranging adequate cleaning of soiled carpet and carpet contaminated with body fluid had become obvious such that they had initiated a program of carpet replacement throughout the facilities which was going to take a long time and be very costly.

Armed with this information, the ICP raised the issue of carpet at every stakeholder meeting attended, and in the background had personal discussions with as many nurse unit managers as possible, pointing out the problems with carpet and providing real examples of the issues it would likely cause. The result was that at every stakeholder meeting many voices were raised against the use of carpet in clinical areas and the project leads realised carpet was not an acceptable option for clinical areas. It was agreed that carpet could be used in public spaces and so the concept of 'front of house versus back of house' was applied to the new facility. In other words, where patients were to be accommodated or treated would be considered back of house and carpet would only be laid in offices, whereas public areas where visitors presented would be considered front of house and carpet could be laid as appropriate. For example, although considered front of house, carpet was not laid in areas where food was prepared and consumed as it was considered inappropriate.

The critical success factors for the ICP in this case were identifying the arguments the designers had in favour of carpet and then gathering the necessary information to debunk these arguments; lobbying the nurse unit managers who had overall responsibility for the wards and patient areas and were well aware of the risks of body fluid contamination of carpet and the cleaning challenges even if carpet squares were used; and having multiple voices raised against laying carpet in clinical areas in stakeholder meetings.

Floor coverings are one of multiple considerations associated with a project. While the initial focus is on the type of services to be provided and the footprint of each service, once the initial plan is developed and agreed the project moves into more detailed design where decisions need to be made around a host of issues common to all areas of the project.

24.6 General considerations

There are a number of general considerations that apply to all building and renovation projects including the furniture and fabrics to be used in the facility, the surfaces and fixtures and storage solutions. They will need to be appropriate to the context, fit for purpose, durable and maintainable.

24.6.1 Furniture and fabrics

If the ICP is to ensure the design supports infection control principles, they must provide input into virtually every element of the design process. Consider the furniture to be purchased. Where will it be placed and who will use it? If it is likely to be used by patients, it needs to be fluid-impervious and easily cleaned. In areas where food is consumed, if used, fabric must be fluid-impervious and robust enough to cope with high use and regular cleaning. There are a range of products on the market with new products and technologies developed all the time (Fig 24.4). The ICP needs to look at as many products as possible before making any recommendations. Where possible, the ICP should obtain the details of other facilities where the fabric has been used and contact those facilities to see whether the product has performed as expected. Curtains are another issue. The options are reusable curtains that need to be removed and laundered intermittently; disposable curtains that have an expiry date and need to be removed and replaced when that is reached; or design out the curtains altogether. This can be achieved in many instances where window curtains are replaced with blinds that can be wiped over during the regular patient discharge cleaning process. Integrated venetian blinds are another option—although they are expensive, they may be warranted in specific circumstances.

24.6.2 Surfaces

Surfaces on counters, reception desks, work benches and similar areas must also be able to withstand the rigors of use and be cleanable, fluid impervious and scratch resistant. Consider also the edges of walls and the walls themselves where trolleys used to move patients, supplies and equipment may be stored or traverse. It is very common to see metal reinforcing exposed on wall edges where trolleys have struck the surface while negotiating

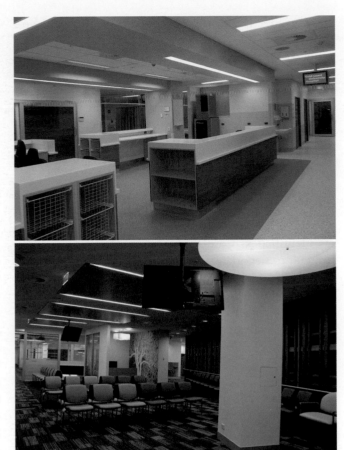

FIGURE 24.4 Furniture, fabrics and surfaces—public versus clinical spaces

a turn, or large scrapes or holes in walls where trolleys have been changed over in the trolley bay but struck the wall with high impact in the process. Consideration of additional surfacing materials to absorb the impact or protect the edges can save on maintenance in the long run. Staff are often reluctant to report maintenance issues, believing that it is not their job, being unaware how to do it, or not wanting the cost of repairs taken from their budget. Poorly maintained surfaces and fittings cannot be cleaned appropriately and may lend themselves to the accumulation of dust and debris, and/or become ideal habitats for vermin.

24.6.3 Fixtures

Other considerations are numerous but include light fittings (will they harbour dust? can they be cleaned?); ceiling tiles; headboards containing gases, suction and electrical outlets; taps, handbasins, sinks and bathrooms; and horizontal surfaces such as shelves and storage solutions.

Consider the context to determine the most appropriate choice. For example, handbasins come in a range of sizes and types.[19] Think about the way each handbasin will be used in the specific environment. Think about their location in terms of supporting appropriate workflow, and also the type of patients accommodated within that specific environment. The handbasin needs to be accessible to staff, but not close enough to patients to pose an infection risk through splashing or aerosolisation of any pathogens colonising the drain.[4]

24.6.4 Floor coverings

As identified in Case study 2, floor coverings can be difficult to negotiate. Consider the purpose of the area, what kind of service will be provided, the level of contamination to which the floors will be exposed and the frequency of such exposures. The ICP needs to negotiate their way through competing considerations such as the impact of flooring on noise levels in the area; the risk of injury associated with patient falls versus the ability to clean the flooring; and the need to be able to prevent staff injury when moving trolleys, beds and wheelchairs when transferring patients or moving stores and equipment.

24.6.5 Storage

Storage is another vexing issue. There are multiple storage requirements including sterile reusable medical devices, medications (controlled drugs, medications requiring refrigeration, antivenoms and others), equipment, sterile clinical consumables such as dressing packs and intravenous solutions.

Storage of sterile instruments must comply with the relevant Australian Standard (AS/NZS 4187:2014)[28] including HEPA filtered air, temperature and humidity controls that are monitored. It must also incorporate restricted access as well as protect the items stored from light, dust and vermin. Less prescriptive requirements are associated with the storage of clinical consumables, but complexity is again applied when it comes to the various types of medication storage. Look at the storage solutions used in your current facility and note their attributes and deficits and then think about what new storage solutions might be available and what they need to offer. One example is to consider the use of wire baskets instead of shelves for clinical consumables where appropriate, as they reduce the accumulation of dust and facilitate cleaning. However, they must be able to hold the items stored therein, so check the gauge of

the gaps in the wire when considering what the basket will store.

Consider storage of food, not only in the kitchen but also in the wards and departments where staff will need access to refrigeration to store their lunches and milk for coffee and tea. What is the plan for storage of breast milk in maternity? Where will waste be stored on the wards and where will it be stored while awaiting collection by external contractors? Where will equipment such as intravenous therapy pumps, wheelchairs, shower chairs, air mattresses, and trolleys be stored? Where will clean linen be stored and where will the soiled linen be stored while awaiting removal? Where will bins be stored? Is the storage space sufficient and is the space appropriate? Is access restricted where necessary? Does the space contain/control odour and moisture?

The range of items requiring ICP input and advice is virtually endless, and the examples provided are not designed to be detailed or exhaustive, but they do serve to demonstrate the importance of a structured approach to the project.

24.7 Patient accommodation: room classes

Until recently the design of Australian hospitals has focused on a mix of single rooms and multi-bed bays, especially in the public health system. Generally, the ICP is asked to consider the number of single rooms required for isolation purposes, and existing guidance documents outline how this might be calculated based on endemic rates of MRO infections, gastrointestinal infection and the incidence of airborne infections such as tuberculosis or varicella. The configuration of the remaining patient beds is decided based on the number of beds allocated to each ward and department grouped into double or multi-bed bays. This approach is considered cost effective because it saves space and limits the number of patient bathrooms required. Where single rooms are included, they will generally have their own ensuite bathroom or a shared bathroom between two single rooms. From an infection control perspective this generally results in the need for bed moves as patients are newly diagnosed with infections and have to be moved from shared accommodation into single room accommodation. In the meantime, the other patients in the shared space have potentially been exposed to the patient with the infection. This has been clearly demonstrated during the recent SARS-CoV-2 pandemic.[13]

Decisions about single room ratios also need to consider the type of single rooms required. There are four types or classes of single room:

1. *Class S* is a standard single room with a dedicated ensuite bathroom. This room is suitable for general isolation purposes, such as for patients with infections requiring contact transmission-based precautions (Fig 24.5).

2. *Class P* is a single room with a dedicated ensuite bathroom, but it also has special air-handling arrangements aimed at protecting the patient accommodated in the room. The air entering the room passes through a HEPA filter and is therefore cleaned of particulate matter. The air enters the room under positive pressure such that the clean air enters above the patient's bed and air leakage is directed out of the room and into the adjacent corridor. This positive pressure room is designed to accommodate patients who are severely immunocompromised and at high risk of infection, such as those undergoing haematopoietic stem cell transplantation (HSCT) where the aim is to push air from the 'clean' interior of the room towards the less clean external corridor area.

3. *Class N* is a single room with a dedicated ensuite bathroom and an anteroom. This room is the opposite of Class P rooms in that the infection risk is the patient inside the room, so the air is actively exhausted from the patient room and the direction of air movement or leakage is from outside the room into the room. This negative pressure differential increases from space to space: the anteroom is in negative pressure compared to the outside corridor, the patient room is in negative pressure compared to the anteroom, and the ensuite bathroom is in negative pressure compared to the patient room. Air inside the room is exhausted directly outside the facility and does not recirculate. The doors to the anteroom and patient room need to be closed to maintain the negative pressure. The purpose of the anteroom is to prevent air from the patient room leaking out directly into the corridor when the patient room door is opened to allow entry or egress.

In the patient room it is important to ensure there is no 'short-circuiting' of the airflow. This means that the inlet duct providing the clean air coming into the room should be in the ceiling away from the head of the patient's bed. In this way, the HCWs and others entering the room are exposed to the cleanest air. The

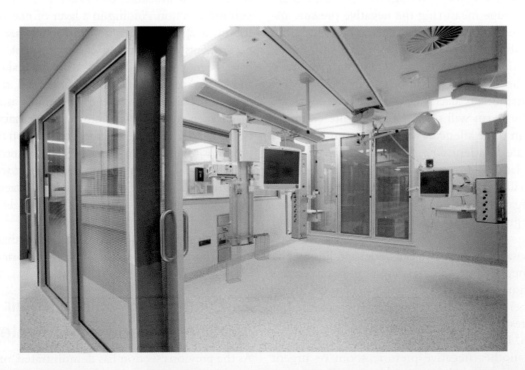

FIGURE 24.5 Patient room in ICU allowing natural light, accommodating technology and providing space

exhaust duct should be located behind the head of the patient's bed so that the clean air flows into the room and across the patient, where it becomes contaminated and is then removed from the room. If the inlet and exhaust are located in close proximity, the clean air may not circulate but instead be drawn out of the room immediately via the exhaust.

Exhaust ducts usually contain lint filters due to the fire risk associated with the accumulation of lint within the duct. Lint filters need to be changed regularly or the exhaust vent grill will become blocked and the negative pressure differential in the room will be lost. The air collected in the exhaust duct will be handled separately from the remaining air-handling system in the ward or department so that it is not recirculated into adjacent areas. Generally, the air from negative pressure isolation rooms will be exhausted separately and released on the roof of the facility, away from air intake systems and at a height designed to ensure the contaminated air is well diluted before it can be inhaled by anyone.

Negative pressure isolation rooms can, and are, often used to accommodate patients who do not require negative pressure. In this case the doors to both the anteroom and patient room are usually left open. The negative pressure functionality is lost when this occurs and it is important that HCWs in the ward/department understand that when the negative pressure functionality is required, the doors to both rooms must remain closed. The gauge measuring the negative pressure inside the patient room is located outside the anteroom and should be checked regularly—every shift when accommodating a patient requiring negative pressure—to ensure the negative pressure is functioning. Most monitors include an alarm; however, if the doors are left open the alarm will sound, so it is quite common for the alarm to be silenced when the room is used to accommodate a patient who does not require negative pressure isolation. This practice results in the risk that the alarm will remain silenced when the room is being used for negative pressure isolation, hence the importance of regularly checking the negative pressure of the room.

It is advisable to have a clear understanding of the minimum negative-pressure reading required to ensure the protection the room is designed to provide. If the reading is below that required, it may indicate the lint filter requires replacing or there is a problem with the exhaust fan. In any case, the patient may need to be moved to another negative pressure room or urgent maintenance may be required. It is also advisable to ensure the exhaust fan is connected to the essential power supply. If not, in the event of a power outage, negative pressure functionality will be lost and staff in the area will need to be aware of and mitigate the subsequent transmission risks.

In recent years there has been a move to reduce the size of the anteroom so that only ambulant patients can enter, and the bed needs to gain access to the room via an alternate route which is usually a door that opens directly into the corridor. This means that if the patient needs to leave the room on the bed for a procedure or some other reason, the air in the patient room can escape directly into the corridor while the door is open. In addition, the more doors into the room, the more door seals that must be maintained for adequate functioning of the negative pressure.

4. *Class Q* is a negative pressure isolation room as described previously. However, in this room the anteroom acts as an air lock and the doors to the anteroom and patient room cannot be opened simultaneously. This class of room is generally used to accommodate patients with highly infectious conditions such as viral haemorrhagic fevers and pneumonic plague and are usually limited for inclusion into one hospital per state or territory designated as the quarantine facility.

From an infection control perspective, the more single rooms available, the easier it is to prevent and control infection. Adding in a layer of negative pressure rooms at appropriate ratios and in a range of wards/departments would, prior to the SARS-CoV-2 pandemic, have been considered more than adequate. However, those working in infection control and related fields have come to recognise the importance and necessity of an adequate supply of single and negative pressure isolation rooms, as well as the urgent need for new approaches to air handling that will allow sections or entire wards and departments to be switched to isolated or negative pressure air handling when patient numbers overwhelm available resources during extraordinary events, such as an outbreak or pandemic.[13,29] Of course, facility planning has to consider more than infection control and there are always competing priorities.

24.8 Heating, ventilation, air conditioning and water systems

As the previous section has demonstrated, management of airflow is an important element in preventing and controlling infections along with the air temperature, humidity and purity. Engineers with expertise in heating, ventilation and air conditioning (HVAC) systems should be available to provide advice to and support the ICP when planning the facility. Considerations should include the positioning of air supply and return grilles to facilitate cleaning, and the location of air intakes in relation to cooling towers.

24.8.1 Cooling towers

Cooling towers are part of the air-handling and air-conditioning systems of healthcare facilities and are designed to cool water that becomes heated during industrial processes such as air conditioning. The heated water is pumped to the cooling towers where it cascades down a vertical surface, thereby expanding the surface area of the water and exposing the maximum amount of water to air. As a result, some of the water evaporates and the remainder is cooled and recirculated back into the air-conditioning system.

Over time the cooling tower will collect dirt and debris which tends to settle and can form sludge and biofilm. This creates an environment conducive to bacterial growth, including *Legionella* spp., which can then contaminate the water recirculated through the system or, if the water vapour is contaminated with *Legionella* spp. and allowed to drift, there is a risk that the contaminated water vapour could be drawn into the air-handling system via air intake valves if they are located near the cooling towers. Modern cooling towers and air-handling systems are designed to mitigate these risks through design elements, such as by installing high efficiency drift eliminators and ensuring air intake valves are located as far from the cooling towers as possible.

In addition to clever design, cooling towers must be cleaned and maintained regularly. This includes collecting water samples from the towers which then undergoes microbiological testing to ensure there is no *Legionella* detected and heterotrophic colony counts are within acceptable parameters in accordance with the Australian Standard.[19,30] Regular dosing of the cooling towers with biocide helps to prevent microbial growth but is only successful if the towers are cleaned and maintained because the build-up of sludge and development of biofilm can reduce the effectiveness of the biocide. Maintenance of cooling towers is conducted monthly and includes cleaning and checking the performance of the biocide dosing mechanisms. Microbiological sampling and testing acts as a quality assurance process to ensure the risk mitigation strategies are effective.

CASE STUDY 3

Recurrent Legionella detection in cooling tower samples

Recurrent positive Legionella detections in cooling tower samples need to be investigated. Two cases of recurrent positive microbiological samples results occurred at different facilities at different times and are described below.

1. Legionella was detected in recurrent water samples from cooling towers despite remediation after the first positive sample. The usual processes were implemented including additional maintenance, extra biocide dosing and maintenance of biocide pumps and monitors. All were found to be in good working order. Ongoing investigation identified the problem to be significant additional bioburden caused by construction of a stadium adjacent to the facility. The work included significant earthworks which generated large plumes of dust that drifted onto the cooling towers and contaminated the water.

2. Legionella was detected in recurrent water samples from cooling towers and, although follow-up testing demonstrated that remediation had been successful, Legionella was detected again shortly thereafter. Investigation identified that the problem was related to significant rainfall that diluted the water in the cooling towers and affected the biocide dose. Additional dosing was undertaken, and the problem resolved; however, careful monitoring of biocide levels continues whenever there is significant rainfall.

24.8.2 Water quality management

Water quality management includes filtration to remove specific chemicals such as calcium and magnesium, which is important in relation to water used in haemodialysis and water used in steam generation for instrument reprocessing. It also incorporates temperature and chemical controls to prevent the growth of pathogenic microorganisms. In this section of the chapter, water quality management will be discussed in terms of minimising the risk of an environment that supports the growth of pathogenic organisms such as *Legionella* spp.

A number of mechanisms are used to control microbial growth in water systems in health facilities, including filtration, chlorine dosing, temperature and circulation.

24.8.3 Filtration

Filtration is usually the responsibility of the water provider and is undertaken before the water reaches the health facility. Additional filtration occurs within the health facility through reverse osmosis processes which are usually limited to the water supplied for haemodialysis and to supply steam for instrument reprocessing. These are discussed in other chapters.

24.8.4 Chlorine dosing and circulation

Chlorine is commonly used to control microbial growth in water supplies. Again, this will be the responsibility of the water provider. However, as chlorine levels are influenced by time, temperature and light, health facilities have a chlorine monitoring and dosing system that monitors chlorine levels in the water as it enters the health system and adds chlorine where levels are inadequate to control microbial growth. The further the end point (e.g. tap or shower) from the entry point, the greater the risk that chlorine levels will be inadequate.

Since microbial growth control requires a consistent chlorine level, and chlorine degrades when the water is stagnant, a constant water flow is required to maintain adequate chlorine levels. Thus, when taps and showers are unused for periods of time, the chlorine levels fall and the risk of biofilm development increases. Biofilm provides an environment conducive to bacterial growth, including *Legionella* spp., and outbreaks of Legionellosis resulting in patient morbidity and mortality have been reported.[1,6,11] As a result, health facilities are required to meet jurisdictional requirements in relation to water quality management, including maintenance, monitoring and reporting. These requirements are detailed in the jurisdictional Public Health Acts and regulations as well as the national infection control guidelines.[31-33]

24.8.5 Temperature

Water temperature has an effect on microbial growth. For example, Legionella has a preferential temperature range between 37–46°C so maintaining water temperature outside this range inhibits the proliferation of Legionella. Thermostatic mixing valves (TMV) are routinely installed in health facilities to prevent patients from scalding themselves when exposed to hot water. The TMV can become a focus for microbial contamination and will need to be accessible for maintenance.

Refurbishment initiatives, especially those designed to repurpose an existing area, can lead to the removal of plumbing fixtures such as handbasins, and result in the creation of a 'dead-leg' which is a piece of plumbing pipe contained within a wall or cavity and no longer connected to an outlet such as a tap. These dead-legs provide a perfect environment for water to stagnate, biofilm to form and bacteria to multiply. Over time, particles of biofilm break away and move through the system, potentially carrying pathogenic microorganisms that may not be exposed to sufficient levels of chlorine to make them impotent. When reviewing plans for refurbishment, consider the likelihood of dead-leg formation.

Maintenance of water quality requires the development of a water quality management plan that includes detailed design plans of the water reticulation system; chlorine monitoring at the point of supply to the facility; regular water sampling plans to check chlorine levels; and microbiological sampling to ensure water management strategies are effective. Management plans may also include tap and shower flushing schedules for end points with minimal or infrequent use.

Apart from the planning and design considerations already discussed, there are many areas that will have special requirements and some of these are outlined in Table 24.1.

The areas listed in Table 24.1 are merely a representation of the variety of areas requiring special consideration, each with their own patient cohort and associated procedures and equipment. Thus, there is a need for ongoing consultation with all the various stakeholders and collaboration with the project team and the expertise they bring.

Conclusion

This chapter has demonstrated the role of the built environment in preventing and controlling healthcare-associated infection and the importance of careful and thoughtful planning and design. The hallmark of a successful project is a finished product that facilitates delivery of excellent patient-centred care in an environment that supports and promotes infection control practice and protects patients, staff and visitors from infection.

TABLE 24.1 Areas for special consideration

Area	Special considerations
Operating theatre	Air handling, workflows, sterile storage, anaesthetic requirements
Central sterilising department	Workflows, water, HEPA filters air handling, steam production, all forms of reprocessing and associated space and equipment
Pathology department	Air handling (exhaust hoods, stem cell labs), phlebotomy
Intensive care unit	Isolation facilities, space for the technology, location of water sources relative to patients, adequate space to allow for procedures at the bedside
Neonatal intensive care units	Facilities to isolate neonates and allow family members to spend time to bond. Space to allow procedures cot-side
Birth suites	Balance between the needs of the birthing woman and support person(s) and clinical needs and priorities. Consider water births and other patient expectations
Pharmacy	Clean rooms for medical and chemotherapy production
Maternity units	Privacy needs as well as space for support person(s) and families to visit. Breast milk expressing equipment and storage. Baby rooming-in with mother. Cots, baby bath
Endoscopy suites	Cleaning and reprocessing and scope storage area. Negative pressure suite(s) for bronchoscopy and recovery of suspected or confirmed tuberculosis patients
Haemodialysis units	Reverse osmosis water filtration, dialysis machine cleaning and storage, isolation facilities for patients with infections or infectious conditions, reprocessing facilities for ultrasound probes used in cannulation
Paediatrics	Co-accommodation for parents, isolation facilities for infectious diseases and conditions as well as protective accommodation for immunocompromised patients and long/frequent stay patients
Outpatients	Consider negative pressure isolation capacity in outpatients as well as adequate space in waiting rooms for patients and support person(s), reprocessing facilities or alternate arrangements for nasoendoscopes, plaster rooms and imaging for orthopaedic outpatients, facilities for wound assessment and dressings. Consider patients eating and drinking while waiting. Consider children attending outpatients with parents
Medical imaging	Reprocessing (ultrasound probes), interventional suites, different modalities
Palliative care	Consider family visiting and wanting to spend extended time with patients, the balance between comfort and clinical care
Oncology/haematology	Isolation facilities, immunocompromised patients
Food services	Workflow, ventilation, work surfaces, flooring, refrigeration, storage, hand hygiene facilities
Supply department	Storage facilities and ability to separate goods—sterile versus non-sterile—equipment, cleaning facilities, hand hygiene
Public areas	Food court, hand hygiene facilities, waiting rooms, bathrooms
Staff areas	Bathrooms, dishwashers, sinks, hand hygiene facilities, food storage
Meeting rooms	Consider flooring—will food/drink be consumed? Fabrics on chairs—comfort versus cleanability

References

1. Bartley PB, Ben Zakour NL, Stanton-Cook M, Muguli R, Prado L, Garnys V, et al. Hospital-wide eradication of a nosocomial Legionella pneumophila serogroup 1 outbreak. Clin Infect Dis. 2016;62(3):273–279.
2. Cummins M, Ready D. Role of the hospital environment in norovirus containment. J Infect Dis. 2016;213 Suppl 1: S12-14.
3. Endres BT, Dotson KM, Poblete K, McPherson J, Lancaster C, Bassères E, et al. Environmental transmission of Clostridioides difficile ribotype 027 at a long-term care facility; an outbreak investigation guided by whole genome sequencing. Infect Control Hosp Epidemiol. 2018;39(11):1322-1329.
4. Marmor A, Daveson K, Harley D, Coatsworth N, Kennedy K. Two carbapenemase-producing Enterobacteriaceae outbreaks

detected retrospectively by whole-genome sequencing at an Australian tertiary hospital. Infect Dis Health. 2020;25(1):30-33.

5. National Health and Medical Research Council. Australian Guidelines for the Prevention and Control of Infection in Healthcare 2019. Canberra: NHMRC, 2019. Available from: https://www.nhmrc.gov.au/about-us/publications/australian-guidelines-prevention-and-control-infection-healthcare-2019#block-views-block-file-attachments-content-block-1.

6. Centers for Disease Control and Prevention and Healthcare Infection Control Practices Advisory Committee. Guidelines for environmental infection control in health-care facilities (2003, updated July 2019) [internet]. Atlanta, Georgia: CDC/HICPAC; 2003. Available from: https://www.cdc.gov/infectioncontrol/pdf/guidelines/environmental-guidelines-P.pdf

7. Breathnach AS, Cubbon MD, Karunaharan RN, Pope CF, Planche TD. Multidrug-resistant Pseudomonas aeruginosa outbreaks in two hospitals: association with contaminated hospital waste-water systems. J Hosp Infect. 2012;82(1):19-24.

8. Hopman J, Meijer C, Kenters N, Coolen JPM, Ghamati MR, Mehtar S, et al. Risk assessment after a severe hospital-acquired infection associated with carbapenemase-producing Pseudomonas aeruginosa. JAMA Netw Open. 2019;2(2):e187665.

9. Xiong L, Sheng G, Fan Z-M, Yang H, Hwang F-J, Zhu B-W. Environmental design strategies to decrease the risk of nosocomial infection in medical buildings using a hybrid MCDM Model. J Healthc Eng. 2021;2021:5534607.

10. Australian Commission on Safety and Quality in Health Care. Preventing and controlling infections standard 2021 [internet]. Sydney: ACSQHC, 2021. Available from: https://www.safetyandquality.gov.au/standards/nsqhs-standards/preventing-and-controlling-infections-standard.

11. Department of Health, Victoria. Legionella risk management 2020 (updated 2 Feb 2022) [internet]. Melbourne: State Government of Victoria, 2020. Available from: https://www.health.vic.gov.au/water/legionella-risk-management

12. Suleyman G, Alangaden GJ. Nosocomial fungal infections: epidemiology, infection control, and prevention. Infect Dis Clin North Am. 2021;35(4):1027-1053.

13. Zhou J, Otter JA, Price JR, Cimpeanu C, Meno Garcia D, Kinross J, et al. Investigating severe acute respiratory syndrome coronavirus 2 (SARS-CoV-2) surface and air contamination in an acute healthcare setting during the peak of the coronavirus disease 2019 (COVID-19) pandemic in London. Clin Infect Dis. 2021;73(7):e1870-e1877.

14. Berry L, Palmer T, Wells F, Williams E, Sibal B, Timms J. Nosocomial outbreak of measles amongst a highly vaccinated population in an English hospital setting. Infect Prev Pract. 2019;1(2):100018.

15. Swaminathan N, Perloff SR, Zuckerman JM. Prevention of mycobacterium tuberculosis transmission in health care settings. Infect Dis Clin North Am. 2021;35(4):1013-1025.

16. Yang J, Liu J, Xing F, Ye H, Dai G, Liu M, et al. Nosocomial transmission of chickenpox and varicella zoster virus seroprevalence rate amongst healthcare workers in a teaching hospital in China. BMC Infect Dis. 2019;19(1):582.

17. Ye G, Lin H, Chen S, Wang S, Zeng Z, Wang W, et al. Environmental contamination of SARS-CoV-2 in healthcare premises. J Infect. 2020;81(2):e1-e5.

18. Escombe AR, Ticona E, Chávez-Pérez V, Espinoza M, Moore DAJ. Improving natural ventilation in hospital waiting and consulting rooms to reduce nosocomial

tuberculosis transmission risk in a low resource setting. BMC Infect Dis. 2019;19(1):88.

19. Australasian Health Infrastructure Alliance. Australasian health facility guidelines 2020 [internet]. Available from: https://healthfacilityguidelines.com.au/.

20. Otter JA, Yezli S, Salkeld JA, French GL. Evidence that contaminated surfaces contribute to the transmission of hospital pathogens and an overview of strategies to address contaminated surfaces in hospital settings. Am J Infect Control. 2013;41(5 Suppl):S6-11.

21. Mitchell BG, Dancer SJ, Anderson M, Dehn E. Risk of organism acquisition from prior room occupants: a systematic review and meta-analysis. J Hosp Infect. 2015;91(3):211-217.

22. Safe Work Victoria. The hierarchy of control 2022 [cited March 2022]. Available from: https://www.worksafe.vic.gov.au/hierarchy-control.

23. Department of Health, Victoria. Infection control principles for the management of contruction renovation repairs and maintenance within health care facilities 2014. [internet]. Melbourne: State Government of Victoria, 2014. Available from: https://www.health.vic.gov.au/publications/infection-control-principles-for-the-management-of-construction-renovation-repairs-and.

24. Department of Health, Western Australia. Communicable disease control directorate guideline: microbiological air sampling of operating rooms in Western Australian healthcare facilities 2021. [internet] Perth: Government of Western Australia, 2021. Available from: https://ww2.health.wa.gov.au/Articles/A_E/Communicable-disease-control-guidelines

25. Macbeth D. Silent practices: imperatives of a culture of urgency. Australian Infection Control. 2002;7(4):120-126.

26. Llanos-Torres KH, Pérez-Orozco R, Málaga G. Nosocomial infections in emergency observation units and their association with overcrowding and ventilation. Revista peruana de medicina experimental y salud publica. 2020;37(4):721-725.

27. Bao J, Li J. The effect of type of ventilation used in the operating room and surgical site infection: a meta-analysis. Infect Control Hosp Epidemiol. 2021;42(8):931-936.

28. Standards Australia. AS/NZS 4187: 2014 Reprocessing of resuable medical devices in health service organisations: Standards Australia, 2014. Available from: https://infostore.saiglobal.com/en-au/standards/as-nzs-4187-2014-111440_saig_as_as_233112/?source=predictive.

29. Cheng VC, Wong SC, Chan VW, So SY, Chen JH, Yip CC, et al. Air and environmental sampling for SARS-CoV-2 around hospitalized patients with coronavirus disease 2019 (COVID-19). Infect Control Hosp Epidemiol. 2020;41(11):1258-1265.

30. Australia S. AS/NZS 3666.4:2011 Air-handling and water systems of buildings - microbial control performance-based maintenance of air-handling systems (ducts and components): Standards Australia, 2011. Available from: https://infostore.saiglobal.com/en-au/standards/as-nzs-3666-4-2011-126857_saig_as_as_267806/.

31. Department of Health, Victoria. Legionella risk management 2022. Melbourne: State Government of Victoria, 2022. Available from: https://www.health.vic.gov.au/water/legionella-risk-management.

32. Public Health Act 2005 (Qld).

33. Queensland Health. Prescribed Legionella water tests 2017. Brisbane: Queensland Government, 2017. Available from: https://www.health.qld.gov.au/public-health/industry-environment/environment-land-water/water/risk-management/plan/implement/prescribed-legionella-water-tests.

CHAPTER 25

Blood-borne viruses

Dr MYONG GYU KIM[i]

ASSOCIATE PROFESSOR MARK W. DOUGLAS[i-ii]

Dr SUSAN MADDOCKS[i]

Chapter highlights

- Blood-borne viruses of importance in the healthcare setting
- How transmission of blood-borne viruses may occur in healthcare settings
- Preventing transmission of blood-borne viruses
- Managing exposures to blood-borne viruses in healthcare settings and the principles of post-exposure prophylaxis

i Centre for Infectious Diseases and Microbiology, Westmead Hospital, Sydney, NSW

ii Storr Liver Centre, The Westmead Institute for Medical Research, The University of Sydney and Westmead Hospital, Sydney, NSW

Introduction

Blood-borne viruses (BBVs) are pathogenic viruses which can be transmitted between individuals through direct contact with blood or other body fluids.

The BBVs of primary concern globally, including in the Australian healthcare setting, are the human immunodeficiency virus (HIV), hepatitis B virus (HBV), and hepatitis C virus (HCV)—all of which can demonstrate a chronic or persistent viraemia in infected individuals. These viruses are responsible worldwide for most occupationally acquired infections[1] and have the potential to cause significant morbidity and mortality. BBVs may also be transmitted in semen, vaginal secretions, breast milk and other body fluids contaminated with blood.

Exposure to blood and infected body fluids, with the attendant potential for transmission of BBVs, can occur in a variety of healthcare settings through percutaneous exposure from needlestick and other sharps injuries, mucous membrane exposure, or skin exposures through open wounds. The aim of infection prevention and control (IPC) guidelines is to minimise the chance of transmission of BBVs occurring in healthcare settings, considering the risk of transmission events occurring from infected patient to healthcare worker (HCW), from infected HCW to patient, between patients or between HCWs, and to provide clear guidance for the management of those infected with or exposed to BBVs.

25.1 Characteristics of blood-borne viruses

25.1.1 Hepatitis B virus

Hepatitis B virus (HBV) is an hepatotropic virus which can cause persistent, chronic infection and lead to liver cirrhosis and hepatocellular carcinoma (HCC).[2] In countries of high HBV endemicity (Western Pacific, Africa, Asia and parts of Central and Eastern Europe),[3] infection typically occurs in infancy or early childhood leading to lifelong, chronic infection in the majority, while only 5% of those infected in adulthood develop chronic infection. Chronic infection is defined serologically as the presence of hepatitis B surface antigen (HBsAg) in serum 6 months after infection. The persistence of hepatitis B 'e' antigen (HBeAg) correlates with a high level of viral replication and increased infectivity. In endemic settings, HBV is most commonly spread

from mother to child, or horizontally in the first 5 years of life,[4] but transmission also occurs via exposure to infected blood or body fluids through unprotected sex, the sharing of needles, tattooing, and the reuse of contaminated sharps. For healthcare workers, the risk of exposure to HBV occurs wherever there is direct contact with infected blood or body fluids, but occupational HBV transmission occurs mainly through percutaneous and mucosal exposure to blood.[1]

HBV is highly infectious and is efficiently transmitted through percutaneous or mucous membrane exposure to infectious fluids, with the risk of percutaneous infection estimated to be 6–30% depending on the immune status or viral load of the source.[5-7] HBV is relatively stable in the environment, remaining viable and infectious for prolonged periods on surfaces.[8]

In Australia, the burden of chronic HBV infection lies within particular populations, including migrants from high prevalence countries, men who have sex with men (MSM), people who inject drugs (PWID), and Aboriginal and/or Torres Strait Islander people.[9,10] In 2020, it was estimated that 222,566 people were living with chronic hepatitis B (CHB) in Australia, of whom 70% were born overseas, 23% were Australian-born non-Indigenous, and 7% were Aboriginal and/or Torres Strait Islander people.[9] Of those living with CHB, only 11% were estimated to be receiving antivirals in 2020.[10]

Australia has a National HBV Strategy which details targets for the diagnosis and management of those living with CHB.[9] These include childhood vaccination targets of 95%, the reduction of newly acquired infections by 50%, and, for those currently living with CHB infection, that 80% are diagnosed, 50% are receiving care, and 20% are receiving antiviral treatment.

Oral antivirals are available for the treatment of CHB and lead to improved survival, slower progression of cirrhosis, and reduced HCC incidence; however, they do not lead to cure. Inducing immunity against infection through vaccination, which is 98–100% effective,[4] remains the mainstay of infection prevention. Protection following vaccination lasts at least 20 years but is probably lifelong. In Australia, universal neonatal vaccination for hepatitis B was introduced in 2000, and those at occupational risk of HBV exposure are recommended to be screened for immunity or chronic carriage, and to receive vaccination against hepatitis B if not immune. This includes all HCWs, carers of people with developmental disabilities, police and emergency workers, armed forces personnel, people who work in correctional or detention facilities, embalmers, tattooists and body-piercers, and funeral workers.[11] Hepatitis B vaccination also prevents infection with hepatitis D virus (HDV)*. For those who are non-immune and are exposed to HBV, administration of HBV-specific immunoglobulin (HBIG) is recommended, ideally within 72 hours of exposure or 48 hours if the exposure is perinatal, followed by a full course of hepatitis B vaccination.[12]

25.1.2 Hepatitis C virus

Hepatitis C virus (HCV) is another hepatotropic virus which can cause both acute and chronic infection and may lead to cirrhosis and hepatocellular carcinoma. HCV is present across all regions of the world, with the highest burden of disease in the Eastern Mediterranean and European World Health Organization (WHO) regions, followed by South-East Asia and the Western Pacific.[4] While 30% of those infected will spontaneously clear the virus, 70% will develop chronic infection, with 15–30% of those developing cirrhosis within 20 years.[13] Most infections occur through exposure to blood from unsafe injecting practices (including nosocomial practices, acupuncture, tattooing), injecting drug use, unscreened blood transfusions, and less commonly through sexual or vertical transmission. Active HCV infection is diagnosed by the detection of HCV RNA in an infected person's blood.[14]

Preventative strategies to reduce exposure to HCV include the safe use of injections with safe handling and disposal of sharps, harm-reduction strategies for PWID, screening of blood products, and avoidance of exposure to blood during sex. The estimated risk of infection following occupational exposure is 1.8%, significantly less than for HBV.[15-18] While there is no vaccine or post-exposure prophylaxis available following exposure to HCV, effective, direct-acting antiviral therapies (DAAs) have been available in Australia since March 2016. In Australia in 2018, an estimated 143,580 people were living with chronic HCV infection, of whom 12% received specific antiviral therapy.[19] Although treatment is highly effective (94% of those treated in 2018 were cured), the National Hepatitis C Strategy target of increasing the cumulative proportion of those living with HCV who have initiated treatment with DAAs to 65% is yet to be reached.[20] Between 2016–20, 47% of those living with chronic HCV infection received antiviral treatment; however, the proportion of infected individuals receiving treatment declined by 25–35% each year in that period, with COVID-19 thought to have had particular impact on treatment uptake in 2020.[10]

25.1.3 Human immunodeficiency virus

Human immunodeficiency virus (HIV) is the cause of the acquired immunodeficiency syndrome, or AIDS. The virus targets CD4 T-cells, part of the body's immune system, reducing their numbers significantly over time and predisposing infected individuals to opportunistic infections and some cancers. In 2020, there were an estimated 37.7 million people living with HIV globally,[21] with an estimated 29,090 in Australia.[22,23] The virus is transmitted through blood and body fluids, including breast milk, semen and vaginal secretions, and can be transmitted from mother to child during pregnancy and delivery. Risk factors for acquisition of HIV include unprotected sex, sharing contaminated injecting equipment, receiving unscreened blood products or contaminated injections, and accidental body fluid splashes to mucosae or penetrating skin injuries in HCWs.

In most cases of infection people develop antibodies to the virus within 4 weeks, and HIV diagnosis is usually made through combination antigen/antibody detection and confirmed by further antibody or nucleic acid detection. While viral antigens and HIV RNA are detectable earlier than antibody and can reduce the diagnostic window to as little as 2 weeks post-exposure, a negative antibody test at 12 weeks post-exposure confirms definitive lack of infection. Although there is no available vaccine or cure for HIV infection, effective antiretroviral therapies (ART) are available and are recommended to be commenced as soon as possible following diagnosis.[24] The aim of treatment is to reduce viral replication to levels such that HIV RNA is no longer detectable in blood, as this significantly reduces mortality and morbidity from HIV infection and prevents transmission of infection to others.[25] ART may also be used as pre-exposure prophylaxis (PrEP) for individuals engaging in high-risk behaviours. Prompt initiation of ART as post-exposure prophylaxis (PEP) given within 72 hours following accidental virus exposure remains the mainstay of secondary prevention following occupational, and non-occupational, exposures.

As with other BBVs, occupational transmission of HIV may be influenced by several factors—volume of blood, procedure type and depth of percutaneous penetration—but overall HIV has the lowest risk of transmission of the three BBVs discussed, at 0.3%.[26-28]

---

*Note: HDV causes infection only in those who have active HBV infection. HDV infection can occur either as co-infection with HBV or as superinfection of someone with CHB. As HDV depends on an HBV-infected host for replication, prevention of HBV infection by immunisation will also prevent HDV infection.

Some individuals will be infected with more than one BBV and all three viruses (HBV, HCV, HIV) must be considered when assessing occupational exposures to BBVs. WHO estimates that while 1% of people living with HBV infection globally are also infected with HIV, 7.4% of those living with HIV are thought to have HBV co-infection, and 6.2% have evidence of previous or current HCV infection.[4]

25.2 Transmission of BBVs in the healthcare setting

Blood-borne pathogens can be transmitted in the healthcare setting by percutaneous injury, human bites, cuts and abrasions, or through mucocutaneous exposure to an infected patient's fluids, with the commonest source of transmission being accidental percutaneous injury from needles or other sharps.[1] Healthcare-associated procedures that are invasive, associated with high volumes of blood and urgency of care present high exposure risk. HCWs in surgery, emergency medicine, critical care, labour and delivery, and dialysis units are most prone to occupational exposure. Other occupations with exposure risk include mortuary and funeral services, hospital maintenance workers and waste disposal workers.[1]

Most occupational exposures, however, do not result in infection. The overall risk of transmission is dependent on several factors, including the type and size of the inoculum, duration of exposure, the titre of the BBV, the prevalence of active infection in the population, the immunity of the recipient, and availability and effectiveness of PEP. While reporting of needlestick injuries (NSIs) is advised in most healthcare settings, underreporting remains significant and estimates of the numbers of sharps injuries can be difficult to obtain. There are an estimated 400,000 sharp injuries per year in the hospital setting in the United States; however, underreporting is estimated to be between 18–70%.[29] Globally, sharps injuries were estimated to cause approximately 66,000 HBV, 16,000 HCV and 200–5000 HIV infections among HCWs in the year 2000; with the fractions of HBV, HCV and HIV infections in HCWs attributable to sharps injuries being 37%, 39% and 4.4% respectively.[30]

25.3 Preventing transmission of BBVs in the healthcare setting

While transmission of hepatitis in the healthcare setting was first identified as a problem in the 1940s,[31] it was the HIV epidemic in the 1980s that brought attention to the

risk of occupational infection between HCWs and patients. The first known case of needlestick-transmitted HIV[32] led to increased awareness about the risk to HCWs from sharps injuries.

Prior to this, hospital isolation practices were based on categories related to the disease present and its transmission route, and included enteric precautions (for diarrhoeal illnesses), wound and skin precautions (for ulcers, burns and skin infections), and blood precautions (for those with known chronic hepatitis B carriage) among others. The rise of nosocomial infections, multidrug-resistant organisms (MROs) and new pathogens led to the publication in 1983 of the CDC Guideline for Isolation Precautions in hospital.[33] Blood precautions were expanded to include other body fluids, and the guidelines included more disease-specific precautions, but these required having a clear diagnosis before implementation.

In 1985, due to the HIV epidemic, a major change in isolation practices occurred globally with the introduction of universal precautions (UP). These were developed out of a concern to protect HCWs from blood-borne pathogens, with a focus on preventing patient-to-HCW transmission. Acknowledging that many patients with BBVs were asymptomatic, undiagnosed and unrecognised, UP emphasised applying blood and body fluid precautions to all persons *regardless* of their presumed infection status.[34] UP emphasised the prevention of needlestick injury, the use of barrier protection with gloves and gowns, and included the use of masks and eye protection to prevent mucous membrane exposures during procedures.[35]

In 1996, isolation precautions were further updated to include a single set of precautions to be used for the care of all patients in healthcare settings, regardless of their presumed infection status. These were termed 'standard precautions' and included three additional categories based on transmission risk—contact precautions, droplet precautions and airborne precautions—to be used in addition to standard precautions as empiric or temporary measures until a diagnosis is confirmed.[36]

Standard precautions are meant to reduce the risk of transmission of blood-borne and other pathogens from both recognised and unrecognised sources and apply to blood, all body fluids and excretions (except sweat), non-intact skin and mucous membranes. Standard precautions incorporate:
- hand hygiene
- the use of personal protective equipment (PPE) guided by risk assessment and the extent of contact anticipated with body substance or pathogens
- the safe use, cleaning and maintenance of patient care equipment

- environmental controls related to cleaning and disinfection
- management of contaminated linen
- prevention of NSI (avoidance of recapping, and availability and use of sharps bins)
- the use of needle-less devices
- the use of mouthpieces/ventilation bags for resuscitation; and
- recommendations for single room use for patients unable to comply with safe self-toileting or hygiene practices.

While isolation precaution guidelines have been further updated since 1996, standard precautions—with the additional of transmission-based precautions of contact, droplet and airborne—remain the basis of our infection prevention and control (IPC) policies today.[37] (For more information about standard precautions, see Chapter 13.)

In Australia, anyone who works in a healthcare setting has a responsibility to comply with IPC principles (code of conduct) and to communicate any breaches of IPC, whether made by themselves or others.[38] All workplaces employing HCWs are also required to have a framework for mitigating BBV exposure events in the workplace, with the focus being on prevention. This includes ensuring:

- that records of hepatitis B vaccination status for staff are kept, and access to vaccination is provided if needed
- that appropriate staff education and training regarding IPC requirements and practices are provided
- that standard precautions are adhered to and promoted, facility-wide
- training in hand hygiene is provided
- there is availability of, access to and training in the proper use of PPE and that basic PPE, gloves, gowns and masks are readily available and worn whenever there is potential for contact with bodily fluids and/or contaminated equipment
- there is availability of and training in the appropriate use of needle-less devices
- there is ready access to puncture-resistant, closeable, leakproof sharps containers
- there are correct storage and disposal mechanisms for contaminated waste and other hazardous substances; and
- that additional equipment, such as face shields, is readily available where additional exposure risk is anticipated, e.g. for wound irrigation.

Accessible, standardised protocols for the management of any BBV exposure events that do occur, including immediate first aid, appropriate clinical review and follow-up, must also be available to all staff. The implementation of such measures is expected to significantly reduce the exposure of HCWs to BBVs in the occupational setting. Breaches of these guidelines can occur, however, resulting in HCW exposures, and patients may remain at risk from HCWs who themselves are infected with a BBV.

25.4 Managing BBV exposures in the healthcare setting

Any HCW who experiences an occupational exposure to blood or body fluids should receive *immediate* first aid followed by careful evaluation of the exposure and the exposure source by an appropriately trained and designated person. There should be clear documentation of the management undertaken, including any commencement of chemoprophylaxis, and follow-up arrangements. Healthcare organisations should have a clear, accessible policy outlining the procedure HCWs are to follow in the event of an exposure, including the referral pathway for immediate expert review for exposure assessment and management. This may be through an on-call roster incorporating ED staff, a staff health officer, infectious diseases or infection control officers, a local sexual health clinic, or via an appropriately serviced hotline. Further details regarding the management of an occupational exposure are outlined in Box 25.1, and Tables 25.1, 25.2 and 25.3.

25.4.1 Immediate management

First aid is site and injury-dependent—wounds, NSIs and cuts that are in contact with blood or body fluids should be washed with soap and water and appropriate care of any wounds undertaken. Alcohol-based hand rub (ABHR) may be used on skin in situations where water is not readily available. Mucous membranes should be flushed with clean water; eyes should be irrigated with clean water or sterile saline (remove contact lenses first); the mouth rinsed with water several times. Contaminated clothing should be removed, and showering allowed if needed.

25.4.2 Risk assessment

Following an exposure incident, a risk assessment regarding the likelihood of BBV transmission for the given exposure should be made. This includes a review of both the injury type and the body fluid involved.[39] Injuries may be assessed as follows.

BOX 25.1 Algorithm for management of occupational exposure to blood/body fluids

In the event of an occupational exposure with the potential for BBV transmission, local guidelines should be followed; those outlined here serve as an example only.

1. **Immediate first aid**
   a. Wash skin injuries with soap and water. ABHR can be used on skin where water is unavailable.
   b. If the injury is bleeding, allow it to bleed but do NOT squeeze to make a non-bleeding injury bleed.
   c. Exposed mucous membranes should be flushed with clean water; eyes should be irrigated with clean water or sterile saline (remove contact lenses first); the mouth rinsed with water several times. Contaminated clothing should be removed, and showering allowed if needed.

2. **Assess injury risk**
   a. Higher risk:
      i. deep percutaneous injury
      ii. injury from a sharp/needle visibly contaminated with blood
      iii. injury from a needle that has directly accessed a blood vessel (e.g. venepuncture, arterial blood gas draw)
      iv. prolonged exposure of broken skin or mucous membranes to large amount of blood
      v. parenteral exposure to laboratory specimens containing high titre of virus
   b. Lower risk:
      i. exposure is to broken skin or to mucous membrane (via splash)
      ii. injury is from an old, discarded sharp
      iii. no visible blood contaminating needle/sharp
      iv. needle not directly used to access a blood vessel (e.g. needle used for suturing, BSL measurement)
   c. No risk:
      i. exposure occurs to intact skin, or skin is not breached
      ii. injury is from a sharp/needle that has not been used on a patient prior to exposure
   → *No further action is required for no risk injuries*

3. **For higher and lower risk injuries, assess the infectious risk of the body fluid involved**
   a. Infectious (known risk of BBV transmission following occupational exposure):
      i. blood
      ii. visibly bloody body fluids
   b. Potentially infectious (risk of BBV transmission following occupational exposure is unknown):
      i. amniotic fluid
      ii. cerebrospinal fluid
      iii. human breast milk
      iv. pericardial, peritoneal, pleural, synovial fluid
      v. saliva in association with dentistry (likely to be contaminated with blood even when not visibly so)
      vi. semen
      vii. tissue fluid from burns or skin lesions
      viii. vaginal secretions
   c. Not infectious (secretions not associated with transmission of BBVs (unless visibly bloody):
      i. nasal secretions
      ii. saliva (non-dentistry associated)
      iii. sputum
      iv. stool
      v. sweat
      vi. tears

PEP is generally recommended for all higher risk injuries involving infectious or potentially infectious body fluids. PEP is most effective when administered early, preferably **within 1–2 hours of exposure**, but before 72 hours post-exposure. The commencement of PEP should not be delayed awaiting the results of serological testing of the source or exposed HCW. The need to continue with PEP can be reconsidered, however, once these results are available.

4. **Assess HCW HBV immunity**
   a. If known to be immune (HBsAb $\geq$10mIU/mL), or HBcAb positive—no need for HBV PEP, and source does not need to be tested for HBV.
   b. If immunity not known—assume non-immunity while awaiting confirmation and provide PEP if indicated by risk assessment.
   c. If HBsAb $\leq$10 and HBcAb is negative—HCW is non-immune and at risk of infection.

BOX 25.1 Algorithm for management of occupational exposure to blood/body fluids—cont'd

5. **Based on 2, 3, 4, decide whether to initiate PEP for HBV and/or HIV**
   a. HIV PEP (see Table 25.3)—2 or 3 antiretroviral drugs given for 28 days
   b. HBV PEP (see Table 25.3)—HBV immunoglobulin 400 IU IM within 72 hours of exposure + HBV vaccination course

6. **Assess BBV status of source**
   a. If unknown, with their consent, the source should be tested for:
      i. combined HIV antigen/antibody immunoassay (4th generation test)
      ii. HBsAg (if HCW is non-immune or immunity is unknown)
      iii. HCV Ab (HCV RNA testing should be considered if the source is considered at risk of hepatitis C infection as they may be antibody negative in acute infection and can remain negative for up to 12 months if immunocompromised).
   b. If source infection with a BBV is confirmed:
      i. viral load (VL—quantitative HIV RNA, HBV DNA, and/or HCV RNA PCR), should be measured
      ii. HBeAg should also be measured if the source tests positive for HBsAg.

Note 1: A source who tests positive for any BBV should be referred for appropriate specialist review if previously undiagnosed.

Note 2: Should the source test negative for BBVs but describe risk behaviours that place them at high risk of infection (within the preceding 3 months for HIV, or 6 months for HBV/HCV) the HCW should be managed as for exposure to a positive source until infection in the source can be excluded. The source should be advised to be retested at 6 and 12-weeks for HIV/HBV/HCV, and again at 24 weeks for HBV/HCV, and to seek medical review in the meantime if they develop symptoms consistent with acute HIV infection or hepatitis. Healthcare workers need not refrain from performing exposure prone procedures (EPPs) pending follow up of occupational exposure to a BBV infected source.

c. High risk of transmission[39] if source:
   i. is known to be infected with a BBV, or
   ii. is known to have a detectable viral load, or
   iii. is known to have advanced or untreated BBV infection, or
   iv. has known risk factors for infection (e.g. injecting drug use, MSM, unprotected sexual intercourse with a partner from an area of high BBV (HIV, HBV or HCV) prevalence).

→ *Counsel HCW, continue PEP and arrange follow-up testing*

d. Lower risk of transmission from source if source:
   i. is infected with a BBV but known to have a fully suppressed viral load, or
   ii. is receiving long-term antiviral therapy and is known to be adherent, or
   iii. has recent blood tests for BBVs that have been negative but source is known to have ongoing risk behaviours.

→ *Counsel HCW; may continue PEP or discontinue depending on perceived risk, and arrange follow-up testing*

e. No risk:
   i. recent bloods demonstrate no infection with BBVs and no recent risk behaviours

→ *Cease PEP in HCW; no further follow-up is required*

7. **Baseline testing of HCW**

Although not urgent, HCWs are encouraged to undergo baseline serological testing to determine if there is preexisting infection with BBVs, and it is important for workers compensation claims in the event of infection occurring following the exposure event. Testing may be done externally to work (e.g. through local medical officer). Recommended testing depends on whether HBV immune status is known or not:

a. HCW HBV immunity unknown:
   i. HBsAg, HBsAb, HBcAb
   ii. HIV Ag/Ab immunoassay
   iii. HCV antibody
b. Known to be HBV immune:
   i. HIV Ag/Ab immunoassay
   ii. HCV antibody

Sources:[39,40,45,46]

TABLE 25.1 Testing requirements post-occupational exposure

BBV	Blood tests required post-exposure	Advice during follow-up*
HIV	Combined HIV Ag/Ab test at 6 wks and 12 wks post-exposure (HIV RNA levels may be checked earlier in high-risk exposures)	Avoid donating plasma, blood, body tissue, breast milk or sperm Adopt safe sexual practices (use of condoms) Seek expert medical advice regarding pregnancy and/or breastfeeding
HBV	HBsAg at 6 wks, 12 wks, and 24 wks post-exposure Check serology at 4–8 weeks following completion of vaccination course	Avoid donating plasma, blood, tissue, breast milk, sperm Avoid pregnancy if possible No restrictions on breastfeeding, or on sexual practices provided timely PEP administered
HCV	HCV RNA at 6 wks HCV Ab at 6 wks, 12 wks, 24 wks	Avoid donating plasma, blood, body tissue, or sperm Avoid pregnancy if possible No restrictions on breastfeeding, or on sexual practices

Source: [40,45]

*Modification of work practices (including avoidance of exposure-prone procedures) is not required on the basis of an occupational HIV, HBV or HCV exposure.

TABLE 25.2 Occupational BBV transmission risks

		Risk of transmission following occupational exposure
HIV	Overall[47]	0.3% (0.2–0.5%)
	Mucous membrane[27]	0.09% (0.006–0.5%)
	Risk increase (Odds Ratio (O.R)[48]:	
	—Deep penetration	O.R 15 (6–41)
	—Sharp contaminated with visible blood	O.R 6.2 (2.2–21)
	—NSI associated with vessel puncture	O.R 4.3 (1.7–12)
HBV[49]	HBsAg positive + HBeAg positive source	Risk of clinical hepatitis 22–31%
		Risk of seroconversion 37–62%
	HBsAg positive, HBeAg negative source	Risk of clinical hepatitis 1–6%
		Risk of seroconversion 23–37%
HCV	Increased risk with increased VL in source[15–18]	Risk of seroconversion 1.8% (0–7%)

Source: [15–18,27,47,48]

- *Higher risk*—there is a deep percutaneous injury; visible blood on sharps; NSI from a needle used on source's blood vessels
- *Lower risk*—there is a superficial injury; exposure through broken skin; mucosal exposure (usually splashes to the eye or mouth); old, discarded sharps; no visible blood on sharps; needle not used on blood vessels, e.g. suturing; subcutaneous injection needles; or
- *No risk*—the skin is not breached; contact of body fluid with intact skin; needle (or other sharp object) not used on a patient before the injury.

Body fluid type is assessed for its potential infectiousness. Infectiousness can be categorised as follows.
- *Infectious fluids*—there is good evidence of BBV transmission following occupational exposure (blood and visibly bloody body fluids)
- *Potentially infectious fluids*—the risk of BBV transmission following occupational exposure is unknown (e.g. amniotic fluid, cerebrospinal fluid, human breast milk, pericardial fluid, peritoneal fluid, pleural fluid, saliva in association with dentistry—is likely to be contaminated with blood even when not visibly so—semen, synovial

TABLE 25.3 Recommendations for PEP for occupational exposure to BBV

	Exposure	Source	Recommended PEP	Potential ARV adverse effects
HIV	Sharps/NSI/mucous membrane/broken skin	VL ND	TDF/3TC or TDF/FTC for 28 days	TDF: renal failure, N/V/D/Fatigue Fanconi's Syndrome RAL: Rhabdomyolysis *Review potential for drug interactions with other medications HCW may be on. **β-HCG test to exclude pregnancy in females of child-bearing age. Seek expert advice if pregnancy confirmed.
	Sharps/NSI/mucous membrane/broken skin	Not on ARV treatment, or has detectable VL, or VL is unknown	TDF/3TC or TDF/FTC + DTG (or RAL, or RPV) for 28 days	
HBV	Percutaneous or mucous membrane exposure in a non-immune, non-infected HCW, or immunity unknown	Unknown or HBsAg positive ± HBeAg positive	HBIG 400IU IM within 72 hours of exposure + HBV Vaccination course: Dose 1: can be administered same time as HBIG but at separate site, or within 7 days of exposure Dose 2: 1 month Dose 3: 6 months	*HBIG is obtained through the local hospital blood bank
HCV	Deep, percutaneous injury with blood-contaminated needle of most risk. Transmission related to mucous membrane exposures/broken skin are rare	HCV RNA detectable	No available PEP or vaccine Effective antiviral therapy is available if infection occurs	

Source: [12,40,45]
*Recommendations for PEP may change as guidelines are updated. Please check updated local guidelines before implementing.
**TDF Tenofovir disproxil fumarate; 3TC Lamivudine; FTC Emtricitabine; DTG Dolutegravir; RAL Raltegravir; RPV Rilpivirine; HBIG HBV. immunoglobulin; VL Viral Load; VK ND Viral Load Not-Detectable

fluid, tissue fluid from burns or skin lesions, vaginal secretions); and

- *Not infectious fluids*—unless visibly bloodstained, there is no risk of BBV transmission following occupational exposure (nasal secretions, saliva—non–dentistry associated—sputum, stool, sweat, tears, urine, vomit).

25.4.3 Post-exposure prophylaxis

Following an assessment of the degree of risk of the injury and the body fluid involved in the exposure, and incorporating—if available—knowledge of the HCW's HBV immunity status, a decision may be made to commence or not commence PEP for HBV and/or for HIV. PEP for HIV and/or HBV (for non-immune HCWs) is recommended for all higher risk injuries involving infectious or potentially infectious body fluids. Should the HCW's HBV immune status

be unclear, they should be assumed to be non-immune and therefore susceptible to infection. PEP should commence immediately and should not be withheld while awaiting blood results. PEP is more effective the earlier it is administered, ideally within 1–2 hours of exposure,[40] and should be commenced within 72 hours of exposure. If the HCW is known to be immune to HBV, there is no requirement to test the source for HBV infection and HBV-specific PEP is not indicated.

The BBV status of the source should also be reviewed and their risk of being BBV-positive assessed. Currently, testing of the source for evidence of infection may only occur with their consent. No testing of the source is required if the injury or body fluid exposure is deemed to be of no risk. Should the source test positive for a previously undiagnosed BBV, they should be offered immediate referral for appropriate specialist care. Should the source test negative for BBVs but describe recent risk factors that could place them at high risk for acquiring infection, they should be advised to seek medical review if they develop symptoms of infection and should be retested for BBVs at 6 and 12 weeks, and at 24 weeks for HCV/HBV. Risk factors may include injecting drug use, MSM, or unprotected sex with a partner from an area of high BBV prevalence.★[3,41-44]

Once a risk assessment of the source is made, the HCW can be further counselled regarding the risk of transmission, and a decision made to continue PEP, or to discontinue PEP (if the source is confirmed to be of no risk, or of low risk). Baseline bloods should be collected from the HCW to determine if they were infected pre-exposure, to assess their immunity if unknown, and are important for workers compensation claims should seroconversion secondary to the exposure occur. These bloods can be collected externally to work, for example by the HCW's local doctor.

Modifications to work practices (including avoidance of exposure-prone procedures—see section 25.5 HCWs living with a BBV and Box 25.2) are not required for occupational HIV, HBV or HCV exposures. However, any HCW on PEP, or who is undergoing follow-up, should be advised to seek medical attention for any acute illness or symptoms consistent with acute HIV infection (i.e. fever, rash, myalgia, fatigue, malaise, lymphadenopathy, anorexia), or hepatitis (anorexia, vague abdominal discomfort, nausea and vomiting, fatigue and/or jaundice). Any occupational exposure that results in an HCW developing a BBV infection should be reported to the local public health unit (PHU) and the HCW referred for appropriate specialist medical follow-up.

Finally, in some exposure events, the source patient may also be exposed to the HCW's blood. In this scenario there is a potential of BBV transmission from HCW to patient, and the patient and their treating team must be informed, the incident reported, and the same assessment process outlined above applied, with testing of the HCW as the source.

In Box 25.1, a detailed exposure management algorithm, BBV-dependent transmission risks, appropriate PEP and follow-up requirements are outlined. These are further described in Tables 25.1, 25.2 and 25.3.

BOX 25.2 Exposure-prone procedures

- Cardiothoracic surgery
- Dental, maxillofacial and oral surgery
- Gynaecological surgery
- Neurosurgery
- Obstetric surgery and midwifery procedures
- Open abdominal, thoracic, urological surgical procedures
- Orthopaedic surgery
- Head and neck surgery
- Plastic surgery
- Trauma
- Endoscopic, endovascular or robotic procedures that have the potential to escalate to open procedures
- Emergency or trauma situations that have the potential to escalate to open procedures

25.5 HCWs living with a BBV

HCWs may themselves be living with a BBV infection. National guidelines for the management of HCWs living with BBVs, and in particular for those who perform exposure-prone procedures (EPPs) are available.[50] EPPs are those procedures where the HCW is at higher risk of acquiring a BBV from a patient and of transmitting a BBV to a patient due to the nature of the procedure. EPPs include those procedures where sharp instruments, needle tips, bone spicules or teeth may come into contact with an HCW's hands during procedures where the hands and fingers may not be always clearly visible.[51] (See Box 25.2.)

The national guidelines outline the monitoring and testing requirements that HCWs with BBVs, and those who perform EPPs, are expected to comply with in order to practise safely.[50] A primary principle underlying the guidelines is that all HCWs (including students) have an ethical and professional responsibility to know their BBV status.

★Areas reporting high (>1%) HIV prevalence[41] include Sub-Saharan Africa, parts of the Caribbean and Asia. Areas reporting high hepatitis C prevalence[42,43] include South and East Asia, Eastern Europe, North Africa, the Middle East and Sub-Saharan Africa. Areas reporting high hepatitis B prevalence[3,44] include most of East and Southeast Asia (except Japan), Pacific Island groups, parts of central Asia and the Middle East, the Amazon Basin and Sub-Saharan Africa.

The risk of BBV transmission from an HCW to a patient remains extremely low provided standard IPC principles are applied. The risk of transmission is considered highest for HCWs who perform EPPs. In the past any HCW with a BBV infection was prohibited from performing EPPs due to this risk. Given the effectiveness of antiviral medications now available for the treatment of HBV, HCV and HIV infections, HCWs living with a BBV are no longer excluded from performing EPPs. However, all HCWs who perform EPPs are required to know their BBV status, to get tested for BBVs every 3 years, and to undergo appropriate testing if potentially exposed to a BBV either within or outside the workplace (i.e. including following any non-occupational exposures that may occur). Confirmation of compliance with these guidelines is required when HCWs who perform EPPs apply to renew their registration annually.

Despite the best infection control practices, however, there remains a very low but real risk of transmission from a HCW with a BBV to a patient. Lookback analyses of documented cases of occupational transmission outlined in the national guidelines, suggest that the risk of transmission from HCW to patient for HBV is between 0.2–13.2%,[50] for HCV, 0.04–4.4%,[50] and for HIV, 0.0000024–0.000024%.[52] Thus, BBV-infected HCWs must not perform any EPPs unless they comply with the regular testing and management criteria outlined in the guidelines.[50] When diagnosed with a BBV infection, HCWs must immediately cease performing EPPs and seek appropriate management. They may return to practising EPPs once they have been formally cleared according to guideline-specified criteria.

HBV-infected individuals must:

- demonstrate they are under ongoing medical care
- demonstrate that their HBV DNA level is <200 IU/mL (and has been on two consecutive tests at least 3 months apart); and
- agree to be tested for HBV DNA levels 6-monthly if on treatment, or 3-monthly if not on treatment.

HCV-infected individuals must:

- demonstrate they are under ongoing medical care
- demonstrate that their HCV RNA level is not detectable following either spontaneous clearance or through antiviral treatment (confirmed 12 weeks following treatment completion)
- agree to ongoing testing with a repeat viral load at 12 months; and
- if still negative, may revert to the routine guideline requirements for EPP-performing HCWs (testing

3-yearly, or after any exposure risk) but using HCV RNA detection for testing as HCV antibody will remain positive in these individuals.

HIV-infected individuals must:

- demonstrate they are under ongoing medical care
- demonstrate that they are on effective ART or are elite controllers (an HIV-infected person who is not on ART but maintains an HIV viral load that is non-detectable for at least 12 months confirmed by three separate viral load tests)
- demonstrate that their HIV RNA level is <200 copies/mL on at least 2 consecutive tests taken a minimum 3 months apart; and
- agree to be tested for HIV RNA levels 3-monthly.

All viral load testing must be performed through a National Association of Testing Authorities (NATA)/ Royal College of Pathologists of Australasia (RCPA)-accredited laboratory. HCWs with a BBV who practise EPPs are expected to be compliant with treatment, have regular viral load testing as indicated, and to seek review if their condition changes in any way that may affect their fitness to practice.

As HCWs may be infected unknowingly and be asymptomatic, all HCWs are advised to undergo regular testing to monitor their BBV status because early diagnosis enables early initiation of appropriate treatment; allows for appropriate changes in work practices to be made where necessary; reduces disease progression and transmission risk; and improves health outcomes.

It is vital that HCW confidentiality be maintained and employers of HCWs living with BBV infection must consider the rights of the HCW in the context of privacy, equal employment opportunity, anti-discrimination and industrial relations legislation when implementing their duty of care to patients and to staff. The healthcare system is expected to support a HCW living with a BBV by providing appropriate retraining or supervision, counselling and a work environment that will reduce any risk of cross-infection or acquisition of other BBVs. The healthcare facility is also expected to provide an environment in which a HCW living with a BBV knows their privacy and confidentiality will be respected and maintained.[50]

Failure of a HCW to comply with testing requirements and measures outlined in the guidelines, however, is expected to be reported to AHPRA and/or the relevant jurisdictional health department in order to protect the public. To support decision making around the practice of EPPs by HCWs living with a BBV, and particularly for complex situations regarding testing or treatment compliance, or ongoing risk factors, jurisdictional expert advisory committees, public health authorities, and the National Expert Reference Panel (NERP) are available to provide advice and guidance. The roles and responsibilities of these bodies are outlined in the national guidelines.[50]

25.6 Other viruses with the potential for blood-borne transmission

Human T-cell leukaemia virus-1 (HTLV-1) is a distant relative of HIV and is endemic in many countries, predominantly Japan, the Caribbean and central Africa. In Australia, the virus is present particularly in Central Australia, with an estimated prevalence in the Indigenous population there of up to 14%.[53]

Two diseases have been specifically associated with HTLV-1 infection: adult T-cell leukaemia/lymphoma and HTLV-associated myelopathy/tropical spastic paraparesis.[54] While only a small proportion of HLTV-1 carriers will develop disease, there is no treatment available for chronic HTLV-1 infection. There is also evidence of other HTLV-associated complications in the Australian Indigenous population, including elevated risk of bacterial infection, bronchiectasis, crusted scabies and Strongyloides hyperinfection. There has been no documented case of HTLV-1 transmission from an NSI in the healthcare setting anywhere in the world. Nevertheless, given the higher prevalence of HTLV-1 in the Northern Territory, HTLV-1 antibodies are tested at baseline following nosocomial exposure occurrence. There have been no studies to date of antiviral therapy used as post-exposure prophylaxis to prevent HTLV-1 transmission.

25.7 Screening of blood donors for BBVs

The Australian Red Cross Lifeblood organisation implements mandatory testing of donors of fresh blood components for the following viral infections—HBV, HCV, HIV and HTLV-1. Donations used for plasmapheresis are tested for HIV, HCV and HBV only. In the decade 2010–19, from more than 11 million total donations, 1803 tested positive for at least one of these viruses.[55]

To assess the risk of donors having other viral infections or exposures, donors are required to complete a comprehensive questionnaire prior to each donation following which their risk of having a transfusion-transmissible infection and their eligibility to donate is reviewed. This includes questions regarding travel. Lifeblood maintains a close liaison with the Australian Government communicable disease control teams and reviews potential emerging infections both within Australia and overseas that may present a threat to the safety of the blood donations. For example, the risks of transmission of Zika virus from donors returning from endemic areas or from close contacts of hepatitis A virus infections are managed by deferring donation for an appropriate period.[55] Other viruses that may be transmitted through blood transfusions, albeit very rarely and are thus managed through deferral of donation, include dengue virus, hepatitis E virus and West Nile virus. From March 2020, in response to the COVID-19 pandemic, Lifeblood deferred all donations from donors returning from overseas for 28 days from their return. This regulation, coupled with existing geographical deferrals, further mitigated any potential risks from overseas outbreaks to blood product safety in Australia.

Conclusion

Blood-borne virus transmission risk remains an important concern in the healthcare setting. HIV, HBV and HCV in particular can lead to chronic viraemia and can cause significant morbidity and mortality in infected individuals. Occupational exposures typically involve direct contact with blood or infected body fluids through percutaneous exposure from needlestick and other sharp injuries or mucous membrane exposures. The primary objective of the IPC guidelines is to minimise BBV transmission risk in the healthcare setting for both patients and HCWs, and to facilitate management of those living with, or exposed to, BBVs.

Useful websites/references

- Australian Government Department of Health and Aged Care. Australian national guidelines for the management of healthcare workers living with, or exposed to, blood-borne viruses. www.health.gov.au/resources/publications/australian-national-guidelines-for-the-management-of-healthcare-workers-living-with-or-exposed-to-blood-borne-viruses?language=en.

- Australasian Society of HIV Medicine. Post-exposure prophylaxis after non-occupational and occupational exposure to HIV 2016. www.pep.guidelines.org.au.
- NHMRC/ACSQHC. Australian guidelines for the prevention and control of infection in healthcare (2019). www.nhmrc.gov.au/about-us/publications/australian-guidelines-prevention-and-control-infection-healthcare-2019.

References

1. Denault D, Gardner H. OSHA Blood-borne pathogen standards. Treasure Island FL: StatPearls Publishing, 2021. Available from: https://www.ncbi.nlm.nih.gov/books/NBK570561/.
2. Maynard JE, Kare MA, Alter M. Viral hepatitis and liver disease. Zuckerman AJ, ed. New York: Alan R Liss Inc., 1988.
3. Schweitzer A, Horn J, Mikolajczyk RT, Krause G, Ott JJ. Estimations of worldwide prevalence of chronic hepatitis B virus infection: a systematic review of data published between 1965 and 2013. Lancet. 2015;386(10003):1546-1555.
4. World Health Organization. Global hepatitis report 2017. Geneva: WHO, 2017.
5. Grady GF, Lee VA, Prince AM, Gitnick GL, Fawaz KA, Vyas GN, et al. Hepatitis B immune globulin for accidental exposures among medical personnel: final report of a multicenter controlled trial. J Infect Dis. 1978;138(5):625-638.
6. Werner BG, Grady GF. Accidental hepatitis-B-surface-antigen-positive inoculations. Use of e antigen to estimate infectivity. Ann Intern Med. 1982;97(3):367-369.
7. Seeff LB, Wright EC, Zimmerman HJ, Alter HJ, Dietz AA, Felsher BF, et al. Type B hepatitis after needle-stick exposure: prevention with hepatitis B immune globulin. Final report of the veterans administration cooperative study. Ann Intern Med. 1978;88(3):285-293.
8. Bond WW, Favero MS, Petersen NJ, Gravelle CR, Ebert JW, Maynard JE. Survival of hepatitis B virus after drying and storage for one week. Lancet. 1981;1(8219):550-551.
9. The Kirby Institute. Tracking the progress 2020: national hepatitis B strategy. Sydney: UNSW, 2020.
10. MacLachlan J, Stewart S, Cowie B. Viral hepatitis mapping project: national report 2020. Darlinghurst, NSW: Australasian Society for HIV, Viral Hepatitis, and Sexual Health Medicine (ASHM), 2020.
11. Australian Technical Advisory Group on Immunisation (ATAGI). Vaccination for people at occupational risk. Canberra: Australian Government, 2018. Available from: https://immunisationhandbook.health.gov.au/vaccination-for-special-risk-groups/vaccination-for-people-at-occupational-risk.
12. Australian Technical Advisory Group on Immunisation (ATAGI). Hepatitis B. 2018. In: The Australian Immunisation Handbook [Internet]. Canberra: Australian Government, 2018. Available from: https://immunisationhandbook.health.gov.au/vaccine-preventable-diseases/hepatitis-b.
13. Seeff LB. The history of the "natural history" of hepatitis C (1968-2009). Liver Int. 2009;29 Suppl 1(0 1):89-99.
14. Schillie S, Wester C, Osborne M, Wesolowski L, Ryerson AB. CDC Recommendations for hepatitis C screening among adults - United States, 2020. MMWR Recomm Rep. 2020; 69(2):1-17.
15. Mitsui T, Iwano K, Masuko K, Yamazaki C, Okamoto H, Tsuda F, et al. Hepatitis C virus infection in medical personnel after needlestick accident. Hepatology. 1992;16(5):1109-1114.
16. Lanphear BP, Linnemann CC, Jr., Cannon CG, DeRonde MM, Pendy L, Kerley LM. Hepatitis C virus infection in healthcare workers: risk of exposure and infection. Infect Control Hosp Epidemiol. 1994;15(12):745-750.
17. Puro V, Petrosillo N, Ippolito G. Risk of hepatitis C seroconversion after occupational exposures in health care workers. Italian study group on occupational risk of HIV and other blood-borne infections. Am J Infect Control. 1995;23(5):273-277.
18. Alter MJ. Epidemiology of hepatitis C. Hepatology. 1997; 26(3 Suppl 1):62s-65s.
19. The Kirby Institute. National update on HIV, viral hepatitis and sexually transmissible infections in Australia: 2009–2018. Sydney: UNSW, 2020.
20. The Kirby Institute. Tracking the progress 2020: national hepatitis C strategy. Sydney: UNSW, 2020.
21. World Health Organization. HIV-AIDS Factsheet. Geneva: WHO, 2022. Available from: www.who.int/news-room/fact-sheets/detail/hiv-aids.
22. The Kirby Institute. Tracking the progress 2019: national HIV strategy. Sydney: UNSW, 2019.
23. Grulich A, Bavinton B, Stoové M, Wright E, Treloar C. Agenda 2025: ending HIV transmission in Australia. Technical paper on science, trends and targets. Sydney: Australian Federation of AIDS Organisations, 2021.
24. National Institutes of Health. Guidelines for the use of antiretroviral agents in adults and adolescents with HIV. US Department of Health and Human Services, 2021.
25. Australasian Society for HIV, Viral Hepatitis and Sexual Health Medicine. U=U: ASHM guidance for healthcare professionals [Internet]. ASHM, 2020. Available from www.ashm.org.au/resources/uu-ashm-guidance-for-healthcare-professionals.
26. Henderson DK, Fahey BJ, Willy M, Schmitt JM, Carey K, Koziol DE, et al. Risk for occupational transmission of human immunodeficiency virus type 1 (HIV-1) associated with clinical exposures. A prospective evaluation. Ann Intern Med. 1990;113(10):740-746.
27. Ippolito G, Puro V, De Carli G. The risk of occupational human immunodeficiency virus infection in health care workers. Italian multicenter study. The Italian study group on occupational risk of HIV infection. Arch Intern Med. 1993;153(12):1451-1458.
28. Gerberding JL. Incidence and prevalence of human immunodeficiency virus, hepatitis B virus, hepatitis C virus, and cytomegalovirus among health care personnel at risk for blood exposure: final report from a longitudinal study. J Infect Dis. 1994;170(6):1410-1417.
29. Rapiti E, Prüss-Üstün A, Hutin Y. Sharps injuries: assessing the burden of disease from sharps injuries to health-care workers at national and local levels. Environmental burden of disease series No. 11. Geneva: WHO, 2005.
30. Prüss-Üstün A, Rapiti E, Hutin Y. Estimation of the global burden of disease attributable to contaminated sharps injuries

among health-care workers. Am J Ind Med. 2005;48(6): 482-490.

31. Murphy HM. The transmission of infectious hepatitis by blood transfusion. Gastroenterology. 1945;5:449-456.

32. Needlestick transmission of HTLV-III from a patient infected in Africa. Lancet. 1984;2(8416):1376-1377.

33. Garner JS, Simmons BP. Guideline for isolation precautions in hospitals. Infect Control. 1983;4(4 Suppl):245-325.

34. Recommendations for preventing transmission of infection with human T-lymphotropic virus type III/lymphadenopathy-associated virus in the workplace. MMWR Morb Mortal Wkly Rep. 1985;34(45):681-686, 691-695.

35. Update: universal precautions for prevention of transmission of human immunodeficiency virus, hepatitis B virus, and other blood-borne pathogens in health-care settings. MMWR Morb Mortal Wkly Rep. 1988;37(24):377-382, 387-388.

36. Garner JS. Guideline for isolation precautions in hospitals. Part I. Evolution of isolation practices, Hospital Infection Control Practices Advisory Committee. Am J Infect Control. 1996;24(1):24-31.

37. Clinical Excellence Commission. Infection prevention and control practice handbook. Sydney: CEC, 2020.

38. National Health and Medical Research Council. Australian guidelines for the prevention and control of infection in healthcare (2019). Canberra: Australian Government, 2019.

39. Riddell A, Kennedy I, Tong CY. Management of sharps injuries in the healthcare setting. BMJ. 2015;351:h3733.

40. Health Protection NSW. HIV, hepatitis B and hepatitis C – management of health care workers potentially exposed. Sydney: NSW Health, 2017.

41. UNAIDS. AIDSInfo, Global data on HIV epidemiology and response. Geneva: WHO, 2022. Available from: https://aidsinfo.unaids.org/.

42. Messina JP, Humphreys I, Flaxman A, Brown A, Cooke GS, Pybus OG, et al. Global distribution and prevalence of hepatitis C virus genotypes. Hepatology. 2015;61(1):77-87.

43. Centers for Disease Control and Prevention. CDC yellow book 2020: health information for international travel. New York: Oxford University Press, 2020. Available from: https://wwwnc.cdc.gov/travel/yellowbook/2020/travel-related-infectious-diseases/hepatitis-c#5521.

44. Centers for Disease Control and Prevention. CDC yellow book 2020: health information for international travel. Chapter 4 Travel-related infectious diseases: Hepatitis B. [cited 21 April 2022]. New York: Oxford University Press, 2020. Available from: https://wwwnc.cdc.gov/travel/yellowbook/2020/travel-related-infectious-diseases/hepatitis-b.

45. Australasian Society of HIV Medicine. Post-exposure prophylaxis after non-occupational and occupational exposure to HIV. Australian national guidelines. 2nd ed. ASHM, 2016. Available from: https://www.ashm.org.au/hiv/hiv-management/pep/.

46. Victorian Government, Department of Health. Managing exposures to blood and body fluids or substances. Melbourne: State Government of Victoria, 2015. Available from: https://www.health.vic.gov.au/infectious-diseases/managing-exposures-to-blood-and-body-fluids-or-substances.

47. Bell DM. Occupational risk of human immunodeficiency virus infection in healthcare workers: an overview. Am J Med. 1997;102(5b):9-15.

48. Cardo DM, Culver DH, Ciesielski CA, Srivastava PU, Marcus R, Abiteboul D, et al. A case-control study of HIV seroconversion in health care workers after percutaneous exposure. Centers for Disease Control and Prevention Needlestick Surveillance Group. N Engl J Med. 1997; 337(21):1485-1490.

49. Panlilio AL, Cardo DM, Grohskopf LA, Heneine W, Ross CS. Updated U.S. Public Health Service guidelines for the management of occupational exposures to HIV and recommendations for postexposure prophylaxis. MMWR Recomm Rep. 2005;54(Rr-9):1-17.

50. Communicable Diseases Network Australia. CDNA national guidelines for healthcare workers living with blood-borne viruses and healthcare workers who perform exposure prone procedures at risk of exposure to blood-borne viruses. Canberra: Australian Government, 2018. (Updated 2019). Available from: https://www.health.gov.au/resources/publications/cdna-national-guidelines-healthcare-workers-living-with-blood-borne-viruses-perform-exposure-prone-procedures-at-risk-of-exposure-to-blood-borne-viruses?language=en.

51. Recommendations for preventing transmission of human immunodeficiency virus and hepatitis B virus to patients during exposure-prone invasive procedures. MMWR Recomm Rep. 1991;40(Rr-8):1-9.

52. Bell DM. Human immunodeficiency virus transmission in health care settings: risk and risk reduction. Am J Med. 1991;91(3b):294s-300s.

53. Schierhout G, McGregor S, Gessain A, Einsiedel L, Martinello M, Kaldor J. Association between HTLV-1 infection and adverse health outcomes: a systematic review and meta-analysis of epidemiological studies. Lancet Infect Dis. 2020;20(1):133-143.

54. Verdonck K, González E, Van Dooren S, Vandamme AM, Vanham G, Gotuzzo E. Human T-lymphotropic virus 1: recent knowledge about an ancient infection. Lancet Infect Dis. 2007;7(4):266-281.

55. The Kirby Institute and Australian Red Cross Lifeblood. Transfusion-transmissible infections in Australia: 2020 Surveillance Report. Sydney: UNSW, 2020.

CHAPTER 26

Infection prevention and control for staff health and occupational exposure

Dr DEBOROUGH MACBETH[i]

Dr JOHN GERRARD[ii]

Chapter highlights

- An overview of staff health issues relevant to infection prevention and control
- Specific advice in relation to pre-employment screening of healthcare workers
- Detailed information regarding the management of occupational exposure to blood and body fluid
- Case studies on Evolve that demonstrate practical applications of the theory in the workplace

i   Gold Coast Hospital and Health Service, Southport, QLD
ii Infectious Diseases, Gold Coast University Hospital, Brisbane, QLD

Introduction

Every health service is entirely reliant on its employees to provide the service. Healthcare workers (HCWs) have a right to expect that they will be protected from exposure to health risks, including infection, while providing healthcare services. In accordance with the relevant jurisdictional legislation, employers are required to ensure the safety of all employees through a range of strategies that include:

- education and training
- competency assessment
- safe work systems
- policies and procedures to support safe systems
- quality assurance measures to ensure compliance with policies and procedures; and
- additional strategies where new risks are identified or current strategies are deemed ineffective.

There are various points of intersection between infection prevention and control (IPC) and staff health. When a patient is diagnosed with an infectious disease, such as varicella or measles, identifying the staff members who may have been exposed prior to the implementation of appropriate precautions and checking their immune status usually becomes the responsibility of IPC. Outbreaks of gastroenteritis in health facilities may involve employees as well as patients. This means that IPC needs to identify all cases and provide the relevant advice regarding exclusion periods as well as, potentially, arrange testing of affected staff to confirm diagnosis. HCWs can also be the cause of infection for patients and other staff, so IPC needs to ensure there are robust mechanisms in place to ensure that HCWs maintain their immunisations, both when onboarding as new employees and on an ongoing basis for conditions such as pertussis and influenza.

While the responsibilities of the health service are well established, the responsibility of the individual HCW is not always so well defined. Vaccine hesitancy amongst HCWs is well documented.[1,2] The issue can be resolved by mandating vaccination—which can be successful if vaccination is a condition of employment, so the prospective HCW makes their decision before applying for a position within the organisation. However, mandating vaccination on an ongoing basis where there is a need for regular booster doses of vaccines (e.g. pertussis), annual vaccination (e.g. influenza), and new vaccines can be a more challenging prospect. Recent experience with vaccines developed to protect against severe acute respiratory syndrome coronavirus 2 (SARS-CoV-2) has demonstrated that there is distrust among HCWs regarding the efficacy of the vaccines and their safety—given the speed with which they were developed—as well as concerns about potential side effects.[2-4]

Mandating vaccinations for HCWs does raise ethical issues, however, as the right of the individual to self-determination and autonomy in relation to decision making is removed. Arguably, HCWs have a moral imperative to be vaccinated against infectious diseases to remove or reduce the risk of transmission which is a risk to their own health and safety, and also to prevent themselves becoming a source of infection for patients in their care who are already vulnerable due to existing medical conditions or as a result of medical interventions such as chemotherapy or other immunosuppressive therapies.[5]

HCWs are first and foremost human beings and therefore susceptible to all the usual fears, concerns and prejudices of any human being. This is evident in the barriers identified as negatively influencing the HCW's decision to be vaccinated. These include a low perception of the risk of a particular infection to the individual, denial of the social benefits of vaccination, a negative attitude to vaccines in general, lack of vaccine-specific knowledge, concerns about the side effects of vaccines, and concerns around vaccine safety.[1,6]

Successful vaccination campaigns rely on a combination of strategies including education and awareness campaigns that address the specific concerns around vaccination and highlight the benefits, such as self-protection and protection for family members. Making vaccines available and accessible, and removing practical and administrative barriers, will also help increase uptake. Regular feedback regarding vaccine uptake by HCW category and by department can also improve uptake by increasing social pressure to be vaccinated.[1] A strong marketing campaign will aid communication and improve awareness amongst HCWs of the importance and benefits of vaccination.[7] The role of the infection control professional (ICP) in supporting vaccination is critical to promote vaccine uptake, protect HCWs and patients, and successfully undertake contact tracing amongst staff in the event of any potential outbreak of vaccine-preventable disease.

The IPC department also plays a role in occupational blood and body fluid exposure management, which will vary from facility to facility based on the available resources. In some facilities, the service is provided by the occupational health department and in other facilities, the IPC department may provide specific services.

The level of involvement of IPC in staff health may be limited to screening for immunity to vaccine-preventable diseases (VPD) such as hepatitis B, measles, mumps and rubella, and provision of vaccination services. The IPC department will likely have some role in occupational exposure to blood and body fluids, even if that role is limited to data collection and reporting. Analysis and monitoring of reliable, comprehensive data on exposure incidents can assist the ICP to identify trends and, like all surveillance, serve as a basis for the introduction or enhancement of rational control measures including product evaluation, policy development and review, and targeting educational initiatives.

Many IPC departments offer an annual influenza vaccination program for HCWs (Fig 26.1). Influenza is one of a range of pathogens to which HCWs may be exposed while providing healthcare services[8-10] and, in turn, the HCW may become a potential source of infection for colleagues, patients and visitors.[11] The SARS-CoV-2 pandemic has clearly demonstrated the potential vulnerability of HCWs as well as their potential role in transmission to colleagues, patients and visitors.[12-15]

Protection from infection exposure can be achieved through appropriate use of personal protective equipment (PPE), hand hygiene practices aligned with the '5 Moments for Hand Hygiene' campaign[16] and the application of standard and transmission-based precautions. However, immunisation against vaccine-preventable diseases also has a place in protecting the HCW from infection. The Australian Government has provided clear advice regarding HCW immunisation and Australian jurisdictions have implemented policies regarding healthcare worker immunisation.[17,18]

Apart from the specific roles already mentioned, the IPC department may have additional responsibilities for staff health including:

- providing advice in relation to exclusion periods relating to infectious diseases and conditions
- pre-employment screening and immunisation
- maintaining immunisation throughout employment
- surveillance and other roles relating to occupational exposure to blood and body fluids; and
- providing advice regarding occupational infection risks specific to pregnancy.

This chapter will discuss these staff health issues and the role of IPC, as well as the resource requirements associated with each element.

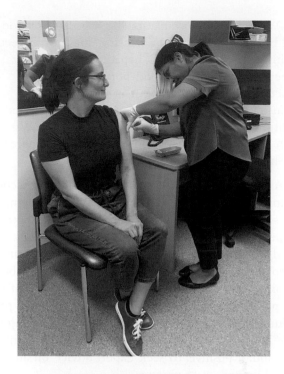

FIGURE 26.1 Staff vaccination clinic

26.1 Vaccine-preventable diseases and pre-employment screening

As previously discussed, immunisation is regarded as a key strategy in protecting HCWs from specific VPDs and preventing transmission to patients and other HCWs. Initially, screening for and immunising against tuberculosis (TB), as well as immunisation against polio, diphtheria, pertussis and tetanus, were considered necessary for clinical HCWs. However, over time the number of vaccines included in recommendations for HCW protection has increased—mainly as a result of the success of immunisation programs and the development of new vaccines such as varicella and measles, mumps, rubella vaccines.

26.1.1 Pre-employment immunisation and screening

Blood-borne pathogens: In the 1980s, with the recognition of a new pathogen—human immunodeficiency virus (HIV)—the risk of blood-borne virus transmission to HCWs through exposure to blood and body fluids was seen as something to be avoided and, along with the introduction of universal precautions (now standard precautions), immunisation against hepatitis B was recognised as essential for

HCWs potentially occupationally exposed to blood and body fluids. While this vaccine does not protect against HIV or hepatitis C, hepatitis B is the most infectious of the three blood-borne pathogens of concern. The development of vaccines to protect against a range of infectious conditions has resulted in additional immunisation requirements for HCWs with evidence of vaccination or immunity required as a condition of employment.[17,18]

Although there is no vaccine to provide protection against hepatitis C or HIV, there are some requirements for screening of HCWs if they perform exposure-prone procedures. These are procedures broadly defined as procedures requiring the HCW to manage sharp implements or be exposed to spicules of bone within a confined body cavity where visibility of the sharp is poor. HCWs performing exposure-prone procedures are required to undertake annual screening for HIV, hepatitis B (if not immune) and hepatitis C infection and, if positive, to seek expert advice on any required limitations to practice.[18,19]

Airborne pathogens: Highly infectious conditions transmitted via the airborne route have been included in immunisation requirements because of their propensity to spread from person to person quickly, resulting in infection outbreaks.[10,20] Screening for immunity to, or evidence of immunisation against, measles and varicella is an example of the airborne pathogen screenings that are routinely included in HCW onboarding processes. Evidence of immunity to measles and varicella may consist of documentation of age-appropriate vaccination courses where immunity is subsequently assumed, or serological test results demonstrating immunity. Tuberculosis screening and vaccination is more complex and discussed separately.

Pathogens transmitted via droplet: According to the Australian Government, pertussis, rubella and mumps immunity is also recommended for HCWs and thus vaccination against these diseases is also required for frontline HCWs. These are transmitted through contact with droplets of respiratory secretions either via direct contact or contact with contaminated environmental surfaces. Influenza is also transmitted via droplet; however, the ability of the virus to mutate means that annual vaccination is required and therefore influenza vaccination will be discussed separately and, similarly, pertussis immunisation requires booster doses at specific intervals, and boosters to maintain pertussis immunity, and will also be discussed separately.

Context and role-specific vaccine requirements: Some additional immunisation requirements are specific to either the HCW role or the context of the healthcare service. For example, hepatitis A immunisation is recommended for plumbers because of their likely occupational exposure to raw sewage, and hepatitis A vaccination is also recommended for HCWs working with children where there is a high proportion of First Nation patients because of the high endemicity of hepatitis A among First Nations peoples and the fact that asymptomatic carriage of hepatitis A is relatively common among children.

Tuberculosis: There are two main circumstances where HCW infection with TB may come to the attention of the ICP: TB infection in the new employee and a new acquisition of TB by an HCW in the work environment.

Following initial infection with *Mycobacterium tuberculosis*, the majority of individuals will contain the organism—that is, it is either cleared or becomes latent. Most are unaware that they are carrying the organism but there is an ongoing risk of reactivation that is both harmful to the HCW and becomes a transmission risk. The lifetime risk of reactivation of disease after infection is estimated to be about 5–10%, with a 5% risk in the 2–5 years following infection and another 5% risk over the remaining lifetime.[21]

Latent infection in HCWs is identified through either a tuberculin skin test (TST or Mantoux test) or an interferon gamma release assay (IGRA) blood test. In HCWs with a positive TST or IGRA test, active infection must be excluded through a careful history to elicit TB symptoms and chest x-ray.

The rationale for pre-employment screening for TB in HCWs is threefold:[22]

1. to identify active TB that is a risk to the HCW and their contacts

2. to identify latent TB infection (LTBI) that may warrant treatment; and

3. to obtain a baseline test result in those staff that may be at risk for infection at work.

As well as obtaining a history of symptoms in new employees, it is important to identify those at high risk of LTBI. High-risk employees are those who:

1. were born or worked for more than 3 months in a country with higher TB incidence (>40 per 100,000)

2. have a known past history of contact with TB (work or personal).

The above information may be obtained through a pre-employment screening questionnaire. Staff who screen positive on a TST or IGRA should undergo further assessment for active TB infection, including performing a chest radiograph. Active infection must be treated in an appropriate specialist setting. Staff members with latent infection (no active disease) should also be assessed in a specialist setting. Whether they are offered treatment will depend on a number of factors including their age and underlying medical status.[23] In some specific circumstances it may be useful to perform baseline screening before employment and then on a recurrent basis. This might apply to HCWs working in areas of very high risk of TB exposure, such as TB clinics and mycobacterial laboratories.

26.1.2 Acquisition of TB by an employee in the work environment

Contact tracing for TB among HCWs may occasionally be required when accidental exposure has occurred. This may happen when a patient with undiagnosed active pulmonary TB is admitted to hospital without appropriate infection control measures in place. Which HCWs are tested depends on a number of factors, including the nature of the infectious patient's accommodation, ventilation and the degree of exposure of the HCW. Appropriate treatment can be initiated when infected HCWs are identified.

Immunisation maintenance: The specific requirements for HCW immunisation pre-employment have been discussed; however, in certain instances, there are requirements for maintaining the protection that immunisation provides. Specifically, pertussis and influenza require booster doses of vaccine to maintain protection.

Pertussis: Protection against pertussis is reliant not only on completion of the initial course administered throughout childhood in Australia, but booster doses of the vaccine are required every 10 years. Pre-employment screening will require evidence that the individual has had a dose of a pertussis-containing vaccine within 10 years of commencing employment.

Influenza: The ability of the influenza virus to mutate means that small changes to the virus occur regularly and more significant changes intermittently. The minor changes that occur relate to genetic mutations that result in changes to the proteins on the surface of the virus: neuraminidase and haemagluttinin. These surface proteins are antigens that are targeted by most influenza vaccines. Therefore, changes in these proteins can result in the influenza vaccine being less effective or ineffective against a specific influenza virus. Changes like this occur frequently due to virus replication and can result in increased morbidity and mortality during the influenza season in a specific year. These minor changes are referred to as 'antigenic drift'.[24]

Each year the influenza vaccine is formulated to try to ensure protection against the circulating influenza viruses. In Australia, the vaccine formulation takes into consideration the influenza strains and sub-types that have been circulating and caused the greatest morbidity and mortality in the winter season just ending in the northern hemisphere. This is why annual influenza vaccination is so important.

The other kind of change in influenza virus is 'antigenic shift' and reflects a major change in the virus. These major changes can result in a new influenza sub-type and antigenic shift can result in influenza pandemics as the entire human population is susceptible to this new sub-type.[24]

Resource requirements: The health service requires systems and processes to support immune status verification and immunisation history verification and recording on employment. It is vital that these systems provide the ICP with absolute confidence that all HCWs meet the requirements, or if unable to meet requirements—such as hepatitis B vaccine non-responders—the matter is flagged and the staff member is aware of what is required if exposed to the pathogen. In the absence of absolute confidence in the verification of immune status, which is difficult to guarantee, it is useful for the IPC department to have access to the immune status and vaccination records of staff in the event that HCWs are occupationally exposed to VPD or blood-borne pathogens so that immune status can be verified at the time of the exposure and prophylaxis offered where appropriate.

In addition to the needs associated with immune status and vaccination when onboarding new employees, the health service requires a mechanism for recording the administration of booster doses of a pertussis-containing vaccine every 10 years for each HCW. The most useful system is one that provides reminders to the individual HCW that booster vaccination is required, and records when it has been completed or notifies an appropriate person, such as the HCW manager, if the deadline passes and evidence of booster vaccination has not been supplied. A mechanism with the ability to seamlessly and automatically update immunisation records at the time the vaccine is administered would be the most effective and efficient. The health service needs policies and procedures to support pre-employment screening and booster immunisation requirements and the escalation of non-compliance, while also complying with confidentiality and privacy regulations and requirements.

26.2 Occupational exposure to blood and body fluids

The very nature of healthcare provision means that HCWs are exposed to blood and body fluid. The risk associated with potential exposure is largely mitigated by the application of standard precautions and the appropriate use of personal protective equipment (PPE); however, HCWs do not always don the PPE as recommended or, where sharp instruments or objects are involved, the PPE can be penetrated, along with the HCW's skin, resulting in exposure.

When discussing occupational exposure to blood and body fluid, the focus is on blood-borne pathogens—specifically hepatitis B and C and HIV—so the disease transmission concerns relate to blood and body fluids containing blood, and exposure that allows these body fluids access to the HCW's bloodstream. This means the body fluid must enter the HCW's bloodstream either through a penetrating injury such as a needlestick, or through contact with the HCW's mucous membranes or non-intact skin.

The management of occupational blood and body fluid exposures is quite complex and requires:

- baseline assessment
- informed consent for testing
- hepatitis B and antiretroviral prophylaxis
- source identification and testing
- notification of results; and
- consideration of associated issues.

26.2.1 Baseline assessment

The nature and circumstances of the exposure will need to be assessed, including the type of exposure—percutaneous (penetrating the skin), or non-percutaneous (where blood or body fluid has had contact with the HCW's mucosa or non-intact skin). In either circumstance, the type and amount of fluid are important, as is the duration of the exposure. A percutaneous exposure also requires consideration of the sharp involved, and if a needle, whether it was solid or hollow-bore

and whether it was in a blood vessel immediately prior to the exposure. This information in totality assists in assessing the level of exposure and associated risk of transmission.

The baseline assessment includes the hepatitis B immune status of the HCW at the time of the exposure. If non-immune, hepatitis B immunoglobulin should be administered prophylactically and within specific timeframes.

Gathering detailed information at the time of the baseline assessment provides the best basis for rational decision making in relation to the affected HCW and provides information that can assist further downstream in terms of education, procedure review and product evaluation. The information should also be considered in terms of assisting the HCW involved to identify factors that contributed to the exposure and strategies that can be employed to prevent a recurrence.

26.2.2 Informed consent for testing

Following baseline assessment of the exposure, baseline testing for hepatitis B, C and HIV would be undertaken where the exposure is deemed to represent a transmission risk. Such testing should be undertaken following discussion with the affected staff member regarding the type of test, the reason for the test, what the test result will demonstrate, and when and how results will be made available.[25] It is important that the HCW understands that baseline testing merely establishes their status in relation to HIV, hepatitis B and C at the time of the exposure and further testing may be required to determine the outcome of the exposure.

Other issues that need to be discussed as part of the consenting process include the fact that in the event of a positive result, contact tracing would be required and notification of the positive result for HIV, hepatitis B and C is required because they are all notifiable conditions, although notification can be coded. It is important to ensure the HCW understands that notification aims to track the epidemiology of these blood-borne infections rather than focus on the individual. Further, in general terms, notification helps to identify where there is need for additional resources, such as education programs, needle and syringe exchanges and so forth, although this generally relates to transmission patterns within a community rather than in the healthcare setting.

The affected HCW must be provided with information about where they can access additional information and support as required. The HCW must be provided with all the information necessary to enable informed consent for testing, and mechanisms to maintain the confidentiality and privacy of the affected HCW should be in place.

26.2.3 Prophylaxis following possible occupational exposure to blood-borne viruses

Hepatitis B: Hepatitis B is the most infectious of the known human blood-borne viruses. The risk of transmission from an infected source patient to a non-immune HCW via a blood-contaminated needlestick injury exceeds 20%.[26] It was shown during the 1970s that non-immune HCWs exposed to blood carrying hepatitis B virus could be partially protected from infection through the administration of hepatitis B immunoglobulin (HBIG) given within a few days of exposure.[27] HBIG is made from human plasma known to contain a high concentration of antibodies to hepatitis B surface antigen (HBsAb). The release of the first commercial hepatitis B vaccine in 1981 radically improved the safety of HCWs exposed to human blood. Healthcare workers who have received the vaccine and have immunity to hepatitis B documented (HBsAb $\geq$ 10 IU/ml) can be considered at negligible risk of infection following exposure to body fluid at any time in the future.[28] Hepatitis B prophylaxis is therefore not required if body fluid exposure occurs. It is therefore critical that HCWs receive proper immunisation with 3 doses of hepatitis B vaccine prior to employment and that resultant immunity is properly documented through antibody testing. The HCW should be made aware of the results of this test. In a well-run health service where hepatitis B immunisation of HCWs is strictly enforced, the need for post-exposure HBIG in HCWs should be a rare event. There are two unusual circumstances where post-exposure HBIG might be considered for an HCW:

1. The HCW has failed to develop antibodies after receiving 6 doses of hepatitis B vaccine (non-responder) and then is exposed to blood from a source known to be a hepatitis B carrier. In this case a dose of HBIG should be administered within 72 hours of the event.

2. The rare occasion where an unvaccinated (or partially vaccinated) HCW is exposed to blood from a source known to be a hepatitis B carrier. This should not occur, but system failures are not unknown. In this case a dose of HBIG

should be administered within 72 hours of the event and a course of vaccination commenced within 7 days.[26]

When the infection status of an exposure source is unknown, the decision to administer HBIG should be made in consultation with expert medical advice.

Hepatitis C: Since the publication of its discovery in 1989, the hepatitis C virus has been shown to occasionally infect HCWs through percutaneous exposure to infected blood products. The risk of HCW infection following such an exposure is very much less than hepatitis B—as low as 0.1%.[29] There are no published studies addressing the question as to whether antivirals might reduce this risk even further. Given the rarity of such transmission, it would be very difficult to perform such a study. The use of antivirals post-exposure is not recommended.

Human immunodeficiency virus: Transmission of HIV to the HCW through exposure to infected blood can occur but is very rare. The main risk is from percutaneous exposure to blood from an infected patient who is not on treatment (probability of transmission estimated at around 0.227%).[30] Exposure of open wounds or mucous membranes to infected blood is associated with very much smaller risk (<0.01%). The risk from exposure to other fluids is smaller still and impossible to quantify. Furthermore, because we know that effective antiretroviral therapy significantly reduces the risk of sexual transmission, it is likely that blood from a treated patient is also much less likely to transmit infection by percutaneous exposure.

Although the risk of transmission of HIV to HCWs is exceedingly small, the consequences are very great, so, much attention has been aimed at reducing the risk further. One way is through the use of post-exposure antiviral medications. A case control study published in 1997 showed that taking zidovudine after exposure to HIV-infected body fluids was associated with a significantly lower risk of transmission.[31] As a result, taking antiretroviral therapy following significant occupational exposure is considered the standard of care. Although animal studies suggest that the benefits are greatest if PEP is started within 24–36 hours, the interval after which no benefit is gained is unknown. So, it is common practice to give PEP up to about a week after exposure. It is usual to give 4 weeks of therapy based on the 1997 case control study. The most effective PEP drug regimen is unknown, so guidelines arbitrarily balance

TABLE 26.1 PEP recommendations after occupational exposure to a known HIV-positive source

Type of exposure with known HIV-positive source	Estimated risk of HIV transmission per exposure if source not on antiretroviral treatment	PEP recommendation	
		Source not on treatment or on treatment with detectable or UNKNOWN viral load	Source viral load KNOWN to be undetectable
NSI or other sharps exposure	1/440	3 drugs	Consider 2 drugs
Mucous membrane and non-intact skin exposure	<1/1000	3 drugs	Consider 2 drugs

Source: Australasian Society for HIV/ASHM. Post-exposure prophylaxis for HIV: Australian National Guidelines 2020.

known drug toxicities against the known effectiveness of drug regimens and the risk of a specific exposure. Monotherapy is not recommended any longer because of both reduced effectiveness and the greater possibility of resistance. On the other hand, full three-drug regimens are not used for lower risk exposures because of the increased risk of toxicity. So current guidelines for post-exposure prophylaxis against HIV in the occupational setting suggest giving just two drugs if the source patient is known to have an undetectable viral load (see Tables 26.1 and 26.2). If the source patient is known to carry a virus that is resistant to one of these antivirals, the regimen can be tailored by a physician with appropriate expertise.

TABLE 26.2 Currently recommended antiretroviral regimens

Two-drug regimens^:
Tenofovir disoproxil fumarate 300mg with lamivudine 300mg (Daily)*
    OR
Tenofovir disoproxil fumarate/emtricitabine 300mg/200mg (Daily)
Three-drug regimens:
Your preferred two-drug regimen PLUS
    dolutegravir 50mg (Daily)
    OR
    raltegravir 400mg (Daily)
    OR
    rilpivirine 25mg (Daily)

Source: Australasian Society for HIV/ASHM. Post-exposure prophylaxis for HIV: Australian National Guidelines 2020.
^Zidovudine, in combination with lamivudine, can be used in two-drug PEP combinations. The benefits of cheaper zidovudine cost are offset by the need for a twice-daily treatment regimen, higher incidences of gastrointestinal side effects, myalgia and headaches in comparison to the recommended regimens.
*TGA-approved generic lamivudine may be used to reduce cost.

Tetanus prophylaxis: In the event of a penetrating injury as the cause of the exposure, consideration should be given to tetanus prophylaxis if the HCW's tetanus vaccination status is unknown or not current.[30]

26.2.4 Source identification and testing

Where possible the source patient associated with the occupational exposure should be identified and asked to consent to testing for HIV, hepatitis B and C. The usual conditions for informed consent apply and, therefore, it is inappropriate for the affected HCW to consent the source patient for testing. Generally, source patients are willing to assist especially given most occupational exposures are accidental. The source patient needs to be advised of their test results. The status of the source patient is relevant to the management of the affected HCW and therefore the system of source testing must be efficient and allow rapid testing turnaround time. It is worthwhile noting that in some occupational exposures the source patient cannot be identified or tested. When this occurs, the information gathered during the exposure assessment will be the basis for decision making in relation to post-exposure prophylaxis requirements.

26.2.5 Notification of results

If possible, it is best to advise the affected HCW of their results in person. This ensures the appropriate people can be present, especially if results of any of the tests are positive. The individual's privacy and confidentiality can be maintained, and time allowed to adequately discuss the results, what they mean, any follow-up that is required and any other issues raised by the affected HCW. When notifying the HCW of the test results it is important to once again explain what the tests mean and their limitations. This is also the time to reinforce the strategies previously identified to mitigate a recurrence of this type of exposure.

26.2.6 Associated issues

Occupational exposure to blood and body fluid can be a very stressful event for individual HCWs when they consider the risk of acquiring an infectious disease, and the implications for their own health, their relationships and their professional life. Those involved in the assessment, management and follow-up of affected HCWs must have excellent communication skills and have a sound knowledge of the blood-borne diseases, transmission risks and modes, and prophylaxis and treatment options. The information needs to be targeted specifically to the individual, including options for further advice and counselling as required. Apart from managing the occupational exposure, ICP involvement enables the collection of de-identified data for analysis. Analysis of the data can inform a range of activities including education, procedure review and development, product evaluation and awareness campaigns.

Exclusion periods: The safety of patients and HCWs can be at risk if HCWs attend work and provide care when they are unwell. The impact of infection outbreaks involving HCWs has been well documented.[10,12,20,32] In one Norwegian study, norovirus alone accounted for more than 20,000 cases of infection in healthcare facilities and residential aged care facilities (RACF) over a 13-year period. The 965 outbreaks comprising these cases included more than 7000 HCWs.[32] These studies demonstrate that HCWs can acquire infection while providing care to patients, and can transmit infection to patients and colleagues while infectious.

Where the infection is vaccine-preventable, the obvious approach is to ensure HCWs are immunised; however, once infected—due to vaccine failure, non-immunisation or where there is no vaccine available to prevent the infection—it is imperative that HCWs remain absent from work until they have recovered and are no longer infectious. The length of time HCWs need to remain away from work (exclusion period) varies with each disease. Common infectious diseases and conditions and their respective exclusion periods are listed in the Australian Guidelines for the Prevention and Control of Infection in Healthcare.[18]

The ICP may be contacted by individual HCWs or their managers seeking guidance on exclusion periods

from work. Some HCWs make contact seeking advice about whether they should attend work when one of their household members has an infectious disease. The ability to provide appropriate advice will often be based on the ICP having access to the immune status of the individual staff member and/or having access to the relevant information on which to base the advice. The Australian Immunisation Handbook lists the VPD and their respective periods of communicability and is a useful resource for ICPs. The Communicable Diseases Network Australia (CDNA) provides detailed information regarding specific infectious diseases and conditions, including the infectious period for the condition, in its Series of National Guidelines (SoNGs).[33]

Pregnant and vulnerable healthcare workers: There are a number of special circumstances where HCWs require consideration in relation to infection risks. Pregnant HCWs, those with specific conditions such as cystic fibrosis or immunocompromised status, and those living with HIV or other blood-borne viruses may require advice and support.

It is not uncommon for HCWs who have been working in health for some years to develop some anxiety when they are pregnant. Pregnant HCWs from all disciplines will contact the ICP seeking advice regarding their infection risks in relation to multi-resistant bacteria and contact with patients who may be infectious. The development of a policy or procedure that provides information for pregnant HCWs can be useful because it is available constantly, even though the ICP may only be available during specific hours.

It is hoped the pregnancy was planned and the HCW included a review of her immunisation status so that any required vaccines or booster doses could be administered before the pregnancy. This is not always the case and HCWs, like any other prospective parents, want to ensure the safety of the fetus. Reiteration of the basic principles of infection control is important at this time, as well as providing support in terms of information and advice.

HCWs with cystic fibrosis, and those who are immunocompromised or have blood-borne viruses, may seek advice regarding the safety of vaccines, their ability to perform their role in certain circumstances, and/or their increased vulnerability to infection. They should be advised to seek specialist advice from their consultant medical officer but should also be supported by the organisation and the ICP. Advice regarding immunisation for people with special circumstances is available in the Australian Immunisation Handbook.

HCWs living with blood-borne viruses may need support and advice, especially in relation to their role if it involves performing exposure-prone procedures. Information is available through national guidelines published by Communicable Diseases Network Australia (CDNA).[19]

Conclusion

There are many points of intersection between IPC and staff health, as discussed in this chapter. The ICP is not expected to replace medical assessment and advice and often the best advice the ICP can offer the individual HCW is to seek medical advice. Nevertheless, there are many opportunities for the ICP to provide advice and support to HCWs which is an opportunity to improve public relations, market the work of the IPC department and serve as a basis for building working relationships.

The extent of IPC department involvement in the staff health elements discussed in this chapter will depend upon the resources available. Often, the responsibility is shared between the IPC, occupational health, and human resource departments. Shared responsibility can work well if there are clearly defined areas of responsibility, excellent communication between the various departments, and a mutual respect and recognition of what each department brings to the issue at hand. In any event, the presence of the IPC department at a time of crisis for individuals or departments, as described in the case studies, is both welcome and valued. For the ICP, involvement in these interactions provides significant opportunities for growth and professional development as long as the ICP is willing to listen, learn and reflect.

Useful websites/resources

- Australian Society for HIV Medicine (AHSM). https://ashm.org.au/
- Communicable Diseases Network Australia (CDNA). Australian Government Department of Health and Aged Care. https://www.health.gov.au/resources/collections/cdna-series-of-national-guidelines-songs.
- The Australian Immunisation Handbook, Australian Government Department of Health and Aged Care. https://www.health.gov.au/resources/publications/the-australian-immunisation-handbook.

References

1. Dini G, Toletone A, Sticchi L, Orsi A, Bragazzi NL, Durando P. Influenza vaccination in healthcare workers: a comprehensive critical appraisal of the literature. Hum Vaccin Immunother. 2018;14(3):772-789.
2. Biswas N, Mustapha T, Khubchandani J, Price JH. The nature and extent of COVID-19 vaccination hesitancy in healthcare workers. J Community Health. 2021;46(6):1244-51.
3. Kara Esen B, Can G, Pirdal BZ, Aydin SN, Ozdil A, Balkan, II, et al. COVID-19 Vaccine hesitancy in healthcare personnel: a university hospital experience. Vaccines (Basel). 2021;9(11).
4. Berry SD, Johnson KS, Myles L, Herndon L, Montoya A, Fashaw S, et al. Lessons learned from frontline skilled nursing facility staff regarding COVID-19 vaccine hesitancy. J Am Geriatr Soc. 2021;69(5):1140-1146.
5. Galanakis E, Jansen A, Lopalco PL, Giesecke J. Ethics of mandatory vaccination for healthcare workers. Euro Surveill. 2013;18(45):20627.
6. Schmid P, Rauber D, Betsch C, Lidolt G, Denker ML. Barriers of influenza vaccination intention and behavior - a systematic review of influenza vaccine hesitancy, 2005–2016. PLoS One. 2017;12(1):e0170550.
7. Maltezou HC, Ioannidou E, De Schrijver K, François G, De Schryver A. Influenza vaccination programs for healthcare personnel: organizational issues and beyond. Int J Environ Res Public Health. 2021;18(21):11122.
8. Schulz-Stübner S, Reska M, Schaumann R. Affected healthcare workers during outbreaks: a report from the German consulting center for infection control (BZH) outbreak registry. Infect Control Hosp Epidemiol. 2018;40(1):113-115.
9. Kellie SM, Makvandi M, Muller ML. Management and outcome of a varicella exposure in a neonatal intensive care unit: lessons for the vaccine era. Am J Infect Control. 2011;39(10):844-848.
10. Orsi A, Butera F, Piazza MF, Schenone S, Canepa P, Caligiuri P, et al. Analysis of a 3-months measles outbreak in western Liguria, Italy: are hospitals safe and healthcare workers reliable? J Infect Public Health. 2020;13(4):619-624.
11. Maltezou HC, Botelho-Nevers E, Brantsæter AB, Carlsson RM, Heininger U, Hübschen JM, et al. Vaccination of healthcare personnel in Europe: update to current policies. Vaccine. 2019;37(52):7576-7584.
12. Piapan L, De Michieli P, Ronchese F, Rui F, Mauro M, Peresson M, et al. COVID-19 outbreak in healthcare workers in hospitals in Trieste, North-east Italy. J Hosp Infect. 2020;106(3):626-628.

13. Nguyen LH, Drew DA, Graham MS, Joshi AD, Guo CG, Ma W, et al. Risk of COVID-19 among front-line health-care workers and the general community: a prospective cohort study. Lancet Public Health. 2020;5(9):e475-e483.

14. Van Praet JT, Claeys B, Coene A-S, Floré K, Reynders M. Prevention of nosocomial COVID-19: another challenge of the pandemic. Infect Control Hosp Epidemiol. 2020;41(11): 1355-1356.

15. Wander PL, Orlov M, Merel SE, Enquobahrie DA. Risk factors for severe COVID-19 illness in healthcare workers: too many unknowns. Infect Control Hosp Epidemiol. 2020;41(11):1369-1370.

16. Australian Commission on Safety and Quality in Health Care. National Hand Hygiene Initiative 2019. ACSQHC, 2019. Available from: https://www.safetyandquality.gov.au/our-work/infection-prevention-and-control/national-hand-hygiene-initiative.

17. Australian Technical Advisory Group on Immunisation (ATAGI). Australian immunisation handbook. Canberra: Australian Government Department of Health, 2018.

18. National Health and Medical Research Council, Australian Commission on Safety and Quality in Health Care. Australian guidelines for the prevention and control of infection in healthcare (2019). In: Health Do, ed. Canberra: NHMRC/ACSQHC, 2019.

19. Australia CDN. Australian national guidelines for the management of healthcare workers living with blood borne viruses and healthcare workers who perform exposure prone procedures at risk of exposure to blood borne viruses 2020. Canberra: Australian Government Department of Health, 2020. Available from: https://www1.health.gov.au/internet/main/publishing.nsf/Content/cda-cdna-blood-borne.htm.

20. Biskupska M, Małecka I, Stryczyńska-Kazubska J, Wysocki J. Varicella - a potential threat to maternal and fetal health. Ginekologia Polska. 2017;88(1):13-19.

21. Comstock GW. Epidemiology of tuberculosis. Am Rev Respir Dis. 1982;125(3 Pt 2):8-15.

22. Waring J, Waring J. National tuberculosis advisory committee guideline: management of tuberculosis risk in healthcare workers in Australia. Commun Dis Intell Q Rep. 2017;41(3):E199-e203.

23. Australia CDN. Tuberculosis (TB): CDNA National guidelines for the public health management of TB. Canberra: Australian Department of Health, 2015. Available from: http://www.health.gov.au/internet/main/publishing.nsf/Content/D140EDF48C0A0CEACA257BF0001A3537/$File/TB-2.0-april2015.pdf.

24. Prevention CfDCa. How the flu virus can change: "drift" and "shift" 2019. Available from: https://www.cdc.gov/flu/about/viruses/change.htm.

25. Australasian Society for HIV VHaSHM. Informed consent for HIV testing 2020. Available from: http://testingportal.ashm.org.au/national-hiv-testing-policy/informed-consent-for-hiv-testing/.

26. Kuhar DT, Henderson DK, Struble KA, Heneine W, Thomas V, Cheever LW, et al. Updated US Public Health Service guidelines for the management of occupational exposures to human immunodeficiency virus and recommendations for postexposure prophylaxis. Infect Control Hosp Epidemiol. 2013;34(9):875-892.

27. Seeff LB, Wright EC, Zimmerman HJ, Alter HJ, Dietz AA, Felsher BF, et al. Type B hepatitis after needle-stick exposure: prevention with hepatitis B immune globulin. Final report of the Veterans Administration Cooperative Study. Annals Int Med. 1978;88(3):285-293.

28. Bruce MG, Bruden D, Hurlburt D, Zanis C, Thompson G, Rea L, et al. Antibody levels and protection after hepatitis B vaccine: results of a 30-year follow-up study and response to a booster dose. J Infect Dis. 2016;214(1):16-22.

29. Egro FM, Nwaiwu CA, Smith S, Harper JD, Spiess AM. Seroconversion rates among health care workers exposed to hepatitis C virus-contaminated body fluids: the University of Pittsburgh 13-year experience. Am J Infect Control. 2017;45(9):1001-1005.

30. Australasian Society for HIV/ASHM. Post-exposure prophylaxis for HIV: Australian national guidelines 2020. Available from: https://www.ashm.org.au/products/product/978-1-920773-47-2.

31. Cardo DM, Culver DH, Ciesielski CA, Srivastava PU, Marcus R, Abiteboul D, et al. A case-control study of HIV seroconversion in health care workers after percutaneous exposure. Centers for Disease Control and Prevention Needlestick Surveillance Group. N Eng J Med. 1997;337(21):1485-1490.

32. Espenhain L, Berg TC, Bentele H, Nygård K, Kacelnik O. Epidemiology and impact of norovirus outbreaks in Norwegian healthcare institutions, 2005-2018. J Hosp Infect. 2019;103(3):335-340.

33. Australia CDN. Series of National Guidelines (SoNGs) 2020. Canberra: Australian Government Department of Health, 2020. Available from: https://www1.health.gov.au/internet/main/publishing.nsf/Content/cdnasongs.htm.

CHAPTER 27

Infection prevention and control in emergency care settings

PROFESSOR RAMON Z. SHABAN[i-iv]

Dr SHIZAR NAHIDI[v-vi]

Dr CATHERINE VIENGKHAM[i,ii]

Chapter highlights

- An overview of healthcare-associated infections (HAIs) and infectious disease in the emergency care setting
- Discussion of the essentials of infection prevention and control (IPC) practices in emergency care in Australia
- Context-specific challenges that interfere with proper IPC practice in Australian emergency care
- Practical guidance on existing IPC practices to reduce the risk of HAI in emergency care

i   Susan Wakil School of Nursing and Midwifery, Faculty of Medicine and Health, University of Sydney, Sydney, NSW
ii Sydney Infectious Diseases Institute, Faculty of Medicine and Health, University of Sydney, Sydney, NSW
iii Public Health Unit, Centre for Population Health, Western Sydney Local Health District, Westmead, NSW
iv New South Wales Biocontainment Centre, Western Sydney Local Health District, Westmead, NSW
v   Latrobe Regional Hospital (LRH), Traralgon, VIC
vi Faculty of Medicine, Nursing and Health Sciences, Monash University, VIC

Introduction

This chapter presents an introduction to infectious diseases and healthcare-associated infection in the context of emergency care. The chapter also describes emergency-specific challenges that interfere with IPC practices and renders the key elements in standard IPC practice in emergency care in Australia.

27.1 Characteristics and contexts of emergency care in Australia

There is no universal definition for the term 'emergency care', and the meaning varies in different contexts. Emergency care is an essential element of the health system and the first point of contact in circumstances where rapid intervention is required to protect the health and wellbeing of individuals and to prevent or minimise morbidity or mortality. It incorporates a multitude of inpatient and outpatient hospital services necessary to prevent the death or serious long-term impairment of the health of a patient who is affected by a sudden or unexpected illness or injury.[1,2] As such, the recipients of emergency care encompass the patients presenting with a broad range of medical conditions ranging from minor to major trauma, acute to chronic diseases, and those with critical, life-threatening illnesses. In most healthcare systems, emergency care services involve a large team of healthcare professionals from different disciplines who assemble to deliver care for patients in varying pre-hospital and facility-based settings. Delivery of standard emergency care is a shared responsibility across nurses, doctors, allied health professionals and many other clinical and non-clinical support staff.[3]

The World Health Organization (WHO) recognises emergency, trauma and acute care as an essential part of the health system and a fundamental part of universal health coverage.[4] In Australia, provision of standard and good quality emergency care is recognised as a right for all citizens.[5] Emergency care services have mainly been funded and are jointly supported and managed by state, territory and local governments. Given the socio-cultural characteristics and geographical landscape of Australia, the structure, resources and operation of emergency care services may be subject to slight variations across metropolitan, urban and remote settings. Even within a given health service network, the role and functions of emergency care services differ from one Facility to another.[2,6] For example, in some hospitals, there are adjacent 24-hour general practice clinics

which admit and manage low-severity patients so as to help emergency departments (EDs) with overcrowding and surge of presentations. In rural and remote health facilities, designated treatment rooms provide limited resuscitation practices and the role of nurses in managing emergency patients is more dominant. In contrast, most healthcare facilities in metropolitan and regional areas have a designated ED with continuous cover of medical officers and specialist nurses, and ongoing access to emergency diagnostic, allied health and intensive care and surgical operating services. In the metropolitan areas of major cities (e.g. Sydney, Melbourne and Brisbane) a two-tiered pre-hospital response system exists of basic life support (BLS) and advanced life support (ALS) paramedics. But small towns have a one-tier system or fall in the catchment of a neighbouring system. These variations exemplify the diverse practice environments and service designs where emergency care is delivered.

27.1.1 The Australian emergency care environment

In the pre-hospital settings, patients conventionally start to receive initial emergency care either from their general practitioner or from an attending paramedic, respectively highlighting the crucial role, and sizeable contribution of, primary healthcare and ambulance paramedic services in the Australian emergency care system. Urgent primary care provision is mainly instituted via either centres for out-of-hours care (e.g. GP-type 24-hour clinics); or home-visit services (e.g. various GP home-visit service providers).[6]

Australia has an emergency call centre (number: 000 or 112), which offers an over-the-phone triage and coordinates rescue activities of the emergency medical services (EMS). After an initial triage, call handlers or emergency medical dispatchers will alert the ambulance station (see Fig 27.1). The pre-hospital emergency care in Australia is provided by state ambulance services, which are a division of each state or territory government, and by St John Ambulance in both Western Australia and the Northern Territory. These services are largely offered and facilitated by four organisations: the land ambulance services, the air ambulance services, first responders, and firefighter emergency medical responders.[7]

Emergency departments are the conventional key entry points for patients entering the hospital system and are considered an essential component of Australia's healthcare system. The Australasian College of Emergency Medicine (ACEM) defines EDs as dedicated

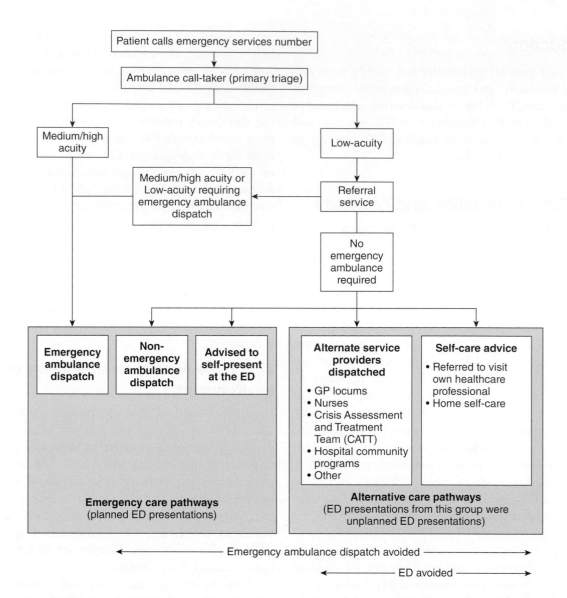

FIGURE 27.1 Case flow from the call to the emergency services to referral service outcome
Source:[10]

hospital-based facilities specifically designed and staffed to provide 24-hour emergency care for patients who require urgent medical, surgical or other urgent attention.[2,3] The role of EDs is to assess, diagnose, treat and manage patients who present with an acute or serious illness or injury. Given the importance of timely care, Australian EDs provide unremitting access to medical and nursing staff, blood products, laboratory and radiology, and access to specialist medical, surgical and support services.[8] Most public hospitals in Australia have an ED. While most EDs accept all emergencies, some are specialised to deliver care for specific cohorts of patients. For instance, there are EDs attached to children's hospitals, women's hospitals, and there are a few that operate

in eye and ear hospitals. During 2020–21, Australians received emergency services in 292 public and 41 private hospitals (Table 27.1).[9]

Patients presenting to Australian EDs are seen in the order of medical urgency. Since 1994, all Australian EDs have used a system of triage, known as the national triage scale (NTS), which is implemented to ensure that the patients who present with most urgent need for help are attended to and treated before the less acute ones. Upon arrival in the ED, patients are assessed by a clinician (usually a triage nurse) against NTS to prioritise patients on the basis of illness or injury severity and need for medical and nursing care. All patients are assigned a triage score which is a subjective ranking

TABLE 27.1 Number of Australian public and private hospitals providing emergency services during 2020–2021

Australian States/ Territories	Number of public hospital EDs	Number of private hospital EDs
New South Wales	172	4
Victoria	40	12
Queensland	26	17
Western Australia	24	3
South Australia	17	3
Tasmania	4	2
Australian Capital Territory	2	–
Northern Territory	6	–
Total	291	41

Source: AIHW, 2021.[9]

TABLE 27.2 National Triage Scale (adopted by the Australian Council on Healthcare Standards in 1994)

Score	Severity	Immediacy of care
1	Resuscitation	Patient needs treatment immediately
2	Emergency	Patient needs treatment within 10 minutes
3	Urgent	Patient needs treatment within 30 minutes
4	Semi-urgent	Patient needs treatment within 1 hour
5	Non-urgent	Patient needs treatment within 2 hours

Source: ACEM, 2016.[12]

from one to five, with one being the most urgent and five being non-urgent (Table 27.2).[11] During the treatment phase of their time in the ED, patients are assessed by a clinician (or a group of clinicians), a diagnosis is made and treatment is given, if required. In the majority of patients, one or a combination of the following six scenarios may conclude their ED journey:

- be admitted to hospital
- remain in ED pro tem to be observed and/or treated

- finish treatment with stitches, dressings, a plaster cast or have surgery
- be discharged (with or without prescribed medicines) for follow-up by patients' general practitioner (GP)
- referred to an outpatient clinic or a specialist service
- be transferred to another hospital for treatment.

Most state and territory health jurisdictions commit to provide Australian people with access to timely, safe and quality emergency care, and to ensure that patients presenting to the public hospital EDs can safely leave the ED for admission to hospital, be referred to another hospital for treatment or be discharged within 4 hours.[13] An ideal ED patient journey (Fig 27.2) necessitates a supportive collaboration between EDs, and the whole of hospital and relevant community health services.[14]

27.1.2 Characteristics of presentations in Australian emergency departments

As a snapshot of the Australian ED activities, during 2020–21, Australian public hospitals managed 8,808,357 presentations of acute and emergency patients in their emergency reception areas.[9,16] Over 52% of ED presentations were assigned to the three most urgent triage categories—Resuscitation, Emergency and Urgent. During this period, most patients left the ED after receiving proper treatment (62%) and almost one-third (31%) were admitted or referred to another hospital for admission for further workup or advanced care.

Children under 4 years of age accounted for 10% of presentations, and patients aged 65 and over accounted for 21% of presentations. In terms of the timeliness of care, over 70% of patients received care on time, which is inclusive of almost all of those requiring immediate care (NTS Grade 1 – Resuscitation) and 71% of those requiring care within 10 minutes (NTS Grade 2 – Emergency). According to the Australian Institute of Health and Welfare, 50% of all ED presentations in 2020–21 were attended and seen within 18 minutes, and 90% of patients were seen within 1 hour and 42 minutes.

With regard to the case-mix, the most common principal diagnosis of ED presentations comprised of those affected by injury, poisoning or the consequence of external causes, which accounted for almost 24% of cases. Disease of the respiratory system was the next

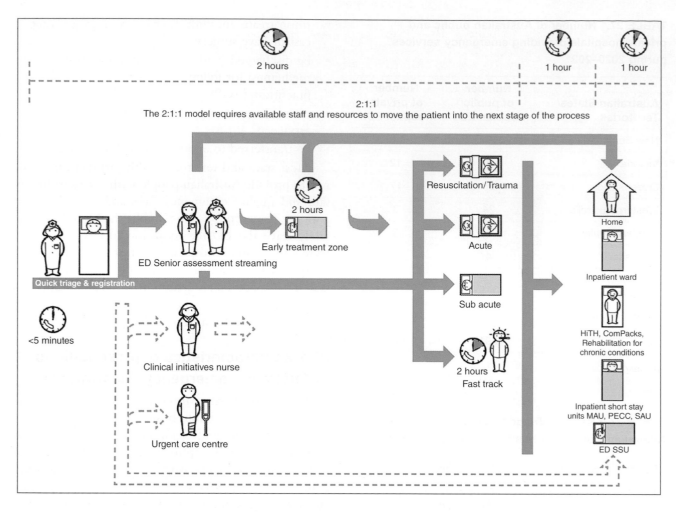

FIGURE 27.2 The ideal emergency department patient journey
Source: NSW Health.[15]

most frequent, followed by factors influencing health status and diseases of the digestive system, which all accounted for approximately 5–6% of cases respectively. A summary statistical profile of emergency presentations in Australian public hospitals (2020–21) is presented in Tables 27.3 and 27.4.

27.1.3 Emergency care workforce

Australian emergency care services largely employ a multidisciplinary team approach to manage workflow and sustain service delivery in the most efficient and effective way possible.[3] Given the contextual dimensions of emergency care services, most EDs need to work closely with a broad range of diagnostic, specialist and allied health services (Table 27.5). In metropolitan urban hospitals, the collaborative dynamic between EDs and these services plays a crucial role in ensuring the quality, safety and timeliness of the

emergency care, and is therefore critical in determining patient outcomes.

Furthermore, the intrinsic arrangements within EDs, which are predominantly influenced by local demand, presentation figures and patient case-mix, also contribute to shape the patient's journey through the ED.[8] For example, staff ratio in EDs is often adjusted to the rates and acuity of presentations and local needs. Over the last two decades, a persistent focus has been placed on endeavours to address key issues in workforce planning, staff ratios and redesign of work practices, in order to improve ED patient outcomes and key performance indicators. However, the complexity of the ED environment, together with the uniqueness of characteristics of each ED and the diversity of staff, make it difficult to tailor universal solutions. Among all these, the ED workforce is commonly acknowledged as a major resource and crucial infrastructure that can largely sustain ED services' delivery.

TABLE 27.3 Statistical summary profile of Australian emergency department presentations during 2020–2021*

State/Territory	Count	Proportion (%)
New South Wales	3,068,572	34.8
Victoria	1,772,359	20.1
Queensland	1,887,381	21.4
Western Australia	997,816	11.3
South Australia	580,575	6.6
Tasmania	170,287	1.9
Australian Capital Territory	153,713	1.7
Northern Territory	177,654	2.0

Sex	Count	Proportion (%)
Females	4,461,284	50.6
Male	4,345,063	49.3

Triage category	Count	Proportion (%)
Resuscitation	68,811	0.8
Emergency	1,256,584	14.3
Urgent	3,297,859	37.4
Semi-urgent	3,293,576	37.4
Non-urgent	888,635	10.1

Remoteness of area of usual residence	Count	Proportion (%)
Major cities	5,534,493	62.8
Inner regional	1,944,809	22.1
Outer regional	911,302	10.3
Remote	190,316	2.2
Very remote	114,729	1.3

Age	Count	Proportion (%)
0–4	895,702	10.2
5–14	829,389	9.4
15–24	1,149,955	13.1
25–34	1,237,774	14.1
35–44	1,007,616	11.4
45–54	935,858	10.6
55–64	858,939	9.8
65–74	798,834	9.1
75–84	677,057	7.7
85–89	240,280	2.7
90–94	134,516	1.5
95+	39,973	0.5

Episode end status	Count	Proportion (%)
Admitted to this hospital	2,572,282	29.2
Departed without being admitted or referred	5,500,450	62.4
Referred to another hospital for admission	150,318	1.7
Did not wait	331,775	3.8
Left at own risk	200,235	2.3
Died in emergency department	4,837	<0.1
Dead on arrival	2,172	<0.1
Registered, advised of another healthcare service and left without being attended to	45,521	0.5
Not reported	767	<0.1

Proportions have been rounded and may not necessarily add up to 100%
Source: AIHW, 2021.[9]

TABLE 27.4 The 20 most common principal diagnoses for emergency department presentations based on ICD-10-AM

ICD-10 Coding	Principal diagnosis	Proportion (%)
A00–B99	Certain infectious and parasitic diseases	4.5
C00–D48	Neoplasms	0.3
D50–D89	Diseases of the blood and blood-forming organs and certain disorders involving the immune mechanism	0.5
E00–E90	Endocrine, nutritional and metabolic diseases	0.9
F00–F99	Mental and behavioural disorders	3.5

Continued

TABLE 27.4 The 20 most common principal diagnoses for emergency department presentations based on ICD-10-AM—cont'd

ICD-10 Coding	Principal diagnosis	Proportion (%)
G00–G99	Diseases of the nervous system	1.4
H00–H59	Diseases of the eye and adnexa	1.3
H60–H95	Diseases of the ear and mastoid process	1.1
I00–I99	Diseases of the circulatory system	3.9
J00–J99	Diseases of the respiratory system	5.9
K00–K93	Diseases of the digestive system	5.1
L00–L99	Diseases of the skin and subcutaneous tissue	3.1
M00–M99	Diseases of the musculoskeletal system and connective tissue	5.1
N00–N99	Diseases of the genitourinary system	3.9
O00–O99	Pregnancy, childbirth and the puerperium	1.2
P00–P96	Certain conditions originating in the perinatal period	0.1
Q00–Q99	Congenital malformations, deformations and chromosomal abnormalities	0.0
R00–R99	Symptoms, signs and abnormal clinical and laboratory findings, not elsewhere classified	24.1
S00–T98	Injury, poisoning and certain other consequences of external causes	23.8
U06.0 & U07.1	Emergency use of codes U06.0 [COVID-19, ruled out] and U07.1 [COVID-19]	1.6
U50–Y98	External causes of morbidity and mortality	0.1
Z00–Z99	Factors influencing health status and contact with health services	5.2
—	Not reported	3.2

Source: AIHW, 2021.[9]

TABLE 27.5 Diagnostic, specialist and allied health services collaborating with EDs to deliver emergency care services in Australia

Diagnostic services	X-ray (Portable and fixed), CT scanner, magnetic resonance imaging (MRI), angiography, positive emission tomography (PET), haematology, biochemistry, microbiology, cytology, histology
Specialist services	Medical assessment units (MAU), psychiatric emergency care centres (PECC), neurosurgery, orthopaedic surgery, surgical services, trauma, cardiology, cardiac catheter lab, neonatal, paediatric, obstetrics, urology, respiratory, oncology, ear nose and throat, mental health, geriatrics, palliative care
Allied health services	Physiotherapy, social work, occupational therapy, pharmacy, play therapy, care coordination, aged care services emergency team (ASET)

In most EDs, the emergency doctors have the primary role of assessing, treating and managing patients.[3] Emergency nurses are similarly involved in patient assessment, initiating interventions and prioritising and managing nursing care for patients, and their roles continue to evolve as the health system grows larger and becomes more complex.[17] ED support staff often assist clinicians with patient management, admission and/or discharge processes, and have a key role in releasing clinical staff from non-clinical tasks. While varying across EDs, the support staff may include clerical staff, administrative staff, clinical and communication support staff, orderlies, transport/transfer staff and cleaners.

In pre-hospital emergency settings, the role of paramedics has been crucial in the timely institution of care by conducting initial assessment and administering basic treatments before and during transport to a medical facility. They implement and oversee the transfer of the patient in connection with transport. They provide assistance in acute situations, implement lifesaving emergency measures, and monitor the performance of the transportation process.[18] Over recent decades, paramedics' scope of practice has been expanded significantly, with the performance of invasive medical procedures being more commonplace (e.g. intravenous cannulation, intubation, fracture reduction and suturing).[19] There are different types of paramedics in Australia—ranging from an ambulance paramedic, through to critical and intensive care paramedics. As shown in Table 27.6, the roles of paramedics are generally classified into the three streams of Professional, Technical and Ambulance communications.[20]

In Australia, emergency care practices are guided by various professional and government bodies which include the Australian Health Practitioner Regulation Agency (APHRA), Medical Board of Australia (MBA), Nursing and Midwifery Board of Australia (NMBA), Australian Nursing and Midwifery Federation (ANMF), Australasian College of Emergency Medicine (ACEM), College of Emergency Nursing Australasia (CENA), Council of Remote Area Nurses of Australia (CRANA), Australasian College of Paramedicine (ACP), Emergency Care Institute of NSW (ECI), Paramedics Australasia (PA), state and territory ambulance services and local, state, territory and federal governments.

27.2 Healthcare-associated infections and infectious diseases in emergency care

As emergency care services are one of the main gateways to Australian hospitals, it is well anticipated that patients may arrive presenting with a constellation of signs and symptoms suggestive of an infectious disease. Over the last decade, between 4.5% to 5.1% of Australian emergency presentations across all age groups had the ICD-10-AM principal diagnosis of 'certain infectious and parasitic diseases' (Fig 27.3).[9,16,21-25] These figures, although not seemingly prodigious, are likely an underestimate of the possible infections that can coexist beneath more obvious presentations of disease and act to further exacerbate patient deterioration.[26] For example, medical conditions such as meningococcal septicaemia and sepsis require swift identification and early intervention to minimise the risk of morbidity and mortality.[26-28] Furthermore, some may

TABLE 27.6 Australian paramedicine streams

Stream	Clinical roles
Professional	Paramedic Intensive care paramedic Retrieval paramedic General care paramedic
Technical	First responder Patient transport attendant – Level 1 Patient transport attendant – Level 2 Basic life support medic
Ambulance Communications	Emergency medical dispatch support officer Emergency medical dispatcher

Source: Paramedics Australasia, 2009.[20]

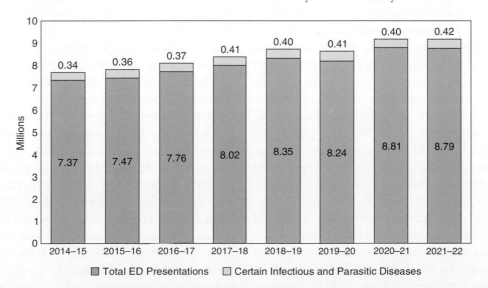

FIGURE 27.3 Emergency presentations across all age groups who had principal diagnosis of 'certain infectious and parasitic diseases' (ICD-10-AM) during 2014-2022

Sources:[9,16,21-25]

present with acute illness or injury while being asymptomatic for a concurrent infectious disease, and therefore carry a great risk of spreading an infection.[29-32] There are also patients at an increased risk to acquire new infections associated with the care they receive.[33,34] The clinical competence and ability of emergency clinicians to recognise infections and to determine their severity plays a critical role in what constitutes quality care in emergency care.[26,27,32]

Emergency care services host a broad variety of infectious disease patients, some of which will be managed in EDs and some being admitted to the hospital for further workup. Training programs and guidelines have, therefore, been implemented to help reduce the risks associated with communicable infectious diseases in pre-hospital and in-hospital emergency care settings.[29] However, it is important to note that increasing trends in the rate and complexity of emergency presentations together with the shortage of skilled workforce in Australian EDs add to the workload of the clinicians working in emergency settings.[35,36] Unexpected national health threat events, such as the COVID-19 pandemic, impose drastic and rapid changes to the health-seeking behaviour of the general public, as well as introduce additional complications to healthcare providers, such as the accessibility to limited supplies of PPE and the quarantining of large portions of the workforce when outbreaks and potential infections are identified. Emergency departments frequently deploy and implement new models of care, in which clinicians are often expected to embark on new roles, extending their clinical practice accountability and scope of practice.[13,37] These changes continue to generate additional challenges for emergency healthcare workers to meet professional practice standards, address their education and training requirements and keep up with current clinical policies and procedures introduced to ensure governance, quality and safety.[38]

Furthermore, the time pressure and the unpredictable nature of working in the emergency care setting precipitates a common concern to emergency care personnel regarding the risk of acquisition of infectious diseases and the transmission of healthcare-associated infection.[39] Paramedics and other emergency care clinicians may be exposed to the body fluids and respiratory droplets of their patients, which are associated with high risks of transmission of blood-borne or airborne infectious diseases respectively. Blood-borne viruses such as hepatitis B, hepatitis C and HIV can be transmitted from a needlestick injury, whereas respiratory diseases like tuberculosis, influenza and COVID-19

can affect emergency care clinicians during the management of patients both outside and inside the healthcare setting.[40-43]

The incidence of HAIs in Australian emergency care varies according to different data sources. Australian states and territories possess and administer their own data systems, and therefore, collect and report different types of HAI epidemiological data. There is no national surveillance system for HAIs, and there are very limited aggregate data sets at the national level.[44-46] As such, there is no figure advising on the national incidence rate of HAIs in emergency care settings or more broadly in healthcare facilities. At the present time, the HAI epidemiological data are collected and can be sourced mainly through three streams:

1. **HAI hospital-acquired complication (HAI HAC)**—data are collected by the Independent Hospital Pricing Authority (IHPA). Access to these data can be granted upon request

2. **State and territory jurisdiction surveillance data**—availability of data on different types of HAI varies significantly across jurisdictions

3. **Data reported in the peer-reviewed literature**—data are limited to specific infections, with significant heterogeneity in adopted HAI definition and methodological approach.

There are significant differences between the figures reported in each stream, necessitating an endeavour to collate the surveillance HAI data sets to report the epidemiology of HAIs in Australian emergency care settings.[47] Taking these limitations into account, a likely incidence of HAIs in Australian acute healthcare facilities is estimated to be around 165,000 cases per annum, which makes HAIs the most common complication affecting patients in hospitals.

Our knowledge of the prevalence rates of HAIs in Australian emergency care is quite limited, as there has been no study to determine the true percentage of HAIs that are directly attributable to pre-hospital and hospital-related emergency care. A recent point prevalence study of HAIs in 19 acute care public hospitals in Australia suggests an overall HAI prevalence of patients with an HAI of 9.9% (363 HAIs in 273 patients; 95% CI: 8.8-11.0) ranging from 5.7% to 17.0%. This study revealed a significant association between HAI and acute care settings. According to Russo et al, out of 273 patients with HAI, 230 patients were admitted through non-elective emergency admissions, accounting for 84.2% of the total HAI presentations.[46]

Notwithstanding, HAIs are known to be associated with increased mortality and morbidity, increased length of stay, and increased risks of antimicrobials resistance.[44,48] Those who acquire an infection during their journey through healthcare facilities will need to bear substantial health costs, which is estimated to be an increase of 8.6% to the cost of a patient's admission.[49] Globally, HAIs generate excessive anguish and discomfort for patients, their families and the healthcare staff involved in caring for these patients.[44,50]

Though HAIs are generally characterised to be preventable adverse events of patients' exposure to microorganisms, the challenges for their control and prevention grow as populations grow and comorbidities increase globally. The current evidence highlights the importance of implementing national surveillance systems for HAI, as well as having consistent, high-quality and safe strategies for IPC across all healthcare settings.[45,51] Implementation of national surveillance systems for HAI, together with effective IPC practices in hospital and pre-hospital emergence care settings, can contribute to warrant high-quality healthcare for patients and a safe working environment for all groups of emergency healthcare workers.[52]

27.3 Infection prevention and control in emergency care

As outlined earlier, the emergency healthcare taskforce is required to provide clinical care to patients where there is often a serious, unprecedented or potentially dangerous situation mandating immediate action to deliver efficient and effective care to warrant patient safety. The complex combination of time pressure and high-stakes care makes emergency care quite unique in the sense that rapid and aggressive interventions should be instituted for patients who often present with complex clinical pictures, injuries or life-threatening conditions. As such, the emergency care settings harbour a unique set of characteristics which may constitute a special context-specific risk profile for HAI, which may differ from that found in non-acute healthcare settings.

Infection prevention and control programs described in Chapters 4 and 7 are critical to the sustained IPC practices across all healthcare facilities, including emergency care. These programs consist of formal processes, measures and structures that collectively aim to break the chain of infection and reduce the risk of transmission of infectious disease. However, there are variations to be expected in implementing the programs at local levels, on the ground of the legislative and statutory differences between states and territories.[5] Australian emergency care is supplied by several national standards, guidelines and policies which render the infection prevention principles and priority areas for action (Table 27.7).[5,29,53-55]

Healthcare facilities are required to develop and implement an infection control management plan (ICMP), a formal and systematic clinical governance process that enables healthcare facilities to meet their IPC obligations in accordance with their corporate missions and visions. Emergency care facilities, managerial stakeholders and emergency clinicians benchmark their IPC protocols and processes against these to tailor management plans specific to their local settings. Successful implementation of ICMP in emergency care settings is founded upon the principles outlined under the IPC systems criteria in NSQHS Preventing and Controlling Infections Standard.[5] All emergency clinicians, whether in pre-hospital or in the hospital settings, must adjust their practice such that they are in accord with the two-tiered system of standard precautions and transmission-based precautions.[5,29,53]

27.3.1 Standard precautions

Standard precautions describe the basic IPC practices to be followed by clinical and non-clinical healthcare workers involved in patient care. These involve a set of universal precautions to be performed for all patients, regardless of their diagnosis and potential risk of infection.[53] The following standard precautions should always be used when providing emergency care in any emergency care facility (e.g. in an ambulance or in a hospital ED).

Hand hygiene: Hand hygiene must be performed in accordance with the '5 Moments for Hand Hygiene'.[56] This includes before touching a patient, before a procedure, after a procedure or body-fluid exposure risk, after touching a patient, and after touching a patient's surroundings. Hands should be washed with soap and water when visibly dirty. This includes the circumstances when hands are contaminated with proteinaceous material, or visibly soiled with blood or other body fluids, or if exposure to potential spore-forming organisms is strongly suspected or proven, or after using the bathroom. For all emergency clinical situations where hands are visibly clean, alcohol-based hand rubs containing at least 70% ethanol or equivalent solutions should be

TABLE 27.7 Key IPC program resources supporting the Australian emergency care professionals

Guidelines	Developed by	Aim and scope
Australian Guidelines for the Prevention and Control of Infection in Healthcare[53]	National Health and Medical Research Council (NHMRC), Australian Commission on Safety and Quality in Health Care (ACSQHC)	Renders a nationally agreed-upon approach to infection prevention and control and incorporates core principles and priority areas for action for healthcare workers and healthcare facilities
The National Safety and Quality Health Service (NSQHS): Preventing and Controlling Infections Standard[5]	Australian Commission on Safety and Quality in Health Care (ACSQHC)	Describes the systems and strategies to prevent infection, effectively manage infections, confine the development of antimicrobial resistance through effective antimicrobial stewardship, and promote use of infection prevention and control resources
Series of National Guidelines for Communicable Diseases or SoNGs[55]	Communicable Diseases Network Australia (CDNA), Australian Heath Protection Principal Committee (AHPPC)	Provides nationally consistent guidance to public health units in responding to a notifiable disease event. The guidelines are disease-specific and provide comprehensive, up-to-date information and protocols informed by health professionals, experts and available research
Guidelines to reducing the spread of communicable infectious disease in the emergency department[29]	Australasian College for Emergency Medicine (ACEM)	Outlines the Australasian College for Emergency Medicine's recommendations and guidelines for ED staff to reduce the likelihood of spreading communicable infectious diseases in the emergency department (ED)

used. Hand hygiene must also be performed after removal of gloves.[53]

Personal protective equipment (PPE): Examples of PPE include, but are not limited to, gloves, goggles, face masks, face shields, impervious gowns and overalls, leggings, shoe covers, boots and earplugs. Non-sterile single-use medical gloves should be used whenever there is a potential for exposure to blood or any bodily substances, or when the condition necessitates contact with patients' non-intact skin or mucous membranes. This equipment is commonly used on ambulances and in EDs for processes and procedures such as venepuncture, general medical examination, examining and dressing abrasions and minor cuts, advancing a naso-gastric tube and emptying a urinary catheter.[57]

Sterile gloves must be used for aseptic procedures and contact with sterile sites (e.g. any surgical procedure, wound examination and dressing if direct contact with wound is anticipated, insertion and changing of intravascular access devices, urinary catheterisation and lumbar puncture). Gloves must be changed between patients and after every episode of individual patient care.

Aprons or gowns should be clean and fit for purpose. All paramedics and emergency clinicians in EDs should wear aprons or gowns whenever there is a risk of contamination of skin, uniforms, scrubs or other clothing

with patients' blood, bodily substances and other potentially infectious materials. They should be worn for a single procedure or during an episode of patient care. A face mask, face shield or goggles must be worn during procedures that generate aerosols, splashes or sprays of blood, bodily fluids, secretions or excretions into the face and eyes.[53,58]

All emergency care professionals should be well trained and be competent in the procedures and sequences of donning and doffing in any emergency care settings, as depicted in Chapter 13 and Chapter 14.

Aseptic technique: Aseptic technique consists of a set of specific infection prevention practices and procedures performed under carefully controlled conditions to protect patients during clinical procedures by using infection prevention measures that minimise the presence of microorganisms. Aseptic techniques include two main types: *standard* (also known as aseptic non-touch technique—ANTT) and *surgical*, and both are employed in emergency care settings (further detailed in Chapter 13).[59-61] Both types of aseptic techniques assert that no direct contact should be made between any sterile items that are to be administered on patient and the healthcare workers' hands or the surrounding environment (e.g. clothing, bedding or bedside table).[62] In general, aseptic techniques consist of five essential components:[53]

- *Sequencing:* To ensure efficient, logical and safe order of procedure events, the practice should be sequenced. Practice guidelines should be used to advise on the correct order of actions for any given procedure.
- *Environmental control:* Emergency clinicians must identify and address any avoidable environmental risks prior to performing an aseptic procedure (e.g. patient bed curtains, cleaning of the trays, trolleys and bedside and bed making).
- *Hand hygiene:* Performing effective and proper hand hygiene before and after glove use.
- *PPE selection:* Correct PPE should be selected and used for the task.
- *Maintenance of aseptic fields:* Clinicians must determine the aseptic field required for a given procedure. Depending on the procedure, the aseptic field may need to be extended by draping the patient. A single-use antiseptic skin solution should be used where skin antisepsis is required to prepare a patient for an emergency aseptic procedure, such as a peripheral intravenous cannulation, a central line insertion or a lumbar puncture.
- *Non-touch techniques:* All ED clinicians should adhere to safe injection practices and avoid touching the sterile components of equipment (e.g. needle hubs, syringe tips, dressing packs and bungs).

It is equally imperative to review aseptic technique competence and audit compliance on an ongoing basis, and use performance measure in IPC through the review of healthcare records, at the point of care, or both.[61]

Safe handling and disposal of sharps: Needles must not be re-sheathed, broken, bent or disassembled after use. Handing of sharp equipment should be kept to a minimum and sharps must not be passed from hand to hand. The person who is using the sharp is responsible for its immediate safe disposal. Used sharps must be discarded into an approved sharps container at the point of use. Overfilling the sharp containers (above the mark that indicates that three-quarters of the container is full) should be avoided.[53,60]

Sterile instruments and devices: Sterile items in emergency care mainly include reusable medical devices (RMDs) sterilised within the healthcare facility and the sterile items supplied by commercial suppliers. All these items shall be stored and handled in a manner that maintains the integrity of packs, and therefore prevents contamination. RMDs must be adequately reprocessed between patients to mitigate the risk of indirect contact transmission.[5] Critical equipment used in direct clinical care or resuscitation ought to be cleaned and disinfected or sterilised between each patient use according to the manufacturer's instructions. Above and beyond the ED practices, a comprehensive sterilisation program should be implemented by hospitals and ambulance services to warrant the consistency of sterilisation practices.[53,63] Common methods for reprocessing RMD in emergency care are described in Chapters 15 and 16.

Routine environmental cleaning and disinfection: Frequently touched surfaces must be cleaned with detergent solution at least daily, or after every conspicuous contamination. General surfaces and fittings must be cleaned when visibly soiled and immediately after spillage. Shared clinical equipment should be cleaned with detergent solution between patient uses. Clinical surfaces (including equipment) that are touched frequently with gloved hands during the delivery of patient care must be protected with surface barriers. The same rule applies to surfaces that are likely to become contaminated with patient blood or other body substances, or are difficult to clean.[53,64]

Cleaning spills of blood or other body substances or any infectious materials is important in prevention and control of HAIs in emergency care. Cleaning must be carried out immediately upon detection by practising the following sequence:[53]

(a) wear utility gloves and other task-appropriate PPE

(b) confine and contain spill

(c) clean visible spill and discard the consumed cleaning materials into appropriate waste streams

(d) clean the area with detergent solution. Choice of chemical disinfectant is based on risk assessment of transmission of infectious agents from that spill.

27.3.2 Transmission-based precautions

Transmission-based precautions are additional IPC interventional practices in situations where standard precautions alone are deemed insufficient to prevent transmission. These specific interventions are applied to patients suspected or confirmed to be infected, aiming to control infection by interrupting the transmission of an infection agent. The application of transmission-based precautions in healthcare is more broadly described in Chapter 14.

Australian emergency departments operate such that they can identify and assess any patients presenting with potential infectious diseases at their triage (hazard identification).[29,54] A common practice called 'syndromic surveillance' refers to exploring febrile patients at the triage stage for a certain combination of symptoms (e.g. fever and rash, fever and respiratory illness, or fever and gastrointestinal illness) to stratify their risk and take appropriate and timely measures (e.g. isolating affected patients).[27,29,65] Additional travel surveillances operate at triage in all cases of actual or reported fever. Consideration will be given to isolating the patients harbouring a high risk for infectious diseases.

Furthermore, Australia has an established national system of surveillance, the National Notifiable Diseases Surveillance System (NNDSS), which was established in 1990. The system operates to record and track the control and prevention of infectious diseases for which transmission-based precautions have been employed.[66,67] It coordinates surveillance of over 50 infectious diseases by generating notifications to the relevant state or territory health authorities under the provisions of the jurisdictional public health legislation. At time of writing, the NNDSS is in the process of being decommissioned and replaced but continues to publish fortnightly disease surveillance reports under the CDNA. Australian emergency services have had, and will continue to have, an active role in such surveillance systems to ensure timely reporting of notifiable diseases to relevant national and state or territory health authorities.[66]

Recent research has argued in favour of characterising transmission modes and their recommended precautions along a continuous spectrum, as opposed to the discrete categories of 'contact', 'droplet' and 'airborne'. Specifically, this model aims to dispose of the arbitrary cut-off currently differentiating droplet and airborne transmissions based on particle size. Furthermore, the advent of COVID-19 has highlighted that diseases can be transmitted via multiple pathways and that combinations of measures must also be carefully considered and exercised when appropriate. Nevertheless, in emergency care the precautions distinguished for contact, droplet and airborne transmitted diseases are still endorsed in most active standards and guidelines. The following guidelines summarise the precautions described in both the NSQHS Standards' 'Preventing and Controlling Infections Standard', and the Australasian College for Emergency Medicine's guideline, 'Reducing the spread of communicable infectious disease in the emergency department'.[29,53]

Contact precautions: Ambulance services and EDs must implement contact precautions in addition to standard precautions when they have a presentation of a patient confirmed or suspected to be infected with agents that are known to spread via direct or indirect contact with the patient or the patient's environment. When working with patients who require contact precautions, all emergency care clinicians must perform hand hygiene (e.g. washing hands with soap and water, pat drying with single-use towels, and using alcohol-based hand rubs). Hand sanitiser dispensers are readily available and accessible within the ED, and at the ED front counter and entrances. Adequate resourcing of hand hygiene devices and regular auditing take place to ensure hand hygiene compliance.[29,53]

Protocols for gloves and proper PPE donning and doffing must be adhered to so to ensure that clothing and skin is not at risk of being contaminated via contact with environmental surfaces. Disposable single-use patient-care equipment (e.g. blood pressure cuffs or stethoscope) or patient-dedicated equipment are to be used whenever possible and such equipment must be disposed of into appropriate waste streams after use.[53]

Consideration should be given to patient placement, particularly in an ED setting. Depending on the resources and existing arrangements, a single-patient room is recommended to isolate patients who require contact precautions. If isolation is not possible, cohorting of patients may be considered in consultation with infection control professionals.[29,54] As per the existing recommendations, patient beds should be separated by approximately one metre or more to minimise the risk of inadvertent sharing of items between patients.[68] If common use of equipment for multiple patients is unavoidable, clean the equipment and allow it to dry before use on another patient. It is generally advised to limit the transfer of patients on contact precautions to reduce the risk of environmental contamination within the healthcare facility. When these patients are transferred within emergency care settings (e.g. from ambulance to ED), or to other facilities (e.g. admitted from ED to wards), the colonised/infected areas of the patient's body must be contained and covered.

Droplet precautions: Droplet precautions must be implemented in addition to standard precautions for patients confirmed or suspected to be infected with agents spread by large respiratory droplets that are generated by coughing, sneezing, talking or during suctioning. Similar patient placement measures as to those outlined for contact precautions are applicable to patients put on droplet precaution (isolation and cohorting). Emergency care staff should explain to the patients on droplet precautions the importance of respiratory hygiene and appropriate cough etiquette and need to consider patients' ability to perform these practices. All emergency clinicians and support staff must put on a surgical mask when coming into contact with those patients.[53]

When transferring a patient on droplet precautions within or between healthcare services or facilities, it is necessary to ask the patient to wear a fluid resistant surgical mask and adhere to respiratory hygiene and cough etiquette while they are being transferred. In the paediatric emergency setting, it is important to provide children with a correctly fitting mask and monitor their oxygen saturation.[53,54]

Airborne precautions: Airborne precautions must be implemented for patients confirmed or suspected to be infected with agents transmitted by increasingly small respiratory droplets or airborne particles (Fig 27.4). As previously mentioned, guidelines have differentiated airborne and droplet transmission based on a hard cut-off in droplet size. While this cut-off distinction is debatable, it remains critical for emergency workers to exercise additional precautions for infectious disease with droplets small enough to travel and remain suspended in the air for extended periods. Clinical and non-clinical staff who come into contact with these patients must wear a correctly fitted P2 (N95) respirator. Patients on airborne precautions must be placed in negative-pressure rooms or in a room from which the air does not circulate to other areas. Patients should also be asked to wear a surgical mask while not in a single room, until advised to remove it by attending emergency staff.

The use of nebulisers is preferably to be avoided in ED patients presenting with fever and lower respiratory tract symptoms, or those suspected of having an infectious disease with the potential of airborne or droplet

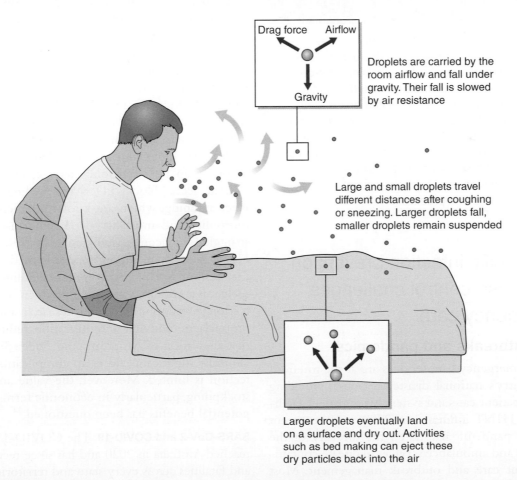

Drag force   Airflow

Gravity

Droplets are carried by the room airflow and fall under gravity. Their fall is slowed by air resistance

Large and small droplets travel different distances after coughing or sneezing. Larger droplets fall, smaller droplets remain suspended

Larger droplets eventually land on a surface and dry out. Activities such as bed making can eject these dry particles back into the air

FIGURE 27.4 Respiratory droplets vary in size, which affects how far the droplets travel when expelled and how long they remain suspended in the air

transmission. If nebulisers are administered, patients should be treated in a room isolated from other patients, with attending staff undertaking appropriate precaution measures.[53,68] Diagnostic procedures such as nasopharyngeal swabs and aspirates can be performed in ED provided that the staff are wearing appropriate PPE.

Visitors should be restricted, but if needed, they must be screened by emergency nursing staff and their details should be recorded.[29,53] Patients should be asked to wear a correctly fitted surgical mask when their transfer outside the negative pressure room is necessitated. During the transfer, the patient ought to follow respiratory hygiene and cough etiquette. To reduce the risk of cross-transmission, any skin lesions associated with the condition (e.g. shingles or chickenpox) should be covered safely.[29]

PRACTICE TIP 1

TAKING CARE WITH TRANSMISSION-BASED PRECAUTIONS

Applying transmission-based precautions may generate unintended adverse psycho-behavioural effects. Some patients who are receiving emergency care and are put on transmission-based precautions may experience anxiety, mood disturbances and/or perceptions of stigma. To alleviate these effects and establish rapport with the patient, it is critical to clearly explain to the patient why these precautions are applied and how they help to maintain the safety of patients and staff, and to answer questions they may have about those practices.

27.4 Specific infection prevention and disease control challenges in emergency care

27.4.1 Outbreaks and pandemics

Australia's emergency care services are at the forefront of the country's national disaster response, providing immediate patient care and system-wide patient facilitation. The H1N1 influenza in 2009 and the recent COVID-19 pandemic illustrated the diversity of the roles of EDs and ambulance services in disease containment, patient care and outbreak management. Most Australian EDs operate over capacity, and are therefore prone to be overwhelmed during large-scale disease outbreaks. Adding to this are the taskforce shortages which may be further aggravated by quarantine requirements when staff are found to be exposed to suspected or confirmed infected patients.[41,69,70]

Influenza: Influenza is a contagious and acute viral infection that attacks the respiratory system. Multiple strains of influenza have been encountered globally. The pathogenicity of avian influenza changes as the virus mutates and spreads between host populations and can result in severe disease. Those strains with the highest mortality rates are referred to as 'highly pathogenic avian influenza' (HPAI) and are thought to have evolved from the 2003 strain (H5N1) found in Asia that spread to most parts of the world through migratory birds and the poultry trade. An outbreak of H5N1 can cause severe and sometimes fatal infections in humans, and if significant enough, could have devastating economic and social impacts on Australia.

The 2009 H1N1 influenza outbreak demonstrated the diversity of roles of EDs in disease containment and management, but also provided an opportunity to describe the extended clinical impact of pandemic disease. Public awareness of H1N1 influenza 2009 led to many patients presenting with flu-like illnesses to both EDs and primary healthcare (including general practitioners), leading to a greater workload of EDs and ambulance services. This impact occurred at a time when Australian emergency care was confronting continual problems of overcrowding associated with access block and growing demand. Some states reported up to a ten-fold increase, resulting in increased access block, ED overcrowding and ambulance ramping, which are known to increase patient morbidity and mortality.[71,72] Furthermore, hospitals struggled to acquire sufficient supplies to care for H1N1 patients, including transport media for laboratory testing, masks, N95 respirators, disinfectant wipes, oseltamivir (Tamiflu) and other products needed for infection prevention.[73] While research indicates that prophylactic antiviral administration reduces time to first alleviation of symptoms, the evidence supporting clinically significant effects on complications from infection is limited. Moreover, the value and utility of stockpiling, particularly in economic terms, relative to potential benefits has been questioned.[74]

SARS-CoV-2 and COVID-19: The COVID-19 pandemic reached Australia in 2020 and has since recorded cases and fatalities across every state and territories.[75] Due to restrictions on mobility, and public hesitation and fear of visiting hospitals, the early months of the pandemic saw a decline of 1.4% in ED presentations compared to the same period in the previous year.[9] However, EDs were still constantly challenged, having to rapidly adapt their responses and procedures as new information on the novel virus and its spread emerged. During this time, studies observed ambulances showed longer response and case times, in addition to greater hospital delays, which were likely the result of ED crowding and limited capacity during lockdown.[76,77] Furthermore, healthcare workers were found to be at a significantly higher risk of infection compared to the general public.[78,79] This was particularly serious when PPE was inadequately donned, or reused, a practice which was further exacerbated by the fear of supply shortages during the beginning of the pandemic.[78,80,81] Additionally, outbreaks within the healthcare workforce were common and especially devastating. Quarantine and self-isolation was the first line of defence in preventing virus spread and this resulted in considerable reductions in the workforce.[82]

Frontline workers were prioritised during the first national rollout of COVID-19 vaccines in early 2021.[82] However, response to the virus must continue to adapt to the new and emerging variants and the waning protection offered by existing vaccinations over time.[83] The easing of restrictions upon reaching vaccination thresholds in late 2021 was met with record case numbers and fatalities, along with an increasing resurgence of ED presentations in 2020–21.[9,84]

Effective management of pandemics requires whole-of-hospital and whole-of-healthcare involvement, which necessitates the integration of ED plans into both. To enhance the preparedness of emergency care in Australia and New Zealand, the Australasian College of Emergency Medicine has developed guidelines to assist emergency clinicians with decisions about planning and redesigning appropriate healthcare in EDs during the COVID-19 pandemic and outbreaks of future emerging infectious diseases.[8] The guidelines suggest ED-centred measures that align with 'Australian Health Sector Emergency Response Plan for Novel Coronavirus COVID-19' and 'Australian Government, Emergency Response Plan for Communicable Disease Incidents of National Significance: National Arrangements', and are recommended to be implemented in conjunction with state and territory plans.[85] In preparation for a pandemic, EDs and other emergency care services are required to take context-specific measures to address four goals (Table 27.8):[54]

(a) To decrease service demands

(b) To increase service capacity

(c) To maintain healthcare system flow

(d) To advance communications.

The COVID-19 pandemic highlighted the necessity of initiating clinical redesign processes to change the layout and flow of emergency care services in preparation for managing outbreaks or pandemics. In response to the COVID-19 pandemic, EDs developed clear risk assessment processes to identify and isolate patients who may be a source of disease transmission.[8,86] Figure 27.5 illustrates an example of a simple risk stratification system linked to IPC procedures in the context of the COVID-19 pandemic.

TABLE 27.8   ED-specific measures in preparation for and response to a pandemic of emerging infectious diseases

Type of measures	Recommendations and advocacy
Measures to decrease ED demand	1. Health services develop clear agreement with external stakeholders and ambulance services regarding transport and reception of patients (especially special populations such as frail older persons) 2. Hospitals develop procedures to defer patients to alternative health services (e.g. private hospitals) or defer time of presentation (e.g. electives) 3. Hospitals redeploy non-ED staff (within their scope of practice) to assess acute, low-risk COVID-19 patients outside the ED (e.g. in clinics, in the community or on wards) 4. Hospitals support early redirection of patients seeking public health screening with mild respiratory symptoms to screening clinics 5. Hospitals improve telehealth support for a range of clinical services 6. Use of preexisting social and traditional media avenues (e.g. mobile apps) to inform patients of appropriate use of emergency services 7. Other specialties urgently develop processes for patients to be reviewed without transit through the ED 8. Algorithms of pre-hospital services are redirected away from the ED (e.g. 13 Health)

Continued

TABLE 27.8 ED-specific measures in preparation for and response to a pandemic of emerging infectious diseases—cont'd

Type of measures	Recommendations and advocacy
Measures to increase ED capacity	1. Urgent measures are required to increase ED staff, equipment and treatment spaces in the short term 2. Health services actively increase work hours of existing staff for those willing to do so who are not full time and recruit additional healthcare staff in the short term 3. Health services utilise other non-ED staff in the low-risk COVID-ED for suitable cases (e,g, orthopaedic registrars for limb injuries, gynaecology registrars for early pregnancy bleeding) 4. Health services consider changing or increasing the footprint of EDs and short stay units to meet demand 5. Health services optimise patient flow in preparation for increased presentations. This is especially important for ICU and respiratory cases 6. Tertiary paediatric hospitals take paediatric presentations away from other hospitals in order to increase capacity to treat unwell adults in those hospitals
Measures to maintain healthcare system flow	1. 'Hub' hospitals maintain their support of, and accountability to, surrounding smaller facilities, although specifics of that support will change with each pandemic phase 2. There are agreed methods of medical evacuation of COVID-19 and non-COVID-19 patients from hub hospitals back to smaller facilities or community services 3. Communication is improved between hospitals and health services and key community services including RACFs and primary care 4. There is collaboration with private hospitals and other healthcare facilities 5. Non-essential education and clinical support time is re-purposed to contribute to the pandemic response 6. Health services assess their capacity to provide non-critical elective surgery during the pandemic 7. Health services assess their capacity to provide non-critical outpatient clinics during the pandemic 8. There is escalation to hospital management or public health unit if there are obstacles to transfer of care on the basis of infection control concerns
Measures to advance communication	1. A single 'point of truth' for rapid communication and dissemination of reliable clinical information that applies at state and national levels 2. Coordination and clear lines of communication in critical care networks at a local, regional, statewide and national level 3. Agreed clinical pathways and thresholds for intervention are shared between all critical care services 4. Agreed referral and communication (including telehealth) pathways between rural, regional and larger metropolitan sites 5. Agreed communication pathways between frontline clinicians and governance networks to inform of rapidly changing policy 6. Agreed public and private healthcare network communication strategies to coordinate response

Source: ACEM, 2020.[54]

In the event of an outbreak of an infectious disease, EDs must consider structural changes to triage, reception, waiting areas and in the interest of patient and staff safety. Specific measures can be implemented to stream patients into dedicated 'high-risk' treatment zones or cohorting the patients, depending on the infrastructural capacity of the ED. Prioritisation of treatment spaces should be based on IPC needs relevant to the infectious agents.[8,54] A hierarchy of isolated treatment spaces in ED can be used, factoring in the mode of transmission and the level of risk the patient poses (Fig 27.6).

In some health emergencies, such as outbreaks of highly transmissible infectious diseases, clinical processes may be subject to rapid and frequent change as information emerges for the safety of emergency care staff and other patients. The experience from COVID-19 illustrates that healthcare workers, especially those undertaking critical care procedures, are at a significant risk of contracting infection.[87] To maintain the safety of the emergency care professionals, clinical guidelines and algorithms for critical patients, such as trauma patients or those needing resuscitation, should be reviewed against appropriate IPC guidelines and practices.[88,89] Figure 27.7 illustrates an example of a CPR algorithm proposed and used in Royal Hobart Hospital in Tasmania during the COVID-19 pandemic.

Acute severe respiratory illness or anticipated to need aerosol-generating procedure	• PPE for aerosol-generating procedures • Negative pressure room if available, otherwise single room
Clinical and/or epidemiological risk factors	• PPE for droplet precautions • Single room wherever possible, otherwise cohorted with patients of similar risk
Other patients	• Usual ED care in low-risk zone or other designated area

Note that risk stratification may change as the pandemic progresses

FIGURE 27.5 Example of a simple risk stratification system in EDs during pandemic
Source:[54]

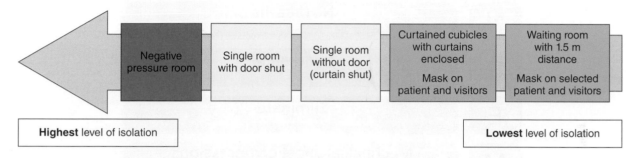

| Negative pressure room | Single room with door shut | Single room without door (curtain shut) | Curtained cubicles with curtains enclosed

Mask on patient and visitors | Waiting room with 1.5 m distance

Mask on selected patient and visitors |

Highest level of isolation   **Lowest** level of isolation

FIGURE 27.6 Hierarchy of isolated treatment spaces in the context of COVID-19 pandemic
Source:[54]

IPC PRECAUTIONS FOR RESPIRATORY EMERGENCIES

Paramedics and ambulance first responders who become involved in assessing or treating self-quarantined or isolated patients with COVID-19 must apply the following measures:

• Use contact and droplet precautions for routine care of patients

• Use contact and airborne precautions when performing aerosol-generating procedures, including intubation and cardiopulmonary resuscitation (CPR)

• Provide advance notice to the receiving destination to clarify transfer of care arrangements

27.4.2 High-consequence infectious diseases in emergency care

High-consequence infectious diseases (HCIDs) are defined as acute infectious diseases that have a high case mortality, are highly communicable, and are difficult to prevent, contain and treat (see Chapter 23). When a

patient is suspected of having an HCID, EDs should consider activating their disaster plan to reduce the risk of transmission. The hospital needs to be involved to prioritise the adequate isolation of the patient, which may involve safe transfer to a proper isolation facility elsewhere in the same hospital or at another hospital. During the transfer of these patients, consideration should be given to clearing corridors of unnecessary traffic, clearing the ED of access-blocked patients, and moving waiting patients to other designated areas. Managing HCID patients should be done by those who are sufficiently trained and have PPE appropriate for the purpose.[29]

INDICATIONS FOR IMMEDIATE SOURCE ISOLATION

Patients presenting with the following symptoms should be actively considered for source isolation in single rooms or areas:

• Fever and rash, or

• Fever and respiratory illness, or

• Fever and gastrointestinal illness

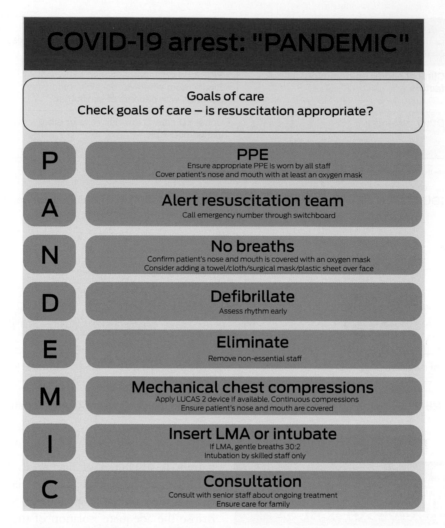

FIGURE 27.7 Resuscitation algorithm during COVID-19 pandemic (Royal Hobart Hospital, Tasmania)

Source: Craig, S., Cubitt, M., Jaison, A., Troupakis, S., Hood, N., Fong, C., ... & Cameron, P. A. (2020). Management of adult cardiac arrest in the COVID-19 era: consensus statement from the Australasian College for Emergency Medicine. Medical Journal of Australia, 213(3), 126–133.[88]

Viral haemorrhagic fever (VHF) is the term for an infectious and life-threatening syndrome of acute and severe febrile illness caused by a large group of viruses from four families, namely Arenaviridae, Bunyaviridae, Filoviridae and Flaviviridae.[90,91] There are four VHFs of primary concern, none of which occur naturally in Australia: Lassa fever, Marburg virus haemorrhagic fever, Crimean–Congo haemorrhagic fever, and Ebola virus disease (EVD).[92] Further details about the symptomatology and epidemiological characteristics of these diseases are provided in Chapter 23.

VHFs are zoonotic diseases where humans accidentally or incidentally contract the virus and subsequently spread it via human-to-human contact. Transmission occurs via contact with mucous membranes or non-intact skin contacting blood or any bodily fluids or organs of an infected patient. Materials and surfaces soiled with those fluids (e.g. clothing, bedding) can also contribute in indirect transmission of VHFs.[91,93] In the clinical setting, inoculation through percutaneous injury or aerosolisation (potentially during procedures such as bronchoscopies, endotracheal intubation and ventilation) can lead to transmission of virus to healthcare staff. Particular attention should be paid to additional risks associated with non-invasive ventilation and mechanism to reduce exposure.

Emergency care professionals may come into contact with patients with suspected or confirmed VHF, with paramedics being potentially the first-hand contact involved in transferring a confirmed case. ED staff may be heavily involved in caring for VHF patients, especially if they are critically ill.[91] Healthcare workers who have followed the infection control recommendations, including wearing the appropriate PPE, are not considered to have exposure to EVD. A study of Australian emergency nurses' perceptions of preparedness for managing EVD stressed the importance of organisational planning for an appropriate response and the necessity of regular training in PPE use.[94] In addition to these, the psychological concerns that frontline healthcare workers would commonly encounter should be properly addressed. For example, concerns that emergency care professionals might inadvertently put themselves or their family members at risk of contracting infection when they are involved in the care of an HCID patient can be ameliorated by the implementation of active counselling and psychological support services.

27.4.3 Bloodstream infection and bacteraemia related to vascular devices

Bloodstream infections (BSI) account for significant morbidity and mortality in Australian healthcare facilities.[47] A recent Australian national point prevalence study of 19 acute care hospitals found 10.0% of HAIs are identified in association with bloodstream infections.[46] Staphylococcus aureus bacteraemia (SAB) is commonly associated with medical procedures, and is identified as a key performance indicator of quality of care across all acute hospitals in Australia.[95]

One of the common procedures used in emergency and critical care is the point of care ultrasound (PoCUS) percutaneous cannulation. While there is a growing body of evidence supporting the efficacy and safety of this practice,[96,97] there are significant risks to patients, especially for BSI and associated sepsis.[98] A recent study of an outbreak of Burkholderia cenocepacia bacteraemia in 11 patients in Australian EDs and ICUs identified contamination of sterile ultrasound gels that were used for central line insertion and other sterile procedures within four hospitals across Australia.[99]

Measures to protect patients from bacteraemia associated with invasive diagnostic or treatment procedures have not been as forthcoming as the popularity of these procedures. Emergency services must adhere to meticulous cleaning and decontamination practices to maintain the safety of semi-critical equipment.[53,100] Implementing the recommendations rendered in 'Guidelines for Reprocessing Ultrasound Transducers' can help emergency clinicians to limit the risk of HAI in EDs.[64] Furthermore, emergency clinicians should meet formal accreditation requirements in the use of PoCUS, especially since the PoCUS percutaneous cannulation is becoming a recognisable core skill in emergency practice. Training in PoCUS should include knowledge and skills for preventing and controlling the risk of HAIs.[100]

27.4.4 Bioterrorism

In general terms, bioterrorism involves the use, or threat of the use, of biological agents to create deliberate harm or fear to leverage a political, religious or other agenda.[101] Bioterrorism is widely recognised as an emerging public health issue of the 21st century, creating significant challenges for the entire healthcare system, including emergency care services. Responding to bioterrorism requires a high level of public health preparedness at an individual, healthcare system and societal level.

The anthrax threat that occurred in Australia in 2001 highlighted the necessity of multidisciplinary approaches to engage security and health intelligence to enable effective management of bioterrorism and biological emergencies.[102] Australia's biosecurity planning is built on several disease and disaster surveillance systems. Australia's federal system fosters integrative collaboration between the Commonwealth and state and territory governments. Emergency Management Australia coordinates the emergency service responses. Public health units and agencies work closely with emergency services and collaborate via the CDNA and the Public Health Laboratory Network (PHLN) to coordinate diagnostic activities and public health responses.[103-105]

The List of Security Sensitive Biological Agents (SSBA) and the SSBA Regulatory Scheme was established in the National Health Security Act 2007 and regulates the handling of biological agents and toxins that pose potential severe security risks and health impacts.[106,107] The agents on this list were rated highly across two risk assessment criteria: health impact and security threat. Health impact assessed human health outcomes, such as the morbidity, mortality, transmissibility and difficulty of treating the disease caused by the agent. Security threat assessed the level of interest in an agent for use by terrorist, criminal or issue-motivated groups of concern in Australia, and the feasibility and ease with which such groups could access and disseminate the agent. The most pernicious potential bioterrorism threats are expected to be in relation to smallpox, anthrax, botulism, plague and viral haemorrhagic fevers.[103,108]

Protocols informing public health unit responses exist in the form of national guidelines for diseases caused by several of these agents, such as smallpox and Ebola virus disease.[109,110] Emergency care clinicians must be provided with adequate resources and ongoing opportunities for clinical education and training in bioterrorism preparedness and management for these dangerous diseases.[101] Paramedics, emergency nurses and emergency physicians should be trained in how to seek specialist advice and guidance from relevant public health authorities at local and state levels. They must be well trained and capable of determining the nature of various biological threats, and should actively participate in preparing and implementing plans to manage these threats at their local facility.[111,112]

27.4.5 Infection in frail and vulnerable populations

Elderly: Elderly populations are more vulnerable for the acquisition of infections than the younger population. They are at an increased risk of infection-related morbidity and mortality as a result of the physiological changes associated with normal ageing.[113,114] Impaired cell-mediated and/or humoral immune responses result in defective host defences, and therefore a declination in the elderly's immune system function, which undermines their response to immunisations and medications. Other impaired physiological functions such as diminished cough reflex, urinary incontinence and reduced wound healing make them more prone to infections. Additional contributors include increased rate of comorbidities (e.g. diabetes, cancer and dementia) and use of multiple medications and medical devices.[115,116] Cognitive changes and/or impairment in mental status make it increasingly difficult to ensure older individuals adhere to all prophylactic measures.

For clinicians working in emergency care, the accurate and timely diagnosis of infections and HAIs in elderly individuals is not always straightforward. Typical signs of infection could be absent or obscured and emergency clinicians should be prepared to encounter non-classical presentation of infections in older patients. For example, patients may present with blunted or no fever, or with no productive cough or sputum despite having pneumonia, or without dysuria or other urinary symptoms of urinary tract infections.[116-118] Furthermore, dissociations in the observed vital signs in many elderly patients can mimic the signs of infection. Alterations in cognitive functioning and behavioural changes generate further barriers to establishing rapport and efficient communication. However, these conditions can be the only signs indicating infection in an older individual.[119]

The COVID-19 pandemic highlighted the disproportionate impact HAIs have on older people.[120] At time of writing, Australians over 60 years of age

comprise less than 10% of cases, yet account for over 90% of deaths.[84] Outbreaks in aged care facilities have been particularly devastating due to the close proximity of residents to each other and to care workers that were mobile within the general community.[82] While pandemic response guidelines for health and emergency care workers were available, inconsistency in preparation, training and execution resulted in multiple outbreaks across facilities and, subsequently, in many fatalities within this vulnerable population.[121] The clinical competence of emergency clinicians, especially in early recognition of infections and HAIs, and timely treatment have crucial importance in reducing the morbidity and mortality associated with HAI in this age group.

Children: A child's immune system is not as advanced and matured as that of an adult, hence putting them at a relatively increased risk for infections. Especially in younger children, the risk of vaccine-preventable infections is still high.[122] Children's dependency upon their parents or their adult caregivers has a direct impact on whether they are adhering to proper hygiene. Similar to adults, children are at risk from HAIs and immunocompromised children or those suffering from immunodeficiency syndromes are at a particularly greater risk, especially during an outbreak or an extended hospital admission.[123] Preparedness of emergency care for infection prevention in paediatric patients is a crucial element in ensuring patient safety and mitigating the risk of HAI in this group. EDs need to be equipped, and clinicians appropriately trained, with medical devices and supplies (such as intravenous kits, needles, endotracheal tubes), as well as the medication dosages that are specific to children.[5]

27.4.6 Issues for pre-hospital emergency care: ED–ambulance interface

In 2015, a paramedic in Queensland who was infectious with measles was on duty transporting patients between four major hospitals and several public locations.[124] The incident led to widespread contact tracing, screening and isolations to control the spread of the disease. Often, the care of a patient suffering from an emergency medical condition starts in a non-hospital setting, where paramedics arrive on-site and are the first to provide the emergency intervention. This practice imposes a high variability in the type of environment paramedics work in, which can frequently be unpredictable and potentially dangerous.[18,43,125] Furthermore, the advancing scope of practice and the evolving roles of paramedics applies additional pressure on paramedics when providing safe and quality care in the early stages of emergency care.[19] Performance of medical procedures in different, and often mobile, settings complicates the implementation of and adherence to standardised IPC practices.[42,126]

A recent Australian study of paramedics suggested that several factors can influence ICP practices in paramedic settings (Table 27.9), and further highlighted the need for the development of national IPC guidelines and audit tools for ambulance services, such that the idiosyncrasies and peculiarities of the paramedic work setting are recognised.[42]

Regardless of the setting and the degree of urgency, all paramedics should endeavour to identify the transmission risk factors as part of their patient assessment and safety measures.[53] Generally, four categories of transmission risk factors could be considered in ambulance settings:

1. *Procedure-related risks:* performing an invasive procedure makes a patient susceptible to contract infections

2. *Environment-related risks:* poor environmental hygiene and cleanliness may undermine the application of aseptic technique in ambulance settings

3. *Risks associated with medical equipment:* some equipment and stock must be used only if they are sterile. The risk of HAI may increase if maintenance of stock's sterility in a crowded, mobile and temperature labile environment is not assured

4. *Risk associated with reprocessing of equipment:* failure to reprocess reusable equipment after its use will increase the risk of indirect transmission to patients.[60]

Ambulance services and all agencies involved in patient transfer and transport must exercise standard precautions during the transfer and transport of any patient. When arranging for transferring or transporting a patient, all agencies involved in the activity should be notified of any patient with an identified infection risk prior to the transfer or transport of the patient.[5,63] Processes for communicating a patient's infectious status should be in place whenever a decision is made to transport a patient with a known or suspected infectious disease. Careful management of the transition between pre-hospital emergency care providers and ED can reduce the risk of infection in both the emergency care task force and admitted patients in the facility. To maintain the high standards of clinical care, ambulance services and EDs must work hand-in-hand to streamline the triaging and admission of patients who carry the risk of infection, and to minimise the delays in handover and exposures in ED corridor or in ambulance ramping areas.[54]

Conclusion

The issue of infectious diseases and healthcare-associated infections permeates all facets of the Australian healthcare system, including emergency care. In this chapter, we identified the key principles and practices of IPC specific to the context of emergency care and with respect to the characteristics, commonalities and idiosyncrasies across emergency care professionals. Specifically, we highlighted the importance of recognising potential risks for disease transmission in varying emergency care settings, and

TABLE 27.9 IPC practice challenges reported by Australian paramedics

Hand hygiene challenges	• Restricted ability to perform correct hand hygiene in some difficult clinical cases • Overuse of gloves, thereby affecting correct hand hygiene
Difficulties in environmental hygiene	• Varying cleaning standards among paramedic staff • Difficulties in the management of clinical waste • Difficulties in the cleaning of portable medical equipment such as computers, cardiac monitors/defibrillators and stethoscopes • Difficulties in cleaning the materials used to house patient care equipment • Advice about and surveillance of home laundering of uniforms • Difficulty with cohorting patients in multi-stretcher vehicles
Issues with vehicles and patient care equipment	• Operating in a confined space with recirculated air, particularly when transporting patients with respiratory conditions • Air conditioners with filters and UV lights to treat recirculated air, especially in the setting of droplet and aerosol transmission of pathogens due to extended periods of time involved with a patient in a closed environment • Difficulty in transporting contaminated equipment and linen safely • Contamination of mobile patient care equipment

Source: Barr N et al., 2017.[42]

stressed that all emergency patients should be assessed against potential risks for being infectious. Furthermore, it is imperative that emergency care professionals demonstrate sufficient clinical competence in using standard precautions and implementing appropriate transmission-based precaution measures to minimise the risk for disease transmission and HAI. We explained the dominant IPC challenges within emergency care and provided context-specific recommendations and practice advice that can help emergency care professionals provide safe and quality care.

Useful websites/resources

- Reducing the spread of communicable infectious disease in the emergency department guidelines. https://acem.org.au/getmedia/8c142867-8286-4294-b096-b463e771a669/G26-Guidelines-for-Infectious-Disease-and-Biohazard-Exposure-in-the-ED-v03.aspx
- Clinical Guidelines for the management of COVID-19 in Australasian emergency departments (v5.0). https://acem.org.au/getmedia/78105c4b-5195-43f6-9c91-25dda5604eaf/Clinical-Guidelines
- ACEM's Position Statement re cleaning and disinfection of ultrasound transducers. https://acem.org.au/getmedia/850165eb-0b9b-4aab-82f6-da91b737e406/S686_v1_Statement_Cleaning_Ultrasound_Transducers

References

1. Schneider SM, Hamilton GC, Moyer P, Stapczynski JS. Definition of emergency medicine. Academic Emergency Medicine. 1998;5(4):348-351.
2. Independent Hospital Pricing Authority (IHPA). Emergency care [cited 28 March 2022]. Available from: https://www.ihpa.gov.au/what-we-do/emergency-care.
3. The Australasian College for Emergency Medicine (ACEM). Responsibility for care in emergency departments. In: ACEM, editor. Policy P182020.
4. World Health Organization (WHO). Emergency care - Overview [cited 28 March 2022]. Available from: https://www.who.int/health-topics/emergency-care#tab=tab_1.
5. Australian Commission on Safety and Quality in Health Care (ACSQHC). National safety and quality health service standards. 2nd ed. – version 2. NSQHS. Sydney, Australia: ACSQHC, 2021.
6. Baier N, Geissler A, Bech M, Bernstein D, Cowling TE, Jackson T, et al. Emergency and urgent care systems in Australia, Denmark, England, France, Germany and the Netherlands - analyzing organization, payment and reforms. Health Policy. 2019;123(1):1-10.
7. Eastwood K, Smith K, Morgans A, Stoelwinder J. Appropriateness of cases presenting in the emergency department following ambulance service secondary telephone triage: a retrospective cohort study. BMJ Open. 2017;7(10):e016845.
8. The Australasian College for Emergency Medicine (ACEM). Emergency department design guidelines (v3.0). 2014.
9. Australian Institute of Health and Welfare (AIHW). Emergency department care 2020–21 data tables Canberra, Australia: AIHW, 2021 [cited 25 March 2022]. Available from: https://www.aihw.gov.au/reports-data/myhospitals/sectors/emergency-department-care.
10. Eastwood K, Morgans A, Smith K, Hodgkinson A, Becker G, Stoelwinder J. A novel approach for managing the growing demand for ambulance services by low-acuity patients. Australian Health Review. 2015;40(4):378-84.
11. Forero R, Nugus P. Australasian College for Emergency Medicine (ACEM) literature review on the Australasian triage scale (ATS). Institute of Health Innovation, 2012.
12. The Australasian College for Emergency Medicine. Guidelines on the implementation of the Australasian Triage Scale in emergency departments. Melbourne, Australia: ACEM, 2016.
13. Nahidi S, Forero R, Man N, Mohsin M, Fitzgerald G, Toloo G, et al. Impact of the Four-Hour Rule/National Emergency Access Target policy implementation on emergency department staff: a qualitative perspective of emergency department management changes. Emergency Medicine Australasia. 2019;31(3):362-71.
14. NSW Government Department of Health. Emergency Department Care 2021 [cited 28 March 2022]. Available from: https://www.health.nsw.gov.au/Performance/Pages/emergency.aspx.
15. New South Wales Health. Emergency Department Care New South Wales, Australia: New South Wales Health, 2021 [cited 28 March 2022].
16. Australian Institute of Health and Welfare (AIHW). Emergency department care 2019–20 data tables Canberra: Australia: AIHW, 2020 [cited 05 June 2021]. Available from: https://www.aihw.gov.au/reports-data/myhospitals/sectors/emergency-department-care.
17. Fry M. Overview of emergency nursing in Australasia. International Emergency Nursing. 2008;16(4):280-6.
18. O'Meara P, Reynolds L. Paramedics in Australia. Frenchs Forrest, NSW: Pearson, 2009.
19. Long DN, Lea J, Devenish S. The conundrum of defining paramedicine: more than just what paramedics 'do'. Australasian Journal of Paramedicine. 2018;15(1).
20. Paramedics Australasia. Paramedicine role descriptions. Paramedics Australasia, 2009.
21. Australian Institute of Health and Welfare (AIHW). Emergency department care 2015–16: Australian hospital statistics. Canberra: Australia: AIHW, 2016.
22. Australian Institute of Health and Welfare (AIHW). Emergency department care 2016–17: Australian hospital statistics. Canberra: Australia: AIHW, 2017.
23. Australian Institute of Health and Welfare (AIHW). Emergency department care 2017–18: Australian hospital statistics. Canberra: Australia: AIHW, 2018.

24. Australian Institute of Health and Welfare (AIHW). Emergency department care 2014–15: Australian hospital statistics. Canberra: Australia: AIHW, 2015.

25. Australian Institute of Health and Welfare (AIHW). Emergency department care 2018–19 data tables Canberra: Australia: AIHW, 2019 [cited 5 June 2021]. Available from: https://www.aihw.gov.au/reports-data/myhospitals/sectors/emergency-department-care.

26. Burrell AR, McLaws ML, Fullick M, Sullivan RB, Sindhusake D. SEPSIS KILLS: early intervention saves lives. Med J Aust. 2016;204(2):73.

27. Patocka C, Turner J, Xue X, Segal E. Evaluation of an emergency department triage screening tool for suspected severe sepsis and septic shock. Journal for Healthcare Quality. 2014;36(1):52-61.

28. Lelubre C, Vincent JL. Mechanisms and treatment of organ failure in sepsis. Nat Rev Nephrol. 2018;14(7):417-27.

29. The Australasian College for Emergency Medicine (ACEM). Guidelines for reducing the spread of communicable infectious disease in the emergency department. v5. The Australasian College for Emergency Medicine (ACEM), 2019.

30. Talan DA. Infectious disease issues in the emergency department. Clinical Infectious Diseases. 1996:1-12.

31. Bouzid D, Zanella M-C, Kerneis S, Visseaux B, May L, Schrenzel J, et al. Rapid diagnostic tests for infectious diseases in the emergency department. Clinical Microbiology and Infection. 2021;27(2):182-91.

32. Atamna A, Shiber S, Yassin M, Drescher MJ, Bishara J. The accuracy of a diagnosis of pneumonia in the emergency department. International Journal of Infectious Diseases. 2019;89:62-65.

33. Stephens RJ, Liang SY. Central nervous system infections in the immunocompromised adult presenting to the emergency department. Emergency Medicine Clinics of North America. 2021;39(1):101-121.

34. Buchan SA, Daneman N, Wang J, Garber G, Wormsbecker AE, Wilson SE, et al. Incidence of Hospitalizations and emergency department visits for herpes zoster in immunocompromised and immunocompetent adults in Ontario, Canada, 2002–2016. Clinical Infectious Diseases. 2019;71(1):22-29.

35. Forero R, Hillman KM, McCarthy S, Fatovich DM, Joseph AP, Richardson DB. Access block and ED overcrowding. Emergency Medicine Australasia. 2010;22(2):119-135.

36. Richardson DB, Mountain D. Myths versus facts in emergency department overcrowding and hospital access block. Medical Journal of Australia. 2009;190(7):369-374.

37. Wylie K, Crilly J, Toloo G, FitzGerald G, Burke J, Williams G, et al. Emergency department models of care in the context of care quality and cost: a systematic review. Emergency Medicine Australasia. 2015;27(2):95-101.

38. Nahidi S, Forero R, McCarthy S, Man N, Gibson N, Mohsin M, et al. Qualitative analysis of perceptions and experiences of emergency department staff in relation to implementation and outcomes of the Four-Hour Rule/National Emergency Access Target in Australia. Emergency Medicine Australasia. 2019;31(3):378-386.

39. Nugus P, Holdgate A, Fry M, Forero R, McCarthy S, Braithwaite J. Work pressure and patient flow management in the emergency department: findings from an ethnographic study. Academic Emergency Medicine. 2011;18(10):1045-1052.

40. Suwantarat N, Apisarnthanarak A. Risks to healthcare workers with emerging diseases: lessons from MERS-CoV, Ebola, SARS, and avian flu. Current Opinion in Infectious Diseases. 2015;28(4):349-361.

41. Li C, Sotomayor-Castillo C, Nahidi S, Kuznetsov S, Considine J, Curtis K, et al. Emergency clinicians' knowledge, preparedness and experiences of managing COVID-19 during the 2020 global pandemic in Australian healthcare settings. Australasian Emergency Care. 2021.

42. Barr N, Holmes M, Roiko A, Lord W. A qualitative exploration of infection prevention and control guidance for Australian paramedics. Australasian Journal of Paramedicine. 2017;14(3).

43. Maguire BJ, O'Meara PF, Brightwell RF, O'Neill BJ, Fitzgerald GJ. Occupational injury risk among Australian paramedics: an analysis of national data. Medical Journal of Australia. 2014;200(8):477-80.

44. Mitchell BG, Shaban RZ, MacBeth D, Wood C-J, Russo PL. The burden of healthcare-associated infection in Australian hospitals: a systematic review of the literature. Infection, Disease & Health. 2017;22(3):117-128.

45. Russo PL, Cheng AC, Richards M, Graves N, Hall L. Healthcare-associated infections in Australia: time for national surveillance. Australian Health Review. 2015;39(1):37-43.

46. Russo PL, Stewardson AJ, Cheng AC, Bucknall T, Mitchell BG. The prevalence of healthcare associated infections among adult inpatients at nineteen large Australian acute-care public hospitals: a point prevalence survey. Antimicrobial Resistance & Infection Control. 2019;8(1):114.

47. Shaban RZ, Mitchell B, Russo P, Macbeth D. Epidemiology of healthcare-associated infections in Australia: Elsevier Health Sciences, 2021.

48. Mitchell BG, Ferguson JK, Anderson M, Sear J, Barnett A. Length of stay and mortality associated with healthcare-associated urinary tract infections: a multi-state model. J Hosp Infect. 2016;93(1):92-9.

49. Independent Hospital Pricing Authority (IHPA). Pricing framework for Australian public hospital services 2018-19, Sydney, Australia: IHPA, 2017.

50. Stone PW. Economic burden of healthcare-associated infections: an American perspective. Expert Review of Pharmacoeconomics & Outcomes Research. 2009;9(5):417-422.

51. Mitchell BG, Russo PL. Preventing healthcare-associated infections: the role of surveillance. Nursing Standard (2014+). 2015;29(23):52.

52. Carter EJ, Pouch SM, Larson EL. Common infection control practices in the emergency department: a literature review. American Journal of Infection Control. 2014;42(9):957-962.

53. National Health and Medical Research Council (NHMRC) and Australian Commission on Safety and Quality in Health Care (ACSQHC). Australian guidelines for the prevention and control of infection in healthcare. Canberra: Australian Government, 2019.

54. The Australasian College for Emergency Medicine (ACEM). Clinical guidelines for the management of COVID-19 in Australasian emergency departments (v5.0). 2020.

55. Australian Government Department of Health. Series of National Guidelines (SoNGs). Canberra, Australia: Commonwealth of Australia, 2020 [cited 28 March 2022]. Available from: https://www1.health.gov.au/internet/main/publishing.nsf/Content/cdnasongs.htm.

56. Sax H, Allegranzi B, Pittet D. My five moments for hand hygiene. Hand hygiene: a handbook for medical professionals. 2017:134-143.

57. Holland M, Zaloga DJ, Friderici CS. COVID-19 Personal Protective Equipment (PPE) for the emergency physician. Vis J Emerg Med. 2020;19:100740-.

58. Siegel J, Rhinehart E, Jackson M, Chiarello L. Health Care Infection Control Practices Advisory C. 2007 Guideline for Isolation Precautions: Preventing Transmission of Infectious Agents in Health Care Settings. 2019.

59. Hart S. Using an aseptic technique to reduce the risk of infection. Nursing Standard (through 2013). 2007;21(47):43-48.

60. Clinical Excellence Commission. Infection prevention and control practice handbook. Sydney, Australia: Clinical Excellence Commission, 2020.

61. Australasian College of Infection Control and Prevention (ACIPC). Aseptic technique resources 2015 [cited 28 March 2022]. Available from: https://www.acipc.org.au/aseptic-technique-resources/.

62. Lee G, Bishop P. Microbiology and infection control for health professionals: Pearson Higher Education AU, 2012.

63. Australian Government Department of Health. Coronavirus (COVID-19) information for paramedics and ambulance first responders. 2020.

64. Basseal J. Guidelines for reprocessing ultrasound transducers. Aust J Ultrasound Med. 20(1): 30–40. 2017.

65. Chen H, Zeng D, Yan P. Infectious disease informatics: syndromic surveillance for public health and bio-defense: Springer Science & Business Media, 2010.

66. Australian Government Department of Health. Introduction to the National Notifiable Diseases Surveillance System 2015 [cited 28 March 2022]. Available from: https://www1.health.gov.au/internet/main/publishing.nsf/Content/cda-surveil-nndss-nndssintro.htm.

67. Communicable Diseases Network Australia. National Notifiable Diseases Surveillance System - current CDNA fortnightly report. Canberra, Australia: Commonwealth of Australia, 2022 [cited 08 March 2022]. Available from: https://www1.health.gov.au/internet/main/publishing.nsf/Content/cdnareport.htm.

68. Siegel JD, Rhinehart E, Jackson M, Chiarello L, Health Care Infection Control Practices Advisory C. 2007 Guideline for isolation precautions: preventing transmission of infectious agents in health care settings. American Journal of Infection Control. 2007;35(10 Suppl 2):S65-S164.

69. FitzGerald GJ, Shaban RZ, Arbon P, Aitken P, Considine J, Clark MJ, et al. Pandemic (H1N1) 2009 influenza outbreak in Australia: impact on emergency departments: Queensland University of Technology, 2010.

70. Mitchell R, Banks C. Emergency departments and the COVID-19 pandemic: making the most of limited resources. Emergency Medicine Journal. 2020;37(5): 258-259.

71. Fitzgerald GJ, Shaban RZ, Arbon P, et al, editors. Emergency department impact and patient profile of H1N1 influenza 09 outbreak in Australia: a national study. H1N1 Influenza 09 Canberra: Urgent Research Forum, 2009.

72. Lowthian JA, Curtis AJ, Jolley DJ, Stoelwinder JU, McNeil JJ, Cameron PA. Demand at the emergency department front door: 10-year trends in presentations. Medical Journal of Australia. 2012;196(2):128-32.

73. Rebmann T, Wagner W. Infection preventionists' experience during the first months of the 2009 novel H1N1 influenza A pandemic. American Journal of Infection Control. 2009;37(10):e5-e16.

74. Jefferson T, Jones M, Doshi P, Spencer EA, Onakpoya I, Heneghan CJ. Oseltamivir for influenza in adults and children: systematic review of clinical study reports and summary of regulatory comments. BMJ. 2014;348.

75. Australian Government. Coronavirus (COVID-19) at a glance – 20 December 2020. In: Department of Health, editor. Canberra, Australia: Department of Health, 2020.

76. Andrew E, Nehme Z, Stephenson M, Walker T, Smith K. The impact of the COVID-19 pandemic on demand for emergency ambulances in Victoria, Australia. Prehospital Emergency Care. 2021:1-7.

77. Dinh MM, Berendsen Russell S. Overcrowding kills: how COVID-19 could reshape emergency department patient flow in the new normal. Emergency Medicine Australasia. 2021;33(1):175-177.

78. Chou R, Dana T, Buckley DI, Selph S, Fu R, Totten AM. Epidemiology of and risk factors for coronavirus infection in health care workers: a living rapid review. Annals of Internal Medicine. 2020;173(2):120-136.

79. Quigley AL, Stone H, Nguyen PY, Chughtai AA, MacIntyre CR. Estimating the burden of COVID-19 on the Australian healthcare workers and health system during the first six months of the pandemic. International Journal of Nursing Studies. 2021;114:103811.

80. Li C, Sotomayor-Castillo C, Nahidi S, Kuznetsov S, Considine J, Curtis K, et al. Emergency clinicians' knowledge, preparedness and experiences of managing COVID-19 during the 2020 global pandemic in Australian healthcare settings. Australasian Emergency Care. 2021;24(3): 186-196.

81. Nguyen LH, Drew DA, Graham MS, Joshi AD, Guo C-G, Ma W, et al. Risk of COVID-19 among front-line health-care workers and the general community: a prospective cohort study. The Lancet Public Health. 2020;5(9):e475-e483.

82. Australian Institute of Health and Welfare (AIHW). The first year of COVID-19 in Australia: direct and indirect health effects. Canberra, Australia: AIHW, 2021.

83. Tenforde MW, Self WH, Naioti EA, Ginde AA, Douin DJ, Olson SM, et al. Sustained effectiveness of Pfizer-BioNTech and Moderna vaccines against COVID-19 associated hospitalizations among adults—United States, March–July 2021. Morbidity and Mortality Weekly Report. 2021;70(34): 1156.

84. Australian Government Department of Health. Coronavirus (COVID-19) case numbers and statistics. Canberra, Australia: Department of Health, 2022 [cited 05 March 2022]. Available from: https://www.health.gov.au/health-alerts/covid-19/case-numbers-and-statistics.

85. Australian Government Department of Health. Australian Health Sector Emergency Response Plan for Novel Coronavirus (COVID-19). Canberra, Australia: Commonwealth of Australia, 2020.

86. Govindasamy LS, Hsiao KH, Foong LH, Judkins S. Planning for the next pandemic: reflections on the early phase of the Australian COVID-19 public health response from the emergency department. Emergency Medicine Australasia. 2021;33(4):759-761.

87. Tran K, Cimon K, Severn M, Pessoa-Silva CL, Conly J. Aerosol generating procedures and risk of transmission of acute respiratory infections to healthcare workers: a systematic review. PLoS One. 2012;7(4):e35797.

88. Craig S, Cubitt M, Jaison A, Troupakis S, Hood N, Fong C, et al. Management of adult cardiac arrest in the COVID-19 era: consensus statement from the Australasian College for Emergency Medicine. Medical Journal of Australia. 2020; 213(3):126-133.

89. England N, Improvements N. Clinical guide for the management of trauma and orthopaedic patients during the coronavirus pandemic. 2020. Apr; 2020.

90. Leligdowicz A, Fischer WA, Uyeki TM, Fletcher TE, Adhikari NK, Portella G, et al. Ebola virus disease and critical illness. Critical Care. 2016;20(1):217.

91. Organization WH. Ebola virus disease: Fact sheet: WHO, 2020 [cited 28 March 2022]. Available from: www.who.int/en/news-room/fact-sheets/detail/ebola-virus-disease.

92. New South Wales Ministry of Health. NSW Contingency Plan for Viral Haemorrhagic Fevers. GL2016_002. Communicable Diseases Branch, Ministry of Health NSW.

93. New South Wales Health. Communicable Diseases. Ebola virus disease control guideline: New South Wales Health, 2018 [cited 28 March 2022]. Available from: www.health.nsw. gov.au/Infectious/controlguideline/Pages/ebola-virus.aspx.

94. Baduge MSP, Moss C, Morphet J. Emergency nurses' perceptions of emergency department preparedness for an ebola outbreak: a qualitative descriptive study. Australasian Emergency Nursing Journal. 2017;20(2):69–74.

95. Collignon P, Cruickshank M, Dreimanis D. Staphylococcus aureus bloodstream infections: an important indicator for infection control. Chapter 2: Bloodstream infections–an abridged version. Healthcare Infection. 2009;14(4):165–171.

96. Simon EM, Summers SM. Vascular access complications: an emergency medicine approach. Emergency Medicine Clinics. 2017;35(4):771–788.

97. Hoffman T, Du Plessis M, Prekupec MP, Gielecki J, Zurada A, Tubbs RS, et al. Ultrasound-guided central venous catheterization: a review of the relevant anatomy, technique, complications, and anatomical variations. Clinical Anatomy. 2017;30(2):237–250.

98. Spelman T, Pilcher D, Cheng A, Bull A, Richards M, Worth L. Central line-associated bloodstream infections in Australian ICUs: evaluating modifiable and non-modifiable risks in Victorian healthcare facilities. Epidemiology & Infection. 2017;145(14):3047–3055.

99. Shaban RZ, Maloney S, Gerrard J, Collignon P, Macbeth D, Cruickshank M, et al. Outbreak of health care-associated Burkholderia cenocepacia bacteremia and infection attributed to contaminated sterile gel used for central line insertion under ultrasound guidance and other procedures. American Journal of Infection Control. 2017;45(9):954–958.

100. Westerway SC, Basseal JM. Advancing infection control in Australasian medical ultrasound practice. Australasian Journal of Ultrasound in Medicine. 2017;20(1):26–29.

101. McCall BJ, Looke D. The infection control practitioner and bioterrorism: threats, planning, preparedness. Healthcare Infection. 2003;8(2):37–41.

102. Smallwood RA, Merianos A, Mathews JD. Bioterrorism in Australia. The Medical Journal of Australia. 2002;176(6): 251–252.

103. Mathews JD, Smallwood RA. Australian responses to threats of bioterrorism. Microbiology Australia. 2003;24(2):11–13.

104. Bratberg J, Deady K. Development and application of a bioterrorism emergency management plan. Prehospital and Disaster Medicine. 2005;20(S3):s158–s159.

105. Flowers LK, Mothershead JL, Blackwell TH. Bioterrorism preparedness. II: the community and emergency medical services systems. Emergency Medicine Clinics of North America. 2002;20(2):457–476.

106. Australian Government Department of Health. Review of biological agents of security concern. In: Department of Health, editor. Canberra, Australia: Commonwealth of Australia, 2016.

107. National Health Security Act 2007 (Commonwealth).

108. Australian Government Department of Health. Overview of biological agents that could be used in a terrorist act Canberra: Australian Government, 2018 [cited 28 March 2022]. Available from: www1.health.gov.au/internet/ main/publishing.nsf/Content/health-pubhlth-strateg-bio-agents.htm.

109. Communicable Diseases Network Australia. Ebola Virus Disease (EVD): CDNA National Guidelines for Public Health Units. In: Department of Health, editor. Canberra, Australia: Communicable Diseases Network Australia, 2014.

110. Communicable Diseases Network Australia. Smallpox: CDNA National Guidelines for Public Health Units. In: Department of Health, editor. Canberra, Australia: Communicable Diseases Network Australia, 2017.

111. Shadel BN, Rebmann T, Clements B, Chen JJ, Evans RG. Infection control practitioners' perceptions and educational needs regarding bioterrorism: results from a national needs assessment survey. American Journal of Infection Control 2003;31(3):129–134.

112. Stevens G, Jones A, Smith G, Nelson J, Agho K, Taylor M, et al. Determinants of paramedic response readiness for CBRNE threats. Biosecurity and Bioterrorism: Biodefense Strategy, Practice, And Science. 2010;8(2):193–202.

113. Brink A, Alsma J, Verdonschot RJCG, Rood PPM, Zietse R, Lingsma HF, et al. Predicting mortality in patients with suspected sepsis at the emergency department; a retrospective cohort study comparing qSOFA, SIRS and National Early Warning Score. PloS One. 2019;14(1):e0211133.

114. Legramante JM, Morciano L, Lucaroni F, Gilardi F, Caredda E, Pesaresi A, et al. Frequent use of emergency departments by the elderly population when continuing care is not well established. PloS One. 2016;11(12):e0165939.

115. Haas LE, Van Dillen L, de Lange D, Van Dijk D, Hamaker M. Outcome of very old patients admitted to the ICU for sepsis: a systematic review. European Geriatric Medicine. 2017;8(5-6):446–453.

116. Boonmee P, Ruangsomboon O, Limsuwat C, Chakorn T. Predictors of mortality in elderly and very elderly emergency patients with sepsis: a retrospective study. West J Emerg Med. 2020;21(6):210–218.

117. Caterino JM, Kulchycki LK, Fischer CM, Wolfe RE, Shapiro NI. Risk factors for death in elderly emergency department patients with suspected infection. Journal of the American Geriatrics Society. 2009;57(7):1184–1190.

118. Fontanarosa PB, Kaeberlein FJ, Gerson LW, Thomson RB. Difficulty in predicting bacteremia in elderly emergency patients. Annals of Emergency Medicine. 1992;21(7): 842–848.

119. Wofford JL, Loehr LR, Schwartz E. Acute cognitive impairment in elderly ED patients: etiologies and outcomes. The American Journal of Emergency Medicine. 1996; 14(7):649–653.

120. Shahid Z, Kalayanamitra R, McClafferty B, Kepko D, Ramgobin D, Patel R, et al. COVID-19 and older adults: what we know. Journal of the American Geriatrics Society. 2020;68(5):926–929.

121. Australian Government Department of Health. First 24 hours - managing COVID-19 in a residential aged care facility. In: Department of Health, editor. Canberra, Australia: Australian Government, 2020.

122. Stein M, Cohen R, Bromberg M, Tasher D, Shohat T, Somekh E. Herpes zoster in a partially vaccinated pediatric population in central Israel. The Pediatric Infectious Disease Journal. 2012;31(9):906–909.

123. Posfay-Barbe KM, Zerr DM, Pittet D. Infection control in paediatrics. Lancet Infect Dis. 2008;8(1):19–31.

124. ABC News. Paramedic visited four Brisbane hospitals while infectious with measles 2015 [cited 28 March 2022]. Available from: https://www.abc.net.au/news/2015-05-19/paramedic-visits-four-brisbane-hospitals-infectious-with-measles/6481864.

125. Sheather R. Challenges in paramedic practice: professionalisation In: O'Meara P, Grbich C, editors. Paramedics in Australia: contemporary challenges of practice. Sydney: Pearson Education Australia, 2009.

126. Shaban R, Creedy D, Clark M. Paramedic knowledge of infectious disease aetiology and transmission in an Australian emergency medical system. Australasian Journal of Paramedicine. 2003;1(3).

CHAPTER 28

Infection prevention and control in intensive and critical care settings

PROFESSOR THEA VAN DE MORTEL[i]

Dr PETA-ANNE ZIMMERMAN[i-ii]

Chapter highlights

- Intensive care unit patient profiles and outcomes have changed substantially in Australia and New Zealand over the last two decades. The proportion of patients requiring ventilation has decreased and patient mortality has nearly halved.
- Healthcare-associated infections in Australian and NZ intensive care units and critical care units include:
  - central-line associated bloodstream infections (CLABSI)
  - non-CLABSI bloodstream infections
  - catheter-associated urinary tract infections (CAUTI)
  - ventilator-associated pneumonia (VAP)
  - multidrug-resistant organisms (MROs); and
  - surgical site infections (SSI).
- HAI risk factors include patient-related, treatment-related and setting-related risk factors
- Evidence-based preventative measures include consistent use of standard and transmission-based precautions, 'bundles' of HAI prevention practices and policies, appropriate staffing and oral care
- Emerging and re-emerging infectious diseases continue to pose a threat to patient and healthcare worker safety

i   School of Nursing and Midwifery Griffith University, Gold Coast, QLD
ii Infection Control Department, Gold Coast Health, Gold Coast, QLD

Introduction

This chapter discusses the characteristics and contexts of intensive care and critical care settings in Australia and New Zealand (NZ), the healthcare-associated infection (HAI) risks associated with those settings, and strategies to prevent and control HAIs in those settings in the Australian and NZ context. The aim is to guide best practice in infection prevention and control (IPC) in these settings, improve the quality of the care delivered, and improve patient outcomes.

28.1 Characteristics and contexts of intensive and critical care settings in Australia and New Zealand

According to the *Critical Care Resources and Activity Report 2018/2019* authored by the Australian and New Zealand Intensive Care Society (ANZICS),[1] in 2019 there were 220 intensive care units (ICUs) across Australia and NZ with 3145 actual beds and 2562 available beds. An available bed is one that is fully staffed

and funded. Table 28.1 illustrates the distribution of beds and admissions across jurisdictions and unit type. One hundred and ninety of these ICUs were based in Australia and the remainder in NZ,[2] two-thirds were based in public hospitals and the remainder were private.[1] Participating ICUs reported 596,534 ICU bed days (n = 182 ICUs), and 223,055 adult and paediatric admissions (n = 209 ICUs).[1] Approximately 43,500 bed days in 2018 were for paediatric patients.[3] Since the previous ANZICS 2017–18 report, actual beds had increased by 2.4%, available beds by 0.6%, admissions by 1%, bed days by 1.4% and expenditure by 11.1%. Over the same period there was a 1.6% decline in the proportion of patients receiving invasive ventilation, continuing a long-term trend[1] illustrated in Figure 28.1, as non-invasive ventilation techniques have become more widely used. In 2018, 36.6% of paediatric patients had at least one episode of intubation, which was a decrease of 2.2% from the previous year.[3]

There are five levels of Australian ICU. Table 28.2 describes these in more detail. Critical care is a broader term that encompasses general ICUs but also high dependency units (HDUs) and specialist ICUs including

TABLE 28.1 Distribution of intensive care unit (ICU) and paediatric intensive care unit (PICU) beds and admissions by jurisdiction, 2018

Location	No. Adult/Mixed ICUs	No. PICUs	Beds	No. Admissions
Australia			8.92/100,000*	676/100,000* 793 adult/100,000 207 child/100,000
New South Wales	67	3	874	58,954
Victoria	45	2	476	42,055
Queensland	36	1	413	32,843
South Australia	12	1	188	13,252
Western Australia	12	1	162	13,282
Tasmania	4	1	50	2,116
Australian Capital Territory	5		44	4,619
Northern Territory	2		22	1,825
Location	**No. Adult/Mixed ICUs**	**No. PICUs**	**Beds**	**No. Admissions**
New Zealand			5.14/100,000*	338/100,000* 369 adult/100,000 219 child/100,000
	29	1	251	16,515

Source: The Australian & New Zealand Intensive Care Society (ANZICS) Centre for Outcomes & Resource Evaluation (CORE). http://www.anzics.com.au.
*Based on population estimates on June 30, 2018.

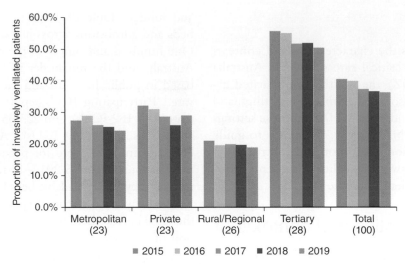

Data from 100 consistently contributing ICUs.

FIGURE 28.1 Trend in proportion of intensive care unit admissions undergoing invasive ventilation
in Australian and New Zealand[1]
Source: The Australian & New Zealand Intensive Care Society (ANZICS) Centre for Outcomes
& Resource Evaluation (CORE). http://www.anzics.com.au.

TABLE 28.2 **Types of ICU in Australia**

Type	Description
Adult Level 3	Capable of providing complex multisystem support for an indefinite period Tertiary referral centre
Adult Level 2	Capable of providing complex multisystem life support for at least several days
Adult Level 1	Capable of providing basic life support for up to 24 hours
PICU	Capable of providing complex multisystem support for an indefinite period to paediatric patients Tertiary referral centre
NICU Level 3	Capable of providing complex multisystem support for an indefinite period to neonates

Source: Australian Institute of Health and Welfare. Intensive Care Unit:
Identifying and definitional attributes 2018. [Available from: https://
meteor.aihw.gov.au/content/index.phtml/itemId/327234.
PICU: paediatric intensive care unit; NICU: neonatal intensive care unit.

neurosurgical, neonatal ICU (NICU), paediatric (PICU), cardiothoracic, surgical and medical ICUs. ANZICs do not provide specific data on HDUs or the proportion of specialty units other than an indication of PICUs.

The median proportion of registered nurse (RN) full-time equivalents in each unit with a critical care qualification was 55.5% in 2018/9.[1] The majority of medical specialists working in Australian and NZ ICUs are fellows of the College of Intensive Care Medicine (FCICM) and the proportion of FCICM has increased by 72% in the last decade.[6] ANZICS[1] report that a range of IPC-specific activities are conducted in Australian and NZ units. For example, 67% of units undertake rounds with a microbiologist or infectious diseases specialist and 72.5% with a pharmacist, and 85.3% of units have an antibiotic stewardship (AMS) program.

Public hospitals are more likely to conduct these safety and quality activities. For example, 98% of tertiary hospital units report conducting rounds with an infectious disease specialist versus 90.6% for metropolitan units, 55.3% for rural and regional units, and 32.7% of units in private hospitals.[1] Similarly, units in private hospitals are less likely to have daily rounds with a pharmacist. Intensive care units in private hospitals also have nearly double the RN vacancy rate compared to the national rate (11% vs 6%), which potentially impacts on safe delivery of care.[1]

Overall, across both countries and in tertiary facilities, approximately half of all admissions are planned, although in non-tertiary public facilities the majority (~70%) are unplanned while in the private sector the majority (~75%) are planned[1] (Fig 28.2). In PICUs the rate of unplanned admissions was 67.7% in 2018.[3] The lower unplanned admission rates in the private sector reflect the for-profit nature of private hospitals that focus on planned surgical cases[7] while the higher

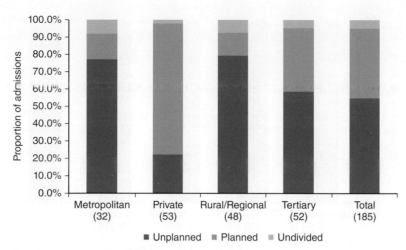

Data from 185 contributing ICUs.

FIGURE 28.2 Proportion of planned and unplanned intensive care admissions 2018–19 by classification[1]

Source: The Australian & New Zealand Intensive Care Society (ANZICS) Centre for Outcomes & Resource Evaluation (CORE). http://www.anzics.com.au.

unplanned admissions in the public sector reflect public hospitals' role in managing emergency and higher acuity cases (Fig 28.3). Overall, approximately half of admissions are to ICUs, about 30% to high dependency units (HDUs), and the remainder to 'other'.[1] Tertiary hospitals and private hospitals have a higher proportion of ICU admissions (Fig 28.4).

In adult ICUs the most common specific reasons for admission are gastrointestinal (16%), respiratory (15%), cardiological (13%), neurological (13%), cardiac surgical (11%), sepsis (8%) and trauma (4%).[6] In PICUs and mixed adult and paediatric ICUs, the most common

reasons for paediatric admission are respiratory conditions (46% of non-PICU admissions, and 25.5% of PICU admissions), followed by surgical conditions (non-cardiac) (15.4% of non-PICU admissions, and 27.2% of PICU admissions).[3] Other less common paediatric diagnoses are, in order from most to least common: cardiovascular, miscellaneous, neurological, injury, and gastrointestinal/renal.[3] Bronchiolitis was the most common cause of paediatric admissions in 2018, followed by pneumonia.[3]

Observed and predicted mortality rates have declined in adult ICUs since 2009 from an observed

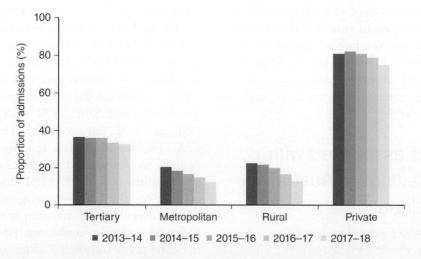

FIGURE 28.3 Elective surgical planned admission by hospital classification—5-year trend[7]

Source: The Australian & New Zealand Intensive Care Society (ANZICS) Centre for Outcomes & Resource Evaluation (CORE). http://www.anzics.com.au.

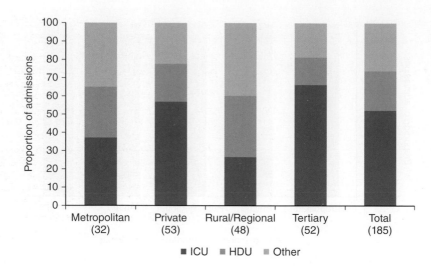

FIGURE 28.4 Proportion of intensive care (ICU) and high dependency (HDU) admissions 2018–19 by classification[1]
*Source: The Australian & New Zealand Intensive Care Society (ANZICS) Centre for Outcomes
& Resource Evaluation (CORE). http://www.anzics.com.au.*

mortality rate of 11% in 2009 to one of just under 8% in 2018,[4] and between 1995 and 2018 mortality has nearly halved.[6] Rates have remained stable since 2016. Both observed mortality (7.7% vs 10.4%) and predicted risk of death (7.7% vs 9.4%) are lower in Australia than NZ.[4] Observed and predicted paediatric mortality in both countries are lower than adult rates at 2.2% and 2.3%, respectively.[3]

In summary, based on the most recent published data there were 220 ICUs across Australia and NZ with 3145 actual beds, the majority of which are adult beds. Over the past two decades ICU patient mortality rates have nearly halved and the proportion of patients undergoing invasive mechanical ventilation has declined. This is despite the proportion of admissions for elective surgery declining. The patient profile differs between the public and private sectors; public patients are more likely to be unplanned admissions and undergo non-elective surgeries (both of which tend to increase the risk profile), while private facilities are more likely to have unfilled staff vacancies.

28.2 HAI risks associated with critical care settings in Australia and New Zealand

Admission to an intensive or critical care unit is a major risk factor for HAI. According to the Centers for Disease Control and Prevention (CDC) National Healthcare Safety Network, just under two-thirds of HAIs in a

12-month period in the USA were reported in critical care settings[8] despite the fact that ICU and critical care admissions typically make up a very small proportion of overall hospital admissions. For example, in Australia in 2016–17 only 1.4% of hospital admissions were to an ICU.[9] A global point prevalence study in 2017 of 15,202 adult patients from 1150 centres in 88 countries demonstrated that 22% had an ICU-acquired infection and when compared to community-acquired infection, an HAI was associated with a higher risk of mortality ([OR], 1.32 [95% CI, 1.10-1.60]; P = .003).[10] In Australia, a point prevalence study determined that 15% of patients who had an HAI were in a medical ICU, compared to 5% of patients who did not.[11] The latter demonstrates that patients with an HAI are more likely to be in ICU.

Typical HAIs seen internationally and in Australian and New Zealand intensive and critical care settings include central line-associated bloodstream infections (CLABSI) (or catheter-related bloodstream infection, CRBSI), non-CLABSI bloodstream infections, ventilator-associated pneumonia (VAP), surgical site infections (SSI), and catheter-associated urinary tract infections (CAUTI).[12-14] Multidrug-resistant organisms are particularly problematic.[15] Chapter 22 details risk factors for antimicrobial-resistant (AMR) infections; however, in brief, in the ICU environment, risk factors include increased overall risk of infection in this cohort, exposure to broad-spectrum antibiotics, poor prescribing practices, and previous hospital admissions.

Limited data are available from the Australian and NZ context on the incidence of specific types of HAI.

In 2017–18 the average CLABSI rate in Australian and NZ ICUs was 0.46 per 1000 line-days.[14] This compares well to the 1 per 1000-line day benchmark.[14] Data extracted from the ANZICS Adult Patient Database[12] over a 6-year period examined the records of 10,034 ICU patients. There were 221 ICU-acquired cases of bacteriuria/candiduria (6·4±0·8 episodes/1000 ICU-days). *Escherichia coli* was the most common bacteria (29%), and *Candida* spp. were responsible for 55% of ICU-acquired positive urine cultures, although the presence of bacteria or yeasts in the urine are not necessarily indicative of infection. Patients with ICU-acquired candiduria had greater illness severity at ICU admission than those with ICU-acquired bacteriuria (APACHE III score 79±25 vs. 66±31, P=0·0015). Other common pathogens included Enterobacteriaceae (*Klebsiella pneumoniae*, *Proteus mirabilis*, *Enterobacter cloacae*, *E. aerogenes*), *Pseudomonas aeruginosa*, Enterococci (*E. faecalis*, *E. faecium*) and *Streptococcus* spp. The VAP rate in 10 Australian and NZ ICUs in 2013 based on the checklist developed by the Quality and Safety (Q&S) Committee of the Australian and New Zealand Intensive Care Society and clinician diagnosis was 25.9 and 26.7 per 1000 mechanical ventilator-days respectively.[16] A single site study in NSW in 2010–11 listed in a systematic review of HAIs in Australia, reported a VAP incidence of 7.02/1000 ventilator-days in a paediatric ICU population.[17] No specific data on SSI incidence in Australian and NZ ICUs have been reported in recent years.

To provide a point of comparison with international ICUs, the European Centre for Disease Prevention and Control in its 2017 report of surveillance data from 14 European countries and 1480 ICUs reported 1.7 to 4.8 episodes of VAP per 1000 ventilator-days, 2.4 urinary tract infections per 1000 patient-days, and CLABSI rates of 1.8 infections/1000 device-days.[18] The difficulty in making comparisons with other countries is that the definitions used and underlying patient acuity may differ, which can influence rates, as does whether the country is high, middle or low income. For example, according to the World Health Organization[19] ~30% of patients in ICUs in high-income countries acquire at least one HAI, while the frequency in low- to middle-income countries is two to three times higher.

Clostridioides difficile is an infectious organism that is not specifically associated with wounds or devices; however, the risk factors for *C. difficile* are likely to be present at a higher rate in ICU populations, for example, broad-spectrum antimicrobial use. There are no specific incidence data from Australian or NZ ICUs.[17] A 41-country study, however, demonstrated a substantially increased incidence of *C. difficile* infection in ICU patients compared to whole-of-hospital statistics (11.08 per 1000 admissions vs 2.24 per 1000 admissions).[20] Australian data from 2018 show that the incidence of severe *C. difficile* infection has been increasing since 2012.[21] Given the above factors, this is an infection of concern in ICU patients.

There are a range of factors intrinsic to critical care patient demographics and the setting that increase HAI risk. Some are modifiable and some are non-modifiable. These risk factors can be grouped into patient-related, treatment-related and setting-related risk factors.

28.2.1 Patient-related risk factors

Patients in critical care units are disproportionately at extremes of age,[15] predominantly either elderly or very young, and both groups tend to have less robust immune systems: the very young because the immune system is still developing until the age of seven or eight,[22] and the elderly because of immuno-senescence. For example, the elderly exhibit reduced numbers of naïve T-cells, reduced B-cell numbers, reduced B- and T-cell receptor diversity, and reduced B- and T-cell proliferation ability, reducing their capacity to generate immune memory to new antigens.[23] The innate immune system is also impaired; phagocytosis—a key factor in a robust immune response—declines with age.[23]

Patient acuity and the presence of chronic disease are also risk factors for HAI. Adult ICU patients are more likely to have a history of complex chronic health conditions that adversely impact immunity—for example, type 2 diabetes—given the median age of ICU admissions in Australia and New Zealand is 65.[6] For example, while 4.9% of the total Australian population have diabetes mellitus, 19.4% of the over 85 age group have it.[24,25] A proportion of ICU patients are also post surgical or post trauma;[6] breaks to skin integrity provide additional portals of entry for pathogens. The APACHE II score—a measure of patient acuity in ICU patients—is an independent risk factor for Gram-negative infection[26] and a predictor of mortality. The higher the score, the higher the infection risk.

Smoking history also influences risk of infectious illness and outcomes from ICU stays. One Victorian study found 23% of patients admitted to ICUs were current smokers.[27] This is double the percentage of Australian adults in the general population (11.6% in 2019) who smoke regularly.[28] Smoking predisposes patients to infection through both immunological and structural/pathophysiological mechanisms.[29] Smoking damages alveolar walls and bronchioles making them floppy and prone to collapsing on expiration. When combined with decreased function of the mucociliary elevator, smokers have a reduced ability to clear respiratory secretions and pathogens from the lungs. Smoking also adversely influences cell-mediated and humoral immunity[29] so smokers are more likely to acquire an infection and to suffer adverse outcomes from those infections. For example, smokers have an up to four-fold increased risk of invasive pneumococcal disease and are more likely to require mechanical ventilation.[29]

28.2.2 Treatment-related risk factors

Various treatments that are comparatively common in ICUs increase the risk of one or more types of HAI. Patients in critical care units disproportionately have invasive procedures and devices that provide portals of entry for pathogens[15] as ICUs provide mechanical ventilation, invasive cardiac monitoring and extracorporeal renal support for critically ill patients.[5] Thus, CLABSI, CAUTI and VAP are a risk for critical care patients, as are SSIs for post surgical patients as described previously. Total parenteral nutrition (TPN) may be used to maintain nutrition in critically ill patients who are unable to receive enteral feeding. TPN is associated with an increased risk of *Klebsiella* CLABSI.[26] Antimicrobial drugs, used to treat a range of infectious organisms, are associated with an increased risk of *C. difficile* infection as the reduction in normal flora can lead to pathogen overgrowth.[20]

28.2.3 Setting-related risk factors

There are a range of setting-related factors that increase the risk of HAIs. As critical care units have a greater proportion of HAIs, infected patients and the ICU environment can act as reservoirs of pathogens that increase the risk of infection transmission to others. In addition, various studies have demonstrated that critically ill patients have fragmented and poor sleep through a combination of factors such as environmental noise, extended exposure to artificial light (suppresses melatonin and disrupts circadian rhythms), pain, stress, frequent disturbance for patient care interactions, impaired cognition, and patient–ventilator dysynchrony.[30,31] Peak noise levels in ICUs are often almost twice the recommended decibel level for hospital settings, and sleep deprivation is one of the top three stressors for ICU patients.[30] Lack of sleep has been demonstrated to have complex impacts on the components and functioning of the immune system and thus infection risk.[30,32]

ICU staffing levels and staff workloads also impact on infection risk. For example, a systematic review of 35 studies examining the impact of nurse-to-patient ratios in ICU/critical care specialty units found that higher staffing levels were associated with significantly lower incidence of infection, including pneumonia.[33] Similarly, an analysis of six years of data from specialty units in a large American hospital system found that patients on units that were understaffed across two shifts were significantly more likely to develop an HAI two days later.[34] Spelman[13] indicated that medical specialist staffing levels in Australian and NZ ICUs were inversely associated with CLABSI risk. The higher the sessional medical specialist staffing levels, the lower the CLABSI risk. Nursing staffing was not associated with CLABSI risk in this study, probably because central lines are inserted by medical staff.

This section has provided evidence of a range of risk factors that increase the risk of developing an HAI in the ICU/critical care setting. These can be grouped into patient-related risk factors (extremes of age, patient acuity, chronic disease, smoking, wounds), treatment-related risk factors (invasive devices and procedures, antimicrobial therapy, TPN) and setting-related risk factors (sleep disruption related to noise and light exposure, a reservoir of pathogens, and staffing and workloads).

Reducing the incidence of HAIs in critical care patients is critically important as HAIs in this group are associated with greatly increased length of stay, healthcare costs and mortality.[35] For example, data from 9.6 million medical and pharmacy claims of ICU patients in the United States with *Staphylococcus aureus* or *P. aeruginosa* infection compared with patients (controls) without these infections had a:

- 'longer mean hospital stay (37.9 or 55.4 vs 7.2 days, P < .001)
- longer ICU stay (6.9 or 14.8 vs 1.1 days, P < .001)
- higher rate of mechanical ventilation (62.6% or 62.3% vs 7.4%, P < .001)
- higher mortality (16.0% or 20.2% vs 3.1%, P < .001)
- higher total mean hospitalisation costs ($146,978 or $213,104 vs $33,851, P < .001).'[35]

The following section discusses strategies to reduce infection risk in intensive and critical care settings.

28.3 Prevention and control of HAI in critical care settings

As we have seen previously, there are a number of risks for patients in acquiring an HAI in intensive and critical care settings related to patient, treatment and setting risk factors. Specific types of HAI include VAP, CLABSI (or catheter-related bloodstream infection, CRBSI), CAUTI and AMR infections. How we prevent and control these in practice is based on breaking the chain of infection plus governance strategies, through the use of 'bundles' of care. What is central to any of this is the consistent use of standard precautions and asepsis (Chapter 13) and transmission-based precautions (Chapter 14) to prevent HAI in both patients and healthcare workers. In addition to these are specific practices and bundles that can further assist in prevention of HAI in these settings

The use of bundles of prevention interventions has become a common strategy to mitigate HAI risk in any type of intensive and critical care setting, using a standardised approach of evidence-based interventions with multidisciplinary input. [36] The use of these bundles has demonstrated improvements in patient outcomes, including decreases in HAI in intensive and critical care units across the world. The following sections will focus on two areas:

1. specific practices to prevent HAI; and

2. bundles of interventions that target intensive and critical care-related infections such as VAP.

28.3.1 Ventilator-associated pneumonia

Specific to VAP is the prevention of micro-aspiration of respiratory secretions that may be colonised either with the patient's own endogenous flora or those acquired from the healthcare environment via contaminated equipment or the hands of healthcare workers.[37] The Institute for Healthcare Improvement[38] recommends a bundle of interventions to prevent ventilator-associated events, including VAP. This bundle has been used worldwide and has been adopted by Australian intensive and critical care settings.[39] In Australia, however, there appears to be a lack of consensus regarding a VAP definition, which some researchers believe has led to a lack of knowledge of prevention methods in nursing staff.[39,40] The key aspects of the VAP prevention bundle are detailed in Box 28.1.

Chlorhexidine oral care: Performing oral hygiene on ventilated patients is an accepted and important care task. What has been disputed over time, however, is what solution(s) should be used in the process and what impact they have on VAP incidence. The most recent Cochrane Review performed in 2016 indicates that chlorhexidine, used as either a mouth rinse or gel, can reduce the rate of VAP from 24% to approximately 18%.[45]

BOX 28.1 Key features of a ventilator-associated pneumonia prevention bundle of care[38,41–44]

Non-Pharmaceutical Interventions

Patient positioning

- Semi-recumbent position (≥30°) may reduce incidence of VAP compared to a supine position[41]

Endotracheal/oropharyngeal suctioning

- Suctioning as required reduces secretions (and subsequent colonisation) that can be aspirated by the patients, thus reducing risk of VAP[42,43]

Endotracheal tube cuff pressure checks

- At least once every eight hours reduces the risk of micro-aspiration[44]

Daily oral care with chlorhexidine

- Dental plaque can be colonised with respiratory secretions and become a reservoir for pathogens causing VAP. Use of chlorhexidine in oral care

reduces this colonisation[38] (see below for further discussion on this)

Pharmaceutical Interventions

Peptic ulcer disease prophylaxis

- Oesophageal reflux can result in aspiration of gastric contents; prophylaxis can reduce the risk of aspiration due to unprotected airway[38]

Daily sedative interruption and assessment of readiness to extubate

- Daily interruption reduces time requiring mechanical ventilation and decreases incidence of VAP[38]

Deep vein thrombosis prophylaxis

- No clear DIRECT link with reduction of VAP, but when full bundle is implemented there is reduction in the incidence of VAP[38]

As we have seen above, oral hygiene is an extremely important aspect of care for mechanically ventilated patients and has been proven to reduce VAP. In reality, though, the literature has demonstrated that Australian nurses are not performing this care consistently and are putting patients at risk of acquiring VAP.[39,40] When observing practice in the intensive or critical care environments or reviewing the incidence of VAP as part of your surveillance program, consider whether the staff are performing routine oral care and using chlorhexidine as a mouth cleanser.

28.3.2 Central line-associated bloodstream infection/Catheter-related bloodstream infection

Prevention of CLABSI or CRBSI is primarily based on stopping endogenous patient or exogenous health-care facility flora entering the bloodstream via an inserted vascular device. All aspects—from insertion and maintenance to removal of the device—may lead to one of these HAIs. It is therefore imperative that all aspects are performed carefully with a focus on asepsis and the reduction of the risk of introduction of potentially harmful pathogens.

A recent review of available literature identified the most important evidence-based measures to prevent CLABSI/CRBSI at various points of the catheter's life span (Box 28.2).

Chlorhexidine gluconate bathing: The most recent systematic review of the literature examining the role of bathing patients with chlorhexidine gluconate to decolonise the skin, thus presumably reducing the risk of HAI, was performed in 2019.[50] This study identified a lack of quality evidence to support the practice and the possibility that it actually causes harm to patients due to skin irritation. There is also the question of the spectrum of effectiveness on Gram-positive versus Gram-negative pathogens.[51] The ultimate conclusion is that there is no certain evidence to support this practice at this time, yet there is no certain evidence to the contrary either. This has been disputed elsewhere but the importance of focusing on the behavioural aspects of implementing

---

BOX 28.2 Best practice in intravenous catheter insertion and care to prevent HAI[46-49]

Insertion

- Monitoring hand hygiene practice and compliance
- Preventing unnecessary catheter insertion
- Careful selection of type of catheter
- Using a peripheral intravenous catheter for short-term vasopressor infusions
- Aseptic technique
- Preparation of the insertion site with 2% alcoholic chlorhexidine gluconate
- Subclavian site insertion

Catheter care

- Remove catheters as soon as unnecessary
- Daily visual inspection of site
- Documentation of dressing changes
- Consider chlorhexidine gluconate impregnated dressings
- Replace tubing no more frequently than every four days, but no less frequently than seven days
- Do not leave dressing in place if unstuck, soiled or damp
- Do not use catheter locks
- Consider routine bathing of patients with chlorhexidine gluconate

Implementation strategies (for consideration)

- Multi-modal
- Vascular access teams (daily audits and point-of-care education)
- Multidisciplinary leadership line care rounds
- Unit-based safety programs
- Translation of research into practice
- Clinical governance and accountability

and performing such care, as with oral hygiene, has been highlighted as this will lead to better patient outcomes.[52]

CASE STUDY 1

Central line management

Situation:

On review of the latest central line surveillance data from the ICU you notice that there appears to be an increase in the length of dwell time for the lines compared to previous months, with what appears to be delayed removal. You know that this is a potential cause of CLABSI in ICU patients, though your ICU has had no increase in incidence in the same time period. On discussion with the nurse unit manager of the ICU you find that there has been increased sick leave due to stress in the unit. This has meant a decrease in ICU trained nursing staff to remove catheters in a timely fashion.

Question:

How might you assist in the timely removal of central lines?

- With the ICU NUM and staff, review policy and evidence to support removal of lines and maximum dwell times
- Review available evidence on best practice care bundles for centrally inserted catheters
- Report concerns and evidence to IPC and Clinical Governance Committees.

28.3.3 Catheter-associated urinary tract infection

Risk of acquiring a CAUTI in any setting is higher for specific patient populations, as seen previously. There are, however, common prevention practices that can, and have been, bundled to prevent CAUTI in all patients. The first is to reduce the use of catheters and the time that catheters are in situ.[53] Some practices that are used, such as chlorhexidine gluconate bathing to decolonise skin, described previously, remain controversial.

Clinical decision making on when a urinary catheter can be removed can be improved. A recent Australian study investigated the role of the nurse in this process and the effect on the use of urinary catheters in intensive and critical care settings.[54] This study demonstrated a reduction in catheter use. Although not specifically measured in this study, reduced catheter use is associated with reduced CAUTI incidence.[53] The most common practices bundled to prevent CAUTI in intensive and critical care are listed in Box 28.3.

BOX 28.3 Practices to prevent CAUTI in intensive and critical care settings[53,55,56]

Catheter placement

- Insertion only when indicated:
  - acute urinary retention or bladder outlet obstruction
  - accurate measurements
  - perioperative use for selected surgical procedures
  - assist healing of open sacral or perineal wounds in incontinent patients
  - prolonged immobilisation
  - comfort for end-of-life care
  - clot retention associated with gross haematuria
- Use of alternatives to catheters
- Aseptic technique
- Document catheter insertion and indication
- Latex-free catheters
- Appropriate size catheter for patient
- NOT as a substitute for nursing care of patient with incontinence
- NOT as means to obtain a urine sample or for diagnostic tests if the patient is continent
- NOT for prolonged postoperative duration
- Antimicrobial prophylaxis only for high-risk patients (unplanned surgery, elevated risk of endocarditis with recent UTI, immunosuppression)

Catheter care

- Maintain asepsis and closed system while catheter in situ
- Only collect urine specimens for culture or other diagnostic tests if indicated and maintain asepsis
- Secure catheter to the patient

Continued

BOX 28.3 Practices to prevent CAUTI in intensive and critical care settings—cont'd

- Ensure no kinks or loops in catheter or drainage tubing
- Empty drainage device when ¾ full
- Empty into a single patient use receptacle (do not go from patient to patient)
- When draining, do not allow contact between the device outlet and the receptacle
- Clean device outlet with alcohol wipe after drainage
- Ensure drainage device is below level of the bladder but off the floor
- Maintain a closed system
- Perform insertion site and periurethral care (antiseptic agents not required)
- Assess the need for the catheter daily
- Routine changes are not recommended unless the closed system has been breached, drainage has been obstructed, or a CAUTI is identified
- Document all care

Catheter removal

- Remove the catheter as soon as it is no longer needed: is there a documented or clinical indication for the catheter to remain in situ?
- Aseptic technique
- Clean and dry genital area after removal
- Document removal

PRACTICE TIP 2

MICROBIOLOGY RESULTS

When reviewing microbiology results don't forget to place these in the context of an overall clinical picture of the patient. Identifying a pathogen in a urine sample (or any other sample for that matter) may not indicate infection. Take into consideration signs and symptoms of infection, comorbidities of the patient, and where and how the sample was collected. Contamination of samples or colonisation rather than infection may be occurring. Collecting these data builds a better clinical picture and assists in identifying whether a patient truly has acquired an HAI.

28.3.4 Antimicrobial resistance

As discussed, a significant risk to patients in any healthcare setting, and particularly intensive and critical care settings, is the acquisition of an antimicrobial-resistant organism.[57] Prevention of colonisation or infection with these organisms comes down to sustained compliance with a comprehensive antimicrobial stewardship program (Chapter 22) as well as standard precautions and asepsis (Chapter 13) and transmission-based precautions (Chapter 14).[58] Key features of these are described in Box 28.4.

Screening for antimicrobial resistance: It is generally accepted practice to screen patients admitted to intensive and critical care units for the presence of, or colonisation or infection by, an AMR organism. The National Health and Medical Research Council (NHMRC) Australian Guidelines for the Prevention and Control of Infection in Healthcare[59] recommend patient screening as described in Table 28.3. Please note that your own facility may have different guidelines based on the local epidemiology of antimicrobial-resistant organisms and the wider surveillance program.

BOX 28.4 Primary interventions in reducing antimicrobial-resistance impact in intensive and critical care settings[58]

1. Enforce infection prevention and control practices
   a. Focus on hand hygiene
   b. Provide feedback on adherence
2. Develop an antimicrobial stewardship program
   a. Multidisciplinary approach including team meetings/rounds
   b. Adapt to local organisational aspects, multi-resistant organism rates and resources
3. Apply smart antibiotic dosing
   a. Adapt to patient physiology and local epidemiology
4. Review antimicrobial use daily
   a. De-escalate when susceptibility allows
   b. Withdraw when infection not confirmed
   c. Cease after 7 days for most therapies

TABLE 28.3 Antimicrobial-resistant organism screening recommended for intensive care settings

Organism	Screen	Sample
MRSA	• On admission • On discharge • Weekly	Multiple sites including nose and another mucosal surface Reasonable sites include: • Anterior nares • Skin lesions/wounds • Catheter sites • Catheter urine • Ostomy sites • Groin/perineum • Tracheostomy • Any skin breaks • Sputum (if productive)
VRE	Endemic VRE: • On admission • On discharge • Weekly	Multiple sites including rectal or perianal Reasonable sites include: • Groin • Wounds • Ostomy sites • Respiratory secretions • Tracheal aspirates
MRGN, ESBLs, plasmid-mediated AmpC, MR-*Pseudomomas aeruginosa*, MRAB, CPE	On admission OR Temporary measure during an outbreak	Multiple sites including rectal or perianal Reasonable sites include: • Groin • Wounds • Ostomy sites • Respiratory secretions • Tracheal aspirates

Source: National Health and Medical Research Council. Australian Guidelines for the Prevention and Control of Infection in Healthcare. Canberra: Australian Government; 2019.
MRSA: methicillin-resistant Staphylococcus aureus
VRE: vancomycin-resistant Enterococci spp.
MRGN: multi-resistant Gram-negative organisms
ESBL: extended spectrum beta-lactamase-producing organisms
MRAB: multi-resistant Acinetobacter baumannii
CPE: carbapenemase-producing Enterobacteriaceae

28.3.5 Environmental cleaning in critical care units

As we saw in Chapter 13 Standard precautions and asepsis, Chapter 14 Transmission-based precautions, Chapter 15 Environmental cleaning, and Chapter 16 Disinfection and sterilisation the role of the environment in transmission of HAI cannot be forgotten. Critical care environments are problematic for this, in particular due to the amount of equipment required to treat and manage patients in these settings. While a large number of consumable items are used (single use or single patient use) there remains equipment that must be cleaned in between patients, including the environment the patients occupy. It is therefore important that all surfaces that are frequently touched in this environment are cleaned as per facility guidelines and to ensure that enhanced cleaning is implemented when caring for—or after discharge of—a patient requiring transmission-based precautions.[53]

PRACTICE TIP 3

CLEANING THE CRITICAL CARE SPACE

Next time you are in a critical care patient space observe the staff caring for their patients. Watch what they are touching in the course of their duties and consider the following:

• Is hand hygiene performed as per the '5 Moments of Hand Hygiene'?

Continued

- Is equipment cleaned before leaving a patient care space?
- What are the most frequently touched surfaces in the patient care space?
- Is hand hygiene performed after removal of gloves?

By doing this you will begin to understand the importance of cleaning the critical care space, what items are easily contaminated, what needs to be cleaned more often, and where the potential for breaches in IPC practice can exist.

28.3.6 Staffing and a multidisciplinary approach

As discussed, there is evidence of poor patient outcomes related to inappropriate staffing and workload allocation in critical care settings.[27] Working to prevent such adverse events for patient and healthcare worker safety requires a solid clinical governance structure and support from leadership.[27,43,52,53]

When looking at the prevention of HAI in any setting including intensive and critical care, a multidisciplinary approach has been reported to be essential in numerous studies and guidelines.[43,46,53,54,58,59] This team approach has demonstrated important improvements in patient outcomes and a reduction in the incidence in HAI in intensive and critical care settings. Review Section 1 Principles, for more information on a team approach as part of a comprehensive IPC program.

28.4 Novel respiratory infections: a new threat

In 2020 we saw the true impact of a pandemic-level novel respiratory infection on intensive and critical care settings in the form of COVID-19 or severe acute respiratory syndrome coronavirus 2 (SARS-CoV-2). This has been a challenge at all levels of healthcare delivery. COVID-19 presents like many other severe acute respiratory infections, including other novel diseases like severe acute respiratory syndrome (SARS) and Middle East respiratory syndrome (MERS). As we have seen in Chapter 8 Infection Prevention and Control for One Health, we will continue to see these novel infectious diseases, potentially from zoonotic sources, arising in our community and spreading rapidly.[60] The level of morbidity and mortality associated with these infections puts an even greater strain on existing pressured intensive and critical care environments. It is with this in mind that we must reinforce and sustain our standard precautions and asepsis (Chapter 13) and transmission-based precautions (Chapter 14) to protect patients and healthcare workers alike.

As we have seen, there are multiple practices that are best used as a comprehensive suite or bundle of care interventions to prevent the acquisition and transmission of HAI in critical care settings. These interventions are supported by a multidisciplinary approach to care and appropriate human resource allocation to support the implementation of practices. Having a solid basis in all aspects of IPC throughout healthcare provision will strengthen the capacity for dealing with emerging and re-emerging infectious diseases that continue to threaten the global community.

Conclusion

The prevention of HAI in modern healthcare is becoming more critical than ever, with our communities developing greater risks of morbidity and mortality due to lifestyle factors; our ageing population; emerging and re-emerging infectious diseases; antimicrobial resistance; and our increased use of invasive interventions to treat disease. This is particularly true of our critical care settings where we see the most vulnerable of our community requiring a high burden of interventional therapy. This places patients at a greater risk of HAI and therefore we must be aware of the patient, treatment, and setting risk factors with their associated preventative interventions and practices to mitigate the transmission or acquisition of HAI in these settings. By considering the comprehensive components of an IPC program, including infection prevention strategies and robust IPC governance involving the multidisciplinary team, you will be better prepared to improve patient and healthcare worker safety outcomes.

Useful websites/resources

- Australian and New Zealand Intensive Care Society (ANZICS) Publications. https://www.anzics.com.au/publications/
- Australian College of Critical Care Nurses (ACCCN) Publications. https://acccn.com.au/publications/
- Australian Guidelines for the Prevention of Infection in Healthcare. https://app.magicapp.org/#/guideline/Jn37kn

References

1. Australian and New Zealand Intensive Care Society. Centre for Outcome and Resource Evaluation intensive care resources and activity report 2018/19. Melbourne, 2020.
2. Litton E, Bucci T, Chavan S, Ho Y, Holley A, Howard G, et al. Surge capacity of Australian intensive care units associated with COVID-19 admissions. Med J Aust. 2020;212(10):463-467.
3. Australian and New Zealand Intensive Care Society. Australian and New Zealand paediatric intensive care registry activity report 2018. ANZICS, 2020.
4. Australian and New Zealand Intensive Care Society. Centre for outcome and resource evaluation report 2018. Camberwell: ANZICS, 2018.
5. Australian Institute of Health and Welfare. Intensive care unit: identifying and definitional attributes 2018. Canberra: AIHW, 2018. Available from: https://meteor.aihw.gov.au/content/index.phtml/itemId/327234.
6. Warrillow S, Raper R. The evolving role of intensive care in health care and society. Med J Aust. 2019;211(7):294-297.
7. Australian and New Zealand Intensive Care Society. Adult Patient Database Activity Report 2017/2018. ANZICS, 2019.
8. Ziakas PD, Zacharioudakis IM, Zervou FN, Mylonakis E. Methicillin-resistant Staphylococcus aureus prevention strategies in the ICU: a clinical decision analysis. Crit Care Med. 2015;43(2):382-393.
9. Australian Institute of Health and Welfare. Australia's hospitals 2016–17 at a glance. Canberra: AIHW, 2018.
10. Vincent J-L, Sakr Y, Singer M, Martin-Loeches I, Machado F, Marshall JC, et al. Prevalence and outcomes of infection among patients in intensive care units in 2017. JAMA. 2020;323(15):1478-1487.
11. Russo PL, Stewardson AJ, Cheng AC, Bucknall T, Mitchell BG. The prevalence of healthcare associated infections among adult inpatients at nineteen large Australian acute-care public hospitals: a point prevalence survey. Antimicrob Resist Infect Control. 2019;8:114.
12. Aubron C, Suzuki S, Glassford N, Garcia-Alvarez M, Howden BP, Bellomo R. The epidemiology of bacteriuria and candiduria in critically ill patients. Epidemiol Infect. 2015;143:653-662.
13. Spelman T, Pilcher DV, Cheng AC, Bull AL, Richards MJ, Worth LJ. Central line-associated bloodstream infections in Australian ICUs: evaluating modifiable and non-modifiable risks in Victorian healthcare facilities. Epidemiol Infect. 2017;4:1-9.
14. Australian and New Zealand Intensive Care Society. Central line associated bloodstream infection (CLABSI) report 2017/18. Camberwell: ANZICS, 2018.
15. Zahar J-R, Blot S. Dilemmas in infection control in the intensive care unit. Intensive Crit Care Nurs. 2018;46:1-3.
16. Elliott D, Elliott R, Burrell A, Harrigan P, Murgo M, Rolls K, et al. Incidence of ventilator-associated pneumonia in Australasian intensive care units: use of a consensus-developed clinical surveillance checklist in a multisite prospective audit. BMJ Open. 2015;5.
17. Mitchell BG, Shaban RZ, Macbeth D, Wood C-J, Russo PL. The burden of healthcare-associated infection in Australian hospitals: a systematic review of the literature. Infect Dis Health. 2017;22:117-128.
18. European Centre for Disease Prevention and Control. Healthcare-associated infections acquired in intensive care units annual epidemiological report for 2017. Stockholm: ECDC, 2019.
19. World Health Organization. Health care-associated infections: Fact sheet. Geneva: WHO, n.d.
20. Balsells E, Shi T, Leese C, Lyell I, Burrows J, Wiuff C, et al. Global burden of Clostridium difficile infections: a systematic review and meta-analysis. J Global Health. 2019;9(1).
21. Australian Commission on Safety and Quality in Health Care. Clostridium difficile infection: monitoring the national burden of Clostridium difficile. Sydney; ACSQHC: 2018.
22. Kloc M, Ghobrial RM, Kuchar E, Lewicki S, Kubiak JZ. Development of child immunity in the context of COVID-19 pandemic. Clin Immunol. 2020;217:108510.
23. Erickson MA, Banks WA. Age-associated changes in the immune system and blood–brain barrier functions. Intl J Molecular Sciences. 2019;20.
24. Australian Institute of Health and Welfare. Older Australia at a glance. Canberra: AIHW, 2018.
25. Australian Institute of Health and Welfare. Diabetes. Canberra: AIHW, 2020.
26. Sahutoglu S, Savran Y, Comert B. Risk factors for resistant gram negative infections in intensive care unit. Turkish J Med Surg Intensive Care Med. 2020;11(1):21-27.
27. Polmear CM, Nathan H, Bates S, French C, Odisho J, Skinner E, et al. The effect of intensive care unit admission on smokers' attitudes and their likelihood of quitting smoking. Anaesth Intensive Care. 2017;45(6):720-726.
28. Australian Institute of Health and Welfare. National Drug Strategy Household Survey 2019. Canberra: AIHW, 2020.
29. Alroumi F, Azim A, Kergo R, Lei Y, Dargin J. The impact of smoking on patient outcomes in severe sepsis and septic shock. J Intensive Care. 2018;6.
30. Kamdar BB, Needham DM, Collup NA. Sleep deprivation in critical illness: its role in physical and psychological recovery. J Intensive Care Med. 2011;27(2):97-111.
31. Zhang Q, Gao F, Zhang S, Sun W, Li Z. Prophylactic use of exogenous melatonin and melatonin receptor agonists to improve sleep and delirium in the intensive care units: a systematic review and meta-analysis of randomized controlled trials. Sleep and Breathing. 2019;23:1059-1070.
32. Irwin M. Sleep and inflammation: partners in sickness and in health. Nat Rev Immunol. 2019 Nov;19(11):702-715.
33. Driscoll A, Grant M, Carroll D, Dalton S, Deaton C, Jones I, et al. The effect of nurse-to-patient ratios on nurse-sensitive

patient outcomes in acute specialist units: a systematic review and meta-analysis. Eur J Cardiovasc Nurs. 2018; 17(1):6-22.

34. Shang J, Needleman J, Liu J, Larson E, Stone P. Nurse staffing and healthcare-associated infection, unit-level analysis. JONA: The Journal of Nursing Administration. 2019;49(5):260–265.

35. Kyaw M, Kern D, Zhou S, Tunceli O, Jafri H, Falloon J. Healthcare utilization and costs associated with *S. aureus* and *P. aeruginosa* pneumonia in the intensive care unit: a retrospective observational cohort study in a US claims database. BMC Health Serv Res. 2015;15:241

36. Dawson D, Endacott R. Implementing quality initiatives using a bundled approach. Intensive Crit Care Nurs. 2011;27(3):117-120.

37. Hellyer TP, Ewan V, Wilson P, Simpson AJ. The intensive care society recommended bundle of interventions for the prevention of ventilator-associated pneumonia. J Intensive Care Soc. 2016;17(3):238-243.

38. Institute for Healthcare Improvement. How-to-guide: prevent ventilator-associated pneumonia. Cambridge, MA: IHI, 2012.

39. Madhuvu A, Endacott R, Plummer V, Morphet J. Nurses' knowledge, experience and self-reported adherence to evidence-based guidelines for prevention of ventilator-associated events: a national online survey. Intensive Crit Care Nurs. 2020;59:102827.

40. Ciampoli N, Bouchoucha S, Currey J, Hutchinson A. Evaluation of prevention of ventilator-associated infections in four Australian intensive care units. J Infect Prev. 2020; 21(4):147-154.

41. Wang L, Li X, Yang Z, Tang X, Yuan Q, Deng L, et al. Semi-recumbent position versus supine position for the prevention of ventilator-associated pneumonia in adults requiring mechanical ventilation. Cochrane Database Syst Rev. 2016(1).

42. Wen Z, Zhang H, Ding J, Wang Z, Shen M. Continuous versus intermittent subglottic secretion drainage to prevent ventilator-associated pneumonia: a systematic review. Crit Care Nurse. 2017;37(5):e10-e17.

43. American Association for Respiratory Care. AARC Clinical Practice Guidelines. Endotracheal suctioning of mechanically ventilated patients with artificial airways 2010. Respir Care. 2010;55(6):758-764.

44. Maertens B, Blot K, Blot SI. Prevention of ventilator-associated and early post-operative pneumonia through tapered endotracheal tube cuffs: a sytematic review and meta-analysis of randomized control trials. Crit Care Med. 2018;46(2):316-323.

45. Hua F, Xie H, Worthington HV, Furness S, Zhang Q, Li C. Oral hygiene care for critically ill patients to prevent ventilator-associated pneumonia. Cochrane Database Syst Rev. 2016(10).

46. Buetti N, Tabah A, Timsit J, Zingg W. What is new in catheter use and catheter infection prevention in the ICU. Curr Opin Crit Care. 2020;26(5):459-465.

47. Eggimann P, Pagani J-L, Dupuis-Lozeron E, Ms BE, Thévenin M-J, Joseph C, et al. Sustained reduction of catheter-associated bloodstream infections with enhancement of catheter bundle by chlorhexidine dressings over 11 years. Intensive Care Med. 2019;45(6):823-833.

48. Tian DH, Smyth C, Keijzers G, Macdonald SP, Peake S, Udy A, et al. Safety of peripheral administration of vasopressor medications: a systematic review. Emerg Med Australas. 2020; 32(2):220-227.

49. Timsit J-F, Rupp M, Bouza E, Chopra V, Kärpänen T, Laupland K, et al. A state of the art review on optimal practices to prevent, recognize, and manage complications associated with intravascular devices in the critically ill. Intensive Care Med. 2018;44(6):742-759.

50. Lewis SR, Schofield-Robinson OJ, Rhodes S, Smith AF. Chlorhexidine bathing of the critically ill for the prevention of hospital-acquired infection. Cochrane Database Syst Rev. 2019(8).

51. Patel A, Parikh P, Dunn AN, Otter JA, Thota P, Fraser TG, et al. Effectiveness of daily chlorhexidine bathing for reducing gram-negative infections: a meta-analysis. Infect Control Hosp Epidemiol 2019;40(4):392-399.

52. Musuuza JS, Guru PK, Horo JC, Bongiorno CM, Korobkin MA, et al. The impact of chlorhexidine bathing on hospital-acquired bloodstream infections: a systematic review and meta-analysis. BMC Infect Dis. 2019;19:NA.

53. Meddings J, Rogers MAM, Krein SL, Fakih MG, Olmsted RN, Saint S. Reducing unnecessary urinary catheter use and other strategies to prevent catheter-associated urinary tract infection: an integrative review. BMJ Qual Saf. 2014;23(4):277.

54. Giles M, Graham L, Ball J, King J, Watts W, Harris A, et al. Implementation of a multifaceted nurse-led intervention to reduce indwelling urinary catheter use in four Australian hospitals: a pre- and postintervention study. J Clin Nurs. 2020;29(5-6):872-886.

55. Calpe N, Wennberg L, Llaurado M. Efficacy of urinary catheter securement in the reduction of urinary tract infection, urinary meatus injuries and discomfort, in the critically ill patient: preliminary results. Intensive Care Medicine Experimental. 2019;7.

56. Clinical Excellence Commission. Adult urethral catheterisation for acute care settings. Sydney: New South Wales Government, 2015.

57. Johani K, Abualsaud D, Costa DM, Hu H, Whiteley G, Deva A, et al. Characterization of microbial community composition, antimicrobial resistance and biofilm on intensive care surfaces. J Infect Public Health. 2018;11(3):418-424.

58. De Waele JJ, Akova M, Antonelli M, Canton R, Carlet J, De Backer D, et al. Antimicrobial resistance and antibiotic stewardship programs in the ICU: insistence and persistence in the fight against resistance. a position statement from ESICM/ESCMID/WAAAR round table on multi-drug resistance. Intensive Care Med. 2018;44(2): 189-196.

59. National Health and Medical Research Council. Australian Guidelines for the Prevention and Control of Infection in Healthcare. Canberra: NHMRC, 2019.

60. Arabi YM, Murthy S, Webb S. COVID-19: a novel coronavirus and a novel challenge for critical care. Int Care Medicine. 2020;46(5):833-836.

CHAPTER 29

Infection prevention and control in residential aged care settings

ASSOCIATE PROFESSOR NOLEEN BENNETT[i-ii]

LYN-LI LIM[iii]

Chapter highlights

- Characteristics of Australian residential aged care facilities (RACFs)
- Aged care residents and infections:
  - infection risk in the elderly
  - healthcare-associated infection
  - multidrug-associated organisms
  - antimicrobial use
- IPC organisational support and work practices in Australian RACFs:
  - core requirements
  - clinical assessment

i   VICNISS Coordinating Centre, The Peter Doherty Institute for Infection and Immunity, Melbourne, VIC

ii Department of Nursing, Melbourne School of Health Sciences, The University of Melbourne, Melbourne, VIC

iii Department of Infectious Diseases, University of Melbourne, Parkville, VIC

Introduction

The Australian federal government has primary responsibility for the aged care system. The development and implementation of aged care policy and funding are the domain of the Commonwealth Department of Health, and ensuring that approved providers meet their responsibilities in relation to quality of care is overseen by the independent Aged Care Quality and Safety Commission (Commission).[1]

The Australian aged care system provides three main subsidised service types for persons who have diminished capacity to care for themselves. These are:

1. Commonwealth Home Support Programme (CHSP; entry level support)

2. home care packages (for those who have complex care needs and require support beyond what CHSP can provide); and

3. respite or permanent care in residential aged care facilities (RACFs).

Home support and home care packages provide the assistance required to maintain independent living. RACFs, also variously known as 'nursing homes', 'aged care homes' and internationally 'long-term care facilities' (LTCFs), deliver 24-hour services to those assessed as needing higher levels of care than can be provided in their own home. In Australian RACFs, services include hotel-like packages (e.g. bedding, furniture, toiletries, cleaning, meals, laundry); personal care (e.g. showering, dressing, assisting with toileting); clinical care (e.g. medical, nursing and allied health services); and social care (e.g. recreational activities, emotional support).[2] While mostly older persons use the Australian aged care system, access is determined by assessed need and not by age.[3]

In 2019, a Royal Commission into Aged Care Quality and Safety undertook 10,574 public submissions, 6800 telephone calls and 99 hearings; these were conducted across a range of urban, rural and remote areas and included 12 community forums. Participants included consumers, family members or carers, aged care workers, peak bodies, advocates and experts. Many examples of substandard care were outlined, including deviations from expected infection prevention and control (IPC) standards. Concerns such as inadequate IPC training and limited access to personal protective equipment (PPE) were raised.[4]

Since early 2020, the Australian aged care system has faced an extraordinary and traumatising period with the COVID-19 pandemic.[5] As of December 2022, there have been 108,793 confirmed resident cases and 3430 related deaths.[6] In a special Royal Commission COVID-19 report (October 2020),[7] the following three recommendations related to IPC—which the Commonwealth has since accepted and implemented—were outlined:

1. The Australian Government should establish a national aged care plan for COVID-19 through the National Cabinet in consultation with the aged care sector.

2. All residential RACFs should have one or more trained infection control officers as a condition of accreditation. The training requirements for these officers should be set by the proposed aged care advisory body.

3. The Australian Government should arrange with the states and territories to deploy accredited IPC experts into residential RACFs to provide training, assist with the preparation of outbreak management plans and assist with outbreaks.

In March 2021, the Royal Commission's final report recommended appropriate amendment of the Aged Care Quality Standards to provide sufficient detail on requirements related to best-practice IPC.[4]

This chapter highlights the unique IPC-related challenges faced by Australian RACFs and outlines some recommendations for IPC practices and organisational support specific to RACFs. Note, however, that if implemented in other residential settings, the recommendations may need to be adapted because of potential differences in populations, disease and transmission risks, levels of acuity and technology.

29.1 Characteristics of Australian residential aged care facilities

29.1.1 Number and type of residential aged care facilities

As at 30 June 2021, 830 approved providers operated 2704 RACFs with 219,105 operational residential aged care places. Not-for-profit, private and government providers operated 56.9%, 34.5% and 8.6% of the RACFs respectively.[2] Most RACFs were located in NSW (32.2%), Victoria (28.0%) and Queensland (17.6%) and almost two-thirds (62.7%) were in metropolitan areas.[3] RACFs were classified as small (70.6%, 1–60 beds), medium (16.3%, 61-100 beds) or large (13.1%, ≥101 beds).[3]

29.1.2 Aged care facility residents

While the numbers vary by country, approximately 2–5% of the developed world's older population resides in some type of LTCF.[8] In Australia, approximately 1% of Australia's population reside in an RACF.[3] At 30 June 2021, there were 183,894 people (66% women, 34% men) receiving permanent residential care; during 2020–21, 244,117 people received permanent residential aged care respectively at some time during the year. Almost two-thirds (64%) of the women were aged 85 years and over, compared with 47% of the men. English was not the preferred language for about one-tenth (9%) of residents.[3] In 2019–20, 54% of residents living in permanent residential aged care were reported as having dementia.[9]

29.1.3 Workforce

The RACF workforce[1] includes anyone employed, hired, retained or contracted (directly or via an external agency) to provide maintenance or administration, or care and services under the control of the RACF. It also includes volunteers who primarily help with social activity support, companionship and planned group activities providing care and services.[10] It does not include:

- visiting medical practitioners, pharmacists and other allied health professionals and services a resident has asked for, but which the RACF does not contract
- tradespersons independently contracted who do not work under the control of the RACF, for example, plumbers, electricians or delivery people who work on a needs basis.

Direct care (and other) workers: The most recent (2020) National Aged Care Workforce Census and Survey[10,11] found there were an estimated 277,671 aged care workers employed in RACFs. Most (n=208,903) were direct care workers; personal care workers (70%), nurses (23%) and allied health professionals (7%). These direct workers predominantly (70%) held permanent part-time positions. Of the remaining 68,768 staff, 76.8% worked in ancillary roles such as cleaners, cooks and laundry assistants. The other staff were in management and administrative roles (20.4%) and pastoral care and educational roles (2.8%). COVID-19 appeared to have had a significant effect on volunteers, with levels (n=11,980) during the last fortnight of November 2020 approximately half of those during the same time in 2016.

About one-third (35%, n=49,475) of the direct care workers identified as being from a culturally and linguistically diverse distribution (CALD) background.

Two-thirds (66%) of personal care workers held a Certificate III or higher in relevant direct care field, with a further 2% studying at the time. IPC was the most commonly reported specialist skill amongst direct care workers. Managers were most likely to come from a nursing (as opposed to business) background.[10]

29.1.4 IPC in Australian residential aged care facilities

Although more studies with sound methodology are required to support the benefit of IPC programs in RACFs,[15,16] a national survey found most (92.4%) RACFs had a documented IPC program. About one-fifth (22.9%) had a specific IPC committee on-site, while 77.1% reported their IPC was encompassed by a different committee, for example, a quality and safety committee.[17] Most RACFs continuously collect and analyse data for common infections.[17-19] The adoption of antimicrobial stewardship (AMS) programs has been slow. Antimicrobial prescribing is mostly the role of general practitioners (GPs), whose main practice is off-site.[18]

RACFs have numerous differences to other settings that impact on how IPC might be approached. These differences can be categorised as resident, workforce, infrastructure and service related.

Residents

- The RACF is a home for residents and hence comfort, dignity, rights and IPC principles must all be addressed.[20]
- Residents may be frequently exposed to colonised and infected persons due to a complex traffic of people between the community, hospitals, other establishments and RACFs.[21]
- Residents are especially intrinsically vulnerable to acquiring infections.
- It can be more difficult in residents to determine whether an infection is present or, if an infection is present, the site and specific etiologic agent.[20] Clinical presentations of elderly residents differ from those in younger populations because of higher prevalence of chronic symptoms of comorbid illness,[20] and dementia or cognitive impairment.[22] Residents may not be able to reliably express signs and symptoms of infection. Diagnostic tests may not be obtained because residents cannot cooperate.
- Goals and outcomes of interventions may differ from those in other populations. For example, for permanent residents, length of stay is not a useful measure of effectiveness of an intervention but

maintenance of functional status likely is. Mortality will sometimes be a humane outcome, such as in the severely functionally impaired demented person who develops pneumonia.[20]

Workforce

- The aged care workforce is currently understaffed and undertrained.[4,10]

- There are few resources in IPC expertise.[7] From late 2020, all Australian aged care providers were required to have a dedicated, on-site IPC lead.[12] (See Box 29.1). IPC personnel employed in RACFs usually have multiple other responsibilities.

BOX 29.1 Aged care infection prevention and control leads

In late 2020, the Australian Government announced that funding would be provided to RACF providers to assist with the engagement of an aged care IPC lead.[12] At time of writing in 2023,[13] the specified requirements of an aged care IPC lead are that they *must*:

- be employed by and report to the provider

- be a member of the nursing staff

- work on-site and be dedicated to a facility

- have successfully completed an IPC focused and assessed course (level AQF8) delivered by a recognised education or training provider; and

- complete at least the minimum requirements of the Department's COVID-19 focused and specified training modules.

The position of aged care IPC lead may be filled by someone who has a broader role in the facility and could be an existing member of the nursing staff. The requirements of this role are to:

- observe, assess and report on the IPC of the service

- help develop procedures; and

- provide advice within the service; and be a key infection control contact.[13]

Providers can determine what level of engagement or workload is required of their IPC leads. To ensure IPC programs are effectively coordinated, larger RACF providers especially may determine that a full-time IPC lead or a number of IPC leads is appropriate.[14]

They may not have a level of training equivalent to that of those similarly employed in acute care facilities, and time allocated to attend IPC education is insufficient.[16]

- Significant barriers for off-site GPs to provide high-quality medical care to RACF residents have been identified, including a lack of recognition of their role as a resident's nominated GP, inadequate clinical and administrative support, clinical complexity of the population, time pressures and poor remuneration.[23]

- Off-site prescribers are often heavily reliant on inexperienced or inadequately trained RACF staff to assess residents for possible infections.[8,24]

- Pharmacists have traditionally performed either dispensing or consultancy roles remotely or in a visitational capacity.[25]

- Access to expert advice when needed, such as a microbiologist or epidemiologist, is limited.[16,17]

Infrastructure

- RACFs are often ill designed for IPC. Larger facilities have been found to experience respiratory or gastrointestinal disease outbreaks more commonly, with a 71% increase in risk per 100-bed increase in size.[26] The communal style of living creates difficulties in adhering to physical distancing. There may be a lack of conveniently placed handwashing basins, an absence of single rooms, shared bathrooms and deficiencies in ventilation systems.[21]

- Access to computers and secretarial support may be limited.

- Medical records may not be useful for infection identification.

- Diagnostic tests may be delayed or not undertaken because of lack of accessibility (e.g. on-site chest radiography).

Service

- There is no national coordinated approach to surveillance activities that promotes the use of standardised criteria, benchmarking and target thresholds.[19]

- Accomplishing high-quality environmental cleaning in RACFs is not always simple. Spills, incontinence and other similar issues are relatively common. Cleaning is mostly undertaken during daylight hours which means continuously navigating variable elements, such as workers, elderly residents, visitors and any objects or equipment they are using or interacting with.

29.2 Residential aged care residents and infections

29.2.1 Intrinsic risk of infections in the elderly in residential aged care facilities

Compared to the younger population, the elderly (especially those in RACFs) are at significantly higher intrinsic risk of morbidity and mortality due to many common infections. This is related to predisposing factors such as physiological changes that accompany ageing and the frequent presence of comorbid conditions (Table 29.1).

29.2.2 Healthcare-associated infections

The term 'healthcare-associated infection' (HAI) is applied to infections acquired in RACFs as well as acute care hospitals. This is because the main elements leading to a nosocomial (or healthcare-associated) infection are the infectious agent, a susceptible host, and a means of transmission. These elements are present in RACFs as in hospitals. Most HAIs are assumed to be preventable—or at least the risk of acquiring an HAI can be reduced by adequate IPC measures—and timely identification of infected persons may help stop transmission. It is recognised that the elderly can present with infections in a different way to younger adults; atypical presentations, including a blunted febrile response, can lead to delayed recognition of infection, including severe infection.[27]

There are many reservoirs for infectious agents in RACFs. Most infections are thought to be endogenous, resulting from the resident's own flora of the perineum, skin or nasopharynx.[21] Infected or colonised residents may serve as reservoirs for certain infectious agents such as methicillin-resistant *Staphylococcus aureus* (MRSA) and extended-spectrum beta-lactamase-producing Enterobacterales (such as *Escherichia coli*). Staff and visitors can also serve as important reservoirs for agents such as influenza and SARS CoV 2 viruses. Endemic infections most commonly reported include respiratory, skin and soft tissue and urinary tract infection (UTI).[28] Epidemic infections most commonly reported include respiratory, gastrointestinal and skin and soft tissue infections[18,19] (Table 29.2).

Respiratory tract: RACF residents are at high risk of respiratory complications from viral respiratory tract infections such as influenza, respiratory syncytial virus (RSV), human metapneumovirus (HMPV), parainfluenza and COVID-19 infections; these infections are generally mild in other populations but can cause significant morbidity and mortality in elderly RACF residents where outbreaks are also common.[29]

Reported infectious diseases outbreaks suggest that that the median attack rate of influenza outbreaks in

TABLE 29.1 Predisposing intrinsic factors for infection

Predisposing factor	Potential outcome
Immunosenescence, related to declines in cell-mediated immunity and antibody responses that affect the body's response to pathogenic organisms and vaccination	Reactivation risk of latent infections
Decreased gastric acid	Viral and bacterial gastroenteritis[44]
Chronic lung and heart disease	Pneumonia
Diabetes mellitus and poor wound healing	Chronic *infected* ulcers
Depressed mental status and swallowing disorders from neurological conditions such as cerebrovascular diseases and dementia	Aspiration pneumonia and pressure ulcers
Inadequate oral hygiene and dental plaque	Pneumonia
Urinary incontinence from neurological or urological conditions	Skin breakdown and fungal skin infections
Incomplete bladder emptying from neurological or urological conditions (e.g. bladder outlet obstruction)	Urinary tract infection
Use of indwelling catheters	Catheter-associated urinary tract infection and *E. coli* bacteraemia
Antimicrobial exposure	Multidrug-resistant organism colonisation and infection

TABLE 29.2 Most common infections in residential aged care facilities

Body system	Endemic	Epidemic (pandemic)
Respiratory	Common cold syndrome or pharyngitis Bronchitis or tracheo-bronchitis Pneumonia Tuberculosis reactivation	Influenza COVID-19
Skin and soft tissue	Cellulitis Fungal skin infections (e.g. tinea) Group A Streptococcus skin and soft tissue infection MRSA skin and soft tissue infection Herpes zoster	Scabies
Urinary	Urinary tract infection	–
Gastrointestinal	Bacterial (e.g. Salmonella spp.)	Viral gastroenteritis (e.g. norovirus) Toxin-related (e.g. *C. perfringens*) *C. difficile* infection

residents was 33% (range 4%–94%) in the elderly in long-term care facilities.[30]

Pathogens are similar to causes of community-acquired pneumonia, with *Streptococcus pneumoniae* the most common; however, atypical bacterial pathogens (e.g. *Mycoplasma pneumoniae*) are less common.[31]

Vaccination against COVID-19, influenza and pneumococcal pneumonia is effective in reducing mortality in the elderly. There is emerging data that vaccination against COVID-19 may be effective in reducing the effects of long COVID in the elderly, especially those living in RACFs.[32] In high-risk populations such as RACF residents, antivirals active against COVID-19 and influenza are recommended to reduce risk of severe complications and death.[33] Currently, nirmatrelvir and ritonavir and molnupiravir are available oral COVID-19 antiviral treatments.[34] Neuraminidase inhibitors (NAIs), oseltamivir and zanamivir, are authorised for the treatment and prophylaxis of influenza in many countries, including Australia. Where antivirals are available, treatment of symptomatic residents is generally recommended to be started immediately. For influenza outbreaks, prophylaxis should be provided for all residents in facilities experiencing an outbreak, regardless of vaccination status.[35,36]

Skin and soft tissue: Cellulitis can occur on intact skin or at the site of a skin break. *Streptococcus pyogenes* (Group A Streptococcus or GAS) followed by *Staphylococcus aureus* are the most common causes of cellulitis. Outbreaks of GAS infections in RACFs have been described, presenting as cellulitis, pharyngitis, pneumonia or septicaemia.[37]

Crusted (Norwegian) scabies infestations are particularly problematic for older people, people who are immunosuppressed and those who are frail and weak.

Urinary tract: In most surveys conducted in LTCFs, UTIs are leading causes of infection and antibiotic prescribing in facilities.[38,39] Indwelling urinary catheters (IDCs), bladder and/or bowel incontinence contributes to risk of UTI. UTI may perhaps be the most over-diagnosed infection in RACF, related to asymptomatic bacteriuria (ASB) misdiagnosed as UTI.[40] ASB is common in the elderly, those living in facilities, and those with IDCs, and is not associated with increased risk of UTI.[41] Catheter-related bacteriuria is ever-changing and not amenable to prophylactic antibiotics; these factors make it inappropriate to screen asymptomatic residents for bacteriuria or to treat asymptomatic bacteriuria.[42] However, the presence of an indwelling urinary catheter increases the risk of both UTIs and bacteriuria. For example, approximately 3–7% of RACF residents with an indwelling urinary catheter will acquire a UTI each day the catheter remains in place. By day 30 following catheter insertion, the prevalence of bacteriuria is almost 100%.[43] Hence it is important to review the need for catheters and remove if not required.

Gastrointestinal: Norovirus is a leading cause of gastroenteritis outbreaks in RACFs. Outbreaks are incredibly difficult to control because of their infectivity and environmental persistence; the virus can be detected in residents' stool samples an average of 28 days after cessation of symptoms.[44]

Clostridium perfringens and salmonellosis have been associated with foodborne outbreaks. *Clostridioides difficile* infection, related to recent antibiotic exposure, can also cause outbreaks. Several studies report the prevalence of *C. difficile* colonisation in LTCF residents to range between 4% and 20% in endemic settings and 30% in the context of an outbreak. A significant proportion of residents may already be carrying *C. difficile* on admission to the LTCF, and an additional 10–20% may acquire the organism during their stay in a LTCF.[45] Admission to a LTCF has been identified as an independent risk factor for CDI; along with having ≥ 3 comorbidities, presence of a feeding tube, faecal incontinence and use of proton-pump inhibitors.[45]

Other infections: Other infections in RACFs include reactivation of infections such as tuberculosis and shingles. Older people (especially those over 70 years) are more likely to have shingles complicated by post-herpetic neuralgia, a chronic pain syndrome and other complications. Zoster vaccination of people aged 70–79 years is estimated to prevent about 41% of cases of shingles and two-thirds of post-herpetic neuralgia.[46]

Bacteraemia may be primary or related to an infection at a secondary site, most commonly the urinary tract. Conjunctivitis in residents may be sporadic or uncommonly related to outbreaks. Many are non-specific (e.g. related to allergy) or viral; *S. aureus* is the most common bacterial cause. Transmission may occur by contaminated eyedrops or by hand cross-contamination.

29.2.3 Multidrug-resistant organisms (MROs)

RACFs have been identified as an important reservoir of MRSA and extended spectrum β-lactamase-producing Enterobacterales (ESBLE) by prevalence and incidence studies conducted in different European countries.[47] Recently, there have also been several reports of infection and/or colonisation by other MROs such as carbapenemase-producing Enterobacterales (CPE) and vancomycin-resistant Enterococci (VRE) amongst residents.

Point prevalence studies in RACFs suggest that up to half of residents are colonised with MRO, most commonly MRSA[39] and ESBL-producing organisms.[48,49] Australian Passive AMR Surveillance using laboratory isolates reported MRSA rates in 2017 to be higher in RACFs compared to overall national rates. For MRSA, rates in RACFs were 32.1% compared to 22.5% and for fluoroquinolone-resistant *E.coli* isolates 18.1% compared to 10.2%.[50]

29.2.4 Antimicrobial use

Rates of antibiotic use are higher in RACF residents compared to the general population.[51] Seven of every 10 residents receive at least one antibiotic a year,

with a median of three antibiotic prescriptions dispensed over a year. There has been a 39% increase in total consumption of systemic antibiotics between 2005–06 to 2015–16.[52] The most common antibiotics dispensed are cefalexin, amoxicillin-clavulanic acid, trimethoprim or trimethoprim-sulfamethoxazole and amoxillin. There is also a wide variation in systemic antibiotic utilisation across RACFs—a greater prevalence of GP hours accessed after-hours is associated with higher antibiotic use.[53]

Estimates suggest that up to half of antimicrobial use is either unnecessary or inappropriate in LTCFs.[54,55] The 2019 Australian Aged Care National Antimicrobial Prescribing Survey[28] highlighted the following ongoing issues of concern which require urgent attention:

- prolonged duration of antimicrobial use
- high rates of PRN (as required) prescriptions for antimicrobials
- high rates of topical antimicrobial use, particularly for PRN administration
- prolonged prophylaxis for conditions that are not recommended by guidelines
- poor documentation of indication, review and stop dates for antimicrobial prescriptions.

29.3 Infection prevention and control organisational support and work practices

RACFs are expected to have governance systems that assess, monitor and drive improvement in the quality and safety of the care and services they provide. This includes having an effective IPC program in place that aims to:[1,20]

- decrease morbidity/mortality attributable to infections in staff, residents and visitors
- prevent and control infection outbreaks
- limit costs of care attributable to infections
- maintain an optimal social environment for residents; and
- comply with legislation, regulation and jurisdictional requirements.

The Australian Guidelines for the Prevention and Control of Infection in Healthcare (2019) outline a nationally accepted systematic programmatic approach that can be applied to RACFs and assist RACFs to achieve the above aims. In its current form, these guidelines focus on core principles and priority areas for action and are underpinned by a risk-management framework. It is recognised that the type of risk differs for different settings, such as RACFs, and hence the implementation of any recommendations should be considered as part of a risk assessment.[56] A 'mini guideline' about IPC in residential care that was based on the previous version of the IPC national guidelines has been rescinded and is now publicly available for historical and research purposes only.[57] Other national aged-care-specific recommendations, advice or guidelines that should be referenced have been developed by the Aged Care Quality and Safety Commission,[58] Australian Commission on Safety and Quality in Health Care[59] and the Infection Control Expert Group.[60]

As part of an RACF IPC program, staff (administrators and clinicians), residents and visitors all have roles and responsibilities that should be clearly defined. It is recommended that all stakeholders are empowered to work together in order to effect change and achieve the best possible IPC outcomes.

A multidisciplinary committee that includes the aged care IPC lead should regularly meet to ensure that current, readily available and accessible organisational policies and procedures are in place to cover IPC priority areas for action.[61] The application of hospital IPC policies and procedures may be inappropriate and/or unrealistic because of the differences that exist between hospitals and RACFs. The committee should have a formal mechanism for considering feedback from all stakeholders. Importantly, the committee should oversee a communication strategy that facilitates the routine implementation of the IPC program and which can be immediately escalated in response to an incident or outbreak.

transmission risk and allows for prompt management of infected residents. Enhanced clinical assessments of RACF residents is encouraged to reduce delays in recognition, diagnosis and management of infection signs and symptoms. The regular use of a valid and reliable clinical screening tool that specifically addresses the pathophysiological changes in ageing and recognises the known atypical presentations of illness in older people is recommended.[62] In addition to typical signs (e.g. coughing, vomiting and rash) and symptoms (e.g. nausea and pain) of infection, residents should be observed for atypical signs (e.g. seeming unwell, being upset and sleeping more). It is important that staff are familiar with what is and is not normal for each resident, and that residents are asked how they are feeling. It is essential that there is staff capability and equipment available to accurately measure vital signs (body temperature, heart rate, respiratory rate and blood pressure) and oxygen saturation (using a pulse oximeter). Any new infection signs and symptoms should be documented and promptly reported to a clinical supervisor. To address the issue of antibiotic overprescribing in Australian RACFs, the Aged Care and Quality Commission has adapted from Therapeutic Guidelines: Antibiotic,[63] a clinical pathway to help staff recognise symptoms and signs of UTI in residents and to avoid the pitfalls of over-interpreting urine dipstick testing.[58]

PRACTICE TIPS 1

CORE REQUIREMENTS OF AN RACF IPC PROGRAM

- Develop, implement and document an IPC program that is aligned with national IPC guidelines.

- Develop IPC policy and procedure documents and action plans that include risk assessment and management strategies, and clear instructions for staff.

- Include in the IPC communication strategy how an infectious status is to be clearly and sensitively communicated to staff, residents and visitors should it be necessary.

29.3.1 Clinical assessments

In the setting of a suspected or known outbreak, a valid and reliable clinical screening process reduces

---

PRACTICE TIPS 2

CLINICAL ASSESSMENT APPROACHES TO IDENTIFY AND MANAGE RESIDENT INFECTIONS

- Utilise a resident clinical screening tool that addresses age-related changes and atypical presentations and thereby identifies any deterioration early.

- Update care and service plans to detail possible or actual infections and any individual and RACF-wide precautions that have been implemented.

- Ensure the list of infectious diseases notifiable to government authorities is periodically checked and updated as necessary.

- Instruct staff and visitors not to come to work if acutely unwell.

- Instigate processes for routinely screening staff and visitors on entry to an RACF where there is a risk of an infectious disease being introduced to the RACF.

- Complete the goals of care for every resident (including respiratory support and ventilation) so their expectations and wishes can be met.

29.3.3 Standard and transmission-based precautions

As for other settings, standard precautions in RACFs are basic first-line IPC practices that are applied to everyone, regardless of their perceived or confirmed infectious status. These precautions include personal hygiene practices (particularly hand hygiene), appropriate use of personal protective equipment, safe use and management of sharps, environment control (e.g. cleaning and spillage management), practising respiratory hygiene and cough etiquette, using aseptic technique and appropriate waste management and handling of linen (see Chapter 14).

Transmission-based precautions are applied where standard precautions may not be sufficient on their own to effectively manage infectious agents; specific interventions are required to interrupt the mode of transmission until the signs and symptoms of infection have resolved or according to IPC guidelines specific to the infectious agent. Types of transmission-based precautions include contact, droplet and airborne precautions (see Chapter 15).

PRACTICE TIPS 3
IMPLEMENTATION OF IPC PRECAUTIONS

- Ensure all staff, residents and visitors understand that IPC precautions are in place to protect everyone from infection.
- Support staff, residents and visitors to apply standard precautions at all times.
- If necessary, instigate transmission-based precautions in addition to standard precautions.

- Allow time for residents to especially practise hand hygiene after toileting and before and after meals.
- Remind residents not to feel offended or afraid if staff use PPE (e.g. gloves, gowns, masks and eye protection) when providing care.
- Ensure PPE and other safety equipment (e.g. safety engineered needles) is available at all times.

29.3.4 Cleaning

Cleaning practices in RACFs are not dissimilar to other settings (see Chapter 15). A risk assessment should identify low- and high-touch surfaces and if routine, preventative or deep-decontamination cleaning is required, the methods, thoroughness and frequency will vary accordingly. High-touch surfaces are those touched often by multiple hands and are at risk of being contaminated (Table 29.3).

PRACTICE TIPS 4
CLEANING

- Document arrangements for cleaning the internal and external service environment. This includes removing general and hazardous waste.
- If third party contractors are used, document arrangements and the systems in place to make sure any safety, cleaning or maintenance of the service environment is delivered as arranged.
- Ensure cleaning equipment is never left unattended or when not in use is locked away from residents.

29.3.5 Resident placement

When a resident is colonised or infected and transmission to other residents may occur, it may be necessary to move the resident or the roommate to another room. If a private single room is not possible, the next best

TABLE 29.3 Examples of high-touch surfaces in residential aged care facilities

Communal areas		Shared bathrooms and toilets
• door handles • light switches • safety railings • lift buttons • counters • dining tables • seat arms and backs • water fountain buttons	• hot desks • shared phones and computer keyboards • shared office equipment • sign-in touchscreens	• door handles • door locks and push plates • basin and shower tap handles and benches • soap dispenser buttons • hand dryer buttons • toilet and urinal flush buttons • toilet lid and seat front

option is to cohort—or group—residents together that are infected with the same confirmed pathogen.

The decision to transfer residents with highly infectious diseases to hospital should be made case by case, taking into account the resident's medical needs and advance care plan, the advice of public health experts, whether the RACF has the capability to provide appropriate care, and local jurisdictional healthcare system arrangements. Ambulance services and hospitals must be advised in advance if a resident is being transferred from an RACF in the midst of an outbreak.

29.3.6 Outbreak management

Guidelines are available to support RACFs to prepare, detect and respond to disease outbreaks, including respiratory, such as COVID-19,[66] and gastroenteritis.[67] Many lessons, as listed below, have been learned about outbreak management in RACFs (Box 29.2). The Aged Care

---

BOX 29.2 Key lessons learnt about outbreak management in RACFs[5,68,69]

- Strong and decisive leadership is critical. Many providers utilise a command and control structure that provides clear reporting lines and defined roles.

- An outbreak management plan, tailored to individual RACF requirements, provides clear triggers for activation by on-site shift leaders, including reporting lines and defined roles, and enables escalation dependent on community transmission and severity.

- Stress-testing the outbreak management plan with staff to clarify their roles and responsibilities and identify and address gaps is recommended.

- Shift leaders should be able to easily access up-to-date staff and resident lists, visitor logs, floorplans and information required for pathology requests.

- Templates can be useful in collecting supportive documentation in the event of an outbreak to support notification to public health and contact tracing. These include the initial report template, outbreak management checklist, and line lists to record the details of residents affected by the outbreak.

- The RACF layout should be checked for cohort 'zones', entry and exit points, access for external amenities, staff rooms, donning and doffing stations, waste management, delivery of food and laundry services, and maintenance of access to outside for all residents. Some providers use coloured tape and clear signage to demarcate different zones. A number of providers create designated areas within which residents can wander safely.

- Resources such as hand hygiene stations, PPE stations and clinical waste bins need to be secure, sufficient and suitable.

- Options for secure storage of large PPE stocks on-site should be identified.

- A staff contingency plan is required to maintain an adequate workforce. Many additional staff with expertise may be required to provide proper care (especially if cohorting is implemented and for residents with wandering and aerosol-generating behaviour); services (such as hospitality, cleaning and laundry); and operation management (e.g. communication). Staff will experience fatigue, increased tasks and workload in outbreak settings. Staff domestic arrangements and ability/willingness to work on-site during an outbreak must be known. A number of providers now have arrangements in place for secondary external (e.g. waste management) providers.

- Screening, monitoring and testing processes for staff and residents should be instigated. Some providers organise testing using existing connections with pathology services.

- Staff policies for sick leave need to ensure staff who stay home because they are unwell are not disadvantaged.

- Early, frequent and ongoing IPC education and training for all staff is necessary to reinforce outbreak management messages and minimise complacency.

- Processes should be in place to induct new staff, including agency or temporary, to include orientation procedures and activities, handover processes, care planning, resident preferences, and PPE requirements.

- Processes should be in place to ensure new and temporary staff are able to access electronic systems if required.

- It is important that communication with staff, residents and their families, external service providers and government agencies is early, regular, consistent and comprehensive. Providers that establish a communication team and prepare strategies, tools and templates find it easier to manage the needs of different stakeholders.

Quality and Safety Commission reflected back to the sector those lessons learned by Australian providers that experienced a COVID-19 outbreak at their RACF(s).[5] In general, these providers felt you could not over-prepare for an outbreak, as once it occurred there was little time to spare.

PRACTICE TIPS 5

OUTBREAK MANAGEMENT IN RACFs

- Document and *stress-test* a comprehensive, tailored outbreak management plan, such as for COVID-19, influenza or gastroenteritis, that explains how the RACF will prepare for, identify and manage any outbreaks. Include in the plan a floor diagram that clearly outlines possible cohort zones, resource requirements, staff continency plans, and education and communication strategies.
- Nominate a senior team to ensure the plans are periodically checked and are up to date.
- Educate staff, residents and visitors about the outbreak management plan and their roles and responsibilities.

29.3.7 Education and training

Education and training tailored for staff (e.g. nurses, PCAs, cleaning, kitchen and laundry staff), residents (if possible) and visitors (as appropriate) is critical to effective IPC in RACFs.[4,70] The basis for this teaching should be information contained in the national IPC guidelines, with an emphasis on standard and transmission-based precautions.[56] The aged care accreditation standards specifically require an RACF to educate relevant members of the workforce in antimicrobial resistance and strategies to reduce the risk of increasing resistance to antimicrobials.[1]

A variety of strategies can be used to improve IPC knowledge. For example, RACFs have successfully implemented:

- having staff demonstrate certain IPC competencies (such as hand hygiene and PPE use) using the 'train the trainer model' to distribute knowledge
- providing task checklists
- showing instruction videos to staff with limited English
- using a buddy system to check each other's practices on-site

- sending text messages to remind staff of certain requirements
- encouraging open feedback loops; and
- having IPC 'spotters' on-site for every shift.[71]

Repetition and interactivity have both been shown to be important factors in RACF behaviour change that is sustained.[15,56] Job-specific strategies should be delivered as part of orientation, annually or more frequently as required,[1] for example when there is a risk of an outbreak because of increased community transmission of a highly infectious disease. Competency should be assessed and records of participation maintained.[1]

PRACTICE TIPS 6

IPC EDUCATION AND TRAINING

- Support access to formal and informal relevant IPC training and education for staff (at all levels), residents and visitors.
- Inform all staff about the rights and responsibilities of residents and how to apply this understanding in the way IPC is delivered.
- Record orientation and ongoing IPC training delivered.
- Post visual signage that assists in instructing how to implement IPC precautions.

29.3.7 Surveillance

Surveillance in RACFs has been shown to be a valuable component of an IPC program (see also Chapter 10). In the Netherlands, between 2009 and 2015, 30 LTCFs participated in the national sentinel surveillance network for three years or more, 16 LTCFs for two years and the remaining 12 LTCFs for one year. Physicians reported weekly the number of cases of influenza-like illness, gastroenteritis, (probable) pneumonia, urinary tract infections (UTIs) and all-cause mortality. Adjusted for calendar year and season, a statistically significant decrease in the incidence of influenza-like illness (odds ratio (OR) = 0.8, P <0.01) and (probable) pneumonia (OR = 0.8, P <0.01) for each extra year an LTCF participated was observed.[72]

All Australian RACFs are strongly encouraged to at least participate in the Aged Care National Antimicrobial Prescribing Survey (NAPS). Aged Care NAPS, first piloted in 2015, was modelled on the European Centre for Disease Prevention and Control Healthcare-Associated Infection in Long Term Care Facilities

(HALT) study. It is an annual standardised point prevalence survey which monitors infections and assesses antimicrobial prescribing practices in RACFs. It can be officially undertaken on any single day between June and December.

The Centers for Disease Control (CDC) LTCF surveillance module provides guidance for standardised surveillance methodology that can be used in Australian RACFs. Protocols, training materials, data collection forms, instructions, and other supporting materials are provided for the following three modules:

1. healthcare-associated infection: UTIs

2. laboratory-identified events: *C. difficile* infection and MRO

3. prevention process measures: adherence to hand hygiene and/or adherence to gown and glove use when caring for residents infected or colonised with MROs or *C. difficile.*

Although their applicability to Australian RACFs has been questioned,[73] most use the McGeer et al surveillance definitions to define infections. These international definitions were developed in 1991. In 2012, an expert panel modified the definitions on the basis of a structured evidence-based literature review. Significant changes were made to the criteria defining urinary tract and respiratory tract infections. New definitions were added for norovirus gastroenteritis and *C. difficile* infections.[74]

PRACTICE TIPS 7

INFECTION SURVEILLANCE

- Collect, analyse and report surveillance data to monitor infections and the effectiveness of the IPC program.

- Do not apply infection surveillance definitions to guide clinical care.

- As a minimum, consider participating in the annual Aged Care NAPS.

29.3.8 Antimicrobial stewardship

The implementation of an antimicrobial stewardship (AMS) program in an RACF is widely recognised as necessary; the new aged care accreditation standards require RACFs to demonstrate appropriate antibiotic prescribing and use to support optimal care and reduce the risk of increasing resistance to antibiotics.[1]

The CDC outlines core elements which are necessary for implementing a successful AMS program in an RACF. The core elements include leadership commitment, accountability, drug expertise, action, tracking, reporting and education. For each core element, RACFs are encouraged to work in a step-wise fashion, adopting one or two AMS strategies to start and gradually adding new strategies over time.[75]

RACF management may initially choose, for example, to demonstrate leadership commitment by sharing with staff, residents and carers endorsed policies that reflect a resource commitment to AMS as a quality and safety initiative. In time, stewardship-related duties may be included in job-position descriptions. Nursing staff with the support of PCAs who deliver the most resident direct care can influence AMS programs by providing input on clinical assessments when prescribers are initiating or changing antibiotics.[8,24]

The RACF pharmacist may be able to assist using medication management software to create in-depth reports on the use of antimicrobials by class and by indication for incorporation in AMS audits, and feedback and education in QUM activities.[76] An accredited pharmacist when requested to do so by a referring medical practitioner can undertake Residential Medication Management Reviews (RMMR), a comprehensive assessment of a resident's medications and medication-related healthcare interventions.

To address action, criterion-based pathways or cognitive interventions to limit urine testing (urine dipstick and culture) may be initiated. Studies suggest that a substantial number of antibiotic starts for unnecessary treatment of asymptomatic bacteriuria can be reduced by introducing these strategies.[77]

PRACTICE TIPS 8

CORE ELEMENTS OF AMS PROGRAMS IN RACFS

- Develop AMS policies and processes that support appropriate antimicrobial use. This may include care strategies for common infections such as UTIs with and without indwelling catheter, respiratory tract infection and skin and soft tissue infection.

- Inform staff, including nurses, PCAs, and visiting GPs and pharmacists about the RACF's expectations regarding their AMS-specific roles and responsibilities.
- Provide education to staff, residents and visitors about antimicrobial resistance and appropriate antimicrobial use.
- Use shared decision-making tools[58] to support discussions with residents and families on using antibiotics when appropriate, ceasing them in a timely fashion when not required, and the risks and harms of excessive exposure to antimicrobials to the person and environment.

29.3.9 Vaccination programs

RACF providers are required as a minimum to have a vaccination program in place which:

- provides staff and volunteers access to a free annual influenza vaccination either on-site or by making arrangements for staff to access the vaccine at a local GP or chemist. RACFs that reported providing access to influenza vaccine under their programs had higher rates of staff vaccination as compared with those who only encouraged staff to go to an external provider[1]
- actively promotes the benefits of a vaccination program, including COVID-19
- keeps records evidencing the workforce influenza immunisation program, up-to-date records of staff flu vaccinations, and evidence of methods to promote the benefits of vaccination to staff.[1]

RACFs should aim for at least 95% of all staff and residents to be vaccinated prior to the commencement of each influenza season.[35]

At the time of admission, the resident's immunisation history should be reviewed. In Australia, it is currently recommended that all persons aged ≥65 receive an adjuvanted influenza vaccine annually. It is also recommended that all persons aged ≥70 receive a single dose 13-valent pneumococcal conjugate vaccine and all persons aged ≥60 receive a single dose of zoster vaccine.[78] RACF residents were prioritised to receive COVID-19 vaccine and boosters in Australia's rollout strategy.[79]

> **PRACTICE TIPS 9**
>
> ### STAFF AND RESIDENT VACCINATION
>
> - Document and implement recommended vaccination policies for staff and residents.
> - Keep up-to-date records of staff and resident vaccinations.
> - Document methods used to promote the benefits of staff and resident vaccination.

29.3.10 RACF design

There is an urgent need to examine architectural design models that balance IPC and quality of life for existing and proposed RACFs (Chapter 25). Early research has suggested smaller, more autonomous RACFs may improve IPC outcomes. The 'Green House model' is an example of these households; it typically has 10 to 12 residents, private bedrooms and bathrooms (as is preferable) that surround a central living area and open kitchen, access to a protected outdoor space and is serviced by a small number of dedicated staff. Outbreaks can be managed in one household without affecting adjacent or co-located settings.[80]

Most RACFs will not have airborne ventilation rooms. Creating a slightly negative pressure room involves installing supplemental exhaust ventilation, upgrading filters and keeping doors closed to maintain the negative pressure.

> **PRACTICE TIPS 10**
>
> ### IPC CONSIDERATION IN IPC DESIGN
>
> Seek expert advice on IPC considerations during the planning, design and construction of an RACF.

Conclusion

Delivering quality IPC to vulnerable residents in RACFs requires comparative formal, structural and organisational commitment. Consideration of the unique characteristics of RACFs and aged care residents is required before implementing key and specific work practices.

Useful websites/resources

- Royal Commission into Aged Care Quality and Safety. Aged care and COVID-19: a special report. Link: https://agedcare.royalcommission.gov.au/publications/aged-care-and-covid-19-special-report
- Royal Commission into Aged Care Quality and Safety. Final Report: Care, Dignity and Respect. Link: https://agedcare.royalcommission.gov.au/publications/final-report
- Aged Care Quality and Safety Commission. IPC Online Tool. Link: https://www.agedcarequality.gov.au/providers/ipc-online-tool
- Aged Care Quality and Safety Commission. Guidance and resources for providers to support Aged Care Quality Standards. Link: https://www.agedcarequality.gov.au/resources/guidance-and-resources-providers-support-aged-care-quality-standards
- Australian Institute of Health and Welfare. GEN Aged Care Data. Link: https://www.gen-agedcaredata.gov.au/
- Australian Government Department of Health and Aged Care. Strengthened Aged Care Quality Standards – Pilot Program. New aged care standards (draft). Link: https://www.health.gov.au/resources/publications/strengthened-aged-care-quality-standards-pilot-program

References

1. Aged Care Quality and Safety Commission. Guidance and resources for providers to support the Aged Care Quality Standards. Canberra: Australian Government, 2021.
2. Australian Government Department of Health and Aged Care. 2020-21 Report on the operation of the Aged Care Act 1997. Canberra: Australian Government, 2021.
3. Australian Institute of Health and Welfare. GEN aged care data. AIHW; May 2022. Canberra: Australian Government, 2021. Available from: https://www.gen-agedcaredata.gov.au/Topics.
4. Royal Commission into Aged Care Quality and Safety. Final report: care, dignity and respect. Canberra; Commonwealth of Australia, 2021. Available from: https://agedcare.royalcommission.gov.au/publications/final-report.
5. Aged Care Quality and Safety Commission. Lessons learned by aged care providers experiencing outbreaks of COVID-19 in Victoria, Australia. April 2021. Canberra: Commonwealth of Australia, 2021. Available from: https://www.agedcarequality.gov.au/media/89099.
6. Australian Government Department of Health and Aged Care. COVID-19 outbreaks in Australian residential aged care facilities, March 2023. Canberra: Australian Government, 2023. Available from: https://www.health.gov.au/resources/collections/covid-19-outbreaks-in-australian-residential-aged-care-facilities.
7. Royal Commission into Aged Care Quality and Safety. Aged care and COVID-19: a special report, 2020. Canberra; Commonwealth of Australia, 2020. Available from: https://agedcare.royalcommission.gov.au/publications/aged-care-and-covid-19-special-report.
8. Crnich CJ, Jump R, Trautner B, Sloane PD, Mody L. Optimizing antibiotic stewardship in nursing homes: a narrative review and recommendations for improvement. Drugs and Aging. 2015;32(9):699-716.
9. Australian Institute of Health and Welfare. Dementia in Australia. AIHW; May 2022. Canberra: Australian Government, 2022. Available from: https://www.aihw.gov.au/reports/dementia/dementia-in-aus/contents/aged-care-and-support-services-used-by-people-with-dementia/residential-aged-care.
10. Australian Government Department of Health and Aged Care. Aged care workforce census report, 2020. Canberra: Australian Government, 2020.
11. Australian Government Department of Health and Aged Care. National Aged Care Workforce Census and Survey - The Aged Care Workforce, 2016. Canberra: Australian Government, 2017.
12. Senator The Hon Richard Colbeck. Letter to aged care service providers about infection prevention and control leads. In: Residential aged care service provider, editor. Canberra: Australian Government, 2020.
13. Australian Government Department of Health and Aged Care. Infection prevention and control leads, May 2021. Canberra: Australian Government, 2021. Available from: https://www.health.gov.au/initiatives-and-programs/infection-prevention-and-control-leads#:~:text=Residential%20aged%20care%20facilities%20must,including%20COVID%2D19%20and%20influenza.
14. Aged Care Quality and Safety Commission. Infection prevention and control leads. Updates for providers. Canberra: Australian Government, 2021.
15. Lee MH, Lee GA, Lee SH, Park YH. Effectiveness and core components of infection prevention and control programmes in long-term care facilities: a systematic review. J Hosp Infect. 2019;102(4):377-393.
16. Shaban RZ, Sotomayor-Castillo C, Macbeth D, Russo PL, Mitchell BG. Scope of practice and educational needs of infection prevention and control professionals in Australian residential aged care facilities. Infect Dis Health. 2020;25(4):286-293.
17. Mitchell BG, Shaban RZ, MacBeth D, Russo P. Organisation and governance of infection prevention and control in Australian residential aged care facilities: a national survey. Infect Dis Health. 2019;24(4):187-193.
18. Stuart RL, Marshall C, Orr E, Bennett N, Athan E, Friedman D, et al. Survey of infection control and antimicrobial stewardship practices in Australian residential aged-care facilities. Intern Med J. 2015;45(5):576-580.

19. Bennett NJ, Bradford JM, Bull AL, Worth LJ. Infection prevention quality indicators in aged care: ready for a national approach. Aust Health Rev. 2019;43(4):396-398.

20. Nicolle LE. Infection control in long-term care facilities. Clin Infect Dis. 2000;31(3):752-756.

21. Smith PW, Bennett G, Bradley S, Drinka P, Lautenbach E, Marx J, et al. SHEA/APIC guideline: infection prevention and control in the long-term care facility, July 2008. Infect Control Hosp Epidemiol. 2008;29(9):785-814.

22. Brown L, Hansnata E, La HA. Economic cost of dementia in Australia 2016–2056. Melbourne: Alzheimer's Australia, 2017.

23. Royal Commission into Aged Care Quality and Safety. Statement of Associate Professor Mark Morgan (2019). Canberra; Commonwealth of Australia, 2021.

24. Lim CJ, Kwong MW, Stuart RL, Buising KL, Friedman ND, Bennett NJ, et al. Antibiotic prescribing practice in residential aged care facilities – health care providers' perspectives. Med J Aust. 2014;201(2):98-102.

25. Sluggett JK, Ilomaki J, Seaman KL, Corlis M, Bell JS. Medication management policy, practice and research in Australian residential aged care: current and future directions. Pharmacol Res. 2017;116:20-28.

26. Milazzo A, Tribe IG, Ratcliff R, Doherty C, Higgins G, Givney R. A large, prolonged outbreak of human calicivirus infection linked to an aged-care facility. Commun Dis Intell Q Rep. 2002;26(2):261-264.

27. Norman DC. Fever in the elderly. Clin Infect Dis. 2000;31(1): 148-151.

28. National Centre for Antimicrobial Stewardship and Australian Commission on Safety and Quality in Health Care. Antimicrobial prescribing and infections in Australian residential aged care facilities: results of the 2019 Aged Care National Antimicrobial Prescribing Survey. Sydney: ACSQHC, 2020.

29. Lansbury LE, Brown CS, Nguyen-Van-Tam JS. Influenza in long-term care facilities. Influenza Other Respir Viruses. 2017;11(5):356-366.

30. Loeb M, McGeer A, McArthur M, Peeling RW, Petric M, Simor AE. Surveillance for outbreaks of respiratory tract infections in nursing homes. CMAJ. 2000;162(8): 1133-1137.

31. Fukuyama H, Yamashiro S, Tamaki H, Kishaba T. A prospective comparison of nursing- and healthcare-associated pneumonia (NHCAP) with community-acquired pneumonia (CAP). J Infect Chemother. 2013;19(4):719-726.

32. Mansell V, Hall Dykgraaf S, Kidd M, Goodyear-Smith F. Long COVID and older people. Lancet Healthy Longev. 2022;3(12):e849-e54.

33. Therapeutic Guidelines Limited Melbourne. Therapeutic Guidelines, March 2023. Available from: https://www.tg.org.au.

34. Australian Government Department of Health and Aged Care. Updated eligibility for oral COVID-19 treatments, March. 2023. Canberra: Australian Government, 2023. Available from: https://www.health.gov.au/health-alerts/covid-19/treatments/eligibility.

35. Communicable Diseases Network of Australia (CDNA). Guidelines for the prevention, control and public health management of influenza outbreaks in residential care facilities in Australia. Canberra: Australian Government, 2017.

36. Centers for Disease Control and Prevention. Interim guidance for influenza outbreak management in long-term care and post-acute care facilities. [cited May 2022]. Atlanta GA: CDC, 2020. Available from: https://www.cdc.gov/flu/professionals/infectioncontrol/ltc-facility-guidance.

htm#:~:text=All%20long%2Dterm%20care%20facility,for%20laboratory%20confirmation%20of%20influenza.

37. Smith PW, Rusnak PG. Infection prevention and control in the long-term-care facility. SHEA Long-Term-Care Committee and APIC Guidelines Committee. Am J Infect Control. 1997;25(6):488-512.

38. Nicolle LE. Urinary tract infection in long-term-care facility residents. Clin Infect Dis. 2000;31(3):757-761.

39. Montoya A, Mody L. Common infections in nursing homes: a review of current issues and challenges. Aging Health. 2011;7(6):889-899.

40. Lim LL, Bennett N. Improving management of urinary tract infections in residential aged care facilities. Aust J Gen Pract. 2022;51(8):551-557.

41. Australian Commission on Safety and Quality in Health Care. Asymptomatic bacteriuria: reducing inappropriate antimicrobial prescribing for aged care facility residents. Sydney: ACSQHC, 2020.

42. Australian Commission on Safety and Quality in Health Care. Asymptomatic bacteriuria: reducing inappropriate antimicrobial prescribing for aged care facility residents. Sydney: ACSQHC, 2020.

43. Warren JW, Tenney JH, Hoopes JM, Muncie HL, Anthony WC. A prospective microbiologic study of bacteriuria in patients with chronic indwelling urethral catheters. J Infect Dis. 1982;146(6):719-723.

44. Kirk MD, Veitch MG, Hall GV. Gastroenteritis and food-borne disease in elderly people living in long-term care. Clin Infect Dis. 2010;50(3):397-404.

45. Chopra T, Goldstein EJ. Clostridium difficile infection in long-term care facilities: a call to action for antimicrobial stewardship. Clin Infect Dis. 2015;60 Suppl 2:S72-76.

46. National Centre for Immunisation Research and Surveillance. Herpes zoster vaccine for Australian adults. NCIRS, 2017.

47. Bonomo RA. Multiple antibiotic-resistant bacteria in long-term-care facilities: an emerging problem in the practice of infectious diseases. Clin Infect Dis. 2000; 31(6):1414-1422.

48. McKinnell JA, Miller LG, Singh RD, Gussin G, Kleinman K, Mendez J, et al. High prevalence of multidrug-resistant organism colonization in 28 nursing homes: an "iceberg effect". J Am Med Dir Assoc. 2020;21(12):1937-43e2.

49. Aliyu S, Smaldone A, Larson E. Prevalence of multidrug-resistant gram-negative bacteria among nursing home residents: a systematic review and meta-analysis. Am J Infect Control. 2017;45(5):512-518.

50. Australian Commission on Safety and Quality in Health Care (ACSQHC). Australian Passive Antimicrobial Resistance Surveillance (APAS) First report: multi-resistant organisms. Sydney: ACSQHC, 2018.

51. Chen Y, Kirk MD, Stuart R, Cheng AC, Pearson SA, Hayen A, et al. Socio-demographic and health service factors associated with antibiotic dispensing in older Australian adults. PLoS One. 2019;14(8):e0221480.

52. Sluggett JK, Moldovan M, Lynn DJ, Papanicolas LE, Crotty M, Whitehead C, et al. National trends in antibiotic use in australian residential aged care facilities, 2005-2016. Clin Infect Dis. 2021;72(12):2167-2174.

53. Sluggett JK, Moldovan M, Lang C, Lynn DJ, Papanicolas LE, Crotty M, et al. Contribution of facility level factors to variation in antibiotic use in long-term care facilities: a national cohort study. J Antimicrob Chemother. 2021; 76(5):1339-1348.

54. Dyar OJ, Pagani L, Pulcinic C. Strategies and challenges of antimicrobial stewardship in long term care facilities. Clin Microbiol Infect. 2015;21(1):10-9.

55. Stuart RL, Wilson J, Bellaard-Smith E, Brown R, Wright L, Vandergraaf S, et al. Antibiotic use and misuse in residential aged care facilities. Intern Med J. 2012;42(10):1145-1149.

56. National Health and Medical Research Council. Australian guidelines for the prevention and control of infection in healthcare. Canberra: NHMRC, 2019.

57. Australian Government Department of Social Services and National Health and Medical Research Council (NHMRC). Prevention and control of infection in residential and community aged care 2013. Canberra: Australian Government, 2013.

58. Australian Government Aged Care Quality and Safety Commission. AMS clinician resources April 2022. Canberra: Australian Government, 2021. Available from: https://www.agedcarequality.gov.au/antimicrobial-stewardship/clinician-resources#clinical-pathway-for-suspected-urinary-tract-infections.

59. Australian Commission on Safety and Quality in Health Care. Antimicrobial stewardship in Australian health care. Sydney ACSQHC, 2018.

60. Australian Government Department of Health and Aged Care - Infection Control Expert Group. Coronavirus (COVID-19) guidelines for infection prevention and control in residential care facilities. Canberra: Australian Government, 2020.

61. The Royal Australian College of General Practitioners. RACGP aged care clinical guide (Silver Book) Part B. Collaboration and multidisciplinary team-based care. RACGP, 2019.

62. Gnanasambantham K, Aitken G, Morris B, Simionato J, Chua EH, Ibrahim JE. Developing a clinical screening tool for identifying COVID-19 infection in older people dwelling in residential aged care services. Australas J Ageing. 2021;40(1):48-57.

63. Antibiotic Expert Group. Therapeutic guidelines: antibiotic. Version 16. Melbourne: Therapeutic Guidelines Ltd, 2019.

64. Cassell JA, Middleton J, Nalabanda A, Lanza S, Head MG, Bostock J, et al. Scabies outbreaks in ten care homes for elderly people: a prospective study of clinical features, epidemiology, and treatment outcomes. Lancet Infect Dis. 2018;18(8):894-902.

65. Lay CJ, Wang CL, Chuang HY, Chen YL, Chen HL, Tsai SJ, et al. Risk factors for delayed diagnosis of scabies in hospitalized patients from long-term care facilities. J Clin Med Res. 2011;3(2):72-77.

66. Communicable Diseases Network Australia. National guidelines for the prevention, control and public health management of COVID-19 outbreaks in residential care facilities in Australia. Canberra: Australian Government, 2021.

67. Australian Government Department of Health and Ageing. Management of outbreaks in aged-care facilities. Canberra: Australian Government, 2010.

68. Communicable Diseases Network of Australia (CDNA). COVID-19 outbreaks in residential care facilities. National guidelines for the prevention, control and public health management of COVID-19 outbreaks in residential care facilities. 5th ed, Canberra: Australian Government, 2022.

69. National Health and Medical Research Council. Australian guidelines for the prevention and control of infection in healthcare. Canberra: Australian Government, 2019.

70. Richards MJ, Stuart R.L. Principles of infection control in long-term care facilities. UpToDate, 2019.

71. Aged Care Quality and Safety Commission. Lessons learned by aged care providers experiencing outbreaks of COVID-19 in Victoria, Australia. Canberra: Australian Government, 2021.

72. Haenen APJ, Verhoef LP, Beckers A, Gijsbers EF, Alblas J, Huis A, et al. Surveillance of infections in long-term care facilities (LTCFs): the impact of participation during multiple years on health care-associated infection incidence. Epidemiol Infect. 2019;147:e266.

73. Bennett NJ, Johnson SA, Richards MJ, Smith MA, Worth LJ. Infections in Australian aged-care facilities: evaluating the impact of revised McGeer criteria for surveillance of urinary tract infections. Infect Control Hosp Epidemiol. 2016;37(5): 610-612.

74. Stone ND, Ashraf MS, Calder J, Crnich CJ, Crossley K, Drinka PJ, et al. Surveillance definitions of infections in long-term care facilities: revisiting the McGeer criteria. Infect Control Hosp Epidemiol. 2016;37(5):610-612.

75. Centers for Disease Control and Prevention. The core elements of antibiotic stewardship for nursing homes. Atlanta GA: CDC, 2015.

76. NPS MedicineWise. Antibiotics for urinary tract infections 2017. [cited 2021 May]. Available from: https://www.nps.org.au/cpd/activities/antibiotics-for-urinary-tract-infections.

77. Meddings J, Saint S, Krein SL, Gaies E, Reichert H, Hickner A, et al. Systematic review of interventions to reduce urinary tract infection in nursing home residents. J Hosp Med. 2017;12(5):356-368.

78. Australian Technical Advisory Group on Immunisation (ATAGI). Australian immunisation handbook. Canberra: Australian Government, 2018.

79. Australian Government Department of Health and Ageing. Information for aged care providers, workers and residents about COVID-19 vaccines 2021. [cited May 2021]. Canberra: Australian Government, 2021. Available from: https://www.health.gov.au/initiatives-and-programs/covid-19-vaccines/information-for-aged-care-providers-workers-and-residents-about-covid-19-vaccines.

80. Cohen LW, Zimmerman S, Reed D, Brown P, Bowers BJ, Nolet K, et al. Collaborative TR. The green house model of nursing home care in design and implementation. Health Serv Res. 2016;51.S1:352-377.

CHAPTER 30

Infection prevention and control in oncology and immunocompromised patient settings

Dr PRIYA GARG[i]

Dr NICOLE GILROY[ii]

Chapter highlights

- An overview of the characteristics and contexts of the oncology and immunocompromised patient in Australia
- Detailed description of the healthcare-associated risks, opportunistic pathogens and management challenges associated with the care of the oncology and immunocompromised patient
- A review of current infection prevention and control strategies employed in the care of the oncology and immunocompromised host

i   Infectious Diseases, Westmead Hospital, Sydney, NSW
ii Centre for Infectious Diseases & Microbiology, Westmead Hospital, Sydney, NSW

Introduction

This chapter presents an introduction to the characteristics of oncology and immunocompromised patients within Australia and broadly defines the disease and treatment-related mechanisms of immunosuppression. It further outlines their specific infectious disease related risks within the healthcare setting, encompassing a broad range of pathogens of bacterial, fungal, viral and parasitic aetiology, and the challenges faced in the management of these. In addition, it provides a structured approach to current strategies of infection prevention and control (IPC) practice within healthcare facilities, delivering care to patients at both an individual and population level. Further opportunities for harnessing novel technological solutions for IPC in the future within the immunocompromised and oncological cohort are also discussed.

30.1 Characteristics and contexts of oncology and the immunocompromised in Australia

The term 'immunocompromised' is broad and ever-expanding in an era of enhanced diagnostic capacity, transplant opportunity, novel immunosuppressive therapies and prolonged patient survival. It can, however, roughly be defined as a host with an increased susceptibility to infection from organisms with a naturally low virulence, or an unusually severe infection from a common pathogen—usually termed an 'opportunistic infection'.[1] They also face an accelerated progression of chronic infection and the reactivation of latent or dormant pathogens.[2] The state of immunocompromise occurs through an impairment of the host defence system, which can be primary or secondary. Oncology patients can be affected both through disease and as a consequence of treatment.

30.1.1 Mechanisms of action in the immunocompromised

Primary immunocompromise: Primary immunodeficiency disorders are defined as a diverse group of conditions in which single or multiple genetic defects cause an alteration in immune function affecting components of the innate or adaptive host immune system (Table 30.1). Innate host mechanisms tend to be rapid and have a predictable response to broad groups of pathogens, leading to activation of the

TABLE 30.1 Examples of primary immunodeficiency disorders and associated infections

Host defence disorder	Disease	Associated infections
Cell-mediated immunity	Chronic mucocutaneous candidiasis, DiGeorge syndrome, X-linked lymphoproliferative disease	Broad range of opportunistic pathogens (including pneumonia—pyogenic bacteria, *pneumocystis jiroveci*), gastrointestinal (viruses), skin and mucous membranes (fungi)
Antibody and cell-mediated	Severe combined immunodeficiency (SCID)	Muco-cutaneous candidiasis; *Pneumocystis jirovecii* pneumonia; chronic diarrhoea; severe and potentially fatal infection from common viral pathogens (herpesviruses; respiratory viruses; rotavirus, adenovirus, norovirus)
Antibody	X-linked agammaglobulinemia, common variable immunodeficiency (CVID), selective IgA deficiency, Wiskott- Aldrich syndrome	Sinopulmonary (pyogenic bacteria and viruses), gastrointestinal (enterovirus/giardia)
Phagocytosis	Congenital neutropenia, Chronic granulomatous disease Leukocyte adhesion deficiency, Chediak-Higashi syndrome	Skin and reticuloendothelial system (staphylococcal infections/fungi/mycobacteria/enteric organisms)
Complement pathway	Deficiencies in: Classical pathway (C1q,r,s; C2-C4 deficiency) Alternative pathway Mannose-lectin binding pathway Terminal components (C5,6,7,8 9)	Sepsis (streptococcal/pneumococcal/ *N. meningitidis*)

Source: Dropulic, L. K., & Lederman, H. M. (2016). Overview of infections in the immunocompromised host. Diagnostic microbiology of the immunocompromised host, 1-50.

complement cascade and phagocytosis. The adaptive immune system, although slower, utilises a specific antigen response which can be enhanced with repeated exposures, and allows for the formation of immunological memory. Components of adaptive immunity include T- and B-cell lymphocytes and antibodies. Disorders of host defence can affect any of these mechanisms—cell-mediated immunity, the complement pathway, phagocytosis and antibody response, increasing the risk for opportunistic infection.[3] (See Fig 30.1.)

Current prevalence of primary immunodeficiency in Australia is estimated to be 5.6 per 100,000, of which most are antibody-related disorders (77.4%), with combined variable immunodeficiency being the most frequently diagnosed disease.[4]

Other genetic syndromes not strictly defined as primary immunodeficiencies, but frequently associated with immunocompromise and increased risk of infection, include the inborn errors of metabolism such as congenital disorders of glycosylation, branched chain amino acidurias and lysinuric protein intolerances. Individuals with a diagnosis of Trisomy 21 may also suffer from an increased risk of infection due to an abnormal expression of interferon-related genes. Low T- and B-cell populations have also been found in patients with Turner Syndrome (monosomy XO). Cystic fibrosis patients with CFTR mutations also classically suffer from altered mucociliary transport and abnormal immune function, leaving them prone to opportunistic infection.[5]

Secondary immunocompromise: Secondary immunocompromise occurs due to factors extrinsic to the immune system and encompasses a wide array of disease- and treatment-related causes.[6] At its most basic it can simply happen at extremes of age—in the neonate this has been attributed to an immaturity of the adaptive and innate immune system, and in the elderly to immunosenescence affecting immune cell functioning.[5] Comparable with most high-resource settings, the Australian population is ageing as life expectancy increases and fertility rates drop. It is predicted that 22.5% of Australia's population will be 65 years and over by 2050.[7]

Pregnancy has also been implicated in altered host defence through the placental immune response modulating maternal susceptibility to, and severity of, certain infections.[8]

30.1.2 Human immunodeficiency virus (HIV)

Acquired immunodeficiency syndrome (AIDS) caused by human immunodeficiency virus (HIV) is one of the most well-documented secondary causes of immunocompromise, of which a quantitative and qualitative reduction in total CD4 T-lymphocyte count is a defining feature.

The advent of effective highly active antiretroviral therapy (HAART) has significantly reduced the morbidity and mortality among patients living with HIV through viral control, particularly in high-resource settings. However, the persistence of inflammation and

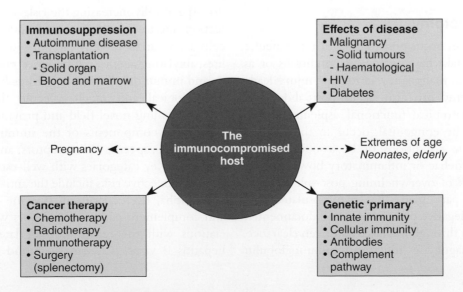

FIGURE 30.1 The immunocompromised host

immune dysfunction in people living with HIV through changes to the adaptive and innate immune system is thought to contribute to non–AIDS-related immunocompromise from the increased development of comorbidities such as diabetes mellitus.[9]

In Australia, the estimated prevalence of HIV among individuals over 15 years is estimated at 0.14%; however, changes in risk over time have shown increasing notifications from heterosexual exposures, and among Aboriginal and Torres Strait Islander population subgroups.[10]

30.1.3 Diabetes

One of the most frequently diagnosed secondary causes of immunocompromise among the Australian population is diabetes mellitus—occurring in almost 1 in every 20 individuals.[11] It is a disease defined by disordered insulin secretion or action and associated with an increased risk of infection through altered immune function. This is caused by a reduction in neutrophil function and T-lymphocyte responses alongside downregulation of pro-inflammatory cytokine secretion. A hyperglycaemic environment has also been postulated to increase the susceptibility of cells to oxidative stress and lead to apoptosis of protective polymorphonuclear cells.[12] A lowered environmental pH found in conditions such as diabetic ketoacidosis is also associated with an increased susceptibility to severe fungal infections such as mucormycosis due to an impairment of phagocytic cell functioning. Furthermore, aberrant iron metabolism in an acidic environment promotes the release of free iron which supports fungal growth.[13] Glycation of immunoglobulins is also thought to occur in proportion to a higher HbA1c which may affect antibody functioning.[12]

30.1.4 Splenectomy

Spleen removal can occur post trauma, as a therapeutic procedure in certain haematological conditions or as treatment for local malignancy. Iatrogenic injury leading to splenectomy can also occur post abdominal intervention. Anatomical/functional asplenia or hyposplenism may be congenital, occur in the context of certain genetic conditions or be associated with diseases such as coeliac or inflammatory bowel disease. An increased risk of overwhelming post-splenectomy infection (OPSI) particularly due to encapsulated bacteria and Gram-negative pathogens is well documented in this population through impaired pathogen clearance, opsonisation, phagocytic function, immunoglobulin

production and antibody activity. Additionally, systemic inflammatory pathways are thought to be attenuated leading to further immunocompromise.[14]

30.1.5 Autoimmune disorders and their treatments

Immune-based diseases are defined by intrinsic immune alteration, autoantibody production and chronic, often multi-organ, inflammation. Common disorders include rheumatoid arthritis (RA), systemic lupus erythematosus (SLE), multiple sclerosis (MS) and inflammatory bowel disease (IBD). Patients with these diseases are prone to opportunistic infection from the disease itself whereby autoantibodies affect routine protective cellular functioning mechanisms and the clearance of pathogens, as well as through disease management via immune suppression.[12] The burden of autoimmune disease is increasing nationally in Australia with SLE thought to disproportionately affect the Indigenous population, unlike other autoimmune conditions.[15]

Corticosteroids alongside biological, non-biological disease modifying drugs and small-molecule therapies are used in the treatment of these disorders. Corticosteroids have well-recognised, potent immunosuppressive effects through the suppression of macrophage differentiation, cytokine production, neutrophil migration and activity, and lysosomal enzyme release. Additionally, they cause significant lymphopenia through inhibiting interleukin signalling and inducing apoptosis of maturing T-lymphocytes.[16]

Traditional immunosuppressants similarly employ a broad range of strategies to dampen the immune response including the suppression of cell replication, inhibition of cell signalling and antagonism of cytokines and their receptors, with the consequence of non-specifically increasing the risk of opportunistic infection due to damage to a multitude of key immune cells. They can be broadly categorised into antimetabolites, alkylating agents, inhibitors of nucleotide synthesis and immunophilin-binding drugs.[17]

Biological and small-molecule therapies are an ever-expanding novel field and provide more targeted therapy to components of the immune system such as cytokines, specific cell-receptors, and pathways (see Fig 30.2). Key categories with well-established specific increased infective risks include the anti–CD20/52 drugs, TNF-alpha, IL-17, Bruton's tyrosine kinase, integrin and complement pathway inhibitors which have associations with the reactivation of latent tuberculosis, hepatitis B virus, JC virus, profound CD4 depletion,

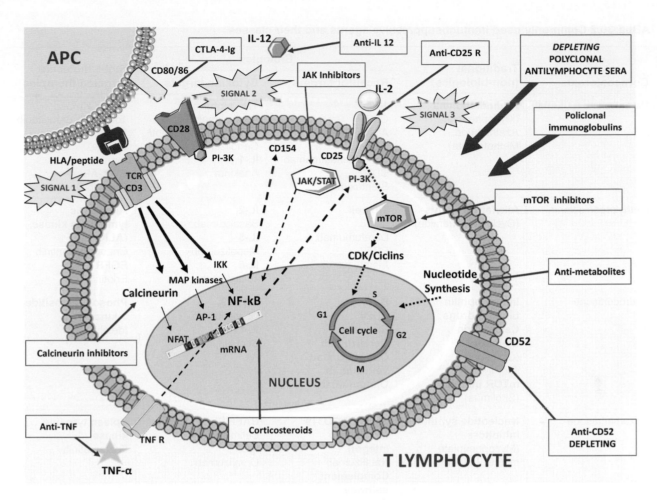

FIGURE 30.2 Major actions of common immunosuppressants on T-cells and antigen-presenting cells
Source: Adapted from the book: Hernando Nefrología Clinica, Panamericana.

mucocutaneous candidiasis, invasive fungal disease, and *Neisseria* spp. infections (Table 30.2).[18]

30.1.6 The oncology patient—solid organ malignancy

Unsurprisingly, oncology patients are highly susceptible to opportunistic infection. Australia has one of the highest incidences of cancer globally, with an increase in the overall age-standardised cancer incidence from 350.7/100,000 population in 1995 to 364.4/100,000 in 2015.[20] Additionally, large increases in age standardised incidence rates have been projected in liver, colorectal and female lung cancer over the next 9 years.[21]

Chemotherapy involves the use of a drug or chemical to lead to tumour cell death. Agents can be subdivided into classes according to their mechanism of

action, with the main groups being alkylating agents, antimetabolites, topoisomerase and mitotic spindle inhibitors.[22] These agents can have potent effects on cellular and humoral immunity, affecting key components such as immunoglobulin production, T-lymphocytes, the complement cascade and macrophages/monocytes, alongside causing profound and often prolonged neutropenia (see Table 30.3).[23]

Additional risk factors for immunocompromise during chemotherapeutic cycles include malnutrition, asplenia, the use of prosthetic devices such as central venous catheters, and injury to skin and mucosal surfaces.[24]

Radiotherapy is considered one of the stalwarts of cancer treatment. Ionising radiation in the form of electro-magnetic waves is delivered in fractions leading to DNA damage, cell death and tumour control.

TABLE 30.2 Commonly used immunosuppressive agents and their classes

| Corticosteroids | Traditional (non-biologics) | Biologics | | Small molecule targeted therapies |
		Receptor targets	Cytokine targets	
Prednisolone	**Antimetabolites** (Mycophenolate, Azathioprine, Methotrexate)	**T cell** CD2 Alefacept CD3 OKT3/Blinatumomab CD30 Brentuximab	**TNF alpha** Adalimumab/ Infliximab/Etanercept/ Certolizumab **IL-1** Anakinra	**Janus Kinase** Tofacitinib/Baracitanib **Bruton's tyrosine kinase** Ibrutinib **BCR-ABL** Imatinib/Dastinib
Methylprednisolone	**Alkylating agents** (Cyclophosphamide)	**T/B cell** CD38 Daratumumab CD52 Alemtuzumab	**IL-2** Basalizumab **IL-5** Mepolizumab **IL-6** Tocilizumab	**Anaplastic lymphoma kinase (ALK)** Crizotinib/Ceritinib **EGFR** Erlotinib
Hydrocortisone	**Immunophilin-binding drugs Calcineurin inhibitors** (Ciclosporin/ Tacrolimus) **mTOR inhibitors** (Sirolimus)	**B cell** CD20 Rituximab **Ocrelizumab Obinutuzumab Veltuzumab Ofatumumab**	**IL12/23** Ustekinumab **IL-17a** Secukinumab	**Phosophoinositide-3-kinase** Idelalisib
Dexamethasone	**Nucleotide synthesis inhibitors** (Mycophenolate mofetil, Leflunomide)	**SLAMF7/CD319** Elotuzumab **Integrin** Natalizumab **Complement pathway** Eculizumab	**BAFF/BLyS** Belimumab **IgE** Omalizumab	**Spleen tyrosine kinase** Fostamatinib

Source: Data from Davis JS, Ferreira D, Paige E, Gedye C, Boyle M. Infectious Complications of Biological and Small Molecule Targeted Immuno-modulatory Therapies. Clin Microbiol Rev. 2020;33(3)

TABLE 30.3 Commonly used chemotherapeutic agents and their mechanisms of action

Class	Subclasses	Example agents
Alkylating agents	Oxazsaphosphorines Nitrogen mustards Platinum agents	Cyclophosphamide/Ifosfamide Melphalan/Temozolomide Cisplatin/Carboplatin/Oxaliplatin
Antimetabolites	Pyrimidine antagonists Purine antagonists Purine analogues Antifolates Ribonucleotide reductase inhibitors	Cytarabine/5-fluorouracil Fludarabine 6-mercaptopurine/azathioprine Methotrexate Hydroxyurea
Topoisomerase inhibitors I & II	Topoisomerase I Topoisomerase II Anthracyclines	Irinotecan Etoposide Idarubicin/Doxorubicin
Mitotic spindle inhibitors	Taxanes Vinca alkaloids	Paclitaxel Vincristine/Vinblastine
Others	Enzymes Antibiotic	L-asparaginase Bleomycin

Source:[22]

However, radiation therapy can also cause the direct depletion of circulating lymphocytes and their progenitors in lymphoid organs, lead to an enhancement of cytokine mediated immunosuppressive pathways and activate myeloid-derived suppressor cells.[25]

The last few decades have also seen the advent of novel targeted immunotherapy agents termed 'checkpoint inhibitors' allowing for directed immune activation to specific cancer cells. The key molecules in immune checkpoint signalling include programmed cell death protein 1 (PD-1), its ligand (PD-L1) and cytotoxic T-lymphocyte associated antigen 4 (CTLA-4).[26] These are increasingly combined with another newer agent in the oncology treatment armoury—ALK inhibitors. ALK inhibitors target the ALK receptor tyrosine kinase pathway relating to cell proliferation and are largely used in the treatment of non-small-cell lung cancer.

Little immunocompromise has been associated with the use of immune checkpoint inhibitors to date, with the incidence of cytopenia post treatment reported to be <1%. Likewise, there is no clear evidence that ALK inhibitors increase the risk of immunocompromise. Nonetheless, longitudinal data on both, including combination therapies, is yet to come.[18]

30.1.7 Haematological malignancies

Haematological malignancies also drive vulnerability to infection through the disease itself or use of antineoplastic therapies—often with profound and prolonged myelosuppressive side effects.

Patients with myeloid cell line malignancies commonly have dysfunctional granulocyte activity despite apparently normal peripheral counts. Chronic lymphocytic leukaemia and B-cell neoplasms are frequently associated with immunoglobulin dyscrasias, affecting antibody-dependent cellular cytotoxicity, phagocytosis, pro-inflammatory cytokine release and activation of complement cascade.

Similar to the autoimmune and oncology population, the use of targeted biological therapy has also expanded significantly over the last decade in the treatment of haematological disease. Important agents include monoclonal antibodies, bispecific T-cell engagers, tyrosine/brutons tyrosine kinase inhibitors, janus-associated kinase inhibitors and B-cell lymphoma 2 inhibitors. These have a host of immune-related complications—including prolonged B-cell depletion, hypogammaglobulinemia, neutropenia and effects on T, NK and dendritic cell functioning—leading to defects in the mechanisms of innate and adaptive immunity.[18,27]

Novel cellular treatments have also become more frequently used in the haematology cohort including T-cell depletion, donor leukocyte infusions and genetically engineered chimeric antigen receptor (CAR) T-cell therapy, with a current paucity of data on their overall long-term risks. The use of preceding lymphodepleting therapy alongside cytokine-related cytopenias, B-cell depletion and hypogammaglobulinemia have all been associated with CAR T-cell therapy related immunocompromise so far, however.[28] Additionally, the requirement for immunosuppressive therapy such as high-dose corticosteroids and IL-6 inhibitors to treat the common complications of CAR T-cell therapy—such as cytokine release syndrome and immune effector cell neurotoxicity—in turn increases the risk of opportunistic infection.[29]

30.1.8 The transplant population—solid organ transplant (SOT)

In 2021, there were 1173 SOT recipients in Australia.[3] Excluding the impact of the COVID-19 global pandemic, since 2009 deceased organ donations have increased by 82% across Australia and were most recently estimated at 20.8 donations per million population.[31]

Agents used in the treatment of autoimmune disorders are similarly employed in the SOT population, with the same consequences of immunocompromise. Additional infectious risks among this cohort also include the transmission of an infectious disease from organ donor to recipient. If anticipated, strategies such as monitoring, prophylaxis or treatment can be used.[32] Strict pre-transplant screening of both donor and recipient pre-transplant across Australia and New Zealand aims to reduce the risk of unexpected pathogen transmission to an acceptable level; however, this risk can never be eliminated.[33]

SOT-specific risks also involve time post-transplant. Surgical-complication related infections generally occur within the first month after transplant and opportunistic infection risk is highest in the first six months where intensive immunosuppression is employed to prevent acute graft injection. Beyond the first six months, defined as the late transplant period, although chronically immunosuppressed, recipients are noted to overall suffer from the same infectious complications as the general community.[34] However, if chronic graft rejection occurs, this is again high risk for opportunistic infection due to the requirement for augmented immunosuppression to prevent graft loss.[35]

30.1.9 Haematopoietic stem cell transplantation (HSCT)

Haematopoietic stem cell transplantations are often used in the management of haematological malignancy, of which infection is a well-recognised complication and a higher risk in those with an allogeneic rather than an autologous transplant. Susceptibility is affected by patient factors including age, obesity, comorbidities, and immunity to previous opportunistic infections. Disease factors such as malignancy type, disease stage and previous chemotherapy regimens also affect risk. Transplant-specific factors include choice of conditioning and immunosuppressive therapy, multiple transplants and the degree of human leukocyte antigen mismatch between donor and recipient.[36,37]

The rates of HSCT over 8 years between 2005 and 2013 increased by 25% in Australia, and 52% in New Zealand, with the major indications being acute myeloid leukaemia (AML), acute lymphoblastic leukaemia (ALL), plasma cell disorders and non-Hodgkin lymphoma.[38]

A total of 725 allogeneic and 1480 autologous HSCT were performed in Australasia in 2020. Infection-related complications contributed to a significant proportion of transplant-related mortality in the first 100 days after autologous and allogeneic transplant.[39]

The early pre-engraftment phase post-HSCT is associated with often profound and prolonged neutropenia, mucositis, and device-related infection risks due to the need for foreign indwelling lines and ports. Following this, the development of graft vs host disease (GvHD) can occur with associated impaired cell and humoral immunity. Occurring within the first 100 days it is termed acute GvHD (aGvHD), while chronic GvHD (cGvHD) is recognised as a risk for late transplant opportunistic infection.[40] Hypogammaglobulinemia may also be found in individuals suffering from intestinal tract GvHD through protein-losing enteropathy.[41] Functional

hyposplenism may be an additional sequalae of cGVHD, whereby rates of invasive pneumococcal disease are noted to be significantly higher compared to the background population.[42]

Increasing evidence has also implicated alterations in the gut microbiome in patients with malignancy and post-transplant, leading to the promotion of bacterial and fungal translocation from the gastrointestinal tract, and invasive infection.[43]

CASE STUDY 1

Unusual cutaneous infection in a renal transplant patient, Sydney

Situation:

A 65-year-old Tongan taxi driver with a preceding renal transplant presented with a slow growing lesion over his left thumb. He described a possible scratch to the thumb while gardening in his vegetable patch several months prior:

- He was immunosuppressed on oral mycophenolate mofetil 1g twice daily, tacrolimus 1.5/1g and prednisolone 10 mg daily

- He had also had a SARS-CoV-2 infection a month before presentation—receiving high-dose steroids, baracitanib (JAK inhibitor) and tocilizumab (IL-6 inhibitor)

- Diabetic screening was unremarkable (HbA1c 5%)

Questions:

What risk factors does this patient have for opportunistic infection? Which organisms would you consider?

- Methenamine silver and periodic acid Schiff (PAS) staining on histopathological specimens from his left thumb lesion revealed oval spores and septate fungal organisms. Tissue and fluid samples from the lesion identified the fungus *Phaeacremonium parasiticum*.

Would you perform any further tests for this patient?

- An MRI of the hand revealed a large multi-loculated cyst at the site of the original lesion and multiple cystic lesions within the carpal bones.

- In the context of a headache, a CT brain and CSF sampling was performed. Due to a persistent dry cough

---

PRACTICE TIPS 1

CAUSES AND CONSEQUENCES OF IMMUNOCOMPROMISE

- Immunocompromise can be broadly caused by innate disease (such as malignancy) and treatment-related factors, all of which predispose patients to infectious risks

- Alongside traditional immunosuppression, chemo and radiotherapy, the broader use of novel biological and small molecule therapies is likely to also cause a significant impact on the risk of opportunistic infection within this cohort

- The effects on innate and adaptive immune mechanisms predispose patients to a variety of differing opportunistic pathogens, some attributable to the pathway affected

and complaints of dyspnoea a CT chest and TTE were also requested to exclude disseminated disease with no positive findings.

- The patient received treatment with oral antifungals (4mg/kg BD voriconazole). Surgical debridement was planned.
- Invasive infections with unusual pathogens are a risk in the immunocompromised patient.

30.2 Healthcare-associated infection risks associated with care in oncology and the immunocompromised in Australia

Healthcare-associated infections (HAIs) are defined as those occurring within a healthcare facility either after the first 48 hours of admission or within 30 days post discharge. Healthcare facilities encompass a wide variety of settings where the immunocompromised and oncology cohort may access treatment including acute hospitals, clinics, ambulatory care centres and hospital-in-the-home.[44] Within acute hospitals alone, 1 in 10 Australians are estimated to experience an HAI. This has further associated effects of increasing morbidity, mortality, length of stay, antimicrobial resistance and additional health costs.[45] Although specific infectious risks may differ among the spectrum of clinical settings, a basic understanding of the types of pathogens and how infections occur is integral to implementing effective control and reducing complications among this population group.[46]

Immunocompromised patients are recognised to be at particular risk of nosocomial infection, relating to their poor immune defences and thus increased propensity for infections of low pathogenicity to cause invasive or fulminant disease. In addition, the frequent requirement for these patients to have instrumentation and indwelling devices (peripheral and central venous access devices, nasogastric tubes and urinary catheterisation), blood products for supportive care, prolonged and frequent healthcare encounters and broad antimicrobial exposures all compound the risk of the transmission of multidrug-resistant organisms (MROs), blood-borne and respiratory viruses and gastrointestinal pathogens. The difficulty in controlling and resolving communicable respiratory and gastrointestinal infections can also present a risk at a

unit level, when patients may be colocated or attending outpatient services.[44]

30.2.1 Bacteria

Bacteria can originate from endogenous and exogeneous settings to cause HAIs, particularly in the immunocompromised. Frequently implicated endogenous pathogens include skin, oropharyngeal and enteric colonisers such as *staphylococci*, *streptococci*, *enterococci* and *Enterobacteriaceae*, notably *E. coli*, *Klebsiella* and *Enterobacter* spp., which under the correct environment can cause invasive disease in a susceptible host.[47]

Exogeneous bacterial pathogens survive in the environment, contaminating hands, surfaces and equipment, whereby the healthcare setting acts as a reservoir for their propagation and transmission. This includes MROs such as methicillin-resistant *Staphylococcus aureus* (MRSA), vancomycin-resistant *Enterococcus* (VRE) and multidrug-resistant Gram-negative bacilli (MDR-GNB). Organisms such as *Enterobacteriaceae* can also persist in biofilms in difficult to clean areas such as drains or equipment, which increases the complexity of eradication.[48,49]

MRSA, *Pseudomonas aeruginosa*, *Acinetobacter* spp. and *Clostridium difficile* are also notable for their ability to thrive in the hospital environment.[47] The invasive nosocomial spread of virulent Gram-negatives has also been associated with exposure to contaminated solutions such as antiseptics and disinfectants, such as in the case of *Burkholderia cepacia*.[50] Immunocompromised patients in particular also experience a high rate of infection and recurrence with *Clostridium difficile*, due to their frequency of antimicrobial use, healthcare exposures and a higher prevalence of gut colonisation.[51]

Moist environments within a healthcare setting can further serve as conduits for hydrophilic organisms such as *Legionella* spp. and nontuberculous mycobacteria (NTM).[52] In 2017, the first case of disseminated *Mycobacterium chimaera* was reported in Australia following cardiothoracic surgery, linked through whole genome sequencing to contamination of a heater-cooler unit used at time of intervention.[53] Whole genome sequencing has also been effectively employed in investigations of *Legionella pneumophilia* outbreaks in Australian hospitals to link cases to the healthcare facility's hot-water supply.[54]

The nosocomial transmission of the soil- and water-based organism *Burkholderia pseudomallei* has also been described in the context of contaminated saline irrigation fluid causing a cluster outbreak among multiple individuals. Melioidosis is a disease endemic to Northern and Western Australia with significant clinical manifestations, particularly in the immunocompromised, including skin and soft tissue infection, pneumonia, often fatal sepsis and meningoencephalitis.[55]

Although Australia has one of the lowest incidences of *Mycobacterium tuberculosis* (MTB) globally (5.8 cases per 100,000 population), this is still a pathogen of significance, particularly in the healthcare environment due to transmission risks from airborne spread in those with symptomatic untreated pulmonary disease. The immunocompromised host has both a greater risk of reactivation of latent infection (particularly among the SOT, HSCT groups or those on treatment with TNF-alpha antagonists) or of disseminated and severe disease.[56]

Interventions such as surgery, prosthesis and the use of medical devices such as peripheral and central intravenous lines, urinary catheters and mechanical ventilation are known risk factors for an invasive bacterial HAI.[44]

Among the Australian population, the most common bacterial HAIs identified in a recent national point prevalence study within the acute care public hospital setting were *Staphylococcus aureus* and *Escherichia coli* spp.[45]

30.2.2 Fungal

The spectrum of nosocomial disease caused by fungal infection is broadening, with outbreaks linked to pathogens such as *Aspergillus* spp., *Candida* spp., *Fusarium* spp., *Mucorales* and other moulds such as *Lometospora prolificans* and *Scedosporium* spp. Clinically significant and occasionally life-threatening disease occurs predominantly in the immunosuppressed, often linked to the duration and severity of neutropenia.[57,58,3]

Aspergillus and *Candida* spp. are noted to cause the majority of fungal HAI in Australia, of which the *albicans* isolates are the predominant cause of candidaemia.[59] Host colonisation, the use of broad-spectrum antimicrobials and disruption of skin or gut barrier all increase the risk of disseminated candida infection.[58] The widespread use of azole prophylaxis and treatment, and more recently echinocandins, have been implicated in the rise in drug-resistant Candida HAIs, alongside other yeasts, particularly among the immunocompromised.[60]

The drug-resistant yeast *Candida auris* has also recently been identified in the last few decades as an HAI of threat, responsible for multiple large-scale outbreaks

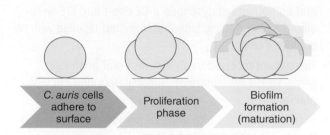

FIGURE 30.3 Schematic displaying the rapid formation of *C. auris* biofilm on surfaces over 24 hours
Source: Kean R, et al.[66]

overseas, and with a notably high propensity for direct transmission between individuals (see Fig 30.3). This is thought to be in part due to its ability to act as a long-term coloniser on human skin, the environment and medical devices, and form a fungal biofilm.[61] Although the disease is now endemic in geographical areas such as South Africa and India, sporadic imported cases have been reported in Australia.[62]

Construction work within hospitals has been linked with the acquisition of airborne fungal HAI such as *Aspergillus*, due to the dispersion of spores. Renovation activities to a lesser extent have been associated with the Zygomycetes. Pseudo-outbreaks have also been reported due to equipment contaminated by dust leading to *Sporothrix* infections.[63]

Within Australia, nosocomial outbreaks with the respiratory pathogen *Pneumocystis jiroveci* have also been described in clusters within multiple renal transplant centres, mediated by airborne droplet spread from infected patient to patient.[64]

Although human-to-human transmission is incredibly rare, the nosocomial transmission of *Cryptococcus* spp. has also been described in multiple settings within the immunocompromised cohort, with hypotheses centred around the inhalation of fungus from contaminated medical instruments.[65]

30.2.3 Viral

Respiratory-borne viruses: The transmission of common community-acquired respiratory viruses such as respiratory syncytial virus (RSV), influenza, parainfluenza, adenovirus, rhinovirus, coronaviruses, human metapneumovirus and bocavirus within a healthcare environment is common, particularly due to the ease of droplet-based spread. Once acquired they can cause a variety of complications, particularly in the immunocompromised host, with a greater likelihood of significant lower respiratory tract pathology and potential dissemination. Secondary pneumonia is a well-recognised complication, whether viral, bacterial, fungal or mixed.[67]

The recent severe acute respiratory syndrome coronavirus 2 (SARS-CoV-2) pandemic has been particularly significant for those who are immunocompromised. Defects in humoral immunity are associated with poor vaccine responses and incomplete immune control due to inadequate functional neutralising antibody production leading to prolonged shedding.[68] Patients also have a greater risk of more significant respiratory pathology with an increased risk of co-infection with invasive fungi such as mucormycosis and pulmonary aspergillosis, alongside prolonged intensive care stays.[69,70] A total of 36 hospital outbreaks alone with SARS-CoV-2 were identified within the Australian setting within 6 months in 2020.[71]

Nosocomial infection with other well-recognised respiratory viral pathogens, including measles, mumps, rubella and varicella zoster virus (VZV), has also been documented. Severe measles infection in the immunocompromised host has been associated with an increased risk of giant cell pneumonia and a case fatality rate of up to 70%. VZV infection in the adult also tends to be of higher severity in those who are immunosuppressed, with a greater risk of pneumonitis, encephalitis and death.[72] The use of live-attenuated vaccines against measles, mumps, rubella and varicella is contraindicated in those with significant immunocompromise, further increasing their vulnerability to these viral pathogens.

Gastrointestinal viruses: Nosocomial gastroenteritis has been documented with a variety of viral pathogens such as rotavirus, Norwalk virus, the caliciviruses (including norovirus), toroviruses, enteric adenoviruses, enteroviruses, astroviruses and paraechovirus. These are predominantly transmitted through the faecal-oral route, alongside occasional aerosol and fomite spread.[72] More prolonged and severe infection is described in the immunosuppressed, associated with significant weight loss, malnutrition, dehydration, and alteration of the intestinal mucosal barrier.[73]

Norovirus is one of the most frequent causes of outbreaks in the healthcare setting due to its ability to produce high and prolonged shedding titres, low

infectious dose, and stability in the environment with resistance to common disinfectants.[74]

The non-polio enteroviruses are also of particular interest in those with impaired immunity, leading to dissemination to secondary target tissues after infecting the GI epithelium, with differing tissue tropism depending on the sub-species. Complications include acute flaccid myelitis, myocarditis, hepatitis, pancreatitis and death.[75] Meningoencephalitis has also been noted, particularly in those with B-cell immunodeficiency.[76]

Blood-borne viruses: Nosocomial outbreaks from the major blood-borne viruses (hepatitis B, C and HIV) occurring through exposure to contaminated body fluids have all been reported whether through patient–patient contact, healthcare worker (HCW)–patient or vice versa. Major risk factors include inadequate instrument decontamination and poor infection control measures, particularly during exposure-prone procedures.[72]

Transfusion-transmitted viral infection has also been described, although careful donor screening and newer technology including nucleic acid testing has meant this is now increasingly rare.[77] The transfer of human T-lymphotropic virus type 1 (HTLV-1) has also been reported to have occurred through the use of contaminated blood products, although limited data is available. Now endemic to Central Australia, the virus is associated with significant complications including myelopathy and adult T-cell leukaemia/lymphoma.[78,79]

Immunocompromised patients are disproportionately affected in their risk of nosocomial blood-borne viruses due to increased hospital encounters, procedures, and use of blood products.

Herpesviridae: The herpesvirus family includes herpes simplex virus (HSV), varicella zoster virus (VZV), Epstein Barr virus (EBV), Cytomegalovirus (CMV), Human herpesvirus-6 (HHV-6), human herpesvirus-7 (HHV-7) and human herpesvirus-8 (HHV-8). Patients may be affected through reactivation of latent virus in the context of immunosuppression, acquisition of the virus from a seropositive donor after transplant, or through primary infection. The transmission of herpesviruses occurs most frequently through contact with infectious bodily fluids.

CMV infection is common after haematological or solid organ transplant. In the HSCT cohort, infection frequently occurs within the first 30–100 days and often alongside GvHD. The risk of significant disease is increased in cases where lymphocyte depleting therapy has been used. Invasive CMV is associated with pneumonitis, gastrointestinal disease including colitis, hepatitis and encephalitis.[80]

Infection with EBV can present with hepatitis, haemolytic anaemia and be a driver for haemophagocytosis. EBV is also a risk factor for the development of early post-transplant lymphoproliferative disorder (<1 year post transplant), particularly in the younger, EBV serologically mismatched allograft recipient.[32]

Donor-derived HSV infection has also been described, predominantly causing mucocutaneous disease; however, systemic infection including fulminant liver failure has been documented.[81] A report of suspected donor-derived HSV-2 infection was reported in a kidney/pancreas transplant patient in 2017 in Australia, with death at day 9 post-transplant associated with ischaemic hepatitis, and a subsequent cluster outbreak likely related to the transplantation of infected organs to new recipients.[82]

The unanticipated transmission of HHV-6 has also been documented in two kidney transplant patients, associated with hepatitis and bone marrow suppression. HHV-6 has also been reported to cause pneumonitis, encephalitis and myelitis in the immunocompromised host.[33]

Neurotropic viruses of transplant significance:
Neurotropic JC polyomavirus (JCV), the causative agent of progressive multifocal leukoencephalopathy, is associated with profound neurological sequelae including motor weakness, cognitive dysfunction, gait, vision and speech disturbance, and is another opportunist among immunocompromised individuals. Although yet to be fully understood, it occurs through reactivation of the virus within the CNS, usually in the context of immunosuppression, AIDS, haematological malignancy, lymphoproliferative disease or among SOT patients.[83]

Unrecognised donor infections with rabies, lymphocytic choriomeningitis (LCMV) and LCMV-related arenavirus have also been linked to SOT recipients.[33] In 2008, a cluster of donor-derived arenavirus-associated encephalitis and early post-transplant deaths occurred in three SOT transplant recipients (2 kidney, 1 liver) in Australia. The donor had travelled prior to his demise, and the organism identified by means of high throughput sequencing of amplified RNA samples post-mortem.[84]

30.2.4 Parasites

Parasitic infection is also thought to play a role in nosocomial infection, either via donor-to-recipient transmission in the case of transplants, the transfusion of blood products, acquired from environmental sources, or through recrudescence of dormant disease in the context of immunosuppression, whether innate or acquired.[85]

Donor-to-recipient parasitic infection risks include the protozoa *Toxoplasma gondii*, associated with chorioretinitis, myocarditis, pneumonitis and fatal encephalitis. More commonly reported in the cardiac and lung transplant population, it is also noted as a significant risk for kidney and HSCT recipients.[86] There is additionally a theoretical transfusion-related risk of the transfer of *Toxoplasma gondii*, although there is very limited data on its incidence in the Australasian population.[87]

Another organism relevant to the Australian setting is the intestinal nematode *Strongyloides stercoralis*, which in the immunocompromised host can lead to a hyperinfection syndrome caused by a rapid proliferation of larvae with migration through the bowel wall. Complications include acute pulmonary distress syndrome, bowel obstruction and secondary sepsis through the translocation of intestinal pathogens. The parasite can be transferred either through transplant, or, more frequently, disseminated disease occurs as a progression of a chronic intestinal infection present prior to transplant and unmasked by immunosuppression. Defects in cell-mediated immunity and glucorticoids are well-recognised triggering factors.[88]

Although the transfer of the metacyclic trypomastigotes of *Trypanosoma cruzi* through transplant have been documented worldwide, there is little evidence for this in Australia. However, in an increasingly global population, the potential risk has recently been highlighted. Complications include oesophageal dysfunction and cardiomyopathy. Infections in the immunocompromised tend to progress more rapidly with a higher risk of mortality.[89]

Reports of transfusion-associated *Plasmodium* spp. are documented, although the last Australian case of transfusion-associated malaria occurred in 1991.[87,90]

Water sources additionally remain a relevant risk for outbreaks of parasitic infection including *Cryptosporidium* spp., an agent of fulminant diarrhoea in those with impaired function, alongside causing pulmonary and biliary tract disease, and *Giardia* spp. *Acanthamoeba* spp. have also been previously isolated from hospital water

Table 30.4 Donor-transmitted infection and methods of screening in SOT Australia (routine vs considered)

Viruses	• HIV-1/HIV-2 Ab combination assay • Hepatitis B sAg/cAb/sAb (+/-NAT) • Hepatitis C Ab (+/ NAT) • CMV IgG Ab • EBV capsid IgG Ab • HTLV-1/2 Ab • SARS-CoV-2 PCR • Influenza NAT if suspected • West Nile Virus/Zika/other arboviruses (if compatible symptoms/travel to endemic or outbreak area <4 weeks prior) • Viral encephalitis (other than HSV/VZV contraindicated)
Bacteria	• Syphilis serology (specific treponemal Ab test) • Urine microscopy and culture (particularly for kidney transplant) • Blood cultures (if suspicion of bacteraemia) • Respiratory tract sampling if lung donor or respiratory tract infection suspected • Consider MDRO screening • Consider diagnostic testing for Mycobacterium tuberculosis in cases with clinical and epidemiological risk factors
Fungi	• Fungal colonisation of donor airway in lung transplantation—consider prophylaxis/pre-emptive therapy
Parasites	• Toxoplasma gondii serology (IgG) • Plasmodium malaria serology/NAT if spent >3 months in an endemic area • Strongyloides serology if spent >3 months in an endemic area • Trypanosoma cruzi screening if spent >3 months in Mexico/South or Central America
Other	• Risk factors for transmissible spongiform encephalopathy (prion disease)—exclude as donor

Source: Data From Zealand TTSoAaN. Clinical Guidelines for Organ Transplantation from Deceased Donors V. 1.52021.

samples in Tasmania, associated with severe encephalitis and keratitis.[91]

30.2.5 Prions

There have been almost 500 incidents of the iatrogenic transmission of prion diseases (transmissible spongiform encephalopathies) reported worldwide, mostly in the context of contaminated cadaveric growth hormone and dura mater grafts, but also through blood products and surgical instrumentation (see Table 30.4). Although still poorly understood, they are thought to be resistant to conventional decontamination methods (see Fig 30.4).[92] So far two cases of CJD (Creutzfeldt–Jakob disease), a rapidly progressive and inevitably fatal neurodegenerative disorder caused by infection with mutated prion proteins, have been reported in transplant recipients (liver and kidney); however, both without clear evidence for tissue transfer (see Fig 30.5). Regardless, one remains mindful that the risk exists, particularly among the immunocompromised population for whom these interventions may more frequently occur.[93,94]

PRACTICE TIPS 2

RELATIONSHIPS BETWEEN IMMUNOCOMPROMISE AND HAIs

• HAIs are of particular importance in Australia among the immunocompromised and oncology cohort, causing significant morbidity and mortality

• Immunocompromised patients are at particular risk of nosocomial infection due to poor immune defence, frequent instrumentation and use of indwelling devices, blood products, multiple healthcare encounters and broad antimicrobial exposures

• Nosocomial infection may be divided into those occurring from bacterial, fungi, viruses, parasites and prions

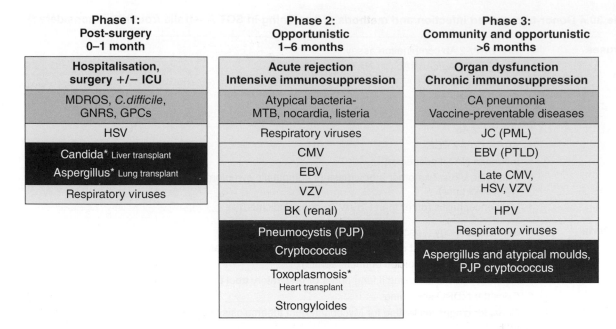

FIGURE 30.4 Examples of infectious risks post-SOT

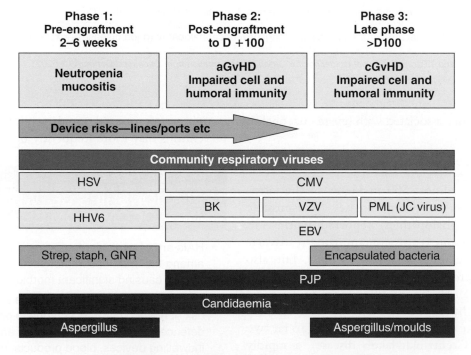

FIGURE 30.5 Examples of infectious risks post-HSCT

Disseminated infection in a patient with COVID-19 and diabetes[96]

Situation:

A 68-year-old Ecuadorian man presented with myalgia, headache, cough, nausea and chills. His past medical history included type 2 diabetes mellitus. His occupational history included work on farms and timber construction.

- SARS-CoV-2 RNA was identified on a nasopharyngeal swab.
- In the context of hypoxic respiratory failure requiring mechanical ventilation, he was administered high-dose steroids and tocilizumab.

Questions:

What causes of opportunistic infection would you ideally screen this patient for given the risk factors detailed above? Is he at risk of any particularly invasive conditions?

- He subsequently developed fevers and was noted to have a peripheral eosinophilia.

Would these symptoms and signs change your management?

- Sputum cultures were sent. Gram and iodine staining revealed larvae consistent with *Strongyloides* spp.
- Strongyloides serology was positive (IgG). Three stool cultures sent for ova, cyst and parasite identification were unremarkable.

- He received treatment with oral ivermectin, then additional albendazole.
- He was also screened for HIV and HTLV-1 and 2.
- Additional screening for hepatitis B, C and *Mycobacterium tuberculosis* may be considered.
- The reactivation of latent disease as well as new opportunistic infection must be considered in the immunocompromised host.

Based on Lier AJ, Tuan JJ, Davis MW, Paulson N, McManus D, Campbell S, et al. Case Report: Disseminated Strongyloidiasis in a Patient with COVID-19. Am J Trop Med Hyg. 2020;103(4):1590-2.

30.3 Prevention and control of HAIs associated with care in oncology and the immunocompromised in Australia

With the advent of enhanced diagnostics and advanced therapeutics, the proportion of the Australian population with an oncological diagnosis or immunocompromise is rising. Within healthcare settings this comes with a host of potential nosocomial complications, including the acquisition and spread of MROs, procedural and device-related infections, and an ever-widening range of opportunistic pathogens. In 2020, SARS-CoV-2 emerged as one of the most significant global pandemics from a respiratory viral pathogen in recent history. Thus, the role for infection prevention and control (IPC) in healthcare for the protection of the immunocompromised host has never been more important.

Effective infection control (see Fig 30.6) involves a wide array of individual and healthcare-based strategies

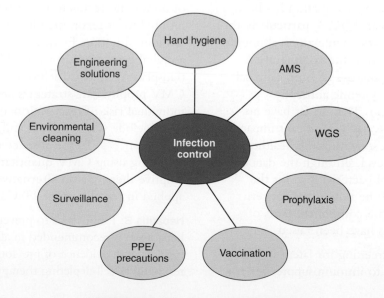

FIGURE 30.6 Infection control strategies

including screening and surveillance techniques, anti-microbial prophylaxis and stewardship, immunisation, personal protective equipment (PPE), hand hygiene, and disinfection and cleaning. Novel mechanisms of engineering and environmental controls have also more recently been integrated into the design of modern healthcare facilities, with many hospitals undergoing extensive renovations in light of SARS-CoV-2. Whole genome sequencing (WGS) has also been key in outbreak investigation and understanding the pathways for transmission of infection.[97]

30.3.1 Infection control strategies

Frequent hospitalisation, the use of broad-spectrum antimicrobials, intensive care stays and overseas travel to areas with high endemicity of MROs are all well-recognised risk factors for colonisation. Although guidelines on the timing and frequency of active surveillance differ between health districts, screening can occur through direct swabbing of individuals for colonisation using axillary/nose and groin swabs for MRSA, and rectal swabs for VRE and multidrug-resistant Gram-negative bacteria (MDR–GNB). Identification of these organisms can help inform future practices at an individual level, including the use of appropriate barrier precautions, hand hygiene, enhanced environmental cleaning and antimicrobial stewardship.[97] From a population perspective, pre-emptive screening is also a helpful strategy to understand the baseline MRO rate within an area and transmission risks within facilities. Screening for *Candida auris* is also recommended for those who have undergone treatment in an overseas facility using groin and axillary swabs.[98]

Decolonisation: Targeted decolonisation has been employed for patients with MRSA, particularly for those suffering from recurrent infections, although is more frequently utilised in the community. A classic regimen involves the use of a topical nasal antimicrobial alongside systemic antiseptic bodywashes and shampoos. Data so far have not shown evidence that this has a significant impact on the transmission of MRSA within the healthcare setting or at a broader level, although the data do support the reduction of bacterial load for the individual. It should also be noted that concerns regarding resistance to the component parts of decolonisation regimens have been raised.[99]

Pathogen screening: Screening for latent infection frequently occurs prior to immunosuppression for patients, and in the context of transplants or blood products, of donors as well. Organisms commonly screened for include the blood-borne viruses (HIV/hepatitis B and C) alongside serological testing for exposure to CMV, EBV, *Toxoplasmosis gondii* and *Treponema pallidum*. Donors may also be screened for exposure to HTLV-1 and 2 depending on the jurisdiction. Screening for immunity to measles, mumps, rubella and varicella may also be performed.

Patients at risk of reactivation of *Mycobacterium tuberculosis* (particularly those receiving high-dose glucocorticoids, or TNF–alpha inhibitors such as Infliximab) should be assessed for exposure to the organism using a QuantiFERON-gold test. Additionally, in those with travel to endemic areas, *Strongyloides stercoralis* screening should be considered.[33]

Molecular testing: The role of molecular testing in the evaluation and screening for infectious aetiology on serum is also more broadly being employed, particularly in the undifferentiated, unwell immunocompromised host with an appropriate clinical history. Molecular diagnostics may be utilised to screen for organisms such as aspergillus, the herpesviruses including EBV, CMV, HHV-6, and adenovirus. Other pre-emptive detection strategies for opportunistic pathogens include the use of cryptococcal antigen and galactomannan assays.[100]

30.3.2 Antimicrobial prophylaxis—viral

Herpesviruses: Herpes simplex reactivation occurs in 80% of allogeneic HSCT patients, CMV in 75% of seropositive patients and VZV in 30–55% within the first 12 months post-transplantation. Given high rates of donor and recipient exposures, universal prophylaxis is recommended in Australia rather than serological testing. Frequently used HSV and VZV antiviral prophylaxis for both HSCT and solid-organ transplant recipients includes aciclovir and valaciclovir. CMV prophylactic strategies are frequently tailored to individual risk of reactivation, or acquisition. Agents used include valganciclovir and, in certain centres, letermovir.[101,95] In the absence of prophylaxis, regular screening using CMV quantitative PCR and pre-emptive therapy is an alternative strategy generally applied in the allogeneic HSCT setting.[102]

Hepatitis B: Prophylaxis to prevent the reactivation of hepatitis B is recommended in all immunocompromised patients with evidence of previous hepatitis B infection receiving B-cell depleting therapy. Moderate risk treatments where prophylaxis should also be considered include anti-CD20 monoclonals, high-dose corticosteroids, anthracyclines, systemic chemotherapy, cytokine-based therapies and when receiving inhibitors of TNF-alpha—immunophilin, tyrosine-kinase, proteasome, and histone deacetylase. Tenofovir and entecavir are the most frequently used antiviral agents.[103]

Among the transplant cohort, hepatitis B surface antigen (HBsAg)-positive donors have the highest risk of transmission of hepatitis B to naïve recipients. Transplantation from HBsAg-negative but core antibody-positive donors has a lesser but still possible risk of transmission, thought to be greatest in liver transplantation.[33,95]

Hepatitis C: The transplant of solid organs from hepatitis C nucleic acid test (NAT) positive donors to negative recipients is currently considered only in exceptional circumstances. Post-transplant direct acting antiviral therapy for the recipient has so far, however, been found to have a highly effective cure rate.[95]

30.3.3 Fungal

In the haematology setting, mould active antifungal prophylaxis is recommended in those with acute myeloid leukaemia (AML) and acute lymphoblastic leukaemia (ALL) undergoing induction chemotherapy, and in those with high-grade myelodysplastic syndromes. It is also suggested in settings of prolonged neutropenia, high-dose steroid use, among the allogeneic transplant group and in those with extensive or severe GvHD. For those deemed lower risk, candida prophylaxis is recommended as first line, such as in the autologous transplant cohort, in allogeneic transplants with a duration of neutropenia of <14 days, and in lymphoma. Prior episodes of invasive fungal infection (IFI) may also dictate future risk and prophylactic strategies.

Targeted and immunomodulatory drug therapies for haematology and oncology patients can also increase the risk of invasive fungal disease, although likelihood differs depending on the number of lines of therapy used, whether single or combination therapy is administered, and whether mucositis or significant neutropenia is expected. There has also been a greater recognition of the association between certain drug classes, for example the Bruton's tyrosine kinase inhibitors, and the risk of IFIs.[104]

30.3.4 Pneumocystis jiroveci pneumonia (PJP)/Toxoplasmosis

Pneumocystis jiroveci pneumonia prophylaxis using oral cotrimoxazole is recommended for all allogeneic

and some autologous BMT patients for at least the first 6 months post-transplant and continued in those receiving ongoing immunosuppressive therapy or suffering from GvHD. It is similarly employed in the organ transplant population, and is notably protective against infection with *Toxoplasmosis* spp.[102,95]

30.3.5 Bacterial

Antibacterial prophylaxis against invasive pneumococcal infection is widespread in the setting of cGvHD post-transplant, for individuals with low IgG levels, and for splenectomy patients. Oral penicillin is preferred; however, local pneumococcal resistance patterns should be used to guide individual choice.

In the setting of adult BMT, some guidelines and centres also recommend the use of widespread antimicrobial prophylaxis for Gram-negative sepsis with fluroquinolone for those with neutropenia of greater than 7 days. However, controversy exists with concerns for the development of hypervirulent bacterial opportunists (such as *C. difficile*) and emerging antimicrobial resistance.[102]

Antimicrobial stewardship (AMS): Optimisation of the duration, choice, dose and route of antimicrobial therapy through stewardship helps reduce unnecessary overuse and resistance and increases safety. This is particularly important in the immunocompromised patient due to their frequent use of both empiric and targeted broad-spectrum antimicrobials, high rates of opportunistic infection and risk of MROs as well as *C. difficile*. Strategies used in these settings include the use of a multidisciplinary AMS service to provide regular prescriber education and support, computer-based governance programs, and antimicrobial restriction and cycling techniques.[97] Australian-based tools such as the National Antibiotic Prescribing Survey (NAPS) also help regularly audit antimicrobial practice. Pharmacokinetic monitoring and adjustment programs, and selective or cascade reporting of antibiotic susceptibility testing, may also assist with appropriate drug choice, dosing and avoiding toxicity.[49]

Vaccination: Pre-emptive vaccination is another weapon in the armoury against the acquisition of infection within the healthcare setting. Although vaccinations are commonly received through the childhood immunisation schedule, HSCT recipients and splenectomy patients require re-vaccination post-procedure. Other vaccines recommended for the immunocompromised include the annual influenza,

COVID-19, and pneumococcal schedule. Hepatitis A and varicella zoster vaccination may also be considered.[102] It is important to remember, however, that live vaccines are contraindicated in the immunosuppressed. Encouraging staff compliance with vaccinations for highly transmissible diseases such as influenza and COVID-19 is also of importance in reducing the spread of communicable disease.

30.4 Infection control—healthcare setting

Hand hygiene: Hand hygiene is one of the central pillars of infection control. It is the single most important practice to prevent and control HAIs according to the World Health Organization (WHO), and is crucial in an oncology and immunocompromised host setting. HCWs are encouraged to comply with the '5 moments for hand hygiene', namely cleaning hands prior to touching a patient and before aseptic procedures, after procedures or body fluid exposure, touching a patient and their surroundings.[44] Alcohol-based products have generally shown superiority to routine soap and water in antimicrobial activity, except in the case of *C. difficile* and norovirus.[97]

A longitudinal study performed over 105 hospitals across Australia after the implementation of the National Hand Hygiene Initiative (NHHI), a culture change program designed to encourage compliance with WHO guidance, found that for every 10% increase in hand hygiene compliance, the incidence of hospital-acquired *Staphylococcus aureus* bacteraemia decreased by 15%.[106] (See Figs 30.7 and 30.8.)

30.4.1 PPE/Barrier precautions

PPE such as gloves, gowns, face masks, eyewear and face shields may be employed by HCWs in the protection of themselves and the patient from transmission of pathogens, and varies according to organism, exposure and other risks. The use of face masks, however, is ubiquitous across Australian healthcare settings since SARS-CoV-2, with fluid-resistant surgical masks employed to reduce the droplet spread of pathogens, and P2/N95 masks frequently used in higher-risk settings to limit airborne spread. The oncology and immunocompromised patients are particularly vulnerable to the spread of communicable disease and frequently cohorted in closed units. Previous studies looking at universal surgical-mask wearing year-round in stem-cell transplant units displayed a significant decrease in respiratory viral infection for both allogeneic and autologous patients in the post-mask period, complementing existing infection control measures.[108]

The optimal application and sustainability of other barrier precautions such as gowns and gloves versus standard precautions in curtailing the spread of HAIs, for example MROs, outside of high-risk units is unclear and weighed against significant environmental and financial costs. However, this differs in the immunocompromised.[49]

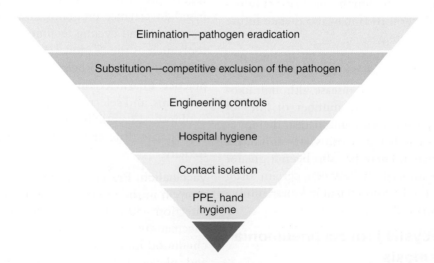

FIGURE 30.7 HAI healthcare setting management strategies (hierarchy of controls)
Source: Dalton KR, et al.[105]

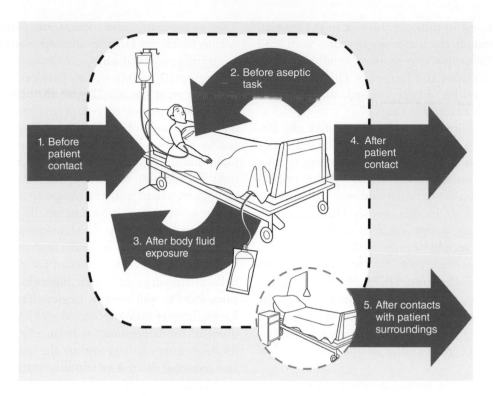

FIGURE 30.8 5 moments for hand hygiene
Source: Sax H, et al.[107]

30.4.2 Hospital hygiene

Healthcare facilities are a rich environmental niche for the acquisition and spread of pathogens, thus cleaning and sterilisation are key in decreasing the transmission of HAIs. Survival of various pathogens on dry and inanimate objects has been reported as several days for viruses, months for MRSA and up to 36 months for VRE.[97]

C. difficile is one of the most common HAIs in Australia and can be both severe and recurrent in the immunocompromised host. Spread through the aerosolisation of spores which can survive desiccation, live on hard surfaces, and resist routine disinfectants such as quaternary ammonium compounds (QATs), the detection of *C. difficile*, isolation of patients and cleaning is key in preventing ongoing spread.[49]

Disinfectant agents such as hypochlorous acid, hydrogen peroxide and paracetic acid are frequently used in the hospital setting, although manual cleaning, including of high-touch surfaces, is unpredictable depending on staff education and technique. Automated enhanced technologies such as microcondensation systems have been effectively employed in providing extra support for decontamination, although they are time-consuming and expensive. Pulsed UV light devices have also been reported to be helpful.[97] Fluorescent marker gels and adenosine triphosphate (AT) bioluminescence assays have been used to assess the thoroughness of cleaning, accepting that visual inspection is an unreliable marker; however, established standardised guidelines, even for facilities with immunocompromised patients, are still lacking.[49]

30.4.3 Engineering controls

The environment is an important reservoir for nosocomially acquired infection in the immunocompromised host.[102] Point source outbreaks of nosocomial infection have been associated with contaminated air, water, fomites and food. Nosocomial outbreaks may be further propagated if the pathogen has the potential for person-to-person transmission.

Ubiquitous airborne organisms such as *Aspergillus fumigatus* and other environmental moulds of intrinsic low pathogenicity may cause invasive or semi-invasive disease in those with prolonged and profound deficiencies of innate immunity, notably neutropenia. HSCT recipients, patients with acute leukaemia and those with primary immunodeficiency states such as chronic granulomatous disease are at heightened risk of aspergillosis and opportunistic mould infections. Engineering measures employed to mitigate this risk in the hospital environment include the use of single rooms with ≥12 air exchanges/hour, positive pressure ventilation with respect to the corridor and the use of High-Efficiency Particulate Air (HEPA) filters to block the ingress of particles down to a size of 0.3 μm.[109]

The regular maintenance of HEPA filters and air-handling systems—in addition to protecting the integrity of window and door seals, and protecting roofing and walls from dust and water damage—is of importance in preventing nosocomial outbreaks of aspergillosis and other environmental moulds. During periods of hospital building, construction or remediation, additional measures should be employed to reduce exposure to environmental moulds. Dustproof barriers around areas of construction, HEPA filtration of recirculated air, cleaning of contaminated surfaces, and the use of N95 personal respirators for those at greatest risk when moving around a hospital when construction is taking place, may confer an additional level of protection.[110]

The surveillance for mould infections in immunocompromised populations at risk during construction, and air sampling in high-risk areas during construction work is a further quality assurance measure for the identification of airborne environmental contamination.[109]

Mould infections may additionally be associated with organic matter brought into the patient's environment. Contaminated equipment such as wooden tongue depressors used as arm splints, or poorly stored linen, have been implicated in outbreaks of cutaneous *Rhizopus* spp. infections in immunocompromised children.[111,112] Flowers and fresh fruit, at risk of decay, are generally prohibited in haem-oncology wards.[102]

Water quality and contaminated water-handling systems have been implicated in outbreaks of bacteria, including multi-resistant *Pseudomonas* spp., other multi-resistant Gram-negative infections, *Legionella pneumophila*, non-tuberculous mycobacteria and moulds such as fusariosis.[113-115] Cryptosporidium, a parasite, has also been described in an HIV ward outbreak, following the index case handling ice, used in drinks, from an ice machine.[116]

Nosocomially acquired *Legionella pneumophila* (serogroup 1) infections are of particular concern in the immunocompromised host given the risks of severe pneumonia. The risk of Legionella proliferation in water distribution systems is increased where free residual chlorine falls below 0.5mg/L. This may occur where a healthcare facility is further downstream from the point of disinfection in a town water distribution network.

The engineering and design of plumbing systems within healthcare facilities are important for preventing Legionella proliferation.

Legionella growth occurs between temperatures of 20–45°C with maximal growth between 37–43°C. Poorly designed water systems that promote heat transfer include hot and cold pipes in close proximity, pipes within poorly insulated spaces such as roof cavities, or pipes that are inadequately concealed and in direct sunlight.[117] Plumbing network systems that have 'dead legs' or pockets where water can stagnate and form biofilms are an additional risk for Legionella proliferation and nosocomial acquisition.[114] Maintenance to prevent the build-up of biofilms, sediment and materials that may impede water flow is important for preventing Legionella colonisation of water networks. Water temperatures ≥60°C will control Legionella growth. As such, having temperature mixing valves (TMVs) close to the point of use is optimal for balancing the requirement for high temperatures within the distribution system and reducing the risk of scalding at the point of use.

Maintenance of water systems should include a schedule of testing residual disinfectant; cleaning, replacing or repairing water storage, tanks or distribution systems with a build-up of sediment; ensuring temperature controls throughout the water distribution system are maintained; periodic cleaning and maintenance of downstream TMVs, tap outlets, shower heads and hoses; and replacing filters according to industry specifications.

Healthcare facilities can further mitigate Legionella and other waterborne exposures by not incorporating water features such as waterfalls or fountains in their design; avoiding the use of mist-generating devices such as air humidifiers in patient zones; and using taps and shower heads that are designed to reduce aerosol generation. The design of sinks and taps is also important for reducing splash-back and environmental colonisation with MDR-GNB.[113]

30.4.4 Whole genome sequencing (WGS)

WGS can be used within healthcare facilities to investigate nosocomial outbreaks and help focus infection control interventions and resources. Phylogenetic analysis alongside epidemiological data can pinpoint transmission events through the identification of highly related patient isolates and monitor their spread. These techniques have been effectively employed during the SARS-CoV-2 pandemic, and also used to reduce the spread of MROs. A prospective genomics study across eight Australian hospitals over 15 months found that

30.8% of patients with an MRO acquired it within hospital (majority VRE). This had major impacts on identifying outbreak clusters, super-spreaders, unexpected transmissions, and led to new strategies for risk mitigation including a review of patient movements and placement, intensive cleaning and enhanced surveillance.[118]

In the oncology and immunocompromised setting, harnessing these tools will be invaluable in aiming to reduce the risk of HAIs.

PRACTICE TIPS 3

EFFECTIVE IPC FOR ONCOLOGY AND IMMUNOCOMPROMISED PATIENTS

- Effective ICP among the immunocompromised and oncology population can be thought of on an individual and population level
- Strategies include screening for infection and colonisation, early recognition of disease and rapid diagnostics, including the use of molecular techniques, antimicrobial prophylaxis, vaccination, governance and antimicrobial stewardship
- Facility level mechanisms include careful hand hygiene, PPE, hospital hygiene, engineering and environmental controls and whole genome sequencing for outbreak management

---

CASE STUDY 3

PJP outbreak within a renal transplant facility, Sydney[119]

Situation:

Fourteen patients over a period of 10 months within a renal transplant unit were noted to have signs, symptoms (and in 11, identification of the organism from microbiological specimens) of *pneumocystis jiroveci* pneumonia (PJP) infection. This led to the suspicion of a cluster outbreak. Inter-human PJP is known to be transmitted by airborne droplet spread.

Questions:

What strategies would you employ in helping determine the risk factors at an individual and cohort level? What are the individual risk factors to be aware of?

- Contact tracing and a transmission map helped in identifying possible routes of spread.
- Whole genome sequencing allowed for genotype analysis and determination of a common cluster and mutations from the original outbreak.
- Individual risk analysis was performed outlining susceptibility to infection including years post-transplantation, HLA mismatch, rejection episodes, lymphodepleting therapy, recent steroid use and dosing, the use of PJP prophylaxis, preceding infection with invasive CMV, degree of immunosuppression and smoking.
- Patients were isolated in single rooms until complete clinical response.
- Sampling of ambient air within multiple common areas did not identify evidence of PJP.
- Oropharyngeal rinses were also taken from HCWs working within the unit to identify PJP on PCR, all results returned negative.

How might your findings change practice within the healthcare facility?

- A policy of extended PJP prophylaxis from 6 to 12 months was implemented for all recent recipients and restarted in those asymptomatic but potentially exposed. Individual risk factors could be used to assess ongoing risk.
- Education on the need for rapid identification and early case isolation may help prevent spread within a closed unit.
- A variety of infection control strategies can be employed at all stages in assessing the risk, transmission, and management of opportunistic infection in the immunocompromised host.

Conclusion

The medical advances of the 20th century have allowed for the increased diagnostic capacity of primary as well as secondary causes of immunocompromise, including malignancy. Combined with increased patient survival, transplant opportunity, global travel and the use of novel interventions and therapeutics, the threat of opportunistic infection within this cohort is ever expanding.

Healthcare facilities are also themselves a major risk for the acquisition and spread of disease among these patients. In this chapter we identify the key aetiological agents of communicable disease among the main sub-classes of the immunocompromised host and the challenges faced in infection prevention within the healthcare facilities looking after this specific population. Furthermore, we identify multiple preventative and active infection control measures which can take place at both an individual and population level to minimise the risk for disease transmission and HAIs, as well as identifying areas for future capacity building.

Useful websites/resources

- Management guidelines providing evidence-based recommendations in preventing infectious complications amongst bone marrow transplant patients: Tomblyn, M et al. (2009) Guidelines for preventing infectious complications among hematopoietic cell transplantation recipients: a global perspective. https://www.ncbi.nlm.nih.gov/pmc/articles/PMC3103296/

- Australasian consensus guidelines on the management of invasive fungal infection and use of antifungal agents in haematology and oncology patients: Chang CC et al. (2021). Introduction to the updated Australasian consensus guidelines for the management of invasive fungal disease and use of antifungal agents in the haematology/oncology setting. https://onlinelibrary.wiley.com/doi/10.1111/imj.15585.

- Australia and New Zealand Clinical guidelines for organ transplantation including screening for communicable infectious disease and management: The Transplantation Society of Australia and New Zealand (2021). Clinical Guidelines for Organ Transplantation from Deceased Donors Version 1.5. https://tsanz.com.au/storage/documents/TSANZ_Clinical_Guidelines_Version-17.pdf.

- Infection prevention and control handbook detailing the mechanisms of healthcare associated infection, risk assessment and management in the Australian setting: National Health and Medical Research Council in collaboration with the Australian Commission on Safety and Quality in Health Care (2019). Australian Guidelines for the Prevention and Control of Infection in Healthcare. https://www.nhmrc.gov.au/sites/default/files/documents/infection-control-guidelines-feb2020.pdf.

References

1. Riccardi N, Rotulo GA, Castagnola E. Definition of opportunistic infections in immunocompromised children on the basis of etiologies and clinical features: a summary for practical purposes. Curr Pediatr Rev. 2019;15(4):197-206.
2. Xunrong L, Yan AW, Liang R, Lau GK. Hepatitis B virus (HBV) reactivation after cytotoxic or immunosuppressive therapy—pathogenesis and management. Rev Med Virol. 2001;11(5):287-299.
3. Dropulic LK, Lederman HM. Overview of infections in the immunocompromised host. Microbiol Spectr. 2016;4(4):10.1128/microbiolspec.DMIH2-0026-2016.
4. Abolhassani H, Azizi G, Sharifi L, Yazdani R, Mohsenzadegan M, Delavari S, et al. Global systematic review of primary immunodeficiency registries. Expert Rev Clin Immunol. 2020;16(7):717-732.
5. Tuano KS, Seth N, Chinen J. Secondary immunodeficiencies: an overview. Ann Allergy Asthma Immunol. 2021;127(6):617-626.
6. Chinen J, Shearer WT. Secondary immunodeficiencies, including HIV infection. J Allergy Clin Immunol. 2010;125(2 Suppl 2):S195-203.
7. McPake B, Mahal A. Addressing the needs of an aging population in the health system: the Australian case. Health Syst Reform. 2017;3(3):236-247.
8. Mor G, Cardenas I. The immune system in pregnancy: a unique complexity. Am J Reprod Immunol. 2010;63(6):425-433.
9. van der Heijden WA, Van de Wijer L, Keramati F, Trypsteen W, Rutsaert S, Horst RT, et al. Chronic HIV infection induces transcriptional and functional reprogramming of innate immune cells. JCI Insight. 2021;6(7):e145928.
10. Smith DE, Woolley IJ, Russell DB, Bisshop F, Furner V. Trends in practice: attitudes and challenges in the diagnosis, treatment and management of HIV infection in Australia. Intern Med J. 2020;50 Suppl 5:5-17.
11. Davis WA, Peters KE, Makepeace A, Griffiths S, Bundell C, Grant SFA, et al. Prevalence of diabetes in Australia: insights from the Fremantle Diabetes Study Phase II. Intern Med J. 2018;48(7):803-809.
12. Maddur MS, Vani J, Lacroix-Desmazes S, Kaveri S, Bayry J. Autoimmunity as a predisposition for infectious diseases. PLoS Pathog. 2010;6(11):e1001077.
13. Ibrahim AS, Spellberg B, Walsh TJ, Kontoyiannis DP. Pathogenesis of mucormycosis. Clin Infect Dis. 2012;54 Suppl 1(Suppl 1):S16-22.
14. Luu S, Spelman D, Woolley IJ. Post-splenectomy sepsis: preventative strategies, challenges, and solutions. Infect Drug Resist. 2019;12:2839-2851.

15. Nikpour M, Bridge JA, Richter S. A systematic review of prevalence, disease characteristics and management of systemic lupus erythematosus in Australia: identifying areas of unmet need. Intern Med J. 2014;44(12a):1170-1179.

16. Youssef J, Novosad SA, Winthrop KL. Infection risk and safety of corticosteroid use. Rheum Dis Clin North Am. 2016;42(1):157-176, ix-x.

17. Trevillian P. Immunosuppressants – clinical applications. Experimental and Clinical Pharmacology. 2006:102-108.

18. Davis JS, Ferreira D, Paige E, Gedye C, Boyle M. Infectious complications of biological and small molecule targeted immunomodulatory therapies. Clin Microbiol Rev. 2020; 33(3).

19. Meneghini M, Bestard O, Grinyo JM. Immunosuppressive drugs modes of action. Best Pract Res Clin Gastroenterol. 2021;54-55:101757.

20. Luo Q, Steinberg J, O'Connell DL, Grogan PB, Canfell K, Feletto E. Changes in cancer incidence and mortality in Australia over the period 1996-2015. BMC Res Notes. 2020;13(1):561.

21. Cameron JK, Baade P. Projections of the future burden of cancer in Australia using Bayesian age-period-cohort models. Cancer Epidemiol. 2021;72:101935.

22. Bukowski K, Kciuk M, Kontek R. Mechanisms of multidrug resistance in cancer chemotherapy. Int J Mol Sci. 2020;21(9).

23. Vento S, Cainelli F. Infections in patients with cancer undergoing chemotherapy: aetiology, prevention, and treatment. Lancet Oncol. 2003;4(10):595-604.

24. Seo SK, Liu C, Dadwal SS. Infectious disease complications in patients with cancer. Crit Care Clin. 2021;37(1):69-84.

25. Khalifa J, Mazieres J, Gomez-Roca C, Ayyoub M, Moyal EC. Radiotherapy in the era of immunotherapy with a focus on non-small-cell lung cancer: time to revisit ancient dogmas? Front Oncol. 2021;11:662236.

26. Ross JA, Komoda K, Pal S, Dickter J, Salgia R, Dadwal S. Infectious complications of immune checkpoint inhibitors in solid organ malignancies. Cancer Med. 2022;11(1):21-27.

27. Little JS, Weiss ZF, Hammond SP. Invasive fungal infections and targeted therapies in hematological malignancies. J Fungi (Basel). 2021;7(12).

28. Stewart AG, Henden AS. Infectious complications of CAR T-cell therapy: a clinical update. Ther Adv Infect Dis. 2021; 8:20499361211036773.

29. Sheth VS, Gauthier J. Taming the beast: CRS and ICANS after CAR T-cell therapy for ALL. Bone Marrow Transplant. 2021;56(3):552-566.

30. Australia and New Zealand Organ Donation Registry. Snapshot of deceased organ donation activity in Australia and New Zealand. Registry AaNZOD, 2022.

31. O'Brien Y, Chavan S, Huckson S, Russ G, Opdam H, Pilcher D. Predicting expected organ donor numbers in Australian hospitals outside of the donate-life network using the ANZICS adult patient database. Transplantation. 2018; 102(8):1323-1329.

32. Nam H, Nilles KM, Levitsky J, Ison MG. Donor-derived viral infections in liver transplantation. Transplantation. 2018; 102(11):1824-1836.

33. White SL, Rawlinson W, Boan P, Sheppeard V, Wong G, Waller K, et al. Infectious disease transmission in solid organ transplantation: donor evaluation, recipient risk, and outcomes of transmission. Transplant Direct. 2019;5(1):e416.

34. Patel R, Paya CV. Infections in solid-organ transplant recipients. Clin Microbiol Rev. 1997;10(1):86-124.

35. Cippà PE, Schiesser M, Ekberg H, van Gelder T, Mueller NJ, Cao CA, et al. Risk stratification for rejection and infection after kidney transplantation. Clin J Am Soc Nephrol. 2015; 10(12):2213-2220.

36. Sahu KK. Infectious disease in hematopoietic stem cell transplantation. Ther Adv Infect Dis. 2021;8: 20499361211005600.

37. Styczyński J, Tridello G, Koster L, Iacobelli S, van Biezen A, van der Werf S, et al. Death after hematopoietic stem cell transplantation: changes over calendar year time, infections and associated factors. Bone Marrow Transplant. 2020;55(1):126-136.

38. Nivison-Smith I, Bardy P, Dodds AJ, Ma DDF, Aarons D, Tran S, et al. A review of hematopoietic cell transplantation in Australia and New Zealand, 2005 to 2013. Biol Blood Marrow Transplant. 2016;22(2):284-291.

39. Australasian Bone Marrow Transplant Recipient Registry. Annual data summary 2020. Registry ABMTR, 2020.

40. Srinivasan A, Wang C, Srivastava DK, Burnette K, Shenep JL, Leung W, et al. Timeline, epidemiology, and risk factors for bacterial, fungal, and viral infections in children and adolescents after allogeneic hematopoietic stem cell transplantation. Biol Blood Marrow Transplant. 2013;19(1): 94-101.

41. Safdar A, Armstrong D. Infections in patients with hematologic neoplasms and hematopoietic stem cell transplantation: neutropenia, humoral, and splenic defects. Clin Infect Dis. 2011;53(8):798-806.

42. Torda A, Chong Q, Lee A, Chen S, Dodds A, Greenwood M, et al. Invasive pneumococcal disease following adult allogeneic hematopoietic stem cell transplantation. Transpl Infect Dis. 2014;16(5):751-759.

43. Koh AY. The microbiome in hematopoietic stem cell transplant recipients and cancer patients: opportunities for clinical advances that reduce infection. PLoS Pathog. 2017;13(6):e1006342.

44. Haque M, Sartelli M, McKimm J, Abu Bakar M. Health care-associated infections – an overview. Infect Drug Resist. 2018;11:2321-2333.

45. Russo PL, Stewardson AJ, Cheng AC, Bucknall T, Mitchell BG. The prevalence of healthcare associated infections among adult inpatients at nineteen large Australian acute-care public hospitals: a point prevalence survey. Antimicrob Resist Infect Control. 2019;8:114.

46. Valentine JC, Hall L, Verspoor KM, Worth LJ. The current scope of healthcare-associated infection surveillance activities in hospitalized immunocompromised patients: a systematic review. Int J Epidemiol. 2019;48(6):1768-1782.

47. Wohrley JD, Bartlett. AH. The role of the environment and colonization in healthcare-associated infections. In Healthcare-Associated Infections in Children. 2018; Jul 16: 17-36

48. Russotto V, Cortegiani A, Fasciana T, Iozzo P, Raineri SM, Gregoretti C, et al. What healthcare workers should know about environmental bacterial contamination in the intensive care unit. Biomed Res Int. 2017;2017:6905450.

49. Fernando SA, Gray TJ, Gottlieb T. Healthcare-acquired infections: prevention strategies. Intern Med J. 2017;47(12): 1341-1351.

50. Mann T, Ben-David D, Zlotkin A, Shachar D, Keller N, Toren A, et al. An outbreak of Burkholderia cenocepacia bacteremia in immunocompromised oncology patients. Infection. 2010;38(3):187-194.

51. Revolinski SL, Munoz-Price LS. Clostridium difficile in immunocompromised hosts: a review of epidemiology, risk factors, treatment, and prevention. Clin Infect Dis. 2019; 68(12):2144-2153.

52. Suleyman G, Alangaden G, Bardossy AC. The role of environmental contamination in the transmission of nosocomial pathogens and healthcare-associated infections. Curr Infect Dis Rep. 2018;20(6):12.

53. Bursle E, Playford GE, Coulter C, Paul G. First Australian case of disseminated *Mycobacterium chimaera* infection post-cardiothoracic surgery. Infect Dis Health. 2017;22(1):1-5.

54. Graham RM, Doyle CJ, Jennison AV. Real-time investigation of a Legionella pneumophila outbreak using whole genome sequencing. Epidemiol Infect. 2014;142(11): 2347-2351.

55. Merritt AJ, Peck M, Gayle D, Levy A, Ler YH, Raby E, et al. Cutaneous melioidosis cluster caused by contaminated wound irrigation fluid. Emerg Infect Dis. 2016;22(8).

56. Coorey NJ, Kensitt L, Davies J, Keller E, Sheel M, Chani K, et al. Risk factors for TB in Australia and their association with delayed treatment completion. Int J Tuberc Lung Dis. 2022;26(5):399-405.

57. Bougnoux ME, Brun S, Zahar JR. Healthcare-associated fungal outbreaks: new and uncommon species, new molecular tools for investigation and prevention. Antimicrob Resist Infect Control. 2018;7:45.

58. Perlroth J, Choi B, Spellberg B. Nosocomial fungal infections: epidemiology, diagnosis, and treatment. Med Mycol. 2007; 45(4):321-346.

59. Slavin M, Fastenau J, Sukarom I, Mavros P, Crowley S, Gerth WC. Burden of hospitalization of patients with Candida and Aspergillus infections in Australia. Int J Infect Dis. 2004;8(2): 111-120.

60. Chapman B, Slavin M, Marriott D, Halliday C, Kidd S, Arthur I, et al. Changing epidemiology of candidaemia in Australia. J Antimicrob Chemother. 2017;72(4):1103-1108.

61. Lionakis MS, Hohl TM. Call to action: how to tackle emerging nosocomial fungal infections. Cell Host Microbe. 2020;27(6):859-862.

62. Keighley C, Garnham K, Harch SAJ, Robertson M, Chaw K, Teng JC, et al. Diagnostic challenges and emerging opportunities for the clinical microbiology laboratory. Curr Fungal Infect Rep. 2021:1-11.

63. Kanamori H, Rutala WA, Sickbert-Bennett EE, Weber DJ. Review of fungal outbreaks and infection prevention in healthcare settings during construction and renovation. Clin Infect Dis. 2015;61(3):433-444.

64. Chen S, Brian N, Carolina F, Kathy K, Debbie M, Peter M, et al. Hospital-acquired Pneumocystis pneumonia: a renewed concern? In Microbiology Australia. CSIRO Publishing, 2014, p. 57-59.

65. Wang CY, Wu HD, Hsueh PR. Nosocomial transmission of cryptococcosis. N Engl J Med. 2005;352(12):1271-1272.

66. Kean R, Delaney C, Sherry L, Borman A, Johnson EM, Richardson MD, et al. Transcriptome assembly and profiling of Candida auris reveals novel insights into biofilm-mediated resistance. mSphere. 2018;3(4):e00334-18.

67. Englund J, Feuchtinger T, Ljungman P. Viral infections in immunocompromised patients. Biol Blood Marrow Transplant. 2011;17(1 Suppl):S2-5.

68. Gordon CL, Smibert OC, Holmes NE, Chua KYL, Rose M, Drewett G, et al. Defective severe acute respiratory syndrome coronavirus 2 immune responses in an immunocompromised individual with prolonged viral replication. Open Forum Infect Dis. 2021;8(9):ofab359.

69. Soni S, Namdeo Pudake R, Jain U, Chauhan N. A systematic review on SARS-CoV-2-associated fungal coinfections. J Med Virol. 2022;94(1):99-109.

70. Machado M, Valerio M, Álvarez-Uría A, Olmedo M, Veintimilla C, Padilla B, et al. Invasive pulmonary aspergillosis in the COVID-19 era: an expected new entity. Mycoses. 2021; 64(2):132-143.

71. Quigley AL, Stone H, Nguyen PY, Chughtai AA, MacIntyre CR. Estimating the burden of COVID-19 on the Australian healthcare workers and health system during the first six months of the pandemic. Int J Nurs Stud. 2021;114:103811.

72. Aitken C, Jeffries DJ. Nosocomial spread of viral disease. Clin Microbiol Rev. 2001;14(3):528-546.

73. Bok K, Green KY. Norovirus gastroenteritis in immunocompromised patients. N Engl J Med. 2012; 367(22):2126-2132.

74. Barclay L, Park GW, Vega E, Hall A, Parashar U, Vinjé J, et al. Infection control for norovirus. Clin Microbiol Infect. 2014; 20(8):731-740.

75. Wells AI, Coyne CB. Enteroviruses: a gut-wrenching game of entry, detection, and evasion. Viruses. 2019;11(5).

76. Dunn JJ. Enteroviruses and parechoviruses. Microbiol Spectr. 2016;4(3).

77. Dwyre DM, Fernando LP, Holland PV. Hepatitis B, hepatitis C and HIV transfusion-transmitted infections in the 21st century. Vox Sang. 2011;100(1):92-98.

78. Hewagama S, Krishnaswamy S, King L, Davis J, Baird R. Human T-cell lymphotropic virus type 1 exposures following blood-borne virus incidents in central Australia, 2002-2012. Clin Infect Dis. 2014;59(1):85-87.

79. Einsiedel L, Pham H, Talukder MR, Taylor K, Wilson K, Kaldor J, et al. Very high prevalence of infection with the human T cell leukaemia virus type 1c in remote Australian Aboriginal communities: results of a large cross-sectional community survey. PLoS Negl Trop Dis. 2021;15(12): e0009915.

80. Azevedo LS, Pierrotti LC, Abdala E, Costa SF, Strabelli TM, Campos SV, et al. Cytomegalovirus infection in transplant recipients. Clinics (Sao Paulo). 2015;70(7):515-523.

81. Arana C, Cofan F, Ruiz P, Hermida E, Fernández J, Colmenero J, et al. Primary herpes simplex virus type 1 infection with acute liver failure in solid organ transplantation: report of three cases and review. IDCases. 2022;28:e01485.

82. Macesic N, Abbott IJ, Kaye M, Druce J, Glanville AR, Gow PJ, et al. Herpes simplex virus-2 transmission following solid organ transplantation: donor-derived infection and transplantation from prior organ recipients. Transpl Infect Dis. 2017;19(5).

83. Harypursat V, Zhou Y, Tang S, Chen Y. JC Polyomavirus, progressive multifocal leukoencephalopathy and immune reconstitution inflammatory syndrome: a review. AIDS Res Ther. 2020;17(1):37.

84. Palacios G, Druce J, Du L, Tran T, Birch C, Briese T, et al. A new arenavirus in a cluster of fatal transplant-associated diseases. N Engl J Med. 2008;358(10):991-998.

85. Barsoum RS. Parasitic infections in transplant recipients. Nat Clin Pract Nephrol. 2006;2(9):490-503.

86. Fürnkranz U, Walochnik J. Nosocomial infections: do not forget the parasites! Pathogens. 2021;10(2).

87. Molan A, Nosaka K, Hunter M, Zhang J, Meng X, Song M, et al. First age- and gender-matched case-control study in Australia examining the possible association between toxoplasma gondii infection and type 2 diabetes mellitus: the Busselton health study. J Parasitol Res. 2020;2020: 3142918.

88. Roxby AC, Gottlieb GS, Limaye1 AP. Strongyloidiasis in transplant patients. Clin Infect Dis. 2009;49(9):1411-1423.

89. Jackson Y, Pinto A, Pett S. Chagas disease in Australia and New Zealand: risks and needs for public health interventions. Trop Med Int Health. 2014;19(2):212-218.

90. Stickland JF, Roberts AN, Williams V. Transfusion-induced malaria in Victoria. Med J Aust. 1992;157(7):499-500.

91. Bradbury RS, French LP, Blizzard L. Prevalence of Acanthamoeba spp. in Tasmanian intensive care clinical specimens. J Hosp Infect. 2014;86(3):170-181.

92. Bonda DJ, Manjila S, Mehndiratta P, Khan F, Miller BR, Onwuzulike K, et al. Human prion diseases: surgical lessons learned from iatrogenic prion transmission. Neurosurg Focus. 2016;41(1):E10.

93. Sharma N, Wang L, Namboodiri H. Creutzfeldt-Jakob disease following kidney transplantation. Cureus. 2022;14(1):e21632.

94. Molesworth A, Yates P, Hewitt PE, Mackenzie J, Ironside JW, Galea G, et al. Investigation of variant Creutzfeldt-Jakob disease implicated organ or tissue transplantation in the United Kingdom. Transplantation. 2014;98(5):585-589.

95. The Transplantation Society of Australia and New Zealand. Clinical guidelines for organ transplantation from deceased donors. Version 1.5, 2021.

96. Lier AJ, Tuan JJ, Davis MW, Paulson N, McManus D, Campbell S, et al. Case report: disseminated Strongyloidiasis in a patient with COVID-19. Am J Trop Med Hyg. 2020;103(4):1590-1592.

97. Ariza-Heredia EJ, Chemaly RF. Update on infection control practices in cancer hospitals. CA Cancer J Clin. 2018;68(5):340-355.

98. Fasciana T, Cortegiani A, Ippolito M, Giarratano A, Di Quattro O, Lipari D, et al. An overview of how to screen, detect, test and control this emerging pathogen. Antibiotics (Basel). 2020;9(11).

99. Henderson A, Nimmo GR. Control of healthcare- and community-associated MRSA: recent progress and persisting challenges. Br Med Bull. 2018;125(1):25-41.

100. Krishna NK, Cunnion KM. Role of molecular diagnostics in the management of infectious disease emergencies. Med Clin North Am. 2012;96(6):1067-1078.

101. Henze L, Buhl C, Sandherr M, Cornely OA, Heinz WJ, Khodamoradi Y, et al. Management of herpesvirus reactivations in patients with solid tumours and hematologic malignancies: update of the Guidelines of the Infectious Diseases Working Party (AGIHO) of the German Society for Hematology and Medical Oncology (DGHO) on herpes simplex virus type 1, herpes simplex virus type 2, and varicella zoster virus. Ann Hematol. 2022;101(3):491-511.

102. Tomblyn M, Chiller T, Einsele H, Gress R, Sepkowitz K, Storek J, et al. Guidelines for preventing infectious complications among hematopoietic cell transplantation recipients: a global perspective. Biol Blood Marrow Transplant. 2009;15(10):1143-1238.

103. Loomba R, Liang TJ. Hepatitis B reactivation associated with immune suppressive and biological modifier therapies: current concepts, management strategies, and future directions. Gastroenterol. 2017;152(6):1297-1309.

104. Rajapakse P, Gupta M, Hall R. Invasive fungal infection complicating treatment with ibrutinib. Cureus. 2021;13(6):e16009.

105. Dalton KR, Rock C, Carroll KC, Davis MF. One Health in hospitals: how understanding the dynamics of people, animals, and the hospital built-environment can be used to better inform interventions for antimicrobial-resistant gram-positive infections. Antimicrob Resist Infect Control. 2020;9(1):78.

106. Grayson ML, Stewardson AJ, Russo PL, Ryan KE, Olsen KL, Havers SM, et al. Effects of the Australian National Hand Hygiene Initiative after 8 years on infection control practices, health-care worker education, and clinical outcomes: a longitudinal study. Lancet Infect Dis. 2018;18(11):1269-1277.

107. Sax H, Allegranzi B, Uçkay I, Larson E, Boyce J, Pittet D. 'My five moments for hand hygiene': a user-centred design approach to understand, train, monitor and report hand hygiene. J Hosp Infect. 2007;67(1):9-21.

108. Sung AD, Sung JAM, Thomas S, Hyslop T, Gasparetto C, Long G, et al. Universal mask usage for reduction of respiratory viral infections after stem cell transplant: a prospective trial. Clin Infect Dis. 2016;63(8):999-1006.

109. Chang CC, Ananda-Rajah M, Belcastro A, McMullan B, Reid A, Dempsey K, et al. Consensus guidelines for implementation of quality processes to prevent invasive fungal disease and enhanced surveillance measures during hospital building works, 2014. Intern Med J. 2014;44(12b):1389-1397.

110. Sehulster L, Chinn RY, CDC, HICPAC. Guidelines for environmental infection control in health-care facilities. Recommendations of CDC and the Healthcare Infection Control Practices Advisory Committee (HICPAC). MMWR Recomm Rep. 2003;52(RR-10):1-42.

111. Mitchell SJ, Gray J, Morgan ME, Hocking MD, Durbin GM. Nosocomial infection with Rhizopus microsporus in preterm infants: association with wooden tongue depressors. Lancet. 1996;348(9025):441-443.

112. Duffy J, Harris J, Gade L, Sehulster L, Newhouse E, O'Connell H, et al. Mucormycosis outbreak associated with hospital linens. Pediatr Infect Dis J. 2014;33(5):472-476.

113. Kizny Gordon AE, Mathers AJ, Cheong EYL, Gottlieb T, Kotay S, Walker AS, et al. The hospital water environment as a reservoir for carbapenem-resistant organisms causing hospital-acquired infections-a systematic review of the literature. Clin Infect Dis. 2017;64(10):1435-1344.

114. Bartley PB, Ben Zakour NL, Stanton-Cook M, Muguli R, Prado L, Garnys V, et al. Hospital-wide eradication of a nosocomial legionella pneumophila serogroup 1 outbreak. Clin Infect Dis. 2016;62(3):273-279.

115. Nucci M, Anaissie E. Fusarium infections in immuno-compromised patients. Clin Microbiol Rev. 2007;20(4):695-704.

116. Ravn P, Lundgren JD, Kjaeldgaard P, Holten-Anderson W, Højlyng N, Nielsen JO, et al. Nosocomial outbreak of cryptosporidiosis in AIDS patients. BMJ. 1991;302(6771):277-280.

117. enHealth. Guidelines for legionella control in the operation and maintenance of water distribution systems in health and aged care facilities. Canberra: Australian Government, 2015.

118. Sherry NL, Gorrie CL, Kwong JC, Higgs C, Stuart RL, Marshall C, et al. Multi-site implementation of whole genome sequencing for hospital infection control: a prospective genomic epidemiological analysis. Lancet Reg Health West Pac. 2022;23:100446.

119. Phipps LM, Chen SC, Kable K, Halliday CL, Firacative C, Meyer W, et al. Nosocomial pneumocystis jirovecii pneumonia: lessons from a cluster in kidney transplant recipients. Transplantation. 2011;92(12):1327-1334.

CHAPTER 31

Infection prevention and control in mental health and psychiatric practice settings

Dr SHIZAR NAHIDI[i-ii]
Dr CATHERINE VIENGKHAM[iii-iv]

Chapter highlights

- An overview of psychiatric and mental health care in Australia, including the key characteristics of Australian mental health services
- Discussion of healthcare-associated infections (HAIs) and infectious disease in Australian psychiatric and mental health services
- Essentials of infection prevention and control (IPC) practices in psychiatric and mental health practice settings
- Practical guidance and context-specific solutions on the current IPC practices to minimise the risk of HAI in mental health care

i Latrobe Regional Hospital (LRH), Traralgon, VIC
ii School of Rural Health, Faculty of Medicine, Nursing and Health Sciences, Monash University, VIC
iii Sydney Infectious Diseases Institute, Faculty of Medicine and Health, University of Sydney, NSW
iv Susan Wakil School of Nursing and Midwifery, Faculty of Medicine and Health, University of Sydney, NSW

Introduction

Mental health and psychiatric facilities 'deliver care to' individuals with mental health problems and advance their social support networks. In these settings, implementing optimal infection prevention and control (IPC) measures can be complex and challenging. This chapter describes the overall contexts of mental health care in Australia and outlines the risks of infectious diseases and HAIs in those settings. The chapter also explains the key elements in standard IPC practices that are specific to mental health and psychiatric care.

31.1 Overview of mental health services in Australia

31.1.1 The early psychiatric institutions

The first psychiatric facilities in Australia were introduced in the early 1800s as a short-term solution to the country's rapidly growing penal population. Overcrowding caused by the combined detainment of both convicts and the mentally ill led to the establishment of Australia's first mental asylum in Castle Hill, New South Wales (NSW) in 1811.[1] The asylum itself was a haphazardly assembled initiative that repurposed a poorly maintained convict barrack, was managed by a non-medical superintendent and utilised a primarily convict staff.[2] Eventually this facility also became overcrowded, and infrastructural neglect and ongoing conflict between managing authorities saw the asylum adopt an increasingly custodial approach to the treatment of its mentally ill occupants.[3-5] The mistreatment of the mentally ill and the mismanagement of mental asylums was eventually recognised, and would subsequently result in the gradual transition to a medical approach with a greater focus on treatment and rehabilitation. The 1900s marked an influx in treatment facilities with dedicated psychiatric wards and services for voluntary patients, with the first of these houses opening in Victoria and NSW in 1907 and 1908, respectively.

Notably, the revolution in the treatment and prevention of infectious diseases initiated by advances in medicine and the discovery of antimicrobial drugs also catalysed substantial improvements in psychiatric healthcare.[3,6] During this time, conditions in asylums were prime conduits for infectious disease, with hygiene and sanitation in both dedicated mental institutes and hospital-based treatment wards maintained to a considerably lower standard compared to general practice settings. The arrival of penicillin and antibiotics came with the added benefit of treating diseases such as syphilis, which was associated with the manifestation of neurological symptoms. The decades that followed World War II saw major advancements in psychopharmacology, leading to the introduction and rapid dissemination of tranquillisers and psychotropic drugs that radically transformed psychiatric practices.[6] For example, the discovery of chlorpromazine, an antipsychotic medication, revolutionised the treatment of schizophrenia. The ability to stabilise and manage the symptoms of psychosis and mood disorders enabled patients to embark on programs of rehabilitation that included therapeutic, vocational and recreational activities, and offered hope of discharge from the asylums. As a result, psychiatric nurses were able to establish therapeutic relationships with clients, and from the 1950s to the 1980s there were rapid changes within the psychiatric industry which dramatically promoted the practice of nursing.

31.1.2 Deinstitutionalisation and the mainstreaming of mental health services

For most of the 20th century, general and mental health services were organised and funded by separate government entities. While the federal government contributed funding and support for state-run public hospitals, the primary responsibility for mental health services rested with state governments until the 1970s. Before then, mental health services were almost exclusively provided through long-term institutionalisation in state mental.[7,8] Following a period of immense change in mental health reform and policy, formal government action to rectify the years of neglect of mental health care began in earnest in 1992 with the endorsement of the National Mental Health Strategy.[9]

Central to the strategy was the gradual process of deinstitutionalisation whereby specialised psychiatric institutions were replaced with community mental health services that were less isolated and more readily accessible to the general population.[10] Moreover, the scope of mental health treatment also shifted, from one with a narrow focus on the treatment of mental illness to one which also sought to prevent mental illness and promote mental wellbeing. Part of this strategy also aimed to reduce the stigmatisation and discrimination against mentally ill patients. As a result, the preferred model of care in recent years has been transitioned towards community-based care in a process known as 'mainstreaming', which encourages mentally ill individuals to actively participate in community life and reduces the prominence of inpatient settings and long-term institutionalisation. The introduction of mainstreaming drastically expanded the mental healthcare workforce—which now involves and subsidises mental health services sought at general practitioners (GPs)—increased the scope of services provided, and vastly facilitated consumer access to these services.

31.1.3 Mental health services in the 21st century

Today, the settings in which mental health services are provided are highly heterogeneous. Deinstitutionalisation means that mental health services can now be found within general healthcare facilities that are not solely dedicated to the treatment of mental health patients. Mental health care can be broadly divided into inpatient and outpatient (or ambulatory) care; however, there is also a distinction between inpatient facilities that provide long-term care for the chronically ill, and short-term hospital services for the acutely unwell.

Different levels of government oversee various mental health-related services.[11] The federal government funds several initiatives which allow access to specialist medical practitioners, psychiatrists, psychologists and other allied health practitioners. Additionally, state and territory governments provide mental health services through public hospitals, emergency departments, and residential and community mental healthcare services. Non-government organisations (NGOs) also play a key role in providing mental health care, particularly in the form of mental health crisis and support services.[11] The common settings in which mental health care is provided are listed in Table 31.1, and are further detailed in the following sections.

Inpatient mental healthcare services: Inpatient psychiatric services remain an essential component of mental healthcare. Deinstitutionalisation precipitated a substantial shift in the provision of inpatient services towards *general public* and *private hospitals*, many of which now include dedicated wards where patients are able to receive specialised psychiatric care. Hospital-based psychiatric wards typically have 20–30 beds and are staffed by health professionals with specialist mental health qualifications or training. In 2019–20, mental health-related hospitalisations accounted for 6.4% of all overnight hospitalisations,

TABLE 31.1 Mental health and psychiatric services in Australia

Inpatient mental healthcare services	Psychiatric hospitals—public and private Psychiatric wards in general and private hospitals Substance abuse units Residential mental healthcare services: Sub-acute residential mental health services Non-acute residential mental health services Specialist dementia care units Alcohol and drug withdrawal and rehabilitation services Forensic mental health units
Ambulatory mental healthcare services	**Hospital-based ambulatory services** Ambulatory mental health services in emergency departments (EDs) Psychiatric emergency care centres (PECC) Hospital-based outpatient clinics Dedicated mental health day clinics **Primary mental healthcare services** General practitioners Primary health networks Medicare-subsidised psychiatrist services Medicare-subsidised psychologist services Allied mental health services (provided by occupational therapists, social workers, and mental health nurses) **Community and/or home-based services** Hospital in the home (HITH) Acute and post-acute care teams Mobile intensive treatment teams Mobile mental health clinics Hospital Admission Risk Program (HARP) Specialised outpatient mental health services* Outpatient rehabilitation and support services Non-government organisations (NGO) Online mental health services and programs

* Specialised outpatient services include electroconvulsive therapy (ECT) clinics, perinatal infant mental health services (PIMHS), Aboriginal and Torres Strait Islander services, outpatient vocational rehabilitation services, and support services for families and primary carers.

with depressive episodes (15.4%) and schizophrenia (13.4%) being the most common principal diagnoses averaged across all hospital types.[12] The use of public acute hospitals and private hospitals in place of dedicated psychiatric hospitals for admitted mental health care has been on a steady increase over the past decade (Fig 31.1). However, the average length of stay in psychiatric hospitals remains considerably longer

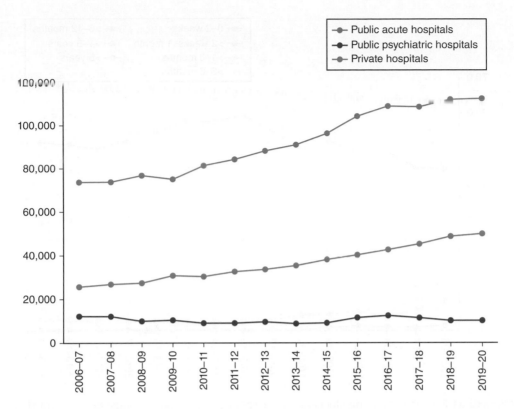

FIGURE 31.1 Overnight mental health-related hospitalisations with specialised psychiatric care, 2006–2020.
Source: AIHW[12]

(49.4 days) compared to public acute (15.3 days) and private hospitals (19.1 days). The Australian Institute of Health and Welfare (AIHW) also appreciates the distinction between mental health-related admissions where both specialised healthcare and non-specialised healthcare is provided. For example, the majority of mental health presentations that do not mandate hospitalisation for specialised psychiatric care corresponds to those who present with mental and behavioural disorders due to alcohol and drug use, or those with organic mental disorders related to brain damage or disease. In such cases, patients could be admitted to other hospital units (such as *substance-abuse units* for alcohol and drug rehabilitation and detoxification procedures) or may be referred to residential aged care facilities.

Residential mental healthcare services provide specialised care within a domestic-style environment, which also serves as accommodation for patients needing long stays.[13] In 2019–20, there were approximately 6617 users of residential mental healthcare facilities, with the most common principal diagnoses being schizophrenia (26.2%), personality disorders (13.8%), schizoaffective

disorders (9.7%) and depressive episodes (9.4%). Services are commonly classified into *sub-acute services* and *non-acute services*, which is differentiated based on the treatment provided and the duration of patient stay.[14] Sub-acute residential services primarily focus on rehabilitation and reconditioning for the purpose of improving patients' mental health functioning and facilitating patient discharge. Non-acute services involve the provision of care and support for the purpose of maintaining patient health and this may last indefinitely. Generally, over 80% of residential mental healthcare users are discharged within a month of admission, and around 3% will require a stay longer than a year (Fig 31.2). Residential units are generally staffed on a 24-hour basis by health professionals with specialist mental health qualifications.

In addition, there are highly specialised residential care settings that target specific vulnerable or disadvantaged groups and those with specific needs, such as patients with brain injury or neuropsychiatric disorders. These include *specialist dementia care units*, which provide palliative, end-of-life care to older people experiencing severe cognitive deterioration and who cannot be adequately cared for in mainstream aged care

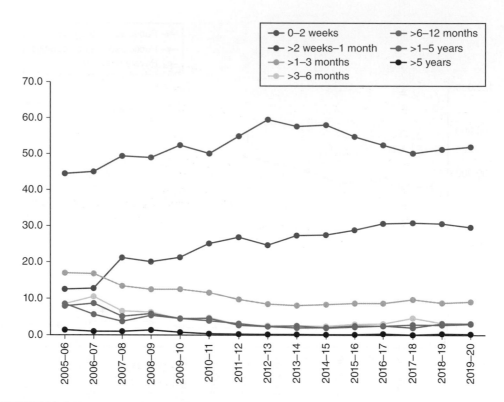

FIGURE 31.2 Proportion of mental health care episodes by length of completed residential stay, 2006–2020.

Source: AIHW[13]

services.[15] *Alcohol and drug withdrawal and rehabilitation services* offer a short-term residential environment for people experiencing withdrawal symptoms, those experiencing more severe forms of substance use disorder, or patients who are unable to overcome addiction via community-based and outpatient services.[16] *Forensic mental health units* are dedicated facilities for holding and providing mental health treatment to offenders and correctional patients.[17,18] Forensic patients are typically characterised by a higher rate of mental disorders compared to the general population, as well as a greater incidence of comorbidities, such as substance use, mood and personality disorders. The majority of forensic patients include offenders who have been found 'Not Guilty by reason of Mental Illness' (NGMI), those found to be unfit to plead, and/or sentenced prisoners who require mental health treatment in a secure setting.

Primary mental healthcare services: The Australian Government also funds Medicare-subsidised consultations via the Medicare Benefits Schedule (MBS) for a range of mental health conditions. These give eligible Australians access to the mental health services provided by GPs, mental health specialists and allied health services. Of these, GPs are the most

common point of contact, with 8.8% of Australians receiving Medicare-subsidised mental health-specific services from a GP. While GPs are capable of providing a range of mental health services (e.g. arranging a mental health care plan or supervising therapy sessions), they are also the primary form of contact for referring the patient to more specialised services.[19]

With respect to specialist consultations, psychologists are the most commonly utilised specialist service, with 5.1% of Australians utilising mental health services through clinical psychologists. Similar to community mental health services, consultations may be provided in several settings, including hospitals, consulting rooms, home visits, or via telehealth (e.g. telephone consultations or videoconferencing).[21] Medicare-subsidised mental health-related services are also provided by psychiatrists and other allied mental health professionals, namely mental health nurses, occupational therapists, social workers and Aboriginal health workers.

Ambulatory mental health services: Mental health services are now more commonly delivered within community-based and general healthcare settings on an outpatient basis. The transition to ambulatory mental health care was a key objective of the inaugural National Mental Health Strategy and aimed to promote greater public accessibility to mental health services while emphasising the ability of users to continue living and working within the greater community.[23,24] Ambulatory mental health services are designed to be widely accessible to the general population and are also flexible in where and how the services are delivered. They offer assessment, treatment, rehabilitation and/or care for patients via hospital-based, community-based or home-based services. These services typically include a multidisciplinary team, involving psychologists, psychiatrists, mental health nurses and social workers.[11]

Hospital emergency departments (EDs) continue to play a vital role in providing ambulatory mental health services, with mental health-related presentations accounting for 3.8% of all ED presentations in 2019–20.[25] EDs offer an initial (and sometimes only) point of contact for many people experiencing acute mental health episodes and are widely accessed due to their after-hours availability.[26] Approximately 38% of ED presentations are subsequently admitted to hospital or referred to another hospital for admission. Disorders due to psychoactive substance use (28.2%) and neurotic, stress-related and somatoform disorders (27.0%) are the two most common principal diagnoses in EDs. Although mental health presentations to EDs have been on a

gradual incline, many EDs are not adequately equipped with the resources and staffing to provide immediate specialised mental healthcare services.[26] Lack of resources, understanding of mental illness, and discriminatory treatment may be the cause of the lengthy delays in assessment and treatment experienced by mental health patients.[27](See Fig 31.3.)

A recent development in emergency mental health services is *psychiatric emergency care centres* (PECC), which are mental health short-stay units typically located within or adjacent to hospital EDs that facilitate quick access to urgent specialised mental health care.[28,29] The first PECC opened in the Royal Brisbane and Women's Hospital in 1983, with more states and facilities adopting the PECC model of care in recent decades.[28] Similar to EDs, these units have 24-hour access, dedicated specialised staffing and enforce a maximum 48-hour length of stay, after which the patient must be discharged, transferred to another mental health facility or admitted to an acute inpatient ward.[30] The introduction of PECCs has been successful in both reducing the length of stay in ED and streamlining the admission of patients requiring specific mental health care, such as those expressing suicidality.[31]

Ambulatory mental health services also include a broad range of specialised outpatient services. These include facilities that offer specific therapies like *electroconvulsive therapy* (ECT),[32,33] and services targeted at specific groups, such as children and adolescents, older

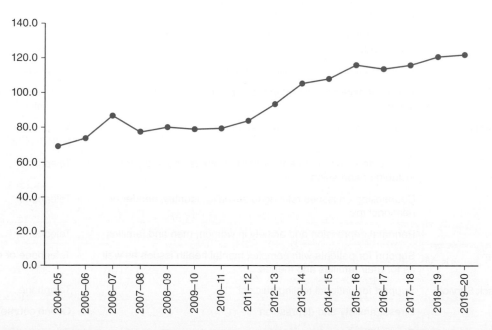

FIGURE 31.3 National rate (per 10,000 population) of mental health-related emergency department presentations in public hospitals, 2004–2005 to 2019–2020
Source: AIHW[25]

people, and Aboriginal and Torres Strait Islander peoples. For example, *perinatal infant mental health services (PIMHS)* provide support for women struggling with perinatal depression (i.e. maternal major and minor depression during pregnancy and/or during the first year postpartum).[36,37] Outpatient rehabilitation and support services are also available for those with substance use disorders and those released from correctional facilities. For forensic patients, these services are used by both those who are mandated by courts to engage in community-based mental health services in place of prison time, and by those who are transitioning back into the community after being institutionalised. These services play a key role in facilitating recovery and providing support, and primarily aim to reduce the risk of relapse or reoffending.[17,18]

Finally, non-government organisations (NGOs) fulfil a vital role in delivering community-based programs to people with mental illnesses. They provide supported accommodation services, vocational rehabilitation programs, consumer self-help services, employment services, and support services for families of mental health patients and/or their primary carer. In addition to providing a wide array of services, they are also an important resource for connecting the wider community to available services. Many NGOs target disadvantaged and hard-to-reach population groups, including Aboriginal and Torres Strait Islander communities, homeless people or those at risk of homelessness, people with intellectual disabilities and former prisoners. Additionally, online and digital mental health services offer low-cost and less resource-intensive mental health services, mainly on psychological counselling and advice. There are several organisations that provide support and education for people with mental illness, their families and carers throughout Australia via mental health telephone helplines (Table 31.2).

TABLE 31.2 Current online and digital mental health services in Australia

Online/digital mental health services	Area of service	Mode of communication
Beyond Blue	Depression and anxiety and reducing stigma	Telephone or online chat
Blue Knot Foundation Helpline	Adult survivors of childhood trauma and abuse	Telephone and email
Black Dog Institute	Self-help programs and resources for people with mood disorders, anxiety and stress.	Online help
Butterfly Foundation	Counselling and treatment referral for people with eating disorders and body image issues	Telephone, online chat and email
eheadspace	General counselling to young people 12–25 and their families and friends	Telephone, online chat and email
Kids Helpline	Counselling service for children and young adults aged 5–25	Telephone
Lifeline	Crisis counselling, support groups and suicide prevention services	Telephone, text message and online chat
MensLine Australia	Counselling service for male Australians	Telephone or online (video) chat
MindSpot	Assessment and treatment for anxiety, stress, mood disorders including depression	Telephone
QLife	Counselling on issues relating to sexuality, identity, gender or relationships	Telephone
PANDA	Perinatal depression and anxiety in women, men and families	Telephone
SANE Australia	Support for patients with complex mental health issues as well as for their families and friends	Telephone or online chat
Suicide Call Back Service	Support for patients feeling suicidal	Telephone
This Way Up	Stress, anxiety and depression	Online courses
Open Arms	Counselling for veterans and anyone who has served at least one day in the ADF, including their families	Telephone

31.1.4 National mental health performance framework and key performance indicators

Australia developed the first National Mental Health Performance Framework (NMHPF) in 2005, which was motivated by the key goal 'to improve all health outcomes for Australians living with mental illness and ensure sustainability of the Australian health system'.[39] The Framework includes three core dimensions:

1. *Determinants of health* examines the factors that influence good health, whether they are changing, and if they are changing for everyone. These include health behaviours, personal biomedical factors, personal history, environmental factors and socio-economic factors.

2. *Health system* examines the preventive capability of the health system. It is characterised by the sub-dimensions of effectiveness, safety, appropriateness, continuity of care, accessibility, efficiency and sustainability. The performance of mental health services is measured by a number of key performance indicators (KPI).

3. *Health status* examines the health of Australians and identifies opportunities for improvement. It is measured in terms of health conditions, human function, wellbeing and deaths.

The KPIs for Australian mental health services are reported by all Australian states and territories, allowing for cross-jurisdictional comparisons and assessment of state mental health services against the national benchmarks (Table 31.3). Performance data of publicly funded mental health services have been collected through NMHPF, and are analysed and published by the AIHW up to 2022.[39]

31.1.5 Characteristics of mental health services

Facility design—communal and safe environments: Communal and domestic-style environments are a key component of residential mental healthcare facilities.[40] These facilities typically include shared spaces, such as dining rooms, activity rooms, lounge rooms and outdoor areas, to encourage participation in social activities and provide opportunities to interact with staff and other residents. Patient bedrooms may also house more than one person and offer a dormitory-style layout to further facilitate opportunities for interaction. However, most facilities will have a mix of single and multi-patient rooms, as well as private spaces, depending on patient needs and mental health indicators. People with mental illnesses often stay longer in psychiatric facilities compared to patients in general hospitals.[41] Ensuring facility safety is essential, and must take into consideration both the safety hazards associated with caring for people with mental illness and the unique problems this presents for infection and outbreak control.

The role of mental healthcare worker: Inpatient and residential facilities are typically used by individuals presenting with more severe mental illness. This is particularly pertinent for residential facilities, which may accommodate patients for a significant period or even indefinitely. These facilities employ a multidisciplinary workforce, including registered nurses, personal care providers, psychologists, psychiatrists, social workers and other allied health professionals. Many patients with severe mental disabilities may be highly dependent on healthcare workers (HCWs) for performing day-to-day activities like personal grooming, bathing and eating.[42,43] Regular maintenance of essential activities is integral to maintaining the therapeutic relationship, and disruption to routine may cause severe distress to the patient.

Restrictive practices: Restrictive practices in clinical settings encompass any actions or interventions that restrict the rights or freedom of a person. These are performed in mental health settings to prevent patients from harming themselves or others, or to ensure that essential medical treatment can be safely administered.[44] Restraint can be achieved through physical, mechanical or pharmacological means. Physical restraint is usually applied by the healthcare workforce and involves the hands-on immobilisation of a patient. Mechanical restraint is the application of devices, such as belts, harnesses, manacles, sheets and straps, to a person's body to restrict their ambulation. Pharmacological restraint involves the administration of tranquillising medications to chemically subdue the patient.

Seclusion is the isolated confinement of a person in a room or area from which the patient is prevented from leaving. The AIHW specifies that the 'purpose, duration, structure of the area and awareness of the person are not considered in determining what constitutes seclusion'.[45] Seclusion is not necessarily always involuntary, and the

TABLE 31.3 National Mental Health Performance Framework and Mental Health Services Key Performance Indicators 2021

KPIs	Description
Change in mental health consumer's clinical outcomes	Percentage of episodes of mental health care where significant improvement, significant deterioration or no significant change was identified between baseline and follow-up
Mental health readmissions to hospital	Percentage of in-scope overnight separations from the mental health service organisation's acute psychiatric inpatient unit that are followed by readmission to the same or to another public-sector acute psychiatric inpatient unit within 28 days of discharge
National Mental Health Service Standards compliance	Percentage of the mental health service organisation's services (weighted by expenditure) that has been reviewed against the National Standards for Mental Health Services
Average length of acute mental health inpatient stay	Average length of stay of in-scope overnight separations from acute psychiatric inpatient units managed by the mental health service organisation
Average cost per acute mental health admitted patient day	Average cost of a patient day within acute psychiatric inpatient units managed by the mental health service organisation
Average treatment days per 3-month community mental health care period	Average number of community treatment days per 3-month period of ambulatory care provided by the mental health service organisation's community mental health services
Average cost per community mental health treatment day	Average cost per community treatment day provided by the organisation's ambulatory mental healthcare services
Population access to specialised clinical mental healthcare	Percentage of consumers who reside in the state/territory and received care from a state/territory specialised mental health service (including admitted patient mental healthcare services, ambulatory mental healthcare services and residential mental healthcare services)
Mental health new client index	Percentage of new clients under the care of the mental health service organisation's mental health services
Comparative area resources	Per capita recurrent expenditure by the organisation on mental health services for the target population within the organisation's defined catchment area
Admission preceded by community mental healthcare	Percentage of admissions to the mental health service organisation's acute psychiatric inpatient unit(s) for which a community mental health service contact, in which the consumer or their carer/support person participated, was recorded in the 7 days immediately preceding that admission
Post-discharge community mental healthcare	Percentage of separations from state/territory public acute admitted patient mental healthcare service unit(s) for which a community mental health service contact, in which the consumer or their carer/support person participated, was recorded in the 7 days following that separation
Mental health consumer outcomes participation	The percentage of episodes of ambulatory mental healthcare with completed consumer self-assessment outcomes measures
Outcomes readiness	Proportion of mental health care episodes with completed clinical outcome measures at both baseline and follow-up. No longer reported
Seclusion rate	Number of seclusion events per 1000 patient days within public acute admitted patient specialised mental health service units
Restraint rate	Number of restraint events per 1000 patient days within public acute admitted patient specialised mental health service units
Involuntary treatment and patient days	Percentage of separations with specialised mental healthcare days or percentage of admitted patient specialised mental healthcare patient days where the consumer has a mental health legal status of 'involuntary'

term extends to individuals who agree to or request confinement. However, if they maintain the liberty to leave at any time they choose, it is no longer considered seclusion. State and territory mental health-related legislation specifies the conditions under which restrictive practices may be used. However, minimising the use of seclusion and restraint in mental health services is a national key focus across multiple sectors—including consumers, carers, governments and services.[46]

Patient rights and involuntary admission: The reception, admission and treatment of a mental health patient is highly complex and may often require the involvement of multiple legal and emergency services. In all Australian states and territories, a person can be involuntarily detained and treated if they are found to be mentally ill following a mental health assessment (Box 31.1). Involuntary contacts account for 14.7% of all community mental healthcare contacts and 19.9% of all residents in residential mental healthcare facilities.[11] All Australian jurisdictions have adopted the policy position that enables involuntary treatment to be authorised (usually by the treating physician) in view of the patient's refusal of treatment. The highest proportion of contacts involving a patient with an involuntary admission was seen in patients with schizoaffective disorders (39.2%), schizophrenia (35.0%), bipolar affective disorder (21.7%), depressive episode (2.8%) and reaction to severe stress and adjustment disorders (2.4%).[45]

> **BOX 31.1 Criteria shared across all states and territories for involuntary commitment and treatment**
>
> In all Australian states and territories, the decision to order involuntary commitment and treatment under the Australian act can be made if a person meets, at the minimum, the following criteria:
>
> (a) The person has a mental illness, and
>
> (b) They are likely to cause serious harm to themselves or to others and/or they are clearly experiencing severe mental or physical deterioration and/or they require immediate treatment; and
>
> (c) There is no less restrictive means of ensuring safe and effective care is provided and/or the person does not have the capacity to give informed consent.

31.2 Infectious diseases and HAIs in mental health and psychiatric practice settings

Infectious diseases and HAIs lead to high morbidity and mortality across all healthcare settings, including mental health and psychiatric practice settings. Unfortunately, both global and Australian HAI data in psychiatric hospitals are scarce. There are only a few long-term surveillance studies that have provided data on the prevalence of HAIs in psychiatric settings. An example is a study from Switzerland of HAIs involving an 18-year surveillance in a university psychiatric hospital, which estimated the prevalence of HAI to vary from 1.0 and 3.7%.[47] In Australia, the data on HAIs are collected by the Independent Hospital Pricing Authority (IHPA), an independent government agency established under Commonwealth legislation. However, these HAI data are not publicly available and alternative sources published in peer-reviewed literature about the incidence and prevalence rates of HAIs in Australian mental health services remain limited.

Despite the small body of evidence to advise on the magnitude of the impact of HAIs on Australian mental health services and patients, there has been a promising level of awareness about IPC practice gaps and the necessity of providing clinical services to ensure the safety of care and patient outcomes are maintained. To address this, the National Standards for Mental Health Services (NSMHS) was first introduced in 1996 to guide the development of appropriate mental health practices in the country, and to gauge continuous quality improvement in Australian psychiatric and mental health services. NSMHS renders ten domains of standards and a number of key criteria within each standard. NSMHS Standard 2 – 'Safety' remarks that all Australian mental health services must comply with IPC requirements to ensure mental health activities and environments are safe for healthcare consumers and their families, healthcare providers and the community more broadly.[48]

31.2.1 Mental health patients and risks of infection and HAIs

Mental health patients are known to harbour increased risks for acquiring HAIs, due to a number of inherent risk factors. Many of these risk factors may also necessitate adjustments to standard IPC procedures.[49] The following section describes several attributes that may be more commonly observed in patients presenting with mental illness compared to the general population, and to what degree these might exacerbate the likelihood of contracting an HAI or inhibit the optimal performance of IPC practices.

Poor physical health and comorbidities: Physical health and mental health are closely linked. People with mental illness are more likely to develop physical comorbidities and vice versa. Some of the factors that increase this risk include greater engagement in poor health choices (e.g. use of alcohol and tobacco, poor nutrition and lack of physical activity), adverse side effects of complex pharmacological treatments, socioeconomic disadvantages, and broader systemic factors such as social stigma and negative experiences from interacting with the healthcare system.[50,51] Moreover, irregular or poor medication compliance can lead to poor physical health outcomes in people with mental health conditions.

Patients with severe mental illness are more susceptible to cardiovascular diseases, respiratory diseases, diabetes and cancer.[23,52] Common physical comorbidities for people with mental illness are listed in Table 31.4. Consequently, people with mental illnesses may have decreased resistance to infection and the increased prevalence of underlying medical conditions means those who are infected may experience more severe disease and have poorer outcomes.[53] On average, people with

serious mental illnesses are estimated to live between 10–32 years less than the general population.[51,54]

Alcohol and substance abuse: A large proportion of patients who are hospitalised in acute inpatient care services are diagnosed with some form of substance abuse disorder.[11] People who had been diagnosed or treated for a mental health condition are at greater risk of alcohol dependence and more likely to have used illicit drugs for non-medical purposes compared to the general population.[56] Excessive substance use is a predictor of the development of physical comorbidities in people with mental illness, such as cancer, cirrhosis and cardiovascular disease.[50,51] Secondly, the use of these substances can also worsen mental health conditions, particularly if patients are presenting at services intoxicated or experiencing withdrawal symptoms. These patients are often unable to communicate effectively with HCWs and unable to follow instructions. Finally, patients with a history of substance use are generally at an increased risk for certain infectious diseases. In particular, intravenous drug users are at high risk of blood-borne disorders (from non-sterile needle use and needle sharing) and sexually transmitted diseases.[57-59]

Reduced cognitive capacity and non-compliance: Impaired cognitive function is observed in several mental health disorders, and habitually leads to high-risk health behaviours, poor hygiene or non-compliance with preventive measures. Patients may be unaware of their physical symptoms, as a result of cognitive deficits or reduced pain sensitivity. Neglected personal hygiene practices present additional avenues for infection spread.[60] These patients often have trouble communicating with healthcare professionals and care providers. While some patients have a trusted advocate or guardian that may be authorised to receive information and make decisions and consent on their behalf, these avenues of communication may also be inhibited by IPC measures, such as the lockdowns introduced in response to pandemic-level emergencies, such as during COVID-19.

Patients with reduced cognitive capacity may have issues adhering to complex infection control practices, like disinfecting, masking, social distancing and mobility restrictions.[61-63] Failure to comply with IPC practices can be related to the patient's illness. Patients with delusions, hallucinations or cognitive impairment may find it difficult to fully comprehend the importance of following infection control measures, or find such practices

TABLE 31.4 Chronic conditions of people with and without mental illness in 2017–2018

Selected chronic condition	Persons with mental illness (%)	Persons without mental illness (%)
Arthritis	23.3	13
Asthma	18.2	9.5
Back problems	27.7	13.5
Cancer (malignant neoplasms)	2.6	1.6
Chronic obstructive pulmonary disease	5.2	1.8
Diabetes mellitus	6.7	4.4
Heart, stroke and vascular disease	7.1	4.2
Kidney disease	1.9	0.8
Osteoporosis	6.3	3.2

Source:[55]

uncomfortable or distressing. Additionally, some basic IPC measures may present sources of external risk to patient health and safety. For instance, the use of alcohol-based hand rubs (ABHR), especially in circumstances where care is provided to patients with a history of excessive alcohol consumption, carries the risk of intentional ingestion.[64] Other IPC practices, such as patient isolation, are often difficult, especially when a patient has acute psychiatric symptoms or behavioural dysregulation (e.g. mania and psychosis).[65]

Some mental illnesses predispose patients to increased antagonistic behaviour towards HCWs, substantially inhibiting their willingness to comply with infection control behaviours.[66] Aggression has been seen more frequently in individuals with substance abuse disorder, bipolar disorder, certain personality disorders and psychotic disorders such as schizophrenia.[67] Aggressive behaviours can also be exacerbated by distress, frustration and anger in the setting of uncertainty, negative interactions between patients and healthcare providers, and perceived figures of authority.

Physical and social environment: Many mental health services are delivered in communal living environments, which is inherently a risk factor for acquiring HAIs and infectious diseases. The closed environment of psychiatric units, their population densities, and the emphasis on recreational activities and group therapies increases the risk for transmission of infectious diseases and the potential for outbreaks within the facilities. Most long-term inpatient and residential facilities feature and encourage the use of communal spaces, such as dining rooms, activity rooms, lounge rooms, seclusion rooms, smoking areas, laundry, toilet and shower facilities. Furthermore, many of the safety features of these facilities may indirectly limit conventional IPC procedures, such as the lack of openable windows to support room ventilation. The close staff-patient contact also poses a significant dilemma for IPC. It is conventional practice for patients and clinical staff to have multiple interactions in a single day, during therapy sessions, examinations and rounding. Clinical staff's failure to adhere to IPC measures (e.g. social distancing or PPE guidelines) can facilitate the transmission of HAIs in mental health facilities.[65]

Self-harm: Self-harm is commonly linked with mental illnesses such as depression, anxiety, schizophrenia, substance abuse and eating disorders.[68] In 2019–20, there were almost 29,000 hospitalisations due to

self-harm in Australia.[69] Rates of self-harming behaviours were the highest among young people aged 15–19, and it is a strong predictor of long-term mental illness and suicide.[70] Approximately 12% of all self-harm hospitalisations were caused by contact with sharp objects, with the extent of the injury varying in severity—ranging from small wounds to much larger injuries.[71] Most self-harm patients are initially treated in EDs, where it is imperative for clinical staff to treat the wounds and establish a positive relationship with the patient.[72] However, the risk of continued intentional self-harming behaviours for these patients during and after admission must be considered, which could also call for adjustments in wound care protocols for mental health patients. Furthermore, the type of personal protective equipment (PPE) used in mental health facilities must also be carefully considered.[73] Certain types of equipment may have the capacity to be repurposed for self-harm and need to be independently vetted prior to use.

31.2.2 Specific HAIs attributed to mental health and psychiatric care

People with mental health illness are recognised as vulnerable patients. Based on their risk profile and predisposing factors, they are at an increased risk for specific types of infectious diseases, whether in the hospital or in the community. As an inpatient, they could be affected by certain HAIs and outbreaks of infectious diseases within mental health services.

Pneumonia and respiratory tract infections: Respiratory tract infections (RTIs), including bacterial and viral pneumonias, typically account for most outbreaks in psychiatric settings. There is compelling evidence for this worldwide, with reports of outbreaks of RTIs—including those caused by influenza, adenovirus and SARS-CoV-2—in psychiatric facilities and services.[74-76] Like other infectious diseases, RTIs can exacerbate the mental health conditions of psychiatric patients, especially in those affected by psychosis, depression, anxiety, insomnia and suicidal ideation.[77]

Multiple factors contribute to predispose psychiatric patients to RTIs. As discussed in previous sections, people with mental illness are more likely to experience adverse health outcomes, largely due to suboptimal self-care, unhealthy lifestyle, and social and environmental circumstances such as loneliness, homelessness, and poor housing. In inpatient settings, context-specific social and environmental characteristics pose additional risks for transmission of RTIs via patient-to-patient and patient-to-provider contact, largely because psychiatric patients are more ambulatory compared to other patients.[78]

High-risk health behaviours are common in people with mental health conditions.[79] Alcohol consumption, smoking and substance abuse, which are frequently seen in patients with mental health issues, are known risk factors for RTI. Additionally, the effect of psychiatric conditions on behavioural and cognitive functions can compromise patients' ability to recognise the symptoms of RTI, to seek care in a timely manner, and to efficiently adhere to medical advice and recommendations. Mental health patients are often found to be less compliant to infection control measures, mainly due to cognitive deficits, behavioural dysregulation and poor insight. Atypical presentation of symptoms (including chest pain and headache) and varied perception of pain are reported in people with severe mental disorders, which can further undermine effective help-seeking. This can lead to delayed recognition of an RTI, resulting in life-threatening infection. A linkage study in the UK showed that people admitted to hospital for severe mental health disorders had an increased risk for lobar pneumonia, pneumococcal pneumonia and pneumococcal septicaemia, which is more in association with their psychiatric disorder than with their hospitalisation.[80]

Continuous and long-term pharmacological therapy is a common mode of treatment in psychiatric patients. Some of these agents have side effects that may undermine respiratory and immune system functioning. Atypical antipsychotics are known to increase the risk of pneumonia due to the anticholinergic action (causing dry mouth and impaired oropharyngeal bolus transport) and blockade of histamine-1 receptor (excessive sedation and decreased swallowing reflex). Patients who take dopamine receptor blocker medications (e.g. haloperidol, fluphenazine or pimozide) are at an increased risk of aspiration pneumonia due to dysphagia resulted from the extrapyramidal effect of these medications.[81,82]

Gastrointestinal infections: Patients in mental health facilities have a significantly higher vulnerability to gastrointestinal (GI) infections and have increased opportunity for transmission of infectious agents. Outbreaks of gastroenteritis in psychiatric services have been reported from around the world,[83,84] and

are acknowledged to be the second most common type of outbreak in mental health facilities.[74] Infections have been reported to be caused by bacteria (e.g. *Salmonella* species, *Shigella sonnei*, *Vibrio cholera* and *Clostridium perfringens*), viruses (norovirus, group A rotavirus, sapovirus) and parasites (*Entamoeba histolytica* and *Trichuris trichiura*).[83,85,86]

The communal nature of mental health care and the patient's underlying psychiatric problem hinder the control of outbreaks in psychiatric facilities. Poor food-handling and suboptimal infection control or cleaning practices, especially in shared facilities, can result in outbreaks of gastroenteritis due to food poisoning.[87] Poor hygiene practice, including hand hygiene, is a challenge that is difficult to overcome. Frequent group therapies and integrative social contact between patients can prolong the outbreak duration in psychiatric settings.[83] As such, controlling and managing the outbreaks of GI infections may require more stringent infection control interventions and reinforced precaution measures.

Like outbreaks of other infectious disease, outbreaks of GI infections interfere with the ordinary functions of mental health services, and place a great burden on clinicians, staff and executives. An outbreak of gastroenteritis in the Psychiatry Department at the Royal Hobart Hospital in 2011 led to the shutdown of the Department of Psychological Medicine and Psychiatric Intensive Care Unit, paused all patient admissions, and limited visitor numbers.[88]

Skin infections: Studies report that comorbidity rates for skin diseases and mental health disorders are as high as 71.5% in primary psychiatric patients.[89-91] Infectious skin diseases are the most common skin dermatological problems among psychiatric patients, with parasitic dermatoses (i.e. scabies and *Pediculosis capitis*) and fungal infections (pityriasis versicolor and tinea) being the more dominant types of infections reported in the literature (Table 31.5).[89,92]

Patients with severe mental illnesses (e.g. schizophrenia and depression) are often impaired in their capability to perform daily personal hygiene. Furthermore, studies suggest that some psychiatric disorders are associated with decreased immune system functioning, leading to increased susceptibility to infectious skin diseases.[91] Chronic psychological stressors are known to be associated with suppression of natural killer cell cytotoxicity and decreased lymphocyte proliferation which can precipitate the risk of skin infections.[94]

TABLE 31.5 Skin diseases among patients with psychiatric disorders

Infectious skin diseases	Non-infectious skin diseases
Parasitic • Pediculosis capitis • Scabies **Fungal** • Pityriasis versicolor • Tinea pedis • Tinea corporis • Tinea circinata • Candidal intertrigo • Onychomycosis **Bacterial** • Acne vulgaris • Pyogenic infections (boils) **Viral** • Verruca vulgaris • Herpes simplex labialis	**Psychogenic** • Delusion of parasitosis/infestation[93] • Trichotillomania • Neurotic excoriation **Non-psychogenic** • Eczema • Pruritus • Psoriasis • Post-inflammatory hyperpigmentation • Freckles • Skin tags • Xerosis • Melasma • Acne

Psychiatric patients are not only susceptible to infectious skin diseases, but also to colonisation with multidrug-resistant organisms (MROs).[95] Reports of methicillin-resistant *Staphylococcus aureus* (MRSA) in psychiatric wards highlights the importance of accounting for predisposing factors, such as illicit drug use and alcoholism, in hospitalised psychiatric patients. Special consideration should be given to the impact of long-term admissions on spread of potentially hazardous clones and outbreaks of infectious skin diseases in inpatient and residential psychiatric settings.[96]

Another practical aspect of skin health in mental health settings is in relation to wound care. In acute psychiatric situations where a patient is suffering from self-induced injury and suicide, special consideration should be given to wound care and management. Likewise, if a patient has undergone surgery, the diminished mental and physical capabilities of patients should be considered to minimise the risk of surgical site infections (SSI).

Blood-borne viruses: Certain mental health conditions may precipitate an individual's engagement in behaviours that put them at an increased for risk of blood-borne viruses (BBVs). Evidence suggests that unprotected sex (e.g. multiple partners, sex work or sex trading), and intravenous drug are seen more frequently in association with severe mental illness such as acute psychosis and mania.[97] Intoxication due to substance misuse can lead to engagement in high-risk sexual behaviours. Additionally, sharing personal equipment (e.g. toothbrushes or razors) among patients who live in shared accommodations increases the risk of transmission of BBVs, such as hepatitis B (HBV) and hepatitis C (HCV).

Australian data, although limited, show that the prevalence of BBVs is increasing among psychiatric patients, and is higher when compared with those reported in the general population.[98] A recent study of patients at a mental health service in eastern Sydney suggests the seroprevalence of HCV is 7.2%, which is up to five times higher compared to the general Australian population.[99] The reported prevalence rates were more than twice what was reported in Australian inpatient psychiatry settings about a decade ago.[100] Data from Western Australia show that viral hepatitis is the second most common cause of hospitalisation across all infectious diseases among the recipients of mental health services. HCV, in particular, increased the hospitalisation of mental health patients by five times more than expected.[101]

Mental healthcare providers must be vigilant about the risks of BBVs and take necessary precautions when working with people with mental health illness, especially those known to harbour a high risk for BBV congregation (e.g. IV drug users). Routine discussion about the risks for blood-borne viruses with people who have serious mental illness, and offering testing and treatment for those at high risk, should be an essential component of IPC practices in these settings.

Sexually transmitted infections: Sexual health is an important contributor to health outcomes in patients with severe mental health illness, such as schizophrenia, schizoaffective disorder, bipolar affective disorder (BPAD) and major depressive disorder (MDD). The rates of sexually transmitted infections (STIs) are higher among mental health patients than those in the general Australian population.[102] Infections, such as gonorrhoea, syphilis, trichomoniasis, chlamydia, human papillomavirus (HPV) and herpes simplex virus type 2 (HSV-2), can cause significant health impacts in mental health patients. These infections may result in infertility, genital and cervical cancer, epididymitis and urethral damage can lead to additional health service consumption and substantial financial costs. The psycho-emotional stress associated with these medical conditions can cause additional morbidity and further compound psychiatric problems.

Mental health patients may exhibit a high predisposition for risky sexual behaviours such as having multiple sexual partners, inconsistent use of protections, and transactional sexual acts. The behaviour frequently presents in tandem with substance misuse, which can lower inhibition and compromise decision-making skills before, during or after sexual intercourse. It is estimated that between 30–50% of people with serious mental illness have substance misuse disorders, a substantial proportion of whom are sexually active and have intimate relationships, and are therefore at higher risk of contracting STIs.[103,104] Increasing awareness about the sexual health of mental health patients is a stepping stone in providing access to assessment, screening and education for STIs in psychiatric patients.

PRACTICE TIP 1

MENTAL HEALTH PATIENTS: A HIGH-RISK POPULATION

Mental health patients should be considered a high-risk group for infectious diseases and HAIs. IPC programs and policies should factor in the unique characteristics of psychiatric patients and fit the specific needs of the mental health services.

31.3 IPC in mental health settings in Australia

Australian psychiatric services play a fundamental role in the treatment, care and rehabilitation of mental health patients while ensuring a physically and psychologically safe environment. Despite implementing a multitude of safety measures, these services are still vulnerable to the emergence and spread of infectious diseases, including HAIs.

The National Safety and Quality Health Service Standards (NSQHS) – Preventing and Controlling Infections Standard describes the systems and key strategies to prevent, manage and control infections (see Chapter 6). The four criteria outlined under the Standard set consistent benchmarks for all Australian healthcare services—including psychiatric services—to implement preventive IPC measures to reduce the risk of patients and HCWs acquiring infections and to ensure good health outcomes are achieved for patients (Table 31.6). The strategies proposed in the NSQHS Standard, together with NSMHS and the Australian Guidelines for the Prevention and Control of Infections in Healthcare (2019), were used to tailor IPC

TABLE 31.6 Australian Commission on Safety and Quality in Health Care standards for IPC

Criteria of the NSQHS Preventing and Controlling Infections Standard	Domains of strategies
1. Clinical governance and quality improvement systems are in place to prevent and control infections, and support antimicrobial stewardship and sustainable use of IPC resources	• Integrating clinical governance • Applying quality improvement systems • Partnering with consumers • Surveillance
2. IPC systems	• Standard and TBP • Hand hygiene • Aseptic technique • Invasive medical devices • Clean and safe environment • Workforce screening and immunisation • Infections in the workforce
3. Reprocessing of reusable equipment and devices	• Healthcare organisations' processes for reprocessing reusable equipment and devices
4. Antimicrobial stewardship	• Healthcare organisations' antimicrobial stewardship programs

policies, strategies and procedures to Australian mental health and psychiatric services.

31.3.1 Clinical governance and quality improvement systems

Australian mental health services must ensure they have governance systems in place to promote and support IPC strategies. The COVID-19 pandemic further highlighted the crucial importance of having a clear governance structure that enables the effective implementation, execution and monitoring of IPC practices and outbreak management strategies. Due to the heterogeneity of mental health services, the means by which HAIs and their associated risks are identified and managed vary widely. For example, acute inpatient care services generally have both structures for reporting processes and an established connection with the hospital's IPC committee (e.g. a mental health representative in the IPC committee).

In some healthcare facilities, new roles have been developed to promote and facilitate the implementation and monitoring of IPC practices, policies and guidelines in mental health services. An example is the introduction of infection control link nurses (ICLNs), which is a portfolio responsibility delegated to a registered or enrolled nurse to assist with IPC management at a local mental health unit or site.[105] Mental health ICLNs assist with the promotion of IPC policies and procedures within a given mental health facility, undertake a range of IPC auditing activities, and act as a liaison between the IPC committee and the department or unit. They also promote IPC education and up-skilling of mental health professionals, and play a supporting role in the risk assessment and management of HAIs and outbreaks. ICLNs are considered by some Australian health jurisdictions to be a key component in governance arrangements for IPC systems.

Provision of mental health care is multifaceted and at times quite complex. Establishing professional partnerships with a wide range of care and support services contributes to generating the best outcomes for patients. Psychiatric services collaborate with a range of services that include, but are not limited to, staff health, pharmacy, pathology services, capital works, Aboriginal and Torres Strait Islander support services, consumer liaison services and cleaning services. Effective partnership with these services can foster sustainable and efficient use of IPC resources.

31.3.2 IPC systems

Standard and transmission-based precautions: Like other health services in Australia, mental health services will apply standard precautions and transmission-based precautions (TBP) in accordance with current IPC guidelines and jurisdictional legislation and policies. However, our knowledge of the compliance of the mental health workforce in the appropriate use of precautions is limited, partly due to the heterogeneity of mental health services, and variations in processes to audit compliance and assess competence in the appropriate use of standard and TBP.

Hand hygiene: Hand hygiene remains an important IPC strategy in psychiatric settings, particularly where communal facility designs are in place and IPC measures, such as isolation, may be detrimental to patient wellbeing.[106] While patients are encouraged to perform regular hand hygiene, some patient-related factors such as lack of cooperation and motivation—resulting from cognitive limitations or severe mental illness—may prevent consistent or correct compliance with this behaviour. As a result, there is a great onus on healthcare staff and volunteers to ensure hand hygiene protocols (i.e. My 5 Moments for Hand Hygiene) are met prior to and after interacting with patients.[107] Psychiatric facilities are responsible for ensuring the routine delivery of hand hygiene education and resources to staff, as well as audits to assess understanding and compliance.[108]

Alcohol-based hand rubs are recommended for hand hygiene in standard healthcare practices.[107] However, there are specific risks associated with their use in mental health settings, particularly in regard to patient safety, which necessarily restrict access to dispensers or require additional staff supervision.[109] The wall-mounted hand sanitisers may carry risk for certain groups of patients, such as those with substance dependence disorders or those who present with self-harming behaviours. The Australian Commission on Safety and Quality in Health Care (ACSQHC) recommends specific engineering controls to minimise the risk of ABHR ingestion and deliberate or unintentional misuse.[110] These controls include the explicit and careful design of hand dispensers—such as lockable dispenser holders, metered dose bottles, labels that de-emphasise alcohol content or warn against consumption, and additives to make the product unpalatable. Furthermore, the use of personal pocket ABHRs by staff in place of mounted dispensers is highly encouraged.[111-113]

PRACTICE TIP 2

A CHALLENGE IN HAND HYGIENE PRACTICE

ABHRs containing more than 60% alcohol must be used carefully in psychiatric facilities. They should not be placed in patients' rooms or in locations where the patients are unsupervised. Alternative solutions include the provision of pocket-sized ABHRs for staff and encouraging frequent hand-washing with soap and water.

Aseptic technique and wound care: The practice of good aseptic technique, particularly during the administration of procedures like IV-line insertion and wound care, is especially critical in the context of psychiatric patients. Prior to undertaking any procedures that require aseptic technique a thorough assessment of the patient and their context must be performed. Patient characteristics that should be taken into account include their immune status (i.e. whether they are immunocompromised), age, medication, nutritional status and presence of an acute or chronic skin condition.[114] The patient's compliance is equally crucial for maintaining asepsis. Where possible, anticipated procedures should be reviewed and described to patients before administration to facilitate collaboration during treatment and good infection control and recovery post-treatment.[115]

Collaboration with mental health patients on wound care presents some unique challenges. Patients in psychiatric wards have an increased risk of skin injuries, such as pressure ulcers, diabetic ulcers, vascular ulcers, partial thickness burns, skin damage, wounds caused by self-injury and abscesses related to intravenous drug use.[116,117] Existing wounds may also be poorly managed and have prolonged recovery times as a result of low motivation, deliberate self-harm, medication side effects and non-adherence to wound care recommendations.[118] Regardless, quality wound management and optimal asepsis in mental health patients require a holistic approach which should incorporate the entirety of the patient's physical and mental health characteristics.[115]

Safe injections and use of sharps: Intramuscular (IM) and intravenous (IV) injections remain common alternative routes of administration of medications to mental health patients, especially for medications like sedatives, antiemetics, hormonal agents and analgesics.[119] Both IV and IM injections must be done carefully to avoid infection, patient pain and additional complications.[120] Best practices for safe injections remain applicable in mental health settings, both in preventing infections in the recipient of the injection and in needlestick injuries to the healthcare provider. These include:

- single use equipment
- single dose vials
- a safe and sterile work environment
- the appropriate preparation and disinfection of equipment and patient's skin
- appropriate hand hygiene and PPE prior to administration; and
- safe collection and disposal of used needles.[107,121]

Involuntary treatment and non-compliance are common challenges faced in mental health settings, leading to agitated or aggressive patients who may physically resisting the treatment. These situations harbour the risk of improper injections that may cause injury and infection to both the patient and HCWs. If non-compliance or aggression is anticipated, HCWs are required to implement measures such as the use of a retractable needle or restraining strategies to prevent patient movement. Furthermore, all psychiatric care facilities must ensure the establishment of appropriate policies for the management of injuries and incidents where HCWs or patients are exposed to blood or other body substances.

Personal protective equipment: Using PPE is challenging in psychiatric settings, partly because therapy sessions are commonly delivered in the form of group settings and in communal spaces.[122] Prior to the COVID-19 pandemic, poor adherence to PPE guidelines and TBP was observed in mental HCWs within inpatient and residential psychiatric facilities. While organisational factors (such as a lack of access, training and management) contributed to low compliance with PPE guidelines, factors relating to the patient–carer relationship also interplayed. PPE can have an unpredictable adverse effect on interactions with mental health patients, with some workers noting that PPE frightens patients, inhibits rapport building or interferes with thorough mental state examinations.[122,123]

PPE forms the last line of defence against outbreaks and infectious diseases. However, it should always be readily available for staff to don prior to entering high-risk areas for infectious diseases.[107] In addition to the routine training of mental health staff in appropriate PPE donning, additional advice may also be required in the use of gestures, body language, expression through the eyes and eyebrows, and vocal intonation and prosody to facilitate important elements of communication that PPE may otherwise obscure.[124] Other strategies include the use of face shields or social distancing in lieu of masking during introductory sessions.[125]

Environmental hygiene and cleaning: Given the communal nature of most psychiatric inpatient facilities, the routine disinfection of the environment (including the frequently touched surfaces) is paramount to infection control and outbreak management.[111,126,127] Some of the supportive therapies and modules administered to address the special needs of mental health patients use specific tools and equipment which are subject to stringent cleaning and disinfection measures. For instance, shared or communal sensory tools that are used to reduce the need for seclusion and restraint in mental health services should be regularly cleaned by neutral detergents, or detergent-impregnated cleaning cloths after each use. Staff should follow the manufacturer's instructions on cleaning of items, and must be trained to ensure cleaning equipment is not left unattended.[128]

Published research indicates that contaminated surfaces are heavily implicated in the high frequency of outbreaks in inpatient and residential psychiatric settings.[129,130] The risk of infection via contamination may be further compounded in certain psychiatric populations that generally maintain a low standard of self-care, have repetitive and compulsive behaviours, and display non-adherence to hygiene protocols. The methods and frequency of cleaning for different surfaces are independently determined by each facility' based on the risk assessment informed by the patients' characteristics and the facility's infrastructures and resources.

PRACTICE TIP 3
HOW TO MAKE IT SAFER FOR EVERYONE

Patients with the following medical conditions should be prohibited from using shared or communal sensory equipment:

- Vomiting or diarrhoea
- Skin conditions such as abscesses, boils, open wounds, scabies or lice infestations
- Unexplained, acute onset of fever or fever with accompanying cough
- Current infections (viral, bacterial, parasitic or fungal)

Staff vaccination and occupational exposures:
Immunisation against common vaccine-preventable diseases provides the first-line defence against the introduction of infectious diseases and outbreaks in mental health services. A substantial number of infectious diseases that can affect mental health patients and HCWs have viable and widely available vaccines. Most healthcare facilities require staff to go through a pre-employment assessment of their immunisation status based on the risks of exposure. The aim of immunisation is twofold: to minimise

the risk of infection in HCWs, and to ensure patient biosafety, especially in those who are immunocompromised or have an otherwise weakened immune system. Occupational exposures in mental health settings can occur through interaction with patients in the group settings, or through needlestick injuries, and are more common with aggressive patients (e.g. scratching and biting, which carry the risk of the transmission of BBVs).

31.3.3 Reprocessing of reusable equipment and devices

Reprocessing of critical and semi-critical medical devices and equipment encompasses a number of processes and procedures in relation to cleaning, disinfection, sterilisation and storage.[131]

A major challenge in meeting IPC standards for the reprocessing of reusable equipment and devices lies with the heterogeneity of mental health services. In the inpatient setting, reprocessing practices are largely regulated in accordance with the facility's universal standards and protocols. Nonetheless, in community-based and ambulatory settings, the processes to reuse and reprocess single use medical devices may vary remarkably. The adherence of these services to the standard national benchmarks remains essentially unknown, and as such there is a potential risk of HAI and outbreaks of infectious diseases in relation to medical equipment and devices.

31.3.4 Antimicrobial stewardship

The National Antimicrobial Prescribing Survey (NAPS) was first introduced in 2013 as a standardised auditing tool to assist all Australian healthcare facilities to assess the patterns and characteristics of antimicrobial prescribing. Our understanding of psychiatric services' compliance with guidelines and the appropriateness of prescribing antimicrobial agents is quite limited, given the limited data available from these facilities—out of 248 participating hospitals and healthcare facilities in NAPS 2014, there was only one psychiatric hospital which presented only 11 prescriptions.[132]

An Australian study of residential aged care facilities where specialised mental health care has been provided suggests a high rate of antimicrobial prescribing and inappropriate antibiotic use. While their findings cannot be generalised to other mental health services in Australia, it highlights the importance of implementing antimicrobial stewardship programs in psychiatric settings.[133]

PRACTICE TIP 4

REDUCING THE RISK OF HAI IN MENTAL HEALTH SERVICES

Risk of HAIs in mental health services can be largely controlled by effective social distancing, adherence to PPE guidelines and compliance with infection prevention policies.

31.3.5 Challenges of IPC practices in psychiatric settings

As discussed previously, psychiatric services experience unique challenges in the prevention and control of infectious disease, mainly due to the limitations of the clinical setting and the unique characteristics of psychiatric services and its patients. The implementation of IPC measures in psychiatric institutions is gravely influenced by factors at the patient, professional, healthcare context and organisational level (Fig 31.4).

Residential and inpatient psychiatric services have inherent risk factors that generate specific challenges both for patients and for mental healthcare providers with regard to the emergence and spread of infections, including HAIs. The communal living environments, inpatient population, patient turnover, and patient–patient or staff–patient contacts can undermine the effectiveness and efficiency of IPC measures, such as social distancing, PPE usage, hand hygiene and self-isolation.

The specific characteristics of mental health patients can pose a challenge in implementing IPC measures in

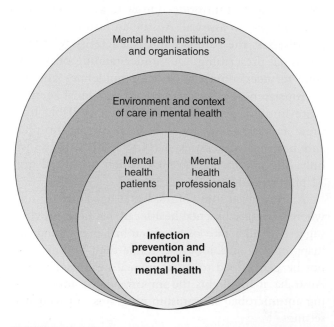

FIGURE 31.4 Factors influencing infection prevention and control in mental health settings

psychiatric settings. Impaired cognitive function, high-risk health behaviours and non-compliance interfere with effective infection prevention and hinder the implementation of preventive measures that are set at local, jurisdictional and national levels. Regular practices for hand hygiene and PPE use may be associated with safety risks for patients and could interfere with routine mental health care.

Practising in mental health often carries a diagnostic dilemma, where clinicians must distinguish whether a patient's symptoms are part of their psychiatric condition or a manifestation of a medical condition or infection. Constitutional symptoms, such as fever, weight loss, fatigue, body pain or altered consciousness, in those suffering from substance use could easily be interpreted as clinical signs of intoxication, which can delay investigations for, or diagnosis of, a masquerading or contemporaneous life-threatening infection. Impaired judgement and insight into severe mental health illnesses could further complicate patient–staff communications, and therefore undermine the timely identification and management of infectious diseases. Fear of stigma and perceived discrimination, especially among patients in rural areas, can further perplex timely help-seeking and effective communication with mental healthcare providers.[21,134] Furthermore, comorbid physical and mental conditions are commonly diagnosed and attended to separately, and the identification of one condition may overshadow the other. Psychiatrists often consider that their primary task is to exclusively treat psychiatric illnesses, thereby may possibly overlook signs of physical disease.[54] Furthermore, an understanding of effective IPC procedures and the importance of IPC is often lower among mental health professionals compared to other healthcare professionals.

Factors that hamper IPC practices may also be related to mental health institutions and professional organisations. At the time of writing, there is a growing awareness at the national level of the importance of IPC practices in the mental health setting. However, a large degree of variability is present at the institutional level. In addition, active and ongoing support of IPC programs by directors of healthcare facilities and mental health services is crucial for successful outcome of IPC practices. Lack of organisational attention, and assigning less priority to IPC, could translate into an inadequacy of IPC resources. Varying and sporadic IPC education and training opportunities in mental health settings mainly focus on disseminating the content of current guidelines, but do not necessarily address specific IPC needs and considerations in mental healthcare. Healthcare organisations have the key leadership role in establishing the clinical governance structures for IPC, and as such need to proactively engage resources to conduct quality improvement activities (e.g. audits) and surveillance to support and improve IPC systems in mental health settings.[65,131]

Conclusion

The last century has seen a drastic shift in how and where mental health services are provided and accessed by Australians. The process of deinstitutionalisation and mainstreaming saw a substantial decline in dedicated psychiatric facilities and mental institutions, and the subsequent emergence of a diverse variety of mental health services being offered in the community, within general public and private hospital settings, and in a range of inpatient and outpatient facilities. The heterogeneity of modern mental health settings necessitates equally diverse and adaptable considerations for IPC. This is further exacerbated by the inherent challenges presented by mental health patients, who are likely to be more susceptible to poor health and infectious complications, and more resistant or non-compliant towards infection control practices. This chapter presented an overview of these unique challenges and of the common HAIs and their associated risks in mental health settings. It also described the current IPC practices and considerations for Australian psychiatric and mental health services.

Useful websites/resources

- Australian Bureau of Statistics. National Study of Mental Health and Wellbeing. https://www.abs.gov.au/statistics/health/mental-health/national-study-mental-health-and-wellbeing/latest-release

- HealthDirect. Australian mental health services. https://www.healthdirect.gov.au/australian-mental-health-services

- Australian Commission on Safety and Quality in Care. NSQHS Standards User guide for health services providing care for people with mental health issues. https://www.safetyandquality.gov.au/publications-and-resources/resource-library/nsqhs-standards-user-guide-health-services-providing-care-people-mental-health-issues

- Australian Institute of Health and Welfare. National Mental Health Performance Framework 2020. https://meteor.aihw.gov.au/content/721188

References

1. Parkinson JP. The Castle Hill lunatic asylum (1811–1826) and the origins of eclectic pragmatism in Australian psychiatry. Aust N Z J Psychiatry. 1981;15(4):319-322.
2. Cummins CJ. A history of medical administration in NSW 1788–1973. 2nd ed: NSW Department of Health, North Sydney, 2003.
3. Lewis MJ. Managing madness: psychiatry and society in Australia, 1788–1980. Canberra: AGPS Press, 1988.
4. Dunk J. Authority and the treatment of the insane at Castle Hill Asylum, 1811–25. Health and History 2017;19(2):17-40.
5. Coleborne C, Mackinnon D. Psychiatry and its institutions in Australia and New Zealand: an overview. Int Rev Psychiatry. 2006;18(4):371-380.
6. Ban TA. Pharmacotherapy of mental illness-a historical analysis. Prog Neuro-Psychopharmacol Biol Psychiatry. 2001;25(4): 709-727.
7. Dunlop R, Pols H. Deinstitutionalisation and mental health activism in Australia: emerging voices of individuals with lived experience of severe mental distress, 1975–1985. History Australia. 2022;19(1):92-114.
8. Rosen A. The Australian experience of deinstitutionalization: interaction of Australian culture with the development and reform of its mental health services. Acta Psychiatrica Scandinavica. 2006;113(s429):81-89.
9. Rosen A. Australia's national mental health strategy in historical perspective: beyond the frontier. Int Psychiatry. 2006;3(4):19-21.
10. Rosen A. The Australian experience of deinstitutionalization: interaction of Australian culture with the development and reform of its mental health services. Acta Psychiatrica Scandinavica. 2006;113:81-89.
11. Australian Institute of Health and Welfare. Mental health services in Australia. Canberra: AIHW, 2022.
12. Australian Institute of Health and Welfare. Overnight admitted mental health-related care. Canberra: AIHW, 2022.
13. Australian Institute of Health and Welfare. Residential mental health care services. Canberra: AIHW, 2022.
14. Independent Hospital Pricing Authority. Subacute and non-acute care. Available from: https://www.ihpa.gov.au/what-we-do/subacute-and-non-acute-care.
15. Australian Government Department of Health. Specialist Dementia Care Program (SDCP). Canberra: Commonwealth of Australia, 2020.
16. Australian Institute of Health and Welfare. Alcohol and other drug treatment services in Australia: early insights. Canberra: AIHW, 2022.
17. Ellis A. Forensic psychiatry and mental health in Australia: an overview. CNS Spectrums. 2020;25(2):119-121.
18. Mullen PE, Briggs S, Dalton T, Burt M. Forensic mental health services in Australia. Int J Law Psychiatry. 2000; 23(5-6):433-452.
19. Australian Institute of Health and Welfare. Medicare-subsidised mental health-specific services. Canberra: AIHW, 2022.
20. Hickie IB, Davenport TA, Pirkis JE, Blashki GA, Groom GL. General practitioners' response to depression and anxiety in the Australian community: a preliminary analysis. MJA. 2004;181(S7): S15-S20.
21. Aisbett D, Boyd C, Francis K, Newnham K. Understanding barriers to mental health service utilization for adolescents in rural Australia: James Cook University. Rural Remote Health. 2007;7(1):624.

22. Pirkis J, Harris M, Hall W, Ftanou M. Evaluation of the better access to psychiatrists, psychologists and general practitioners through the Medicare benefits schedule initiative. Melbourne, VA: Centre For Health Policy, Programs and Economics, 2011.

23. Australian Government National Mental Health Commission. The Fifth National Mental Health and Suicide Prevention Plan. Canberra: Commonwealth of Australia, 2017.

24. Parliament of Australia. Chapter 9 - Mental health services in the community. Canberra: Parliament of Australia.

25. Australian Institute of Health and Welfare. Emergency department mental health services. Canberra: AIHW, 2022.

26. Weiland TJ, Mackinlay C, Hill N, Gerdtz MF, Jelinek GA. Optimal management of mental health patients in Australian emergency departments: barriers and solutions. Emerg Med Australas. 2011;23(6):677-688.

27. Duggan M, Harris B, Chislett W-K, Calder R. Nowhere else to go: why Australia's health system results in people with mental illness getting 'stuck' in emergency departments. Melbourne: Mitchell Institute, Victoria University, 2020. Available from: https://vuir.vu.edu.au/41956/.

28. Frank R, Fawcett L, Emmerson B. Development of Australia's first psychiatric emergency centre. Australasian Psychiatry. 2005;13(3):266-272.

29. Seymour J, Chapman T, Starcevic V, Viswasam K, Brakoulias V. Changing characteristics of a psychiatric emergency care centre. An eight year follow-up study. Australas Psychiatry. 2018;28(3):307-310.

30. Brakoulias V, Seymour J, Lee J, Sammut P, Starcevic V. Predictors of the length of stay in a psychiatric emergency care centre. Australas Psychiatry. 2013;21(6):563-566.

31. Huber JP, Wilhelm K, Landstra JM. Months of May: mental health presentations and the impact of a psychiatric emergency care centre on an inner-city emergency department. Emerg Med Australas. 2021;33(4):691-696.

32. Leiknes KA, Schweder LJv, Høie B. Contemporary use and practice of electroconvulsive therapy worldwide. Brain and Behavior. 2012;2(3):283-344.

33. Espinoza RT, Kellner CH. Electroconvulsive therapy. New Eng J Med. 2022;386(7):667-672.

34. Read J, Bentall R. The effectiveness of electroconvulsive therapy: a literature review. Epidemiol Psychiatr Soc. 2010; 19(4):333-347.

35. Tharyan P, Adams CE. Electroconvulsive therapy for schizophrenia. Cochrane Database Syst Rev. 2005;(2).

36. Goodman JH. Perinatal depression and infant mental health. Arch Psychiatr Nurs. 2019;33(3):217-224.

37. Myors KA, Schmied V, Johnson M, Cleary M. 'My special time': Australian women's experiences of accessing a specialist perinatal and infant mental health service. Health Soc Care Community. 2014;22(3):268-277.

38. Australian Institute of Health and Welfare. Mental health non-government organisation establishments NBEDS 2015-2014. Canberra: AIHW, 2014. Available from: https://meteor.aihw.gov.au/content/494729.

39. Australian Institute of Health and Welfare. National Mental Health Performance Framework 2020. Canberra: AIHW, 2014. Available from: https://meteor.aihw.gov.au/content/721188.

40. Curtis S, Gesler W, Wood V, et al. Compassionate containment? Balancing technical safety and therapy in the design of psychiatric wards. Soc Sci & Med. 2013;97:201-209.

41. Loewenstein K, Saito E, Linder H. Lessons learned from a mental health hospital: managing COVID-19. JONA. 2020; 50(11):598-604.

42. Higgins R, Hurst K, Wistow G. Nursing acute psychiatric patients: a quantitative and qualitative study. J Adv Nurs. 1999;29(1):52-63.

43. Geurtzen N, Keijsers GP, Karremans JC, Hutschemaekers GJ. Patients' care dependency in mental health care: development of a self-report questionnaire and preliminary correlates. J Clin Psychol. 2018;74(7):1189-1206.

44. Cleary M, Hunt GE, Walter G. Seclusion and its context in acute inpatient psychiatric care. J Med Ethics. 2010;36(8): 459-462.

45. Australian Institute of Health and Welfare. Restrictive practices in mental health care. Canberra: AIHW, 2022.

46. Allan JA, Hanson GD, Schroder NL, O'Mahony AJ, Foster RMP, Sara GE. Six years of national mental health seclusion data: the Australian experience. Australas Psychiatry. 2017; 25(3):277-281.

47. Büchler AC, Sommerstein R, Dangel M, Tschudin-Sutter S, Vogel M, Widmer AF. Impact of an infection control service in a university psychiatric hospital: significantly lowering healthcare-associated infections during 18 years of surveillance. J Hosp Infect. 2020;106(2):343-7.

48. Australian Government. National Standards for Mental Health Services, 2010. Canberra; Australian Government, 2010.

49. Breeze JA, Repper J. Struggling for control: the care experiences of 'difficult' patients in mental health services. J Adv Nurs.1998;28(6):1301-1311.

50. Australian Institute of Health and Welfare. Physical health of people with mental illness. Canberra: AIHW, 2020.

51. Australian Institute of Health and Welfare. Comorbidity of mental disorders and physical conditions, 2007. Canberra: AIHW, 2012.

52. De Hert M, Correll CU, Bobes J, et al. Physical illness in patients with severe mental disorders. I. Prevalence, impact of medications and disparities in health care. World Psychiatry. 2011;10(1):52.

53. Kavoor AR, Chakravarthy K, John T. Remote consultations in the era of COVID-19 pandemic: preliminary experience in a regional Australian public acute mental health care setting. Asian J Psychiatry. 2020;51:102074.

54. Cooper S-A, McLean G, Guthrie B, et al. Multiple physical and mental health comorbidity in adults with intellectual disabilities: population-based cross-sectional analysis. BMC Family Practice. 2015;16(1):110.

55. Australian Bureau of Statistics. National health survey: first results (2017-2018). Canberra: ABS, 2018.

56. Australian Institute of Health and Welfare. National drug strategy household survey 2019. Canberra: AIHW, 2019.

57. Phillips KT, Stein MD. Risk practices associated with bacterial infections among injection drug users in Denver, Colorado. Am J Drug Alcohol Abuse. 2010;36(2):92-97.

58. Mehta SH, Astemborski J, Kirk GD, et al. Changes in blood-borne infection risk among injection drug users. J Infect Dis. 2011;203(5):587-594.

59. Vlahov D, Fuller CM, Ompad DC, Galea S, Des Jarlais DC. Updating the infection risk reduction hierarchy: preventing transition into injection. J Urban Health. 2004;81(1):14-19.

60. Stewart V, Judd C, Wheeler AJ. Practitioners' experiences of deteriorating personal hygiene standards in people living with depression in Australia: a qualitative study. Health & Social Care in the Community, 2021.

61. Mills W, Sender S, Lichtefeld J, et al. Supporting individuals with intellectual and developmental disability during the first 100 days of the COVID-19 outbreak in the USA. J Intellect Disabil Res. 2020;64(7):489-496.

62. Courtenay K, Perera B. COVID-19 and people with intellectual disability: impacts of a pandemic. Irish J Psychol Med. 2020;37(3):231-236.

63. Buonaguro EF, Bertelli MO. COVID-19 and intellectual disability/autism spectrum disorder with high and very high

support needs: issues of physical and mental vulnerability. Advances in Mental Health and Intellectual Disabilities. 2020.

64. Stevens DL, Hix M. Intentional ingestion of hand sanitizer in an adult psychiatric unit. Mental Health Clinician. 2020; 10(2):60-63.

65. Li P-H, Wang S-Y, Tan J-Y, Lee L-H, Yang C-I. Infection preventionists' challenges in psychiatric clinical settings. Am J Infect Control. 2019;47(2):123-127.

66. Pompili E, Carlone C, Silvestrini C, Nicolò G. Focus on aggressive behaviour in mental illness. Rivista di Psichiatria. 2017;52(5):175-179.

67. Pulay AJ, Dawson DA, Hasin DS, et al. Violent behavior and DSM-IV psychiatric disorders: results from the national epidemiologic survey on alcohol and related conditions. J Clin Psychiatry. 2008;69(1):22223.

68. Singhal A, Ross J, Seminog O, Hawton K, Goldacre MJ. Risk of self-harm and suicide in people with specific psychiatric and physical disorders: comparisons between disorders using English national record linkage. J Royal Soc Med. 2014;107(5):194-204.

69. Australian Institute of Health and Welfare. Suicide and self-harm monitoring. Canberra: AIHW, 2022.

70. Beckman K, Mittendorfer-Rutz E, Lichtenstein P, et al. Mental illness and suicide after self-harm among young adults: long-term follow-up of self-harm patients, admitted to hospital care, in a national cohort. Psychol Med. 2016; 46(16):3397-3405.

71. Rogers B, Pease F, Ricketts D. The surgical management of patients who deliberately self-harm. Ann R Coll Surg Engl. 2009;91(1):59-62.

72. Rayner G, Blackburn J, Edward Kl, Stephenson J, Ousey K. Emergency department nurse's attitudes towards patients who self-harm: a meta-analysis. Int J Mental Health Nurs. 2019;28(1):40-53.

73. Katato HK, Gautam M, Akinyemi EO. The danger of face masks on an inpatient psychiatric unit: new protocol to prevent self-harm. The Primary Care Companion for CNS Disorders. 2021;23(5):36551.

74. Fukuta Y, Muder RR. Infections in psychiatric facilities, with an emphasis on outbreaks. Infect Control Hosp Epidemiol. 2013;34(1): 80-88.

75. Strihavkova M, Havlícková M, Tůmová B. An epidemic of type B influenza in the geriatric psychiatry department of a psychiatric hospital. Casopis Lekaru Ceskych. 1990;129(36): 1129-1132.

76. Klinger JR, Sanchez MP, Curtin LA, Durkin M, Matyas B. Multiple cases of life-threatening adenovirus pneumonia in a mental health care center. Am J Respir Crit Care Med. 1998;157(2):645-649.

77. Gobbi S, Płomecka MB, Ashraf Z, et al. Worsening of preexisting psychiatric conditions during the COVID-19 pandemic. Front Psychiatry. 2020;11.

78. Xiang Y-T, Zhao Y-J, Liu Z-H, et al. The COVID-19 outbreak and psychiatric hospitals in China: managing challenges through mental health service reform. Int J Biol Sciences. 2020;16(10):1741.

79. Goff DC, Cather C, Evins AE, et al. Medical morbidity and mortality in schizophrenia: guidelines for psychiatrists. J Clin Psychiatry. 2005;66(2):183-194.

80. Seminog OO, Goldacre MJ. Risk of pneumonia and pneumococcal disease in people with severe mental illness: English record linkage studies. Thorax. 2013;68(2): 171-176.

81. Haga T, Ito K, Sakashita K, Iguchi M, Ono M, Tatsumi K. Risk factors for pneumonia in patients with schizophrenia. Neuropsychopharmacology Reports. 2018;38(4):204-209.

82. Knol W, Van Marum RJ, Jansen PAF, Souverein PC, Schobben AFAM, Egberts ACG. Antipsychotic drug use and risk of pneumonia in elderly people. J Am Geriatr Soc. 2008; 56(4):661-666.

83. Tseng CY, Chen CH, Su SC, et al. Characteristics of norovirus gastroenteritis outbreaks in a psychiatric centre. Epidemiol Infect. 2011;139(2):275-285.

84. Weber DJ, Sickbert-Bennett EE, Vinjé J, et al. Lessons learned from a norovirus outbreak in a locked pediatric inpatient psychiatric unit. Infect Control Hosp Epidemiol. 2005;26(10):841-843.

85. Moffatt CR, Howard PJ, Burns T. A mild outbreak of gastroenteritis in long-term care facility residents due to Clostridium perfringens, Australia 2009. Foodborne Pathog Dis. 2011;8(7):791-796.

86. Galloway A, Roberts C, Hunt E. An outbreak of Salmonella typhimurium gastroenteritis in a psychiatric hospital. J Hosp Infect. 1987;10(3):248-254.

87. Sharp JCM, Collier PW, Gilbert RJ. Food poisoning in hospitals in Scotland. J Hyg (Lond). 1979;83(2):231-236.

88. ABC News. Gastro outbreak hits RHH. 2011. Available from: https://www.abc.net.au/news/2011-05-14/gastro-outbreak-hits-rhh/2715694.

89. Moftah NH, Kamel AM, Attia HM, El-Baz MZ, Abd El-Moty HM. Skin diseases in patients with primary psychiatric conditions: a hospital based study. J Epidemiol Glob Health. 2013;3(3):131-138.

90. Mookhoek E, Van De Kerkhof P, Hovens J, Brouwers J, Loonen A. Skin disorders in chronic psychiatric illness. J Europ Acad Dermatol Venereol. 2010;24(10):1151-1156.

91. Magin P, Sibbritt D, Bailey K. The relationship between psychiatric illnesses and skin disease: a longitudinal analysis of young Australian women. Arch Dermatol. 2009;145(8): 896-902.

92. Manish P, Bijaya K, Dipa R. Skin diseases in patients with primary psychiatric conditions admitted in psychiatry ward. J Psychiatr Assoc Nepal. 2017;6(1):48-53.

93. Tran MMA, Iredell JR, Packham DR, O'Sullivan MVN, Hudson BJ. Delusional infestation: an Australian multicentre study of 23 consecutive cases. Internal Med J. 2015;45(4): 454-456.

94. Segerstrom SC, Miller GE. Psychological stress and the human immune system: a meta-analytic study of 30 years of inquiry. Psychol Bull. 2004;130(4):601-630.

95. Hughes F, Smoyak SA. Antimicrobial resistance (AMR): why psychiatric/mental health nurses need to have AMR in their alphabet. J Psychosoc Nurs Ment Health Serv. 2016;54(7):13-14.

96. Ebner W, Schlachetzki J, Schneider C, Dettenkofer M, Langosch JM. Hand hygiene seems to be sufficient for prevention of MRSA transmission on a closed psychiatric ward. J Hosp Infect. 2010;75(4):334-335.

97. Hughes E, Bassi S, Gilbody S, Bland M, Martin F. Prevalence of HIV, hepatitis B, and hepatitis C in people with severe mental illness: a systematic review and meta-analysis. Lancet Psychiatry. 2016;3(1):40-48.

98. Ellen S, Devlin H, Aizenstros J. HIV, hepatitis B and C virus screening among psychiatry inpatients. Aust NZ J Psychiatry. 2003;37(Suppl):A21.

99. Williams J, Barclay M, Omana C, Buten S, Post JJ. Universal blood-borne virus screening in patients with severe mental illness managed in an outpatient clozapine clinic: uptake and prevalence. Australas Psychiatry. 2020;28(2):186-189.

100. Gunewardene R, Lampe L, Ilchef R. Prevalence of hepatitis C in two inpatient psychiatry populations.

Australasian Psychiatry: Bulletin of Royal Australian and New Zealand College of Psychiatrists. 2010;18(4):330-334.

101. Lawrence D, Jablensky A. Preventable physical illness in people with mental illness. 2001.

102. Stevens M, Ratheesh A, Watson A, Filia K, Donoghue BO, Cotton SM. Rates, types and associations of sexual risk behaviours and sexually transmitted infections in those with severe mental illness: a scoping review. Psychiatry Res. 2020;290:112946.

103. Hercus M, Lubman DI, Hellard M. Blood-borne viral and sexually transmissible infections among psychiatric populations: what are we doing about them? Aust NZ J Psychiatry. 2005;39(10): 849-855.

104. Meade CS, Sikkema KJ. HIV risk behavior among adults with severe mental illness: a systematic review. Clin Psychol Rev. 2005;25(4):433-457.

105. Australia GoW. Infection control link nurse role in governance arrangement for NSQHS Standard 3 Guideline (version 3.0). 2018. Available from: https://www.wacountry.health.wa.gov.au/~/media/WACHS/Documents/About-us/Policies/Infection-Control-Link-Nurse-Role-in-Governance-Arrangement-for-NSQHS-Standard-3-Guideline-Grt-Sth.pdf?thn=0.

106. Hsu S-T, Chou L-S, Chou FH-C, et al. Challenge and strategies of infection control in psychiatric hospitals during biological disasters—from SARS to COVID-19 in Taiwan. Asian J Psychiatr. 2020;54:102270.

107. National Health and Medical Research Council. Australian guidelines for the prevention and control of infection in healthcare. Canberra: NHMRC, 2019.

108. Ahmed K. Audit of hand hygiene at Broadmoor, a high secure psychiatric hospital. J Hosp Infect. 2010;75(2): 128-131.

109. Jorge V, Curet K, Aly R, Gupta S, Gupta S, Hares H. Safety of alcohol-based hand sanitizers in behavioral health facilities. Am J Med Qual. 2021;36(5).

110. Australian Commission on Safety and Quality in Health Care. National safety and quality health service standards: user guide for health services providing care for people with mental health issues. Sydney: ACSQHC, 2018.

111. Cheng V, Wu A, Cheung C, et al. Outbreak of human metapneumovirus infection in psychiatric inpatients: implications for directly observed use of alcohol hand rub in prevention of nosocomial outbreaks. J Hosp Infect. 2007;67(4):336-343.

112. Gilbride SJ, Lee BE, Taylor GD, Forgie SE. Successful containment of a norovirus outreak in an acute adult psychiatric area. Infect Control Hosp Epidemiol. 2009; 30(3):289-291.

113. Bonine CJ. Strategies for promoting hand hygiene compliance on inpatient psychiatric units. J Psychosoc Nurs Ment Health Serv. 2021;59(5):21-24.

114. Pegram A, Bloomfield J. Wound care: principles of aseptic technique: service users may have injuries related to intravenous drug use or self-harm, so nurses need the appropriate skills to provide physical care. Anne Pegram and Jacqueline Bloomfield outline the principles of aseptic procedures. Mental Health Practice. (London). 2010;14(2): 14-18.

115. Samuriwo R, Hannigan B. Wounds in mental health care: the archetype of a 'wicked problem of many hands' that needs to be addressed? Int J Ment Health. 2020;49(1): 81-96.

116. Pegram A, Bloomfield J. Wound care: principles of aseptic technique: service users may have injuries related to intravenous drug use or self-harm, so nurses need the appropriate skills to provide physical care. Anne Pegram and Jacqueline Bloomfield outline the principles of aseptic procedures. Mental Health Practice. 2010;14(2):14-19.

117. Kaba E, Triantafyllou A, Fasoi G, Kelesi M, Stavropoulou A. Investigating nurses' views on care of mentally ill patients with skin injuries. International J Environmental Research and Public Health 2020;17(20): 7610.

118. Hemingway S, Cook L, Stephenson J. Assessing and managing wounds in mental health settings. Wounds UK. 2014;9:34-40.

119. Wynaden D, Landsborough I, McGowan S, Baigmohamad Z, Finn M, Pennebaker D. Best practice guidelines for the administration of intramuscular injections in the mental health setting. Int J Ment Health Nurs. 2006;15(3): 195-200.

120. Ogston-Tuck S. Intramuscular injection technique: an evidence-based approach. Nursing Standard. 2014;29(4).

121. Hutin Y, Hauri A, Chiarello L, et al. Best infection control practices for intradermal, subcutaneous, and intramuscular needle injections. Bull World Health Organ. 2003;81: 491-500.

122. Bojdani E, Rajagopalan A, Chen A, et al. COVID-19 pandemic: impact on psychiatric care in the United States. Psychiatry Res. 2020;289:113069.

123. Pal A, Gupta P, Parmar A, Sharma P. 'Masking' of the mental state: unintended consequences of personal protective equipment (PPE) on psychiatric clinical practice. Psychiatry Res. 2020;290:113178.

124. Mehta UM, Venkatasubramanian G, Chandra PS. The "mind" behind the "mask": assessing mental states and creating therapeutic alliance amidst COVID-19. Schizophrenia Res. 2020;222:503-504.

125. Pamungkasih W, Sutomo AH, Agusno M. Description of patient acceptance of use of mask by doctor at poly out-patient care Puskesmas, Bantul. Review of Primary Care Practice and Education (Kajian Praktik dan Pendidikan Layanan Primer). 2019;2(2):70-75.

126. Alanazi KH, Bin Saleh GM, Hathout HM, et al. Investigation of varicella outbreak among residents and healthcare workers in psychiatric hospital-Saudi Arabia. Arch Environ Occup Health. 2020;76(2):116-120.

127. Deloughery DM, Johns D, Kent D, et al. Challenges of managing a non-invasive gas outbreak on an inpatient psychiatric unit. Am J Infect Control. 2014;42(6): S155-S6.

128. NSW Health. Safe use of sensory equipment and sensory rooms in NSW mental health services. In: Office MHaDaA, editor. GL2015_001;2015.

129. Wu HM, Fornek M, Schwab KJ, et al. A norovirus outbreak at a long-term-care facility: the role of environmental surface contamination. Infect Control Hosp Epidemiol. 2005;26(10): 802-810.

130. Johnston CP, Qiu H, Ticehurst JR, et al. Outbreak management and implications of a nosocomial norovirus outbreak. Clin Infect Dis. 2007;45(5):534-540.

131. Bendall J-A, Woods S, Crossie K, Worthington T, Norring L, Rees G. How difficult is it to develop an audit tool for AS/NZS 4187:2014 Reprocessing of reusable medical devices in health service organizations? Infect Dis Health. 2017;22:S10.

132. Australian Commission on Safety and Quality in Health Care. Antimicrobial prescribing practice in Australian hospitals: results of the 2014 National Antimicrobial Prescribing Survey, 2015. Sydney: ACSQHC, 2015.

133. Stuart RL, Wilson J, Bellaard-Smith E, et al. Antibiotic use and misuse in residential aged care facilities. Internal Med J. 2012;42(10):1145-1149.

134. Griffiths KM, Nakane Y, Christensen H, Yoshioka K, Jorm AF, Nakane H. Stigma in response to mental disorders: a comparison of Australia and Japan. BMC Psychiatry. 2006;6(1):21.

CHAPTER 32

Infection prevention and control in medical, veterinary and scientific laboratory settings

Dr ROSELLE ROBOSA[i]

Dr DAVID H. MITCHELL[i]

Dr CECILIA LI[ii]

PROFESSOR SHARON C.A. CHEN[i]

Dr MATTHEW V.N. O'SULLIVAN[i]

Chapter highlights

- The principles of laboratory biocontainment
- Common laboratory-acquired infections (LAIs)
- Responses to exposure
- Preventative measures, including vaccination

i   Centre for Infectious Diseases and Microbiology Laboratory Services, New South Wales Health Pathology, Institute of Clinical Pathology and Medical Research, Westmead Hospital, Westmead, NSW

ii Infection Prevention and Control, University of Sydney, Sydney, NSW

Introduction

Clinical microbiology laboratories play a critical role in patient care, the detection and management of infectious diseases, and public health surveillance. Laboratory scientists can support ongoing infection prevention and control (IPC) programs, including healthcare-associated infection (HAI) surveillance programs, by providing accessible, timely and detailed laboratory findings to IPC units. As such, trained laboratory scientists with expert knowledge of IPC practices enable efficient and effective coordination with IPC units and experts, and also ensure the safety of laboratory staff by implementing safe laboratory practices that incorporate IPC measures. This chapter details the principles of laboratory biocontainment, common LAIs, responses to exposure, and preventative measures including vaccination.

32.1 Principles of laboratory biocontainment

The response to inadvertent exposures to microorganisms in the laboratory and preventative measures cannot be overemphasised. While measures need to be tailored to the specific exposure, every diagnostic laboratory must have a minimum set of safety and biocontainment strategies to minimise accidents and leaks of infectious pathogens into the environment. In diagnostic laboratories in particular, the nature of organisms received, and their potential for harm, cannot always be predicted. For this reason, all specimens should be handled and treated as potentially infectious. To this end, the joint Australian/New Zealand Standard on Safety in Laboratories[1] has set out the containment procedures for safe laboratory practice in microbiology laboratories. The pertinent concepts for minimising risks to laboratory and other staff are summarised below.

It is essential for all laboratory personnel to understand:

1. the type or level of containment measures; and
2. the differences in safety measures required for the different levels of containment.

Other professional bodies in the USA and United Kingdom, as well as the World Health Organization, outline biosafety precautions similar to those in the Australian/New Zealand Standard.[1-4]

32.2 Containment measure types

Containment of microorganisms involves a combination of:

1. physical structures and engineering functions that form the *skeleton* of a microbiology laboratory
2. equipment and safety structures or *vital components* within the facility; and
3. work practices that *circulate* to handle microorganisms safely.

Physical containment (PC) is the term used to describe the structures and their associated support that are designed to minimise the release of viable microorganisms into the environment. In Australia and New Zealand there are four PC levels—designated PC1 to PC4—assigned for working with organisms.[1]

Viable microorganisms and tissues inoculated with microorganisms from defined risk groups (RG2–RG4) should be used (Chapter 23), stored or housed in corresponding or higher-level containment facilities as appropriate. Typically, microbiological containment may be achieved using three categories of containment—primary, secondary and tertiary measures.[1-4] Optimal microbiological containment is provided by the box-within-a-box principle (Fig 32.1)[1] where the highest hazards are enclosed by multiple containment measures.

32.2.1 Primary containment measures

Primary containment measures refer to the physical constraints immediately surrounding the source of infectious material, for example a biological safety cabinet (BSC) or the leakproof container forming the inner receptacle of an International Air Transport Association (IATA) approved infectious materials transport container. These act as primary barriers to restrict the passage of microorganisms into the immediate environment.

32.2.2 Secondary containment measures

Secondary containment measures refer to the structural aspects and design of a laboratory-specific part of a laboratory, or a device that encloses the component or components of the primary containment. Essential components of secondary containment include the facility design *per se* but, critically, also the engineering build and operations providing air pressure control and directional airflow, and air exhaust supplemented by High Efficiency Particulate Air (HEPA) filtration where required. Smaller in scale but no less important

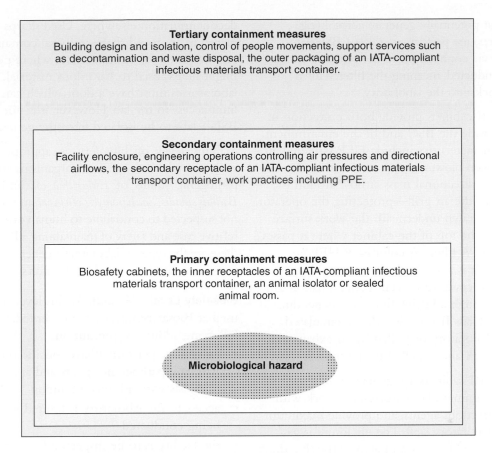

FIGURE 32.1 The three levels of physical containment measures
Source: Image courtesy of courtesy of Standards Australia and Standards New Zealand.

are other features, for example the secondary receptacle of an IATA-approved transport container. In all laboratories, secondary physical containment measures *must* be supplemented by defined work safety practices, including personal protective equipment (PPE).

32.2.3 Tertiary containment measures

Tertiary containment measures aim to protect the wider environment from coming into contact with infectious microorganisms by supporting the secondary containment, for example by:

- controlling the movement of personnel and mitigating against uncontrolled movement
- housing infectious material in a separate or even isolated building
- using the outer packaging of an IATA-approved transport container; and
- providing essential support services, such as decontamination and laundering of clothing, and infectious waste disposal.

32.2.4 Biological safety cabinets

The main objective of a biological safety cabinet (BSC) is to protect the laboratory worker and the surrounding environment from infectious microorganisms. To this end, all exhaust air is HEPA-filtered as it exits the BSC, filtering out bacteria and viruses. This is in contrast to a laminar flow clean bench, which blows unfiltered exhaust air towards the user and is not safe for work with pathogens. In addition, notably, a fume hood is unsuitable for use in protecting the environment. However, many classes of BSCs also have a secondary purpose, which is to maintain the sterility of materials inside the cabinet. There are three main classes of BSCs—I to III.

Class I: Class I cabinets provide personnel and environmental protection but no protection of material inside the BSC from infectious material. In fact, the inward flow of air can contribute to contamination of samples. As such, these BSCs are commonly used to enclose equipment (e.g. centrifuges) or where procedures that potentially generate aerosol (e.g. aerating cultures) are performed. Class I BSCs are either ducted, via connections to the building exhaust network, or unducted, meaning the filtered air is recirculated back into the laboratory.

Class II: Class II cabinets provide both protection of the contents inside the BSC and of the environment. Operational characteristics include HEPA-filtered air and motor-driven blowers (fans) mounted in the cabinet to draw directional mass airflow around the worker and into the air grill—protecting the operator. The air is then drawn underneath the work surface and back up to the top of the cabinet where it passes through the HEPA filters. A column of HEPA-filtered, sterile air is also blown downward over products and processes to prevent contamination. Air is exhausted through a HEPA filter and, depending on the type of Class II BSC, is either recirculated back into the laboratory or pulled by an exhaust fan through ductwork and expelled to the outside.

Class III: Class III cabinets are generally only used in maximum containment laboratories, for work with BSL-4 level infectious agents, and provide maximum protection to laboratory staff. The enclosure is gastight, and all materials enter and leave through a dunk tank or double-door autoclave. Gloves attached to the front prevent direct contact with hazardous materials. These cabinets are often custom-built, often attach into a line, and the equipment contained within them is also custom-selected or built.

32.2.5 Physical containment (PC) classifications

Biosafety Level 1 (BSL-1): Physical containment Biosafety Level 1 (PCBSL-1) facilities are suitable for work with well-characterised agents which do not cause disease in healthy humans. In general, these agents should pose *minimal hazard* to personnel and the environment. Laboratory personnel must wash their hands upon entering and exiting the lab. Research with these agents may be performed on standard open laboratory benches without the use of special containment equipment; however, precautions must be taken to minimise the generation of aerosols when working on an open bench. Eating and drinking are generally prohibited in laboratory areas. Potentially infectious material must be decontaminated before disposal, either by adding a chemical such as bleach or isopropanol, or by packaging for

decontamination elsewhere. Used sharps must be placed in approved sharps disposal containers. PPE is only required for circumstances where personnel might be exposed to hazardous material. BSL-1 laboratories must have a door which can be locked to limit access to the lab. However, it is not necessary for BSL-1 labs to be isolated from the general building.

This level of biosafety is appropriate for work with several kinds of microorganisms including nonpathogenic strains of *Escherichia coli* and *Staphylococcus*, *Bacillus subtilis*, *Saccharomyces cerevisiae* and other organisms not suspected to contribute to human disease. Due to the relative ease and safety of maintaining a BSL-1 laboratory, these are the types of laboratories generally used as teaching spaces for high schools and universities.

Biosafety Level 2 (BSL-2): At this level, all precautions used at Biosafety Level 1 are observed, with the following additional precautions:

- laboratory personnel have specific training in handling pathogenic agents and are directed by scientists with advanced training
- access to the laboratory is limited when work is being conducted
- the facility is to be inspected for containment compliance at least annually
- extreme precautions are taken with contaminated sharp items
- certain procedures in which infectious aerosols or splashes may be created are conducted in BSCs or other containment equipment; and
- contaminated, reusable glassware must be autoclaved or chemically disinfected prior to reuse.

BSL-2 is suitable for work involving agents that is of *moderate potential hazard* to personnel and the environment. This includes various microbes that cause mild disease in humans or that are described as being difficult to contract via aerosol in a laboratory setting. Examples include hepatitis A, B and C viruses, human immunodeficiency virus (HIV), pathogenic strains of *Escherichia coli* and Staphylococcus, Salmonella, *Plasmodium falciparum* and *Toxoplasma gondii*.

Biosafety Level 3 (BSL-3): A Biosafety Level 3 laboratory is intended for working with microbes which cause serious and potentially lethal disease through inhalation. This type of work encompasses that carried out in clinical and diagnostic laboratories as well as that in research or industrial production facilities. Here, the precautions undertaken in BSL-1 and BSL-2 labs are followed, in addition to the following:

- all laboratory personnel are provided medical surveillance and offered relevant immunisations as appropriate to reduce risk of an accidental or unnoticed infection
- all procedures involving infectious material must be done within a *biological safety cabinet*
- laboratory personnel must wear solid-front protective clothing (i.e. gowns that tie in the back). This cannot be worn outside of the laboratory and must be discarded or decontaminated after each use
- dedicated cleaning equipment is to be stored within the facility
- laboratory waste must be decontaminated, preferably by autoclaving, before disposal; and
- a laboratory-specific biosafety manual must be drafted which details how the laboratory will operate in compliance with all safety requirements.

The entrance to the laboratory must be separated from areas of the building with unrestricted traffic. The laboratory must be behind two sets of self-closing doors (to reduce the risk of aerosols escaping). The construction of the laboratory must be such that cleaning is easy. Carpets are not permitted, and any seams in the floors, walls and ceilings are sealed to allow for easy cleaning and decontamination. Windows must be sealed, and a ventilation system installed which forces air to flow from the 'clean' areas of the lab to the areas where infectious agents are handled. Air from the laboratory must be HEPA filtered before it can be recirculated.

Biosafety Level 3 is commonly used for research and diagnostic work involving microbes which can be transmitted by aerosols and/or cause severe disease. Typical examples are *Francisella tularensis*, *Mycobacterium tuberculosis*, *Chlamydia psittaci*, SARS coronavirus, SARS-Cov-2, MERS coronavirus, *Coxiella burnetii*, *Rickettsia rickettsii*, Brucella, Yersinia pestis, and other viruses such as chikungunya, West Nile virus and Japanese encephalitis virus.

Biosafety Level 4 (BSL-4): Biosafety Level 4 is the highest level of biosafety precautions and is required for work with microorganisms that could easily be aerosol-transmitted within the laboratory and cause severe to fatal disease in humans for which there are no available vaccines or treatments. BSL-4 laboratories are generally set up to be either cabinet laboratories or protective-suit laboratories. In cabinet laboratories, all work must be done within a Class III BSC. It follows that materials leaving the cabinet must be decontaminated either by passing through an autoclave or through a tank of disinfectant. The cabinets must have seamless edges to allow for easy cleaning. Additionally, the cabinet and all materials within must be free of sharp edges in order to reduce the risk of glove damage. In a protective-suit laboratory, all work must be done in a Class II BSC by personnel wearing a positive-pressure suit. In order to exit the BSL-4 laboratory, personnel must pass through a chemical shower for decontamination, then a room for removing the positive-pressure suit, followed by a personal shower. Entry into the BSL-4 laboratory is restricted to trained and authorised individuals only and a log of all persons entering and exiting the laboratory is essential.

BSL-4 laboratories must be separated from areas that receive unrestricted traffic. In addition, airflow must be tightly controlled to ensure that air always flows from 'clean' areas of the lab to areas where work with infectious agents is being performed. Airlocks at the entrance to the BSL-4 lab are installed to minimise potential leak of aerosols to outside the laboratory. Prior to leaving the facility all waste, including filtered air, water and trash, must be decontaminated.

In essence, these laboratories are reserved for diagnostic and other work on easily transmitted pathogens which can cause fatal disease. These include a number of viruses known to cause viral haemorrhagic fever such as Marburg and Ebola viruses, and some flaviviruses. Additionally, poorly characterised pathogens which appear closely related to dangerous pathogens are often handled at this level until sufficient data are obtained either to confirm continued work at this level, or to permit working with them at a lower level. This level is also used for work with variola virus, the causative agent of smallpox, currently only performed at the Centers for Disease Control, USA, and the State Research Centre of Virology and Biotechnology in Koltsovo, Russia.

32.3 Common laboratory-acquired infections

Laboratory-acquired infections (LAIs) are occupationally acquired infections of laboratory personnel. Fortunately, modern laboratory practices and laboratory safety make LAIs an uncommon occurrence. However, accidental infection of laboratory staff can occur even with strict biosafety procedures and measures implemented.

Multiple pathogens have been documented to cause LAIs and a wider range have the potential to cause infection. The earliest published LAI was a Brucella infection documented in 1897.[5] Pathogens of particular concern include those in the BSL-3 and BSL-4 categories due to their high pathogenicity and their potential for community transmission. Several LAI cases have been associated with secondary and even tertiary infection or transmission. Data regarding known incidence of LAIs have primarily been collected through surveys and literature reviews of published studies. Australia does not have a national LAI surveillance program. Most extensive surveys have been done in the UK and the United States.

Surveys of LAIs suggest that most common causes of infections are Brucella spp., *Mycobacterium tuberculosis*, arboviruses and Salmonella spp.[6] In the United States, the Laboratory-Acquired Infection Database documents published incidents of LAIs. Extensive studies of LAI occurrence and cause were conducted in the United States by Pike and Sulkin between 1935 and 1978, with a total of 4079 LAIs reported.[7] They concluded that the majority of LAIs were caused by bacteria, with a smaller number of viral and fungal infections. It is interesting to note that the 10 most common LAIs are caused by organisms in biological Risk Group 3 (RG-3), although this may reflect an under-recognition of RG-2 LAIs, as these infections often result in only mild disease, and may be less readily distinguished from community-acquired infection.

More recent surveys show an emergence of *Mycobacterium tuberculosis* and arboviruses as common causes of LAI.[8] Byers and Harding conducted an updated comprehensive literature search of LAIs between 1930–1979 and 1979–2015 and recorded totals of 2168 and 1753 cases respectively. Their most recent survey showed bacteria, in particular Brucella spp., as being the most commonly described LAI, with a lower number of viral infections (Table 32.1).[6] Laboratory Incidence Notification Canada (LINC) surveillance systems monitor laboratory incidents, including exposure incidence to human pathogens, and suspected or confirmed laboratory infections in Canada. In 2018, there was a total of 89 exposure incidents with 235 people exposed, with a subsequent 5 suspected and 1 confirmed laboratory incident.[9] A recent review of the LAIs in the Asia–Pacific region between 1982 and 2016 found the most common pathogens associated with LAIs were dengue virus, the

TABLE 32.1 The 10 most frequently reported laboratory-acquired infections worldwide (1930–1979 versus 1979–2015)

Rank	1930–1979		1979–2015	
	Agent	# LAI	Agent	#LAI
1	Brucella spp.	426	Brucella spp.	378
2	Coxiella burnetti	280	M. tuberculosis	255
3	Hepatitis B	268	Arboviruses	222
4	Salmonella enterica Typhi	225	Salmonella spp.	212
5	Francisella tularensis	225	Coxiella burnettii	205
6	M. tuberculosis	194	Hantavirus	189
7	Blastomyces dermatitidis	162	Hepatitis B virus	113
8	VEE		Shigella spp.	88
9	Chlamydia psittacosis	116	HIV	48
10	Coccicioides immitis	93	N. meningitidis	14

Source: Adapted from Byers K. Laboratory-acquired infections 1979–2013 [https://absaconference.org/pdf56/II930Byers.pdf].

dermatophyte Arthroderma spp., Brucella spp., Mycobacterium spp. and Shigella spp.[10]

The majority of reported LAIs were from high-income countries (HIC) such as the United States, Australia and Japan where laboratories are more likely to comply with international biosafety standards.[10]

32.4 Bacterial LAIs

Bacterial infections comprise the majority of LAIs and are the largest cause of fatal LAIs. This includes 13 fatalities to *N. meningitidis*, 4 aborted foetuses due to *Brucella melitensis*, 3 due to Salmonella spp., 1 due to *Yersinia pestis* and 1 due to attenuated *Yersinia pestis*.

32.4.1 Brucella spp.

Brucella spp. are the predominant cause of reported LAIs, making up to 2% of all human cases of brucellosis.[11] This high risk is attributed to a combination of factors, including genus-specific biological features which makes it easily communicable. Brucella organisms are highly infectious, requiring only a low number of viable organisms to establish an infection (10–100 cells). Furthermore, it is readily aerosolised and can invade the host through various routes that are relevant to standard laboratory work, including the respiratory mucosa, conjunctiva, gastrointestinal tract and impaired skin barrier. However, aerosolised Brucella organisms are the most common route of exposure.[12]

Brucella is uncommon in Australia and often presents with non-specific symptoms which may not lead clinicians to suspect a Brucella infection. Despite laboratory safety measures and post-exposure recommendations, cases of laboratory-acquired brucellosis continue to occur worldwide. In the United States, an average of 120 cases of brucellosis are reported annually. In Australia, a case of laboratory exposure resulted in the follow-up of 44 exposed workers, with 7 high-risk cases receiving prophylaxis. No clinical symptoms or seroconversion to suggest subacute infection developed in any exposure patient. There has been only one published report of laboratory-acquired Brucella in Australia, which occurred in Townsville, Queensland.[13]

A literature review of 167 workers in case reports of laboratory exposure to Brucella spp. found 43% of workers (n = 71) developed laboratory-acquired brucellosis (LAB). The most common activity leading to exposure was manipulation of an organism outside of a BSC, which comprised up to 91% of exposure cases. All LAB cases had either a positive serology or culture with 96% being seropositive and 66% being culture positive. Symptomatic LAB cases developed typical non-specific symptoms including fever, arthralgia, sweats, headache and myalgia. Severe presentations include soft-tissue abscesses, spondylitis or sacroiliitis and neurologic brucellosis. Additionally, 20% (n = 7) of recorded female workers were pregnant at time of exposure with 6 developing LAB. Four of these LAB cases aborted, including 2 spontaneous abortions following onset of fever, malaise and vaginal bleeding. One patient underwent therapeutic termination following a diagnosis of disseminated intravascular coagulation. The fourth patient underwent therapeutic abortion following onset of night sweats after exposure; the reason given was the potential risk to the fetus, although the placental tissue culture was negative.

Management of possible laboratory-associated
Brucella exposure: Brucella is the most often reported laboratory-acquired bacterial infection in clinical microbiology laboratories. The following management principles could be modified to apply to laboratory exposures due to other Risk Group 3 organisms that

have low infectious doses and may be aerosolised during laboratory processing (e.g. *Francisella tularensis*, *Histoplasma capsulatum*, *Coccidioides immitis*).

The ease of international travel means that Brucella species are an expected occasional isolate in clinical microbiology laboratories, even in non-endemic areas. While clinicians would be expected to inform the laboratory that brucellosis was clinically expected when sending specimens this may not always happen. Standard blood culture bottles support the growth of Brucella spp. which usually signal in automated blood culture instruments after 3–4 days of incubation (i.e. well within standard incubation protocols). The systemic manifestations of brucellosis mean that it is an occasional isolate in tissue and fluid specimens as well as blood cultures.

Most Brucella exposure incidents occur when:
* staff work on a Brucella isolate on an open bench
* staff are working in close proximity (<1.5 metres) when a Brucella culture is processed on an open bench even if they have no direct involvement with manipulating the culture; or
* staff are present in the laboratory when a Brucella aerosol-generating incident occurs.

As a general principle, unidentified isolates, especially from blood culture or tissue/fluid specimens, should be processed in such a way that staff exposure to splashes or aerosols is minimised (e.g. performing work in a BSC, wearing of appropriate PPE, using sealed centrifuge cups) until sufficient work-up of the isolate has occurred to confidently exclude a possible Class 3 pathogen.

Assessing laboratory exposure risk level: When a potential exposure incident involving Brucella is recognised, the staff who were present in the laboratory during the at-risk period should be identified (this may include visitors like students or equipment service personnel) and interviewed to determine where they were in relation to the exposure and what they did with specimens/isolates (Table 32.2). This should be done in private and in a professional and non-judgmental manner, preferably by senior medical microbiology laboratory staff.

The key information that needs to be determined during staff interviews includes:
* where they were in the laboratory when relevant specimens/culture were processed
* whether work was performed on clinical specimens (blood, CSF, fluids, tissues) and/or on enriched material, e.g. isolate culture, positive blood culture

TABLE 32.2 Level of infection risk based on degree of exposure to the pathogen

	Description	Action
Minimal risk	• Staff who manipulated specimens/cultures in a BSC, using appropriate PPE and without the occurrence of aerosol-generating events • Other staff present in lab while specimens/cultures were processed as above	• Staff are monitored for the development of fever or other symptoms
Low risk	• Staff who were present in the laboratory when cultures were manipulated on the open bench, but not within 1.5 m of the workbench and if no aerosol-generating events occurred	• Staff are monitored for development of symptoms • Staff have baseline Brucella serology taken • Post-exposure prophylaxis could be offered to pregnant or immunosuppressed staff
High risk	• Staff who manipulated specimens or cultures on an open bench or were within 1.5 m when cultures were manipulated on an open bench • Staff who were present in the laboratory when an aerosol-generating event involving specimens or cultures occurred	• Staff are monitored for symptoms • Baseline and monitoring serology every 6 weeks for 4 months following exposure • Post-exposure prophylaxis recommended

- whether work was performed in a biosafety cabinet or on an open bench
- whether appropriate PPE (gown, gloves, eye protection) was worn
- whether any aerosol-generating events occurred, e.g. centrifuging in unsealed carriers, vortexing, sonicating of specimens/cultures
- whether any accidents occurred during processing, e.g. spillages, splashes, sharps injuries; and
- for low- or high-risk exposures, whether a staff member has underlying health conditions (e.g. immunosuppression, pregnancy) that may increase the risk of complications of infection or influence the choice of post-exposure prophylactic antibiotics (if required).

Following investigations as above, staff can be designated to risk categories and appropriate follow-up monitoring and need for post-exposure prophylaxis determined.

Post-exposure prophylaxis for Brucella: Doxycycline 100mg twice daily + Rifampicin 600mg once daily for 3 weeks.

Co-trimoxazole or ciprofloxacin are alternative agents in patients who cannot take doxycycline.

32.4.2 Burkholderia pseudomallei

Burkholderia pseudomallei is the causative agent of melioidosis, which is endemic in northern Australia and southeast Asia. In 1992, a laboratory in Northern Queensland reported three laboratory workers who tested positive for subclinical melioidosis, despite no record of unsafe laboratory practices. BSL-2 practices are recommended to prevent acquired infections.[14] Principles similar to those used for follow up Brucella exposures in the laboratory should be employed in the event of exposure to *Burkholderia pseudomallei*.[15]

32.4.3 Bacillus anthracis

Bacillus anthracis is of particular concern due to its potential as a bioterrorism agent. A large outbreak of anthrax cases from a military facility in Sverdlovsk, Russia, on 2 April 1979 due to an aerosol leak secondary to neglecting to replace an exhaust filter, resulted in 64 deaths from pulmonary anthrax.[16] In 2002, a US laboratory worker was diagnosed with cutaneous anthrax a day after cutting himself over the right jaw and then handling vials of *B. anthracis* without gloves.[17]

32.4.4 Francisella tularensis

Francisella tularensis is a fastidious Gram-negative coccobacillus and the causative organism of tularaemia. In 2002, 12 microbiology laboratory employees were exposed to *F. tularensis* and the majority received prophylaxis. No subsequent LAIs occurred.[18]

32.4.5 Mycobacterium tuberculosis

Early inspections of the prevalence of laboratory-acquired tuberculosis found that the incidence of tuberculosis in laboratory workers was 3–9 times greater than the general population. However, without a specific accident or incident to which the infection can be traced, it is difficult to state with certainty that tuberculosis was laboratory acquired.[19]

Important risk factors for acquiring tuberculosis are procedures and manipulations which generate aerosols and the bacteria's high infectivity, with relatively low numbers of bacilli required for infection. Acquisition is typically by aerosol spread; however, percutaneous inoculation is also well documented. Use of biosafety cabinets while processing samples, particularly in aerosol-generating procedures (AGPs), is imperative. In laboratories which process >5000 cultures/year or manipulate known MDR stains, PC2 and additional practices such as controlled access, self-closing double door access and negative-pressure airflow is recommended as per the Australian National Tuberculosis Advisory Committee.[20]

32.4.6 Rickettsia typhi and Orientia tsutsugamushi

Twenty-five cases of Scrub typhus caused by *Orientia tsutsugamushi* were documented from 1931–2000 with 8 deaths during the pre-antibiotic era. During the same period there were 35 cases of murine typhus caused by *Rickettsia typhi* without any deaths.[21] They were associated with high-risk activities including working with infectious laboratory animals involving significant aerosol exposures, accidental self-inoculation or bite-related infections.

32.4.7 Neisseria meningitidis

A review of 16 cases of laboratory-acquired meningococcal disease in the US between 1985–2001 was examined by Sejvar et al.[22] The majority of cases (56%) were due to serogroup B and the remainder were due to serogroup C with a 50% fatality rate. Route exposure was most commonly via aerosols, and in 15 of 16 cases procedures performed on the isolates occurred on a laboratory benchtop outside of a biosafety cabinet without protection from droplets. They calculated an attack rate of 13 cases per 100,000 microbiologists compared to 0.3 per 100,000 among the general population.

32.4.8 Enteric bacteria

With respect to enteric bacteria, Salmonella is the most commonly reported pathogen and typhoid is the most frequently reported cause of fatal LAIs. A large survey done by Blaser et al. reported 32 cases of laboratory-acquired typhoid between 1977 to 1980.[13] Concerningly, some infected individuals proceeded to infect their family members, which resulted in one fatality.[13] In Australia, there has been one recorded case of laboratory-acquired typhoid, in Queensland in a worker who was culturing positive stool.[23] ATCC 14028, a commercially available strain of *S. enterica* serovar

Typhimurium, which is widely employed in clinical laboratories including quality control of Salmonella antisera and culture media has been implicated in laboratory-acquired cases in Canada and the multistate cluster of LAIs in the United States.[24,25]

Furthermore, increasing numbers of *Shigella* species causing LAI have also become evident, due to their high virulence and high infectivity rate.

32.5 Viral LAIs

Laboratory-acquired viral infections are rarer than bacterial infections but are an emerging concern due to the growing volume of virological research. A systematic review of articles published between 1930–2008 reviewed the incidence of accidental viral infection in workers or students in research or hospital laboratories and analysed 35 articles relating to 219 laboratory infections.[26]

32.5.1 Hepatitis B

Of the blood-associated viruses, hepatitis B is the most common cause of laboratory-acquired infection. The incidence of hepatitis B infection in healthcare workers in the United States has been surveyed to be 3.5–4.6 infections per 1000 workers, which is 2–4 times that of the general population in 1984.[27]

32.5.2 HIV

Laboratory-acquired HIV infection from exposure to contaminated blood and body fluids is one of the greatest concerns among healthcare and laboratory workers. A prospective study on occupation exposure which enrolled 1534 healthcare workers—and comprised 17% laboratory workers—calculated an infection rate of 0.3%.[28] Surveillance data on this risk of occupationally acquired HIV in the US between 1981–1992 showed that 32 healthcare workers acquired HIV during this period including 25% recorded laboratory workers.[29] The majority of these infections occurred through the percutaneous route with a smaller number via aerosol exposure.

32.5.3 Arboviruses

Arboviruses are a source of considerable fear and fascination to the public and media; however, they only account for a small number of laboratory infections. Of the LAIs, most occurred in research laboratories rather than clinical laboratories.

Pedrosa et al. analysed 16 LAIs caused by alphaviruses including 2 cases of Western equine encephalitis virus, 12 of Venezuelan equine encephalitis virus

(VEEV), 1 case of chikungunya and 1 case of Mayaro virus; and 15 infections by flaviviruses including 4 cases of louping ill virus, 4 of tick-borne encephalitis virus, 3 of Kyasanur Forest disease virus, 3 of West Nile virus and 1 case of St Louis encephalitis virus.[26]

Many of these cases were before the 1980s, including those caused by VEEV that resulted in two laboratory-acquired case clusters in 1943 and 1947, with 8 and 4 cases, respectively. Both incidents were thought to have occurred from inhalation of aerosolised particles. A case of laboratory-acquired chikungunya virus—from a suspension of chikungunya-infected mouse brain—was reported in 1965 in a researcher who was working with infectious mosquitoes through a nylon membrane. Between 2004 and 2014 there were 3 case reports of laboratory staff acquiring dengue LAIs via needlestick injuries, and in one case, from a bite from a laboratory-infected mosquito that escaped during the day during a procedure involving the primary infection of colony mosquitoes with DENV-type-2 in an Australian laboratory.[30] Infection with laboratory-acquired Zika virus has also been reported in a case study of a PhD student who was bitten by a Zika-infected mouse at an animal research lab.[31]

32.5.4 Viral haemorrhagic fever

One of the largest incidents of significant viral laboratory-acquired infection occurred in 1967. In this incident, 31 workers were infected with Marburg virus, a virus which had not previously been encountered, while manipulating tissue specimens from African green monkeys, resulting in 7 deaths. The agent was named Marburg virus after the town where the majority of cases occurred.

32.5.5 Hanta virus

In Japan, in 1985, there were a recorded 126 human cases of laboratory-acquired haemorrhagic fever with renal syndrome (HFRS) related to Hanta virus in primarily laboratory research workers. Acquisition was thought to be due to inhalation of Hantavirus-contaminated air in an animal facility which housed contaminated rats.[32]

32.5.6 Vaccinia virus

Vaccinia virus is the live viral component of smallpox vaccine. There is a report of a laboratory-acquired infection in a 20-year-old man working in a laboratory with VACV and who developed ocular vaccinia.[33] In 2009, one case was reported in Australia in a laboratory worker

who sustained a needlestick injury while inoculating mice with a live attenuated strain of vaccina (Western Reserve) in a research lab.[34]

32.5.7 SARS-CoV

The first case of laboratory-acquired SARS-CoV occurred in 2003 after the initial global outbreak ended. This happened in a 27-year-old microbiology graduate student working with West Nile virus in a BSL-3 laboratory that had been heavily involved in SARS-CoV work. It is interesting to note that the student was not directly involved in handling SARS-CoV.[31] Although the precise mechanism of contamination remains unknown it is thought that SARS-CoV had contaminated the VeroE6 cell culture, as high levels of SARS-CoV were found in the sample of West Nile virus culture. There were a further two reports of laboratory-acquired SARS-CoV-2 both of which occurred in 2004, one in a laboratory researcher in Taiwan and in 8 people in China, including one fatality.[10,35]

32.5.8 SARS-CoV-2

There have been no publications to date implicating the acquisition of SARS-CoV-2 infection from microbiology specimens or cultures in the laboratory. However, like the rest of the population, SARS-CoV-2 infection has been exceedingly common amongst laboratory workers in recent years. In healthcare workers generally, much of the burden of SARS-CoV-2 infection has been from community acquisition and between healthcare workers, and the same is likely to be true for microbiology laboratory workers.

32.5.9 Arenaviruses

A case of laboratory-acquired Sabia virus in a virologist who was working with infected Vero cells containing Sabia virus was likely due to a spill incident. The individual was treated with IV ribavirin and survived.[36]

32.6 Other LAIs

32.6.1 Fungi

Dimorphic fungi such as *Blastomyces dermatitides*, *Coccidiodies immitis* and *Histoplasma capsulatum* are the predominant organisms implicated in laboratory-acquired fungal infection. Most infections are caused by inhalation of aerosolised conidia from the mould form causing pulmonary infection. Requesting clinicians should alert laboratories if they suspect these organisms when referring diagnostic samples for fungal culture. Cutaneous infections due to accidental inoculation of dimorphic fungi have been recorded.

32.6.2 Parasites

Parasites are an uncommon cause of LAI. Pike's 1976 review of 3921 LAIs counted 115 parasitic cases.[37] Herwaldt et al. conducted an extensive review of parasitic LAIs and found approximately 313 cases of parasitic LAI from 1924–1999.[38] In this review, blood and tissue protozoa cases enumerated to 164, including *Trypanosoma cruzi* (65 cases), *Toxoplasma gondii* (47 cases), Plasmodium spp. (34 cases), Leishmania spp. (12 cases) and *Trypanosoma brucei* (6 cases). Intestinal protozoa were even more uncommon with a total of 21 cases, including *Cryptosporidium parvum* (16 cases), *Isospora belli* (3 cases) and *Giardia lamblia* (2 cases). Helminth infections were the most rare, with only 18 recorded cases.[38]

An additional 16 cases of malaria in laboratory workers were reported, with a total of 52 cases. Fifteen cases were caused by *Plasmodium falciparum*, 10 cases by *Plasmodium cynomolgi* and 9 cases were due to *Plasmodium vivax*. The majority of infections occurred in healthcare and laboratory workers rather than in research staff.[38] (Table 32.3).

TABLE 32.3 Common laboratory routes of exposure to infectious agents

Route	Microbiological incident
Inhalation	• Procedures that produce aerosols • Centrifugation • Mixing, sonication, vortexing, blending • Spills and splashes • Pouring/decanting culture fluids • Manipulation of inoculating loop
Inoculation	• Needlestick • Lacerations from sharp objects, e.g. blades, broken glass
Ingestion	• Splashes to the mouth • Placing contaminated articles/fingers in or around the mouth • Consumption of food in the laboratory • Mouth pipetting
Contamination of skin and mucous membranes	• Splashes • Contact with contaminated fomites

32.7 IPC in laboratory settings

32.7.1 Immunisation

In Australia, laboratory safety is overseen by both national and state and territory governments. In most jurisdictions, vaccinations and occupational screening remain the prevailing preventative measure against LAIs. For example, in New South Wales, the policy directive Occupational Assessment, Screening and Vaccination Against Specified Infectious Diseases requires all laboratory staff, students and collaborating researchers working within healthcare facilities to provide evidence of immunity against the following infectious diseases: diphtheria, tetanus, pertussis, hepatitis B, measles, mumps, rubella, varicella and SARS-CoV-2.

In addition, this policy directive states that laboratory staff must undergo regular screening for tuberculosis—the frequency of which is based on an individual risk assessment—and annual influenza vaccination is recommended. All vaccinations must be given in accordance with the recommendations of the current NHRMC Australian Immunisation Handbook, with reference to the indications and contraindications.

However, additional vaccination policies are required for staff working in microbiology laboratories and should be made based on an assessment of their specific occupational risks. Workers must take reasonable steps to protect themselves against occupational infectious disease risks by complying with current laboratory safety procedures, be aware of their own infectious diseases and vaccination status, and minimise the risk of transmitting infectious diseases to patients or other laboratory members. Workers who are pregnant or those who are immunocompromised due to illness or medication use should seek additional medical advice. Workers undertaking specific work that may expose them to the organisms should provide evidence of vaccination against these organisms prior to commencing work (Table 32.4).

Record keeping for workers: Prior to employment or the start of research, potential recruits should provide evidence that they are 'protected' as specified in local requirements. The evidence may be based on immunisation evidence, immunity evidence or assessment evidence, or a combination of all. Each staff member employed should be issued with a record detailing the results of all screening tests and vaccinations administered, including the date, batch number, type and brand name of each vaccine. Pre-vaccination screening

TABLE 32.4 Recommended vaccinations based on the types of laboratory activities to be performed

Staff member duties	Special vaccinations needed*
Processing or handling faeces specimens	Hepatitis A, *Salmonella* Typhi, poliovirus
Sterile site isolate handling, including blood cultures	*Neisseria meningitidis* and *Salmonella* Typhi
Faecal culture isolate handling	*Salmonella* Typhi
Other isolate handling	*Neisseria meningitidis*
Specialised viral culture laboratories, including neutralising antibody testing	Japanese encephalitis, yellow fever, rabies, smallpox/monkeypox, poliovirus
Q fever culture	Q fever

* These vaccinations are in addition to those required by national and jurisdictional legislation.

shall be undertaken by the facility if indicated to determine immunity and/or vaccination status, including the results of previous serological tests. Staff, students and researchers must present the required evidence of immunity (vaccination records or serologic tests) prior to commencement. Employee records should be updated as necessary and maintained by the facility.

Documentation of employee refusal to participate in screening and/or vaccination should also be retained. Where it is refused, their non-participation should be acknowledged in writing and include an understanding of the risks consequent upon non-participation. Furthermore, in such instances consideration should be given to restricting their scope of work.

32.7.2 Special vaccination requirements

Salmonella Typhi: Typhoid fever is a commonly reported laboratory infection, and vaccination is recommended for all laboratory staff who process enteric specimens or who may be involved in the isolation and identification of potential *Salmonella* Typhi isolates. Options for vaccination against *Salmonella* Typhi include intramuscular purified polysaccharide capsule of *Salmonella* Typhi (TY 2 strain) either alone ('Typhim Vi') or as part of a combined hepatitis A/typhoid vaccine (Vivaxim), or else an oral live vaccine consisting of capsules containing an attenuated *Salmonella* Typhi strain. Protection is achieved in 60–80% of vaccinees during the first year and in 50–70% during the next 2 years. It is important to appreciate that protection is not absolute, and that clinical infection may still develop if a high enough inoculum is ingested. The vaccine does not protect against infection with *S.* Paratyphi or

non-Typhi Salmonella. Booster doses are required at 3-yearly intervals.

Hepatitis A virus: Hepatitis A vaccine is recommended for laboratory staff who process faecal specimens. Staff who spent their childhood in endemic countries or who were born before 1950 may already be immune from previous exposure: antibody testing can be performed to determine this. Hepatitis A vaccination is typically performed using an inactivated hepatitis A virus vaccine, which requires two doses, 6 months apart. This provides long-lasting protection and booster doses are not required.

Neisseria meningitidis: Vaccination against *Neisseria meningitis* is recommended for laboratory staff working in laboratories where they may encounter the bacteria in culture. Two vaccines are currently recommended:

1. The quadrivalent (serogroup A, C, W135 and Y) conjugate vaccine (Menveo or Nimenrix). This vaccine has been available since November 2010 and replaces both the previous quadrivalent polysaccharide vaccine that did not provide long-lasting protection (Mencevax or Menomune) and also the monovalent serogroup C conjugate vaccine that does not provide protection against serogroups A, B, W135 or Y (Meningitec, Menjugate or Neis-Vac C). Workers previously vaccinated with Mencevax, Menomune, Meningitec, Menjugate or Neis-Vac C should receive Menveo or Nimenrix.

2. The 4-component conjugate meningococcal serogroup B vaccine (Bexsero). This vaccine requires 2 doses, 1–2 months apart. This is the first serogroup B vaccine licensed in Australia, and has been available since August 2014. Since B is the

serogroup most commonly encountered in the microbiology laboratory, all staff for whom meningococcal vaccination is indicated should also receive this vaccination, regardless of any previous meningococcal vaccines administered.

Staff with ongoing exposure should receive the quadrivalent conjugate vaccine (Menveo or Nimenrix) every 5 years. A single booster dose of serogroup B vaccine (Bexsero) 5 years after the initial 2-dose course is recommended.

Japanese B encephalitis virus: This vaccination should be considered for laboratory staff working with arboviruses. Booster doses are required every 3 years or as determined by antibody titres.

Yellow fever virus: This vaccination is also recommended for laboratory staff working with arboviruses. Yellow fever vaccinations use a live attenuated yellow fever virus strain and require boosters every 10 years or as guided by antibody titres.

Rabies virus: This vaccine provides protection against rabies virus and the closely related Australian bat lyssavirus (ABL) and is strongly recommended for laboratory staff performing rabies or ABL tests. Vaccinations use an inactivated rabies virus vaccine and staff who perform ABL or rabies diagnostic tests should have rabies antibody titres measured every year, and booster doses are necessary when antibody titres fall below 0.5 IU/mL.

Coxiella burnetii (Q fever): *Coxiella burnetii* culture is rarely undertaken in diagnostic laboratories, since culture of this organism is a major hazard for LAI and should only be undertaken by staff who are vaccinated or otherwise have evidence of immunity. Severe adverse reactions to the vaccine can occur in those previously exposed to Q fever. The vaccine is only administered after serological confirmation of an absence of antibodies to Q fever and a negative skin test. The skin test is performed by injecting 0.1ml of diluted *Coxiella burnetii* antigen intradermally and examining the site 7 days later to look for induration.

The presence of any induration indicates a positive skin test and vaccination is contraindicated.

Poliovirus: Staff may rarely be unexpectedly exposed to poliovirus if performing viral cultures or handling faecal specimens, or if performing neutralising antibody testing. All staff performing this work should have had poliovirus immunisation (a primary course or a booster) within the last 10 years. The most readily available vaccines for adults are intramuscular combined diphtheria-tetanus-acellular pertussis-inactivated poliovirus vaccines.

Smallpox/monkeypox virus: With the worldwide emergency of monkeypox (Mpox) infection in 2022, laboratory staff who handle specimens for diagnosis of Mpox, including viral culture, may be at risk of occupational-acquired infection. Third generation smallpox vaccines based on replication deficient vaccinia Ankara strain (e.g. Jynneos vaccine) have been shown to offer cross-protection against monkeypox virus infection. The vaccine is administered as 2 subcutaneous doses at least 28 days apart, with a booster at 10-year intervals if there is ongoing exposure.

Other vaccines: Other vaccines may be recommended for some or all staff in the event of emerging infections or perceived bioterrorist threats (e.g. anthrax). Currently these vaccines are not indicated.

Conclusion

Contemporary IPC systems, processes and activities apply equally to patients and to those who provide their care. Much of this focus is placed on those who are typically referred to as 'front-line' clinical staff, but necessarily includes other staff members who are essential to systems care for patients—and, in particular, laboratory staff. All clinical and other IPC practice relies on both confirming the pathogen or pathogens responsible for infection, and protecting laboratory workers from occupational exposures. This is core to infection prevention and control in any healthcare setting.

Useful websites/resources

- Australian Immunisation Handbook. https://immunisationhandbook.health.gov.au/
- Clinical and Laboratory Standards Institute. M29-A4. Protection of laboratory workers from occupationally acquired infections: Approved guidelines. 4th ed: https://clsi.org/
- OECD Best Practice Guidelines for Biological Resource Centres: https://www.oecd.org/sti/emerging-tech/oecdbestpracticeguidelinesforbiologicalresourcecentres.htm.

References

1. Australian/New Zealand Standard. Safety in laboratories. Part 3: Microbiological safety and containment: Australian/New Zealand Standard, 2010.

2. World Health Organization. Laboratory biosafety manual, 4th ed. Geneva: WHO, 2020.

3. UK Advisory Committee on Dangerous Pathogens. The management, design and operation of microbiological containment laboratories. London: Health and Safety Executive, 2001.

4. US Department of Health and Human Services. Biosafety in microbiological and biomedical laboratories, 5th ed. Washington DC: HHS Publication, 2009.

5. Eddie B & Meyer K. 1941. Laboratory infections due to Brucella. J Infect Dis. 68(1);24-32. Available from: https://academic.oup.com/jid/article/68/1/24/2193349.

6. Byers K. Laboratory-acquired infections 1979–2013. ABSA; 2013. Available from: https://absaconference.org/pdf56/II930Byers.pdf.

7. RM. P. Laboratory-associated infections: incidence, fatalities, causes, and prevention. Annu Rev Microbiol. 1979;33:41-66.

8. Sewell DL. Laboratory-associated infections and biosafety. Clin Microbiol Rev. 1995;8(3):389-405.

9. Lien A, Abalos C, Atchessi N, Edjoc R, Heisz M. Surveillance of laboratory exposures to human pathogens and toxins, Canada 2019. Can Commun Dis Rep. 2020;46(9).

10. Siengsanan-Lamont J, Blacksell SD. A review of laboratory-acquired infections in the Asia-Pacific: understanding risk and the need for improved biosafety for veterinary and zoonotic diseases. Trop Med Infect Dis. 2018;3(2):36.

11. Mesureur J, Arend S, Cellière B, Courault P, Cotte-Pattat P-J, Totty H, et al. A MALDI-TOF MS database with broad genus coverage for species-level identification of Brucella. PLoS Negl Trop Dis. 2018;12(10): e0006874.

12. Traxler RM, Lehman MW, Bosserman EA, Guerra MA, Smith TL. A literature review of laboratory-acquired brucellosis. J Clinical Microbiology. 2013;51(9):3055-3062.

13. Eales KM, Norton RE, Ketheesan N. Brucellosis in northern Australia. Am J Trop Med Hyg. 2010;83(4):876.

14. Ashdown L. Melioidosis and safety in the clinical laboratory. J Hosp Infect. 1992;21(4):301-306.

15. Peacock SJ, Schweizer HP, Dance DAB, Smith TL, Gee JE, Wuthiekanun V, DeShazer D, Steinmetz I, Tan P and Currie BJ. Management of Accidental Laboratory Exposure to Burkholderia pseudomallei and B. mallei. Emerg Infect Dis. 2008 Jul; 14(7): e2. doi: 10.3201/eid1407.071501)

16. Meselson M, Guillemin J, Hugh-Jones M, Langmuir A, Popova I, Shelokov A, et al. The Sverdlovsk anthrax outbreak of 1979. Science. 1994;266(5188):1202-1208.

17. Centers for Disease Control and Prevention. Suspected cutaneous anthrax in a laboratory worker – Texas, 2002. MMWR. 2002;51(13):279-281.

18. Shapiro DS, Schwartz DR. Exposure of laboratory workers to Francisella tularensis despite a bioterrorism procedure. J Clin Microbiol. 2002;40(6):2278-2281.

19. Weinstein RA, Singh K. Laboratory-acquired infections. Clin Infect Dis. 2009;49(1):142-147.

20. Committee NTA. Guidelines for Australian mycobacteriology laboratories. Commun Dis. Intell Q Rep. 2006;30(1):116-128.

21. Blacksell SD, Robinson MT, Newton PN, Day NP. Laboratory-acquired scrub typhus and murine typhus infections: the argument for a risk-based approach to biosafety requirements for Orientia tsutsugamushi and Rickettsia typhi laboratory activities. Clin Infect Dis. 2019;68(8):1413-1419.

22. Sejvar J, Johnson D, Popovic T, Miller JM, Downes F, Somsel P, et al. Assessing the risk of laboratory-acquired meningococcal disease. J Clin Microbiol. 2005;43(9): 4811-4814.

23. Ashdown L, Cassidy J. Successive Salmonella give and Salmonella typhi infections, laboratory-acquired. Pathology. 1991;23(3):233-234.

24. Centers for Disease Control and Prevention. Human Salmonella Typhimurium infections linked to exposure to clinical and teaching microbiology laboratories: CDC, 2014 [cited 30 August 2022]. Available from: https://www.cdc.gov/salmonella/typhimurium-labs-06-14/.

25. Alexander DC, Fitzgerald SF, DePaulo R, Kitzul R, Daku D, Levett PN, et al. Laboratory-acquired infection with Salmonella enterica serovar Typhimurium exposed by whole-genome sequencing. J Clin Microbiol. 2016;54(1):190-193.

26. Pedrosa PB, Cardoso TA. Viral infections in workers in hospital and research laboratory settings: a comparative review of infection modes and respective biosafety aspects. Intl J Infect Dis. 2011;15(6):e366-e376.

27. West DJ. The risk of hepatitis B infection among health professionals in the United States: a review. Am J Med Sci. 1984;287(2):26-33.

28. Beekmann SE, Fahey BJ, Gerberding JL, Henderson DK. Risky business: using necessarily imprecise casualty counts to estimate occupational risks for HIV-1 infection. Infect Control Hosp Epidemiol. 1990;11(7):371-379.

29. Control CfD. Surveillance for occupationally acquired HIV infection – United States, 1981-1992. MMWR. 1992;41(43):823-825.

30. Britton S, van den Hurk AF, Simmons RJ, Pyke AT, Northill JA, McCarthy J, et al. Laboratory-acquired dengue virus infection—a case report. PLoS Negl Trop Dis. 2011; 5(11):e1324.

31. Talon de Menezes M, Rilo Christoff R, Higa LM, Pezzuto P, Rabello Moreira FR, Ribeiro LdJ, et al., editors. Laboratory acquired Zika virus infection through mouse bite: a case report. Open Forum Infect Dis. 2020;7(11):ofaa259.

32. Kawamata J, Yamanouchi T, Dohmae K, Miyamoto H, Takahaski M, Yamanishi K, et al. Control of laboratory acquired hemorrhagic fever with renal syndrome (HFRS) in Japan. Lab Anim Sci. 1987;37(4):431-436.

33. Control CfD, Prevention. Laboratory-acquired vaccinia exposures and infections—United States, 2005-2007. MMWR. 2008;57(15):401-404.

34. Senanayake SN. Needlestick injury with smallpox vaccine. MJA. 2009;191(11):657.

35. Lim PL, Kurup A, Gopalakrishna G, Chan KP, Wong CW, Ng LC, et al. Laboratory-acquired severe acute respiratory syndrome. N Eng J Med. 2004;350(17):1740-1745.

36. Barry M, Russi M, Armstrong L, Geller D, Tesh R, Dembry L, et al. Treatment of a laboratory-acquired Sabia virus infection. N Eng J Med 1995;333(5):294-296.

37. Herwaldt BL. Laboratory-acquired parasitic infections from accidental exposures. Clin Microbiol Rev. 2001;14(4):659-688.

38. Pike RM. Laboratory-associated infections: summary and analysis of 3921 cases. Health Lab Sci. 1976;13(2):105-114.

CHAPTER 33

Infection prevention and control in operating theatre and endoscopy practice

PAUL SIMPSON[i]

Dr CHRISTINE RODER[ii]

PROFESSOR EUGENE ATHAN[iii]

Chapter highlights

- In Australia, one in three healthcare-associated infections (HAIs) is related to surgery.[1] Mitigation practices include skin preparation, aseptic technique, hand hygiene, surgical attire and personal protective equipment (PPE)
- The benefits of care bundles and the responsibility of the surgical team in ensuring high standards of infection prevention practice
- The risks for both surface and air contamination, with a case study of infection transmission as a result of contaminated heater-cooler units
- The management of reusable medical devices, with both surgical and endoscopy unit design

i   Infection Prevention and Control Service, Redcliffe Hospital, Metro North Health, Brisbane, QLD
ii Department of Infectious Disease, Barwon Health, Geelong, VIC
iii Infectious Disease, School of Medicine, Deakin University, Geelong, VIC

Introduction

In the United States, surgical site infection (SSI) accounts for 20% of all healthcare-associated infections (HAIs).[2] Often requiring additional antibiotics, further surgery, or an extended stay or readmission to hospital,[3] it can also be associated with a 2–11 times increase in mortality. The consequence for the US health system is an estimated annual cost of US$3.3 billion.[2] In Australia, a 2019 point prevalence study of 18 hospitals identified almost 1 in 10 inpatients (9.9%) with an HAI. Of these, the most frequently occurring was SSI, accounting for more than a third of all HAIs.[1] The acquisition of an infection is a significant burden on patients, both physically and emotionally,[4] and particularly for elderly patients who face the consequences of a substantially increased risk of mortality.[4,5] Fortunately, clinical infections following an endoscopic procedure are considered rare;[6] however, there is an increasing awareness and recognition of the risks of endoscopy-associated pathogen transmission, with outbreaks linked to duodenoscopes, bronchoscopes and urological scopes.[7]

Patients undergoing surgical and endoscopic procedures are reliant on healthcare workers (HCWs) to safeguard their wellbeing and reduce the risk of infection through strict adherence with infection control principles in their daily practice.[8,9] This chapter explores mitigating practice to reduce infection risks from surgical site skin preparation, aseptic technique, hand hygiene, surgical attire and PPE. It will also review care bundles, surgical team responsibilities, environmental hygiene, reusable medical devices (RMDs), and surgical and endoscopy unit design.

33.1 Historical infection control and surgery

From the earliest development of tools, humans have attempted surgery. Pain, bleeding and infection meant it was always a risky undertaking.[10] The evolution of anaesthetic techniques in the mid-19th century ushered in a rapid rise in, and development of, surgical procedures. However, the constant spectre of postoperative infection challenged public confidence in relation to this burgeoning science.[11]

In 1842, Oliver Wendell Holmes, an American anatomist, investigated 13 deaths due to puerperal fever and concluded that birthing attendants were spreading the disease.[12] Independently, Ignaz Phillip Semmelweis, in Austria, also as an action against puerperal fever, introduced a process of washing hands with chloride of lime solution for medical officers after they attended post-mortems and before entering maternity wards. This resulted in dramatic reductions in postpartum mortality.[13,14] In 1867, Joseph Lister, a British orthopaedic surgeon, pioneered the use of antisepsis and in doing so revolutionised surgery. Lister's epiphany, inspired by Pasteur's aetiology on fermentation, led him to think of carbolic acid—which was used to neutralise the smell from sewage—and make use of those same properties by applying it to disinfect surgical instruments and wounds. This innovative process led to a significant reduction in postoperative infections. Lister had changed the treatment of compound fractures from amputation to limb preservation and opened the way for abdominal and other intra-cavity surgery.[15] Other notable infection control pioneers included Florence Nightingale, the 'Lady of the Lamp', whose endeavours to use epidemiologic principles and strict hygiene practices resulted in a significant reduction in morbidity and mortality due to infection amongst British soldiers during the Crimean War.[16] And this was despite the fact that she rejected germ theory (Table 33.1).

33.2 Mitigating the risk of infection

Today, the most frequent adverse outcome for patients receiving healthcare remains the development of healthcare-associated infection (HAI). Despite the constant evolution and improvement in infection control and prevention (IPC) practice, one-third of patients still develop an HAI associated with surgery.[1-3] This results in a significant increase in the associated risks—increased hospital stay, morbidity and low morale.[17]

In terms of endoscopy, high standards of IPC practice are essential for safe and efficient endoscopic procedures.[6] This has been emphasised in recent years following endoscopy-associated outbreaks.[18,19] There are also concerns regarding the transmission of multidrug-resistant organisms (MROs) such as carbapenemase-producing *Enterobacteriaceae* and *Candida aureus* to name a few, and the use of simethicone during endoscopic procedures. There are several patient and procedure-related risk factors for endoscopy-associated bacteraemia and infection. These include compromised patient immune status, endoscopy procedures involving an infected site, increased risk of bacterial lodgement during bacteraemia, and procedure-induced tissue damage.[6] Mitigation of risk during surgery requires adherence to a number of evidence-based practices including surgical site skin preparation, aseptic technique, hand

TABLE 33.1 Historical pioneers of infection control

Year/s	Pioneer	Infection control practices
1840 1882	Holmes	Applied epidemiology to demonstrate direct transmission of infection by healthcare workers
1844–1861	Semmelweis	Devised a process of washing hands with chloride of lime solution, resulting in a dramatic reduction in postpartum mortality
1854–1890	Nightingale	Campaigned for hospital cleanliness and sanitation during the Crimean War and advanced hospitals
1856–1885	Lister	Used carbolic acid, one of the first agents used as a microbicide, to disinfect surgical incisions and prevent postoperative infections
1890	Halsted	Introduced gloves for surgery
1897	Berger	Introduced face masks into operating theatres
1934	Price	Demonstrated that bacteria on hands were either resident (rarely pathogenic and difficult to remove with routine handwashing) or transient organisms

Source: Adapted from Pitt D, Aubin JM. Joseph Lister: father of modern surgery. Can J Surg. 2012;55(5):E8–E9.

hygiene, surgical attire and the use of PPE. (Endoscopy-related risks are discussed later in this chapter.)

33.2.1 Surgical site skin preparation

Surgical site preparation is the process of preoperative antisepsis for intact skin at the operative site of a patient (Fig 33.1). To be effective, the antiseptic solution must be applied and allowed to dry immediately prior to the surgical procedure commencing.[20] The antiseptic must be applied not only to the intended site of the surgical incision but also to the broader areas of the skin surrounding the intended incision site.[21] The antiseptic solution is intended to cleanse the patient's skin and reduce the microorganisms present on the skin. Organisms found in skin flora targeted by antiseptic solutions include Staphylococci, Diphtheroid organisms, Pseudomonas, and Propionibacterium species, all of which can lead to SSI if allowed to proliferate.[22] (Table 33.2.)

The first use of an antiseptic skin agent in surgery is credited to the British surgeon Joseph Lister. Along with disinfecting surgical equipment, Lister's pioneering skin antisepsis process led to significant reduction in SSIs.[14] In contemporary surgery, skin antiseptics continue to play a significant role in reducing the risk of SSI and is routine practice immediately prior to the surgical incision.[25-29] The most common skin preparation agents used today include products containing alcohol, iodophors, chlorhexidine gluconate (CHG) or a combination of these agents.[30]

CHG offers persistent activity to kill a range of microorganisms such as bacteria,[26] viruses and fungi that reside on the surface of the skin.[27-31] CHG does not become inactivated in the presence of organic material.[31] Iodophors such as povidone-iodine also kill a range of bacteria, viruses and fungi.[27-33] Povidone releases its iodine slowly; the iodine kills bacteria quickly but does not appear to have a residual effect.[31] Unlike CHG, iodine does become inactivated by organic material, so should only be applied to clean skin.[30] As with CHG and povidone-iodine, alcohol kills a range of bacteria and many viruses and fungi.[26-30] Alcohol kills microorganisms rapidly and effectively but unlike CHG it does not have any residual activity.[27-33]

Overall, low to moderate quality of evidence appears to support the use of alcohol-based antiseptic solutions as more effective in reducing SSI when used for surgical site skin preparation compared to aqueous solutions. A meta-analysis of available low quality of evidence indicates alcohol-based CHG is beneficial in reducing SSI rates when compared to alcohol-based povidone-iodine.[25] The British National Institute for Health and Care Excellence (NICE) was unable to make a strong recommendation on the most effective surgical skin preparation, concluding however that available evidence demonstrates CHG in alcohol was associated with the lowest incidence of SSI, whereas aqueous povidone-iodine was associated with the highest incidence of SSI. Therefore, CHG in alcohol is recommended as a first choice for surgical skin preparation.[26] CHG in alcohol is also likely to be a more cost-effective option.[31] Caution is required when using alcohol-based solution containing CHG on premature infants due to the risk of chemical injuries. It is recommended to use minimum amounts required of

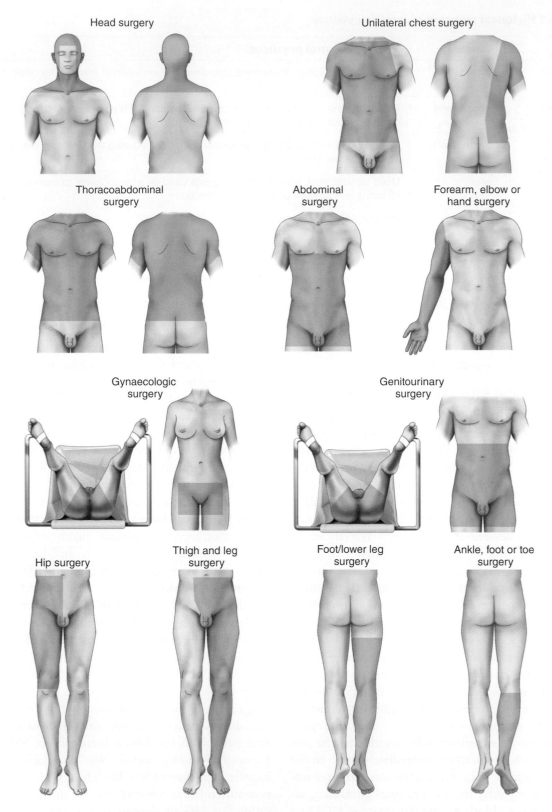

FIGURE 33.1 Skin preparation of common surgical sites

Source: Rebar C, Bashaw M. Concepts of care for perioperative patients (chapter 9).
In: Ignatavicius DD, Workman ML, Rebar CR, Heimgartner NM. Medical-surgical nursing:
concepts for interprofessional collaborative care, tenth edition. Elsevier, 2021.

TABLE 33.2 Surgical skin preparation application technique

Skin preparation application technique
1. Remove all jewellery from the operative site prior to commencing skin preparation
2. Use sterile applicator if available
3. Use single use preparation solutions only
4. The preparation solution should be applied using friction. Commence from the cleanest area, usually the operative and/or incision site and proceed in a concentric fashion to the least clean area. Discard applicator once the edge of the skin preparation area is reached
5. If an area is highly contaminated, where possible, the area of least contamination should be prepared first, followed by the area of higher contamination
6. If both the abdominal and perineal areas require preparation, the preparation should be performed sequentially (not simultaneously). Evidence as to the sequence in which the areas are prepared is not conclusive; whether preparing the perineal area or abdominal first, ensure a new applicator is used for each site, gloves are replaced and hand hygiene is performed between site
7. Preparation solution should be allowed to completely dry naturally
8. Avoid drying the incision site after the application with a swab or sponges as this reduces the efficacy of the preparation solution
9. The prepared area of skin should extend to an area large enough to accommodate potential shifting of the drape fenestration, extension of the incision, potential for additional incisions and all potential drain sites
10. Ensure preparation solution remains in contact with the skin for the required period as per manufacturer instructions

Hazard precautions
• Alcoholic preparations are safe if used correctly. The volume used should be sufficient to thoroughly wet the site for the recommended time as per manufacturer's instructions
• Avoid excessive pooling of preparation on, beneath or around the patient
• Allow adequate contact, drying and vapour dissipation time of preparation solution to prevent skin irritation and to prevent fire or burn injuries
• Areas with excess hair may take longer to dry
• All alcohol preparation solutions are potentially flammable; it is imperative that all preparations are allowed to evaporate completely before electrocautery/diathermy or laser instruments are switched on
• Avoid dripping or pooling of preparation solutions on sheets, padding, positioning equipment, adhesive tape and on or under the patient

Source: Adapted from Surgical skin disinfection guideline, Version 3, October 2015. Queensland Department of Health. [Accessed 05/07/2022. https://www.health.qld.gov.au/__data/assets/pdf_file/0020/444422/skin-disinfection.pdf].

alcohol-based solution containing CHG, not allow pooling, and remove any excessively soaked materials, drapes or gowns from the skin.[34]

33.2.2 Surgical aseptic technique

The term sterile is generally defined as meaning free from all microorganisms; however, due to the persistence of microorganisms in the air, sterility is not achievable within a typical operating theatre environment. Therefore, use of the term sterile technique, or sterile field, should be discouraged. Sterile can be used to describe the state of, for example, sterilised equipment within its package. Once sterile equipment packaging has been opened the contents are exposed to airborne organisms, so cannot truly be considered sterile. Traditionally, the terms 'sterile' and 'aseptic' were often used interchangeably.[35-37] Often there can be an array of terms describing varying degrees of the presence of microorganisms during medical procedures. In the 1990s, in an effort to standardise terms and practices, Rowley developed and implemented a practice framework called 'Aseptic Non-Touch Technique' (ANTT©).[37] ANTT uses the following definitions:

• clean—free from visible marks and stains

• aseptic—free from pathogenic organisms in numbers needed to cause infection

• sterile—free from all microorganisms.

Aseptic technique, which involves actions designed to protect patients from infection when undergoing invasive clinical procedures, is prescribed by guideline makers as a critical component in the prevention of infections—although the mechanics of aseptic technique and how it is applied are not adequately provided within most of these guidelines.[17,25,37] Aseptic technique is best described as a combination of decontamination processes, use of sterilised equipment, and techniques to minimise the potential for transmission of pathogenic microorganisms.[37-40]

While the Australian National Health and Medical Research Council's (NHMRC) IPC guidelines do not directly endorse ANTT, they recognise that it represents an example of best practice in aseptic technique as a set of practices aimed at minimising contamination. ANTT is described as a specific type of aseptic technique with a unique theory and practice framework based on a concept of protecting the procedural equipment 'key-parts' and the patient's 'key-sites' from contamination by microorganisms.[41] In ANTT, asepsis is achieved by identifying and then protecting all key-parts and key-sites through hand hygiene, the use of non-touch technique, using sterilised equipment and cleaning existing 'key-parts' to a standard that renders them aseptic before use.[40,41]

33.2.3 Surgical hand hygiene

Semmelweis has been widely attributed for recognising in the mid-19th century the risk of infection transmission within a healthcare environment via the hands of healthcare workers. Semmelweis concluded that the 'cadaverous particles' acquired during post-mortems, which were then transferred to the women examined in the maternity clinic, played a role in causing 'bed-fever' and increased rates of mortality. Following this revelation, Semmelweis insisted that anyone who had attended a post-mortem wash their hands with a chloride of lime solution before entering the maternity wards.[42] Following this unpopular directive there was a dramatic reduction in postpartum mortality.[43]

During the 19th century, surgical hand hygiene was achieved by washing the hands with antimicrobial soap and warm water, frequently with the use of a brush.[44] By the end of the 19th and start of the 20th century, interest in presurgical disinfection of hands increased, following the previously mentioned pioneering work by Scottish orthopaedic surgeon Joseph Lister.[45] In 1938, laboratory studies conducted by Price established that bacteria on hands were distinguished as resident or transient organisms.[13] Price identified that resident bacteria normally found on skin were rarely pathogenic and that they were difficult to remove through routine handwashing techniques.[14] Over the next 30 or so years, interest in hand disinfection mainly revolved around the hands of surgeons and the mechanisms of reducing bacterial contamination.[46,47] Over the second half of the 20th century, recommendations for surgical hand hygiene duration decreased from 10 minutes to 5 minutes.[48]

The direct benefits of presurgical hand hygiene on patient safety cannot be proven by randomised control trials. This is due to the existence of a large body of indirect evidence supporting presurgical hand hygiene, making it unethical to deny this vital step due to the high risk of subsequent infection.[49] Traditionally, members of the surgical team would perform presurgical hand hygiene or scrub using a surgical hand antiseptic and water. Most common surgical hand preparations were antibacterial soaps containing CHG or povidone-iodine.[50] However, the uptake of alcohol-based hand rub (ABHR) into the wider healthcare environment due to its antimicrobial effectiveness, quick application, availability at the point of care and skin benefits due to emollients has now slowly crossed over into the surgical environment. Both in vitro and in vivo studies have demonstrated ABHR to be superior to antibacterial soaps. Surgical ABHR should meet European Norm (EN) 12791 or equivalent and be registered by the Therapeutic Goods Administration (TGA) for this use in Australia.[51]

The World Health Organization (WHO) recommends that the hands of the surgical team should be clean upon entering the operating department by washing with a non-medicated soap (Fig 33.2). Once in the operating area, repeating surgical ABHR without an additional prior handwash is recommended before switching to the next procedure. It should be kept in mind that the activity of ABHRs may be impaired if hands are not completely dried following handwashing before applying ABHR.[42,52] The Australian College of Perioperative Nurses (ACORN) has also endorsed the use of surgical ABHR when used according to manufacturers' guidelines. In keeping with WHO guidelines, ACORN no longer recommends a preliminary surgical hand preparation with an antimicrobial solution and water, as surgical ABHR alone should be sufficient to eliminate transient flora and reduce resident skin flora on the user's hands.[52] Adverse effects of using surgical hand preparation and water include skin irritation, dryness and irritation. These adverse effects are less likely with surgical ABHR due to it containing emollients.[42]

33.2.4 Surgical attire

Due to the nature of surgery there is a high risk of transferring microorganisms, some potentially pathogenic, that may cause SSI or a blood-borne infection in both the patient and/or the surgical team. This risk may be reduced by the surgical team wearing a protective barrier in the way of appropriate surgical attire and PPE.[25] PPE refers to a variety of barriers, used alone or in combination, to protect mucous membranes, airways, skin and clothing from contact with body fluids

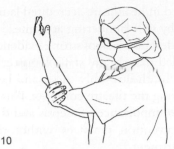

10

Smear the hand rub on the left forearm up to the elbow. Ensure that the whole skin area is covered by using circular movements around the forearm until the hand rub has fully evaporated (10-15 s)

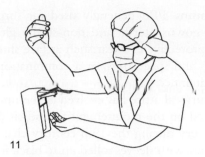

11

Put approximately 5 mL (3 doses) of alcohol-based hand rub in the palm of your left hand, using the elbow of your other arm to operate the distributor. Rub both hands at the same time up to the wrists, and ensure that all the steps represented in Images 12-17 are followed (20-30 s)

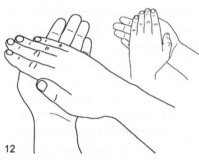

12

Cover the whole surface of the hands up to the wrist with alcohol-based hand rub, rubbing palm against palm with a rotating movement

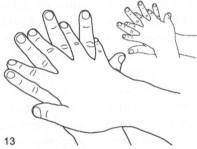

13

Rub the back of the left hand, including the wrist, moving the right palm back and forth, and vice versa

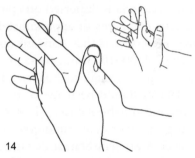

14

Rub palm against palm back and forth with fingers interlinked

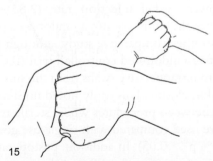

15

Rub the back of the fingers by holding them in the palm of the other hand with a sideways back-and-forth movement

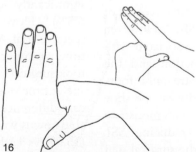

16

Rub the thumb of the left hand by rotating it in the clasped palm of the right hand and vice versa

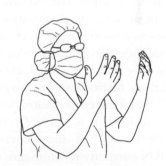

17

When the hands are dry, sterile surgical clothing and gloves can be donned

---

Repeat the above-illustrated sequence (average duration 60 s) according to the number of times corresponding to the total duration recommended by the manufacturer for surgical hand preparation with an alcohol-based hand rub.

FIGURE 33.2 Surgical alcohol-based hand rub technique

Source: World Health Organization. Guidelines on hand hygiene in health care. First global patient safety challenge: Clean care is safe care. Geneva: WHO; 2009.

and microorganisms. PPE generally used for surgery includes sterile gowns, sterile and non-sterile gloves, surgical masks, protective eyewear such as face shields, surgical helmets and space suits, or a combination of several of these items.[53]

The use of surgical attire has evolved as the understanding increased on the requirement for asepsis during surgery. Surgery during the 19th century changed from street clothes, with sleeves rolled up, to black frock coats heavily stained with blood and pus, worn as a badge of honour.[54] In contemporary practice, clean surgical scrubs are an expectation within semi-restricted and restricted areas of the surgical department. Wearing surgical scrubs is likely to ensure cleanliness and reduce the risk of healthcare staff introducing microorganisms to the theatre environment. While no study has directly linked non-sterile surgical attire and increased SSIs, the skin of staff working in the operating theatre is known to be a major source of bacteria dispersed into the air.[55] Bacteria is dispersed on epithelial cells which break into fragments of approximately 20 mm in size as they shed. Given that standard cotton fabric has a pore size of 80–100 mm, these fragments are small enough to pass through such fabrics. Therefore, surgical scrub fabrics should be made of tightly woven, stain-resistant and durable fabric.[56] It is also recommended that surgical scrubs are laundered in laundry facilities that meet Australian Standards rather than staff laundering at home. Accredited laundry facilities follow industry standards for quality control and water quality testing.[57]

In terms of appropriate footwear for surgery there is a lack of evidence to demonstrate the effectiveness of theatre-only footwear in reducing SSIs.[58] However, outdoor shoes have been shown to be associated with significantly more bacterial contamination and the transfer of microorganisms than theatre-only footwear.[59] Alternatives to theatre-only footwear are shoe covers. Again, there is a lack of evidence to demonstrate the effectiveness of shoe covers in reducing SSI. ACORN currently recommends that the surgical staff wear dedicated theatre shoes to prevent bacterial contamination and postoperative infections.[53]

Theatre personnel wear head coverings to contain hair and bacteria, and to help prevent contamination of the sterile field. However, no research has demonstrated that covering the hair lowers the incidence of SSIs.[60] Head coverings may be single use or reusable. In keeping with surgical attire, reusable surgical head coverings should be made of tightly woven and durable fabric.[61] It is also recommended that reusable hand coverings

are laundered in healthcare accredited laundry facilities rather than by staff laundering at home.[62]

Overall, despite a lack of strong evidence it is widely recommended that theatre staff change into laundered surgical scrubs, theatre-only shoes and head coverings before entering the theatre complex. This may serve to reinforce the importance of asepsis and the priority of infection prevention practices within the operating theatre department.[55]

33.2.5 Personal protective equipment (PPE)

Gowns: It is widely accepted practice that sterile surgical gowns are worn over scrubs by the surgical team during procedures to maintain a sterile surgical field and reduce the risk of the transmission of pathogens to both patients and the surgical team.[60] Sterile gowns are generally either sterile, disposable single use non-woven, or sterile reusable woven, although debate continues regarding the benefits and deficits of each type.[61] The benefits of single use gowns include consistent quality and fluid-repellent properties. The deficits include a lack of comfort for the wearer. For reusable gowns, the benefits include being comfortable for the wearer and their adaptability; however, reusable gowns may have inconsistent quality and reduced fluid-repellent properties when compared to single use gowns.[60]

Single use gowns are more costly than reusable gowns.[62] In terms of the reduced risk of SSI, evidence is scarce. One study noted that single use gowns had a significantly lower overall infection rate (2.83% vs 6.5%).[60] However, the study was not a randomised prospective trial. Another comparative study, although this time a prospective randomised controlled trial (RCT), took surgical site intraoperative swabs from the surgical site at time of skin closure. This study noted no significant difference between procedures where sterile reusable gowns were used compared with single use gowns (15.5% vs 13.1% p > 0.05). In addition, postoperative SSI rates were not significantly different between the two groups.[57]

Gloves: To prevent contamination from hand contact during surgery the surgical team wear sterile gloves.[64] Glove use in surgery was first implemented by William Stewart Halsted in 1890, to protect his surgical scrub nurse from dermatitis resulting from contact with sterilisation chemicals rather than to prevent infection.[65] Later, assistants in charge of instruments began to wear gloves, and as these assistants began to perform surgery themselves, they maintained their glove use to protect against harsh antibacterial agents and improve dexterity.[66] The adoption of gloves for surgery to reduce SSI took time, even though it was first postulated in the late 1890s. During the 20th century, studies regarding the use of gloves during surgical procedures initially showed dramatic reductions in SSIs, including a 1931 study that demonstrated the rate of SSI during hernia repairs decreased from 29% to 0.55% when gloves were worn by the entire team.[67] However, the advent of universal glove usage for surgery in recent times has seen debate relating to the following issues:[68]

- whether double gloving reduces SSI
- whether changing gloves intraoperatively reduces SSI; and
- sterile versus non-sterile gloves for minor surgical procedures.

The main aim of wearing an additional glove on each hand during surgery is to provide extra protection against infection. However, a 2006 Cochrane systematic review has suggested there is no evidence to support wearing additional gloves to prevent infection.[64] However, gloves can become perforated and their protective function is then compromised. Perforations usually occur due to injuries from sharps, such as sutures, instruments, bone fragments and through natural wear and tear.[64] A recent study suggests that the high rate of damage even in low impact surgical procedures represents an underestimated problem in soft tissue surgery.[69] The Cochrane review concluded that wearing two pairs of sterile surgical gloves is associated with significantly fewer inner glove perforations.[64] The WHO identified that most surgeons prefer to double-glove due to the risk of bacterial contamination of the surgical field in the event of glove perforation. Also, surgeons may prefer to double-glove for their own protection against injury from sharps and potential blood-borne infections.[21]

Gloves should be changed promptly if punctured; however, the WHO's 2016 guidelines for preventing SSI suggest a periodic change of the outer gloves when double gloves are worn during long surgeries.[21,69] This recommendation is endorsed by a 2020 study finding that when double gloves are worn, the gloves have an increased perforation rate the longer the gloves are worn. To reduce the risk of intraoperative exposure to blood and body fluid and SSI, outer gloves should be changed every 60 to 90 minutes and inner gloves changed every 240 minutes.[69]

Masks and eye protection: The first use of a mask within surgery was described in 1898 with a published study demonstrating reduced droplet spread from a test subject wearing a mask.[67] Since then, many studies have been undertaken comparing various types of masks and how they should be worn and whether they have any impact on the bacterial counts within the operating room or on SSI rates.[70-76] Results are mixed, with limited evidence supporting the wearing of masks to prevent SSI. However, face masks and eyewear are a vital part of PPE protecting surgical teams from blood and body fluid exposure.[77-79]

Research to date does not overwhelmingly support the use of surgical helmets within orthopaedic surgery to reduce the risk of SSI.[80-84] In fact, some studies suggest increased particle and microbiological emission rates when helmets are worn as part of a 'space suit' when compared with standard surgical clothing.[82] However, a 2022 New Zealand study of 19,322 primary total knee arthroplasty suggests surgical helmets were associated with a lower rate of infection when compared with conventional surgical gowning.[84] Some surgical helmets are designed as a powered air-purifying respirator (PAPR), which offers the wearer protection against airborne transmitted pathogens, such as tuberculosis (TB) or SARS-CoV-2. If not designed as a PAPR, standard surgical helmets offer the user no protection against airborne transmitted diseases. Surgical helmets will offer protection from body fluid splash, but this is likely to be comparable protection to surgical masks and eye protection such as face shields.[85]

33.3 A care bundle approach to infection

A care bundle is a set of evidence-based interventions that, when used together, significantly improve patient outcomes.[86] Bundles are structured practices which simplify decisions and aim to reduce errors.[87] Care bundles were first used by intensive care practitioners aiming to improve ventilated patients' outcomes. In a large 2004 multi-centre study, after introducing an evidenced-based bundle, an average of 44.5% reduction of ventilator-associated pneumonia was observed.[88] This bundle approach within intensive care units (ICUs) was extended to include central line-associated bloodstream infection (CLABSI) which was also successful in reducing CLABSI rates and demonstrated the improvement is sustained over time.[89,90]

Bundled approaches have already been widely used within the surgical environment in the form of the WHO surgical safety checklist.[91,92] More recently care bundles have been used within the perioperative environment to reduce the risk of SSI. Although these bundles have consistently demonstrated success, they are currently not consistently or uniformly implemented within Australian healthcare.[87] (Table 33.3.)

33.4 Perioperative surgical and procedural team IPC responsibilities

The surgical team play a crucial role in maintaining a safe environment and ensuring high standards of infection control within the operating theatre. The prevention of harm is a basic tenet of healthcare.[93,94] All healthcare staff within the surgical team generally—including surgeons, anaesthetists, gastroenterologists (endoscopy units), interventional radiologists and nurses and technicians—are bound by the codes of conduct embodied in the requirements of the Australian Health Practitioner Regulation Agency (APHRA) registration.[95,96]

All members of the team must perform their respective roles in accordance with the principles of infection control and must also monitor themselves and their colleagues to identify and intervene to prevent or address any potential infection control breaches. 'Surgical conscience' is the term used to explain this moral obligation to safeguard surgical asepsis and patient safety.[97,98] The intention of surgical conscience is to reduce the risk of preventable adverse outcomes. However, findings from a qualitative study suggest that surgical conscience requires moral courage developed through role-modelling on the journey from novice to expert and optimised by the organisational culture, resourcing, leadership and infrastructure.[99] Clinicians believe that poor surgical conscience may lead to poor patient safety and an increased risk of SSI.[100,101]

33.4.1 Environmental hygiene

Contaminated surfaces: As previously discussed, acquisition of SSI is likely to be complex and multifactorial, and although microorganisms can survive on surfaces for extended periods of time, the risk of microorganisms contaminating the physical environment and reaching an open wound is unknown. However, over the last two decades there has been an increasing awareness of the healthcare environment as a reservoir for pathogenic and MROs. Given the enclosed setting of an operating theatre, in which there are multiple and frequent contacts between the environmental surfaces, the surgical team and patient, there remains the potential to transmit an

TABLE 33.3 Examples of evidence-based surgical bundle interventions

Scrub/scout nurse
1. Removal of hair from the operating site should be avoided unless completely necessary. If the surgeon feels that hair at the surgical site should be removed it is recommended that clipping should be done as close to the commencement of the procedure; however, it should be done outside the operating room
2. Excessive theatre traffic and opening of the operating door increases airborne bacteria, increasing the risk of surgical site infection. A maximum number of door openings should be agreed upon for each speciality of surgery. Measures should be taken to ensure that door openings are kept within this number
3. Incise adhesive drapes, impregnated or not, should not be used for the purpose of preventing surgical site infection. However, they do offer additional benefits which may be considered important in practice
4. Changing of gloves prior to wound closure has been demonstrated as having a significant reduction in surgical site infection incidence

Anaesthetic nurse
1. Active warming via a warming device, as opposed to passive warming, should be used for patients undergoing a surgical procedure
2. Blood glucose levels for both diabetic and non-diabetic adult patients undergoing a surgical procedure should be closely monitored by the anaesthetic team with the aim of reducing surgical site infection
3. Education and monitoring of hand hygiene for anaesthetic staff has been identified as an area of improvement in the operating room. Strategic placement of alcohol-based hand rub and non-sterile gloves may support compliance

Source: Adapted from Proops EM. Implementing a surgical site infection care bundle: implications for perioperative practice. J Periop Nurs. 2019; 32(2):25-28.

organism of concern from the environment to a patient. Therefore, effective cleaning and disinfection of the operating theatre environment is essential.[102-104] Environmental cleaning is discussed in detail in Chapter 15; however, some examples of the range of cleaning requirements and procedures within the procedural environment are outlined in Table 33.4.

Air contamination: In the mid to late 19th century, Nightingale famously hypothesised that miasmas (a perceived gas-like substance) spread infection from wound to wound. During this same era, following Lister's demonstration of the importance of antisepsis, operating theatre design considered potential airborne transmission and sited theatres as far as possible from wards. The 1930s saw renewed interest in the air as a potential source of surgical wound infection. The earliest widely quoted study on the control of airborne bacteria and its influence on wound infection was not published until 1946 and reported the effects of a new system of ventilation in a room used for changing dressings in a burns unit.[106]

Today it is widely understood that the air in operating theatres and procedural areas may contain microorganisms, dust, aerosol, lint, squamous epithelial skin cells and respiratory droplets. The Australasian Health Facility Guidelines state that control of infection is influenced by the design and effectiveness of the air conditioning and ventilation systems. Thus, operating theatres and procedural areas should always be provided with high-quality air.[107] Ventilation systems for operating theatres are designed to:

- create thermal comfort for staff and patient

- maintain consistent air quality by removing aerosols and other particles from the air to reduce the risk of infection; and

- eliminate the transfer of air from one theatre or procedural room to another.

It is recommended that air supply passes through high-efficiency particulate air (HEPA) filters, to remove unwanted air particles. Around 20 air changes per hour are recommended as being optimal to dilute microorganisms generated in the operating theatre and to stop ingress from surrounding areas.[105] Various approaches

TABLE 33.4 Examples of cleaning procedures for operating theatres and procedural areas

Frequency	Responsible	Technique/product	Additional guidance/description

Before first procedure	Shared cleaning possible, peri-operative nursing/clinical staff and cleaning staff	Clean and disinfect:
		• horizontal surfaces
		  ◦ furniture
		  ◦ surgical lights
		  ◦ operating bed
		  ◦ stationary equipment
			Records of previous evening terminal clean required; if not or if no surgeries on the day prior, perform terminal clean (as below)

Before and after every procedure	Shared cleaning possible, peri-operative nursing/clinical staff and cleaning staff	Clean and disinfect: • high-touch surfaces (e.g. light switches, door handles) outside surgical field • any surface visibly soiled with blood or body fluids • all surfaces and noncritical equipment and the floor inside the surgical field	Remove all used linen and surgical drapes, waste (including used suction canisters, ¾ filled sharps containers), and kick buckets, for reprocessing or disposal Portable non-critical (e.g. compressed gas tanks, X-ray machine) equipment should be thoroughly cleaned and disinfected before and after each procedure
After last procedure (terminal clean)	Shared cleaning possible, peri-operative nursing/clinical staff and cleaning staff	Clean and disinfect: • all surfaces and non-critical equipment in the operating room • the entire floor • any surface visibly soiled with blood or body fluids • scrub and utility areas/sinks	Carefully move the operating table and any mobile equipment to make sure that the floor areas underneath are thoroughly cleaned and disinfected Clean and disinfect low-touch surfaces, (e.g. the insides of cupboards and ceilings/walls) on a scheduled basis (e.g. weekly)

Source: Adapted from Centers for Disease Control and Prevention. Environmental cleaning in resource limited settings: appendix b2 – cleaning procedure summaries for specialized patient areas. CDC; 2022.

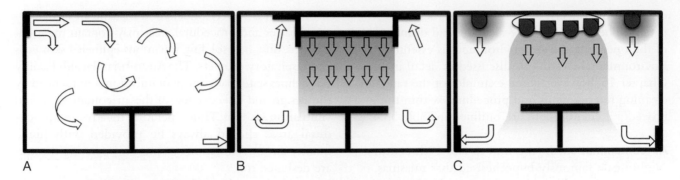

FIGURE 33.3 Diagram of three airflow principles: (a) turbulent mixing airflow; (b) laminar airflow; and (c) temperature-controlled airflow

Source: Alsved M, Civilis A, Ekolind P, Tammelin A, et al. Temperature-controlled airflow ventilation in operating rooms compared with laminar airflow and turbulent mixed airflow. J Hosp Infect. 2018;98:181-190.

to air handling within the theatre environment have been proposed and tested based on different principles. as demonstrated in Fig 33.3.[108-111]

In terms of reducing the numbers of microorganisms in the air, limiting the number of people in the theatre and the traffic in and out during a procedure have been identified as simple and effective strategies.[109-111]

CASE STUDY

Contaminated medical device: heater-cooler units

Within a theatre environment the risk of biofilm formation and transmission of infection from contaminated equipment via air was highlighted by an infection issue experienced worldwide and which was associated with the use of heater-cooler units during cardiac surgery. This case study demonstrates the infection risk within the confines of a closed intraoperative environment when a contaminated medical device is the source of an infection transmitted via aerosols.

Situation:

In 2011, cases of sterile site *Mycobacterium chimaera* (*M. chimaera*) infection were identified in patients undergoing open-chest cardiac surgery.[112-115] *M. chimaera* is a slow growing, non-tuberculosis mycobacterium (NTM). In the environment, it is commonly identified in biofilms, surface water, tap water and soil. Historically, it has been recognised as a cause of pulmonary and disseminated infections among patients who are immunocompromised, have

significant underlying structural lung disease or are susceptible to Mycobacterial infections.[113,114]

Hospitals worldwide including the United States, Canada, the United Kingdom, Switzerland, the Netherlands and Germany were reporting clustered outbreaks of *M. chimaera*.[112-118]

Solution:

An association was found between these cases and a particular model of heater-cooler unit (HCU), Stockert 3T, LivaNova (3T-HCU). At the time this model represented ~70% of HCUs in circulation globally. HCUs are commonly used during cardiac procedures that require extracorporeal cardiopulmonary function during surgery (cardiopulmonary bypass, or CPB). HCUs circulate water through heat exchangers and warm or cool blood passing through the CPB circuits.[112-114]

Based on the hypothesis that patients were infected by contaminated aerosols from the water tanks of HCUs, multiple independent investigations were undertaken to confirm the mode of transmission and identify the source of contamination. Environmental sampling of the hospital operating rooms and associated equipment cultured *M. chimaera* from hospital tap water and the water tanks of most models of HCU, as well as the water tanks of extracorporeal membrane oxygenation (ECMO) devices. Air sampling found contaminated aerosolised particles coming from the exhaust fan of the 3T-HCUs, but not other models.[112-114]

Examination of the 3T-HCUs identified breaches in the tank covers. When the HCU was in operation, contaminated aerosols were released through construction joints on the tank covers into the body of the HCU. These aerosols were then able to move from these areas to the outside environment via the cooling fan at the rear of the HCU.[114] HCUs may be positioned adjacent to the CBP pump, and the exhaust airflow from the HCU may be directed towards the operating field, thus contributing to the risk of *M. chimaera* infection. Laminar flow ventilation was insufficient to prevent aerosols containing *M. chimaera* from dispersing towards the surgical field.[113]

Upon confirmation that a single model of HCU was linked to all cases, and suspicion of a single point of contamination, environmental sampling at the manufacturing site was initiated, with positive *M. chimaera* samples recovered. According to the manufacturer, there may have been environmental mycobacteria present in HCUs manufactured prior to mid-August 2014 at the time of delivery to the hospitals.[113] Whole genome sequencing of *M. chimaera* isolates from infected patients, samples from the 3T-HCUs, other models of HCU, the manufacturing site and unrelated *M. chimaera* isolates from patient and environmental sources was undertaken. Phylogenetic analysis of these sequences found that the isolates from patients, contaminated machines and the LivaNova manufacturing site were the same distinct phylogenetic subgroup, with isolates from other models and unrelated sources more widely distributed in the phylogenetic tree. These findings strongly supported the hypothesis that the cases were related, with a point-source of the contamination being the manufacturing facility.[117]

Recommendations:

Recommended prevention and infection control measures for healthcare institutions include:[112,115]

1. changes in HCU disinfection protocols
2. removal of HCUs from operating rooms or replacement with other models
3. microbiologic testing of HCU water
4. retrospective review for case identification
5. notification of exposed patients
6. education of healthcare providers; and
7. obtaining modified consent from patients undergoing cardiac surgery going forward.

These recommendations come with a number of limitations. There is evidence that decontamination methods may fail, due to the disinfection tolerance of mycobacterial biofilms, and intensified cleaning may damage the HCUs, creating additional risks.[115,117] Removal of the HCU from the operating room may not be feasible due to theatre design. The HCU may be placed in an encasing with controlled air extraction, although it should be noted that these encasings may alter the functioning of the HCU. If HCU exhaust air cannot be reliably separated from the operating room, the HCU should be placed as far away from the

operating field as is possible, with the vent exhaust directed away from the patient and the surgical instruments. This should be considered a temporary measure as the risk of airborne transmission is not eliminated.[116]

Although some regulatory bodies have recommended routine microbiological testing of HCUs,[112,116] there is no standardisation of sampling or laboratory methods used and the degree of device contamination required to generate positive *M. chimaera* cultures from water and air samples is not known. *M. chimaera* is also slow growing, with laboratory cultures taking up to 8 weeks. During this time, potentially contaminated HCUs may still be in use, exposing more patients.[114] Surveillance through case identification is also inappropriate for IPC purposes as infection may take a long time to present. The maximum latency period reported between exposure and disease presentation is 4 years. Patients who may have been exposed to *M. chimaera* due to contaminated HCUs should continue to look for signs of potential infection, and keep in touch with their clinicians, for several years following surgery.[112,114]

Overall, the number of *M. chimaera* cases was low; however, the infection was often severe including endocarditis and disseminated infection, with significant morbidity and mortality.[115] This outbreak provides an example of external sources of contamination that may be present within the operating room, and highlights the importance of investigating and reporting unexplained, rare or unusual infection events. Without the reporting from hospitals worldwide, and the subsequent investigations, both in the hospital environment and the manufacturing site, the source of this outbreak may not have been identified.

33.4.2 Reusable medical devices

Disinfection and sterilisation processes are critical for safeguarding medical and surgical instruments against transmitting infectious pathogens to patients.[119] Examples of the failure to adequately disinfect and/or sterilise surgical instruments and medical devices include an outbreak in a UK hospital where 15 orthopaedic patients developed deep SSI following metal insertion. The subsequent investigation revealed post-sterilisation contamination as the cause of these SSIs.[120]

In another well-documented investigation in the USA, between 2012 and 2015, closed-channel duodenoscopes were linked to at least 25 different instances of antibiotic-resistant infections in at least 250 patients worldwide.[121] Transient bacteraemia following various types of endoscopic procedures are frequently detected but clinical infections are rare. The exceptions to this are peristomal infections following percutaneous endoscopic gastrostomy (PEG) and post-endoscopic retrograde cholangiopancreatography (ERCP) cholangitis.[6] A recent retrospective study reported a 21.9% infection rate following PEG placement.[122] ERCP has the highest rate of serious infections amongst endoscopic procedures and is associated with sepsis and occasional acute cholecystitis, liver abscess and infected pancreatic pseudocyst. Outbreaks of infections following ERCP suggest the major causes are:

- inadequate disinfection of the endoscope
- failure to rinse endoscope channels with alcohol at the end of a session and subsequent drying with forced air
- contamination of water; and
- contamination of disinfecting machines by Pseudomonas species.[6]

Infection transmitted by bronchoscopy is considered low. However, outbreaks have been reported due to lapses in cleaning, contamination, storage and maintenance of bronchoscopes. The risk of transmitting a blood-borne virus related to endoscopy procedures is ever present and requires adherence to prompt and meticulous endoscope cleaning to remove all visible traces of blood and proteinaceous material.[6]

Detailed discussion of the requirements for cleaning, disinfection and sterilisation of reusable medical devices (RMDs) and appropriate storage and handling is provided in Chapter 16. However, the relatively unique association between Creutzfeldt-Jakob disease (CJD) transmission and the theatre environment and biofilm formation on scopes and the use of Simethicone are worth mentioning here.

CJD is an invariably fatal human prion disease belonging to the transmissible spongiform encephalopathies. Although transmission of CJD in the healthcare setting is rare, there is a risk of a contaminated RMD becoming a mechanism for transmission. Minimisation strategies to reduce the risk of CJD transmission can include steps in confinement, containment, safe handling, disinfection, sterilisation and disposal of contaminated materials, tissues and instruments within the operating theatre environment.[123]

Biofilm formation is a process that may enhance the risk of pathogenic organism transmission with RMDs. Biofilm is formed when these bacteria adhere to a surface and secrete large amounts of extracellular polymeric substances to form a protective matrix or film around themselves. These biofilms protect the bacteria against physical (e.g. brushing, fluid flow) and chemical (e.g. disinfectant) forces, making the microorganisms more difficult to remove or destroy.[124] In endoscopy, reducing biofilm formation is a key infection prevention objective.[6] Water quality in an endoscopy unit is vital to reduce the risk of biofilm formation. Many systems to provide high levels of water quality include:

- oxidising agents and line and filter sterilisation— removal of biofilm
- physical agents such as hot water, and chemicals such as chlorine-releasing agents
- high-level disinfectants (HLD), reverse membrane osmosis, and ultraviolet irradiation systems.[125]

Modern automated flexible endoscope reprocessors (AFERs) when correctly designed, installed, maintained and used, provide reliable and effective HLD. AFERs reduce unpopular, time-consuming, arduous and repetitive manual tasks and occupational exposure to irritant chemicals.[6] However, concerns have been raised about the use of simethicone, a defoaming agent that enhances detailed views by reducing bubbles and improving visual assessment of mucosa, which is often delivered via an endoscope channel. Simethicone has been associated with a potential risk of biofilm formation. Currently, no published study has provided data showing that simethicone directly increases the risk of biofilm formation.[126] The Gastroenterological Society of Australia (GESA) states that given the evidence for improved quality of endoscopic imaging and polyp detection, and without definitive evidence of clinical adverse events over decades of use, continued use of simethicone, administered orally or through any endoscope channel, is considered appropriate.[6] (Table 33.5.)

33.4.3 Preparation of sterile instrument trays

Preparation of sterile items and instrument trays should be undertaken as close to the time of the surgery as possible to maintain sterility (Table 33.6). The requirements are that:
- each tray should have a checklist detailing all the instruments held on the tray, and which are to be checked against this list by the scrub and scout staff before each procedure
- each instrument should be inspected to make sure it is in good working order, intact, and free from any contaminants such as dried blood and body tissues; and
- if any damaged or contaminated instruments are present, the entire tray set is to be discarded.

TABLE 33.5 Recommendations on simethicone use

Recommendations on simethicone use
• The continued use of simethicone is considered reasonable as it improves mucosal inspection during gastroscopy and colonoscopy and likely facilitates adenoma detection at colonoscopy
• The smallest effective quantity of simethicone should be added to lavage fluid. A suggested, yet untested, concentration would be 2–3 mL of 120 mg/mL (i.e. 0.24%–0.36% [g/L]) simethicone added to 1 L of sterile water
• Simethicone may be administered orally or through any endoscope irrigating channel
• Strict adherence to instrument reprocessing protocols is essential. The importance of immediate bedside pre-clean endoscope decontamination that includes post-procedure flushing and prompt commencement of manual or machine cleaning is highlighted

Source: Adapted from Australian Commission on Safety and Quality in Health Care. NSQHS Standards 2021 Preventing and controlling infections standard: preventing and controlling infections standard. Sydney, ACSQHC, 2021.

TABLE 33.6 Setting up of the surgical instrument tray

Maintaining sterility of the tray
• Pre-set trays are either perforated or solid. Some trays are modified to house specialty-specific instruments. To maintain the sterility of the instruments, trays are often wrapped with a double lining of either reusable or disposable linen
• Outer layer is opened away from the body first then towards the body by the scout
• Inner sterile layer in the opposite direction, towards the body first then away. If using a trolley set-up system, the trolley should be prepared with a double layer of drapes large enough to cover the surface and sides of the trolley
• The instrument set should be prepared as close to the time of the surgery as possible to maintain sterility
• The scrub or scout should <u>not</u> lean over the instrument tray/trolley set
• The scout nurse should hand over any supplementary instruments and other necessary sundries avoiding any contamination either of the tray or the contents of the pack
• Sharps and heavy instruments should be passed to avoid piercing the tray linen and injury
• The scout should avoid splashes when pouring liquid solutions into tray pots presented by the scrub practitioner
• Wet linen can affect the tray's sterility
• The scrub is responsible for the instrument tray, and once prepared they should always stay with the tray

Source: Adapted from Hughes S, Mardell A. Oxford handbook of perioperative practice. Oxford University Publications, 2009.

Instrument and device traceability is an important element of patient safety and enhances investigation and management of potential infection transmission or outbreaks related to RMDs. A traceability process is required within Australia for critical and semi-critical equipment, instruments and devices. These tracking processes should be capable of identifying the patient, the procedure and RMDs that were used for the procedure.[119,128]

33.5 Surgical and endoscopy unit design

33.5.1 Operating theatre design

In the distant past, operations were carried out in hospital wards. By the 19th century, dedicated operating rooms were built primarily to facilitate teaching of surgery.[106] Historically, operating theatres were created as an amphitheatre with seats surrounding the upper tiers for students and onlookers, hence the continuation of the name theatre into modern times.[129] Despite constant innovation in surgical practice, however, moderately few advances have been made in operating theatre design.[130] According to the Australasian Health Infrastructure Alliance (AHIA), operating departments should be self-contained, physically distinct and an environmentally controlled area. In the past, operating departments were designed with clean and dirty zones with a separate corridor system, one for patients and one for clean and dirty goods. In modern surgical practice, operational policy and procedure (which includes infection prevention) plays a larger role in managing and controlling the different workflows and safety.[131] Infection control and operating staff should be involved early in the design phase; however, there is often a gap between expectations and budgetary constraints for completing builds (Table 33.7).[130]

TABLE 33.7 Operation department design considerations

Operation department design options
General principles for an operating unit to consider
• preoperative phase which includes patient management prior to the surgery or procedure to the point of transfer to the operating room
• intraoperative phase which includes surgery or procedures
• postoperative phase which begins with first stage recovery until a patient is transferred to an inpatient unit or discharged
Single corridor option
• an option where goods, clean and used and all pre- and post-operative patients traverse the one corridor
• option works well when the main circulation corridor is sufficiently wide to permit separation of the passage of patients on beds, goods and waste
• it can also provide an opportunity for natural light within operating rooms
Racetrack design
• this model aims to separate dirty from clean traffic by controlling the use of each corridor
• sterile stock and RMD storage is usually centralised in a sterile 'core' which prevents duplication of supplies and staff
• a central sterile core is a good option for operational efficiency; the use of this approach on a large number of operating rooms means that travel distances to recovery become significant
• first-stage recovery should be located so it is easily accessible from each operating room
• in large units, a sterile core option can be used but for a smaller number of rooms
Clusters and pods:
• a cluster of 2–4 operating rooms with a shared sterile stock store is a model often considered during the planning stages
• clusters of theatres are often grouped around surgical specialities
• the operating costs of providing dedicated staff and stock duplication in this arrangement of operating theatres need to be considered
• this model can add to the corridor space and circulation space and staff may prefer the extra space to be allocated to stock storage
Dedicated operating theatres with fixed equipment:
• this model dedicates particular operating rooms to specific types of surgery using fixed equipment for specialities such as urology with a dedicated table and drainage, and ophthalmology with ceiling-mounted microscopes
• this may be beneficial in larger units where work volumes justify this specialisation
• in smaller units the benefits of flexible use of operating rooms usually outweigh the benefits of specialisation
• fixed equipment can preclude the multifunctional use of the room and if a piece of equipment needs servicing or repair, the theatre cannot be used
• fixed radiology equipment is large and difficult to clean and may not be required for all cases

Source: Based on Ibrahim AM, Dimick JB, Joseph A. Building a better operating room: views from surgery and architecture. Annals of Surgery. 2017, 265(1): 34

Hybrid theatres with integrated imaging: The use of medical imaging in the operating theatre is an innovation that leads towards less invasive procedures. The list of imaging equipment is extensive and includes items such as image intensifiers, general X-ray, ultrasound, video laryngoscopes for tracheal intubation, stereotactic equipment, fixed imaging such as C-arms, angiography, computed tomography (CT), ultrasound and even magnetic resonate imaging (MRI).[131] Mobile versions of this equipment need to be 'parked' in dedicated locations when not in use. This can significantly impinge on space within an operating department, leading to a cramped and cluttered environment. Clutter can also reduce the ability to keep equipment clean, leading to dust and microbial contamination. In hybrid environments, the fixed imaging unit is best designed so that it can be parked away from the sterile field.[131] While advances in technology in theatre present benefits to patients, they also present challenges for IPC practices around maintaining a clean environment. Delicate and expensive equipment must be protected against damage from potentially corrosive disinfection chemicals. It is important that manufacturers' guidance is followed when cleaning and decontaminating delicate equipment, but this must not compromise the clean environment required within an operating theatre.

Robotic surgery: The benefits of robotic surgery include:
- improved mobility
- improved visibility
- an ergonomic position for the surgeon
- smaller surgical incisions
- less-invasive procedures; and
- less blood loss for the patient.[132]

Robotic use in surgery, similar to laparoscopic surgery, reduces the invasiveness of those surgical procedures. It offers greater precision and control than is possible with conventional techniques. Two broad types of systems are used. The first are large robotic units, such the 'DiVinci' which can be difficult to manoeuvre and require one dedicated operating theatre. The second broad type includes haptic robot arms—tactile-feel technology systems that are much more mobile.[131]

As robotic surgery evolves, procedures are increasingly being performed in general, spinal, orthopaedic, cardiac, gynaecological and neurological surgical specialties. The use of robotic surgery can lead to improved patient outcomes. However, robotic surgery has counterintuitively been associated with an increased risk of SSI. Reasons for this may be related to the difficulty of cleaning such complex instruments and equipment. Robotic-assisted procedures also involve a different workflow than non-robotic procedures, which can challenge personnel in space-constrained operating theatres with respect to maintaining good aseptic technique.[133]

33.5.2 Endoscopy unit design

Endoscopy units can also be purposely designed and constructed. Unfortunately, design is necessarily influenced by space constraints.[6] If bronchoscopy procedures are conducted, a negative-pressure air handling system is required in the bronchoscopy suite.[134] GESA suggests the following general principles around optimal infection prevention in endoscopy unit design:
- unidirectional patient flow from arrival in the unit to discharge, with no or minimal interaction between pre- and post-procedure patients

- endoscopic instruments and accessories should proceed in a unidirectional flow from clean areas to dirty areas, without contact between clean and dirty equipment
- pass-through automated flexible endoscope reprocessing systems to facilitate unidirectional flow of dirty to clean in the reprocessing area.[6]

In recent years, the ACSQHC has aimed to improve existing provisions for reprocessing of RMDs within endoscopy units, with a series of advisories detailing the requirements under AS/NZS 4187:2014.[135] In particular, the ACSQHC singles out the following requirements:
- segregation of clean and dirty activities
- adequate sterile stock storage with monitored temperature and humidity
- compliant cleaning, disinfecting and sterilising equipment; and
- monitoring and management of water quality.

As with the design of operating theatres and surgical departments, infection control and endoscopy staff should be involved early in the design phase in order to meet national standards and statutory authority requirements, such as those of the ACSQHC.[128]

Conclusion

The acquisition of an infection following surgery or an endoscopic procedure can affect a patient physically and emotionally, with an increased risk of morbidity and mortality. The financial burden of HAIs on health systems are also great.[1-5] This chapter has reviewed practices to reduce infection acquisition from surgical site skin preparation, aseptic technique, hand hygiene, surgical attire and PPE. Care bundles, surgical team responsibilities, environmental hygiene, the use of reusable medical devices (RMDs), and surgical and endoscopy unit design were reviewed for their impact on infection transmission. Surgical and endoscopy teams must employ the highest standards of contemporary IPC practices to protect patients from the risk of infection.[8,9]

Useful websites/resources

- Australian College of Perioperative Nurses (ACORN). https://www.acorn.org.au/
- Association of periOperative Registered Nurses (AORN). https://www.aorn.org/
- Australasian Health Facility Guidelines (AusHFG). https://healthfacilityguidelines.com.au/

References

1. Russo PL, Stewardson AJ, Cheng AC, Bucknall T, Mitchell BG. The prevalence of healthcare associated infections among adult inpatients at nineteen large Australian acute-care public hospitals: a point prevalence survey. Antimicrob Resist Infect Control. 2019:8(1):1-8.

2. Centers for Disease Control and Prevention. Surgical site infection (SSI) event. Procedure-associated module. CDC; 2022. [Accessed 19/05/2022.] Available from: https://www.cdc.gov/nhsn/pdfs/pscmanual/9pscSSIcurrent.pdf.

3. Australian Commission on Safety and Quality in Health Care. Approaches to surgical site infection surveillance. Sydney: ACSQHC, 2017.

4. Andersson AE, Bergh I, Karlsson J and Nilsson K. Patients' experiences of acquiring a deep surgical site infection: an interview study. Am J Infect Control. 2010;38:711–717.

5. Lee J, Singletary R, Schmader K, Anderson DJ, Bolognesi M and Kaye KS. Surgical site infection in the elderly following orthopaedic surgery. J Bone Joint Surg Am. 2006;88: 1705–1712.

6. Devereaux BM, Jones D, Wardle E. Infection prevention and control in endoscopy 2021. Melbourne: Gastroenterological Society of Australia, 2021.

7. The Lancet Gastroenterology Hepatology, Editorial. Scoping the problem: endoscopy-associated infections. Lancet Gastroenterol Hepatol. 2018;3(7):445.

8. Hughes S, Mardell A. Oxford handbook of perioperative practice. Oxford University Publications, 2009.

9. Herrin A, Loyola M, Bocian S, Diskey A, et al. Standard of infection prevention in the gastroenterology setting. Society of Gastroenterology Nurses and Associates, 2015. [Accessed 24/07/2022.] Available from: https://www.sgna.org/Portals/0/Education/PDF/Standards-Guidelines/Standard%20of%20Infection%20Prevention_FINAL.pdf.

10. Bishop WJ. The early history of surgery. London: Hale,1960.

11. Funk DJ, Parrillo JE, Kumar A. Sepsis and septic shock: a history. Crit Care Clin. 2009:25:83-101.

12. Larson E. A retrospective on infection control. Part 1: Nineteenth century: consumed by fire. Am J Infect Control. 1997:25(3);236-241.

13. Nuland SB. The doctors' plague: germs, childbed fever, and the strange story of Ignac Semmelweis. New York: WW Norton, 2003.

14. Pittet D, Boyce JM. Hand hygiene and patient care: pursuing the Semmelweis legacy. Lancet Infect Dis. 2001;1:9-20.

15. Pitt D, Aubin JM. Joseph Lister: father of modern surgery. Can J Surg. 2012;55(5):E8–E9.

16. Curran E. What can the early infection preventing pioneers teach infection prevention and control teams today? Infect Dis Health. 2022;27:105-11.

17. Yokoe, DS, Calssen D. Improving patient safety through infection control: a new healthcare imperative. Infect Control Hosp Epidemiol. 2008;29(S1):S3-S11

18. Dancer SJ, Stewart M, Coulombe C, Gregori A, Virdi M. Surgical site infections linked to contaminated surgical instruments. J Hosp Infect. 2012;81:231-238.

19. United States Senate Health, Education, Labor, and Pensions Committee, Patty Murray, Ranking Member. Preventable tragedies: superbugs and how ineffective monitoring of medical device safety fails patients. Minority Staff Report January 13, 2016. [Accessed 30/07/2022.] Available from: https://www.help.senate.gov/imo/media/doc/Duodenoscope%20Investigation%20FINAL%20Report.pdf.

20. Boyce JM. Best products for skin antisepsis. Am J Infect Control. 2019;47:A17−A22.

21. World Health Organization. Global guidelines for the prevention of surgical site infection. Geneva: WHO, 2016.

22. Dumville JC, McFarlane E, Edwards P, Lipp A, Holmes A, Liu Z. Preoperative skin antiseptics for preventing surgical wound infections after clean surgery. Cochrane Database Syst Rev. 2015;(4):CD003949.

23. Queensland Department of Health. Surgical skin disinfection guideline, version 3, October 2015. Queensland Government. [Accessed 05/07/2022.] Available from: https://www.health.qld.gov.au/__data/assets/pdf_file/0020/444422/skin-disinfection.pdf.

24. Rebar C, Bashaw M. Concepts of care for perioperative patients (chapter 9). In: Ignatavicius DD, Workman ML, Rebar CR, Heimgartner NM. Medical-surgical nursing: concepts for interprofessional collaborative care, tenth edition. Elsevier, 2021.

25. Webster J, Osborne S. Preoperative bathing or showering with skin antiseptics to prevent surgical site infection. Cochrane Database Syst Rev. 2012;(9):CD004985.

26. National Institute for Health and Care Excellence (NICE). Guideline: surgical site infections: prevention and treatment. NICE, 2019. [Accessed 05/07/2022.] Available from: https://www.nice.org.uk/guidance/ng125.

27. Hemani ML, Lepor H. Skin preparation for the prevention of surgical site infection: which agent is best? Rev Urology. 2009:11(4):190-195.

28. Anderson D, Podgorny K, Berrios-Torres S, et al. Strategies to prevent surgical site infections in acute care hospitals: 2014 update. Infect Control Hosp Epidemiol. 2014;35(6):605-27.

29. Barnett J. Surgical skin antisepsis preparation intervention guidelines. Health Quality and Safety Commission New Zealand, 2014. [Accessed 05/07/2022.] Available from: https://www.hqsc.govt.nz/assets/Our-work/Infection-Prevention-Control/Publications-resources/SSII-skin-antisepsis-preparation-intervention-guidelines-Feb-2014-v2.pdf.

30. Tanner J. Methods of skin antisepsis for preventing SSIs. Nursing Times. 2011;108(37):20-22.

31. Maiwald M, Chan E. The forgotten role of alcohol: a systematic review and meta-analysis of the clinical efficacy and perceived role of chlorhexidine in skin antisepsis. PLoS One. 2012;7(9).

32. Darouiche RO, Wall MJ, Itani KMF, Otterson MF, et al. Chlorhexidine-alcohol versus povidone-iodine for surgical-site antisepsis. N Engl J Med. 2010;362:18-26.

33. Peel TN, Cheng AC, Buising KL, Dowsey MM, Choong PFM. Alcoholic Chlorhexidine or Alcoholic Iodine Skin Antisepsis (ACAISA): protocol for cluster randomised controlled trial of surgical skin preparation for the prevention of superficial wound complications in prosthetic hip and knee replacement surgery. BMJ Open. 2014;4:e005424.

34. Medicines and Healthcare Products Regulatory Agency (MHRA). Chlorhexidine solutions: reminder of the risk of chemical burns in premature infants, 2014. [Accessed 05/07/2022.] Available from: https://www.gov.uk/drug-safety-update/chlorhexidine-solutions-reminder-of-the-risk-of-chemical-burns-in-premature-infants.

35. Weller BF. Encyclopedic dictionary of nursing and health care. London: Bailliere Tindall, 1997.

36. Rowley S, Clare S, Macqueen S, Molyneux R. ANTT v2: An updated practice framework for aseptic technique. Br J Nurs. 2010 (Intravenous Supplement),19(5):S5-S11.

37. Hart S. Using an aseptic technique to reduce the risk of infection. Nurs Standard. 2007;21(47):43-48.

38. Khan S, Shih T, Shih S, Khachemoune A. Reappraising elements of the aseptic technique in dermatology: a review. Dermatol Pract Concept. 2021;11(1):1-6.

39. Rowley S, Clare S. Right asepsis with ANTT® for infection prevention. In: Moureau NL, ed. Vessel health and preservation: the right approach for vascular access. Springer International Publishing, 2019:147-162.

40. Clare S, Rowley S. Implementing the Aseptic Non Touch Technique (ANTT®) clinical practice framework for aseptic technique: a pragmatic evaluation using a mixed methods approach in two London hospitals. J Infect Prev. 2017;19(1):6-15.

41. National Health and Medical Research Council (NHMRC). Australian guidelines for the prevention and control of infection in healthcare. Canberra: NHMRC, 2019.

42. World Health Organization. Guidelines on hand hygiene in health care. First global patient safety challenge: clean care is safe care. Geneva: WHO, 2009.

43. Wenzel, RP. The antibiotic pipeline – challenges, costs, and values. N Eng J Med. 2004:351(6):523-526.

44. Ayliffe GAJ, English M. Hospital infection: from miasmas to MRSA. Cambridge: Cambridge University Press, 2003.

45. Story, P. (1952). Testing skin disinfectants. BMJ. Nov 22: 1128-1130.

46. Lowbury EJL, Lilly HA. Disinfection of the hands of surgeons and nurses. BMJ. 1960;14:1445-1450.

47. Lowbury EJL, Lilly HA, Bull JP. Disinfection of hands: removal of transient organisms. BMJ. 1964;2:230-233.

48. O'Farrell DA, et al. Evaluation of the optimal hand-scrub duration prior to total hip arthroplasty. J Hosp Infect.1994;26:93-98.

49. Tanner J, Swarbrook S, Stuart J. Surgical hand antisepsis to reduce surgical site infection. Cochrane Database Syst Rev. 2008; (1):CD004288.

50. Widmer AF. Surgical hand hygiene: scrub or rub? J Hosp Infect. 2013;83(1):S35-S39.

51. Widmer AF, Pittet D, Voss A, Boyce J, Allegranzi B, Nthumba P, Rotter M. Surgical hand preparation: state-of-the-art. Hosp Infect Soc. 2010;74(2):112-122.

52. ACORN Standards Applied to Practice (ASAP). Why shouldn't hand scrub and alcohol-based surgical hand rub be used sequentially? October 2020.] Available from: [Accessed 06/06/2022.] Available from: https://www.acorn.org.au/asap.

53. Moola S. ACORN Standard S11: Perioperative attire. [Accessed 06/06/2022.] Available from: https://www.acorn.org.au/standards.

54. Britt RC. The glove made from love: a history of surgical attire. Am Surg. 2019;85(9):935-938.

55. Woodhead K, Taylor EW, Bannister G, Chesworth T, Hoffman P, Humphreys H. Behaviours and rituals in the operating theatre. A report from the Hospital Infection Society Working Party on infection control in operating theatres. J Hosp Infect. 2002;51(4):241-255.

56. Mitchell NJ, Gamble DR. Clothing design for operating room personnel. Lancet. 1974;1133-1136.

57. McHugh SM, Corrigan MA, Hill ADK, Humphreys H. Surgical attire, practices and their perception in the prevention of surgical site infection. Surgeon. 2014;12:47-52.

58. Braswell ML, Spruce L. Implementing AORN recommended practices for surgical attire. AORN J.2012;95(1):122-137.

59. Amirfeyz R, Tasker A, Ali S, Bowker K, Blom A. Theatre shoes - a link in the common pathway of postoperative wound infection? Ann R Coll Surg Engl. 2007;89(6):605-608.

60. Gilmour D. Considerations for gown and drape selection in the United Kingdom. AORN Journal. 2010;92(4):461-465.

61. Garibaldi RA, Maglio S, Lerer T, Becker D, Lyons R. Comparison of nonwoven and woven gown and drape fabric to prevent intraoperative wound contamination and postoperative infection. Am J Surg. 1986;152(5):505-509.

62. Baykasoglu A, Dereli T, Yilankirkan N. Application of cost/benefit analysis for surgical gown and drape selection: a case study. Am J Infect Control. 2009:37:215-226.

63. Moylan JA, Kennedy BV. The importance of gown and drape barriers in the prevention of wound infection. Surg Gynecol Obstet. 1980;151(4):465-470.

64. Tanner J, Parkinson H. Double gloving to reduce surgical cross-infection. Cochrane Database Syst Rev. 2006;(3): CD003087.

65. Spirling LI, Daniela IR. William Stewart Halsted — surgeon extraordinaire: a story of 'drugs, gloves and romance'. J R Soc Promot Health. 2002;122:122-124.

66. Blair DM. First use of gloves in surgery. Br Med J. 1933;1:632.

67. Eisen DB. Surgeon's garb and infection control: what's the evidence? J Am Acad Dermatol. 2010;64(1):960-20.

68. Enz A, Kamaleddine I, Grib J, et al. Is single gloving still acceptable? Investigation and evaluation of damages on sterile latex gloves in general surgery. J. Clin. Med. 2021;10:3887.

69. Kobayahi M, Tsujimoto H, Takahata R, et al. Association between the frequency of glove change and the risk of blood and body fluid exposure in gastrointestinal surgery. World J Surg. 2020;44:3695–3701.

70. Tunevall TG. Postoperative wound infections and surgical face masks: a controlled study. World J Surg. 1991;15:383–387.

71. Ritter MA, Eitzen H, French ML, Hart JB. The operating room environment as affected by people and the surgical face mask. Clin Orthop Relat Res. 1975:111:147-150.

72. Humphreys H, Russell AJ, Marshall RJ, Ricketts VE, Reeves DS. The effect of surgical theatre head-gear on air bacterial counts. J Hosp Infect. 1991;9(3):175-180.

73. Bergman BR, Hoborn J, Nachemson AL. Patient draping and staff clothing in the operating theatre: a microbiological study. Scand J Infect Dis. 1985;17:421-426.

74. Mclure HA, Talboys CA, Yentis M, Azadian BS. Surgical face masks and downward dispersal of bacteria. Anaesthesia. 1998;53:624–626.

75. Zhiqing L, Yongyun C, Wenxiang C, et al. Surgical masks as source of bacterial contamination during operative procedures. J Orthop Translat. 2018;14:57-59.

76. Vincent M, Edwards P. Disposable surgical face masks for preventing surgical wound infection in clean surgery. Cochrane Database Syst Rev. 2016;(4): CD002929.

77. Ogo N, Foran P. The effectiveness and compliance of surgical face mask wearing in the operating suite environment: an integrated review. J Periop Nurs. 2020;33(4):e11-e18.

78. Webster J, Croger S, Lister, C, et al. Use of face masks by non-scrubbed operating room staff: a randomized controlled trial. ANZ J Surg. 2010;80(3):169-173.

79. Hemsworth S, Selwood K, van Saene R, Pizer B. Does the number of exogenous infections increase in pediatric oncology patients when sterile surgical gloves are not worn for accessing central venous access devices? Eur J Oncol Nurs. 2007;11:442-447.

80. So E, Juels CA, Seidenstricker C, Walker R, Scott RT. Postoperative infection rates after total ankle arthroplasty: a comparison with and without the use of a surgical helmet system. J Foot Ankle Surg. Article-in-press, 2021.

81. Blomgren G, Hambraeus A, Malmborg AS. The influence of the total body exhaust suit on air and wound contamination in elective hip-operations. J Hosp Infect. 1983;4:257.

82. Vijaysegaran P, Knibbs LD, Morawska L, Crawford RW. Surgical space suits increase particle and microbiological emission rates in a simulated surgical environment. J Arthroplasty. 2018;33(5):1524-1529.

83. Hooper GJ, Rothwell AG, Frampton C, Wyatt MC. Does the use of laminar flow and space suits reduce early deep infection after total hip and knee replacement?: the ten-year results of the New Zealand Joint Registry. J Bone Joint Surg Br. 2011;93:85-90.

84. Rahardja R, Morrie AJ, Hooper GJ, Grae N, Frampton CM. Surgical helmet systems are associated with a lower rate of prosthetic joint infection after total knee arthroplasty: combined results from the New Zealand Joint Registry and Surgical Site Infection Improvement Programme. J Arthroplasty. 2022;37(5):930-935.

85. Temmesfeld MJ, Jakobsen RB, Grant P. Does a surgical helmet provide protection against aerosol transmitted disease? Acta Orthopaedica. 2020;91(5):538-542.

86. McCarron K. Understanding care bundles. Nurs Made Easy. 2011;9(2):30-33.

87. Proops EM. Implementing a surgical site infection care bundle: implications for perioperative practice. J Periop Nurs. 2019;32(2):25-28.

88. Resar R, Pronovost P, Haraden C, Simmonds T, Rainey T, Nolan T. Using a bundle approach to improve ventilator care processes and reduce ventilator-associated pneumonia. Jt Comm J Qual Patient Saf. 2005;31(5):243-248.

89. DePalo VA, McNicoll L, Cornell M, Rocha JM, Adams L, Pronovost PJ. The Rhode Island ICU collaborative: a model for reducing central line-associated bloodstream infection and ventilator-associated pneumonia statewide. Qual Saf Health Care. 2010;19:555-561.

90. Pronovost PJ, Watson SR, Goeschel CA, Hyzy RC, Berenholtz SM. Sustaining reductions in central line–associated bloodstream infections in Michigan intensive care units: a 10-year analysis. Am J Med Qual. 2016;31(3): 197–202.

91. World Health Organization. WHO guidelines for safe surgery 2009: safe surgery saves lives. Geneva: WHO, 2009.

92. Gawande A. The checklist manifesto: how to get things right. London: Profile Books, 2011.

93. National Library of Medicine, National Institutes of Health. Greek medicine. [Accessed 29/07/2022.] Available from: https://www.nlm.nih.gov/hmd/greek/greek_oath.html.

94. NOVA. The Hippocratic Oath: modern version. [Accessed 29/07/2022.] Available from: https://www.pbs.org/wgbh/nova/doctors/oath_modern.html.

95. Medical Board APHRA. Good medical practice: a code of conduct for doctors in Australia, October 2020. Canberra: Australian Government, 2020. [Accessed 29/07/2022.] Available from: https://www.medicalboard.gov.au/Codes-Guidelines-Policies/Code-of-conduct.aspx.

96. Hamlin L. From theatre to perioperative: a brief history of early surgical nursing. J Periop Nurs. 2020;33(4):3.

97. Australian College of Perioperative Nurses. Nursing roles. ACORN, 2022. [Accessed 26/07/2022.] Available from: https://www.acorn.org.au/Nursing-roles.

98. Duff J, Bowen L, Gumuskaya O. What does surgical conscience mean to perioperative nurses: an interpretive description. Collegian. 2022;29(2):147-153.

99. Chambers KL. Patient safety equals: aseptic technique, surgical conscience and time out. Surgical Technologist. March 2013:109-119.

100. Ward SF. Infection prevention and the surgical conscience. Surg Serv Management. 2000;6(3):6.

101. Farley M. Surgical conscience and its role in patient safety and care. ORNAC J. 2022;40(1):15-20.

102. Ledwoch K, Dancer SJ, Otter JA, Kerr K, Roposte D, Rushton L, et al. Beware biofilm! Dry biofilms containing bacterial pathogens on multiple healthcare surfaces; a multi-centre study. J Hosp Infect. 2018;100(3):e47-e56.

103. Mitchell BG, Dancer SJ, Anderson M, Dehn E. Risk of organism acquisition from prior room occupants: a systematic review and meta-analysis. J Hosp Infect. 2015;91(3):211-217.

104. Munoz-Price LS, Birnbach DJ, Lubarsky DA, Arheart KL, et al. Decreasing operating room environmental pathogen contamination through improved cleaning practice. Infect Control Hosp Epidemiol. 2012;33(9):897-904.

105. Centers for Disease Control and Prevention. Environmental cleaning in resource limited settings: appendix b2 – cleaning procedure summaries for specialized patient areas. CDC, 2022. [Accessed 29/07/2022.] Available from: https://www.cdc.gov/hai/prevent/resource-limited/special areas.html#anchor_1585592126579.

106. Stacey A, Humphrey H. A UK historical perspective on operating theatre ventilation. J Hosp Infect. 2002;52:77-80.

107. Australasian Health Infrastructure Alliance. Australasian Health Facility Guidelines Part D - infection prevention and control. 2015 (Update November 2020). Australasian Health Infrastructure Alliance, 2020.

108. Alsved M, Civilis A, Ekolind P, Tammelin A, et al. Temperature-controlled airflow ventilation in operating rooms compared with laminar airflow and turbulent mixed airflow. J Hosp Infect. 2018;98:181-190.

109. Ayliffe GAJ. Role of the environment of the operating suite in surgical wound infection. Rev Infect Dis. 1991; 13(suppl):S800–S804.

110. Sehulster LM, Chinn RYW, Arduino MJ, Carpenter J, et al. Guidelines for environmental infection control in health-care facilities. Recommendations from CDC and the Healthcare Infection Control Practices Advisory Committee (HICPAC). (Updated 2019.) Chicago IL; American Society for Healthcare Engineering/American Hospital Association, 2004.

111. Roth JA, Juchler F, Dangel M, Eckstein FS, et al. Frequent door openings during cardiac surgery are associated with increased risk for surgical site infection: a prospective observational study. CID. 2019;69 290-294.

112. Centers for Disease Control and Prevention. Non-tuberculous Mycobacterium (NTM) infections and heater-cooler devices. CDC, 2015.

113. Haller S, Höller C, Jacobshagen A, Hamouda O, Sin MA, Monnet DL, et al. Contamination during production of heater-cooler units by Mycobacterium chimaera potential cause for invasive cardiovascular infections: results of an outbreak investigation in Germany, April 2015 to February 2016. 2016;21(17):30215.

114. Hasse B, Hannan MM, Keller PM, Maurer FP, Sommerstein R, Mertz D, et al. International Society of Cardiovascular Infectious Diseases Guidelines for the diagnosis, treatment and prevention of disseminated Mycobacterium chimaera infection following cardiac surgery with cardiopulmonary bypass. 2020;104(2):214-235.

115. Garvey M, Ashford R, Bradley C, Bradley C, Martin T, Walker J, et al. Decontamination of heater–cooler units associated with contamination by atypical mycobacteria. J Hosp Infect. 2016;93(3):229-234.

116. Mertz D, Macri J, Hota S, Amaratunga K, Davis I, Johnston L, et al. Response to alert on possible infections with Mycobacterium chimaera from contaminated heater-cooler devices in hospitals participating in the Canadian Nosocomial Infection Surveillance Program (CNISP). 2018;39(4): 482-484.

117. Schreiber PW, Kuster SP, Hasse B, Bayard C, Rüegg C, Kohler P, et al. Reemergence of Mycobacterium chimaera in heater–cooler units despite intensified cleaning and disinfection protocol. 2016;22(10):1830.

118. van Ingen J, Kohl TA, Kranzer K, Hasse B, Keller PM, Szafrańska AK, et al. Global outbreak of severe Mycobacterium chimaera disease after cardiac surgery: a molecular epidemiological study. 2017;17(10):1033-1041.

119. Standards Australia and Standards New Zealand. AS/NZS 4187: 2014 Reprocessing of reusable medical devices in health service organisations (incorporating Amendment No. 1 and 2). Sydney; Standards Australia, 2014.

120. Dancer SJ, Stewart M, Coulombe C, Gregori A, Virdi M. Surgical site infections linked to contaminated surgical instruments. J Hosp Infect. 2012;81:231-238.

121. United States Senate Health, Education, Labor, and Pensions Committee, Patty Murray, Ranking Member. Preventable tragedies: superbugs and how ineffective monitoring of medical device safety fails patients. Minority Staff Report. January 13, 2016. [Accessed 30/07/2022.] Available from https://www.help.senate.gov/imo/media/doc/Duodenoscope%20Investigation%20FINAL%20Report.pdf.

122. Khashab MA, Chithadi KV, et al. Antibiotic prophylaxis for GI endoscopy. Gastrointest Endosc. 2015;81:81-89.

123. Department of Health and Aged Care. Creutzfeldt–Jakob disease – infection control guidelines, 2013. [Accessed 31/07/2022.] Available from: https://www.health.gov.au/diseases/creutzfeldt-jakob-disease-cjd?utm_source=health.gov.au&utm_medium=callout-auto-custom&utm_campaign=digital_transformation.

124. Johani K, Hu H, Santos L, et al. Determination of bacterial species present in biofilm contaminating the channels of clinical endoscopes. Infect Dis Health. 2018;23:189-196.

125. Australasian Health Infrastructure Alliance. Australasian health facility guidelines. Procedure room – endoscopy, 2018. Australasian Health Infrastructure Alliance.

126. Alfa MJ, Singh H. Impact of wet storage and other factors on biofilm formation and contamination of patient-ready endoscopes: a narrative review. Gastrointest Endosc. 2020; 91: 236-247.

127. Devereaux BM, Taylor ACF, Athan E, et al. Simethicone use during gastrointestinal endoscopy: position statement of the Gastroenterological Society of Australia. J Gastroenterol Hepatol. 2019;34:2086-2089.

128. Australian Commission on Safety and Quality in Health Care. NSQHS Standards 2021 Preventing and controlling infections standard: preventing and controlling infections standard. Sydney: ACSQHC, 2021. [Accessed 30/07/2022.] Available from: https://www.safetyandquality.gov.au/standards/nsqhs-standards/preventing-and-controlling-infections-standard.

129. Wengensteen OH, Wengensteen SD. The surgical amphitheatre, history of its origins, functions, and fate. Surgery. 1975;77(3):403-418.

130. Ibrahim AM, Dimick JB, Joseph A. Building a better operating room: views from surgery and architecture. Annals of Surgery. 2017;265(1):34.

131. Australasian Health Infrastructure Alliance. Australasian health facility guidelines part b - health facility briefing and planning 0520 – sterile supply unit (version 4). 2010, Australasian Health Infrastructure Alliance.

132. Hou Y, Hu Y, Song W, Zhang J, Luo Q, Zhou Q. Surgical site infection following minimally invasive lobectomy: Is robotic surgery superior? Cancer Medicine. 2022;11: 2233–2243.

133. Liu WP, Reaugamornrat S, Sorger JM, Siewerdsen JH, et al. Intraoperative image-guided transoral robotic surgery: pre-clinical studies. Int J Med Robot. 2015;11(2) 256-267.

134. Australasian Health Infrastructure Alliance. Australasian health facility guidelines. procedure room – endoscopy, 2018. Australasian Health Infrastructure Alliance, 2018.

135. Australian Commission on Safety and Quality in Health Care. Reprocessing of reusable medical devices in health service organisations, AS18/07 V.8.0. Sydney: ACSQHC, 2021. [Accessed 31/07/2022.] Available from: https://www.safetyandquality.gov.au/sites/default/files/2021-07/nsqhs_standards_advisory_as1807_july_2021.pdf.

CHAPTER 34

Infection prevention and control in dentistry practice

Dr ROSLYN FRANKLIN[i]

Dr HERDEZA VERZOSA[ii]

Dr TONY SKAPETIS[ii]

Chapter highlights

- Dental healthcare professionals (DHPs) and staff require knowledge about potential infectious diseases to be able to protect themselves and their patients in the dental practice setting
- Infection can be transmitted in the dental practice setting via four main pathways: contact, droplet, airborne and a vehicle
- There is limited evidence of transmission of pathogens in dental practice settings due to lack of healthcare-associated infection (HAI) surveillance
- Dental procedures increase the risk of microorganism transmission and to minimise this risk, standard and transmission-based precautions (TBP) are applied
- Dental practice settings should implement a written, comprehensive IPC program to minimise the risk of HAIs among patients, and injuries and illness among DHPs and staff

i   Amalgamate 2020 Pty Ltd, Bunbury, WA
ii Westmead Centre for Oral Health, Westmead, NSW

Introduction

The primary purpose of infection prevention and control (IPC) in the dental practice setting is to eliminate the risk of cross-contamination and the risk of healthcare-associated infections (HAIs) among patients and dental healthcare professionals (DHPs) before, during and after the provision of dental treatment services. The safe delivery of dental treatment requires optimal IPC education to all within dentistry.

This section begins by describing IPC within the dental setting and includes a historical overview and the effect of hepatitis B and HIV/AIDS on IPC development. This is followed by a summary of the dental workforce involved with IPC, the regulatory environment and the practice settings in which dental care is delivered.

34.1 Dentistry and dental practice settings

Dental healthcare professionals are exposed to many occupational hazards and are routinely at an increased risk of cross-infection while providing dental treatment to their patients. DHPs provide a wide range of treatments from simple oral examinations, tooth cleaning and tooth restorations to implant surgery and extensive maxillofacial surgery. Dental practices have a rapid turnover of patients, and it is not uncommon for a general dentist to see 10 or more patients per day. Dental procedures and treatments vary and range in complexity, bringing varying degrees of cross-contamination risk. Unique to the dental practice setting is the close and sustained proximity between the patient and the DHP. Regular and repeated exposure to high concentrations of splatter and aerosols from the patient's saliva, blood and respiratory secretions are generated during the use of dental rotary instruments and ultrasonic scalers as well as during surgical procedures, exposing DHPs and their clinical support staff to a wide range of potentially infectious microorganisms.

Dental healthcare professionals have professional, legal and ethical obligations to meet for their patients, staff and the public. The management of risks associated with the provision of treatment in dentistry is directed at reducing, to an acceptable level, the probability that an infection could be transmitted. Management and control of the risk of cross-infection in the dental practice setting is the subject of this chapter.

34.1.1 A history of Australian dental infection control

Infection prevention and control in dentistry is still a relatively new science. Until the early 1980s, basic infection control information for the DHP was based upon the knowledge of older professionals, trained dental assistants, dental supply company personnel, teachings from universities and state-based guidelines. It was only with the emergence of certain infectious diseases and an accompanying realisation that there was a risk of cross-infection in the dental practice setting that dental-practice-specific IPC recommendations were first published in the 1980s.[1,2] Until the mid-to-late 1980s, most DHPs were 'wet fingered' (an informal term for bare hands), as gloves (and mask and protective eyewear) were not standard (Figs 34.1, 34.2).

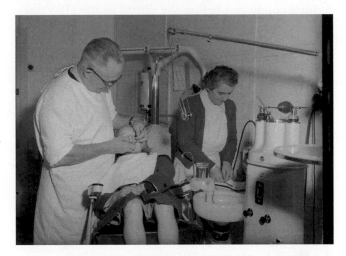

FIGURE 34.1 A typical dental practice surgery room in 1952
Source: https://purl.slwa.wa.gov.au/slwa_b1921972_1

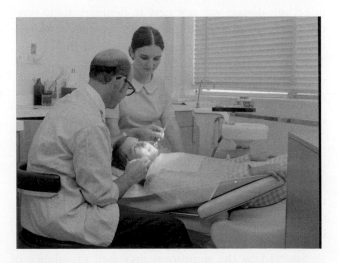

FIGURE 34.2 A typical dental practice surgery room in 1969
Source: https://purl.slwa.wa.gov.au/slwa_b2433566_1

Reusable dental equipment was sterilised in boiling water or via the common method of 'cold sterilisation', in which equipment was placed in disinfectant solutions. The patient's medical history provided the only means of identifying infectious patients.

The recognition of the potential for disease transmission in the dental practice setting was only given cursory attention. Even though the well-established principles and practices of aseptic techniques were practised until the mid to late-1980s, DHPs were at risk of catching certain infectious diseases. Dental healthcare professionals have a significant risk since dental treatment involves the use of sharp instruments. Blood and saliva often present a hazard, especially when the skin on hands is cut or cracked. Diseases such as herpetic whitlow, caused by infection with herpes simplex virus (HSV), and hepatitis B (HBV) are well known. Studies conducted before the arrival of the HBV vaccine indicated many dentists and oral surgeons had serologic evidence of past or current HBV infection several fold higher than the general population. Several clusters of HBV transmission between DHPs and patients were reported.[3-7]

The emergence of various pathogens, including HBV and hepatitis C (HCV), human immunodeficiency virus (HIV) and SARS-CoV-2 in the last 50 years led to a series of dental infection control protocols being developed by various dental professional bodies and government agencies around the world and in Australia.

The emergence of hepatitis B virus: The emergence of the blood-borne virus HBV in the mid-1960s generated an initial concern among healthcare workers about cross-infection. Although concern over infectious disease was not new in dentistry, there was no way to avoid exposure and DHPs appeared to take their chances with perhaps little worry. In the early 1970s, DHPs began to realise the potential for cross-infection in the dental practice setting and promoted some change to everyday IPC practices in dental practice settings. Suggestions and recommendations were put forth that advocated various barrier protections, such as gloves, gowns, surgical masks and protective eyewear, when dealing with infectious patients.[1,8] Awareness started to grow that high numbers of DHPs, including specialists, had evidence of prior HBV infection and recognition that some DHPs might be asymptomatic carriers of HBV.[9-11]

Spurred by the significant increased prevalence of HBV cases in the Australian community, a reappraisal

of the current approach to dental IPC ensued. The National Health and Medical Research Council (NHMRC) produced the first of a series of documents aimed explicitly at DHPs called 'Hepatitis B and Dentists' in 1984.[2] This national document was the first to provide practical information about HBV's risk to dentists, routine and special precautions to be taken and heavily promoted protection of DHPs through vaccination.[1,12-16]

At this time, IPC measures employed hinged on the basis that a patient was either infectious, in a designated high-risk group or non-infectious. For the non-infectious patient, the recommendation was that hands should be washed thoroughly before and after treating patients, but if blood exposure was anticipated, gloves should be worn. More stringent measures were employed if the patient fell into the infectious category—such as wearing full PPE, a gown, cap, surgical mask and eye protection.

Hepatitis B—a personal view by David Robert Booth who acquired hepatitis B from a patient[17]

'The patient ... suffered a Le Fort I fracture of his maxilla and a fractured mandible. The patient showed no signs of acute hepatitis ... but his serology showed he was hepatitis B-antigen positive.

'During the operation to wire Gunning splints in place, I pricked my finger with a wire. I hardly felt it, but there was blood inside the glove after the operation.'

The emergence of human immunodeficiency virus (HIV/AIDS): The human immunodeficiency virus is a blood-borne virus first recognised in 1981. HIV may be transmitted by direct contact with blood or other body substances, through non-intact skin or inoculation and can cause a severe, life-threatening disease called acquired immune deficiency syndrome (AIDS).[18]

While advances in IPC practices and the production of various IPC guidelines had been made over the past decade, it was only due to the AIDS epidemic's arrival in the 1980s that a paradigm shift took place in everyday infection control practices in dental settings towards comprehensive, proactive practices.[2,19,20] This disease captured the attention of the dental profession and challenged DHPs to practise in a safer manner.

The official recognition by the Centers for Disease and Control and Prevention (CDC) in 1987 that all blood and body fluid precautions be consistently used for all patients, regardless of their blood-borne infectious status, was a new approach. This extension of precautions—applied universally to all persons—was known as *universal precautions*.[19,21]

In 1990 the CDC announced the first transmission of HIV from a healthcare worker, a dentist, to a patient which brought dentistry into the spotlight. When Kimberly Bergalis, a young university student, was diagnosed as HIV-positive, subsequent investigations led the CDC to confirm the most likely source of her infection was her dentist, Dr David Acer, who had previously been diagnosed with AIDS. The CDC subsequently reported a further five patients had been infected with HIV by Dr Acer.[22,23]

The real significance of the HIV virus was the awareness it raised through the dental profession. Updated recommendations for infection control practices for dentistry were continuously released and updated by the CDC to deal with the HIV virus and equipped DHPs and staff to deal more effectively with other pathogens, such as HBV and HCV.[24,25]

In the 1990s in Australia, there were still no national guidelines, but rather a collection of guidelines developed by some states, the NHMRC, the Australian National Council on AIDS, and the national dental professional body, the Australian Dental Association (ADA).[26-30] It appears compliance with various guidelines was largely voluntary.

At the end of 1993, the New South Wales Government announced four HIV infection cases had apparently been acquired during minor surgery at an office-based medical practice of a general surgeon.[13] The resulting federal government national review of existing infection control guidelines produced the first, single, non-hospital-setting infection control guidelines in 1994.[31] While there was now a single, national guideline specifically written for office practices, it was written as a companion volume to four of the other current guidelines.[32-35] Other sources of information were available from the ADA.[36]

In 1996, the two-year-old national office practice guide was replaced with another single national guideline that now incorporated hospital and non-hospital settings.[18,37-39] This was particularly important as it was the first time nationally agreed guidelines on IPC had been presented in one single reference. Also, a change in terminology from *universal precautions* to *standard precautions* with *additional precautions* was adopted and incorporated, reflecting the terminology adopted by the CDC in 1996. However, the guidelines concentrated mainly on the principles of infection control rather than a set of guidelines on which to base dental practice protocols.

In 2008, the ADA produced the first, specific dental IPC guidelines.[40-42] At that time, the ADA had no regulatory or enforcement powers and could only make recommendations that may not be accepted or implemented. In 2010, that changed when the Dental Board of Australia included the latest edition of the ADA IPC guidelines as one of three key reference documents in its policies and guidelines.[43]

The 2020 COVID-19 pandemic led to another paradigm shift in everyday IPC practices.[44] During the early stages of the pandemic, challenges on how to operate safely for DHPs, staff and patients emerged due to the ongoing uncertainty about the risk of transmission of this new respiratory-based disease. Review of existing IPC practices in the dental practice setting were undertaken and modifications suggested based on current evidence. Given concerns about aerosol generation, restrictions on all dental treatment across Australia was rapidly implemented and routine dental care was severely limited.[45-47] Resumption of full dental care, including aerosol-generating procedures (AGP), was contingent on risk management by individual practices and subject to enhanced IPC procedures such as screening protocols, plastic screening barriers in waiting rooms, enhanced PPE, introduction of air distribution and filtration systems, and enhanced environmental cleaning practices (Table 34.1).

34.1.2 The dental workforce

A broad group of DHPs and staff, the dental workforce, is involved in the delivery of oral health care. The dental workforce includes five divisions who are formally registered and regulated: dentists, dental prosthetists, oral health therapists, dental hygienists and dental therapists.[48] Other members of the workforce include dental technicians, dental assistants and receptionists, who are not registered.

To practise dentistry, all dental practitioners are required to register with the Dental Board of Australia (DBA). Once registered, practitioners can practise Australia-wide.[49] In 2019, there were just over 24,000 registered dental practitioners.[48]

Dental assistants: Dental assistants are an essential member of the staff and play a central role in IPC. Responsibilities are varied and include direct contact

TABLE 34.1 IPC dental history timeline

1981	HIV recognised.
1981	First specific dental IPC guidelines published by NHMRC
1984	NHMRC publishes *Hepatitis B and Dentists* due to increased HBV community cases; focused on selective precautions for high-risk patients, DHP immunisation, autoclave or disinfection of reusable instruments
1987	NHMRC publishes *Guidelines for Dental Treatment of Patients with Infectious Diseases*; focused on glutaraldehyde disinfectant for environmental cleaning, plastic barriers, single use items, and double gloving
1987	CDC introduces 'Universal Precautions' against blood-borne diseases; recommends gloves, surgical masks and protective eyewear, rubber dam, high volume evacuation, heat sterilised handpiece
1988	NHMRC publishes *Hepatitis B and Clinical Dental Practice*; recommended routine wearing of PPE, including glove use, additional selective precautions for HBV-positive patients, heat sterilisation preferred over chemical means, promoted HBV vaccination
1990	The tragic story appears of 22-year-old Kimberly Bergalis, who contracted HIV from her dentist, and concerns about infection control in dentistry become public news
1996	NHMRC adopts terms 'standard precautions' and 'additional precautions'; practices used in the treatment of every patient regardless of infection status
1998	AS 4187:1998 *Cleaning, disinfecting and sterilizing reusable medical and surgical instruments and equipment, and maintenance of associated environments in health care facilities* released
2001	AS/NZS 4815:2001 *Office-based health care facilities not involved in complex patient procedures and processes – cleaning, disinfecting and sterilizing reusable medical and surgical instruments and equipment, and maintenance of the associated environment* released; first comprehensive guideline for dental practice settings
2003	AS/NZS 4187:2003 *Cleaning, disinfecting and sterilizing reusable medical and surgical instruments and equipment, and maintenance of associated environments in health care facilities* released
2006	AS/NZS 4815:2006 *Office-based health care facilities – reprocessing of reusable medical and surgical instruments and equipment, and maintenance of the associated environment* released; update to 2001 release
2008	The ADA publishes the first comprehensive dental IPC guidelines
2010	DBA established under the Health Practitioner Regulation National Law, publishes inaugural *Guidelines on Infection Control*; first time every dental practice setting, regardless of location, is required to have documented IPC procedures in place
2010	NHMRC releases updated *Australian Guidelines for the Prevention and Control of Infection in Healthcare*; focus is on all healthcare organisations rather than the average dental practice setting
2012	ADA Guidelines for Infection Control, 2nd edition released; focused on incorporating the AS/NZS 4815:2006 and NHMRC 2010 guidelines into a dental-specific guideline
2012	*Australian national guidelines for the management of healthcare workers living with blood borne viruses and healthcare workers who perform exposure prone procedures at risk of exposure to blood borne viruses* released by the CDNA
2015	ADA Guidelines for Infection Control, 3rd edition, released
2019	*Australian national guidelines for the management of healthcare workers living with blood borne viruses and healthcare workers who perform exposure prone procedures at risk of exposure to blood borne viruses* released; focus is on clearer definitions of exposure prone and non-exposure-prone procedures, blood-borne virus testing requirements increased to every 3 years and the ability to return to work if diagnosed with a blood-borne virus
2020	In light of COVID-19 pandemic, the DBA advised all dental practitioners to adopt the triage system published by the ADA and endorsed by the Australian Health Protection Principal Committee
2021	ADA Guidelines for Infection Prevention and Control, 4th edition, released

with patients, patient management, assistance for the DHP during treatments, reprocessing reusable instruments and environmental cleaning.[50] Dental assistants are the largest group of people working in the oral health workforce, with an estimated 31 900 workers in 2020.[51]

Dental assistants are not required to be formally qualified.[50] Therefore, it becomes the responsibility of the dental practice setting to recognise and provide formal training to ensure dental assistants maintain contemporary knowledge of IPC guidelines and operate in compliance. DHPs rely on dental assistants to carry out many of the daily IPC procedures, yet DHPs have the overarching responsibility and accountability.

Dental prosthetists and dental technicians: Dental prosthetists deal directly with the public. They design, construct, repair and fit patient removable prostheses (dentures) and mouthguards for sport. Dental technicians perform the technical work on the order of a dental prosthetist or other DHP. They may deal with the public when taking tooth shades for crowns, bridges, implants or dentures on referral from a DHP.[52,53]

34.1.3 The regulatory environment

The DBA has created several resources to aid dental practitioners in maintaining and enhancing health and safety by preventing or minimising the transmission of infection. These resources include information on how the DBA's regulatory framework relates to IPC, opportunities for practitioners to reflect on their practice and detailed guidance on IPC practices. By using these resources, practitioners can find the information they need to practise in a manner consistent with the DBA's expectations.[54,43]

The DBA handles complaints against practitioners. External oversight of DHP compliance with the DBA guidelines is limited. Monitoring of compliance is generally complaint-driven. The exception is in Queensland and New South Wales where DHPs are co-regulated.[55-57]

Dental practice settings—the business model: Australian dentistry is predominantly a private, small business model with much of the costs of care resting with the individual, and accounts for about 85% of the dental services provided.[58] Private dental practices vary from large group practices, often owned and operated by dentists as partnerships or professional corporations, to a small group or solo practice across single or multiple locations.

Public dental programs are operated by individual states and territories, with service organisations providing a range of treatments and criteria for patient eligibility.[59]

With the introduction of the Australian Health Service Safety and Quality Accreditation Scheme in 2013, health service organisations, including dental practice settings, were provided with a structured set of standards (National Safety and Quality Health Service [NSQHS] Standards) to drive improvements in quality and safety of patient care. Standard 3 addresses the prevention of HAIs, and this includes standards for infection control.[60,61]

The current model of accreditation mandates assessment to the standards for most public dental settings. In contrast, for private dental settings, assessment to the standards is voluntary. Given that participation in accreditation is voluntary, adherence to IPC measures becomes more challenging to monitor within private dental settings. The standards for safety and quality for mobile dental practices must be the same as those for fixed clinics[40] and similarly for denture clinics and dental laboratories. The accreditation scheme is constantly undergoing continuous improvement and evolving to protect patient safety in healthcare. Refer to the Australian Commission on Safety and Quality in Health Care (ACSQHC) for the latest information.

CASE STUDY 1

Risk assessment of the unwell patient

Situation:

A 40-year-old patient has arrived for their scheduled dental appointment, and they are unwell. The patient asks to go ahead with their treatment as they feel it should be fine as everyone wears gloves and masks.

Questions:

1. What questions can be asked to determine if the treatment can or cannot go ahead?
2. What procedures should a practice have in place to handle this situation?
3. Write a sample 'sick patients' policy.

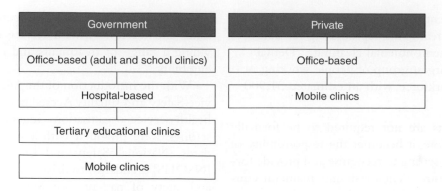

FIGURE 34.3 Dental practice settings

Answers:

1. It is important to determine the type of illness or infection the patient may have. There are risks with treating unwell patients depending on the treatment they are having. Enquire if the patient is contagious or is the patient unwell due to allergies.

2. It is important for a dental practice to have an established policy and procedures for handling and rescheduling unwell patients:

    *   The first point of contact is the reception staff, and they should be suitably trained, understand and follow the practice's policy

    *   Have readily available a supply of masks should you need to provide one to the patient and try to minimise the risk of exposure to other patients

    *   Provide an alcohol-based hand rub for the patient to use

    *   Provide options to conduct screening prior to the appointment e.g. text messaging or phone calls, and a poster or sign listing symptoms and asking patients to identify themselves

    *   Display cough etiquette posters.

3. Example of a sick patient policy:

    We care about the safety and health of our patients and staff. For health and safety reasons, we politely ask our patients to reschedule their appointments if during the last 24 hours you have experienced symptoms such as fever, headache, joint or muscle aches, fatigue, weakness, nausea or diarrhoea. If you experience the symptoms of a mild cold and still want to come, please inform reception so that we can take special precautions to make the appointment safe for everyone.

34.2 HAIs and modes of transmission in the dental practice setting

The oral cavity harbours a diverse and complex community of microorganisms: bacteria, fungi, several species of protozoa and various intracellular viruses.[62] The oral cavity can serve as a portal for pathogens to enter the body. Saliva and blood are frequently encountered in dental treatment and can provide a vehicle for infectious disease transmission.

In contrast to many other healthcare settings, DHPs usually see healthy patients. However, many patients may be asymptomatic carriers of potential infectious diseases. DHPs and staff require knowledge about potential infectious diseases to protect themselves from infectious diseases that may present in the dental practice setting. While HBV in the 1970s may have generated the initial awareness and concern about cross-infection, DHPs in the 2020s have become aware of the threat posed by other infectious diseases.

This section highlights the pathogens which are more relevant to IPC in dentistry, their modes of transmission and HAIs.

34.2.1 Blood-borne pathogens

Blood-borne viruses (BBV) of particular concern for DHPs include HBV, HCV and HIV. Transmission of BBV is possible due to frequent direct and indirect contact with blood or blood-contaminated saliva.

BBV are primarily transmitted through the following routes in the dental practice setting:
*   inoculation through broken or penetrated skin (percutaneously), e.g. needlestick injuries, cuts from dental burs and sharp hand instruments; and

- mucosal (permucosally) contact with infected blood and other body fluids.[63]

The HBV vaccine, available in Australia since the early 1980s, is strongly recommended for all DHPs and staff.[64] Currently, there is no vaccine for HCV and HIV. Dental treatment does not have to be delayed if standard precautions are implemented.

PRACTICE TIP 1

Offer HBV vaccination to all DHPs and staff with a potential occupational exposure to blood and body fluids. Refer to the National Immunisation Handbook for further details.[65]

34.2.2 Respiratory pathogens

The most common and relevant infectious diseases the DHP should be familiar with include the respiratory viral pathogens that cause tuberculosis, influenza, pneumonia, the common cold and COVID-19.[66] DHPs should also be familiar with pathogens that are transmitted by the respiratory route but are not a respiratory pathogen. This includes the viruses that cause chicken pox (varicella) and measles.

34.2.3 Waterborne pathogens

Dental unit waterlines (DUWL) are a complex network of tubes that carry air and water to the dental handpieces, air and water syringes, and ultrasonic scalers. Water acts as a coolant and irrigant for non-surgical procedures such as ultrasonic scaling (teeth cleaning) and tooth restorations. DUWL consist of narrow tubes, with slow water flow rates and recurrent periods of water stagnation providing a favourable environment resulting in the growth of bacteria on the inside of the tubes; a biofilm.

Over 40 different microorganisms have been identified in biofilm, including *Pseudomonas aeruginosa*, *Mycobacterium species* and *Legionella pneumophila*.[67,68] These opportunistic pathogens have the potential to cause infection in DHPs, staff and patients.[69-72]

34.2.4 Other notable pathogens

Herpes simplex virus: Herpes labialis, a common infection, generally appears as a cluster of vesicles on the lips or in the perioral region. Patients can shed HSV in their saliva during periods when the lesions are present and in between recurrences when lesions are not present. DHPs should be aware that the lesions are infectious during the vesicle and ulcer stage. HSV infections are a potential occupational hazard to the DHP, dental team and their patients. Dental care should be delayed until HSV lesions are scabbed over or healed.

Prions: Prions are the causative agents of a group of incurable degenerative disorders of the nervous system called prion diseases. The relevance to dentistry is that prions are extremely difficult to destroy. While dental procedures have not been implicated in the transmission of prions, the level of infectivity in oral and dental tissues is unknown. In Australia, guidelines state single use items should be used when possible and subsequently destroyed by incineration along with disinfection of surfaces.[39]

34.2.5 Modes of transmission[63,73]

The patient's oral cavity can host a multitude of microorganisms which may contain bacteria, fungi and viruses. Saliva and blood are the primary agents of cross-contamination. Risk of transmission and the probability of clinical infection developing will depend on the virulence of pathogens transmitted, frequency or duration of exposure to the infectious material and susceptibility of the host.[74] (See Table 34.2.)

Once the route/s of transmission of a microorganism are understood, the most effective precautions can be taken to prevent or minimise transmission (Fig 34.4). DHPs can train and advise their dental team, and at the same time, reassure their patients of a safe dental visit.

Infection can be transmitted in the dental practice setting by four main modes of transmission or[70,72,75-84] pathways:[85]

1. Contact—direct or indirect
2. Droplet—from nasopharyngeal secretions directly onto broken or intact skin or mucosa
3. Airborne—including through aerosolisation of saliva or blood which may contain microorganisms
4. Vehicle—such as dental unit waterlines.

Contact transmission: Microorganisms may be transmitted via direct contact from one person to another. A significant route of transmission is via a percutaneous injury. Sharps injuries can arise from dental syringe needles, sharp hand instruments, dental burs, and during cleaning and reprocessing of instruments. A spatter or splash of saliva and blood may contaminate the clinical staff's face, particularly the eyes if not wearing appropriate eye protection.

TABLE 34.2 Diseases spread by respiratory/oral fluids

Bacterial diseases	Microorganism
Tuberculosis	*Mycobacterium tuberculosis*
Diphtheria	*Corynebacterium diphtheria*
Pneumonia	*Streptococcus pneumoniae* (most common cause of community-acquired infection)
Viral diseases	Microorganism
Common cold	Rhinoviruses and several others
Influenza	Influenza viruses
Middle Eastern Respiratory Syndrome (MERS-Co-V)	Middle East respiratory syndrome coronavirus (MERS-CoV)
Severe Acute Respiratory Syndrome (SARS)	Severe acute respiratory syndrome coronavirus
COVID-19	Severe acute respiratory syndrome coronavirus 2
Measles	Paramyxovirus
Pneumonia	Multiple viruses can cause pneumonia including MERS-Co-V, human metapneumonovirus, adenoviruses and influenza viruses
Perioral herpes (herpes labialis)	Herpes simplex type 1, herpes simplex type 2
Infectious mononucleosis	Epstein-Barr virus
Chicken pox, shingles	Varicella zoster virus
Rubella	Rubivirus
Mumps	Paramyxovirus

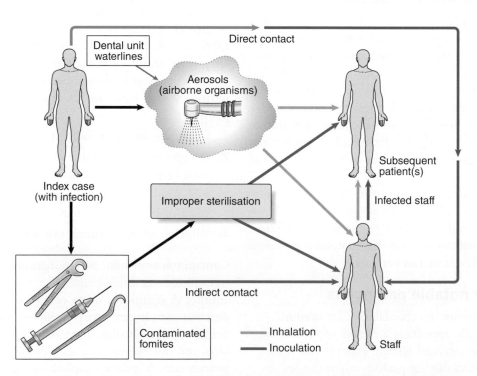

FIGURE 34.4 Routes and modes by which infection may spread in the dental practice

Source: Samaranayake L. Essential Microbiology for Dentistry, 5th edn (978-0-7020-7435-6), Elsevier, 2018.

Indirect contact transmission occurs when microorganisms spread via instruments and equipment or contaminated environmental surfaces.[77] Contaminated hands touching own mucosal tissues can also be a pathway for transmission.

Direct contact transmission is interrupted by hand hygiene, wearing personal protective equipment and careful sharps management.

Indirect contact transmission is interrupted by:

- environmental cleaning of dental chairs, dental equipment and surgery room bench tops/cupboard between patients and throughout the dental practice setting (frequently touched surfaces)
- reprocessing of reusable dental instruments
- cleaning and/or disinfecting laboratory work prior to transport to the dental laboratory and upon laboratory work return.

Transmission from clinical staff to patients can occur through exposure-prone procedures. These are procedures where there is risk of injury to the clinical staff and as a result the patient could potentially be exposed to the blood resulting from the injury sustained by the clinical staff. In dentistry, these include maxillofacial and oral surgical procedures, including extraction of teeth, periodontal surgical procedures, endodontic surgical procedures and implant surgical procedures. One of the suggested recommendations for clinicians who perform exposure-prone procedures is to determine their blood-borne virus status and be tested every 3 years.[86]

Transmission from one patient to another can occur through inappropriately sterilised instruments, contaminated hands, not changing contaminated PPE and inadequate environmental cleaning.

PRACTICE TIP 2

Possible sources of pathogens in the dental practice setting include:

- Patients with infectious diseases—asymptomatic, symptomatic
- Contaminated environmental surfaces
- Dental unit waterlines
- Contaminated instruments
- Sharps
- Splatter and aerosols

Droplet transmission: Droplet transmission occurs when respiratory droplets expelled by coughing,

sneezing or talking come into contact with another person's mucosa (eyes, nose or mouth) either directly or via contaminated hands. These droplets are considered more than 5 microns in size and do not remain suspended in the air for long periods. However, they can land directly on another person's mucosal tissues, or drop to surfaces to contaminate the dental environment.[87]

Airborne transmission: Airborne transmission occurs when aerosolised droplets that are less than 5 microns in size remain suspended for a period and may be transmitted by inhalation.[88] In dentistry, there are two mechanisms by which aerosols are generated:

1. Dental procedures that mechanically produce and disperse aerosols with the use of dental instruments such as high-speed handpieces, ultrasonic scalers, air polishers, and air and water triplex (Fig 34.5).
2. Dental procedures that can induce the patient to cough or gag potentially expelling aerosols containing microbes.[89]

Aerosols contain microorganisms originating from the patient's oral cavity and dental unit waterlines. Because of the frequent aerosol-generating procedures, these aerosols can function as a mode for infection transmission.[84]

Microorganisms transmitted via the respiratory route are of particular concern in the dental practice setting. Use of dental rotary instruments combined with water coolant and saliva creates a large spray and plume composed of a combination of splatter, droplets and aerosols. Saliva is a potential source of respiratory

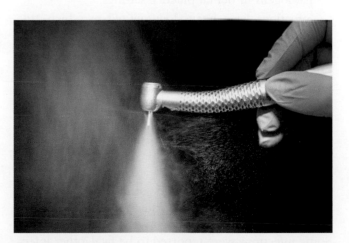

FIGURE 34.5 High-speed handpiece and dental bur use water as a coolant when cutting tooth structure

viral and bacterial pathogens. Patients infected by these pathogens are often in the prodromal or recovery period when presenting for dental treatment.[81]

Vehicle transmission—waterlines: Patients, DHPs and staff are regularly exposed to potentially pathogenic water splatter, splashes and aerosols produced by dental equipment; in addition, patients ingest water during treatment.[67,68,70,72,90]

The DUWL output water often contains multiple bacteria in greater quantities than recommended guidelines of less than 200 CFU/mL.[40] Exposing DHPs and staff to the risks of the output water is not consistent with current IPC practices. The presence of these pathogens is cause for concern due to the growing number of vulnerable individuals, such as the elderly and immunocompromised.

34.3 Prevention and control of HAIs in the dental practice setting

While HAIs have been well documented in the hospital setting, in contrast, the dental practice setting neither systematically surveys nor monitors HAIs. The lack of reporting poses a huge barrier to obtaining an accurate picture of the transmission of infection in dental practice. The information is difficult to obtain because:

- there is complexity in detecting and documenting HAIs in the dental practice setting
- many infectious diseases have long incubation periods and patients can be asymptomatic[74]
- there is limited evidence of transmission of pathogens in dental practice settings.

Situations have been documented in which IPC practice breaches have led to HIV, HBV and HCV transmission from the DHP to their patients, patients to DHP and patient-to-patient transmission.[91,92] There is limited evidence of cross-transmission and infection of herpes simplex virus type 1 (HSV-1).[92] An outbreak of bacterial endocarditis within an oral surgery practice in America was reported and investigated. The outbreak was likely associated with IPC breaches during IV drug administration.[93]

Recent documented cases of *L pneumophila* and *M abscessus* have shown that infectious diseases can be acquired from DUWL during routine dental treatment. Some infections were reported to be fatal, other infections led to substantial morbidity.[69–71,75,94] While the incidence of DUWL infections appears to be minimal,

the risk should not be underestimated. Direct contact with contaminated water during dental treatment, and exposure to aerosolised water from equipment such as dental handpieces and ultrasonic scalers, are the likely sources of infection and present a risk for both DHPs, the dental team and patients. Mitigating risk measures involves reducing microbial contamination of DUWL. The topic of water quality is now addressed in IPC guidelines that provide current recommendations for water quality management.

The potential for transmission of the SARS-CoV-2 virus during dental treatment, although possible, has not been adequately documented in current evidence.[95,96]

34.3.1 Cost of healthcare-associated infections

The cost of HAI related to dentistry is unknown as there is no system of surveillance to monitor these infections at a state or even national level. The true burden and cost of dentally acquired HAI is difficult to estimate.

Dental procedures increase the risk of microorganism transmission and to minimise this risk, standard and transmission-based precautions (TBPs) are applied in practice. Standard precautions (SPs) comprise the minimum level of IPC practices employed, regardless of the patient's infection status. TBPs are additional precautions used when SPs alone are not sufficient to protect from infection and where there is a higher risk of the pathogens being transmitted via contact, droplet or airborne route.[39,97]

This section attempts to highlight several relevant SPs and TBP elements (work practices) for dentistry, and the requirements for a successful IPC program.

34.3.2 Standard precautions

While SPs apply to every patient encounter and procedure, the application of SPs is determined by the task being performed and the type of exposure to pathogens, blood and body fluids that is anticipated.[39]

34.3.3 Hand hygiene

When properly carried out, hand hygiene reduces the number of microorganisms present on hands and is an important measure in preventing HAIs. Exceedingly high compliance with a hand hygiene program can lead to a substantial decline in HAI rates.[98]

For routine dental procedures hand hygiene can be performed using soap and water or an alcohol-based hand rub. When hands are visibly clean, alcohol-based hand rubs can be used. When hands are visibly dirty, soap and water use is preferable.

Clinical indications are:

1. when hands are visibly clean, alcohol-based hand rubs should be used; and

2. when hands are visibly dirty or soiled with blood or body fluids, or exposure to spore-forming microorganisms is suspected or confirmed, or after a visit to the toilet, hands should be washed with soap and water as alcohol has no action against spores.[99]

Every dental practice setting should have a hand hygiene policy and procedure that follows the '5 Moments for Dental Hand Hygiene' (Fig 34.6).[100,101] Some dental practices may choose to participate in a hand hygiene program that involves an audit process. Hand Hygiene Australia recognises that the auditing system for hospitals may not be relevant to the dental setting, hence it provides guidance for dental services including the establishment of dental-specific healthcare worker and department codes for auditing purposes.[102]

For surgical procedures, surgical hand antisepsis with alcohol-based surgical hand rubs, an alternative to the traditional scrub, is gaining popularity among DHPs. In addition to saving time and water, suitable handwashing facilities at many dental practice settings do not have scrub taps and deep sinks.

Gloves do not replace the need for hand hygiene. Hand hygiene should be performed on removal of gloves and hand hygiene should be performed immediately prior to donning new gloves.[78]

34.3.4 Patient hand hygiene

Patients within dental settings should also be aware of their role in minimising risk of disease transmission and should be encouraged to perform basic hand hygiene.[39] The COVID-19 pandemic has emphasised the importance of this measure.

34.3.5 Personal protective equipment

The selection of appropriate PPE is dictated by a risk assessment of the procedure, the patient and degree of patient interaction, probability of exposure to blood substances, and probable type and probable route of transmission of infectious agents. With these factors to consider in the dental setting, it becomes necessary for dental clinical staff to wear PPE that will offer the maximum protection.[39]

To prevent cross-contamination, PPE worn during patient contact should not be worn outside the patient care areas or public areas, and PPE should be replaced before attending to another dental patient. COVID-19 has reinforced the importance of the correct sequence of donning and, in particular, the steps for doffing contaminated PPE.

Gloves: Gloves should be worn when there is anticipated contact with blood, body fluids or mucous membranes. In dentistry, gloves are worn for every dental clinical procedure which involves the patient's face and mouth and exposure to saliva, body secretions or blood. Single use disposable gloves should be used and replaced when torn or heavily soiled. Wearing gloves, however, is not a substitute for hand hygiene. Non-sterile gloves are used for routine dental procedures and sterile gloves should be worn for surgical procedures. Gloves supplied for use in dental practice are required to conform to Australian and New Zealand Standard AS/NZS 4011.[40]

Eye protection: Eyewear designed to protect eyes and surrounding structures from splashes or projectiles should be worn during clinical dental procedures (Fig 34.7). Chemicals—including tooth etchant, disinfectants for root canal procedures and environmental cleaning—as well as tooth and dental material that has become airborne debris provide hazards. Reusable or disposable eyewear for both dental clinical staff and patients is required to conform to Australian and New Zealand Standard AS/NZS 1337:2012 An alternative to protective eyewear is a face shield but this should be worn in conjunction with a surgical mask as on its own, it cannot protect the wearer from inhalation of microorganisms.[40]

Gowns or aprons: The dental uniform should not be considered as a protective gown or apron as it can become contaminated during general dental procedures and when cleaning instruments. Impervious gowns should be worn and should be single use, particularly for aerosol-generating procedures or when there is risk of splatter or splashing. For surgical procedures, disposable sterile gowns are recommended.

Masks: Mask selection will be dependent on a risk assessment. Dental procedures generate large volumes of particles or aerosols near the DHP and staff's breathing zone. Single use, fluid-resistant level 2 or 3 surgical masks should be worn for every dental procedure or patient contact to protect mucous membranes of the nose and mouth. These masks should comply with AS 438.[40]

5 Moments for
HAND HYGIENE

Dental and oral health settings

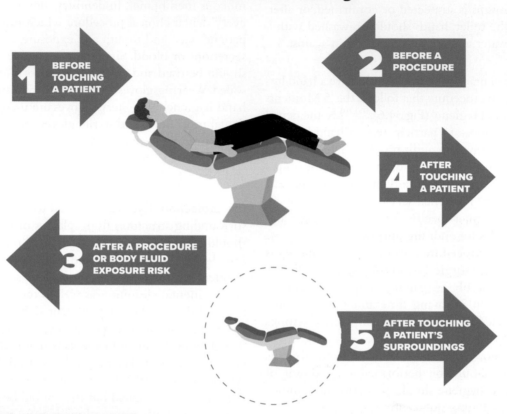

1	**BEFORE TOUCHING A PATIENT**	**When:** Clean your hands before touching a patient and their immediate surroundings. **Why:** To protect the patient against acquiring harmful germs from the hands of the HCW.
2	**BEFORE A PROCEDURE**	**When:** Clean your hands immediately before a procedure. **Why:** To protect the patient from harmful germs (including their own) from entering their body during a procedure.
3	**AFTER A PROCEDURE OR BODY FLUID EXPOSURE RISK**	**When:** Clean your hands immediately after a procedure or body fluid exposure risk. **Why:** To protect the HCW and the healthcare surroundings from harmful patient germs.
4	**AFTER TOUCHING A PATIENT**	**When:** Clean your hands after touching a patient and their immediate surroundings. **Why:** To protect the HCW and the healthcare surroundings from harmful patient germs.
5	**AFTER TOUCHING A PATIENT'S SURROUNDINGS**	**When:** Clean your hands after touching any objects in a patient's surroundings when the patient has not been touched. **Why:** To protect the HCW and the healthcare surroundings from harmful patient germs.

This poster is based on the World Health Organization's My 5 Moments for Hand Hygiene approach, which defines the key moments when healthcare workers should perform hand hygiene.

NHHI
National Hand Hygiene Initiative

AUSTRALIAN COMMISSION
ON SAFETY AND QUALITY IN HEALTH CARE

FIGURE 34.6 Dental 5 Moments for Hand Hygiene

Reproduced with permission from 5 Moments for hand hygiene poster – Dental and oral health settings, *developed by the Australian Commission on Safety and Quality in Health Care (ACSQHC). ACSQHC: Sydney 2022.*

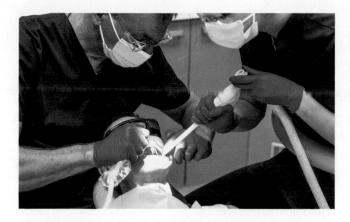

FIGURE 34.7 Appropriate clinical attire consisting of short-sleeved tops, gloves, masks and protective eyewear

Wearing a surgical mask can hamper communication with patients. Rather than pulling the mask temporarily down under the chin, with potentially dirty gloves, remove the mask, and after discussion with the patient, put on a new mask.

34.3.6 Aseptic technique

The terms *clean*, *sterile* and *aseptic technique* are often used interchangeably, but this is incorrect. Clean means the absence of visible dirt while sterile means the complete absence of microorganisms. Aseptic technique is the more appropriate term, which is defined as the range of IPC measures that prevent or minimise the risk of introducing pathogens onto key parts or key sites of the body when undertaking clinical procedures (Figs 34.8, 34.9).[39]

Aseptic technique in dentistry is divided into standard aseptic technique and surgical aseptic technique (Table 34.3).

Each dental procedure must be risk assessed to determine if a surgical aseptic technique is required. Principles of surgical aseptic technique should be applied whenever the procedure performed involves:

- incision into mucosal soft tissues
- surgical penetration of bone or elevation of mucoperiosteal flap
- entry to sterile tissues for removal of fully unerupted teeth
- enucleation of radicular cysts; and
- endodontic surgery and implant placement.[40]

Sharps management: Everyone in the dental practice has a role to play in the prevention of sharps injuries. The person who has used a disposable sharp item, for example scalpels and dental syringe needles, should be the one responsible for its immediate safe management and disposal.[40]

Sharps including wedges and matrix bands should always be contained in a puncture-resistant tray for

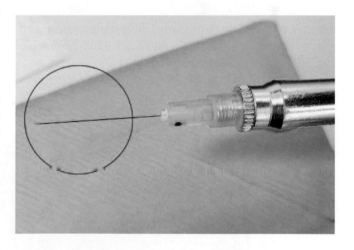

FIGURE 34.8 Example of a key part

TABLE 34.3 Difference between dental standard and surgical aseptic technique

Aseptic technique	Key parts and key sites	Hand hygiene	Gloves	Aseptic fields
Standard e.g. LA delivery, tooth restorations, scale and clean, simple extraction	Small number of key parts or key sites. Small sized key parts or key sites	Standard hand hygiene	Non-sterile	General aseptic fields. Micro-critical aseptic fields
Surgical e.g. Oral surgical procedures including implant surgery	Large number of key parts or key sites. Large-sized key parts or key sites	Surgical hand asepsis	Sterile	Critical aseptic fields. Micro-critical aseptic fields.

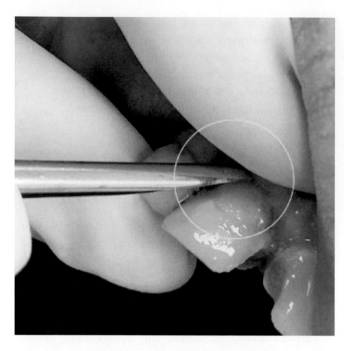

FIGURE 34.9 Example of a key site

transfer, particularly to a clearly labelled puncture-proof sharps container that conforms to AS 4261 if reusable or AS 4301 if non-reusable (Fig 34.10).

Needles should not be re-sheathed following injection; however, most dental settings use dental reusable syringes for local anaesthetic administration, so removal of the anaesthetic cartridge and used needle becomes necessary along with recapping needles. To reduce the risk of sharp injuries the use of safety engineering devices that preclude recapping of needles or removal of sharps from reusable procedural equipment, and that facilitate safe disposal of the sharps, should be considered.[103]

Reprocessing of reusable medical devices: Reprocessing of instruments must be in accordance with AS/NZS 4815 or AS/NZS 4187. Detailed information can be found in Chapter 16.

34.3.7 Waste management

General and clinical: Proper management and disposal of all waste is an important component of IPC practices as dental practices produce a range of contaminated waste. Each state and territory has different definitions of clinical waste and every dental practice setting has a legal requirement to comply with its relevant state or territory's legislation and guidelines. Further guidance can be sourced from AS 3816:2018 As a guide, general and clinical wastes should be segregated at the point of use and there should be dedicated bags or containers for their collection. General wastes include those that cannot

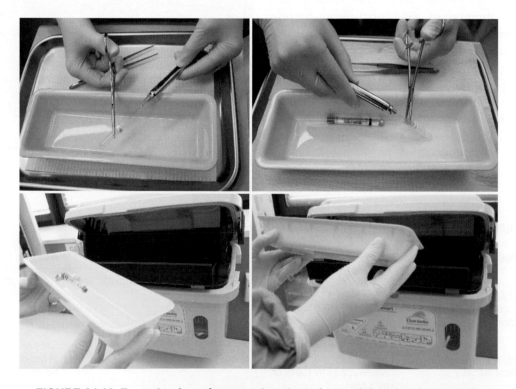

FIGURE 34.10 Example of a safe removal method of a used dental syringe needle

be recycled or reprocessed and must not be heavily soiled with blood or body fluids. Used PPE items without visible blood contamination, such as single use clinical gowns and masks, belong to this waste stream. Clinical wastes have the potential to cause injury or infection and are usually collected in a coloured bag or container and labelled as biohazard or medical waste. Disposable sharps and visibly bloodstained disposable material or equipment are examples of clinical waste.

Amalgam: Dental amalgam, an alloy containing mercury, has long served the dental profession as a successful tooth restorative material. Dental practices are recognised as a source of environmental mercury and reasonable measures should be in place to minimise the discharge of mercury containing amalgam into the general environment. This waste should be recycled as much as possible. Dental clinics must collect and send any amalgam waste to authorised recyclers. This may include amalgam capsules, excess amalgam not placed in restorations, amalgam retained in chair-side suction filters and amalgam separators, and even extracted teeth which have been restored with amalgam (Fig 34.11).[104]

34.3.8 Environmental cleaning

Surgery design and zones: The design of modern dental equipment and cabinetry should facilitate cleaning. The use of disposable plastic barriers is essential for equipment that cannot be cleaned. A dental surgery room is typically divided into two zones based on the potential for contamination. The clean and contaminated zones provide a clear area for workflow once treatment has commenced and facilitates a methodical approach to environmental cleaning after the procedure is completed.

The contaminated zone around the patient must be identified and a useful guide is 1–1.8 m in diameter from the patient's head.[40]

Care must be taken to avoid contaminated instruments, equipment or waste entering the clean zone. Instruments placed in the contaminated zone for a treatment session, but not used, are regarded as contaminated. When moving from the contaminated zone to the clean zone to retrieve instruments or materials, they must not be handled unless gloves have been removed and hand hygiene performed. Alternatively, transfer tweezers (kept separate from other instruments and in the clean area) or over gloves can be used (Fig 34.12).

Environmental surfaces are divided into two categories: clinical contact surfaces and housekeeping surfaces.

Clinical contact surfaces are surfaces within the contaminated zone that can become directly contaminated by gloved hands, instrument contact and dental materials or by direct splatter and aerosols. Examples include the dental chair, the tray table, overhead light handles, suction tubes, and dental assistant work area. These surfaces must be cleaned between each patient or covered with a disposable plastic barrier to prevent contamination (Fig 34.13).

A risk assessment will determine the choice of cleaning products, methods and frequency. A written

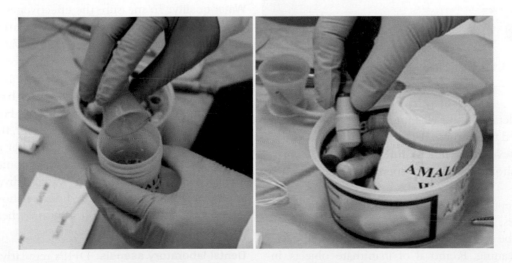

FIGURE 34.11 Disposal of amalgam waste

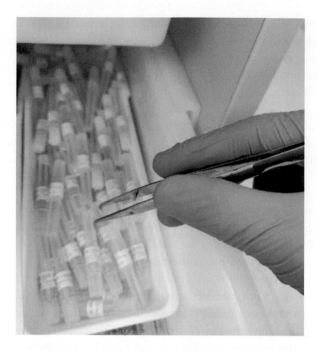

FIGURE 34.12 Using transfer tweezers to retrieve a clean item from drawer

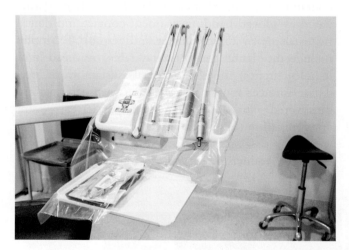

FIGURE 34.13 Example of the use of the disposable plastic barriers

procedure detailing the cleaning order from the least contaminated to the most contaminated areas is important to achieve consistency and facilitate training of staff. PPE should be worn when undertaking these tasks.

Housekeeping surfaces such as waiting room chairs, door handles, light switches and telephone handsets should also be regularly cleaned, and a schedule developed for cleaning. Removal of inanimate objects, including magazines and toys, from waiting rooms, should

be considered as these can act as fomites with the potential to transmit infections via indirect contact.

A process for decontamination after use of equipment such as microscopes and imaging equipment is similarly important.

Other considerations that can assist with environmental cleaning include:

- plastic barriers for equipment that is impossible to decontaminate, such as computer keyboards and mice
- high-volume suction to reduce the amount of aerosols generated during the dental procedure[89]
- rubber dam to reduce droplet and aerosol spread
- dental materials should be stored in cupboards or drawers and prevented from being contaminated during dental procedures.[40]

PRACTICE TIP 3

Use one hand to wipe surface while keeping the other hand 'clean' to enable handling of recently cleaned items

---

Waterline asepsis: Dental unit waterlines are not exempt from microbial contamination and should be cleaned and disinfected based on the manufacturer's instructions. There are several ways of minimising biofilm levels in dental equipment, and these include water treatments using ozonation or electrochemical activation, chemical dosing of water and flushing of waterlines. Flushing lines is recommended after each patient and at the start of the day to reduce the overnight biofilm build-up.[40]

Water quality: To measure the effectiveness of DUWL cleaning and chemical treatments, regularly test the microbial quality of the output water. Water output from handpieces and ultrasonic scalers for non-surgical dental treatment should have <500 colony forming units (CFU)/ml of heterotrophic water bacteria which is the same standard for drinking water. For use in immunocompromised patients, however, the recommendation is <200CFU/ml. Water testing should be conducted periodically to monitor water quality. Sterile saline, or sterile water, delivered appropriately using a dedicated device should be used as coolant or as an irrigation solution when performing oral surgical procedures.[105]

Dental laboratory asepsis: DHPs regularly send clinical materials such as impressions, bite registration records, fixed and removable prostheses, to the dental laboratory. The responsibility for appropriately cleaning lab work lies with the practice. All items must be transported in a clean state to minimise cross infection and protect laboratory personnel. Blood, saliva and other debris must be carefully cleaned from an item by washing under running water as soon as possible before cleaning with a neutral detergent and/or disinfectant as per the practice's policy. Dental laboratories may provide their own disinfection method, and communication between the laboratory and dental practice is important to determine the suitable procedure. All items received from the dental laboratory must undergo cleaning and/or disinfection prior to being delivered to the patient in consultation with the laboratory's recommendations (see Fig 34.14).

34.3.9 Transmission-based precautions

For management of patients who may be infected with certain infectious agents, these additional precautions are applied in addition to standard precautions in order to prevent transmission of such infections. More than one category can be applied at the same time (Table 34.4).

TBPs were developed for the hospital setting. As a result, TBPs must be translated for the office-based setting.

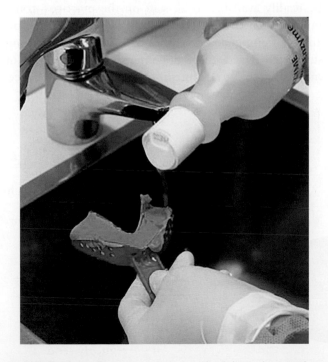

FIGURE 34.14 Cleaning a lower arch alginate impression

TABLE 34.4 Examples of transmission-based precautions work practices in dentistry

Precaution category	Description
Contact	Regular cleaning of frequently touched surfaces Good hand hygiene practice for dental staff and patient
Droplet	Use of fluid-repellent gown Physical distancing
Airborne	Use of P2/N95 surgical respirators Patient treatment in negative pressure rooms

In dentistry, there is some overlap between SP and contact precautions. For example, DHPs and staff routinely don safety eyewear, surgical masks, gloves and a protective gown/apron for every dental procedure. Patient treatment is provided in a single room/cubicle surgery room, and the environment in the dental surgery room is cleaned after every procedure.

Droplet precautions: If a patient requires contact precautions, additional preventive measures include:

- placing the patient in a single dental surgery room promptly on arrival to limit potential spread of infectious agents
- completing screening questions, medical history and other details prior to entering the practice
- asking the patient to wear a mask upon or before arrival
- DHPs and staff donning surgical masks prior to entering the room
- environmental cleaning after treatment procedure using a TGA–registered disinfectant.[106]

Airborne precautions: Most dental practices are unable to provide airborne precautions and must refer patients to an appropriate facility. Dentistry straddles between droplet and airborne transmission as many of the treatments use AGP. This has been highlighted with the COVID-19 pandemic. Traditionally, patients who were too sick would not seek out routine dental care. With the emergence of the new pathogen SARS-CoV-2, it is possible that asymptomatic patients are seeking dental treatment. DHPs and staff must be aware of TBPs and the additional measures that must be taken. The ADA released a series of publications endorsed by the DBA to guide DHPs and risk manage levels of IPC precautions based on patient risk.[107]

34.4 IPC programs and education in dentistry

Dental practice settings should implement a written, comprehensive IPC program to minimise the risk of HAIs among patients, and injuries and illness among DHPs and staff (Fig 34.15).

The framework of a dental IPC program (program) encompasses:

1. system of clinical governance
2. IPC policy
3. IPC management plan
4. IPC procedure manual
5. education and training
6. quality improvement.

The program provides the framework to allow the practice to develop IPC policies and procedures appropriate to their organisation. Every IPC program will be site-specific due to variations in the type of organisation—public or private—and the range of types of clinical services, but the fundamental concepts remain the same. Each setting will need to determine their risks and appropriate actions (a risk management framework) to develop their program. Also, time and financial restraints will affect the structure, implementation and management of the program. A systematic approach to education and training during induction and ongoing throughout employment ensures a systematic approach, so DHPs and the dental team feel safe and confident. The program should also have a valid means of measuring its effectiveness to allow the opportunity to improve. Finally, the success of an IPC program is best achieved when it is embedded in the day-to-day running of a practice.

34.4.1 System of clinical governance

To facilitate a successful IPC program, regardless of the type and size of the dental practice setting, requires effective leadership with a clear vision of the standard required and an ability to communicate this to all dental team members.

In private solo or small practices, the owner is responsible for the IPC program. In a corporate setting, a culture of safety and leadership is provided with leadership at each practice location. In public dental clinics, a culture of safety and leadership is provided through the company with leadership at each practice location. Regardless of the practice setting type, at least one staff member should be designated as the infection control coordinator (ICC). The ICC is responsible for developing and managing the IPC program, and overseeing its implementation and evaluation to provide consistency and accountability.[34,96] The ICC is integral to the success of the IPC program.

First steps in developing an IPC program involve evaluating the practice environment to determine what policies and procedures exist and if any alterations in current IPC practices are required. The plan should be communicated to the staff at regular staff meetings or during morning team huddles. Any education materials should also be presented and tabled. The ICMP must be readily available to all staff on the practice's computer system, and a printed copy can be displayed on any staff noticeboard. Continual audits and training supported by adequate documentation are helpful in motivating staff to maintain a high level of compliance.

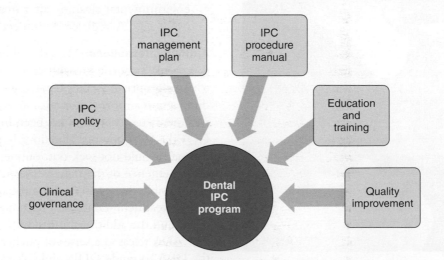

FIGURE 34.15 Framework of a dental IPC program

KEY RESPONSIBILITIES OF THE ICC

Management:
- Manages IPC program
- Serves as a leader and positive role model
- Regular review of related legislation, guidelines, standards and regulations
- Reviews practice's IPC Procedure Manual and ICMP
- Regular review of any reported HAIs

Training:
- Provide and arrange IPC training and support to existing and new DHPs and staff
- Monitor and evaluate IPC compliance as stated in the practice's IPC documentation
- Recognise staff compliance
- Issue non-compliance warnings and provide additional training for non-compliant staff
- Seek feedback from DHPs and staff

Medical and dental history questionnaire:
- Review and ensure medical and dental history questionnaire for patients is current

Immunisation program:
- Manage staff immunisation program

Work health and safety:
- Manage sharps and occupational exposure

Environmental cleaning:
- Evaluate product selections
- Assess staff cleaning effectiveness

Reprocessing (sterilisation) area:
- Oversee reprocessing of reusable instruments
- Manage all sterilisation records and equipment maintenance

34.4.2 IPC policy

The purpose and scope of an IPC policy is to minimise the transmission of infection, effectively manage infections should they occur and ensure compliance by the DHP and staff at a dental practice setting.

Key policy domains
- Governance
- IPC program
- IPC practice manual

- Staff training and compliance
- Immunisation program
- Hand hygiene
- Environmental cleaning
- Work health and safety
- Incident management
- Management of adverse incidents
- Patient communication

34.4.3 IPC management plan

The development of the ICMP is the responsibility of the ICC.[39,108] Upon identifying a risk in the dental practice, appropriate measures to prevent or control the risk are determined using the practice's policies and procedures, relevant guidelines and standards, and related regulatory requirements. During development, measurable goals are determined for the coming year, along with the methods used to achieve those goals. Checklists are used and readily detail the elements not being met. Suitable checklists are available from Hand Hygiene Australia, the DBA and the ADA but can be customised to suit the particular dental setting.

34.4.4 IPC procedure manual

An Infection Prevention and Control (IPC) manual comprises a collection of standard operating procedures (SOPs) that delineate the steps involved in specific tasks. The manual is created in accordance with the prevailing guidelines, standards, and best practices. Having written procedures aids dental healthcare providers and staff in comprehending and visualizing each process, and it promotes accountability, leading to the establishment of behaviours that ensure everyone's safety. The manual should be subject to an annual review or updated earlier in response to new recommendations, products, and regulations.

34.4.5 Education and training

Ongoing education and training for DHPs and staff should be provided during orientation, when new procedures or equipment are introduced, and on a regular ongoing basis. The DBA expects dental practitioners to continue to update IPC knowledge on a regular basis to maintain contemporary knowledge.[109] There are several entities that offer continuing education courses on infection prevention and control such as the Australian Dental Association (ADA), universities and private consultants.

34.4.6 Quality improvement

Evaluation offers the opportunity to improve the effectiveness of the IPC program. The program must be monitored and evaluated for compliance, efficiency and cost-effectiveness. Evaluation should be ongoing, from both a day-to-day assessment and extended to a more comprehensive annual evaluation to determine if the IPC program has been successful.[39,110] Upon reviewing the plan, the ICC can determine if the target goals were reached. Any targets that were not met can be revised and new strategies arranged to meet the targets, such as further education and training. These revisions would be conducted with regard to the current clinical governance structure and ensure that any new IPC practices and revised targets still meet the practice's mission and vision and align with the practice's policies, procedures, relevant guidelines and standards, and related regulatory requirements.

Strategies to use:
- periodic observational assessments
- checklist to document procedures
- routine review of occupational exposures and illnesses (i.e. monitor HAIs).

While the risk of HAIs in the dental practice is low, there is still potential for this to occur. Compliance, commitment and accountability with IPC practices are required of all DHPs and the dental team. An IPC program provides a framework for all staff to follow. This program also establishes a routine for evaluating the existing IPC program to ensure the dental team's adherence to infection control practices and promote an effective IPC program.

Conclusion

While the underlying principles and science are constant across all healthcare disciplines, unique challenges exist for IPC in dentistry. Dental treatment requires a large variety and variability of dental equipment and materials. Achieving a balance between the amount of time spent on infection control procedures versus time spent in the actual clinical care of patients may be difficult for many dental practices. When allocating time and resources towards IPC procedures, economic considerations need to be included, which could potentially compromise patient, DHP and clinical staff safety. The likely unavailability of a dedicated IPC consultant or coordinator within mainly smaller private practices poses significant limitations on the implementation of appropriate IPC measures.

Responsibility lies with the individual practitioner to monitor infection control standards and compliance. Private practitioners rely heavily on professional organisations to provide up-to-date guidelines and infection control awareness through professional publications and professional development courses. Frequently, the responsibility is designated to the lead dentist, oral health therapist, practice manager or even the lead dental assistant. This is an added challenge that requires special training and time to develop comprehensive IPC programs.

Lastly, with the requirement for cleaning and disinfection becoming more stringent, practices are now resorting to the use of more disposable items. The environmental impact of this practice may need to be considered.

The impact of the pandemic on dental IPC has been considerable. Until scientific research can clarify the true risk of SARS-CoV-2 virus as it relates specifically to the dental environment, extensive IPC measures are likely to keep changing. Practices to mitigate the risk of transmission of disease via aerosol generation will be a key focus for the future.[66,79,80,82,83,111,112]

Useful websites/resources

- Dental Board of Australia. www.dentalboard.gov.au.
- Australasian College for Infection Prevention and Control. www.acipc.com.au.
- Australian Dental Association. www.ada.org.au.
- Dental Hygienists Association of Australia. www.dhaa.info.
- Australian Dental and Oral Health Therapists' Association. www.Adohta.net.au.
- Australian Dental Prosthetist Association. www.adpa.com.au.
- Australian Immunisation Handbook. www.immunisationhandbook.health.gov.au.

References

1. National Health and Medical Research Council. Hepatitis B and dentists; summary of recommendations for preventing the spread of Hepatitis B in dental surgeries. Aust Dent J. 1981;26(1):49.

2. National Health and Medical Research Council. Hepatitis B and dentists. Aust Dent J. 1985;30(1):49-54.

3. Mosely JW, Edwards VM, Casey G, Redeker AG, White E. Hepatitis B virus infection in dentists. N Eng J Med. 1975; 293(15).

4. Amerena V, Andrew JH. Hepatitis B virus: the risk to Australian dentists and dental health care workers. Aust Dent J.1987;32(3): 183-189.

5. Smith JL, Maynard JE, Berquist KR, Doto IL, Webster HM, Sheller MJ. From the Centers for Disease Control: comparative risk of hepatitis B among physicians and dentists. J Infect Dis. 1976;133(6).

6. Younai FS. Health care-associated transmission of hepatitis B & C viruses in dental care (dentistry). Clinics in Liver Disease. 2010;14(1):93-104.

7. Manzella JP, Mcconville JH, Valenti W, Menegus MA, Swierkosz EM, Arens M. An outbreak of herpes simplex virus type I gingivostomatitis in a dental hygiene practice. JAMA. 1984;252(15):2019-22.

8. Hribar DLA. Viral hepatitis: a review of clinical, laboratory and research aspects. Aust Dent J. 1977;22(6):471-477.

9. Rimland D, Parkin WE, Miller GB, Schrack WD. Hepatitis B outbreak traced to an oral surgeon. N Eng J Med. 1977;296(17): 953-958.

10. Reingold AL, Kane MA, Murphy BL, Checko P, Francis DP, Maynard JE. Transmission of hepatitis B by an oral surgeon. J Infect Dis. 1982;145(2):262-268.

11. Savage CM, Christopher PJ, Murphy AM, Crewe EB, Lossin C. The prevalence of hepatitis B markers in dental care personnel at the United Dental Hospital of Sydney. Aust Dent J. 1984;29(2):75-0.

12. National Centre for Immunisation Research & Surveillance. Significant events in hepatitis B vaccination practice in Australia 2020. Available from: http://ncirs.org.au/sites/default/files/2019-07/Hepatitis-B-history-July%202019.pdf.

13. National Health and Medical Research Council. Statement on hepatitis B vaccine. Aust Dent J. 1983;28(4).

14. Petersen MS, Goldberg AF. Hepatitis: the risk in hospital dentistry. Special Care in Dentistry. 1981;1.

15. National Health and Medical Research Council. Hepatitis B and clinical dental practice. Canberra: Canberra Publishing and Printing Co, 1988.

16. Reed BE, Barrett AP. Hepatitis B virus carrier groups and the Australian community. Aust Dent J. 1988;33:171-176.

17. Booth DR. Hepatitis B - a personal view. Aust Dent J. 1985; 30(1):47-48.

18. National Health and Medical Research Council. Infection control in the health care setting: Guidelines for the prevention of transmission of infectious diseases. Canberra: Commonwealth of Australia, 1996.

19. Centers for Disease Control and Prevention. Recommended infection-control practices for dentistry 1986. Available from: https://www.cdc.gov/mmwr/preview/mmwrhtml/00033634.htm.

20. Barrett AP, Reed BE, National Health and Medical Research Council, Department of Health, AIDS Task Force. Guidelines for dental treatment of patients with infectious diseases. Canberra: Commonwealth of Australia, 1987.

21. Control. CfD. Recommendations for prevention of HIV transmission in health-care settings. In: MMWR, ed. 1987.

22. Centers for Disease Control and Prevention. Investigations of persons treated by HIV-infected health-care workers - United States 1993. In: US Department of Health, ed. Atlanta, GA: CDC, 1993. Available from: https://www.cdc.gov/mmwr/preview/mmwrhtml/00020479.htm.

23. Ciesielski C, Marianos D, Ou C, Dumbaugh R, Witte J, Berkelman R, et al. Transmission of human immunodeficiency virus in a dental practice. Ann Int Med. 1992;116:798-805.

24. Centers for Disease Control and Prevention. Recommendations for preventing transmission of human immunodeficiency virus and hepatitis B virus to patients during exposure-prone invasive procedures 1991. Available from: https://www.cdc.gov/mmwr/preview/mmwrhtml/00014845.htm.

25. Centers for Disease Control and Prevention. Recommended infection-control practices for dentistry, 1993. In: MMWR, ed. 1993.

26. Australian Dental Association Inc. Blood borne infections - some guidelines. Australian Dental Association Inc News Bulletin. 1986, June:14.

27. Australian Dental Association Inc. Infection control in dentistry. Australian Dental Association Inc News Bulletin. 1986, August:10-1.

28. Association AD. Infection control. Australian Dental Association Inc News Bulletin. 1987, November:11-2.

29. Australian Dental Association Inc. AIDS - is saliva infectious? Australian Dental Association Inc News Bulletin. 1988, September:3-5.

30. Australian Dental Association Inc. Infection control. Australian Dental Association Inc News Bulletin. 1988 May:3-5.

31. Australian National Council on AIDS. Infection control in office practice: medical, dental and allied health. Canberra: Australian Government, 1994.

32. National Health and Medical Research Council, Australian National Council on AIDS. Management guidelines for the control of infectious disease hazards in health care establishments: report of the joint NHMRC/ANCA Working Party on Management guidelines for the Control of Infectious Disease Hazards in Health Care Establishments. Canberra: Australian Government, 1993.

33. National Health and Medical Research Council. Guidelines for the prevention of transmission of viral infection in dentistry. Canberra: Australian Government, 1992.

34. Sterilisation/disinfection guidelines for general practice. 2nd ed. Magennis A, ed. Sydney: Royal Australian College of General Practitioners, 1994.

35. Standards Australia. AS 4187-1994 Code of practice for cleaning, disinfecting and sterilizing reusable medical and surgical instruments and equipment, and maintenance of associated environments in health care facilities. Standards Australia, 1994.

36. Association AD. Practical Guides for Successful Dentistry. 4th ed. Tyas MJ, Atkinson HF, Harcourt JK, eds. New South Wales: Scanagraphics Pty Ltd, 1993.

37. Department of Health and Ageing. Infection control guidelines for the prevention of transmission of infectious diseases in the health care setting. Canberra: Australian Government, 2004.

38. National Health and Medical Research Council. Australian Guidelines for the Prevention and Control of Infection in Healthcare. Canberra: Australian Government, 2010.

39. National Health and Medical Research Council. Australian Guidelines for the Prevention and Control of Infection in Healthcare. Canberra: Australian Government, 2019.

40. Australian Dental Association. Guidelines for infection control, 3rd edn. ADA, 2015.

41. Australian Dental Association. Guidelines for infection control. 1st ed. St Leonards, NSW: ADA, 2008.

42. Association AD. Guidelines for infection control. 2nd ed. St Leonards, NSW: ADA, 2012.

43. Dental Board of Australia. Infection prevention and control. Resources for dental practitioners. Available from: https://www.dentalboard.gov.au/Codes-Guidelines/Infection-prevention-and-control.aspx.

44. World Health Organization. WHO characterizes COVID-19 as a pandemic 2020. Geneva: WHO, 2020. Available from: https://www.who.int/emergencies/diseases/novel-coronavirus-2019/events-as-they-happen.

45. Australian Dental Association. Managing COVID-19 guidelines. St Leonards, NSW: ADA, 2020.

46. Australian Health Protection Principal Committee. Recommendations for managing COVID-19 in dental services 2020. Available from: https://www.health.gov.au/news/australian-health-protection-principal-committee-ahppc-advice-to-national-cabinet-on-25-march-2020.

47. Dental Board of Australia. Urgent alert – Australian Health Protection Principal Committee advice. Dental Board of Australia, 2020.

48. Dental Board of Australia. Dental Board of Australia registrant data. 2020.

49. Australian Government Department of Health. National registration and accreditation scheme (NRAS) 2019. Canberra: Australian Government, 2019. Available from: https://www1.health.gov.au/internet/main/publishing.nsf/Content/work-nras.

50. Australian Dental Association. Dental assistant. St Leonards, NSW: ADA. Available from: https://www.ada.org.au/Careers/Dental-Team/Assistant.

51. Outlook AGJ. Dental assistants. Available from: https://joboutlook.gov.au/Occupation?search=Career&code=4232.

52. Australian Dental Association. Dental prosthetist. St Leonards, NSW: ADA, 2020. Available from: https://www.ada.org.au/Careers/Dental-Team/Dental-Prosthetist.

53. Australian Government Job Outlook. Dental prosthetists 2020. Available from: https://joboutlook.gov.au/occupations/dental-prosthetists?occupationCode=411212.

54. Dental Board of Australia. Code of Conduct. 2022. Available from: https://www.dentalboard.gov.au/Codes-Guidelines/Policies-Codes-Guidelines/Code-of-conduct.aspx

55. Dental Council of New South Wales. Available from: https://www.dentalcouncil.nsw.gov.au/.

56. Health Professional Councils Authority. Available from: https://www.hpca.nsw.gov.au/.

57. Office of the Health Ombudsman. Available from: Office of the Health Ombudsman, QLD.

58. Graham B, Tennant M, Shiikha Y, Kruger E. Distribution of Australian private dental practices: contributing underlining sociodemographics in the maldistribution of the dental workforce. Aust J Prim Health. 2019;25(1):54.

59. Australian Institute of Health and Welfare. Oral health and dental care in Australia. Canberra: AIHW, 2019. Available from: https://www.aihw.gov.au/reports/dental-oral-health/oral-health-and-dental-care-in-australia/contents/dental-workforce.

60. Australian Commission on Safety and Quality in Health Care. National Safety and Quality Health Service Standards. Sydney: ACSQHC, 2011.

61. Australian Commission on Safety and Quality in Health Care. National Safety and Quality Health Service Standards. 2nd ed. Sydney: ACSQHC, 2017.

62. Lamont RJ, Hajishengallis GN, Jenkinson HF. Oral microbiology and immunology. Washington, USA: ASM Press, 2013.

63. Australian Institute of Health and Welfare. Hepatitis B in Australia. Canberra: Australian Government, 2018.

64. Australian Government Department of Health. Australian Immunisation Handbook. Hepatitis B. Canberra: Australian Government. n.d. Available from: https://immunisationhandbook.health.gov.au/vaccine-preventable-diseases/hepatitis-b.

65. Australian Government Department of Health. The Australian Immunisation Handbook. Canberra: Australian Government, 2021. Available from: https://immunisationhandbook.health.gov.au/.

66. Australian Government Department of Health. CDNA National guidelines for public health units 2020. Canberra: Australian Government, 2020. Available from: https://www1.health.gov.au/internet/main/publishing.nsf/Content/cdna-song-novel-coronavirus.htm.

67. Baudet A, Lizon J, Martrette J, Camelot F, Florentin A, Clement C. Dental unit waterlines: a survey of practices in eastern France. Int J Environ Res Public Health. 2019;16(21).

68. Ji X-Y, Fei C-N, Zhang Y, Liu J, Liu H, Song J. Three key factors influencing the bacterial contamination of dental unit waterlines: a 6-year survey from 2012 to 2017. Int Dent J. 2019;69:192-199.

69. Hatzenbuehler LA, Tobin-D'Angelo M, Drenzek C, Peralta G, Crranmer LC, Anderson EJ, et al. Pediatric dental clinic - associated outbreak of *Mycobacterium abscessus* infection. J Pediatr Infect Soc. 2017;6(3):e116-e22.

70. Realpe OJC, Gutierrez JC, Sierra DA, Martinez LAP, Palaciou YYP, Echeverria G, et al. Dental unit waterlines in Quito and Caracs contaminated with nontuberculous mycobacteria: a potential health risk in dental practice. Int J Environ Res Public Health. 2020;17(7):2348.

71. Ricci ML, Fontana S, Pinci F, Fiumana E, Pedna MF, Farolfi P, et al. Pneumonia associated with a dental unit waterline. Lancet. 2012;379:684.

72. Volgenant CMC, Persoon IF. Microbial water quality management of dental unit water lines at a dental school. J Hosp Infect. 2019;103:e115-e118.

73. Lee GM, Bishop P. Microbiology and infection control for health professionals. 6th ed. Melbourne: Pearson Australia, 2016.

74. Laheij AM, Kistler JO, Belibasakis GN, Valimaa H, de Soet JJ, European Oral Microbiology Workshop. Healthcare-associated viral and bacterial infections in dentistry. J Oral Microbiol. 2012;4.

75. Schonning C, Jernberg C, Klingenberg D, Andersson S, Paajarvi A, Alm E, et al. Legionellosis acquired through a dental unit: a case study. J Hosp Infect. 2017;96:89-92.

76. Samaranayake LP. Essential microbiology for dentistry. 5th ed. Elsevier, 2018.

77. Volgenant CMC, de Soet JJ. Cross-transmission in the dental office: does this make you ill? Curr Oral Health Rep. 2018;5(4):221-228.

78. Centers for Disease Control and Prevention. Guidelines for dental settings. In: US Department of Health, ed. Atlanta, GA: CDC, 2019. Available from: https://www.cdc.gov/coronavirus/2019-ncov/hcp/dental-settings.html.

79. Gallagher JE, Sukriti KC, Johnson IG, Al-Yaseen W, Jones R, McGregor S, et al. A systematic review of contamination (aerosol, splatter and droplet generation) associated with oral surgery and its relevance to COVID-19. Br Dent J Open. 2020;6(25).

80. Health CO. Aerosol generating procedures and their mitigation in international guidance documentation 2020. Available from: https://oralhealth.cochrane.org/news/aerosol-generating-procedures-and-their-mitigation-international-guidance-documents.

81. Kumar PS, Subramanian K. Demystifying the mist: sources of microbial bioload in dental aerosols. J Periodontology. 2020;91:1113-11122.

82. Scottish Dental Clinical Effectiveness Programme. Mitigation of aerosol generating procedures in dentistry - a rapid review. 2020.

83. Sergis A, Wade WG, Gallagher JE, Morrell AP, Patel S, Dickinson CM, et al. Mechanisms of atomization from rotatory dental instruments and its migration. J Dent Res. 2021;100(3):261-267.

84. Zemouri C, Bolgenant CMC, Buijs MJ, Crielaard W, Rosema NAM, Brandt BW, et al. Dental aerosols: microbial composition and spatial distribution. J Oral Microbiol. 2020;12(1):1762040.

85. Molinari J A HJA. Cottone's practical infection control in dentistry, 3rd ed. Philadelphia, PA: Lippincott Williams & Wilkins, 2010.

86. Communicable Diseases Network Australia. Australian national guidelines for the management of healthcare workers living with blood borne viruses and healthcare workers who perform exposure prone procedures at risk of exposure to blood borne viruses. In: Department of Health, ed. Canberra: Australian Government, 2019.

87. Ge ZY, Yang LM, Xia JJ, Fu XH, Zhang YZ. Possible aerosol transmission of COVID-19 and special precautions in dentistry. J Zhejiang Univ Sci B. 2020;21(5):361-368.

88. Boswell C, Longstaff J. Health protection scotland aerosol generating procedures (AGPs). In: Scotland HP, ed. Health Protection Scotland Infection Control, 2020.

89. Harrel SK, Molinari J. Aerosols and splatter in dentistry: a brief review of the literature and infection control implications. J Am Dent Assoc. 2004;135(4):429-437.

90. Centers for Disease Control and Prevention. Dental unit water quality. In: US Department of Health, ed. Atlanta, GA: CDC, 2016. Available from: https://www.cdc.gov/oralhealth/infectioncontrol/summary-infection-prevention-practices/dental-unit-water-quality.html.

91. Cleveland J, Gray SK, Harte JA, Robison VA, Moorman AC, Gooch BF. Transmission of blood-borne pathogens in US dental health setting: 2016 update. J Am Dent Assoc. 2016;147(9):729-738.

92. Laheij AMGA, Kistler JO, Belibasakis GN, Valimaa JJ, de Soet JJ. Healthcare-associated viral and bacterial infections in dentistry. J Oral Microbiol. 2011;4.

93. Ross KM, Mehr JS, Greeley RD, Montoya LA, Kulkarni PA, Frontin S, et al. Outbreak of bacterial endocarditis associated with an oral surgery practice. J Am Dent Assoc. 2018;149(3):191-201.

94. Merte JL, Kroll CM, Collins AS, Melnick AL. An epidemiologic investigation of occupational transmission of Mycobacterium tuberculosis infection to dental health personnel. Journ J Am Dent Assoc. 2014;145(5):464-471.

95. Froum SH, Froum SJ. Incidence of COVID-19 virus transmission in three dental offices: a 6-month retrospective study. Int J Periodontics Restorative Dent. 2020;40(6):853-859.

96. Estrich CG, Mikkelsen M, Morrissey R, Geisinger ML, Ioannidou E, Vujicic M, et al. Estimating COVID-19 prevalence and infection control practices among US dentists. J Am Dent Assoc. 2020;151(11):815-824.

97. Molinar JA, Harte JA. Cottone's practical infection control in dentistry. 3rd ed. Lippincott Williams & Wilkins, 2010.

98. Sickbert-Bennett EE. Reduction of healthcare-associated infections by exceeding high compliance with hand hygiene practices. Emerg Infect Dis. 2016;22(9):1628-1630.

99. Centers for Disease Control and Prevention. Hand hygiene in health care. In: US Department of Health, ed. Atlanta, GA: CDC, 2020. Available from: https://www.cdc.gov/handhygiene/index.html.

100. World Health Organization. WHO guidelines on hand hygiene in health care. Geneva: WHO, 2009.

101. Australian Commission on Safety and Quality in Health Care; Initiative NHH. 5 Moments of Hand Hygiene: Dental. Sydney: ACSQHC, 2019.

102. Hand Hygiene Australia. Dental 2020. Available from: https://www.hha.org.au/local-implementation/specific-settings/dental.

103. Queensland Health. Developing a sharps safety program. Brisbane: Queensland Government, 2017. Available from: https://www.health.qld.gov.au/clinical-practice/guidelines-procedures/diseases-infection/infection-prevention/standard-precautions/sharps-safety/sharp-safety-program.

104. Australian Dental Association. Policy statement 6.11 - dental amalgam waste management. St Leonards NSW: ADA, 2020.

105. Centers for Disease Control and Prevention. Dental unit water quality. In: US Department of Health, ed. Atlanta, GA: CDC, 2020. Available from: https://www.cdc.gov/oralhealth/infectioncontrol/summary-infection-prevention-practices/dental-unit-water-quality.html.

106. Australian Dental Association. Transmission-based precautions. St Leonards NSW: ADA, 2020. Available from: https://www.ada.org.au/Transmission-Based-Precautions.

107. Australian Dental Association. ADA COVID-19 risk management guidance. St Leonards NSW: ADA, 2020.

108. Rasslan O. Organizational Structure. In: Friedman C, Newsom W, eds. IFIC Basic concepts of infection control. 2nd ed. Portadown, Ireland: International Federation of Infection Control, 2011.

109. Dental Board of Australia. Your infection control obligations under the National Law. Dental Board of Australia, 2015.

110. Centers for Disease Control. Summary of infection prevention practices in dental setting: basic expectations for safer care. In: US Department of Health, ed. Atlanta, GA: CDC, 2016.

111. Peng X, Xu X, Yuqing L, Cheng L, Zhou X, Ren B. Transmission routes of 2019-n-CoV and controls in dental practice. International Journal of Oral Science. 2020;12(1).

112. Meng L, Hua F, Bian Z. Coronavirus disease 2019 (COVID-19): emerging and future challenges for dental and oral medicine. J Dent Res. 2020;99(5):481-487.

CHAPTER 35

Infection prevention and control in allied health settings–physiotherapy, speech pathology, podiatry and rehabilitation

Dr SUSAN COULSON[i]

Dr TIFFANY DWYER[i]

Dr EMMA CHARTERS[ii]

Dr FIONA HAWKE[iii]

BELINDA C. HENDERSON[iv]

Chapter highlights

- Allied health practitioners are required to practise within their professional codes of conduct which have the common theme of 'minimising risk'
- Prolonged periods of time spent with patients in rehabilitation units and colocation of allied health, nursing and medical professionals in multidisciplinary settings increases the risk of infection spreading among patients and staff
- Treatment plinths and the wide variety of therapeutic equipment used by allied health practitioners require equipment-specific disinfection and decontamination to reduce the risk of cross-infection
- Additional infection control measures are required for the aerosol-generating and particle-generating procedures undertaken by allied health practitioners

i   Discipline of Physiotherapy, Sydney School of Health Sciences, Faculty of Medicine and Health, The University of Sydney, Sydney, NSW

ii Head and Neck, Allied Health, Chris O'Brien Lifehouse, Sydney, NSW

iii College of Health, Medicine and Wellbeing, University of Newcastle, Newcastle, NSW

iv Infection Management Services Princess Alexandra Hospital, Brisbane, QLD

Introduction

Allied health professionals, such as physiotherapists, speech pathologists and podiatrists, are first-contact practitioners who assess and treat patients of all ages in a variety of workplaces, including hospitals and rehabilitation settings. There are a variety of infection risks in allied healthcare workplaces that require identification. In aged care units for example, there is a high prevalence of methicillin-resistant *Staphylococcus aureus* (MRSA), particularly in patients with urinary catheters and chronic wounds.[1,2] Comorbidities and prolonged periods of stay in rehabilitation units increase the susceptibility to healthcare-associated infections (HAIs).[2,3] Compliance with hand hygiene procedures reduces the transmission of HAIs which can spread across, and within, allied health workplaces.[1]

Patients managed by allied health practitioners range from those with minor conditions, to people who require acute care. They are treated one-on-one or in group settings, with the main goal of optimising function and preventing recurrence of injuries or diseases. Practitioners often spend extended time periods in close proximity to their patients which, along with the therapies and medical equipment involved, can increase the risk of transmission of HAIs.[3]

Allied healthcare practitioners are integral members of multidisciplinary teams. Their main goal is to rehabilitate the patient by maximising functional capacity and minimising dysfunction so they can live as independently as possible. The therapies used to achieve this level of function bring practitioners into close physical contact with patients, their families, the community and other healthcare practitioners. The healthcare settings in which allied healthcare clinicians practise have evolved over the past few decades, from strictly hospital and clinical settings to less formal environments such as residential care homes, gyms, sports clubs and community rooms, hydrotherapy pools, schools and commercial workplaces. Telehealth has also become more widely used, particularly since the start of the COVID-19 pandemic.

One area where groups of allied health professionals work closely together to treat patients is in the rehabilitation wards of hospitals and health facilities. In these wards, the focus is on restoring function and optimising the individual patient's independence. In conjunction with the therapies and medical and nursing expertise, patients in this setting are usually encouraged to socialise with each other, and many of the therapy activities are communal in nature. This is relatively unique within health, especially in relation to inpatient units—except for those in mental health—and as such, this setting potentially facilitates infection transmission if infection risks are not identified promptly and managed appropriately.

Although 'hands-on' treatment remains one of the main roles of allied health practitioners, a wide range of equipment is also used. This includes:

- electrotherapeutic machines
- computers and keyboards
- bed-lifters and walking aids such as crutches, sticks and frames
- pillows and towels, swabs, dressings and cotton wool
- tendon hammers and tongue depressors
- video-fluoroscopes, nasendoscopy and functional swallowing examination equipment
- sports tape, compression stockings and bandages
- acupuncture needles, scalpels, stethoscopes and chest suctioning tools
- goniometers and inclinometers
- tape measures
- sports equipment such as exercise bands,, weights, pulleys and resistance machines
- plastering and splitting materials, creams, oils, lotions and gels; and
- children's toys.

Environmental disinfection is challenging when medical equipment is shared, particularly for items such as wheelchairs which have complex designs.[4] Therefore, allied health practitioners are trained to implement infection control procedures across a range of different healthcare and community settings. These include using single use, disposable items such as sports tape, tongue depressors and acupuncture needles, and disinfection to reduce *Clostridium difficile* spores on therapeutic equipment such as wheelchairs.[4]

The surfaces upon which practitioners treat patients include vinyl plinths, linen-covered hospital beds and treatment couches, chairs, stools, bean bags, exercise gyms and gym mats, to name a few. The range of equipment, treatment surfaces, rooms and spaces, as well as the close nature of patient, carer and healthcare professional interactions, provide many potential pathways of infection transmission. Therefore, fastidious and consistent infection control and prevention (ICP) procedures by well-trained practitioners at all points of patient interaction are mandatory to minimise risk of transmission.

Professional regulation: Allied health professions are formally regulated to ensure that practitioners are fit to practise whilst minimising the risk of harm to the general public, including harm caused by infection transmission between practitioners and patients, carers, colleagues and the general community. Physiotherapists and podiatrists are regulated by the Australian Healthcare Practitioner Regulation Agency (AHPRA), and have codes of conduct, with the common themes of 'minimising risk'.[5,6] Speech pathologists are required to practise in line with the Speech Pathology Australia National Code of Conduct. The Speech Pathology National Code of Conduct explicitly states that practice must include *'adopting standard precautions for infection control'*.[7]

Risk management: Allied healthcare workers (HCWs) have a personal responsibility to understand and adhere to the health and safety requirements of the variety of workplaces in which they practise. This includes attending training, following relevant guidelines, and using equipment to protect themselves against exposure to pathogens and potentially infectious materials. They must also understand how to assess risk and prepare infection mitigation strategies in advance of all treatment interactions. This risk assessment also includes identification and containment of potential sources of infection, such as providing masks to patients with respiratory symptoms and separating them from others in treatment and waiting rooms.

To minimise or prevent the transmission of infection, allied health practitioners use a risk management approach including standard precautions (SP) and transmission-based precautions (TBP). SP are required for all patients and clinicians to prevent the transmission of infection.[8] This involves diligent adherence to hand hygiene practices, appropriate use of personal protective equipment (PPE), sharps disposal, environmental cleaning and following procedures for reprocessing reusable equipment. For those patients confirmed or suspected to have infectious diseases or conditions, TBP are required in addition to SP to prevent transmission by airborne, droplet or contact routes.

Allied HCWs are at risk of exposure to blood and body substances, and to infectious diseases; therefore, it is both a personal and an employer responsibility to manage occupational exposure to blood and other body substances. The overall aim is to manage staff health, which is covered in detail in Chapter 26.

35.1 Physiotherapy

Physiotherapists are experts in movement and function who work in partnership with their patients, assisting them to overcome movement disorders which may have been present from birth, acquired through accident or injury, or are the result of ageing or life-changing events. Physiotherapists help people recover from injury, reduce pain and stiffness, increase mobility and prevent further injury. They assess, diagnose and treat a broad range of acute and chronic musculoskeletal, neurological and cardiopulmonary conditions, and often work as an integral member of a multidisciplinary team. They work in hospitals and in private practice consulting rooms, as well as in community settings such as sporting gyms and in people's homes. Standard infection prevention and control (IPC) procedures therefore need to be implemented across these different working environments. In hospital settings, infection control equipment and procedures are usually readily available; however, in private practice and community settings, the onus is on the physiotherapist to plan and instigate the infection control process themselves. For example, when a community physiotherapist visits someone's home, they need to have taken along the appropriate infection control equipment and work in partnership with community members to ensure that high standards are maintained to minimise cross-infection.

35.1.1 Identification of the risks in physiotherapy practice and risk minimisation

The microorganisms most frequently isolated in the physiotherapist's environment are opportunistic pathogens which can negatively affect elderly and immunosuppressed patients or those weakened by chronic diseases. Therefore, physiotherapists need to understand the potential pathways of infection transmission as well as control procedures.[9] These can include clinical treatment surfaces—items such as chairs, floormats and therapeutic equipment—as well as airborne and bodily fluid transmission. While regular, general cleaning regimens and laundry services occur in more formalised hospital and clinical environments, it is the responsibility of the individual physiotherapist to clean and disinfect the treatment surfaces they use for each patient in line with SP (see Chapter 15).

Microbial contamination has been found on treatment surfaces and therapeutic equipment including ultrasound, interferential and transcutaneous electrical stimulation (TENS) machines (discussed in next section), with sponge electrodes found to have very high levels of contamination.[9] Vinyl-covered treatment plinths have been found to harbour pathogenic bacteria such as *Staphylococcus*,[1] therefore, wiping plinths and therapeutic equipment with a detergent disinfectant can significantly reduce the risk of cross-transmission between patients.[1] However, organisms that have been detected on cloth coverings include *S. aureus* and *Propionibacterium*, and allergen-producing moulds including *Candida*, so they should not be left in situ between treatments.[10] Treatment tables with non-removable cloth coverings are not recommended for clinical use as they have been shown to contain pathogenic microbacteria and allergens.[10]

The following section describes the inherent infection risks and mitigation strategies in the types of procedures undertaken by physiotherapists.

35.1.2 Specific physiotherapy assessment and treatment procedures

Hands-on physiotherapy techniques: Physiotherapists are trained to use a number of hands-on therapy procedures to assess and treat musculoskeletal pain and dysfunction, and neurological and cardiopulmonary conditions. However, cross-contamination and transmission of microorganisms has been found to spread via the hands of HCWs.[11] Hands-on treatments are undertaken within close proximity of the patient; therefore, social distancing, which was strongly emphasised during the COVID-19 pandemic, is difficult to implement during the majority of face-to-face assessment and treatment interactions. Mask-wearing, hand antisepsis and handwashing procedures with soap and water or alcohol-based sanitiser are some of the key elements of infection control to reduce cross-transmission,[11] as is the wearing of gloves when there is a risk of body fluid exposure (see Chapter 14). Furthermore, when cuts and abrasions of the hands and forearms are present on the HCW, they should be covered with a waterproof dressing.[12]

Respiratory physiotherapists and aerosol-generating procedures: Specialised respiratory physiotherapists work in a number of clinical settings, including hospitals, outpatient clinics, private practices and in the community. They assess and treat people with chronic lung diseases such as emphysema; acute lung diseases, including pneumonia; after major surgery, for example open-heart surgery; and patients with severe illnesses, such as those in intensive care with sepsis or following trauma such as severe burn injury (see Chapter 18). Many of these patients have bacterial or viral infections, so potentially pose an infection risk to the HCW providing their care as well as to visitors and other patients. In addition to the use of masks and handwashing and other standard procedures,[8] environmental contamination from aerosol-generating procedures (AGPs) requires adequate room ventilation and cleaning to reduce risk of transmission to other patients and HCWs, such as the use of negative pressure, single patient rooms, ideally with high-efficiency particulate air (HEPA) filtration, and thorough cleaning of all contact surfaces after performing any AGP. The assessment and treatment techniques performed by respiratory physiotherapists commonly have additional infection control risks, mainly due to the use of AGPs.

These assessments include:
- lung function testing
- maximal exercise capacity testing
- induced sputum, using an ultrasonic jet nebuliser; and
- any assessment where a patient is prescribed nebulised medication or is on positive pressure ventilation (including high-flow nasal prong oxygen, continuous positive airway pressure [CPAP], non-invasive ventilation [NIV] and if intubated and mechanically ventilated).

Treatments which can generate aerosols include:
- repositioning or mobilising patients who are mechanically ventilated, where there is risk of disconnecting from the ventilator
- all airway clearance techniques
- mechanical insufflation/exsufflation
- suctioning (including nasopharyngeal, oropharyngeal, via tracheostomy or endotracheal tube); and
- manual hyperinflation and inspiratory muscle training for patients who are mechanically ventilated.

The first step in risk minimisation when performing any AGP is to identify the level of risk of infection transmission. If there is no history of viral or bacterial infection, there is a confirmed negative test for current infection, no risk factors were identified during a thorough screening of the patient and there is currently low incidence of community transmission of infections, it would be classified as low risk. In those situations, it is adequate to continue assessment and treatment involving aerosol-generating procedures, while adhering to SPs such as the use of surgical masks, gloves, gown and goggles or face shield (see Chapter 13). It is important to remember, however, that low risk does not mean no risk.

If the patient history, diagnosis or screening identifies a patient as high risk (e.g. MRSA or tuberculosis isolated from a sputum culture) and/or there is a high incidence of community transmission of infections (e.g. swine flu), additional risk minimisation steps need to be taken. First, consider whether the activity is truly necessary or if it could be avoided (e.g. during the COVID-19 pandemic lung function testing was only conducted in medically essential cases, where treatment decisions required lung function results, and required the approval of the patient's treating physician). Other assessment techniques can be modified to minimise risk, such as teaching patients with chronic lung diseases to perform spirometry lung function testing with home-based personal devices. In hospital settings, physiotherapy staff and visitors should wait at least 30 minutes before entering a patient's room after completing nebulised treatment; however, if care is required prior to this time, all HCWs entering the patient bed space are required to adhere to TBPs.

Some treatments can also be modified to avoid risk (e.g. patients can be taught independent airway clearance techniques via TeleHealth and parents can provide respiratory physiotherapy treatments for their children if the child were in a stable condition and the parents performed the treatments as part of the usual home regimen). Medical staff can also consider changing some nebulised medication to metered-dose inhalers with a spacer (e.g. salbutamol) and manual hyperinflation could be substituted by ventilator hyperinflation, to avoid the risks of dispersing aerosols when the ventilator is disconnected for manual hyperinflation.

If the aerosol-generating assessment or treatment is deemed necessary and the risks cannot be avoided, additional PPE is required to include airborne precautions PFR—N95/P2 respirator, gloves, impermeable gown covering to wrists, and goggles or face shield. Modifications to reduce risk include having the patient in a negative pressure and/or single room; maintaining more than 1.5 metres distance whenever possible; not standing in front of the patient when they are doing lung function testing, huffing or coughing; encouraging the patient to have good cough etiquette (coughing

into tissues or elbow, immediately disposing of tissues and cleaning hands afterwards); performing manual techniques of percussion and vibration when standing behind the patient; and only performing suctioning when absolutely necessary, using an inline suction catheter where possible.

35.1.3 Therapeutic equipment and infection risk

Therapeutic ultrasound: Therapeutic ultrasound (US) is applied using US heads and a non-sterile coupling gel which comes into direct contact with the patient's skin, hence increasing the risk of HAIs from cross-contamination between patients.[13] It is used to treat soft tissue injuries of the ligaments, muscle tendons and connective tissues, with some practitioners also applying it to surgical wounds and ulcers.[14] The most common procedure involves direct contact of a transducer head with a non-sterile coupling gel;[15] however, therapeutic US equipment has been found to be a potential fomite for infection transmission between patients.[13] While transducer heads have been found to have relatively low levels of contamination, coupling gels may be heavily contaminated with potentially pathogenic organisms, including *Stenotrophomonas maltophilia*, *S. aureus*, *Acinetobacter baumannii* and *Rhodotorula mucilaginosa*.[14] It has been found that nearly 80% of *S. aureus* placed on US transducer heads in gel survived for 1 hour;[16] hence, US gel should be manually removed from the transducer head prior to cleaning. The transducer should be cleaned using a Therapeutic Goods Administration (TGA) approved disposable cleaning wipe or a freshly made-up solution of cleaning agent at the correct concentration which is then rinsed thoroughly under running water to remove cleaning agent residues before drying using a single use, low linting cloth.[17] If therapeutic US had come into contact with non-intact skin, or was used in body cavities, higher levels of disinfection would be required.

Interferential therapy: Musculoskeletal injuries are treated with interferential therapy machines by some practitioners. These machines use suction cups and water-infused sponges to apply alternating electrical currents to patients. There is also a vacuum device to hold the suction cups onto the skin and a water reservoir which supplies a small volume of water to the rim of the suction cup to facilitate the attachment to the skin surface. Bacteria have been cultured from the sponges used in the suction cups of interferential machines, with 16 out of 20 sponges contaminated with microorganisms including *Pseudomonas*, *Acinetobacter*, *Pasteurella* and *Rhodotorula* species. Water from the reservoir attached to the machine has also been found to be significantly contaminated with *Pseudomonas aeruginosa*.[18] To decrease the likelihood of transmission of microorganisms via interferential therapy machines, it is recommended that disposable electrodes are used and that both the suction cups and sponges are thoroughly cleaned in accordance with manufacturers' guidelines.

Transcutaneous electrical nerve stimulation:
Transcutaneous electrical nerve stimulation (TENS) is commonly used to treat pain and for neurological deficits. Contact electrodes are used to apply the TENS, with bacteria and/or fungi found to be present on the electrodes. Thorough disinfecting between patients and the use of disposable electrodes are recommended to minimise transmission of infection.[19]

35.2 Speech pathology

A speech pathologist is an allied health professional trained to assess and manage communication and swallowing disorders. Speech pathologists study, diagnose and treat communication disorders, including difficulties with speaking, listening, understanding language, reading, writing, social skills, stuttering and using voice. They work with people who have difficulty communicating because of developmental delays, stroke, brain injuries, learning disability, intellectual disability, cerebral palsy, dementia and hearing loss, as well as other problems that can affect speech and language. People who experience difficulties swallowing food and drink safely can also be helped by a speech pathologist. Their practice extends to a wide range of settings including the home, hospital, community health centres, schools, respite and residential care, private clinics, research and university roles.

A speech pathologist works within a broader multidisciplinary team which focuses its care on the patient or client's needs. Their role varies greatly depending on the context of their employment and area of specialty. The workforce covers private and public health settings and the profession is supported by the Speech Pathology Australia (SPA) association, which was established 70 years ago. This association details the ethics, scope and parameters of practice, position statements and clinical guidelines relevant to the Australian Speech Pathology workforce. While membership is not mandated for all graduate clinicians, it is required for any clinician who requires a Medicare provider number and as a condition of employment in some institutions. Eligibility for membership is required for all new-hires in Australia.

35.2.1 Identification of the risks in speech pathology practice and risk minimisation

Risks associated with the speech pathology practice are unique to the specific workload. The Speech Pathology Australia Risk Assessment Tool (SPAR AT COVID-19) was created by SPA to identify the level of risk for COVID-19 transmission associated with a face-to-face clinical interaction. The tool takes approximately 5–10 minutes to complete, with a risk profile generated based on:

- details of the clinician's individual practice, e.g. the number of sites they visit, patients or clients they see, and the types of populations they interact with
- the infection prevention processes in place, e.g. access to training and appropriate infection control resources; and
- patient or client factors, e.g.
  - recent COVID-19 or norovirus test results
  - resistant organism status, such as methicillin-resistant staphylococcus (MRSA) or vancomycin-resistant enterococci (VRE)
  - age
  - transport and proximity to the patient.

While the tool was created for use during the COVID-19 pandemic, it is relevant for any infection control risk evaluation. Risk mitigation has been carried out through the use of replacement services such as telehealth; diligent adherence to institution-specific IPC guidelines including the use of PPE; and relevant task modifications to allow for adequate distancing to minimise the risk of infection transmission.

Schools and preschools: Speech pathologists who specialise in paediatric speech and language in the early childhood and education settings collaborate and interact with the whole school. They often use resources considered to be 'high touch' in their special education programs, particularly for group work where there is little time to carry out disinfection between users. School-based speech pathologists often are contracted by different institutions and hence across a working day can have multiple contacts with different schools or preschools, increasing the risk of infection transmission. In accordance with the National Code of Conduct for HCWs, speech pathologists are expected to adopt SPs, and adhere to IPC policies present in Australian schools.

Hospitals: Speech pathologists cover a wide range of clinical areas in acute and rehabilitation hospitals. Implementation and compliance with an IPC program is fundamental, given the percentage of vulnerable populations present in a hospital and the close proximity required for routine interventions—many of which are considered to be aerosol generating. Specifically, patients referred for a dysphagia assessment following extubation from prolonged mechanical ventilation, with risk factors such as age and impaired cognition, are at risk of silent aspiration—making access to speech pathology and instrumental assessment imperative.[20,21]

Residential aged care facilities: The prevalence of complex comorbidities increases with age. Speech pathologists are routinely called upon to assess and manage communication and swallowing in this population, where up to 68% of residents have dysphagia (swallowing impairment).[22] Considering the risk of infection is higher for those of greater age, with chronic health conditions or compromised immune systems, people residing in aged care facilities are considered vulnerable to both contracting an infection or experiencing a severe illness relating to that infection.[23] Speech pathologists are often contracted with one or more facilities, adding to the risk that any infection they are exposed to will be transmitted across locations.

Risk minimisation: In order to minimise or prevent the transmission of infection, speech pathology services use a risk management approach, including SP and TBPs. Standard precautions are required for all patients and clinicians to prevent the transmission of infection. This involves diligent adherence to hand hygiene practices, appropriate use of PPE, sharps disposal, environmental cleaning and following procedures for reprocessing reusable equipment. For those patients where an infectious disease or condition is confirmed or suspected, TBPs are required, in addition to SPs to prevent airborne, droplet or contact transmission.

Telehealth uses technology to provide health services that allow people in a vulnerable position to receive education, counselling, assessment, intervention and support care remotely.[24] It was first instigated to facilitate equal access to specialised health services for those from regional and remote communities; however, it has now been endorsed by Speech Pathology Australia (SPA) and the American Speech-Language-Hearing Association (ASHA) as a viable option for providing SP services during a pandemic.

The recent COVID-19 pandemic has highlighted the risk of infection associated with communication and swallowing procedures considered to be aerosol generating. High-risk procedures such as tracheostomy cuff deflation, momentary digital occlusion and speaking valve use, laryngectomy care, and management involving stoma care and voice prosthesis changes and cough reflex testing are of particular concern. They are managed by minimising the number of personnel present, appropriate social distancing, adherence to PPE and clinician training.

35.2.2 Specific speech pathology assessment and treatment practices and infection control procedures

Reprocessing of speech pathology equipment: Specialised equipment in different subspecialties of speech pathology practice have different reprocessing requirements based on manufacturers' recommendations and institutional policies. Engaging the correct process is essential for the adequate decontamination and reprocessing of reusable healthcare equipment and preventing the transmission of infective agents. This is done by either cleaning, disinfection or sterilisation, or a combination of all three. All reusable assessment and rehabilitation devices are required to be approved by the TGA. The institution is responsible to follow manufacturers' guidelines relating to the reprocessing of individual pieces of equipment. Every clinician and institution is likely to have its own policies, protocols, constraints and local legislation for different practices and protocols which need to be considered.[8] Standard or routine infection control practices are in place for all patients (or clients) in contexts including, but not limited to, ambulatory care, community clinics, private practice, aged or retirement homes, group homes, private homes and hospital settings. These practices follow the Australian Guidelines for the

Prevention and Control of Infection in Healthcare (2019),[25] with added precautions for those at risk of, or confirmed to have, an infective process transferred by airborne, droplet or contact transmission.

Equipment common for swallow and communication assessment and management is divided into items which are strictly:

(a) single use (single use within a single session)

(b) single patient use (single patient; however, able to be reused over multiple sessions); and

(c) multiple use (multiple patients).

The purpose of such protocols is to prevent transmission of infection using best practice standards. Examples include:

(a) single use items, individually packaged food and fluids, plastic utensils, mouth swabs, cups, tongue depressors and gloves; and

(b) single patient use items including therapy equipment such as a Therabite® (a jaw stretching device), tracheostomy speaking valves, tracheostomy caps, laryngectomy tubes, expiratory muscle strength trainer (EMST), laryngectomy dilators and voice prosthesis cleaning brushes. Typically, these are cleaned daily to allow for use on the same patient over multiple days. Cleaning or disinfection is dependent on the manufacturer and institutional guidelines. Labelling the device so it is only used on the same patient is also important; and

(c) reusable items consisting of:

  critical—flexible and rigid scopes used for endoscopy or stroboscopy in instrumental swallowing and voice assessment. Require cleaning and sterilisation

  semi-critical—surgical forceps used for voice prosthesis changes in patients with a laryngectomy, thermometers and microphones. Require cleaning and disinfection (high level)

  non-critical—examination tables and furniture, toys, books, language and speech testing equipment, computer-assisted materials (headsets, masks), desks, penlights, dishes, head torches and carry bags. Require cleaning with detergent and/or disinfection depending on the item (low level).

Context-specific cleaning and disinfectant practices: The varied scope of practice and areas of sub-specialty necessitates context-specific cleaning practices. Specified infection control practices are mandated for all practising speech pathologists and reinforced through annual or routine training in order to protect clinicians, clients/patients and communities from the spread of infection. IPC processes are required both for the protection of the HCW and the patient as well as any carers present.

Clinical swallowing examination (CSE): Standard cleaning and disinfection precautions are applicable to most routine assessment and management practices, such as a face-to-face communication or a swallowing assessment. This involves hand hygiene, non-sterile single use medical gloves and the donning of context-specific PPE, and regular cleaning of surfaces and equipment. The propensity for CSEs to elicit a cough response raises concerns for any infection transferable via contact or droplets.[26] Specialised cleaning practices are required for equipment involved in advanced scope of practice procedures such as laryngectomy, tracheostomy, voice, instrumental assessments (fibreoptic endoscopic evaluation [FEES] and videofluoroscopy swallow study [VFSS]. This has become particularly relevant post the COVID-19 pandemic where those practices which are considered an AGP require additional diligence.

Laryngectomy: A laryngectomy is the removal of the larynx (voice box) by surgically dividing the oesophagous and trachea. Speech pathologists working in this area need to be aware of the manufacturers' requirements for individual equipment. Gold standard voice restoration involves the insertion of a voice prosthesis, which directs airflow from the stoma through a vibrating neo-pharynx to create speech. The equipment required for voice prosthesis changes and prosthesis maintenance is considered a semi-critical medical instrument and it is recommended that it is sterilised between patient exams according to the specific manufacturer's guidelines. Equipment in this category includes tracheoesophageal dilators, voice prosthesis sizers and mosquito forceps (which can also be designed for single use). For patients without a voice prosthesis, an electrolarynx (artificial larynx) is usually recommended. The device can be pressed to the patient's neck or an intraoral adaptor can be inserted into their mouth, then the vibrations activated by the user. As it does not come into contact with mucous membranes it is considered non-critical and can be used by multiple patients if cleaned and disinfected between uses. Single use items such as eyeglasses, heat moisture exchanges (HMEs), face shields and swabs are disposed of after the session. Any sharps used (e.g. scissors) are disposed of in a designated sharps bin. Single patient use items, such as voice prostheses, are not designed to be shared between patients due to infection risk after coming into contact with mucous membranes. Consultation with manufacturers' guidelines is essential due to different guidelines for different products. One example of this is soft silicone laryngectomy tubes; individually purchased tubes are to be cleaned between each use with purpose-built cleaning brushes, warm water and non-oil-based dish soap or disinfected with 70% ethanol, isopropyl alcohol or 3% hydrogen peroxide then air dried. They are not, however, designed to be sterilised or shared between patients. In contrast, some sizing kits can be reprocessed by sterilisation after removal of visible debris through cleaning. Strict adherence to the reprocessing guidelines for single and multiple patient use is essential given the risk of device degradation if proper procedures are not followed.

Some patients with a laryngectomy or tracheostomy require a nebuliser for humidification of the upper airway. Nebulisers are considered semi-critical medical devices and, to prevent accumulation of bacterial pathogens, require cleaning and disinfection followed by a sterile water rinse and air drying. This reduces the accumulation of the disinfectant agent. Nebulisers are not designed to be shared between patients in the home setting. In the hospital setting, nebuliser masks are either designed to be single use or single patient use. The durability of the mask will be compromised if reprocessing is conducted outside of manufacturers' guidelines.

During the COVID-19 pandemic, speech pathologists postponed, reduced or eliminated non-urgent procedures such as voice prosthesis changes, or changed their practice to minimise risk. In the event a procedure was required (e.g. voice prosthesis changes or management, tracheostomy changes or management, stoma care and nasendoscopy) the following were considered in addition to the standard and droplet precautions:

- particulate filter respirator (PFR) P2/N95 respirator—individually fit checked each time used, reduces the incidence of transmission via aerosol particles
- face shield and protective eyewear—a clear plastic barrier to cover the face and eyes from transmission of droplets or aerosols
- negative pressure room—a specially designed room with a pressure level below that of the surrounding environment, preventing the transmission of aerosols from the room.

Tracheostomy: A tracheostomy can be a temporary or permanent placement of a breathing tube which connects the airway to a stoma (hole) in the neck, to facilitate breathing or ventilation support. Restoration of communication can involve augmentative and alternative communication (AAC) options, speaking valves or capping. The AAC options available vary widely from single use low-tech products such as paper and pen, to high-tech smart tablets with voice banking and picture or text-to-speech capabilities. Tracheostomy management involves specialty equipment specific to the individual's requirements. Portable humidification (Swedish nose) or a nebuliser mask is designed to be a single patient use product, whereas some portable suction devices can be used by multiple patients after sterilisation if the antibacterial filter and tubing is changed. This, however, is subject to the individual unit manufacturer's specifications. Other items frequently used in tracheostomy care, such as cleaning brushes, speaking valves, caps, inner and outer cannulas, are all single patient use and can be cleaned, disinfected, air dried and then reused by the same patient.

Voice: A voice disorder is any problem with a patient's pitch, voice quality or loudness that prevents them from meeting their activities of daily living. The assessment and management of voice disorders often involves the use of specialised acoustic and aerodynamic equipment for voice recording, analysis and biofeedback. This equipment is appropriate for multi-patient use; however, all components require specialised cleaning between patients. Microphones for voice sample recording or sound pressure level analysis require cleaning according to the manufacturer's guidelines. Some microphones have a removable head basket (a metal mesh dome) or foam lining which can then be gently cleaned or replaced. Foam-based microphone cleaners or single use disposable microphone covers are also options, particularly when there is limited time available for cleaning between patients in a voice clinic setting. Alternatively, use of remote recording where patients record their own voices using a smartphone, tablet or downloadable software is an option. Miniature and sub-miniature lavaliers and headsets also will have equipment-specific guidelines; however, generally they can be rinsed in demineralised water then wiped gently with a damp cloth and left to dry. Surfaces of headsets, clips, booms, grids and adaptors can also be cleaned with isopropyl alcohol and water.

Nasometers can typically be dismantled and cleaned with disposable detergent disinfection wipes.

Trismus: Trismus is a condition where jaw opening is restricted. The Therabite® and other devices with a similar purpose are designed for single patient use to stretch the mouth open progressively. Cleaning with soap and warm water is recommended between uses, followed by time to air dry.

Swallowing: *Clinical swallowing examination (CSE):* requires use of non-sterile single use medical gloves and the donning of context-specific PPE and regular cleaning of surfaces and equipment. Specific clinical populations, such as paediatric feeding, may require sterilisation of equipment intended to be used for multiple patients (e.g. bottles, dummies, teats).

Instrumental swallow assessments: considered the gold standard in swallow evaluation. Setting up an assessment in a clinical area should include the use of a surface barrier such as a blue sheet in addition to environmental surface cleaning between patients. For patients with multidrug-resistant organisms (MROs), where the bacteria are resistant to antimicrobial agents—such as MRSA, vancomycin-resistant enterococci (VRE) and Gram-negative bacteria (MRGNs)—specific attention to the high touch and visually soiled environments such as the bed, chair and benchtops is also required.

Videofluoroscopy swallowing study (VFSS): a procedure which examines the anatomy and physiology of the oral and pharyngeal phases of swallowing. The procedure allows for greater physical distancing between the patient and clinicians than fibreoptic endoscopic evaluation (FEES); however, personnel minimisation, use of PPE, patient prioritisation and post-procedure cleaning are still required for those considered an infection risk.

Fibreoptic endoscopic evaluation of swallowing (FEES) and nasendoscopy: examine the anatomy and physiology of the velopharynx, oropharynx and laryngopharynx accessed transnasally using a flexible endoscope. Correct disinfection of nasendoscopes is required to prevent the iatrogenic transmission of infection. Nasendoscopes come into contact with a patient's intact mucous membranes of the upper aerodigestive tract, and are therefore considered by the Centers for Disease Control and Prevention (CDC)[27] and in the Australian Guidelines for the Prevention and Control of Infection in Healthcare (2019)[25] as a semi-critical medical instrument. Sterilisation between patient examinations to prevent infection, cross-contamination and HAIs is recommended.[28]

Surface electromyography (SEMG) (multiple patient use): a type of visual biofeedback which displays the activity of swallowing musculature for the purposes of rehabilitation. The electrodes are single patient use and measure the electrical output of the submental muscles non-invasively, guiding target muscle contraction. Prior to and following application of the electrodes, the patient's skin is disinfected with alcohol wipes.[29]

Expiratory muscle strength trainer (EMST): a single patient use device designed to improve the musculature involved in expiration, cough, swallow and voice. The manufacturer recommends that the mouthpiece is cleaned weekly with warm water and a mild soap, then air dried.

Manometry: the measurement of contractions through the pharynx and oesophageous which propel a bolus towards the stomach. It involves a thin, flexible catheter with pressure sensors inserted transnasally extending to the stomach. A protective sheath (e.g. Manosheath, Sierra Scientific) can be used to preserve sterility of the catheter[30] although this does not preclude the need for cleaning and reprocessing.

Communication: Augmentative and alternative communication (AAC) refers to devices, tools or strategies which replace or assist someone's usual verbal speech. AAC comprises low- and high-tech options and is prescribed based on the individual's needs. AAC options are imperative for those who do not have access to verbal communication due to developmental or acquired conditions. This is often seen in patients with a speech or language disorder preventing them from acquiring verbal speech, or in those who are mechanically ventilated or tracheostomised. Providing a mode of communication for those ventilated or with a tracheostomy allows them to express their concerns, pain and be involved in their healthcare.[31] However, if appropriate infection control processes are not established, the use and safety of AAC are significantly compromised.[32]

Low-tech options, such as a paper and pen or alphabet board, are typically restricted to single patient use. Boogie boards, whiteboards, smart tablets, smartphones and purpose-built speech generating devices can all be used by multiple patients, provided they are cleaned and disinfected between users. Appropriate infection control for these devices typically comprises the use of covers, and device-appropriate disinfection or cleaning between patients.

The NHMRC classifies most types of AAC as non-critical patient care items and encourages protective covers to be used for smartphones, smart tablets, computer keyboards, whiteboards and boogie boards, in order to facilitate cleaning and avoid device degradation by the disinfection process. Cleaning of smartphones and tablets has been examined with the recommended procedure including:

(a) unplugging the phone or tablet from any electrical source

(b) cleaning the device with a soft, slightly damp lint-free microfibre cloth; and

(c) using a disinfecting wipe.[33]

Clinic-based therapy: Toys, learning resources and communication assessment materials can be used across multiple patients or given out on loan for equipment trials and homework activities. Items which are more difficult or unable to be cleaned between sessions are either considered for single use only or not used, such as kinetic sand, play dough and soft toys. An alternative is for patients to bring resources from home, or items are selected based on ease of cleaning. Waiting rooms may also be closed, with staff allowing patient entry to the clinic only at the time of their session and minimising additional visitors to sessions.

35.3 Podiatry

Podiatrists are involved in the prevention, diagnosis, treatment and rehabilitation of medical and biomechanical conditions of the feet and lower limbs. These may result from chronic disease such as diabetes, peripheral vascular disease and arthritides, soft tissue and muscular pathologies, and sports injuries. Podiatrists assess gait, footwear, prescribe physical therapy and orthoses, treat lower limb skin and nail disorders including corns, calluses and ingrown toenails, and manage chronic wounds of the lower limbs.

Clinical services require the skilled use of sterilised instruments and appropriate infection control procedures, along with the appropriate application of pharmacological agents, specialist wound dressings and a variety of physical therapies.

35.3.1 Identification of the risks in podiatry practice and risk minimisation

As with other allied health professions, podiatrists work in diverse settings and perform a wide range of assessments and treatments. Many physical assessments and therapies performed by podiatrists have the same risks as identified previously, for example, as in physiotherapy.

Podiatrists are unique among health professions in treatments involving cutting and filing of nails, and debridement of wounds and thick skin (corns and calluses). For these activities, podiatrists should routinely wear gloves, face mask (PFR if filing), eye protection and gown. Mechanical room ventilation systems are not commonly used. When a patient is known to be immunocompromised or to have lung disease, the patient should also be offered a face mask.[34] Podiatrists routinely use electric drills for the treatment of nail and skin conditions. Nail drills typically have vacuum exhausts which collect dust in dust bags, although nail drills with water spray dust suppression systems are available. An audit of 50 nail dust bags from podiatry clinics in Australia identified 151 colonies of dermatophytes from 43 of the 50 samples, and, in addition, isolated 471 non-dermatophyte moulds, along with some yeasts and bacteria.[35] It is clear that podiatrists are exposed to bioaerosols and organic dust during their daily clinical practice, including toenail dust generated from podiatric nail drills.[36] Toenail dust particles are plate-like in shape and can remain airborne for long periods making them respirable, with 80% of the particles within a 0.8–1.6 μm particle size range. Once inhaled, these particles are able to penetrate the lower lung region[37,38] which potentially increases the likelihood of respiratory diseases such as asthma occurring in podiatrists. Furthermore, the prevalence of methicillin-susceptible *S. aureus* (MSSA) was found to be higher among podiatrists who did not use an aspiration system (32.3%) compared to those who did use one (19.3%; p = 0.0305), and among podiatrists with respiratory diseases (36.8%) compared to those without (20.8%; p = 0.0272).[39]

Fungal pathogens: Fungal pathogens have also been identified in the dust generated by podiatrists. The most common dermatophytes are from the *Trichophyton mentagrophytes/interdigitale* complexes; however, *Trichophyton rubrum*, *Trichophyton tonsurans*, *Trichophyton soudanense* and *Epidermophyton floccosum* have also been found. The three most common genera of non-dermatophyte moulds were Aspergillus, Penicillium and Scopulariopsis, all of which have been implicated in onychomycosis and more general disease. Viable fungal pathogens in the dust could potentially pose a health problem to podiatrists.[35,40]

Risk minimisation: Due to the known risks of using nail drills, many public hospital podiatry departments have banned the use of nail drills. Podiatrists instead reduce the thickness of thickened nail by sharp debridement, filing or not at all if clinically indicated.

Podiatrists working in private practice may feel their patients expect them to use a nail drill to achieve good cosmesis so continue to use nail drills despite being aware of the risk. Nowadays, university students are taught to never drill a nail that shows signs of onychomycosis, though of course, the diagnostic accuracy of using nail appearance to determine infection presence is not ideal. To reduce the incidence of organic particle inhalation within podiatry practices, implementation of respiratory protective equipment, mechanical room air-filtration systems,[41] local exhaust ventilation and nail drills with water spray dust suppression systems (where nail drills are deemed to be necessary) is recommended for daily use in clinical practices, as well as refresher hygiene training for podiatrists. Instruments require decontamination by steam sterilisation, and the use of an ultraviolet (UV) irradiation instrument cabinet may be considered an adjunct to conventional cleaning and disinfection processes.[42] Hollow Load Type A instruments (AS/NZS: 4815 Standards), such as the beaver blade handle, require vacuum sterilisation. It has recently been proposed that the spring in many commonly used nail clippers is hollow so should be vacuum sterilised. This poses a major hurdle for private podiatrists, most of whom sterilise their own instruments and do not own vacuum sterilisers, which are more expensive and labour intensive in their upkeep.

Cleaning, disinfection and sterilisation: As organic material, such as dirt or skin, has the potential to block the action of disinfection or sterilisation processes, equipment such as nail clippers and drill burrs must be manually cleaned as soon as possible after using them before undergoing sterilisation by moist heat between patients to remove organic and inorganic material that can reduce the effectiveness of these processes. Podiatry instruments used in cutting and filing nails and sharp debridement of skin require sterilisation, not just disinfection, as they are classed as 'semi-critical', that is, a medical device that comes into contact with mucous membranes or non-intact skin. Processing must follow these steps:

1. Clean as soon as possible after using.
2. Sterilise by moist heat after cleaning. If a reusable medical device (RMD) will not tolerate moist

heat sterilisation, use a low-temperature sterilisation process or thermal disinfection or disinfection using a high-level instrument-grade chemical disinfectant. If the instruments can tolerate moist heat they must be sterilised.

Hand hygiene should be attended to and gloves worn during all routine procedures, such as clipping nails and debriding calluses and wounds, and then changed and hand hygiene performed between each patient.[43] Open wounds need to be treated with a sterile dressing as they can pose an infection risk and patients should put their shoes back on before they return to the floor from the treatment chair.

35.4 Rehabilitation units

Multidisciplinary approaches are implemented in rehabilitation settings to maximise healthcare outcomes, such as facilitating patients to improve a range of functional abilities to enable them to live as independently as possible. Allied healthcare practitioners and other healthcare staff and patients are often situated in the same physical environment which increases the likelihood of infection spread. Furthermore, socialisation between patients is encouraged by involving them in group activities and encouraging them to eat in the communal dining areas. Group exercise classes are another way that socialising occurs, and these activities bring patients into close proximity with one another which can facilitate transmission of infection by respiratory viruses or where patients experience urinary or faecal incontinence. Vigilance is required by all HCWs to ensure early identification of potential infections, with prompt investigation, diagnosis and treatment as appropriate and potentially the suspension of communal activities until the infection is resolved.

Conclusion

Although different allied healthcare practitioners carry out assessment and treatment practices that are specific to their profession, there are common infection control risks and procedures undertaken by all practitioners. The multidisciplinary team environments require allied health practitioners to maintain high standards of healthcare delivery to minimise the risk of harm to their patients, their colleagues and to themselves.

Useful websites/resources

- Australian Allied Health Leadership Forum. https://aahlf.com/
- Allied Health Professions Australia. Infection Prevention and Control Guidance in Allied Health Practice. https://ahpa.com.au/resources/
- Allied Health Professions Australia. Infection Prevention and Control in Allied Health – In Practice. https://ahpa.com.au/resources/
- Allied Health Professions Australia. Infection Control Checklist for Allied Health – In Home. https://ahpa.com.au/resources/

References

1. Anguelov A, Giraud K, Akpabie A, Chatap G, Vincent J. Predictive factors of acquired methicillin-resistant Staphylococcus aureus in a rehabilitation care unit. Med Mal Infect. 2010;40(12):677-682.
2. Bellaviti G, Balsamo F, Iosa M, Vella D, Pistarini C. Influence of systemic infection and comorbidities on rehabilitation outcomes in severe acquired brain injury. Eur J Phys Rehabil Med. 2021;57:69-77.
3. Tinelli M, Mannino S, Lucchi S, Piatti A, Pagani L, D'Angelo R, et al. Healthcare-acquired infections in rehabilitation units of the Lombardy Region, Italy. Infection. 2011;39(4):353-358.
4. Weppner J, Gabet J, Linsenmeyer M, Yassin M, Galang G. Clostridium difficile infection reservoirs within an acute rehabilitation environment. Am J Phys Med Rehabil. 2021; 100(1):44-47.
5. Podiatry Board. Code of Conduct. Available from: https://www.podiatryboard.gov.au/policies-codes-guidelines/code-of-conduct.aspx.
6. AHPRA. Code of Conduct. Available from: https://www.ahpra.gov.au/Resources/Code-of-conduct/Shared-Code-of-conduct.aspx.
7. Australia SP. National Code of Conduct. Available from: https://www.speechpathologyaustralia.org.au/SPAweb/Resources_for_Speech_Pathologists/Professional_Resources/HTML/National_Code_of_Conduct.aspx?WebsiteKey=fc2020cb-520d-405b-af30-fc7f70f848db.
8. ACSQHC. The National Safety and Quality Health Service (NSQHS) Standards. Canberra: ACSQHC, 2017.
9. Pérez-Fernández T, Llinares-Pinel F, Troya-Franco M, Fernández-Rosa L. Analysis of the microbiota of the physiotherapist's environment. Arch Phys Med Rehabil. 2020;101(10):1789-1795.
10. Evans MW, Campbell A, Husbands C, Breshears J, Ndetan H, Rupert R. Cloth-covered chiropractic treatment tables as a source of allergens and pathogenic microbes. J Chiropr Med. 2008;7(1):34-38.
11. Pittet D, Dharan S, Touveneau S, Sauvan V, Perneger TV. Bacterial contamination of the hands of hospital staff during routine patient care. Arch Int Med. 1999;159(8):821-826.
12. Mercier C, Haig L. Infection control in physiotherapy. Physiotherapy (United Kingdom). 1993;79(6):385-387.
13. Spratt HG, Jr., Levine D, Tillman L. Physical therapy clinic therapeutic ultrasound equipment as a source for bacterial contamination. Physiother Theory Pract. 2014;30(7):507-511.
14. Schabrun S, Chipchase L, Rickard H. Are therapeutic ultrasound units a potential vector for nosocomial infection? Physiother Res Int. 2006;11(2):61-71.
15. Robertson V, Ward A, Low J, Reed A. Electrotherapy explained: principles and practice. London: Elsevier Health Sciences, 2006.
16. Spratt HG, Jr., Levine D, McDonald S, Drake S, Duke K, Kluttz C, et al. Survival of Staphylococcus aureus on therapeutic ultrasound heads. Am J Infect Control. 2019;47(9):1157-1159.
17. Basseal JM, Westerway SC, Juraja M, van de Mortel TF, McAuley TE, Rippey J, et al. Guidelines for reprocessing ultrasound transducers. Australas J Ultrasound Med. 2017; 20(1):30-40.
18. Lambert I, Tebbs SE, Hill D, Moss HA, Davies AJ, Elliott TSJ. Interferential therapy machines as possible vehicles for cross-infection. J Hosp Infect. 2000;44(1): 59-64.
19. Mobin M, de Moraes Borba C, de Moura Filho OF, de Melo Neto AQ, Valenti VE, Vanderlei LCM, et al. The presence of fungi on contact electrical stimulation electrodes and ultrasound transducers in physiotherapy clinics. Physiotherapy. 2011;97(4):273-277.
20. Macht M, Wimbish T, Bodine C, Moss M. ICU-acquired swallowing disorders. Critical Care Med. 2013;41(10): 2396-2405.
21. Marvin S, Thibeault S, Ehlenbach WJ. Post-extubation dysphagia: does timing of evaluation matter? Dysphagia. 2019;34(2):210-219.
22. Steele CM, Greenwood C, Ens I, Robertson C, Seidman-Carlson R. Mealtime difficulties in a home for the aged: not just dysphagia. Dysphagia. 1997;12(1):43-50.
23. Strausbaugh LJ, Joseph CL. The burden of infection in long-term care. Infect Control Hosp Epidemiol. 2000;21(10): 674-679.
24. Mashima PA, Birkmire-Peters DP, Syms MJ, Holtel MR, Burgess LP, Peters LJ. Telehealth. 2003.
25. Committee ICGA. 2010 Australian Guidelines for the Prevention and Control of Infection in Healthcare. ICGA, 2019.
26. Bolton L, Mills C, Wallace S, Brady MC. Aerosol generating procedures, dysphagia assessment and COVID-19. Royal College of Speech & Language Therapists, 2020. Int J Lang Commun Disord. 2020;55(4):629-636.
27. The Centers for Disease Control and Prevention CDC. Available from: https://www cdc gov/dpdx/strongyloidiasis/index.html, 2013.
28. Kramer A, Kohnen W, Israel S, Ryll S, Hübner N-O, Luckhaupt H, et al. Principles of infection prevention and reprocessing in ENT endoscopy. GMS Curr Top Otorhinolaryngol, Head Neck Surg. 2015;14.

29. Moon J-H, Jung J-H, Hahm S-C, Jung K-S, Suh HR, Cho H-y. Effects of chin tuck exercise using neckline slimmer device on suprahyoid and sternocleidomastoid muscle activation in healthy adults. Journal of Physical Therapy Science. 2018;30(3):454-456.

30. Hoffman MR, Mielens JD, Ciucci MR, Jones CA, Jiang JJ, McCulloch TM. High-resolution manometry of pharyngeal swallow pressure events associated with effortful swallow and the Mendelsohn maneuver. Dysphagia. 2012;27(3): 418-426.

31. Salem A, Ahmad MM. Communication with invasive mechanically ventilated patients and the use of alternative devices: integrative review. J Res Nurs. 2018;23(7): 614-630.

32. Mobasheri MH, King D, Judge S, Arshad F, Larsen M, Safarfashandi Z, et al. Communication aid requirements of intensive care unit patients with transient speech loss. Augment Altern Commun. 2016;32(4):261-271.

33. Howell V, Thoppil A, Mariyaselvam M, Jones R, Young H, Sharma S, et al. Disinfecting the iPad: evaluating effective methods. J Hosp Infect. 2014;87(2):77-83.

34. Coggins MA, Hogan VJ, Kelly M, Fleming GT, Roberts N, Tynan T, et al. Workplace exposure to bioaerosols in podiatry clinics. Ann Occup Hyg. 2012;56(6):746-753.

35. Hainsworth S, Hamblin JF, Vanniasinkam T. Isolation of dermatophytes (and other fungi) from human nail and skin dust produced by podiatric medical treatments in Australia. J Am Podiatr Med Assoc. 2015;105(2) :111-120.

36. Burrow J, McLarnon N. World at work: evidence based risk management of nail dust in chiropodists and podiatrists. Occup Environ Med. 2006;63(10):713-716.

37. Abramson C, Wilton J. Inhalation of nail dust from onychomycotic toenails. Part I. Characterization of particles. 1984. J Am Podiatr Med Assoc. 1992;82(2):111-115.

38. Donaldson C, Carline T, Brown D, Gilmour R, Donaldson K. Toenail dust particles: a potential inhalation hazard to podiatrists? Ann Occup Hyg. 2002;46(suppl_1):365-368.

39. de Benito S, Alou L, Becerro-de-Bengoa-Vallejo R, Losa-Iglesias ME, Gómez-Lus ML, Collado L, et al. Prevalence of Staphylococcus spp. nasal colonization among doctors of podiatric medicine and associated risk factors in Spain. Antimicrob Resist Infect Control. 2018;7(1):1-7.

40. Nowicka D, Nawrot U, Włodarczyk K, Pajączkowska M, Patrzałek A, Pęcak A, et al. Detection of dermatophytes in human nail and skin dust produced during podiatric treatments in people without typical clinical signs of mycoses. Mycoses. 2016;59(6):379-382.

41. McLarnon N, Burrow G, Maclaren W, Aidoo K, Hepher M. The use of an air filtration system in podiatry clinics. Int J Environ Health Res. 2003;13(2):215-221.

42. Humphreys PN, Davies CS, Rout S. An evaluation of the infection control potential of a UV clinical podiatry unit. J Foot Ankle Res. 2014;7(1):1-10.

43. Wise ME, Bancroft E, Clement EJ, Hathaway S, High P, Kim M, et al. Infection prevention and control in the podiatric medical setting: challenges to providing consistently safe care. J Am Podiatr Med Assoc. 2015;105(3):264-272.

CHAPTER 36

Infection prevention and control in Aboriginal and Torres Strait Islander Health

Dr VANESSA SPARKE[i]

MARGARET WYMARRA[ii]

The authors of this chapter respectfully acknowledge the Gimuy Walubara Yidinji and Kaurareg Aboriginal traditional owners, elders past, present and emerging of Gimuy (otherwise known as Cairns) and Waibene (otherwise known as Thursday Island) respectively, for the lands we live and work on in Far North Queensland, Australia.

With respect, throughout this chapter the terms 'Aboriginal and Torres Strait Islander' and 'Indigenous Australians' are used interchangeably.

Following suit of the Aboriginal and Torres Strait Islander authors in this text[11] the Torres Strait Islands are intermittently referred to as Zenadth Kes.

Chapter highlights

- Aboriginal and Torres Strait Islander peoples experience a greater burden of infections and infectious diseases than non-Indigenous Australians
- The biomedical model of disease causation and transmission is not necessarily present in the beliefs of Aboriginal and Torres Strait Islander peoples
- The high prevalence of non-communicable disease within the Aboriginal and Torres Strait Islander population influences high rates of infections and infectious diseases
- The interplay between social, cultural and historical determinants of health is complex. This, along with institutional racism, influences treatment-seeking practices and thus health outcomes
- Infection prevention and control (IPC) personnel need to provide culturally capable care, assume respectful dialogue, adopt appropriate health language, and employ strength-based approaches when engaging with Indigenous Australians around healthcare-associated infections and communicable disease prevention and care

i Nursing and Midwifery, James Cook University, Smithfield, QLD
ii ndigenous Education and Research Centre, James Cook University, Ngulaigau Mudh Campus, Thursday Island, QLD

Introduction

For Australia's Aboriginal and Torres Strait Islander peoples, health and illness is intrinsically linked with land, sea, kinship, culture and spirituality. Prior to invasion and subsequent colonisation by the British, Australia's Indigenous peoples lived a life that enhanced their overall health.[2] Following the arrival of the British, not only were they hit hard by diseases to which they had not previously been exposed, the ensuing colonial policies of dispossession and extermination followed by protection and segregation[3] meant that for many, their self-determination was eroded, along with their language, culture, spirituality and worldview.

This chapter provides a background to the overall health of Aboriginal and Torres Strait Islander peoples and insight into the influence that culture and spirituality have on beliefs about illness causation and disease transmission. The relationship between non-communicable and communicable disease is explored, and specific infections commonly experienced by Aboriginal and Torres Strait Islander peoples are discussed in the context of IPC. The chapter concludes with a discussion around ways of delivering culturally appropriate educational messages, with the aim of reducing and preventing healthcare-associated infections (HAIs) both within healthcare facilities and following discharge.

It must be noted that some topics and discussion throughout this chapter not only apply to Aboriginal and Torres Strait Islander peoples, but to many socially disadvantaged and culturally diverse groups.

Background: the health of Aboriginal and Torres Strait Islander peoples: In the 2021 Census of Population and Housing, 812,000 people identified as Aboriginal and/or Torres Strait Islander, which represents 3.2% of the Australian population.[4] Despite popular belief, the majority of Aboriginal and Torres Strait Islander people live in major centres, not in remote areas, with 35% living in capital city areas.[3] The Northern Territory is the only jurisdiction in Australia where only one-quarter of Aboriginal and Torres Strait Islander people live in the capital city area.

Knowledge of this population distribution is significant, as it is often assumed that IPC professionals will only have contact with Aboriginal and Torres Strait Islander peoples in northern Australia or rural and remote areas of the southern Australian states, yet the statistics show otherwise. Therefore, the importance of understanding IPC in the context of an Aboriginal and Torres Strait Islander person or group is fundamental for all IPC professionals.

There are major inequalities in communicable disease burden in Australia, with Indigenous Australians carrying the greatest burden.[5] Despite Australia's status as one of the most privileged countries in the world—boasting government-funded healthcare and education—some populations, including Indigenous Australians, have shorter life expectancy and worse health outcomes than others.[5]

Infections that are more prevalent in Aboriginal and Torres Strait Islander populations are described later in this chapter, and it would be easy to hold a person or their family/kin to account for not taking the preventive advice given by healthcare providers. However, the germ theory of disease causation and transmission is not necessarily present in the knowledge and beliefs of Aboriginal and Torres Strait Islander people, and it is difficult to discuss infectious diseases separately to the social, cultural and historical determinants of health as they are intertwined and influence each other.

36.1 Influencing factors for health and illness in Aboriginal and Torres Strait Islander peoples

36.1.1 Worldviews on health and illness and spirituality

Aboriginal and Torres Strait Islander health and illness is closely tied to kinship, culture and spirituality, and connection to Country on land and sea.[6] As such, Australian Indigenous peoples' interpretation of health, illness and spirituality is markedly distinct in comparison to the dominant Western biomedical model which focuses on the physical factors impacting health and causation of illness and disease transmission.[7]

A plethora of information is written about *cultural competency*; however, the emphasis throughout this chapter will be on the provision of *culturally safe and respectful care*. Consequently, it is imperative for the *culturally safe and respectful practitioner* to have knowledge of the local Country they live and work on as a matter of importance for the delivery of safe and effective healthcare to Aboriginal and Torres Strait Islander clientele.[60]

Indigenous Australians comprise over 500 groups of peoples.[8,9] As such, worldviews on health and illness and spirituality for Aboriginal and Torres Strait Islander

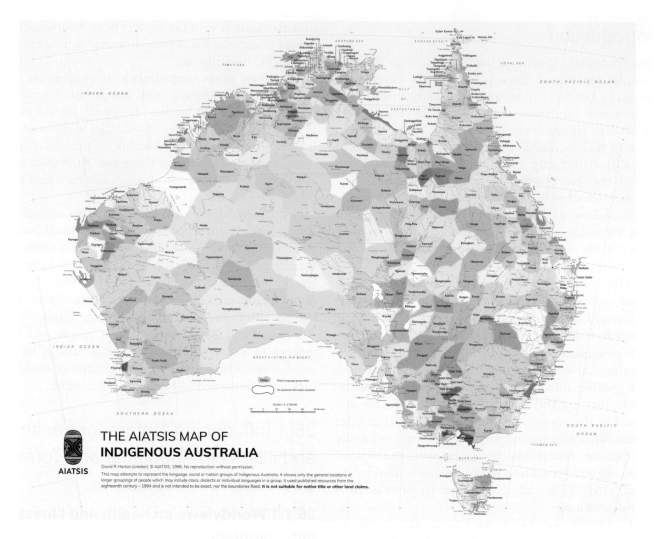

FIGURE 36.1 The AIATSIS map of Australia

Source: This map attempts to represent the language, social or nation groups of Aboriginal Australia. It shows only the general locations of larger groupings of people which may include clans, dialects or individual languages in a group. It used published resources from the eighteenth century–1994 and is not intended to be exact, nor the boundaries fixed. It is not suitable for native title or other land claims. David R Horton (creator), © AIATSIS, 1996. No reproduction without permission. To purchase a print version visit: https://shop.aiatsis.gov.au/.

people are complex subjects to broach. Each Indigenous group varies in its 'languages, histories and cultural traditions'.[9] Furthermore, the AIATSIS Map of Australia (Fig 36.1) shows the nature of diversity among the First Nations peoples of Australia and highlights the fact that the Indigenous Australian landscape is extensive. As a result, the laws and customs are specific and differ for each grouping across the nation.[8] Please note that as specified by AIATSIS, the fringes of the borders on the AIATSIS Map of Australia are not true boundaries; however, they give the reader an approximate guide as to where different tribal groups, customary locations lie.

PRACTICE TIPS 1

REFLECTING ON CULTURAL DIFFERENCES IN PRACTICE

A culturally safe and respectful health practitioner should familiarise themselves with the AIATSIS Map of Australia. (See Fig 36.1.)

Spend some time looking at the AIATSIS Map of Australia. Search and reflect on the land/Country you are currently living on—where you work and where you spend your leisure time. What is the traditional name for your community?

Do you know who the traditional owners are for that region?

If you have lived in various locations around Australia, look up the names of those locations and learn the traditional names for those too.

Zenadth Kes is the traditional name for the Torres Strait Islands, a group of islands scattered over 150 km from north to south that lie between the lower coastline of Papua New Guinea and Pajinka (otherwise known as Cape York Peninsula, Queensland) which is the northernmost point of the Australian continent. A map of Zenadth Kes (Fig 36.2) is provided by the Torres Strait Regional Authority.[12]

It encompasses 48,000 km² of ocean, extends approximately 200 to 300 km from east to west[10] and, although much smaller in area than mainland Australia, the region is complex and multifaceted in its customs, traditional laws and worldviews regarding health, illness and spirituality. More than 200 islands are located in the region, 17 of which are inhabited.[7]

The Indigenous authors, in *Yatdjuligin Aboriginal and Torres Strait Islander Nursing & Midwifery Care*, discuss the return to the use of the local traditional name of Zenadth Kes for the islands.[11] The authors assert that the use of 'the local name instead of the colonial name is an exercise of sovereignty. The reclaiming of places through knowing their local name is an important part of truth telling and decolonising Country'.[11] As a move away from colonial influences on Country, there is currently a paradigm shift among Aboriginal and Torres Strait Islanders to realign the names of their traditional *Countries* to the original names and places of their origin. Since time immemorial, the Torres Strait Islands have been known by the traditional owners as Zenadth Kes. Zenadth Kes is *Ged* or *Lag* meaning 'home' in the two main dialects of Meriam Mir and Kalaw Lagaw Ya. *(Note that in this text the Torres Strait Islands are intermittently referred to as Zenadth Kes.)*

36.1.2 Aboriginal and Torres Strait Islander beliefs around disease causation and transmission

The World Health Organization (WHO) defines health as 'a state of complete physical, mental and social wellbeing and not merely the absence of disease or infirmity'.[13] In contrast, the National Aboriginal Community

Controlled Health Organisation (NACCHO) finds that Aboriginal health is more holistic and is:

> Not just the physical well-being of an individual but refers to the social, emotional and cultural well-being of the whole Community in which each individual is able to achieve their full potential as a human being thereby bringing about the total well-being of their community. It is a whole of life view and includes the cyclical concept of life-death-life.[14]

Other definitions of the Indigenous perspective of health embrace the ecological, referring to the importance of connection to Country, land and sea; the social, being connection to kinship structures; and connection to the spiritual and culture.[11] The WHO's definition of health is inconsistent with the Aboriginal and Torres Strait Islander viewpoint on wellbeing and merely highlights the disparities between the Western worldview and the Indigenous Australian worldview on health, illness and spirituality. For Aboriginal and Torres Strait Islander people, the influence that spiritualty and culture have on beliefs about disease causation and disease transmission is as significant as the accepted scientific germ theory.

So, what does an infection control nurse or practitioner require in order to become more culturally safe and respectful in their practice when working with Aboriginal and Torres Strait Islander clients? Understanding how Indigenous Australians perceive disease transmission is vital when talking with any patient, and in particular when caring for this vulnerable group of the population.

Traditional health beliefs around illness and spirituality are not often shared with non-Indigenous health practitioners by Aboriginal and Torres Strait Islander people. It is almost an unspoken rule to not share cultural information in regard to traditional healing practice or treatments with outsiders as the information is confidential and often privately shared among close family, and decision making is led by the elders of tribal groups. Considering the historical influences of colonisation and the impact of past government policies and the intergenerational trauma that has impacted Indigenous Australians, it is no wonder that Aboriginal and Torres Strait Islander people are reluctant to share their traditional cultural knowledge around disease causation, illness transmission and traditional treatments of various ailments with non-Indigenous health practitioners due to a mistrust of existing mainstream health services. This impacts on the provision of

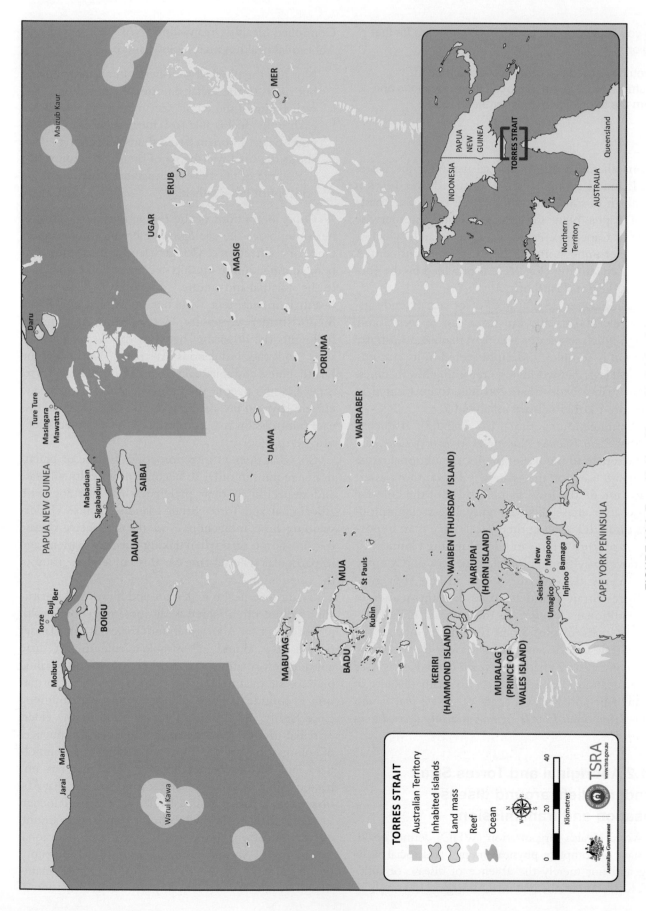

FIGURE 36.2 Zenadth Kes (Torres Strait Islands)
Source: Torres Strait Regional Authority, 2012

care to Aboriginal and Torres Strait Islander patients, as non–Indigenous healthcare professionals often encounter difficulties in their understanding of why they are sick and what treatments are to be given. Unless they are from the same cultural group, frontline healthcare staff have difficulty understanding the role of traditional healers, and reasons around why Aboriginal and Torres Strait Islander people get sick.

Adapting care through culturally responsive interventions

1. Reflect upon your own biases and prejudices about Aboriginal and Torres Strait Islander peoples by considering the following questions:
   - Is the information I know about Aboriginal and Torres Strait Islander people based on evidence?
   - What informs my biases and prejudices?

2. Apply the cultural lens when caring for Aboriginal and Torres Strait Islander people.

3. A culturally safe and respectful healthcare practitioner should recognise and respect the *differences* in Aboriginal and Torres Strait Islander cultures from their own; and

4. A culturally safe and respectful healthcare practitioner should recognise and respect the *similarities* between Aboriginal and Torres Strait Islander cultures and their own.
   - Ask yourself, what have I learned? Who and where are my resources to learn more about Aboriginal and Torres Strait Islander people and cultures?

See Useful websites/resources at the end of this chapter.

36.1.3 Governance

To address the ongoing struggle for social justice and recognition for Aboriginal and Torres Strait Islander peoples, collaborative governance structures are vital.[15] Governance structures have traditionally been dominated by a Western worldview which is in conflict with Indigenous ways of health and wellbeing, including social, emotional, physical and spiritual wellbeing.[16] Institutional racism, generally regarded as the policies, practices, processes and conditions which increase power differentials between ethnic, cultural, racial or religious groups, is the most widespread form of racism,

and impacts strongly on Indigenous people's health and treatment-seeking practices. Institutional racism is now considered by the Australian Government as a significant social determinant of health.[17] Inclusive governance is therefore significant, particularly for communities with diverse cultural populations when aiming to achieve wellbeing.[15] Rather than the colonial 'top-down' approach, inclusive governance in healthcare, which includes IPC, enables a healthcare facility to be more responsive to Indigenous worldviews and knowledges. Embedding Indigenous voices into IPC policy, particularly when including the different worldviews on disease causation and transmission, while still adhering to IPC principles is an important process of clinical governance. As it currently stands, IPC policies and procedures globally are based on the biomedical model of disease causation and transmission, paying little or no heed to Indigenous beliefs, worldviews and cultural processes. Mainstream health services in Australia must acknowledge the importance of Indigenous peoples' contribution to decision making, as the differences between Aboriginal and Torres Strait Islander and non-Aboriginal cultures are vast. This means that a blanket approach to IPC is very likely to be ineffective.[18]

Current health governance and policy, particularly in mainstream healthcare facilities, is very much linear, as Western knowledge systems categorise health into compartments and boxes, which is very different to the holistic model of Indigenous people. Funding for health, which includes HAI, is based on diagnosis, body parts and disease, yet for Indigenous people this does not fit their worldview on health. The ongoing funding of in-hospital and post-discharge care therefore does not take into consideration the cultural obligations an Indigenous person may experience while in hospital or once returning to the community, and nor does it provide for comprehensive primary healthcare.

Capacities and empowerment: Successful and sustainable change in governance requires institutional ownership and relationship building and must be a united responsibility. Strengthening capacity (as opposed to building capacity) is one approach. Strengthening capacity recognises the strengths to thrive, lead and govern which has been in existence in Indigenous communities for generations. As well as leadership capacities, capacities can involve the non-human structures that surround IPC such as infrastructure, resources and equipment.[15] The literature often discusses the need for Indigenous groups to be empowered; however, without supporting governance structures, empowerment is not a reality.

With Indigenous people experiencing higher in-hospital mortality rates for some diseases and higher rates of self-discharge (against medical advice),[19] inclusive governance which includes collaboration with Aboriginal and Torres Strait Islander community-controlled organisations and other services which deliver primary healthcare services[16] may decrease the disparities in health outcomes for Aboriginal and Torres Strait Islander people, both in hospital and in the community.

36.1.4 Culturally appropriate healthcare

Despite Australia's world-class health system, it is not accessed equally by all Australians. Indigenous Australians' need for health service access is 2–3 times higher than for non-Indigenous people, yet is reported to be only 1.1 times higher.[16] Advocacy for culturally capable health services has been growing for several decades. Cultural capability refers to 'the skills, knowledge, behaviours and systems that are required to plan, support, improve and deliver services in a culturally respectful and appropriate manner'.[20] Culture influences Indigenous people's decisions about when and why they seek health services and also influences their treatment-seeking behaviours.[6] The holistic health needs of Indigenous people can be overlooked as a result of social and political invisibility;[21] however, governmental health services, such as Queensland Health under the guidance the Cultural Capability Team,[20] is committing to the provision of accessible clinical services that are culturally safe for Aboriginal and Torres Strait Islander people, thus moving towards a culturally capable, safe and competent mainstream health workforce.

In 2018, CATSINaM, the Nursing and Midwifery Board of Australia (NMBA), the Australian College of Midwives (ACM), the Australian College of Nursing (ACN), and the Australian Nursing and Midwifery Federation (ANMF) published a joint statement, *Cultural safety: Nurses and midwives leading the way for safer healthcare.* This document emphasises the importance of implementation of culturally safe practice to improve the 'health outcomes and experiences for Aboriginal and Torres Strait Islander peoples'.[22] The Code of Conduct for nurses and the Code of Conduct for midwives[23] provide sound practicalities for the *culturally safe and respectful* practitioner to implement when collaborating with Aboriginal and Torres Strait Islander peoples.[24]

As the nation's peak governing body for Aboriginal and Torres Strait Islander nurses and midwives, CATSINaM specified two strategic directions to effectively lead the way in healthcare settings: firstly, by reinforcing their advocacy efforts and thus the efficiency of the provision of culturally safe health services to Indigenous communities; and secondly, by supporting the recruitment and retention of Indigenous Australian nurses and midwives. In alignment with these strategic directives, in 2021 the Queensland Nurses Union (QNU) First Nations Branch collaborated with Indigenous Australian nurses from the Torres and Cape Hinterland Health Service (TCHHS) to support and lead the COVID-19 vaccination rollout in these regions.[25] Following robust consultation with Aboriginal and Torres Strait Islander nurses from TCHHS, the Palaszczuk government supported the QNU's recommendations to amend closed border roadmaps in Indigenous communities to facilitate effective consultation with First Nations peoples appropriately resourced and led by Aboriginal and Torres Strait Islander nurses and midwives.[25] This is a good example of how cultural safety and the delivery of culturally appropriate healthcare can work well as the rollout of COVID-19 vaccination in the TCHHS regions assists in overcoming vaccination hesitancy.[26]

Aboriginal Community Controlled Health Organisations: Aboriginal Community Controlled Health Organisations (ACCHO) were established in the early 1970s in response to the poor care being experienced in mainstream health services by Indigenous Australians.[27] The ACCHO primary health network is comprised of over 550 sites across Australia and includes fixed, outreach and mobile clinics operating in urban, rural and remote settings.[28] ACCHOs across Australia are governed by the national leadership body for Aboriginal and Torres Strait Islander Health in Australia, NACCHO (National Aboriginal Community Controlled Health Organisation). NACCHO has a Secretariat in Canberra which improves the capacity of Indigenous Australians involved in ACCHO to participate in national health policy development.[28] ACCHOs provide a broad range of preventative health and wellbeing programs as well as other community services.[29] ACCHOs are grounded in Indigenous culture and promote Indigenous empowerment and self-determination. Governance structures generally include board members who have expertise in Indigenous health, or are actively chairing

Indigenous-led organisations, and include Indigenous representation. This ensures Indigenous people are instrumental in decision-making processes.[17] Many ACCHOs work closely with other health providers, such as state health departments, mainstream general practices and community-based social health and other support services, to ensure appropriate healthcare across the health system.[17] While ACCHOs have their own governance structures, the foundational premise of IPC according to relevant national IPC guidelines and protocols is followed.

Australian Indigenous healthcare workers: Aboriginal and Torres Strait Islander healthcare workers (HCWs) are crucial members of the health workforce, in both specialised service delivery and a wide range of mainstream healthcare roles.[30] Indigenous HCWs make it possible to bring together the differing understandings of health and healthcare services, and bring the Indigenous perspective to the patient–hospital worker interaction, something that is not completely understood by non-Indigenous staff.[19] Aboriginal and/or Torres Strait Islander healthcare workers and health practitioners are the only culturally based health professions with national training and registration in the world, and are a standalone profession, registered through the Australian Health Practitioner Regulation Agency (AHPRA).[31] Involving Indigenous HCWs in care brings with it the principles of foundational Indigenous knowledge, ease of consultation with family, kin and Aboriginal and Torres Strait Islander community organisations, shows respect for Indigenous conceptions of health and wellbeing, and provides reciprocal learning for both Indigenous and non-Indigenous HCWs.[1]

36.1.5 Social and cultural determinants of health

The social determinants of health (SDoH)—which include housing, education, level of income, food security, geographical location and access—are broadly accepted and understood. Social processes are underpinned by culture, history and government processes, and understanding these helps a HCW recognise the 'causes of the causes', or the social practices which influence the high prevalence of communicable infections experienced by Aboriginal and Torres Strait Islander people.[32] Racism also forms a key SDoH. Racism, both institutional and overt, can deter people from seeking healthcare as it debilitates confidence and self-worth, ultimately leading to poorer health outcomes.[16]

What is not well understood by clinicians is the complex interplay between the historical, social, environmental and cultural determinants that influence health outcomes.[33] Understanding the social, cultural and historical perspectives of communicable disease from Indigenous Australians also informs directions and strategies for care. Clinicians must also be mindful, however, that social determinant models include protective factors, such as social cohesion and social networks.[32]

Housing: Housing is a well-recognised SDoH and is closely linked with social, economic and geographic factors.[29] The spread of infectious diseases within households—such as intestinal infections, eye and ear infections, skin disease and respiratory infections—has long been attributed to inadequate 'health hardware' in unmaintained housing. Health hardware includes equipment and hardware associated with bathrooms, kitchens, laundries and sanitation.[34] Despite popular assumptions around lack of home ownership by Indigenous people, the latest Australian Bureau of Statistics (ABS) data show that approximately 41.3% of Aboriginal and Torres Strait Islander households either owned the property outright or owned it with a mortgage, with 26.9% renting through an estate agent and only 14.1% renting through a state or territory housing authority.[4] The numbers of people renting are disproportionately high in remote or very remote areas, including homes on traditional Country, where there is a higher population of Aboriginal and Torres Strait Islander people, although there are urban areas with lower home ownership than in the broader Aboriginal and Torres Strait Islander population.[29] It is these very areas where malfunctioning health hardware is at the highest, and where the burden of infectious disease, related to housing, is also the highest.[34] Malfunctioning health hardware is largely related to the crowding of houses, and while it has been found that good hygiene within the home is generally valued, the absence of functional health hardware and the crowding of houses impairs residents' ability to perform protective behaviours such as hand hygiene, washing of clothes, and hygienic storage of food.[29,34]

The condition of the houses can also create conditions for infectious disease transmission. The presence of mould and mildew contributes to respiratory and gastrointestinal (GIT) infections, with the more housing problems a child is exposed to, the greater the risk of recurrent GIT infections.[29] Targeted housing repair and maintenance, and improved health hardware, can prevent exacerbation of disease transmission,[34] and has been shown to reduce hospital admissions for many infectious diseases, particularly GIT infections.[29]

36.2 Infection prevention and control for Aboriginal and Torres Strait Islander health

36.2.1 Interconnection between communicable and non-communicable disease

Chronic disease—or non-communicable disease (NCD)—increases host susceptibility to infection. People diagnosed with one or more chronic conditions often have poorer quality of life, complex health needs and die early.[35] The interconnectedness between chronic disease and increased risk of infection was demonstrated in the COVID-19 pandemic where underlying NCDs and their risk factors (e.g. smoking and obesity) influenced the severity of the outbreak by increasing pathogen virulence in affected people.[36] Seasonal and pandemic influenza also affect those with chronic disease more often.[37] A person who has one or more chronic disease is more likely to have contact with a health service, which increases the risk of acquiring an HAI. Indigenous Australians experience potentially preventable hospitalisations (PPH) at rates three times higher than non-Indigenous Australians, with PPH for chronic conditions being twice the rate of a non-Indigenous person.[38]

Colonised Indigenous populations around the world have a higher burden of NCDs.[37] In 2019, 46% of Aboriginal and Torres Strait Islander people were reported to have at least one or more selected chronic conditions, which included arthritis, asthma, chronic back problems, cancer, chronic obstructive pulmonary disease, diabetes mellitus, heart, stroke and vascular disease, mental and behavioural conditions and osteoporosis.[35] Chronic kidney disease (CKD) rates are also higher in Indigenous Australians than in non-Indigenous Australians, with CKD-related deaths in major cities and regional areas occurring at rates twice as high as those of non-Indigenous people, and in outer regional, remote and very remote areas the rate is four-fold. In 2012–13, haemodialysis (or renal replacement therapy) accounted for 48% of hospital episodes in Indigenous Australians.[39] Globally, risk factors for infectious diseases such as TB, including tobacco,

alcohol consumption and diabetes, are in high prevalence in Indigenous populations.[40]

With high rates of chronic disease and hospitalisations, Aboriginal and Torres Strait Islander people are more likely to come into contact with a health service and are more susceptible to HAIs, factors which need to be taken into consideration.

36.2.2 Specific HAIs and communicable diseases considerations

The aim of this section is not to discuss the IPC management of prevalent communicable diseases or HAIs experienced by Aboriginal and Torres Strait Islander people, as infection prevention measures for specific pathogens are discussed in earlier chapters. The aim is to increase awareness of the prevalence of specific infections and highlight the consequences for the person if not detected early or managed effectively.

Gastrointestinal infections: Gastrointestinal (GIT) infections are a leading cause of childhood mortality globally and a public health issue in Australia. While usually mild and self-limiting in developed nations, serious cases can cause dehydration, hospitalisation and death in susceptible populations. Health sequelae of GIT can include a range of cardiovascular, rheumatologic, GIT, neurological, skin and lung conditions. Children with GIT infections are also more likely to experience recurrent skin, ear and chest infections.[29] The link between GIT infections and poor housing is well established, particularly in remote communities; however, while there is also poor housing in urban areas, the link between poor housing and GIT infections in these areas is not well researched.[29]

Infections of the skin: Skin diseases are a common reason for presentation to rural and remote primary healthcare centres in Australia.[41] Skin and soft tissue infections (SSTI) are an increasing cause of hospitalisation, with SSTIs causing up to 10.5% of septic episodes.[42] In the East Arnhem region of Australia, 95% of children had received at least one antibiotic and almost 50% of children had six antibiotic prescriptions during the first year of life[43] for SSTIs. This is not only concerning for health and the potential sequelae of unresolved SSTIs, but also for the ongoing necessity to curb antibiotic misuse and decrease the rate of MRO infections. Skin infections include impetigo (caused by Group A *Streptococcus* or *Staphylococcus aureus*), scabies and fungal infections.[41]

SKIN AND SOFT TISSUE INFECTIONS

Caring for a person presenting with skin and soft tissue infections:

- SSTIs should not be ignored or 'normalised' as the consequences may result in RHD, sepsis or kidney failure

- Where possible, collect samples for microbiological/parasitology testing to ensure targeted treatment

- Seek consultation on antibiotic prescribing based on geographical location of healthcare facility, and where patient 'normally' resides

- Ask the person for their understanding of the causes of their skin infection

- Discuss the practicalities of hand hygiene and antibiotic-taking habits with the person—what are their social/living circumstances—what would work best? Consult the end user!

- Maintain or commence surveillance activities to gauge organism prevalence in the community

Due to their high prevalence, skin infections tend to be 'normalised'. The sequela of this normalisation is that skin infections tend to be underreported and unrecorded, and individuals may not present for care. Serious consequences of skin infection include sepsis, skeletal infection, soft tissue infection, post-streptococcal glomerulonephritis and rheumatic heart disease.[41]

In Central Australia, the annual rate of hospitalisation for cellulitis is more than three and a half times the national average. Interestingly, Central Australia also has the highest rate of bloodstream infections (BSI), although the link between SSTIs and BSIs is not clear.[42] While skin infections are largely linked to household crowding and limited access to health hardware (i.e. functioning water supply and sanitation),[41] the high burden of chronic disease is thought to be the cause of high annual incidence of severe skin and soft tissue infections requiring advanced care.[42]

Group A streptococcal (GAS) infections are the leading cause of impetigo (skin infections) in remote Australian communities, affecting around 45% of Indigenous children at any one time.[44] GAS infections are associated with socio-economic factors and household crowding.[45] Rheumatic fever, a potential consequence of GAS infection (pharyngeal and skin), has a clinical onset approximately 1–4 weeks post-GAS infection and therefore isolating GAS from cultures is not often possible; however, antibiotic therapy for eradication is still recommended.[45]

Scabies is hyperendemic in disadvantaged remote communities, with severe cases causing life-threatening sepsis. Severe or crusted scabies facilitates the establishment of SSTIs caused by Streptococcus and Staphylococcus[46] with subsequent invasive BSIs. Skin infections due to scabies are due to the ectoparasite *Sarcoptes scabei*, transmitted primarily through direct skin-to-skin contact.[47] Untreated scabies causes significant morbidity, ranging from sleep deprivation leading to impaired concentration, through to invasive bacterial infections potentially resulting in death from sepsis.[47] The standard technique for identification of mites is time-consuming and requires access to a laboratory or microscope, and thus diagnosis can be challenging.

Respiratory infections: Respiratory disorders in Indigenous Australians are the most common reason for general practice presentations and the second most common for hospital presentations.[48] While malnutrition, GIT diseases and child mortality have declined over the past 50 years, rates of acute respiratory infections have not followed this trend.[49] Acute and chronic respiratory disease are 10 times higher in Indigenous children than non-Indigenous children, with a hospitalisation rate almost double in the 0–4 age group.[48]

Respiratory syncytial virus (RSV) is the leading cause of lower respiratory tract infections in young children; however, severe cases can present in older adults, particularly those with chronic disease. RSV is now nationally notifiable under legislation;[50] however, it was previously a non-reportable disease and therefore accurate population-based incidence reporting is difficult.[51] Aboriginal and Torres Strait Islander children are at particular risk of hospitalisation for RSV as they are likely to have higher rates of comorbidities (malnutrition, anaemia and GIT illness).[48]

Rates of bronchiolitis and pneumonia are also particularly high in Indigenous children, with hospitalisation rates greater than that of non-Indigenous children. Common causes of pneumonia include *Streptococcus pneumoniae*, Staphylococcus and, in tropical regions, melioidosis. In communities where respiratory infections are common, a chronic cough is often considered normal, yet is probably indicative of a treatable respiratory infection.[49] The sequelae of untreated chronic childhood respiratory infection is adult lung disease.

Indigenous adults with bronchiectasis commonly die in their fourth decade of life.[48,49]

SDoH are linked with respiratory infection in Indigenous populations, so to curb high rates of morbidity and mortality, strategies including high vaccination rates, standard treatment protocols and early identification of suppurative lung disease, along with addressing the SDoH are required.

Tuberculosis: The incidence of tuberculosis (TB) in Australia is low, with the majority of people diagnosed with TB born outside Australia in countries with a high TB incidence. Of people born in Australia diagnosed with TB, Aboriginal and Torres Strait Islander people are disproportionately represented, with the annual notification rate being six times higher than the rate for the non–Indigenous Australia-born population.[40]

The history of TB for Aboriginal and Torres Strait Islander people is connected with European invasion and subjugation.[32] Considered a white man's disease and coming from 'elsewhere', it was the leading cause of illness and death for Australia's First Nations peoples during colonisation. Interestingly (and sadly), TB was not often recognised in Indigenous Australians due to the religious and ethnocentric beliefs of the European invaders and questioning as to whether the disease could 'jump species'.[32]

Caring for an Indigenous person diagnosed with TB can be challenging due to multifactorial influences which include:

- interpretations of illness and wellness (as patients may be asymptomatic)
- knowledge, attitudes and beliefs around treatment
- personal behaviours; and
- influence of family, community and members of the household.

Health service factors, such as staff unfamiliar with diagnosis and treatment of TB, poor access to diagnostic tools and incompatible communication between health services, also add to the burden of TB infections.[52] Ideally treatment should commence within 3 days of active disease to decrease the risk of transmission with a 2-week hospitalisation recommended at the start of treatment.[52] However, the unavailability of diagnostic facilities in remote locations means travel away from home and community is required for further testing. Travelling without family or kin support for cultural safety increases the risk of the person not attending ongoing appointments, which places households and the rest of the community at risk of contracting the disease through treatment failure.

CASE STUDY 1

Adapting care through culturally responsive interventions

Situation:

A middle-aged Aboriginal woman from a remote Cape York Peninsula Indigenous community initially presented to the local primary healthcare centre (PHCC) with cough and fever, at which time a local outpatient chest X-ray demonstrated a new apical lung lesion. Multiple serial X-rays were obtained over a few months which showed persistence of the lesion so a CT radiograph was recommended for definitive diagnosis. The CT required transfer to the closest tertiary hospital, more than 800 km away. The patient did not attend for the scan and was lost to follow-up. The patient re-presented to the PHCC 3 years later and a CT chest radiograph, with findings suggestive of TB, was completed. Sputum sample smears confirmed Mycobacterium tuberculosis 3 months post-CT. Although at this stage she was asymptomatic.

As per guidelines and under the remote supervision of the state-led TB control unit, the patient was admitted to the local remote hospital to commence the first 2 weeks of drug treatment. Attempts at isolating her in hospital for induction treatment proved unsuccessful as the patient self-discharged. The patient continued to engage with the health staff in the community although her adherence to medical treatment and appointments was inconsistent.

To reduce the public health risk, the TB unit advised the patient to cease her welfare/government-supported employment at the local childcare centre. The loss of her work role appeared to precipitate an increase in alcohol and cannabis use, resulting in chaotic social interactions and loss of routine. This complicated the medical management of this patient, with the health service eventually using a modified, directly observed therapy (DOT) approach to optimise medication adherence.

Treatment strategies

Following the initial failed hospital admission, DOT was trialled in the community. Initially, a clinical nurse consultant, with support from an Indigenous health worker (IHW), delivered medication Monday to Friday, with weekend medication left with the patient on a Friday. Locating the patient was problematic. The period directly after diagnosis was the most chaotic for the patient. The patient's loss of a consistent daily routine that would ordinarily support treatment adherence affected the delivery of treatment in the first few months.

Alternative treatment routines were trialled, including 3 times weekly treatment and provision of take-home medications for weekends; however, there remained uncertainty with adherence when self-administering. Finally, in consultation with the patient, the use of a pre-packed medication system (Webster-pak) was trialled. Initially the registered nurse and an IHW observed self-administration of medications from the Webster-pak daily. As the use of the Webster-pak did not require a registered nurse to administer medication, the case management of the patient care was able to be transferred to the IHW, who was able to build a relationship with the patient to facilitate more reliable treatment adherence. Daily visits were short (approximately 5 min).

Through building a medication routine acceptable to the patient, the IHW could gradually reduce the level of support provided to the patient to ensure medication adherence. This short-term intensive support to develop a medication routine had positive unintended consequences, such as improving the consistency of the patient's daily routine, reducing alcohol and improving her nutritional intake. The patient also re-engaged with her employment provider. She ceased medication after 14 months of therapy and thus far is considered cured of TB, for ongoing surveillance.

(Adapted from Miller, Cairns, Richardson and Lawrence, 2020)

Community-acquired methicillin resistant *Staphylococcus aureus* (CA-MRSA): Healthcare-associated methicillin–resistant *Staphylococcus aureus* (HA-MRSA) is a leading cause of life-threatening HAI. Once confined to the hospital environment, methicillin-resistant *Staphylococcus aureus* (MRSA) is now isolated in people with little or no previous exposure to healthcare. Community-acquired MRSA (CA-MRSA) is commonly isolated, particularly in Indigenous Australians, with people residing in remote locations in the Northern Territory, Western Australia and New South Wales, and increasingly, Far North Queensland, showing a higher prevalence.[53] Risk factors for CA-MRSA include the previously

described SDoH, including overcrowding in houses, inadequate health hardware and socio-economic disadvantage. Infection control measures such as hand hygiene are effective in curbing HA-MRSA rates, but this is more difficult in the community setting. A highly mobile population moving between remote locations and larger towns may also explain the presence of CA-MRSA in larger regional healthcare facilities.

36.2.3 Antimicrobial stewardship

As the distance from a major city increases, access to hospital services declines, the population tends to be sicker, and the delivery of healthcare more costly. There also is a greater proportion of Indigenous people in remote Australia.[54] The incidence of sepsis and infection-associated mortality is higher in the Aboriginal and Torres Strait Islander population, along with higher rates of antimicrobial resistance (AMR).[55] AMR stems from a number of causes, including the misuse and overuse of antibiotics—administering antibiotics when not needed, prescribing lengthy courses of antibiotics, and increasing patient expectation to be prescribed antibiotics are all contributing factors.[56]

In 2018, approximately 26% of prescriptions for SSTIs in 10 central Australian clinics were found to be inappropriate, and 44% did not conform to established guidelines.[43] Upstream factors that contribute to inappropriate antimicrobial prescribing include:

- workforce issues
- remoteness and access to healthcare
- a lack of antimicrobial stewardship (AMS) surveillance
- limited rural-specific clinical guidelines on prescribing practices
- a paucity of diagnostic facilities
- the carriage of potentially pathogenic micro-organisms (such as MRSA); and
- suboptimal adherence.[54]

Poor antimicrobial stewardship in the context of Indigenous Australians is also influenced by Aboriginal and Torres Strait Islander treatment-seeking behaviours. Indigenous Australians may not access healthcare when needed for a variety of reasons including being too busy, dislike for the facility, embarrassment, fear, lack of transportation and distance from the facility. There could also be a concern that treatment may require evacuation to a larger centre where they don't have their usual support network, and different beliefs around illness causation could also lead to delays in presentation. The liberal use of antibiotics is more likely to occur when an Indigenous person engages with a health facility with the understanding that follow-up may not occur.[55]

36.3 Communicating the message differently—caring for Aboriginal and Torres Strait Islander people within the IPC context

Collaborative ways of discovering what will work best is important when caring for Aboriginal and Torres Strait Islander people. A different approach—one that incorporates beliefs around health and illness, and the social and cultural influences that affect wellbeing—is required. Treatment strategies are more likely to be successful when using a holistic approach than with the compartmentalised biomedical model.

36.3.1 Respectful dialogue

Engaging in respectful dialogue is crucial when communicating with Aboriginal and Torres Strait Islander people about preventing and controlling infection in the healthcare facility, the community and in the home. Acknowledging that different worldviews exist between Indigenous and non-Indigenous people is the first step in this process.[3] It is also important to understand that for Indigenous people, the person cannot be separated from family and community.

Minimising power differentials between Aboriginal and Torres Strait Islander community members, patients and the healthcare system is necessary for cultural safety in healthcare. It is important for healthcare staff to exchange the detached health-professional voice for yarning and the social-inclusive voice.[40] Communicating with Aboriginal and Torres Strait Islander people and their families about infection prevention measures, such as standard precautions or the more complex nuances of transmission-based precautions, requires an understanding that while social inclusion is important, not all patients and families will want to engage in conversation. Kinship relations, which non-Indigenous people may see as complex, may mean that members of the group may feel uncomfortable speaking out if they are the only Aboriginal or Torres Strait Islander person in the group, or if they are in the close vicinity of certain family members. For example, there is an avoidance relationship between a mother-in-law and a son-in-law.[3] It is not expected that the IPC professional will understand the intricacies around kinship relations and

obligations, but when planning or entering into conversation with an Indigenous person and their family or kin, explain the intent of the conversation and ask, 'Who are the appropriate family members to include in this conversation?'.

36.3.2 Engaging for health education

The pre-eminent Torres Strait Islander academic Professor Martin Nakata, in his seminal work on the Cultural Interface, explores the intersection of Western knowledge systems and the positions and experiences of people of the Torres Strait.[57] Since that work was published, Professor Nakata's research has been used to explore the cultural divide between Indigenous and non-Indigenous knowledge systems in various countries.[58,59] So, what does this have to do with IPC in Aboriginal and Torres Strait Islander health? Historically, Indigenous Australians and their epistemologies have been excluded in Australian higher education.[60] Subsequently, health professional education 'has produced generations of healthcare professionals who are ill-equipped and lack confidence to provide culturally safe care' for Indigenous communities.[60] All the above considered, health practitioners need Indigenous Australian content to be taught that is cognisant of Aboriginal and Torres Strait Islander epistemologies in their respective health courses in higher education in order to further enhance the cultural capability of the health practitioner.[60,61]

Approaches to healthcare education, particularly IPC, which support culture, worldviews and beliefs are paramount as education based on individual behaviour only has a limited effect in all cultures. Participatory approaches, where an Indigenous person takes the lead in their health recovery, supported by community and in partnership with the health service—all with complementary but different expertise—will promote inclusion, self-determination and better overall success in preventing and controlling infection.[40]

Tackling control of TB is an example of a participatory approach to prevention. Considered a social disease, managing and controlling the disease is complex, and there has never been a simple method offered by either biomedical or Indigenous health models. Health models that recognise and embrace the strengths of Indigenous models while still enabling the strengths of biomedical approaches help to embrace the strengths of both cultures to address TB control.[32]

Strength-based approaches have been shown to improve the health of communities with limited resources. Strength-based approaches use the strengths of the community to promote and tailor self-sufficiency, efficiency and empowerment of patients and communities.[43] Strength-based approaches require planning and the commitment of like-minded healthcare professionals and identified community representatives, however, when successfully applied they have been shown to improve treatment of infections such as SSTIs.[43] Strength-based approaches are family- and patient-centred which aligns with culturally appropriate approaches to care for Indigenous Australians.

36.3.3 Use of language

The health field is dominated by the English language. English words and names mean different things to different cultures and can change according to the cultural context. For some Indigenous people the dominant language of English may be a second or third language, which can provide a communication barrier between the IPC professional and the Indigenous person. This difference in language can impede health literacy and is a constraint when providing health education.[18] Engaging a translation service or providing written materials in a local language are often cited as solutions; however, with different conceptual meanings of health, and for cultures that communicate heavily through the spoken word, these other forms of communication can lack depth or change meaning.[18] Strategies that include using visual cues, such as visual pain scales, and that accept culturally appropriate informed consent (e.g. oral consent) need to be considered.[62] However, consulting with family or kin for appropriate language use, introducing your intended conversation, and collaborating with the family and Indigenous HCW is the best way to provide relevant information.

36.3.4 Isolation for infection prevention and control

This chapter has discussed Indigenous Australians' worldviews on health and illness and the cultural nuances that influence these, as well as the importance of kinship and connectedness to family and community, which are all crucial to wellbeing. The challenges faced by young Indigenous Australians—such as racism, social disadvantage and intergenerational trauma alongside concomitant factors such as incarceration and substance use—place them at high psychological distress.[63] The practice of isolation for IPC purposes, both in the community (as during the COVID-19 pandemic) and in healthcare facilities cannot be underestimated and is required to prevent the spread of highly communicable diseases and protect immunocompromised patients. Yet

for Indigenous Australians, isolation from family can increase psychological distress and exacerbate any perceptions about lack of autonomy.

PRACTICE TIPS 3

CONSIDERATIONS WHEN ISOLATING ABORIGINAL AND TORRES STRAIT ISLANDER PATIENTS

When undertaking isolation protocols for IPC purposes, consider the following:

- Is the room large enough to accommodate a number of visitors (within IPC guidelines)?
- Can a family member stay overnight (while accommodating for isolation protocols)?
- Does the room have Indigenous art?
- Does the room promote connection to the outdoors e.g. large windows, views of nature? Can family be seen and heard? Does it allow for yarning?
- Talk to the person about why they are in isolation and what can be done for them to feel less isolated.

The move towards single-patient rooms for newly built or refurbished hospitals is recommended as they are beneficial for IPC, as well as for patient privacy and dignity and staff comfort. However, despite a move towards culturally appropriate health service delivery, hospital designers have given little consideration to the cultural and spiritual wellbeing of Aboriginal and Torres Strait Islander people.[21] Maintaining social relationships and family practices is vitally important as it reinforces cultural identity. The impact of social isolation by being placed in a single room can cause undue distress for an Indigenous person as it can promote a sense of cultural exclusion, feelings of institutional racism, and the belief that without family presence they may succumb to harmful spiritual forces.[21] Being placed in isolation also removes the connectedness to the outside environment.[62] The value of seeing outside for physical, psychological and cultural reasons is important; however, more important is the preference for sitting in the sun and 'yarning' with others, thus deepening a cultural connection.[21]

Conclusion

Aboriginal and Torres Strait Islander people experience a higher burden of infectious diseases than the rest of the Australian population. Beliefs around disease causation and transmission, and institutional racism influence how and when Indigenous people will seek treatment. SDoH, such as inadequate housing and health hardware, increase the risk of infectious disease transmission in a household and due to their high prevalence, many infectious diseases are normalised within some communities. Normalisation of infectious diseases leads to a lack of, or late presentations to, healthcare and potentially inadequate treatment. The consequences of inadequate treatment for an Indigenous person are far more severe than for a non-Indigenous person, resulting in high morbidity rates and early mortality.

Preventing the transmission of infection in a healthcare facility in the Indigenous context requires a culturally aware health system. A collaborative approach which includes all members of an IPC team, including an Indigenous HCW, is vital to prevent self-discharge (against medical advice). Respectful dialogue and appropriate use of language is required to engage an Indigenous person and their family and involve them in their care, and should isolation be required, careful consideration should be given to ensure the most culturally appropriate strategy.

Useful websites/resources

- Cultural Safety Position Statement – Congress of Aboriginal and Torres Strait Islander Nurses and Midwives (CATSINaM) Safety Position Statement. www.secureservercdn.net/198.71.233.110/dgc.5bd. myftpupload.com/wp-content/uploads/2021/01/cultural-safety-endorsed-march-2014-wfginzphsxbz.pdf
- Queensland Health Aboriginal and Torres Strait Islander Cultural Capability Framework 2010 – 2033. www.health.qld.gov.au/__data/assets/pdf_file/0014/156200/cultural_capability.pdf
- Aboriginal and Torres Strait Islander Patient care guideline. www.health.qld.gov.au/__data/assets/pdf_file/0022/157333/patient_care_guidelines.pdf
- Taylor K, Guerin PT. Health Care and Indigenous Australians: Cultural Safety in Practice. Sydney: Bloomsbury Publishing Pty, 2019.
- Queensland Government. (2018, April 20). *Thursday Island (Waiben).* Retrieved March 3, 2023, from Queensland Government: https://www.qld.gov.au/firstnations/cultural-awareness-heritage-arts/community-histories/community-histories-s-t/community-histories-thursday-island.

References

1. Gimuy Walubara Yidinji Elders Aboriginal Corporation. Home 2021. Available from: www.yidinji.com.
2. Best O, Fredericks B, eds. Yatdjuligin – Aboriginal and Torres Strait Islander Nursing and Midwifery Care. 3rd ed. Sydney: Cambridge University Press, 2021.
3. Centre for Cultural Competence Australia. A foundation in Aboriginal and Torres Straight Islander cultural competence. Sydney: CCCA, 2022.
4. Australian Bureau of Statistics. Australia: Aboriginal and Torres Strait Islander population summary 2022. Canberra: Australian Government, 2022. Available from: www.abs.gov.au/articles/australia-aboriginal-and-torres-strait-islander-population-summary.
5. Gibney KB, Cheng AC, Hall R, Leder K. Sociodemographic and geographical inequalities in notifiable infectious diseases in Australia: a retrospective analysis of 21 years of national disease surveillance data. Lancet Infect Dis. 2017;17(1):86-97.
6. Sparke VL. Improving infection control at Atoifi Adventist Hospital, Solomon Islands: a participatory action research approach. James Cook University, 2022.
7. Gan Titui Cultural Centre. Torres Strait n.d. Available from: www.gabtitui.gov.au/torres-strait.
8. The Australian Institute of Aboriginal and Torres Strait Islander Studies. The AIATSIS Map of Indigenous Australia. AIATSIS, 2022.
9. Australian Institute of Health and Welfare. Profile of Indigenous Australians. AIHW, 2021.
10. Wapau H, Kris E, Roeder L, McDonald M. Community-driven health research in the Torres Strait. Aust J Prim Health. 2022;28(4):289-295.
11. Drummond A, Mills Y, Nona F. Torres Strait Islander health and wellbeing. In: Best O, Fredericks B, eds. Yatdjuligin: Aboriginal and Torres Strait Islander nursing and midwifery 3rd ed. Sydney: Cambridge University Press, 2021.
12. Torres Strait Regional Authority. Torres Strait regional map. TSRA, 2012. Available from: www.tsra.gov.au/the-torres-strait/regional-map.
13. World Health Organization. Health promotion glossary of terms 2021. Geneva: WHO, 2021. Available from: www.who.int/publications/i/item/9789240038349.
14. National Aboriginal Community Controlled Health Organisation. Aboriginal Community Controlled Health Organisations (ACCHOs) 2022. Available from: www.naccho.org.au/acchos/.
15. McKivett A, Glover K, Clark Y, Coffin J, Paul D, Hudson JN, O'Mara P. The role of governance in Indigenous medical education research. Rural Remote Health. 2021;21(2):6473.
16. Australian Government Department of Health and Ageing. National Aboriginal and Torres Strait Islander Health Plan 2013-2023. Canberra: Australian Government, 2013.

17. Socha A. Addressing institutional racism against Aboriginal and Torres Strait Islanders of Australia in mainstream health services: insights from Aboriginal Community Controlled Health Services. Int J Indigenous Health. 2021;16(1).

18. Sparke VL, Diau J, MacLaren D, West C. Solutions to infection prevention and control challenges, do they exist? An integrative review. Int J Infect Control. 2020;16(1).

19. Bnads H, Orr E, Clements CJ. Improving the service to Aboriginal and Torres Strait Islanders through innovative practices between Aboriginal Hospital Liaison Officers and social workers in hospitals in Victoria, Australia. Brit J Social Work. 2020;51(1):77-95.

20. Queensland Health. Cultural capability March 2022. Brisbane: Queensland Government, 2022. Available from: www.health.qld.gov.au/public-health/groups/atsihealth/cultural-capability.

21. Nash D, O'Rourke T, Memmott P, Haynes M. Indigenous preferences for inpatient rooms in Australian hospitals: a mixed-methods study in cross-cultural design. HERD: Health Environ Res Design J. 2021;14(1):174-189.

22. Cusack L, Kinnear A, Ward K, Mohamed J, Butler A. Cultural safety: nurses and midwives leading the way for safer healthcare. Melbourne: NMBA, 2018.

23. Nursing and Midwifery Board of Australia. Code of conduct for nurses and code of conduct for midwives 2019. Melbourne: NMBA, 2019. Available from: www.nursingmidwiferyboard.gov.au/Codes-Guidelines-Statements/FAQ/Fact-sheet-Code-of-conduct-for-nurses-and-Code-of-conduct-for-midwives.aspx.

24. Nursing and Midwifery Board. Professional standards 2021. Melbourne: NMBA, 2021. Available from: www.nursingmidwiferyboard.gov.au/Codes-Guidelines-Statements/Professional-standards.aspx.

25. Queensland Nurses and Midwives Union. First Nations members supported to lead the COVID-19 vaccinations rollout 2021. Brisbane: QNMU, 2021. Available from: https://www.qnmu.org.au/.

26. Kaufman J, Tuckerman J, Danchin M. Overcoming COVID-19 vaccine hesitancy: can Australia reach the last 20 percent? Expert Rev Vaccines. 2022;21(2):159-161.

27. Durey A, Thompson SC. Reducing the health disparities of Indigenous Australians: time to change focus. BMC Health Serv Res. 2012;12(1):151.

28. National Aboriginal Community Controlled Health Organisation. About us 2022. Canberra: NACCHO, 2022. Available from: https://www.naccho.org.au/about-us/.

29. Andersen MJ, Skinner A, Williamson AB, Fernando P, Wright D. Housing conditions associated with recurrent gastrointestinal infection in urban Aboriginal children in NSW, Australia: findings from SEARCH. Aust NZ J Public Health. 2018;42(3):247-253.

30. Australian Indigenous HeatlhInfoNet. Aboriginal and Torres Strait Islander health workers and health practitioners n.d. Mt Lawley WA: InfoNet AIH. Available from: https://healthinfonet.ecu.edu.au/key-resources/health-professionals/health-workers/.

31. National Association of Aboriginal and Torres Strait Islander Health Workers and Practitioners. History. NAATSIHWP, 2021. Available from: www.naatsihwp.org.au/history.

32. Devlin S, MacLaren D, Massey PD, Widders R, Judd JA. The missing voices of Indigenous Australians in the social, cultural and historical experiences of tuberculosis: a systematic and integrative review. BMJ Glob Health. 2019;4(6):e001794.

33. Carey M, Clague L, Magick Dennis F, Magick Dennis L. Paediatric nursing in Australia and New Zealand. 3rd ed. Sydney: Cambridge University Press, 2022.

34. Ali SH, Foster T, Nina Lansbury H. The relationship between infectious diseases and housing maintenance in Indigenous Australian households. Int J Environ Res Public Health. 2018;15(12):2827.

35. Australian Bureau of Statistics. National Aboriginal and Torres Strait Islander Survey 2022. Canberra: Australian Government, 2022. Available from: https://www.abs.gov.au/statistics/people/aboriginal-and-torres-strait-islander-peoples.

36. Kostova D, Richter P, Van Vliet G, Mahar M, Moolenaar RL. The role of noncommunicable diseases in the pursuit of global health security. Health Security. 2021;19(3):288-301.

37. Dixit R, Webster F, Booy R, Menzies R. The role of chronic disease in the disparity of influenza incidence and severity between Indigenous and non-Indigenous Australian peoples during the 2009 influenza pandemic. BMC Pub Health. 2022; 22:1-10.

38. Banham D, Chen T, Karnon J, Brown A, Lynch J. Sociodemographic variations in the amount, duration and cost of potentially preventable hospitalisation for chronic conditions among Aboriginal and non-Aboriginal Australians: a period prevalence study of linked public hospital data. BMJ Open. 2017;7(10):e017331.

39. Hoy WE, Mott SA, McDonald SP. An update on chronic kidney disease in Aboriginal Australians. Clin Nephrol. 2020;93(1):124-128.

40. Devlin S, Ross W, Widders R, McAvoy G, Browne K, Lawrence K, et al. Tuberculosis care designed with barramarrany (family): participatory action research that prioritised partnership, healthy housing and nutrition. Health Prom J Aust. 2021(00):1-12.

41. Thomas L, Bowen AC, Ly M, Connors C, Andrews R, Tong SYC. Burden of skin disease in two remote primary healthcare centres in northern and central Australia. Intern Med J. 2019;49(3):396-399.

42. Secombe P, Planche Y, Athan E, Ollapallil J. Critical care burden of skin and soft tissue infection in Central Australia: more than skin deep. Aust J Rural Health. 2019;27(6): 550-556.

43. Cheluvappa R, Selvendran S. Strengths-based nursing to combat common infectious diseases in Indigenous Australians. Nurs Rep. 2022;12(1):22-28.

44. May PJ, Bowen AC, Carapetis JR. The inequitable burden of group A streptococcal diseases in Indigenous Australians. MJA. 2016;205(5):201-203.

45. Ralph AP, Noonan S, Boardman C, Halkon C, Currie BJ. Prescribing for people with acute rheumatic fever. Aust Prescr. 2017;40(2):70-75.

46. Lynar S, Currie BJ, Baird R. Scabies and mortality. Lancet Infect Dis. 2017;17(12):1234.

47. Cox V, Fuller LC, Engelman D, Steer A, Hay RJ. Estimating the global burden of scabies: what else do we need? Br J Dermatol. 2021;184(2):237-242.

48. Basnayake TL, Morgan LC, Chang AB. The global burden of respiratory infections in Indigenous children and adults: a review. Respirology. 2017;22(8):1518-1528.

49. Torzillo PJ, Chang AB. Acute respiratory infections among Indigenous children. MJA. 2014;200:559-560.

50. National Health Security (National Notifiable Disease List) Instrument 2018, (2022).

51. Saravanos GL, Sheel M, Homaira N, Dey A, Brown E, Wang H, et al. Respiratory syncytial virus-associated hospitalisations in Australia, 2006–2015. MJA. 2019; 210(10):447-453.

52. Miller A, Cairns A, Richardson A, Lawrence J. Supporting holistic care for patients with tuberculosis in a remote Indigenous community: a case report. Rural Remote Health. 2020;20(1):5552.

53. Guthridge I, Smith S, Horne P, Hanson J. Increasing prevalence of methicillin-resistant Staphylococcus aureus in remote Australian communities: implications for patients and clinicians. Pathology. 2019;51(4):428-431.

54. Yau JW, Thor SM, Tsai D, Speare T, Rissel C. Antimicrobial stewardship in rural and remote primary health care: a narrative review. Antimicrob Resist Infect Control. 2021; 10(1):105.

55. de Jong J, Speare T, Chiong F, Einsiedel L, Silver B, Gent D, et al. Evaluating antimicrobial prescribing practice in Australian remote primary healthcare clinics. Infect Dis Health. 2021; 26(3):173-181.

56. Dadgostar P. Antimicrobial resistance: implications and costs. Infect Drug Resist. 2019;12:3903-3910.

57. Nakata M. The cultural interface: an exploration of the intersection of Western knowledge systems and Torres Strait Islanders positions and experiences: James Cook University, 1997.

58. Martin G, Nakata V, Nakata M, Day A. Promoting the persistence of Indigenous students through teaching at the cultural interface. Studies in Higher Education. 2017; 42(7):1158-1173.

59. Maakrun J, Maher M. Cultural interface theory in the Kenya context and beyond. Issues in Educational Research. 2016; 26:298-314.

60. Delbridge R, Garvey L, Mackelprang JL, Cassar N, Ward-Pahl E, Egan M, et al. Working at a cultural interface: co-creating Aboriginal health curriculum for health professions. Higher Education Research & Development. 2022;41(5):1483-1498.

61. Laverty M, McDermott DR, Calma T. Embedding cultural safety in Australia's main health care standards. MJA. 2017; 207(1):15-16.

62. Schill K, Caxaj S. Cultural safety strategies for rural Indigenous palliative care: a scoping review. BMC Palliative Care. 2019; 18(1):21.

63. Usher K, Marriott R, Smallwood R, Walker R, Shepherd C, Hopkins K, et al. COVID-19 and social restrictions: the potential mental health impact of social distancing and isolation for young Indigenous Australians. Australasian Psychiatry. 2020;28(5):599-600.

CHAPTER 37

Infection prevention and control in home and community health settings

GARETH HOCKEY[i]

PROFESSOR SUE RANDALL[ii]

Chapter highlights

- Discusses how the context of working in a person's home or a community setting affects infection control
- Explores strategies to maintain infection prevention and control (IPC) in a private home and in community settings

i   Infection Prevention and Control, Prince of Wales Hospital, Randwick, NSW
ii The University of Sydney's Department of Rural Health (Broken Hill) and the Susan Wakil School of Nursing and Midwifery, Faculty of Medicine and Health, Broken Hill, NSW

Introduction

In this chapter we explore IPC in home and community health practice settings. Firstly, we set out the characteristics and contexts of home and community settings in Australia. Specifically, we focus on home (district) nursing, hospital in the home (HITH), acute and post-acute (APAC) services, and community health clinics including sexual health and wound clinics. Secondly, we explore IPC strategies in home and community settings. We then explore the risks, including the risk of healthcare-associated infections (HAI), associated with home and community health settings. Finally, three case studies are presented to demonstrate the application of the practice principles described in this chapter.

37.1 Characteristics and contexts of home and community health settings in Australia

To understand the characteristics and contexts of home and community health settings in Australia, an overview of the Australian healthcare system's lines of responsibility and funding is presented. Governance of healthcare in Australia is a multi-jurisdictional response, with broad relationships between:

- the Commonwealth, state and territory health departments
- patient advocacy stakeholders; and
- healthcare organisations—both not-for-profit bodies and private entities.

The Commonwealth Department of Health (DoH), in conjunction with state and territory services, has a network of 17 agencies and commissions to support the work and key focus areas to ensure safety for all patients in Australia. One example of healthcare governance via these agencies is the activities of the Australian Commission for Safety and Quality in Health Care (ACSQHC). The ACSQHC commenced as an independent statutory authority on 1 July 2011 and is jointly funded by the federal, state and territory governments. The ACSQHC developed eight standards, known collectively as the National Safety and Quality Health Service (NSQHS) Standards.[1] These standards include the Preventing and Controlling Infections[2] and provides details as to how IPC strategies are to be implemented by healthcare organisations and providers. To meet the accreditation and governance standards

required of healthcare organisations, providers must show evidence that IPC is being delivered in accordance with NSQHS Standard 3. These quality standards are inclusive of agreed criteria that include IPC policy and procedures that include, but are not limited to, hand hygiene compliance, consumer engagement, multidrug-resistant organism (MRO) surveillance, and sterilisation and disinfection standard compliance.

The DoH also oversees a range of national health and promotion programs that include Aboriginal and Torres Strait Islander programs, primary and ambulatory care, and health protection. The latter comprises health promotion, public health surveillance, emergency preparedness and responses, and communicable disease control.

State, territory and local governments have the responsibility for the provision and allocation of health funding and managing community services which may operate in clinic settings or where care takes place in a person's home. Meeting the National Safety and Quality Health Service Standards (NSQHS) (2nd edition, 2021) is a mandated requirement for community and ambulatory care setting accreditation, where external auditors, as delegated by the ACSQHC, review all evidence identifying compliance with criterion within the NSQHS Preventing and Controlling Infections Standard.

Working in the community offers a unique set of challenges. Some people live in chaotic environments. For example, a client may be a hoarder, resulting in limited space to move around, difficulty in setting up for a procedure such as a wound dressing, and difficulty in accessing hand washing facilities that may be blocked by rubbish.

Another challenge is the need to provide services to the homeless, either on the street or in hostels. People who inject drugs (PWID) and sometimes the homeless and other clients may exhibit behaviours that impact care delivery and even the personal safety of healthcare workers (HCWs). In addition HCWs may have difficulty in gaining cooperation and concordance with treatment and therapies. The lack of amenities for bathing, laundering and sleeping increases the risks of skin infections, scabies and other parasitic infestations. Finally, the impact of poor nutrition and poor hygiene on health in general can be magnified for vulnerable individuals in the community.

Collectively and individually, these factors can affect the client's health overall and pose significant challenges specific to the community context. Such complexities have an impact on staff who may need to work creatively to deliver a service in line with IPC in the home.

37.2 Prevention and control of HAIs in home and community health settings in Australia

While clear guidance and infection control policies exist, they do not necessarily address the environmental issues that occur in the community and especially in people's homes.[3]

Maintaining infection control principles can be difficult in private homes which may be chaotic due to both personal and environmental factors such as pets, vermin, clutter, poor hygiene and limited resources.[4] Therefore, the client, their family members, pets, living environment and HCWs are all reservoirs of microorganisms that exist in patient home settings,[5] several of which are potential reservoirs that never have to be considered in a hospital or clinic setting.

Raymond (2016) notes that although home environments are not controlled and do not offer hospital standards, this does not mean that IPC measures should be compromised—people in the community are entitled to clean, safe and competent care. IPC is necessary to protect patients from potentially life-threatening infections, not least because many people who have their care managed at home are vulnerable, elderly and at higher risk of infection.[6,7]

37.2.1 Hand hygiene

In reality, examples of challenges that community nurses face include a lack of clean surfaces to use for dressings, and handwashing facilities in households that include bars of soap and towels that are more likely to transmit infection than to control it.[8]

Handwashing basins may be inadequate, dirty or in some cases offer no running water.[3] While handwashing with soap and water was considered to be the gold standard, alcohol-based hand rubs (ABHR) are now the most effective way of removing harmful bacterial load from both the HCW and the individual as long as hands are not visibly soiled. Therefore, ABHR should be available for all healthcare interactions.[9] It should be noted though that there is potential to spread organisms that are resistant to alcohol, for example *Clostridium difficile*. To counter this, traditional soap and water is effective for spore removal and all HCWs must wear gloves when in potential contact with bodily fluids, including faeces.[10]

Swanson and Jeanes[8] note that there is a risk that community staff may develop reduced levels of compliance with hand hygiene due to suboptimal environments, and that the provision of ABHR in all community staff home visit kits provided by health services is supported by mandated completion of IPC education modules annually.

PRACTICE TIPS 1

HAND HYGIENE FOR COMMUNITY AND HOME VISITS

- Always include alcohol based hand rub (ABHR) in home visit kits
- Always be bare below the elbows to reduce uniform or clothing contamination
- Don't leave ABHR in cars (temperature will affect the efficacy of the solutions)
- Ask your patients to perform hand hygiene before contact
- Perform hand hygiene before getting out of the car and before you get back into the vehicle
- Moisturise your hands frequently

The WHO's 5 Moments for Hand Hygiene[11,12] are part of an essential toolkit in clinic and home settings where facilities for effective handwashing are available.

In 2012, the WHO produced a document which showed how the 5 Moments for Hand Hygiene could be translated to fit community settings, including the home.[13] A section has been reproduced that provides an example of managing hand hygiene when undertaking a wound dressing in the home. (See Box 37.1.)

Further precautions for nurses to minimise infection risk pertain to aseptic technique and hand hygiene, and relate to the concept of 'bare below the elbows'— that is, removal of all wrist and hand jewellery (although commonly a plain wedding band is acceptable), no nail varnish, and cuts and abrasions should be covered with an impervious waterproof dressing.[10]

37.2.2 Personal protective equipment (PPE)

HCWs who work in a patient's home or in a community clinic should ensure that they are familiar with the mode of transmission of any infection that could present in a person in their care. This will ensure that

BOX 37.1 The 5 moments for hand hygiene adapted for home and community settings

6b. Home care—wound dressing

Brief explanation

The nurse goes 3 times a week to the home of a disabled patient to change the dressing on an ulcerous leg wound. This care is provided after the patient has been assisted in bathing by an auxiliary nurse. All care items (gauze, antiseptic product, adhesive band, personal protective equipment, alcohol-based hand rub, etc.) are brought by the nurse in a plastic container. The patient and the home environment represent the *patient zone*. The *point/s of care* is/are where the procedures take place. The plastic container and the care items brought by the HCW represent the *healthcare area*. Although the care is delivered at home, the 'My five moments' approach fully applies.

Sequence of care

A. The nurse arrives and goes to the patient's bedroom where he is waiting.

B. The nurse enters the room and puts his medical bag on a chair.

The nurse performs hand hygiene (Moment 1).

C. He then shakes hands with the patient, has a brief conversation, and finally uncovers the patient's leg.

D. The nurse cleans a table close to the bed.

The nurse performs hand hygiene (Moment 4).

E. The nurse takes out a record book and a plastic box from the medical bag.

The nurse performs hand hygiene (Moments 1 & 2 combined).

F. The nurse prepares the sterile dressing set and all other necessary items and dons non-sterile gloves.

G. The nurse removes the wet bandages from the leg and examines the dressing and the wound.

H. The nurse discards the soiled bandages in the waste bin, and removes and discards gloves.

The nurse performs hand hygiene (Moments 3 & 2 combined).

I. Using instruments, the nurse applies antiseptic several times, removes some fibrin with scissors, and applies antiseptic again. All waste is discarded in the bin and the instruments are placed in the plastic container.

J. Using an instrument, the nurse places the gauze with ointment on the wound with other dry gauzes on top, followed by an adhesive bandage.

K. Once the dressing is complete, the nurse clears everything remaining on the table, closes the plastic container and puts it into a plastic bag, and cleans the table with a wipe.

The nurse performs hand hygiene (Moments 3 & 4 combined).

L The nurse records notes on the wound status and procedure and puts the record book in the medical bag.

The nurse performs hand hygiene (Moment 1).

M. The nurse helps the patient to install himself in the kitchen for breakfast, switches on the television, shakes hands with the patient, and leaves.

The nurse performs hand hygiene (Moment 4).

Care sequence features

Likely frequency of the sequence per hour	1
Duration of the sequence	60 minutes
Number of hand hygiene opportunities per sequence	7
Types of hand contact	Intact skin/non-intact skin/body fluids/contaminated items
Use of personal protective equipment	Gloves
Use of disposable items	Yes
Use of sterile items	Yes
Use of shared items	No
Patient zone	The patient and the home environment
Point of care	Where the dressing is performed

Source: Adapted from WHO 2012, 5 Moments for Hand Hygiene.

correct PPE is considered. Chapter 13 and Chapter 14 explore this in detail.

37.2.3 Sepsis

Sepsis is the body's extreme response to an infection; it threatens life and is a medical emergency. Sepsis is responsible for increased rates of morbidity and mortality. People being nursed in their own homes are at high risk of sepsis as many have comorbid chronic conditions, are receiving palliative or end-of-life care, have had recent surgery, or have chronic wounds or an invasive device (e.g. urinary catheters, peripherally inserted central lines and gastrostomies). As such, community, HITH and APAC nurses regularly care for people with infections, and this places them in a good position to monitor for infection and recognise the early signs of sepsis and act accordingly.[14]

PRACTICE TIPS 2

KNOW THE SIGNS OF SEPSIS[15,16]

Infection confirmed or suspected PLUS:

- Temperature >38.3C or <36C (normal temperature does not exclude sepsis)
- Respiratory rate >20/minute
- Heart rate >90/minute
- Acute confusion or decreased level of consciousness
- Hyperglycemia (blood glucose >7.7 mmol/L in patient without diabetes)
- Oliguria (urine output less than 0.5 mL/kg/hour)

Check out your organisation's sepsis pathway.

Apart from the general infection prevention strategies previously outlined it is worthwhile to consider the risks of infection associated with health provision in the home and community setting.

37.3 HAI risks associated with home and community health settings in Australia

While the extent of the prevalence and burden of HAIs within the community and home setting within Australia is not completely known or comprehensively quantified, emerging research indicates that these settings play an integral part in both HAI prevention and transmission risks.[1]

HAIs that are reported in the community disproportionally affect persons who are susceptible to infection, have weakened immune systems and have a preexisting or chronic illness diagnosis as previously described. These individuals typically have frequent episodes of hospitalisation, placing them at a higher risk of infection and complications from those infections.[17]

S. aureus, and multidrug-resistant organisms (MROs) including methicillin-resistant *S. aureus* (MRSA), community-associated methicillin-resistant *S. aureus* (cMRSA), carbarpenemase-producing enterobacterales (CPE) and *Candida auris* occur in community settings as they do in hospital. Detailed information about these organisms can be found in other chapters in this publication.

In a community clinic setting, cleaning of equipment between patients would occur. In a home setting, the end of visit signifies a natural break to an episode of care, resulting in handwashing before travel to the next client. The end of the episode of care is clearer cut than in hospital, where moving to the next patient bed is easier, and may result in less thorough hygiene measures being employed.

The expansion of the delivery of healthcare into the community has resulted in patients with intravenous devices, such as Permacaths, Hickman lines and Portacaths, being managed in the community or in a home setting. In 2020, in NSW, a key performance indicator (KPI) that is reportable to the NSW Ministry of Health (MoH) was updated to include whether intravenous lines, or other invasive devices such as Permacaths, Hickman lines and Portacaths, were implicated in *S. aureus* and MRSA bloodstream infection (bacteraemia) source acquisition.[18] The recognition of the prevalence of the infections clearly indicates the risks that the bacteria pose in a range of home and community settings, particularly where the immunocompromised are receiving intravenous therapies and treatments. Infection risk associated with these IV devices lasts as long as the IV device remains in situ.

37.3.1 Risk assessment within the community health setting

The terminology of 'risk assessment' conjures a variety of associations, particularly within Work Health Safety frameworks, and in its strictest interpretation this is the purpose of the assessment. The intention of the holistic assessment, which is inclusive of IPC, is to help the community health and home settings care provider to identify issues that require planning and interventions for the individual (or individuals) to ensure the impact or potential impact from HAIs is mitigated.[19]

Any infectious agent or resistant pathogen poses a risk of transmission. A description of modes of potential contact transmission risks for community and home healthcare services to consider includes the following list. Note that the list is not exhaustive in relation to infection risk assessment but provides a basis for the development of a risk assessment tool for service delivery in the home and community context (see Table 37.1).

Direct contact: patient-to-patient contact, while unlikely in a home setting, presents risks in community clinics or respite facilities.

Indirect contact: transmission via an HCW with poor hand hygiene adherence; contamination of the environment, including pool cars, following contact with a patient with an infectious or resistant organism; by contaminated environmental surfaces and equipment.

As part of a risk assessment, some individuals with infectious or resistant organisms pose a higher risk of transmission than others. This is, in part, linked to what is sometimes considered the unpredictable nature of community settings. Particular attention is required for patients with:

- diarrhoea, faecal incontinence, stomas
- urinary catheters and ileal conduits or other drainage devices
- respiratory management and support—tracheostomies, CPAP
- feeding tubes—nasogastric and percutaneously endoscopically placed gastrostomy tubes (PEG)
- poorly healing wounds with the presence of exudates
- requirements for an increased level of personal care, i.e. patients with spinal cord injury or other forms of decreased mobility.

When managing patients and individuals with confirmed or suspected infections or resistant organisms the use of transmission-based precautions (TBP) is recommended, that is, full contact—impervious gown, gloves, scrupulous hand hygiene before and during donning and doffing, and eye protection if the intervention identifies the risk of blood and body fluid splash exposure.[20]

37.4 Strategies for infection prevention in patient homes

Identification of the infection risks associated with the patient and the environment; of the social and cultural factors associated with care provision; and the application of general IPC practices, will all help to mitigate infection

risks. However, there are additional specific infection risks associated with care provision in this context. Challenges include:

- the management of invasive devices
- specific infections that are more prevalent in the home and community setting
- cleaning the environment; and
- reprocessing of equipment.

Consumers in this context require specific education tailored to their needs and their own circumstances, and HCWs need to adapt to the context in which they deliver the care while also maintaining standards of practice.

In this section strategies for infection prevention in patients' homes are considered for specific health risks: urinary tract infections (UTIs) and catheter-associated urinary tract infections (CAUTIs), pressure ulcers and respiratory infections. Education and capacity building for healthcare professionals and patients is explored. The following section then discusses strategies to manage sterile stock and shared equipment, environmental cleaning, laundering and segregation, and disinfection and reprocessing.

37.4.1 Urinary tract infections

Catheter-associated urinary tract infections:
Considerable district nursing time is focused on people who have urinary or suprapubic indwelling catheters (IDCs). Data for community prevalence of IDCs is not readily available.

In the hospital setting, CAUTIs account for most HAIs and the WHO identifies that 4% of people with indwelling catheters will develop a CAUTI,[21] so there is no reason to think that the issue has less impact in the community setting. Indication for IDC is poorly documented, and this is an area that should be improved[22] because the best way to avoid CAUTI is to not catheterise at all. Bacteria can enter the bladder during catheterisation. Infection risk increases the longer a catheter remains in situ because the bladder becomes colonised with bacteria that can then cause infection. When a bladder fills and empties naturally, bacteria are flushed out by passing urine. However, catheterisation enables the bacteria to form a biofilm and this sticky, slimy layer offers protection to the bacteria, reducing the effectiveness of antimicrobials and a person's immune system.[22]

Colonisation of the bladder results in cloudy, smelly urine that tests positive for leucocytes and nitrates. This condition is known as asymptomatic bacteriuria (ASB).

TABLE 37.1 Risk assessment considerations

Focus	Consideration	Rationale	Example
Patient/consumer	Reason for health service provision (diagnosis)	Increased risk of infection	Immunosuppressed due to chemotherapy. Infectious condition e.g. TB
	Frequency of service provision	More frequent contact provides more opportunity for exposure to infection	HCW providing service is source of infection e.g. COVID-19 or respiratory viruses in winter even before symptoms declare themselves
	Type of service provided	Invasive procedures and devices increase the potential for infection if asepsis is not maintained	Wound dressings, intravenous infusions, venepuncture
	Recent overseas travel and/or hospitalisation	Increased risk of colonisation with multidrug-resistant organisms	Endemic nature of MRO such as CPE in other countries
	Healthcare supplies and equipment	Need for storage and reprocessing of sterile stock and reusable medical instruments	Poor or absent appropriate storage options in the home. Risk of sterility breaches during transport of sterile items
	Home environment	Water, electricity, lighting, heating, domestic or rural animals, washing machines	Impact on hygiene for the patient and also on the ability of the HCW to maintain asepsis
	Patient factors	Confusion, drugs, language or comprehension difficulties	Inability to understand or comply with treatment requirements may lead to incomplete course of therapy and subsequent antibiotic resistance
	Transport options for treatment	Reliance on community health transport for treatment	Increased risk of transport of patients with infections in same vehicle as non-infectious patients
	Social factors	Drug use, smoking history, aggression, number of persons living within household	Contribute to patient's health and infection risks
Healthcare worker	Known infection risks	Patients posing a risk of infection transmission to HCW	Patient with TB non-concordant with medication poses a risk of multidrug-resistant TB
	Environmental issues	Inability to maintain asepsis	Lack of hand hygiene facilities or clean spaces
	Frequency and timing of visits	Inability to ensure staff safety— may need to consider two staff to visit to ensure safety	Drug use, smoking history, aggression, number of persons living within household
Other considerations	Telehealth and IT access	Improve access to advice and review and reduce travel requirements	Provide opportunity for telehealth reviews, advice and education
	Stakeholders involved	Reduce duplication of efforts and non-essential contact	Create a clear plan of care involving all stakeholders so responsibility is assigned

A culture would return a result showing mixed bacteria; however, in the absence of symptoms in the catheterised person, treatment is not required.[23] UTIs, especially in older people, are overdiagnosed and treated, as both dipsticks and microbiology are unable to distinguish between ASB and CAUTI.

Again, a key role of the nurse in a community setting is to work with patients, family members and carers to maximise knowledge and promote concordance with both prevention strategies and management plans. Effective IPC requires all those involved in the delivery of care to understand and practise according to agreed principles. That community nurses act as role models and educators is central to influencing the behaviour of clients.[8]

This is important in relation to whether a person with an IDC has an infection or not, and therefore careful consideration is required to determine when antibiotics are needed and when they are not.

PRACTICE TIPS 3

HOW TO PREVENT A CATHETER-ASSOCIATED URINARY TRACT INFECTION (CAUTI)[21,22]

- Avoid catheterisation whenever possible
- Perform catheterisation with sterile equipment and using asepsis
- Maintain a closed drainage system
- Do NOT use bladder irrigation or washout
- Do NOT instil antiseptics or antimicrobial agents; none prevent CAUTIs

---

Reducing urinary tract infection: Many people who are nursed at home are elderly and their risk of infection is higher, leading to increased morbidity and mortality. Whether due to ageing and reduction of their thirst reflex or living with one or comorbid chronic conditions, the elderly have an increased risk of dehydration. This in turn can increase the incidence of urinary tract infections (UTIs).[6]

UTIs are known to require hospital admissions as people present with confusion and delirium which makes it unsafe for them to stay at home. With sound preventive care, the incidence of UTIs and subsequent hospital admission can be reduced. Encouraging people to drink 1.5 litres of fluids per day is important.

Ensuring that drinks are available nearby, such as in a thermos, is a simple way to improve oral intake. A referral for home care to assist with buying drinks or filling the kettle may be needed. The need for special drinking cups that can be held when manual dexterity is reduced could be assessed by an occupational therapist. Working with people and their families to enhance their knowledge and understanding may result in increased concordance with a treatment plan.

It is not unusual to hear someone say that they find it hard to get to the toilet, so they drink less to reduce the number of times they must go to the toilet. What is missing is the knowledge that without sufficient fluids, the bladder becomes irritated and increases the urge to urinate. Subsequent reduction in fluids also increases constipation.

37.4.2 Reducing pressure ulcers

Inactivity is a cause of infection in the elderly. Being mobile reduces the risk of pressure ulcers. By increasing heart rate, blood and oxygen perfusion of tissues is increased.[6] Not being mobile enough may lead to pressure ulcers which in turn are prone to becoming infected. Assessing mobility and being able to see the person's home environment offers the community nurse a unique opportunity to collaborate with the person to develop a management plan that can reduce the risk of infection.

37.4.3 Reducing respiratory infections

Inactivity associated with or without other health problems places elderly people at risk of respiratory infection. Similarly, the advent of cooler weather can also be a trigger. As well as encouraging mobility and making appropriate referrals, such as to include a physiotherapist, discussing vaccination is an important infection prevention measure. This discussion should include the importance of pneumococcal vaccination and the annual influenza vaccination.[24] Dispelling myths is important. For example, it is often thought that the fact that the elderly are housebound offers protection from exposure to others. However, if they have carers and family coming in to see them, then their risks of exposure to a respiratory illness may still be quite high.

37.4.4 Education and capacity building for healthcare professionals

Education and capacity building within and external to health should also be considered for staff. Patient elements will be explored later in the chapter. Within health and specifically community settings, strategies such as 'train the trainer' can be used. Leadership in infection control is also critical. Knowledge and understanding of the community demographics, such as language spoken at home, is an important facet in determining how to pitch information and what sort of education might work best.

Outside health, other services contribute to public health. At a macro level, public health units and the media are important players in providing or disseminating health messages. On a meso level, local councils are involved with removal of environmental hazards. These might include clinical waste, or pest and rodent eradication in the case of hoarding. At a micro level, services such as Meals on Wheels may be visiting numerous different people in a community. An understanding of IPC measures is necessary to enhance the safety of individuals, both within these organisations and with the people they visit.

Managing equipment that has been used with clients in either a clinic setting or in someone's own home requires a different consideration in the community and is explored next.

37.5 Sterile stock and shared equipment in the community health and home setting

The management of consumables in all healthcare settings has come under review, not only from an economic and sustainability perspective, but from an infection transmission perspective. Patients and individuals with complex health needs often require months to years of care, and will subsequently require extensive supplies of health consumables and equipment for the duration of their care.[18]

Conditions for storing consumables in a patient's home are not comparable to the storage facilities in hospital. Therefore, judicious and appropriate allocation of consumables and reusable equipment such as wound dressings means that there is less likelihood there will be unused stock. Unused stock may not be returned for redistribution to other clients due to the inability to ensure correct storage conditions were met while outside the clinic/hospital environment. This is irrespective of whether a patient has an MRO or not. Community nurses often carry stock in the boot of their cars to prevent too much being in a person's home. Queries have arisen from families where the person they have been caring for is now deceased and no longer have the need for the equipment. A standard response must be developed and applied consistently.

HITH and community health settings service provision must include storage of all sterile stock in a dedicated area in accordance with the relevant standard. This storage will be separate from patient zones and supplies should only be taken for the intended purpose just as in any hospital.[23]

Decisions about the volume of stock required will be determined based on the service, the intervention and treatment required for the patient/individual's treatment plan (e.g. daily diabetic foot ulcer dressings, PEG or NG feeds for tubing and nutritional supplementation).

Equipment that is rented, borrowed, donated or provided from a centralised service (e.g. crutches, support frames, commodes and patient lifters) must be adequately cleaned prior to their return to the central store or allocation to other patients. Crutches are often issued as single patient use items now due to the fact that the rubber tips often need to be replaced to make them safe to be reissued to another person. Finding someone to do this is often more problematic than simply allocating the items to a single patient.

The cleaning process includes a two-step clean consisting of a neutral detergent and a disinfectant agent approved by the Therapeutic Goods Administration (TGA) of Australia for the purpose. Consideration must also be given to the cleaning instructions provided by the equipment manufacturer in terms of what is compatible and effective for the specific equipment.

Some health service providers may employ a centralised equipment cleaning and tracking process/strategy to ensure this cleaning and disinfection process has been completed for shared care equipment and is an effective strategy of managing and mitigating these risks.

This process/strategy is also utilised for the return of pressure area mattresses and cushions to registered manufacturers and providers.

PRACTICE TIP 4

Consult manufacturers' recommendations for cleaning and disinfection of reusable equipment to ensure compatibility between the disinfectant and the item.

37.5.1 Environmental cleaning

Environmental cleaning where healthcare service is provided is an essential intervention to reduce the risk of transmission of infection and is a basic component of IPC.

The cleanliness of community health facilities should be aligned with best practice principles irrespective of the location, although in some areas access to water may be limited at times and thus a focus on disinfection and cleaning should incorporate the use of chemical agents and include a wipe-based system and microfibre. The provision of often expensive cleaning equipment is an investment for prevention and is an essential component of the risk mitigation bundle for the reduction of HAIs and is often a trade-off over time—'spend now save later'.

All community health and HITH services are strongly recommended to have detailed guidelines for cleaning processes according to the risk rating of the environment in which the services are provided. Considerations include:

- the frequency of cleaning of general locations, including clinic rooms where patients are seen/reviewed, e.g. chairs and beds, and equipment used such as trolleys and venepuncture kits
- the types of clinical procedures undertaken, e.g. cryotherapy tips used for the removal of *Molluscum contagiosum* genital and anal warts; disinfection and sterilisation vs single use tips; and genital speculums
- for reusable items, accessibility to centralised sterilisation service departments and loan sets
- the ultrasound and other diagnostic equipment used in areas, including antenatal imaging and urology clinics, must be cleaned effectively and after use using validated and manufacturer approved cleaning systems
- cleaning required between patients in challenging, resource-restricted and behaviourally challenging populations—despite challenges reported by some areas, a two-step clean with an approved wipe system for areas such as mental health, homeless health and outreach services should be considered
- the barriers used between patients—some areas may use paper and plastic covering in lieu of linen. Barriers of both linen and disposable sheeting may be considered acceptable based on an assessment of the area, ensuring that cleaning is undertaken between patients. More frequent cleaning may be needed where increased soiling potential (blood and fluid) is encountered
- areas that are considered to be extended stay and where patients require invasive treatments or infusions (see dialysis and oncology services) require additional controls. A focus on asepsis and cleaning is essential.

As discussed, significant challenges arise in the provision of services in patient homecare settings including community respite and home dwellings. As there is variation between households, HCWs providing care at these locations must ensure that cleaning of the areas where dressings are undertaken, or IV infusion packs are changed, is optimal to ensure asepsis.

In the absence of optimal cleaning within the household, HITH and other community health services should provide/ensure access to cleaning wipes, hand hygiene solution and sharps containers. Any bags or bogeys should be able to be cleaned.

As demands for space increase in hospital settings, alternative group sessions and simple non-invasive clinics are held in community halls, council spaces and school settings. The same principles apply for the assessment and cleaning of these areas and spaces, including hand hygiene facilities, bathrooms, tables and chairs. Simple cleaning using traditional methods of buckets and mops provided by these services will suffice; cleaning wipes can be used on equipment and environmental surfaces.

Major spills or contamination (incontinence, vomiting and diarrhoea) can be cleaned according to service agreement requirements, with spill kits to absorb and contain these situational problems.

In addition to these locations, some service providers, including homeless health, sex worker outreach programs and drug and alcohol outreach services, use community outreach buses to reach their patient/consumer cohorts. Within these vehicles, blood tests and simple sexual health testing are often undertaken. Again, cleaning principles include the cleaning of surfaces between patients and in the absence of water (as per Ambulance services), cleaning wipes are strongly recommended in addition to single use equipment (including tourniquets), contained sharps disposal (for used FitPacks and blood collection). More information on environmental cleaning can be found in Chapter 15.

PRACTICE TIP 5

Equipment used in community home visits should be purchased after rigorous selection processes including consideration of the cleaning requirements.

37.5.2 Laundering and segregation

Along with the challenges associated with environmental cleaning in the community, an effective laundering process is also key to reducing HAI and MRO transmission, particularly between household members and other occupants of respite and group homes. These considerations are also important for homeless shelters.

Laundering of linen and personal effects requires temperature and detergent controls to remove soil and bacteria and kill parasites such as scabies mites. The impact of scabies infestations is well documented in homeless people.[26,27]

Availability of, and access to, water can impact areas of Australia that are affected by ongoing drought and water restrictions; however, in relation to laundering the following principles should be applied:

- limit the laundry load to items belonging to one individual, e.g. clothing, towels, facewashers
- if linen and clothing from large respite and group homes is sent to a laundry, ensure that the laundry is accredited and compliant with Australian standards
- many hot water systems have temperature controls that reduce heat and may not be hot enough to eradicate lice and scabies—temperature must be able to reach >50 degrees Celsius
- cold wash temperatures in conjunction with detergent action are adequate for normal household laundering
- linen and clothing should be separated into separate bags. Ensure the laundry layout segregates clean from dirty/soiled
- in colder, wetter environments or where outdoor access or space is limited, dryers may be required. Ensure the temperature of dryers is adequate. The same recommendations in relation to separating clothing apply
- laundering of equipment used for mobility, such as slings and hoists, is required where these are in use, such as group homes
- mop heads and other cleaning items should be laundered in separate washing machines and dryers, not those used for laundering clothing and linen, to reduce the risk of cross-contamination.

PRACTICE TIP 6

Community health staff are encouraged to review or visually check the laundry and washing areas of the HITH/community patient to provide helpful and logical advice.

37.5.3 Disinfection and reprocessing

In general, single use disposable items are used in community or homecare settings, as noted previously. If a reusable medical device was required, it must be sent for disinfection and sterilisation at an accredited facility or hospital sterilisation department; these facilities are currently required to implement the current ACSQHC Advisory AS/07 published on 27 February 2020.[28]

While reprocessing reusable medical devices is discussed in detail in Chapter 16, community and health settings within many areas are adopting and have adopted a single use system to move away from any sterilisation requirements; however, this is dependent on the service provided.

As has been discussed throughout the chapter, a comprehensive risk assessment is recommended to detail the types of equipment used and the procedures that are performed when formulating decisions about disinfection and sterilisation. Some examples of reprocessing required in this context include ultrasound-type equipment, including bladder scanners, transvaginal probes and IVC/CVAD siting equipment.

Generally, in community settings non-invasive ultrasound equipment is used as the higher level, and invasive diagnostics are not performed. Cleaning wipes are approved for cleaning; however, it is essential that the cleaning wipe systems are TGA-approved as being effective for the intended use. In addition, the cleaning process carried out by the operator/cleaner must be reviewed to ensure correct application of the chemical system. However, the type and level of reprocessing will change, depending on the type of procedure the ultrasound was used to perform. For example, if the ultrasound was used on broken skin, or where there is access to the bloodstream, the level of reprocessing may need to be elevated to the level appropriate for semi-critical or critical devices as per the Spaulding Scale (see Practice tip) and high-level disinfection or sterilisation would then be required.

PRACTICE TIP 7
THE SPAULDING SCALE

1) **Critical**—Objects which enter normally sterile tissue or the vascular system and require sterilisation

2) **Semi-critical**—Objects that contact mucous membranes or non-intact skin and require high-level disinfection, which kills all but high levels of bacterial spores

3) **Non-critical**—Objects that contact intact skin but not mucous membranes, and require low-level disinfection

Departments and services including sexual health and others (briefly discussed earlier in this chapter) may have specific trays or loan sets for identified procedures including minor skin repairs and/or cryotherapy. These loan sets are provided and reprocessed by a CSSD and therefore the compliance requirements rest with the CSSD under service level agreements (SLAs). These SLAs are usually provided to satellite sites of a larger health service; however, there is economic benefit with this method as it ensures compliance with AS18/07:2019[28] in addition to creating sustainability. Checking the integrity of packaging post-sterilisation should be undertaken and there should be clear evidence that the sterilisation processes were completed, and the specific evidence will be relevant to the type of process used, that is, steam, STERIS and thermal disinfection.

For some community respite and/or group homes where shared utensils, bowls and urinals are used, washer disinfectors may be used. Detergents and disinfection solutions recommendations are made by the manufacturers and can be either self-dosing or manual loading. Staff must ensure these disinfectors are maintained and detergent/disinfection solutions are always used.

Sterile, single use items in any setting should be stored according to Standards, thereby meeting the requirements for temperature and humidity controls, stored away from direct light and stored off the floor. In the home environment, where possible, stock supply should be limited to reduce waste as it cannot be returned to a general inventory/NITH and consideration should be given to storing the stock in a cleanable, rigid-walled container that has a lid and can keep the items safe from exposure to moisture.

PRACTICE TIP 8
BLOOD AND BODY FLUID CONTACT

Consider the extent of potential blood and body fluid contact involved when using any equipment that comes into direct or indirect contact with the patient/consumer.

PRACTICE TIP 9
STAFF MOBILITY

Consider limiting and allocating staff to set patients to reduce potential risk of exposure and exclusion from work due to quarantine requirements—think pandemics, think COVID-19.

37.6 Patient knowledge and education

Social and mental health issues, complex behaviours and relationships can prevent or create barriers for health provision, including IPC. People at risk may belong to culturally and linguistically diverse communities, Indigenous communities, or live in geographical locations that lack resources. Stigma and discrimination can also be barriers to effective prevention and management of infections. Other factors which may function as barriers include misinformation, being too unwell to retain information or having poor health literacy. One advantage of working in a community health setting can be a longer-term relationship and comprehensive knowledge of clients and their circumstances. This offers HCWs in community settings the advantage of knowing their patients and being able to tailor strategies to meet their specific needs. Including clients as partners in care is important.[29] In one initiative, cancer patients at increased risk of infection were encouraged to engage with an interactive website to complete an assessment of their infection risk. After completion, they were provided with specific strategies designed to help them reduce their risk.[30] Another initiative aimed at reducing infection was to send people home with a PaD (photo at discharge) of their wound, thus encouraging them to check their wound against the photo and report changes. The photo could also be shared with other healthcare professionals.[31]

Knowledge deficits are pervasive among the general public; even deficits related to simple activities such as the importance of hand hygiene have been reported. These can be overcome by forging a partnership between health providers and the patient where both parties agree on a sustainable, patient-centred infection prevention strategy. This approach is appropriate and achievable in all healthcare settings and the broader community.[32] Knighton draws on her research and has developed a framework that addresses some of the key issues. The framework is known under the acronym PAPERS (Practical Accessible Preventative Education that's Readable and Seeable). PAPERS addresses health literacy and self-management through empowerment. Information is provided in an easy reading format; visual representation of steps is provided; material is written at a reading age of someone equivalent to 8–11 years old; and the material is checked by people who are not healthcare professionals.[32] Innovative strategies such as these can be helpful in building sustainable patient education that enhances partnerships between healthcare professionals and patients, and empowers people to participate in their own care.

Conclusion

Throughout this chapter, the authors have introduced readers to the nuances of IPC in the home and in community health settings. Key areas that have been addressed include the characteristics and contexts of home and community health settings in Australia; IPC in settings outside hospital; HAI risks specific to community health; risk assessments that are pertinent to the community environment; and strategies to manage the identified risks. Education and capacity building for healthcare professionals and for patients has also been explored.

Useful websites/resources

- Clinical Excellence Commission Infection prevention and control practice handbook. https://www.cec. health.nsw.gov.au
- Australian Commission on Safety and Quality in Health Care. https://www.safetyandquality.gov.au/

References

1. Australian Commission on Safety and Quality in Health Care. National Safety and Quality Health Service (NSQHS) Standards. 2nd ed. Sydney: ACSQHC, 2021.
2. Australian Commission on Safelty and Quality in Health Care. Standard 3, Preventing and controlling healthcare associated infections. Sydney: ACSQHC, 2021.
3. Felemban O, St John W, Shaban RZ. Infection prevention and control in home nursing: case study of four organisations in Australia. Brit J Community Nurs. 2015;20(9):451-457.
4. Kenneley I. Infection control and the home environment. Home Health Care Management Practice. 2010;22(3): 195-201.
5. Raymond L, Regional Wounds Victoria. Importance of preventative hand hygiene practices in community nursing-wound management. Aust Nurs Midwifery J. 2016;24(2):32.
6. Cattini P. Infection prevention in community settings. J Community Nurs. 2018;32(6).
7. Lindh M, Holmstrom I, Perseius K-I, Windahl J. Enhancing adherence to infection control in Swedish community care: factors of importance. Nurs Health Sci. 2016;18:275-282.
8. Swanson J, Jeanes A. Infection control in the community: a pragmatic approach. Brit J Community Nurs. 2011;16(6):282-288.
9. Wyeth J. Hand hygiene and the use of personal protective equipment. Br J Nurs. 2013;22(16):920-925.
10. Palmer SJ. Practising asepsis during dressing changes in community settings. Brit J Community Nurs. 2019;24(12):600-603.
11. Sax H. 'My five moments of hand hygeine': a user centred design approach to understand, train, monitor and report hand hygiene. J Hosp Infect. 2007;67:9-21.
12. World Health Organization. WHO guidelines on hand hygiene in health care. Geneva: WHO, 2009.
13. World Health Organization. Save lives clean your hands. Hand hygiene in outpatient and home-based care and long-term care facilities: a guide to the application of the WHO multimodal hand hygiene improvement strategy and the 'five moments for hand hygiene' approach. Geneva: WHO, 2012.

14. Jones J. Managing sepsis effectively with national early warning scores and screening tools. Brit J Community Nurs. 2017;22(6):278-281.
15. Australian Sepsis Network. Recognising sepsis 2020. Available from: https://www.australiansepsisnetwork.net.au/healthcare-providers/recognising-sepsis.
16. National Institute for Health and Care Excellence. Sepsis: recognition, diagnosis and early management 2016. [updated 2017]. Available from: https://www.nice.org.uk/guidance/ng51.
17. Australian Institute of Health and Welfare. Health expenditure Australia 2014-2015. Canberra: AIHW, 2016.
18. Clinical Excellence Commission. Infection prevention and control practice handbook. Sydney: CEC, 2020.
19. Moore M, Huber K. The inherent safety value of using a dedicated infection control practitioner for infection control risk assessments. Am J Infect Control. 2014;42(6, Supplement): S85.
20. Otter JA, Mookerjee S, Davies F, Bolt F, Dyakova E, Shersing Y, et al. Detecting carbapenemase-producing Enterobacterales (CPE): an evaluation of an enhanced CPE infection control and screening programme in acute care. J Antimicrob Chemother. 2020;75(9):2670-2676.
21. World Health Organization. Advanced infection prevention and control training. Geneva: WHO, 2018.
22. Nazarko L. Catheter-associated urinary tract infections in the community. Reprinted with permission from Independent Nurse: Nazarko L. Brit J Community Nurs. 2020;25(4): 188-92.
23. National Institute for Health and Care Excellence. Urinary tract infection (catheter associated): antimicrobial prescribing 2018. Available from: https://www.nice.org.uk/guidance/ng113.
24. Aziz AM. Winter and the key infection prevention and control practices. British Journal of Community Nursing. 2018;23(11): 530-3.
25. Australian Health Infrastructure Alliance. Australasian health facility guidelines. Sydney: Australian Health Infrastructure Alliance, 2016.

26. Fazel P, Geddes J, Kushel M. The health of homeless people in high-income countries: descriptive epidemiology, health consequences, and clinical and policy recommendations. Lancet. 2014;384:1529-40.

27. Arnaud A, Chosidow O, Detrez M. Prevalences of scabies and pediculosis corporis among homeless people in the Paris region: results from two randomized cross-sectional surveys. Brit J Dermatol. 2016;174(1):104-112.

28. Australian Commission on Safety and Quality in Health Care. Reprocessing of reuseable medical devices in health service organisations. Sydney: ACQSHC, 2020.

29. Randall S, Neubeck L. What's in a name? Concordance is better than adherence for promoting partnership and self-management of chronic disease. Australian J Primary Health. 2016;22(3):181-184.

30. Dunbar A, Tai E, Beauchesne Nielsen D, Shropshire S, Richardson LC. Preventing infections during cancer treatment: development of an interactive patient education website. Clin J Oncol Nurs. 2014;18(4):426-431.

31. Rochon M, Magboo R, Barlow C, Ibrahim S, Carruthers L, Pagett J, et al. Implementing enhanced patient education for surgical site infection prevention in cardiac surgery. Brit J Nurs. 2020;29(17):994-1002.

32. Knighton S. Amplifying infection prevention self-management among patients and people in the community. J Emerg Nurs. 2020;46(6):727-730.

CHAPTER 38

Infection prevention and control in radiology and diagnostic imaging practice settings

Dr JOCELYNE M BASSEAL[i]

Chapter highlights

- Medical imaging (ultrasound, x-ray, CT and MRI) is an essential diagnostic tool used in almost every setting within hospital radiology departments and private diagnostic imaging clinics
- Studies have shown there is a potential risk of transmission of infectious pathogens between patients and practitioners in a medical imaging setting
- Adequate training and education for medical imaging practitioners on basic infection prevention and control (IPC) principles, which is currently lacking, is vital to break the chain of infection

i Sydney Infectious Diseases Institute, Faculty of Medicine and Health, The University of Sydney, Sydney, NSW

Introduction

Medical imaging performed by specialist imaging practitioners in a hospital or private diagnostic imaging practice setting is an essential tool for the diagnosis and management of medical conditions. The field of medical imaging encompasses radiographers, radiologists, sonographers, sonologists, radiation technicians and all practitioners who are directly involved with the medical imaging of a patient. The most common imaging modalities include ultrasound, x-ray, computerised tomography (CT), magnetic resonance imaging (MRI) and interventional radiology. Medical imaging equipment is expensive, and training to operate equipment effectively for diagnostic purposes as well as training in cleaning and disinfection processes are crucial to ensure optimal clinical management and patient safety.

Hospital radiology departments are an integral component of a hospital system, servicing patients from wards as well as outpatients. Due to the high numbers of patients attending the radiology department, many of which may be postoperative or immunocompromised, IPC principles are critical for this setting. Waiting rooms for patients also pose an additional risk for infectious diseases to spread between patients and to staff. Depending on the imaging modality, practitioners may be in close contact with the patient for a prolonged period of time in small, often non-ventilated rooms and are often unaware of the infectious disease status of the patient prior to imaging.

A systematic review of healthcare-associated infectious organisms within radiology departments identified a high risk of pathogen transfer between patients, equipment and professionals, in particular via radiographic cassettes and ultrasound probes.[1] A study sampling medical imaging equipment (x-ray, ultrasound, CT and MRI) revealed high rates of bacterial contamination (85%) on the equipment, with almost half identified on x-ray machines.[2] These included coagulase-negative *staphylococci*, *Pseudomonas aeruginosa* and methicillin-resistant *Staphylococcus aureus* (MRSA). This is consistent with previous studies highlighting that the x-ray tube, control panels and imaging plates showed high rates of bacterial contamination.[3] Imaging consoles and workstations are often neglected in the cleaning process,[4] with several reports of bacterial colonisation, including faecal microorganisms, on ultrasound machine keyboards.[5] Along with cleaning and disinfection, it is well established that hand hygiene practices reduce the risk of infection transmission within a healthcare setting.[6] Staff working within radiology settings have been shown to act as vectors in transmitting pathogens.[7,8]

Barriers to hand hygiene compliance have been studied and a pragmatic risk-based approach for chest x-ray procedures suggested to improve compliance.[9]

For decades, medical imaging safety has been primarily focused on radiation protection, with radiographers and radiologists showing little interest in IPC.[10] A total of 44% of interventional radiologists participated in infection control training prior to initiating practice,[11] highlighting a significant need for improvement in in-service training. The lack of basic IPC knowledge and training for medical imaging practitioners has been well documented.[12] While several education-based articles have attempted to address this gap by providing IPC-specific guidance within a radiology setting,[13-16] there has been no evidence of mandatory IPC training implemented into the training curriculum of medical imaging practitioners in Australia. Upskilling will be crucial as new generation point-of-care devices enter the market allowing for rapid and critical imaging to be performed at the bedside, in the emergency department (ED) and the intensive care unit (ICU).

This chapter outlines healthcare-associated infections (HAIs) specific to each imaging modality (ultrasound, interventional radiology, x-ray and CT/MRI). Key components of cleaning and disinfection pertinent to the medical imaging equipment for each modality will be discussed, including specific challenges and potential solutions. Considerations for medical imaging during an outbreak will also be highlighted and key recommendations presented.

38.1 Ultrasound

Ultrasound is a safe diagnostic imaging tool that is used in almost every area of medicine, from obstetrics, gynaecology, cardiology, breast imaging, vascular, thyroid, small parts and more. It is also an invaluable guide for procedures such as aspiration of fluid, tissue biopsies and injections of joints, tendons and nerves. There have been several reports in the literature of patients who have acquired HAIs following an ultrasound examination. This includes the death of a patient who contracted hepatitis B following a transoesophageal (TOE) examination, whereby the ultrasound probe was not reprocessed effectively.[17] Outbreaks of infections following TOE ultrasound have also been attributed to the use of damaged probes which have prevented adequate reprocessing. A retrospective observational study of patients undergoing cardiac surgery revealed that 20% developed postoperative infection, with particularly high pneumonia incidence (13.8%) from periods where patients were examined using a damaged

TOE probe. During the study period, a beta–lactam resistant strain of *Klebsiella oxytoca* was found in respiratory samples of 22 patients after intraoperative use of a TOE probe; a total of 10 patients acquired *Pseudomonas aeruginosa* of which 3 developed a bloodstream infection and died of septic shock; and 2 patients developed endocarditis with *Enterococcus faecalis* of which one died. All 3 bacteria (*K. oxytoca*, *P. aeruginosa* and *E. faecalis*) were cultured from the damaged TOE probe that had undergone reprocessing.[18] As highlighted by the authors, while probe covers are recommended for TOE examinations, they are impractical, as ultrasound views of the heart are impaired and the covers are not robust enough to maintain integrity during lengthy surgery. This study concluded that if probe covers are not used, visual inspection of TOE probes for any signs of degradation or damage which can affect reprocessing is essential. Other outbreaks attributed to TOE probes include infections with *Enterobacter cloacae*,[19,20] *Escherichia coli*[21] and *Pseudomonas aeruginosa*.[22]

Contamination of ultrasound probes cannot be excluded by visual inspection alone. A study conducted in the EDs of 5 public hospitals in Australia found 61% tested positive for blood contamination and 48% for bacterial contamination. Ultrasound cords and probes had high blood contamination (88% and 57% respectively) and bacterial contamination (62% and 46% on ultrasound probes respectively).[23] Of these, only 51% of blood-contaminated samples were visibly stained. A multi-centre audit of 16 emergency departments in France indicated a compliance rate of 66% (n=85) on ultrasound disinfection practices.[24] In Australia and New Zealand, ultrasound equipment used within the emergency setting may be overlooked in these high-risk and fast-paced environments where equipment may not undergo cleaning and disinfection immediately following the examination (Fig 38.1).

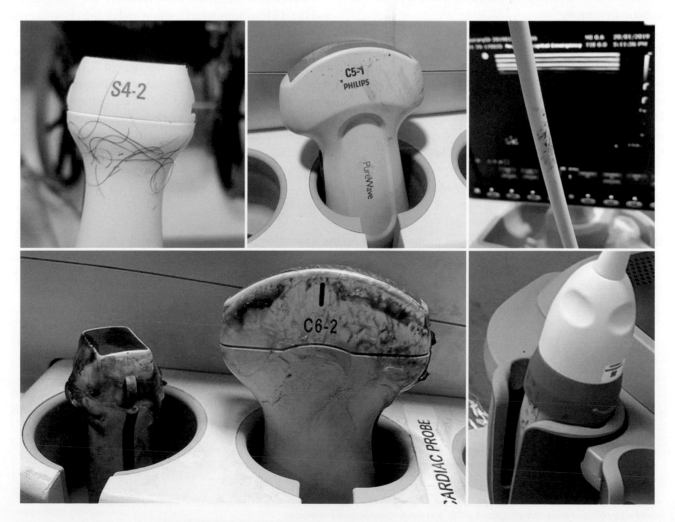

FIGURE 38.1 Contamination of ultrasound probes, cord and hub
Source: Images courtesy of Dr Vijay Manivel, Dr David Herbert and A/Prof Konstantin Yastrebov

Probes used for internal ultrasound present additional challenges, such as blood-borne viruses. The main risk for transvaginal ultrasound is transmission of human papillomavirus (HPV), the leading cause of invasive cervical cancer, as the virus persists on surfaces and can remain viable for long periods of time.[25,26] Early studies showed HPV contamination of transvaginal and transrectal ultrasound probes despite the use of probe covers.[27] This was confirmed by a prospective study sampling for HPV from transvaginal ultrasound probes highlighting a 3.5% contamination rate with HPV following low-level disinfection (LLD), despite the use of probe covers.[28] This was also consistent with another study detecting 7.5% of transvaginal probes positive for HPV DNA.[29] A retrospective cohort study in Scotland, using linked national data sets of patients undergoing transvaginal ultrasound showed that patients were 41% more likely to have positive bacterial cultures and 26% more likely to be prescribed antibiotics in the 30 days after ultrasound compared to the matched controls.[30]

Reprocessing of ultrasound probes is guided by the Spaulding Classification system for reusable medical devices. Within this system, ultrasound probes are reprocessed according to the risk of transmission of microorganisms associated with their use (Table 38.1). Ultrasound probes undergo different levels of disinfection which include:

- low-level disinfection (LLD): kills vegetative bacteria, some fungi and some viruses

- intermediate-level disinfection (ILD): kills vegetative bacteria, Mycobacteria, viruses and most fungi but not bacterial endospores
- high-level disinfection (HLD): kills all microorganisms with the exception of high numbers of bacterial endospores.

Cleaning is the first essential step before disinfection, as any residue, such as ultrasound gel, may bind and inactivate chemical disinfectants. Box 38.1 highlights the key steps for cleaning and disinfection of ultrasound probes. Due to the sensitive nature of ultrasound equipment, it is essential that cleaning and disinfection agents be intended for use on medical devices, and the manufacturer's instructions for use are followed. Care should be taken to follow the manufacturer's labelled conditions for the use of their specific products and directions for use are not interchangeable between formulations from either the same or different manufacturers.[31]

Ultrasound machine manufacturers are obliged to publish a list of approved cleaning and disinfection agents that are validated for use on ultrasound machines. These disinfection agents can vary from manual wipe or soak-based systems to automated chemical or light-based systems. This information is provided at the point of purchase and also available on the manufacturer's website. Any product used for cleaning and disinfection that has not been validated for use by the manufacturer may result in voiding of warranty. This presents a unique set of challenges which includes training, which is sometimes

TABLE 38.1 Disinfection of ultrasound probes based on the Spaulding Classification system

Classification	Definition	Level of disinfection	Use of probe cover	Examples
Non-critical	Ultrasound probes that come into contact with intact skin	Low-level or intermediate-level disinfection	Not required	Transabdominal probes, general external use ultrasound probes
Semi-critical#	Ultrasound probes that come into contact with non-intact skin and/or mucous membranes and have likely had contact with blood/body fluids	High-level disinfection	Single use probe cover	Transvaginal, transrectal, transoesophageal probes
Critical#	Ultrasound probes that are used in intraoperative procedures*	High-level disinfection or sterilisation (depending on ultrasound probe)	Sterile single use probe cover	All probes used in aseptic setting

*For all ultrasound-guided procedures (e.g. biopsies, drainages) skin must be disinfected and the probe used with sterile ultrasound gel. Note appropriate personal protective equipment (PPE) and waste management procedures.
#Probes used for semi-critical and critical examination that undergo high-level disinfection also require a record/log for traceability purposes.

BOX 38.1 How to clean and disinfect ultrasound probes

Step 1: Cleaning

1. Remove the ultrasound gel and clean the probe thoroughly using soft dry paper, a detergent-based wipe system or detergent cleaning solution. Ensure the operative head of the probe is cleaned while protecting the electrical part

2. If the ultrasound probe has grooves or crevices, it may be cleaned with a soft brush following manufacturer's instructions. Rinse under water and dry with a low-linting cloth

Step 2: Disinfection

1. After cleaning, follow manufacturer's instructions for use to disinfect the ultrasound probe. Levels of disinfection depend on the examination performed, i.e. low-level disinfection (LLD), intermediate-level disinfection (ILD) and high-level disinfection (HLD)

2. Disinfection options include manual systems (e.g. disinfectant instrument-grade wipes or liquid disinfectant solutions for soaking) or automated systems (e.g. chemical or light based automated systems)

3. Rinsing is an important step to remove any disinfectant residue or byproduct as per manufacturer's instructions for use

Step 3: Storage

1. After cleaning and disinfection, all ultrasound probes must be stored in an appropriate environment

2. Non-critical probes may be stored on the ultrasound machine mount

3. Semi-critical probes must be protected from environmental contamination and stored in a cupboard or container

4. Critical probes must be stored in sterile boxes

---

difficult in a fast-paced environment such as the ED with high turnover of residents and staff. Furthermore, cleaning ultrasound machines can be complex due to the heterogenous nature of the machine—consisting of mixed parts made from plastic, metal and glass, some of which are fixed and some that rotate. As only specific products may be used on particular parts of the machine, this is further complicated by the assortment of cleaning and disinfection products on the market. Although they are readily available in a healthcare setting, the use of alcohol-based disinfectants, including 70% isopropyl alcohol, is not recommended for the disinfection of probes due to the potential of drying out and destruction of probes.[32] The use of liquid sprays to clean ultrasound machines is not recommended as the liquid can permeate through the grooves and short-circuit the machine.[33]

As with every cleaning and disinfection process, there may be areas of potential IPC breaches. Manual processes rely on the practitioners' ability to follow each cleaning and disinfection step according to the product manufacturer's instructions, paying close attention to contact time required for disinfection. Newer automated technology, such as UV light and chemical-based automation, relies heavily on the effectiveness of pre-cleaning to ensure proper disinfection. Validation processes for automated systems are also crucial to ensure that disinfection cycles have been complete and effective. Any breaches of the manufacturer's instructions will result in negation of proper disinfection. Therefore, the IPC professional plays an essential role in working closely with practitioners and machine manufacturers to ensure all standard operating procedures are aligned and there is adequate training on cleaning and disinfection processes specific to the product used within the department.

As outlined in examples above with TOE, damaged probes may also pose a risk of infection transmission as blood and bodily fluid can enter through degraded probe case seams (Fig 38.2 a–b) which make the device difficult to clean and disinfect (Fig 38.2 c–d).

Apart from the ultrasound probe, the entire ultrasound machine—such as the console, machine handle, keyboard, cords and touchscreen monitor—also requires cleaning. Several studies have reported the presence of microorganisms on the ultrasound machine keyboard, cord and console handles,[5] indicating that these are often neglected in the cleaning process. While ultrasound machine manufacturers stipulate the specific products required for cleaning keyboard, cords and touchscreen monitors, it is essential that cleaning is followed routinely by the practitioners in their daily

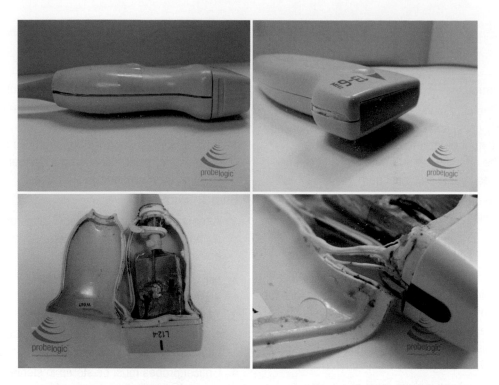

FIGURE 38.2 Damaged ultrasound probes are a risk of infection transmission
Source: Images courtesy of ProbeLogic Pty Ltd

practice. Environmental cleaning and disinfection should also include the patient bed and high-touch areas of the examination room, such as the door handles and light switches. Linen and waste management is also an important consideration as some examinations may involve blood, body fluid and mucous membranes.

Ultrasound gel is an essential requirement for every examination and this is stored in large bottles, single use bottles or as individual gel sachets (Box 38.2). Usage is dependent on the type of ultrasound examination—sterile ultrasound gel is recommended for any procedure where there is broken skin and risk of infection,

---

BOX 38.2 How to use and store ultrasound gel

Current recommendations

- Avoid 'topping up' or refilling single use ultrasound gel bottles as this poses a higher risk of contamination
- Once opened, gel bottles should be labelled with the opening date
- Store gel bottles at room temperature
- If gel warmers are used for patient comfort, only gel bottles for immediate use should be warmed. Use dry gel warmers rather than water baths and ensure these are also cleaned regularly according to the manufacturer's instructions
- Avoid heating and reheating gel bottles due to the risk of multiplication of microorganisms

- Do not leave the lid open on gel bottles when in use
- Avoid storing gel bottles upside down in warmers or in the gel holder as the dispensing tip may become contaminated
- When dispensing, care should be taken to avoid contact of the dispensing tip to the patient, the ultrasound probe or any other potential source of contamination
- Sterile gel is required for all interventional procedures and when scanning broken skin or wounds
- When using sterile ultrasound gel sachets, a new sachet should be opened for every patient

and non-sterile gel is used for all other examinations. Contaminated ultrasound gel has been responsible for a number of infectious disease outbreaks. In 2017, across four hospitals in Australia, an outbreak of *Burkholderia cenocepacia* bacteraemia in 11 patients occurred following central line insertion and was attributed to contaminated ultrasound gel.[34] Other organisms identified in ultrasound gel that have caused outbreaks and patient infections include *Pseudomonas aeruginosa*,[35] *Mycobacterium massiliense*,[36] *Burkholderia cepacia*[37,38] and *Acinetobacter baumannii*.[39] The practice of refilling ultrasound gel bottles and heating bottles, which allows for bacterial growth, has been discouraged.

Ultrasound probe covers are an essential component of any examination involving blood, body fluid or mucous membranes (Box 38.3). As ultrasound probes contain grooves and crevices, probe covers are integral to reduce further soiling of the probe leading to more effective reprocessing post-examination. The use of probe covers does not negate the requirement for cleaning and disinfection of the ultrasound probe which should be performed as soon as the procedure is completed. There has been varied usage in the type and quality of probe covers for internal and interventional ultrasound examinations. Items that are not approved for use on medical devices pose a risk of infection transmission as these have not been tested nor validated for use. Examples include the use of clingwrap/film, adhesive wound care dressings, plastic/food freezer bag and disposable hand gloves as substitute probe covers. Furthermore, the use of condoms as probe covers, although commonly used due to cost-effectiveness, is also questionable as there have been several reports of breakages.[10,12] A study on the integrity of probe covers and condoms post transvaginal ultrasound highlighted that commercial cover breakage rates were not as high as previously reported.[43] This study also illustrated micro-tears and perforations which were not visible to the practitioner after removal post ultrasound, highlighting that visible inspection of covers cannot be relied on. Hence all ultrasound probes used for internal examination must undergo cleaning and high-level disinfection.

38.1.1 Point-of-care ultrasound

Point-of-care ultrasound (POCUS) devices are widely used throughout the hospital setting and are essential for rapid real-time results to aid clinical diagnosis, as well as to guide interventions in anaesthesia and EDs. Other scenarios within an emergency setting for POCUS include trauma, chest pain, cardiac arrest, dyspnoea, pregnancy evaluation and abdominal pain. Compared to using a cart-based machine, POCUS has been useful for imaging infectious patients within an isolation room, whereby the smaller device can be cleaned and disinfected with ease post examination. More recently the technology has been used to monitor disease progression for COVID-19 (coronavirus disease 2019) patients within critical care settings (discussed below). With the increasing use of POCUS across a variety of settings, from emergency to critical care, and contact of the probe with multiple patients, proper IPC measures are vital to ensure these devices are not vectors in the spread of infection.

Depending on the ultrasound examination, POCUS devices are reprocessed according to the Spaulding Classification (Table 38.1). Reported challenges of reprocessing ultrasound probes within an ED include the lack of appropriate high-level disinfection options for probes, the time and resources for reprocessing, high staff turnover and lack of training on how to reprocess devices.[44]

Given the rapid advancement in ultrasound technology and the development of smaller and more efficient POCUS devices, incorporating appropriate IPC measures is critical to ensure patient safety in all healthcare settings. As new disinfection technology also enters the market at a rapid pace, new products and cost-effectiveness need to be reviewed on a regular basis.

BOX 38.3 How to use ultrasound probe covers

Current recommendations

- Ultrasound probe covers should be single use only
- Probe covers are required for all ultrasound examinations where the probe is in contact with non-intact skin, mucous membranes or blood/body fluids
- Sterile probe covers must be used for any interventional examinations
- If the patient is sensitive to latex, ensure non-latex alternatives are available for use
- The probe cover should completely cover the operative end of the probe. Ensure there is no over-stretching to minimise the risk of possible rupture of the cover
- After the examination, care must be taken to remove the probe cover with a gloved hand and discard into clinical waste

38.2 Interventional radiology

Interventional radiology (IR) is a minimally invasive image guided technique that is used for basic diagnostic or therapeutic purposes. This modern area of medicine has several advantages over traditional open surgery procedures including lower rates of morbidity, fast recovery time and cost-effectiveness. However, IR may be considered 'high risk' for the transmission of an HAI and prophylactic antibiotics are often prescribed following high-risk procedures.[45,46] Infection rates vary according to the type of interventional radiology procedure.[47] A study of interventional procedures during a 3-year period showed that overall mortality rate was 0.3% (1/336) with one patient developing a liver abscess and sepsis, treated with ultrasound-guided aspiration and antibiotics.[48] Percutaneous gastrostomies performed using fluoroscopy via radiology highlighted increased risk of local infection and complications compared to an endoscopic procedure.[49] A retrospective analysis of 4800 patients with access site complications after coronary or peripheral angiography identified 45 complications of which the infection rate was 9% (n=4/45).[50]

Reports of infections from interventional ultrasound procedures are limited and suggest incidence is low. A retrospective analysis of 13,534 interventions during a 12-month period revealed a total of 14 infections (0.1%)[51] and another study reporting 4 reported cases of *P. aeruginosa* infections following ultrasound-guided transrectal biopsies attributed to a contaminated needle guide.[52] While a majority of these ultrasound-guided procedures use surface ultrasound probes, there are some cases where an internal probe is required and these need to be reprocessed between patients as per the manufacturer's instructions for use. The use of probe covers for ultrasound-guided procedures has been inconsistent and widely debated, and usage varies according to the type of procedure in different clinical settings. Recommendations include the use of adhesive wound cover dressings as a makeshift barrier for peripheral venous access in EDs,[44] while high-level disinfection with a sterile probe cover is recommended in the critical care setting.[53] Variable and poor IPC practices may result in transmission of infection if ultrasound probes are not covered and do not undergo proper cleaning and disinfection.

Interventional radiology procedures should be carried out in a fit-for-purpose setting to ensure the prevention of surgical site infections (SSIs) and that all infection transmission risks are minimised. In addition, practitioners need to adhere to aseptic practices, wear appropriate PPE, ensure proper hand hygiene and follow cleaning and disinfection procedures that are in line with local guidance for high-risk settings. It is imperative that the patient's skin is disinfected, and any hair at the site is removed prior to the procedure. All interventional radiology procedures must adopt stringent IPC principles in order to prevent the spread of HAIs.

38.2.1 X-ray

X-ray technology has vastly improved over the past decade with the development of faster technology and smaller portable units. Machines consist of several components which include:

- an operating console
- the x-ray cassette
- the x-ray generator and detector
- supporting devices such as a Bucky stand and positioning blocks/devices; and
- other safety devices such as lead aprons.

Patients undergoing an x-ray examination may also require an examination bed with linen, pillows and towels. Portable x-ray units are useful for bedside imaging as well as for the examination of patients who are situated in isolation rooms.

In terms of risk of transmission of infection, traditional x-ray examination does not involve patient blood, body fluids or mucous membranes, and is classified as non-critical. The exception is dental radiology whereby devices are placed inside a patient's mouth and contaminated with blood or saliva. Adherence to cleaning and disinfection, waste management, hand hygiene and appropriate PPE is essential, and described in more detail in Chapter 34.

Within the x-ray examination room, contact with multiple patients from multiple settings poses a risk of transmission of infectious agents from patient to patient. Machine manufacturers provide a comprehensive guide to cleaning and disinfection products that are suitable for each aspect of the x-ray machine and its parts. As this will vary depending on the brand and type of machine, it is essential for the practitioner to adhere to the manufacturer's instructions for cleaning and disinfection.

38.2.2 Computed technology (CT) and magnetic resonance imaging (MRI)

CT and MRI technology has expanded rapidly, along with improved mobile access via smaller machines.

BOX 38.4 X-ray and CT/MRI considerations

After a patient leaves the imaging room

- Change linen/pillowcase on bed (if applicable) and/or clean the bed. Ensure towels are not reused and are laundered as per facility guidelines
- Clean all equipment that had contact with the patient including:
  - for x-ray: x-ray cassette, lead/blocking aprons, bucky stand and any positioning devices
  - for CT/MRI: supporting/positioning devices, gantry and headphones
- Ensure the console undergoes cleaning at the end of the day, including the keyboard, mouse, cords and touchscreens
- Check proper waste management procedures for infectious waste
- For interventional procedures, ensure safe injection practices and aseptic technique

---

Machines consist of several parts, some of which are in contact with the patient and require cleaning and disinfection. These include the gantry and patient bed as well as any supportive positioning devices and headphones. Products used for cleaning and disinfection of these machines must be approved by the machine manufacturer.

Interventional procedures commonly use CT and MRI machines (discussed above under Interventional radiology) and hence these require additional IPC measures. Furthermore, aseptic technique and safe injection practices must be adhered to, along with appropriate waste management. For a detailed explanation of standard precautions refer to Chapter 13.

Aspects to consider for cleaning and disinfection after a routine x-ray, CT and MRI examination are highlighted in Box 38.4.

38.3 Medical imaging during an outbreak

Classified as an essential service, medical imaging is a vital tool during an outbreak. Strict adherence to IPC measures while balancing productivity and workflow with patient safety and staff health are all critical within an already overwhelmed radiology department.

Medical imaging during infectious disease outbreaks involves strict adherence to standard precautions (SPs) and transmission-based precautions (TBPs) as these will vary depending on the nature of the infectious agent. There have been many lessons learnt from medical imaging during outbreaks caused by Ebola virus disease (EVD), severe acute respiratory syndrome (SARS) and more recently from the COVID-19 (coronavirus disease 2019) pandemic.

During EVD, x-ray and ultrasound technology was used as a supportive tool to assess the complications of the infection and as a result several radiology guidelines were published to assist practitioners with IPC.[54,55] Due to the nature of EVD infection, an additional challenge for medical imaging equipment used during the outbreak was the unsealed gaps near moving parts, crevices and hinges that may conceal fluid, making disinfection complex. As such, portable medical imaging equipment wrapped in plastic, as well as supporting devices in fluid-impermeable coverings, were adopted for EVD.[55] These are important aspects for imaging devices when considering contact and droplet precautions.

Respiratory outbreaks pose other challenges such as adequate ventilation for medical imaging suites especially during aerosol-generating procedures (AGPs). Situating dedicated imaging facilities outside the main radiology department was a key lesson from SARS, along with segregation of patients with suspected infection from others to reduce the risk of cross-infection.[56-58]

Noting the importance of medical imaging for COVID-19, the World Health Organization (WHO) published a Rapid Advice Guide that was endorsed by radiological and medical imaging organisations globally.[59] This guide outlined IPC precautions for medical imaging during COVID-19 and covered aspects pertinent to each modality (ultrasound, x-ray and CT). Other medical imaging and radiology organisations also released IPC-specific guidance for COVID-19.[60-62] These guidelines were critical for practitioners who were in close contact with potentially infectious patients, especially during periods of high community transmission.

Despite the plethora of COVID-19 guidance, a cluster of infections from a CT imaging suite in the Qingdao province in China highlighted the importance of vigorous disinfection of medical imaging equipment used on infectious patients.[63] This was the first reported outbreak linking COVID-19 to a CT imaging suite. The time taken to allow for cleaning, disinfecting and adequate air exchange in the CT rooms following chest scans on COVID-19 patients affects workflow within the radiology department. Novel solutions to reduce contamination and facilitate containment include a disposable isolation bag device for use in CT.[64] Medical imaging practitioners play a crucial role in triaging, diagnosing and monitoring patients during COVID-19, and with the significant increase in the number of imaging studies, a mass casualty plan for a hospital radiology department is also crucial.[65] Along with a hospital mass casualty plan which includes radiology departments and mobilisation of resources, specific focus areas for medical imaging departments (outlined in Table 38.2) will assist with planning and preparing for an outbreak.

TABLE 38.2 Focus areas for medical imaging during an outbreak

Focus area	Recommendation
Patient flow	• Ensure a specific route for patient flow to the radiology/imaging department. If patients require transportation from wards to the department, ensure the route is the most direct with minimal exposure to the public
Scheduling patients	• Schedule confirmed infectious patients at the end of the clinic day to allow for extended disinfection • Extend appointment times between imaging scans to allow for cleaning and disinfection • Cancel all non-urgent scans if possible (explore if the imaging examination will change patient management ensuring this does not affect patient management, but do not compromise patient health)
Waiting rooms	• Reduce patients in the waiting room by confirming appointments so there are limited numbers in the room • Ensure appropriate physical distancing, hand hygiene (e.g. alcohol-based hand rub) and masks for patients • Provide visual signage with reminders for respiratory etiquette and hand hygiene
Accompanying people/trainees/students	• Limit accompanying people unless urgent (e.g. paediatric examination, support for elderly) • Use virtual training options for trainees and students
Dedicated imaging room/equipment	• A dedicated room for infectious patients is recommended along with dedicated portable machines to reduce cross-contamination with low-risk patients • Rooms should be decluttered with all non-essential items removed (e.g. extra paperwork, stationery, unused ultrasound probes) • Ensure the imaging room is prepared before the patient arrives with all equipment clean, patient bed prepared and items ready (e.g. gloves, ultrasound probe covers, single use gel sachets)
Contact and non-contact technician/practitioner	• Use a two-person approach for x-ray and CT/MRI whereby one is dedicated to the patient and has direct contact for positioning for scans; the other has no contact with patients and is operating the console for image acquisition
Cleaning and disinfection	• Rigorous measures should be undertaken to clean and disinfect all medical imaging equipment, noting that only approved products should be used
Ventilation	• For respiratory outbreaks, ensure adequate ventilation and time for air exchange following an aerosol-generating procedure
Staff	• Ensure all staff undergo updated IPC training in line with the outbreak. This should include non-clinical staff (e.g. reception area, cleaning staff) and clinical practitioners who are in contact with patients • Monitor staff health daily for signs of infection as well as their mental health and physical wellbeing • Limit all staff interaction including multidisciplinary meetings for discussion of patient results and use video conferencing alternatives • Limit staff numbers in common rooms (e.g. break rooms, lunchrooms)
Communication	• Ensure updated and clear communication to all staff regarding the outbreak (cases in community) and changes to any practices within the imaging department (e.g. mask use). Communicate and confirm required changes to patients via email or telephone if necessary • Provide virtual and online opportunities for staff to liaise with management on any concerns regarding IPC practices or mental health and physical wellbeing

Prior to the COVID-19 pandemic, occupational stress among Australian medical imaging practitioners was well documented.[66] Increased use of chest CT during the COVID-19 pandemic and resulting changes in work practices amplified the anxiety of Australian radiographers and radiation therapists, and this was mainly attributed to shortages of PPE and increased workplace stress.[67] While IPC requirements had contributed to the increased length of time and complexity of procedures, particularly with immuno-compromised patients undergoing radiation therapy, respondents were confident in their understanding of IPC principles during the pandemic (61.9%; n=117/189). This study highlighted the importance of the workplace to mitigate work-related stress during an outbreak by ensuring adequate supplies of PPE and providing psychosocial support to patient-facing medical imaging practitioners. Another Australian study of five public medical imaging departments' insights into the COVID-19 pandemic outlined four pertinent themes: IPC, resources, communication and change management.[68] The study challenged medical imaging departments to rethink and redesign workflows, leveraging lessons learned from COVID-19 to prepare for future events.

38.4 Discussion

Several survey-based studies have highlighted the gap in knowledge of basic IPC in radiology and medical imaging departments, and this can have a dramatic impact on the transmission of HAIs. An Australian survey on IPC practices by ultrasound practitioners (n=395; 60% respondents working in private practice) highlighted the need for updated guidelines and education.[69] The study indicated that practitioners were using non-approved agents (such as Milton's solution) for disinfection of ultrasound probes used for internal ultrasound (16%; n=44 of 270 respondents) and when the probe comes into contact with blood over 13% (n=50 of 361 respondents) do not use an approved high-level disinfectant every time. On-site training of practitioners was also lacking whereby 52% of respondents do not receive training from the machine manufacturer on how to clean probes and 29% of respondents do not receive any training from the product manufacturer on how to use the cleaning product. This is consistent with another international study showcasing a mean knowledge score of 66% (n=100) of radiographer knowledge of IPC.[70] A survey of IPC professionals (n=358) from health facilities in the United States highlighted a high degree of non-compliance between reported practices and recommendations from local ultrasound guidelines.[71] In this study 20% of IPC professionals reported they were aware of instances where the ultrasound probe was used and not correctly reprocessed. Reprocessing failures were attributed to non-compliance with manufacturer's instructions for use; reprocessing was not documented; and storage and transport issues.

There has been increasing evidence that IPC training and education designed specifically for medical imaging practitioners has been overlooked over the past few decades and this has contributed to the gap in knowledge of IPC practices. Poor practices may also be attributed to the complexity of reprocessing reusable medical devices combined with the abundance and variety of cleaning and disinfection agents on the market. On-site training that is contextualised to the workplace (both in public hospitals and private practice settings) may be useful for practitioners to ensure compliance with IPC measures. Champions to drive change within the medical imaging department and provide peer-to-peer support for IPC practices will be valuable. In addition, leadership and management have an important role to play in providing opportunities for continuous professional education and psychosocial support. Surveillance of HAIs, hand hygiene compliance, and audit tools designed specifically for medical imaging departments and diagnostic imaging practices will be essential to mitigate risks and prevent outbreaks. Furthermore, stronger IPC practices, particularly for interventional radiology, resulting in fewer prescriptions of prophylactic antibiotics, may have a profound effect on antimicrobial resistance.

Conclusion

Medical imaging technology is rapidly evolving, with the use of artificial intelligence for accuracy and easing the increasingly heavy workloads of practitioners. The development of smaller and faster point-of-care diagnostic imaging devices designed for mobile phones and tablets has allowed for urgent and critical diagnosis in emergency settings. While the future in medical imaging technology is exciting and dynamic, adherence to IPC principles in medical imaging is more important than ever. The ongoing collaborative efforts of the IPC professional, medical imaging practitioners, leadership and management are vital to reduce the risk of transmission of an HAI from a medical imaging examination.

Useful websites/resources

- The Royal Australian and New Zealand College of Radiologists. Standards of Practice for Clinical Radiology. https://www.ranzcr.com/
- Australasian Society for Ultrasound Medicine. https://www.asum.com.au/
- Australasian Society for Ultrasound Medicine and Australasian College for Infection Prevention and Control. Guidelines for Reprocessing Ultrasound Transducers. https://www.asum.com.au/standards-of-practice-new/safety/
- International Society for Infectious Diseases. Guide to Infection Control in Healthcare Setting - Infection Prevention and Control in the Radiology Department/Service. https://isid.org/guide/hospital/infection-prevention-and-control-in-the-radiology-department-service/

References

1. Picton-Barnes D, Pillay M, Lyall D. A systematic review of healthcare-associated infectious organisms in medical radiation science departments. Healthcare (Basel, Switzerland). 2020; 8(2):80.
2. Getu B. Bacterial contamination of radiological equipment and factors affecting disinfection among radiology health professionals Addis Ababa, Ethiopia. Int J Microbiol Res. 2020;11(1):48-57.
3. Giacometti M, Gualano MR, Bert F, Minniti D, Bistrot F, Grosso M, et al. Microbiological contamination of radiological equipment. Acta Radiologica (Stockholm, Sweden: 1987). 2014;55(9):1099-103.
4. Zhang E, Burbridge B. Methicillin-resistant Staphylococcus aureus: implications for the radiology department. AJR Am J Roentgenol. 2011;197(5):1155-1159.
5. Westerway SC, Basseal JM, Brockway A, Hyett JA, Carter DA. Potential infection control risks associated with ultrasound equipment - a bacterial perspective. Ultrasound Med Biol. 2017;43(2):421-426.
6. Allegranzi B, Pittet D. Role of hand hygiene in healthcare-associated infection prevention. J Hosp Infect. 2009;73(4):305-315.
7. Lin YC, Dong SL, Yeh YH, Wu YS, Lan GY, Liu CM, et al. Emergency management and infection control in a radiology department during an outbreak of severe acute respiratory syndrome. Br J Radiol. 2005;78(931):606-611.
8. Nihonyanagi S, Hirata Y, Akabosi T, Uchiyama Y, Yamaura N, Sunakawa K, et al. [Nosocomial infection by multidrug-resistant Pseudomonas Aeruginosa (MDRP) presumably spread by a radiation technician]. Kansenshogaku Zasshi. 2006;80(2):97-102.
9. Jeanes A, Henderson F, Drey N, Gould D. Hand hygiene expectations in radiography: a critical evaluation of the opportunities for and barriers to compliance. J Infect Prevent. 2019;20(3):122-131.
10. Üstünsöz B. Hospital infections in radiology clinics. Diagnostic and interventional radiology (Ankara, Turkey). 2005;11(1):5-9.
11. Reddy P, Liebovitz D, Chrisman H, Nemcek AA, Jr., Noskin GA. Infection control practices among interventional radiologists: results of an online survey. Journal of Vascular and Interventional Radiology: JVIR. 2009;20(8):1070-4.e5.
12. Westerway SC, Basseal JM, Abramowicz JS. Medical ultrasound disinfection and hygiene practices: WFUMB global survey results. Ultrasound Med Biol. 2019;45(2):344-352.
13. Mirza SK, Tragon TR, Fukui MB, Hartman MS, Hartman AL. Microbiology for radiologists: how to minimize infection transmission in the radiology department.

Radiographics: A Review Publication of the Radiological Society of North America, Inc. 2015;35(4):1231-1244.
14. Nyirenda D, Ten Ham-Baloyi W, Williams R, Venter D. Knowledge and practices of radiographers regarding infection control in radiology departments in Malawi. Radiography (Lond). 2018;24(3):e56-e60.
15. Stogiannos N, Fotopoulos D, Woznitza N, Malamateniou C. COVID-19 in the radiology department: what radiographers need to know. Radiography (Lond). 2020;26(3):254-263.
16. Martini C, Nicolò M, Tombolesi A, Negri J, Brazzo O, Di Feo D, et al. Phase 3 of COVID-19: treat your patients and care for your radiographers. A designed projection for an aware and innovative radiology department. J Med Imaging Radiat Sci. 2020;51(4):531-534.
17. (UK) MaHPRA. Medical device alert: reusable transoesophageal echocardiography, transvaginal and transrectal ultrasound probes (transducers) (MDA/2012/037). United Kingdom Government, 2012.
18. Vesteinsdottir E, Helgason KO, Sverrisson KO, Gudlaugsson O, Karason S. Infections and outcomes after cardiac surgery - the impact of outbreaks traced to transesophageal echocardiography probes. Acta Anaesthesiologica Scandinavica. 2019;63(7):871-878.
19. Kanemitsu K, Endo S, Oda K, Saito K, Kunishima H, Hatta M, et al. An increased incidence of Enterobacter cloacae in a cardiovascular ward. J Hosp Infect.2007;66(2):130-134.
20. Noël A, Vastrade C, Dupont S, de Barsy M, Huang TD, Van Maerken T, et al. Nosocomial outbreak of extended-spectrum β-lactamase-producing Enterobacter cloacae among cardiothoracic surgical patients: causes and consequences. J Hosp Infect. 2019;102(1):54-60.
21. Bancroft EA, English L, Terashita D, Yasuda L. Outbreak of Escherichia coli infections associated with a contaminated transesophageal echocardiography probe. Infect Control Hosp Epidemiol. 2013;34(10):1121-1123.
22. Seki M, Machida H, Yamagishi Y, Yoshida H, Tomono K. Nosocomial outbreak of multidrug-resistant Pseudomonas aeruginosa caused by damaged transesophageal echocardiogram probe used in cardiovascular surgical operations. J Infect Chemother. 2013;19(4):677-681.
23. Keys M, Sim BZ, Thom O, Tunbridge MJ, Barnett AG, Fraser JF. Efforts to Attenuate the Spread of Infection (EASI): a prospective, observational multicentre survey of ultrasound equipment in Australian emergency departments and intensive care units. Crit Care Resusc. 2015;17(1):43-46.

24. Andolfo A, Maatoug R, Peiffer-Smadja N, Fayolle C, Blanckaert K. Emergency ward ultrasound: clinical audit on disinfection practices during routine and sterile examinations. Antimicrobial Resist Infect Control. 2021;10(1):25.

25. Roden RB, Lowy DR, Schiller JT. Papillomavirus is resistant to desiccation. J Infect Dis. 1997;176(4):1076–1079.

26. Ding DC, Chang YC, Liu HW, Chu TY. Long-term persistence of human papillomavirus in environments. Gynecol Oncol. 2011;121(1):148-151.

27. Kac G, Podglajen I, Si-Mohamed A, Rodi A, Grataloup C, Meyer G. Evaluation of ultraviolet C for disinfection of endocavitary ultrasound transducers persistently contaminated despite probe covers. Infect Control Hosp Epidemiol. 2010;31(2):165-170.

28. Casalegno JS, Le Bail Carval K, Eibach D, Valdeyron ML, Lamblin G, Jacquemoud H, et al. High risk HPV contamination of endocavity vaginal ultrasound probes: an underestimated route of nosocomial infection? PloS One. 2012;7(10):e48137.

29. Ma ST, Yeung AC, Chan PK, Graham CA. Transvaginal ultrasound probe contamination by the human papillomavirus in the emergency department. Emerg Med J. 2013;30(6):472-475.

30. Scotland HP. NHSScotland risk based recommendations for the decontamination of semi-invasive ultrasound probes: risk of infection following semi-invasive ultrasound procedures in Scotland, 2010 to 2016. Public Health Scotland, 2017.

31. Australasian Society for Ultrasound in Medicine (ASUM). Guidelines for reprocessing ultrasound transducers. Australas J Ultrasound Med. 2017;20(1):30-40.

32. Koibuchi H, Fujii Y, Kotani K, Konno K, Matsunaga H, Miyamoto M, et al. Degradation of ultrasound probes caused by disinfection with alcohol. J Med Ultrason (2001). 2011;38(2):97-100.

33. Ding J, Fu H, Liu Y, Gao J, Li Z, Zhao X, et al. Prevention and control measures in radiology department for COVID-19. Eur Radiol. 2020;30(7):3603-3608.

34. Shaban RZ, Maloney S, Gerrard J, Collignon P, Macbeth D, Cruickshank M, et al. Outbreak of health care-associated Burkholderia cenocepacia bacteremia and infection attributed to contaminated sterile gel used for central line insertion under ultrasound guidance and other procedures. Am J Infect Control. 2017;45(9):954-958.

35. Chittick P, Russo V, Sims M, Robinson-Dunn B, Oleszkowicz S, Sawarynski K, et al. An outbreak of Pseudomonas aeruginosa respiratory tract infections associated with intrinsically contaminated ultrasound transmission gel. Infect Control Hosp Epidemiol. 2013;34(8):850-853.

36. Cheng A, Sheng WH, Huang YC, Sun HY, Tsai YT, Chen ML, et al. Prolonged postprocedural outbreak of Mycobacterium massiliense infections associated with ultrasound transmission gel. Clin Microbiol Infect. 2016;22(4):382.e1-.e11.

37. Abdelfattah R, Al-Jumaah S, Al-Qahtani A, Al-Thawadi S, Barron I, Al-Mofada S. Outbreak of Burkholderia cepacia bacteraemia in a tertiary care centre due to contaminated ultrasound probe gel. J Hosp Infect. 2018;98(3):289-94.

38. Viderman D, Khudaibergenova M, Kemaikin V, Zhumadilov A, Poddighe D. Outbreak of catheter-related Burkholderia cepacia sepsis acquired from contaminated ultrasonography gel: the importance of strengthening hospital infection control measures in low resourced settings. Le Infezioni in Medicina. 2020;28(4):551-557.

39. Yagnik KJ, Kalyatanda G, Cannella AP, Archibald LK. Outbreak of Acinetobacter baumannii associated with extrinsic contamination of ultrasound gel in a tertiary centre burn unit. Infect Prevent Pract. 2019;1(2):100009.

40. Storment JM, Monga M, Blanco JD. Ineffectiveness of latex condoms in preventing contamination of the transvaginal ultrasound transducer head. South Med J. 1997;90(2):206-208.

41. Milki AA, Fisch JD. Vaginal ultrasound probe cover leakage: implications for patient care. Fertil Steril. 1998;69(3):409-411.

42. Amis S, Ruddy M, Kibbler CC, Economides DL, MacLean AB. Assessment of condoms as probe covers for transvaginal sonography. J Clin Ultrasound. 2000;28(6):295-298.

43. Basseal JM, Westerway SC, Hyett JA. Analysis of the integrity of ultrasound probe covers used for transvaginal examinations. Infect Dis Health. 2020;25(2):77-81.

44. Shokoohi H, Armstrong P, Tansek R. Emergency department ultrasound probe infection control: challenges and solutions. Open Access Emerg Med. 2015;7:1-9.

45. Sutcliffe JA, Briggs JH, Little MW, McCarthy E, Wigham A, Bratby M, et al. Antibiotics in interventional radiology. Clin Radiol. 2015;70(3):223-234.

46. Venkatesan AM, Kundu S, Sacks D, Wallace MJ, Wojak JC, Rose SC, et al. Practice guidelines for adult antibiotic prophylaxis during vascular and interventional radiology procedures. Written by the Standards of Practice Committee for the Society of Interventional Radiology and endorsed by the Cardiovascular Interventional Radiological Society of Europe and Canadian Interventional Radiology Association [corrected]. J Vasc Interv Radiol. 2010;21(11):1611-1630; quiz 31.

47. Halpenny DF, Torreggiani WC. The infectious complications of interventional radiology based procedures in gastroenterology and hepatology. J Gastrointestin Liver Dis. 2011;20(1):71-75.

48. Giorgio A, Tarantino L, de Stefano G, Coppola C, Ferraioli G. Complications after percutaneous saline-enhanced radiofrequency ablation of liver tumors: 3-year experience with 336 patients at a single center. Am J Roentgenol. 2005;184(1):207-211.

49. Silas AM, Pearce LF, Lestina LS, Grove MR, Tosteson A, Manganiello WD, et al. Percutaneous radiologic gastrostomy versus percutaneous endoscopic gastrostomy: a comparison of indications, complications and outcomes in 370 patients. Eur J Radiol. 2005;56(1):84-90.

50. Meyerson SL, Feldman T, Desai TR, Leef J, Schwartz LB, McKinsey JF. Angiographic access site complications in the era of arterial closure devices. Vasc Endovascular Surg. 2002;36(2):137-144.

51. Cervini P, Hesley GK, Thompson RL, Sampathkumar P, Knudsen JM. Incidence of infectious complications after an ultrasound-guided intervention. Am J Roentgenol. 2010;195(4):846-50.

52. Gillespie JL, Arnold KE, Noble-Wang J, Jensen B, Arduino M, Hageman J, et al. Outbreak of Pseudomonas aeruginosa infections after transrectal ultrasound-guided prostate biopsy. Urology. 2007;69(5):912-914.

53. Costello C, Basseal JM, Yang Y, Anstey J, Yastrebov K. Prevention of pathogen transmission during ultrasound use in the intensive care unit: recommendations from the College of Intensive Care Medicine Ultrasound Special Interest Group (USIG). Australas J Ultrasound Med. 2020;23(2):103-110.

54. Bluemke DA, Meltzer CC. Ebola virus disease: radiology preparedness. Radiology. 2015;274(2):527-531.

55. Mollura DJ, Palmore TN, Folio LR, Bluemke DA. Radiology preparedness in ebola virus disease: guidelines and challenges for disinfection of medical imaging equipment for the protection of staff and patients. Radiology. 2015;275(2):538-544.

56. King AD, Ching AS, Chan PL, Cheng AY, Wong PK, Ho SS, et al. Severe acute respiratory syndrome: avoiding the spread of infection in a radiology department. Am J Roentgenol. 2003;181(1):25-27.

57. Gogna A, Tay KH, Tan BS. Severe acute respiratory syndrome: 11 years later—a radiology perspective. Am J Roentgenol. 2014;203(4):746-748.

58. Chen Q, Zu ZY, Jiang MD, Lu L, Lu GM, Zhang LJ. Infection control and management strategy for COVID-19 in the radiology department: focusing on experiences from China. Korean J Radiol. 2020;21(7):851-858.

59. World Health Organization. Use of chest imaging in COVID-19: a rapid advice guide 2020. Geneva: WHO, 2020. Available from: https://www.who.int/publications/i/item/use-of-chest-imaging-in-covid-19.

60. Abramowicz JS, Basseal JM. World Federation for Ultrasound in Medicine and Biology Position Statement: how to perform a safe ultrasound examination and clean equipment in the context of COVID-19. Ultrasound Med Biol. 2020;46(7):1821-1826.

61. Poon LC, Abramowicz JS, Dall'Asta A, Sande R, Ter Haar G, Marsal K, et al. ISUOG Safety Committee Position Statement on safe performance of obstetric and gynecological scans and equipment cleaning in context of COVID-19. Ultrasound Obstet Gynecol. 2020;55(5):709-712.

62. Basseal JM, Westerway SC, McAuley T. COVID-19: Infection prevention and control guidance for all ultrasound practitioners. Australas J Ultrasound Med. 2020;23(2):90-95.

63. Xing Y, Wong GWK, Ni W, Hu X, Xing Q. Rapid response to an outbreak in Qingdao, China. N Engl J Med. 2020;383(23): e129.

64. Amalou A, Turkbey B, Xu S, Turkbey E, An P, Carrafiello G, et al. Disposable isolation device to reduce COVID-19 contamination during CT scanning. Acad Radiol. 2020; 27(8):1119-1125.

65. Myers L, Balakrishnan S, Reddy S, Gholamrezanezhad A. Coronavirus outbreak: is radiology ready? Mass casualty incident planning. J Am Coll Radiol. 2020;17(6):724-729.

66. Singh N, Knight K, Wright C, Baird M, Akroyd D, Adams RD, et al. Occupational burnout among radiographers, sonographers and radiologists in Australia and New Zealand: findings from a national survey. J Med Imaging Radiat Oncol. 2017;61(3):304-310.

67. Shanahan MC, Akudjedu TN. Australian radiographers' and radiation therapists' experiences during the COVID-19 pandemic. J Med Radiat Sci. 2021;68(2):111-120.

68. Eastgate P, Neep MJ, Steffens T, Westerink A. COVID-19 Pandemic − considerations and challenges for the management of medical imaging departments in Queensland. J Med Radiat Sci. 2020;67(4):345-351.

69. Westerway SC, Basseal JM. Advancing infection control in Australasian medical ultrasound practice. Australas J Ultrasound Med. 2017;20(1):26-29.

70. Abdelrahman MA, Alhasan M, Alewaidat H, Rawashdeh MA, Al Mousa DS, Almhdawi KA. Knowledge of nosocomial infection control practices among radiographers in Jordan. Radiography (Lond). 2017;23(4):298-304.

71. Carrico RM, Furmanek S, English C. Ultrasound probe use and reprocessing: results from a national survey among U.S. infection preventionists. Am J Infect Control. 2018;46(8):913-920.

CHAPTER 39

Infection prevention and control in correctional health practice

CATHI MONTAGUE[i]

CHRISTINE FULLER[ii]

SYLVIA GANDOSSI[iii]

Chapter highlights

- Specific infection prevention and control (IPC) contexts and risks exist in the custodial population and environment, with implications for public health
- Individuals in custody retain their human rights to health, wellbeing and safety, yet are wholly reliant on the actions of others to support this
- Multiple stakeholders and responsible agencies are involved in the safety and care of individuals in custody. Clear communication, policy and command-and-control processes support the identification of, and response to, infection risks
- Effective IPC governance is essential to support knowledge, practice and preparedness across all custodial workforces
- Health education supports initiatives to reduce, recognise and respond to infection in the custodial environment, for both individuals in custody and associated workforces. This must incorporate appropriate literacy, language translations, cultural relevance and peer engagement
- Strong vaccination programs are a proven public health measure and reduce vaccine-preventable disease prevalence and disease-related severity for individuals in custody and the associated workforce
- IPC expertise in renovation, design and build teams in the custodial setting reduces infection-related risk and subsequent potential costs of facility remediation or infectious disease response

i   Drug and Alcohol Services South Australia, SA Health, Adelaide, SA
ii Correct Care Australasia, Melbourne, VIC
iii Microbiology, Western Diagnostic Pathology, Jandakot, WA

Introduction

Infection is 'a potentially preventable adverse event'.[1] Globally, custodial populations and environments have common and specific risks relating to health and IPC. Health, safety, security and costs are impacted by population burden of disease, crowding, the built environment, governance structures and operational practices.

A custodial setting is any facility where an individual is held securely with restricted freedoms, through government powers which obligate an associated duty of care. In Australia, this includes:

- police holding cells and watch-houses
- detention centres for youth (also referred to as juvenile justice)
- immigration detention
- forensic psychiatric facilities
- military detention and a sole military criminal correctional centre; and
- criminal correctional settings (including remand centres, prisons, prison work camps and courthouse cells).

The criminal custodial context is generically referred to as the 'correctional setting' and individuals held within the correctional setting are referred to as 'prisoners'. This chapter will more specifically address the correctional context; however, the implications and principles for IPC practice translate across the custodial spectrum.

Right to health

Care and service provision involving custodial populations evokes a range of personal, social and political attitudes.[2,3] Ill health in any population group has significant cost impacts on society. Individuals in all forms of custody retain their human rights to health and access to healthcare, despite their punishment of imprisonment with loss of freedom.[4-6] An individual's ability to access healthcare within the custodial setting is, however, wholly dependent on the actions and interventions of others who are responsible for their care.

39.1 Overview of custodial governance in Australia

Australian jurisdictional states and mainland territories hold individual responsibility for the provision of the majority of custodial services. The federal government holds powers and responsibilities for individuals in immigration detention, as well as legislative powers relating to custody in some external territories.[7,8] There is no federal prison, so federal prisoners are managed through state institutions by arrangement under the federal Constitution.[9,10]

Safe care and health of individuals in custody are inextricably intertwined together, yet jurisdictional legislations for health and custody either do not, or only minimally, reference healthcare for prisoners specifically.

Correctional and health agencies are generally separate, with individual responsibilities for fiscal and operational aspects of security/offender management and prisoner health. In the Victorian correctional system Justice Health operates as a business unit within the Department of Justice and Community Safety. Criminal custodial healthcare is broadly referred to as 'correctional health practice' or 'prison health'. Jurisdictional agencies for criminal custody and security have naming variants of corrective, corrections, custodial or correctional services. Service and purchasing models differ across each jurisdiction and may incorporate public, private and/or non-government sectors.

Australia has approximately 111 criminal justice correctional facilities in urban, peri-urban, regional and remote areas across Australia (excluding juvenile facilities, police and court cells and forensic mental health facilities).[11] Remanded and sentenced prisoners may be held in the same facility. Security classifications range from minimum, restricted minimum, medium, maximum or super-max and there may be a mix of security levels across any one correctional site.

39.1.1 Health standards and performance indicators in correctional health

Australia has no standard mandatory reportable performance indicators for health access or health status of prisoners, and no requirements, guidelines or measures demonstrating the shared responsibilities of correctional services and correctional health for the security and health of prisoners.

The Australian Productivity Commission measures Corrective Services performance indicators which do not include health access or health status measures.[12] National prisoner health data surveys are undertaken by the Australian Institute of Health and Welfare (AIHW); however, jurisdictional, prison and prisoner participation are voluntary.[13] Jurisdictional correctional health services have differing accreditation processes, measures of service delivery assessment and internal epidemiological data review.

Guiding Principles for Corrections in Australia are developed and co-signed by jurisdictional correctional services agencies (rather than as a joint correctional and health agreement) and reviewed intermittently by the Corrective Services Administrators Council.[14] Outcome 4: Health and Wellbeing outlines a series of measures including a broad brushstroke intent to 'protect public health'. The Guiding Principles for Corrections in Australia are not mandatory instructions, nor do they have the requirement for reportable performance standards or measures. They 'represent a national intent' (see page 4) by the correctional system, rather than by all key stakeholders delivering care and services to prisoners. Areas related to health and human rights within these guidelines have been identified for improvement in alignment to the United Nations Mandela Rules, including solitary confinement.[15]

Various bodies have created guidelines that address prisoner health, including the United Nations (UN), the World Health Organization (WHO), the Public Health Association of Australia (PHAA) and the Royal Australian College of General Practitioners (RACGP), among others.[2,5,6,16,17]

39.1.2 Access to federal or private health schemes for prisoners

Federal programs to support population health have significant exclusions or limitations for prisoners, whether they are remanded or sentenced, with implications for aspects of IPC.

Correctional health services and prisoners are not able to access Medicare due to the dichotomy of the federal funding model of Medicare and state responsibility for prisoners.[18] Very limited access to the Pharmaceutical Benefits Scheme (PBS) exists. PBS access has been made available to Schedule 100 (Highly specialised drugs) and only since 2016, Schedule 85 for Direct Acting Antivirals (DAA) to support hepatitis C treatment in prisoners.[19,20(p21),21] Previously, prison health services funded these treatments at full market price with a significant impact on health service budget costs. These funding complexities can add layers to health access navigation for prisoners and contribute to increased morbidity and mortality from a range of causes.[18,22–24]

Over the past decade, increasing clinical research, health advocacy and public health work to improve the health of Australia's prisoners has been undertaken by a variety of individuals and bodies with expertise in public health and prisoner health, with increasing improvements and awareness of prisoner health impacts and costs

to the wider community. The need to better support and utilise health engagement; public health screening together with prevention and management of transmissible disease; healthcare; and medication therapies is leading to increasing calls for prisoner access to specific Medicare and other PBS items.[19,25–29]

National Disability Insurance Scheme (NDIS) access (initially not available to prisoners) may now be possible where specific conditions are met, or responsibility for care support may lie with the justice system.[30] Department of Veterans, Affairs (DVA) healthcare access may be possible in specific conditions, for a small proportion of veteran prisoners.[31] Private healthcare use requires specific correctional services permissions. The prisoner is personally liable for non-covered cost components as well as transport and correctional officer escort costs.

39.2 The justice system custodial population in Australia

In 2021, nearly 43,000 prisoners (sentenced or remanded to custody awaiting trial) were in custody, around a 43% increase since 2013.[32,33] There was a temporary reduction in the numbers of prisoners in custody in 2020, attributed by the Australian Bureau of Statistics (ABS) to government restrictions and practice changes across all states and territories as a result of the COVID-19 pandemic which 'may have had an impact on the criminal activity and the justice system'.[32] This growth has impacted custodial and health service funding and service delivery.[34]

There is ongoing disproportionate representation of Aboriginal and Torres Strait Islander peoples in Australian prison populations across all jurisdictions.[32,35]

2021 ABS prisoner census data shows 30% of the Australian prison population identifies as being Aboriginal and/or Torres Strait Islander peoples. This disproportionate representation has significant implications for the planning and delivery of culturally safe and inclusive healthcare. Correctional services and correctional healthcare have a responsibility to 'close the gap' by addressing health inequity during imprisonment to improve health outcomes.[36,37,44–47,171]

The custodial population spans age ranges from juvenile to elderly or the end of life. Jurisdictions have individual policies and regulations on supporting ongoing maternal care during imprisonment and the co-boarding of babies, infants or young children. South Australia is the only state that does not currently permit this.[38] The care and wellbeing of neonates to young children in the correctional environment brings additional implications for safety, healthcare and IPC.

Cognitive impairment, disability, language barriers, low health literacy, cultural needs, comorbid disease, mental health and learning support requirements must also be considered in service planning and care delivery.

Annual numbers of prisoners reflect 'bed state' rather than prison churn or flow. Similar to a hospital health system, individuals requiring custody, care and services flow in, through and out of the system, often on multiple occasions. Understanding the local context of bed numbers, churn/flow and local population specifics is essential to IPC-related service planning and delivery.

39.3 Correctional context challenges

Correctional facilities share commonalities and risks with other settings where populations are held in close or crowded proximity.[39] Environmental and population risks can challenge innate immunity as well as the early identification and management of infection, infestation and transmissible disease.

39.3.1 Disease prevalence and healthcare

Populations in custody in Australia and globally have over-representation of burdens of disease compared to the general population, including higher rates of comorbidity, infectious and transmissible disease.[29,40–42] This includes morbidity and mortality related to general poor health, mental health conditions, substance use disorders, malnutrition, disability, trauma, cognitive impairment, risk-taking behaviours and ageing.

Aboriginal and Torres Strait Islander peoples have health risks and comorbidities at a younger age-equivalency compared to the general population.[43] Higher rates of incarceration compared to non-Indigenous populations add to health inequality.[44] Considerable challenges continue to exist in the provision of high-quality, culturally safe and responsive healthcare to Indigenous peoples. These challenges can be amplified in the custodial context. Awareness and incorporation of high-performing health system standards for Aboriginal and Torres Strait Islander peoples is essential.[45–54]

Imprisonment can offer significant opportunities to improve public health and reduce the burden of disease and prevalence of infection for all prisoners. Correctional healthcare should incorporate high-performing healthcare principles and be both proactive (through scheduled structured health reviews for screening, assessment and management) and reactive (in response to unanticipated individual or population health changes).

39.3.2 Health assessments in the correctional population

Admission to prison assessment is undertaken by correctional nurses and/or medical officers as close to the time of admission as possible. This includes:

- identification and management of immediate health risks
- identification of the presence of transmissible disease, and whether it is an active infection and/or infestation requiring immediate management or is life threatening
- health comorbidities
- consults and triage for medical and mental health review; and
- prisoner education on health risks in prison and how to access health services.

Focus should be maintained on the clinical safety of the individual throughout the health admission process.[55] Communication with correctional officers is essential to identify and manage immediate risks to the health and wellbeing of the individual prisoner and the wider prison population.

Proactive streaming into scheduled structured health reviews or clinical pathways for specific health needs can help ensure key screenings, assessments, education, treatment responses and continuation of care goals are met while also supporting healthcare work planning and performance, even with prisoner transfers between facilities. Annual general health reviews on their own are not demonstrated to be particularly helpful in populations already engaged with ongoing primary healthcare.[56] However, the correctional population has overall higher health risks and increased disruption or disengagement from consistent healthcare and assessment. In a vulnerable population group, even a small reduction in disease (including infection) prevalence or severity through proactive detection, management and education can be beneficial to the individual and overall health system.[57,58] Reactive healthcare is required for unanticipated or emerging illness, trauma or infectious disease.

Pre-release health planning is essential to support ongoing care and treatment for health conditions. A pre-release health appointment may not always be possible due to custodial or legal processes, or to the engagement of individual prisoners with the process.

Implications for practice

- All health assessments must include consideration for the presence of infection, transmissible disease or infestation, with screening, education, management and treatment as required.

- Initial admission to prison health assessment should occur as soon as practically possible after arrival into custody to support timely health risk assessment; prioritisation of emergent care; medication continuation; assessment for possible contagious disease and/or infestation; and triage of follow-up reviews for more comprehensive health assessment, screening and care. Pre-admission records and prisoner handover may provide essential health information, such as court documents, health letters, hospital transfer information, previous prison health records and custodial transport staff concerns. Induction information and education (verbal and literacy/language appropriate written formats) should include risks, prevention and management of transmissible disease in the custodial setting.

- Education, screening, intervention and care planning is undertaken in partnership with the individual in custody.

- Medication history includes items that the individual has been prescribed but may not be taking or has recently ceased, including transmissible disease-related medications e.g. direct acting antivirals for hepatitis. Continuation of medications and medication education must be supported wherever possible, including through to release from prison medication arrangements.

- Where health staff are not available across all hours, clearly defined processes must be in place for custodial staff to identify, assess and respond appropriately to immediate health and disease risks.

- Discharge/release care planning should commence soon after admission to prison, including the prioritisation and flagging of prisoners at increased risk or with complex needs who may require significant interventions to safely support discharge into ongoing community healthcare.

- Discharge health documentation that includes known follow-up appointments (including health investigations) in the community should be provided, and/or consent sought to communicate with post-release planned primary healthcare

providers.[59] Individuals with highly complex health and/or social needs and risks may require comprehensive care planning ahead of release, including involvement of different agencies to support ongoing care in the community.

39.3.3 Nutritional status and immunity

Malnutrition is seen in prisoners.[3,60] Links between poor nutrition and immunity, infection, disease, cognitive processing, aggression and impulsive behaviours, and increased morbidity and mortality from all causes are clear.[61–66] Individuals with severe malnutrition or underlying severe illness causing metabolic stress may be at risk of 'refeeding syndrome' with resumption of food and fluid intake, for example after admission to prison following a period of poor nutrition, or after hunger-strike.[67,68] Refeeding syndrome is associated with significant and rapid onset of potentially fatal electrolyte and fluid imbalances, and early risk recognition and management is essential.[67–69]

Access to healthy eating choices in prison can be limited, controlled by prison catering and additional purchasing access which may be skewed with high production volume/low nutritional quality meals, convenience and 'junk' foods. Dietary food access or 'special diets' (including diabetic diets or other nutritional support requirements) may require medical practitioner or correctional approval in some locations. Approval of dietary modification fits within the scope of nursing, dietician or speech pathology practice and should be supported unless a clear rationale otherwise exists. Delays in authorisation for appropriate nutrition for specific health conditions can occur while waiting for a clinic appointment, which may have adverse impacts on health including the ability to mount an effective immune response.

Glycaemic control is more challenging in the custodial environment. Variable glycaemic control negatively impacts on immunity and disease response.[70–73] Correctional operations take precedence in the prison system over best health practice with regard to timings of medication and food access. Independent access to non-injectable glycaemic agents, monitoring equipment or overnight food is also dependent on correctional services permissions. Prisoners generally are unable to hold their own insulin due to security risks.

Implications for practice

- Nutritional status assessment is an important component of healthcare in custodial populations, including to support immunity and infection response.[74–77] This should include assessment for malnutrition and deficiency screening where concerns exist. Education, treatment, management and monitoring plans should be developed and implemented for prisoners at risk, including communication and agreed responsibilities by both health and correctional services.[75,77,78] Validated and easy-to-use malnutrition screening tools are readily available.[79] Nutritional screening should be completed upon entry to inform comprehensive health/medical assessment triage urgency; support timely interventions as required; and repeated at intervals for ongoing assessment and monitoring.[67,68,74,77,79]

- Registered nurses can assess nutritional need and dietary modification requirements for prisoners, working with appropriate allied health expertise as required. Timely access to appropriate nutrition for specific health needs will support health and immunity.

- Access to glycaemic control medications at health-appropriate intervals (rather than at permitted correctional access intervals) can be difficult. Health and correctional agencies should have clear processes at site and service levels for communication of risk and responsibility to meet health needs and support safe custody.

39.3.4 Access to healthcare

On-site health services may operate for limited hours, with out-of-hours health support dependent on correctional services officers, medical phone consults or ambulance response.

Prisoners predominantly do not have freedom of movement within prisons to independently access healthcare services, attend appointments or administer their own medications, being dependent on security levels and operational requirements.

Operational and security precedence can cause health access delays. Situations may change rapidly, impacting the ability of the prisoner to attend the correctional health service and for health staff to access prisoners. This is outside of the control of health staff who are required to fit clinics and medication administration in around security priorities, prison regime times and prisoner movements. Correctional services officers are generally required to provide permissions and unlock barriers or cells for all prisoner or staff movements, including in a correctional inpatient setting. Medical emergency response delays can occur waiting for a correctional officer with the relevant authority or keys to provide access for health staff.[80]

Implications for practice

- Correctional healthcare staff require a great deal of flexibility, innovation, rescheduling and communication to negotiate healthcare service provision daily.

- Healthcare delays can have detrimental impacts on the physical and mental health and safety of the individual prisoner, the broader prisoner population as well as for correctional and health staff.

- Communication pathways should be clearly defined for both health and corrections operational staff and line managers to assess and manage risk related to access to health delays. Clear reporting of actual or near-miss adverse incidences should occur and be escalated as required in a timely manner.

- Shared custodial and health processes that assess risk and support access to specific own medications ('in-possession' medications) for administration can reduce dependence on health medication rounds, promote independence and self-management of health, and support optimal physiological responses to treatment, especially for time-critical medications.[81–83]

39.3.5 Telehealth

Prisoners refuse external health appointments for a variety of reasons, including lengthy journey times (even in a metropolitan context); disruption to accommodation and prison employment; and conflicts with other correctional or legal appointments. Off-site secure escorts for health appointments as well as in-reach specialist health providers can be impacted by security, access delays, length of time required and cost considerations.

Video links or teleconferencing facilities in prisons may be available for prisoners to access legal appointments, court appearances or healthcare. There are significant advantages as well as challenges to the widespread adoption of telehealth in every correctional facility.[53,84–88] Increased attention triggered by the ongoing global response to the COVID-19 infection outbreak, together with the associated restrictions and difficulties on movements and in-person attendance at health appointments, has led to further increases in telehealth expansion and uptake across a number of countries.[89]

Telehealth facilities also support workforces across diverse geographic areas to build high-performing teams through education and connectedness.[90]

Implications for practice

- Practical considerations for improving telehealth access include infrastructure, security, consistent network access and speed, and technical support.
- Shared facilities between correctional and health services can be challenging where legal and custodial access is viewed as a priority over health.
- Telehealth can support timely IPC assessment, education and support, with benefits for prisoners, health staff and the correctional workforce alike.

39.3.6 Healthcare-related equipment management in the correctional setting

Contemporary healthcare equipment management principles remain, including appropriate processes and controls for packaging, storage, cleaning and expiry.[91] Blood-borne virus (BBV) prevalence is higher in the correctional population, posing additional risks for reusable equipment items being sterilised or cleaned on-site.

Healthcare equipment, medications and supplies can be misappropriated by prisoners for misuse, trading or weaponising. Stock security and monitoring controls are essential.

Implications for practice

- Reprocessing or sterilisation of medical equipment for reuse is a high-risk procedure and should not occur within a prison unless this process demonstrably meets the specific standards and requirements for instrument sterilisation.[91]
- All healthcare professionals in the correctional environment must remain alert to the very real security risks associated with the provision or misappropriation of healthcare equipment, supplies or medications, however innocuous the item may seem.
- Nothing can be provided to prisoners to retain or take away by health staff without the appropriate security permissions, notifications and adherence to jurisdictional policy—this can include seemingly innocuous items such as wound dressings or medications.

39.4 The built environment considerations for IPC

39.4.1 Facility infrastructure and design

Correctional facilities vary widely, from completely modern new-build or a combination of new and old,

to old and outdated buildings or temporary and portable expansion modules. As in any building project, new builds and renovations do not necessarily imply fit for purpose design, being dependent on the commissioning scope of requirements as well as the priorities and viewpoints of the commissioning team. Many aspects of healthcare may be overlooked in correctional facility builds worldwide, where a predominant focus is on security.

Some correctional facilities have areas still in use dating from the late 1800s, albeit with some upgrades since, remaining far from a contemporary setting. In the majority, security priorities predominate over health or IPC in the built environment. Highly regulated security access requirements, barriers, gates and security screening stations apply to all prisoner and personnel movement in, through and out of correctional facilities.

Healthcare delivery settings within the correctional facility are also widely variable, ranging from newer purpose-built to far older or adapted spaces. Funding, design and maintenance may be through the correctional agency rather than health, bringing challenges where architecture, design and maintenance teams are predominantly security focused. The Australasian Health Facilities Guidelines are generally not referenced or used as a guide in the design, build or renovation of healthcare settings in the correctional context, and do not reference correctional healthcare setting requirements or best practice.[92]

Healthcare occurs anywhere from inpatient style settings, health clinics (purpose-designed or adapted temporary spaces) or use of prisoner facilities such as common rooms. Emergency healthcare may occur anywhere across an entire site, including residential, industrial or agricultural contexts, with support from external emergency services as required. Delays in attendance and access can occur for correctional health staff, as well as incoming emergency response services.

Environmental or facility responsibility lies on many occasions with the correctional agency. Health services may have limited ability to make amendments to healthcare delivery spaces to support best practice requirements for operational and IPC needs.

Implications for practice

- Jurisdictional facility commissioners should have strong engagement and advocacy with designing for health at all stages of the commission, design and build process to deliver a stronger end-product that actively supports worker and custodial population health, manages operational risks, and reduces later on-costs from design amendments or unforeseen design consequences.

- IPC relating to the built environment involves multiple stakeholders and varying agency responsibilities, requiring clear risk management processes for the notification and remediation of concerns.
- The preparedness of the correctional health service to respond and manage common presenting health emergencies and disease outbreak should reflect site location and setting requirements.
- Ready access to appropriate personal protective equipment (PPE) as well as blood and body fluid spill kits for health and correctional staff should be available throughout the facility as well as in emergency response preparedness kits.

39.4.2 Crowding and accommodation

Increasing incarceration rates have caused degrees of crowding across Australian correctional facilities, predominantly managed through increases in cell occupancy (single cells converted to double accommodation, double cells to four, and so on) and reduced space between beds and personal areas. Crowding and associated security, infrastructure and funding challenges can lead to longer daily 'in-cell' times, impacting on prisoner health and disease transmission risks.[3,39,93,94]

Toilet and shower facilities are generally rudimentary even in new-build facilities. In-cell facilities can commonly have an open toilet (no seat lid) with minimal screening, shared between occupants who may also be required to also take meals, sleep or spend most of each day in that confined cell space.[93,94] Placement of facilities within the cell may contribute to the transmission of infection, for example an open toilet immediately next to a small table for meals. Showering facilities or communal areas may be shared by large cohorts of people daily. These close-proximity shared spaces increase the transmission risk of infestation or infectious disease as well as personal safety risk and impact on physical and mental health.[3,93-97]

Implications for practice
- Early identification, robust risk management and limitation of contagion in the crowded prison environment is an essential health and safety measure for correctional and health services.
- Health assessment and screening outcomes should be used to initiate education and treatment as

required; inform accommodation placement by correctional services officers; and triage further health review and health interventions.
- Effective communication, working in partnership for the safety of all and clear processes for the recognition, response and escalation of contagion in a timely and appropriate manner are essential processes.

39.4.3 Isolation facilities

Solitary isolation cells are generally only found in correctional facility areas, housing a small number of prisoners requiring maximum security or constant observation for risk of self-harm or harm from others. There are both physical and mental health risks associated with prolonged periods of isolation in any context.[98-101]

Negative pressure rooms (via heating, ventilation and air conditioning [HVAC] systems or dedicated setup) for IPC purposes are not available. A small number of prisons in each state may have a limited number of purpose-built 'inpatient' style cells or rooms for health monitoring and healthcare delivery; however, these are predominantly not built to healthcare 'isolation room' standards for infectious disease purposes.

Implications for practice
- Ability to effectively isolate individuals with contagion is extremely limited in the correctional environment.
- Communication and planning must occur in advance of any transfer of prisoners with transmissible disease to and from hospital/healthcare, or between correctional facilities, to support the most appropriate transport, placement and the health and safety of all involved.
- Correctional and correctional health services may require some time for this process which can be complex to navigate. Prisoner movements involve custodial, legal, health planning and health access requirements to be assessed and addressed.
- It is never acceptable for an external health service to knowingly return a prisoner with a transmissible disease into the correctional setting without prior communication with the correctional health service in the first instance. A written health provider to health provider clinical discharge summary or other clinical handover documentation must be provided for all prisoners with known transmissible diseases, together with clear written care instructions for correctional services staff where the correctional health service

is not on-site, for example after hours. Reliance on verbal handover via correctional officers is not acceptable.

- Correctional health services have facility and corporate team clinicians who can assist external healthcare services with navigating pathways.

39.4.4 Hygiene

Cleaning can be of variable standards and may be undertaken by prisoners, correctional staff, or contract cleaners. Clothing and bedding may be laundered in-house or on a domestic basis by prisoners, with potential implications for effective removal of infestation or infection.[102,103] Access to commercial laundering standard facilities may not be available. Clothing, footwear and items of personal hygiene equipment including razors, hair grooming equipment or toothbrushes may be shared or contaminated (by choice or by wilful intent from other prisoners). Frequently touched surfaces such as doors, handles or switches can be contaminated by use for purpose, or through wilful intent.

Hand hygiene access including soap, handwashing basins and/or appropriately effective alcohol-based hand rub (ABHR) may not be readily available in all areas. ABHR access may raise concerns around security risks, including ingestion or flammability, despite ABHR being an integral component of infection transmission reduction in a healthcare setting.[39,104–106] Access to ABHR in specific correctional or forensic contexts may be controlled, including where legislative jurisdictional requirements mandate the use of non-ABHR product. Optimal hand hygiene is required to support the control of contact transmitted pathogens.

Health centres may have old, damaged or unsuitable flooring, surfaces and fittings, or inadequate separation of 'dirty' and 'clean' work zones in preparation or treatment areas that impact negatively on the ability to minimise harbouring of infectious agents in the health environment.

Implications for practice

- Cleaning, laundering and personal hygiene equipment sharing are potential contributors to infection risks.
- Hand hygiene education for health and non-health workforce includes specifics and limitations for the appropriateness of handwashing and/or ABHR use to the situation and pathogen of concern.[91,107]
- Education, stock management controls and secure fixtures can assist to promote safe and effective

ABHR access for health, correctional staff and prisoners alike in appropriate facility areas.[91,107]

- Environmental cleaning must be to an acceptable standard, and to a health standard in health facility areas.[108–111]
- Regular environmental auditing from an infection control perspective must be paired with action outcomes and risk management controls to raise or rectify identified concerns.[108]

39.4.5 Ventilation and thermal control

Effective air conditioning and ventilation systems (air filtration and airflow) are essential to support IPC. Old, poorly maintained, or interconnected systems between multiple spaces are a known risk for the harbouring of pathogens or the transmission of infection.[110,112–118]

Thermal stress can impair innate immunity and cause or contribute to death. Deaths in custody related to heat stress occur in Australian and global custodial environments.[119–123]

Thermal comfort principles may not be incorporated into all areas of the correctional facility. HVAC systems may not be present in all prisons or accommodation spaces. Prisoners and workforce staff may be unable to achieve environmental temperature control in weather extremes without the intervention of others.[121,124,125] Natural ventilation can support infection control but may be minimal in cells or communal areas, with secured windows and heavy cell doors restricting airflow.[116] Access to outside areas may be severely restricted, or prisoners may be required to be outdoors during extreme weather events.[125] Transport vans can be sealed spaces, may not have heating or cooling in prisoner compartments, and prisoners can be transported over journey times of several hours.[123] Hydration access during transport may not be freely available, instead being dependent on the provision from correctional staff.

Implications for practice

- Prevention and control of infection related to heating, ventilation and air conditioning (HVAC) systems in the correctional setting requires awareness and understanding of system management, risks and controls. Scheduled maintenance, cleaning and audit programs are necessary to ensure the effectiveness of HVAC systems in reducing pathogen transmission.
- Thermal stress can be rapidly life-limiting and present as a medical emergency. Clear, timely and proactive correctional and health processes must

be available for the management of extreme environmental conditions, as well as early identification, assessment and intervention for prisoners or workforce staff suffering from thermal stress.

- Infective causes of thermal stress must be considered for individuals presenting with extremes of hypothermia or hyperthermia, even in an extreme weather event. Sepsis is a medical emergency that may present as a precursor to heat-stroke, or from an infective source. Correctional health services must have clear protocols and guidelines available for the recognition and early management of sepsis.[126–129]

- Jurisdictional agencies should have processes and protocols in place that include the correctional setting and context (as well as transport) and the management of thermal control, extreme weather events, access to hydration and at-risk vulnerable populations.

39.4.6 Prisoner transport

Prisoner transport is the responsibility of the correctional services agency and occurs frequently across the correctional system for a variety of reasons including sentencing pathways, crowding management, attendance at courts, external health appointments and on discharge from hospital. Transport can occur over long distances or journey times, with groups of prisoners held in proximity in a closed space with limited ventilation and thermal control.

Frequent movement of individuals (within or between custodial facilities, or into and from the general community) creates potential gaps in healthcare assessment, treatment and services, as well as risks for disease progression or transmission.

Implications for practice

- Prisoner transport creates risks for undetected adverse health events as well as pathogen transmission.

- Prisoners with symptoms of respiratory illness should not be transported without prior appropriate health assessment/'fit to travel' clearance. Appropriate PPE for the individual and transport staff must be used, together with the most clinically appropriate transport mode.

- Correctional agencies should have clear protocols for cleaning and disinfection of transport-associated security items, including restraints,

contaminated areas and frequently touched surfaces, to reduce the risk of infection transmission.[91,103,108,130] Where correctional services staff seek input or advice from health staff, this should be provided from an IPC-informed knowledge base and in accordance with operational processes for inter-agency communication of advice.

39.4.7 The outside built environment

Outside time is restricted and limited, dependent at any time on the prison regime, workforce, prison crowding and security risks. Some facility areas may only provide an enclosed paved area with no direct sunlight. Access to daylight and the natural environment supports immunity and overall physical and mental health.[60,93,131–133]

Implications for practice

- Correctional and health staff need to recognise the impact of limited exposure to the outdoor environment and sunlight on health (physical, including immune system health and mental health).

- Screening, assessment and management should occur for prisoners at risk of physical or mental health deterioration. This may include vitamin D supplementation as required, especially for prisoners housed for prolonged periods of time in isolation or with limited access to outside space and sunlight.[60,65]

- Clear risk assessment, communication and risk management should occur between jurisdictional agencies for those individuals evidencing or at greatest risk of health deterioration.

39.4.8 Health promoting prisons

The links between public health, correctional health, custody, safety, wellbeing and risk for individuals in custody and the associated workforces are inextricable. Health for all is a human right.[4,5] The costs of ill health to a taxpayer-funded system are well recognised and understood.[134] Proactive approaches to health for prisoners, correctional and health workforces aim to positively impact population health and reduce burden of disease from all causes.

Built environment design and facility operations can support or hinder physical and mental health, immunity, IPC, self-management of health (including medications) and rehabilitation. Health promoting prisons (HPP) is an approach that recognises this and promotes a salutogenic approach to health in all aspects of prison design, build and operations.[18,95,135–138]

Some newer build facilities across Australia have taken the opportunity to use aspects of health promoting prison design to support health and wellbeing, as well as improve environmental and cultural safety for Indigenous peoples.[139,140]

Implications for practice

- Correctional facility commissioning, design, build, renovation and purchasing activities should include a strong focus on health for all from the outset and at all stages of the process. Design and build teams must include input from health professionals with governance and operational expertise across a broad range of practice. This must include IPC,[141] health facility standards requirements,[92] physiotherapy and occupational therapy, pharmacy, ventilation management, emergency health response and health workflow. Additionally, expertise in disability support, ageing, and Indigenous and cultural health will provide a lens to the finished product that is invaluable. These inclusions will support robust salutogenic design and reduce infrastructure changes, costs or risks in the life of the facility.

39.5 Correctional health staffing

Correctional health is delivered by a range of health professionals who may be employed under differing governance structures depending on service arrangements. These health professionals may bring differing levels of awareness, context and educational needs to IPC in the correctional environment.

Overall, correctional healthcare is a predominantly nurse-led system of care. The correctional or prison health nurse is generally the first health professional seen by an individual prisoner on entry into the system. Correctional nurses work with a range of healthcare disciplines as well as correctional services staff to comprehensively assess and manage prisoner health.[142,143] The health workforce generally has a high level of expertise in the assessment and management of prisoner health, including commonly seen acute and chronic presenting conditions, infectious disease, infestation, vaccine-preventable disease, vaccination and screening programs, patient education, health screening and care-planning. Correctional healthcare nurses are pivotal to inter-professional and inter-agency communication and planning to support prisoner health. Specific nurses may have specialist area or primary nurse portfolios,

including BBV clinics, opioid substitution programs, sexual health, forensic assessment, men's or women's health, antenatal and postnatal care, IPC, chronic disease and more.[144–148]

Nurse–patient staffing ratios do not exist in correctional healthcare. There is generally only a minimal number of nurses on-site to deliver clinic and inpatient healthcare, medication management and emergency response in prisons with a capacity of hundreds of prisoners. Staffing levels often depend on the jurisdiction, contracts and prison size, with some shifts covered with one to two nurses or a full multidisciplinary team for other sites.

Nurse practitioners are not commonly used but certainly have scope in correctional healthcare for minor illness/minor injury; chronic disease management; mental health; BBV/STI/sexual health and opioid substitution programs and other areas.[149,150]

Medical officers generally provide healthcare via general or specialised clinic services, inpatient management depending on the facility, and via telephone consultation. Medical staff work closely with nursing staff in healthcare assessment, planning and delivery.

Aboriginal and Torres Strait Islander Health Workers and AHPRA-registered health practitioners enhance health service delivery for prisoners through culturally safe support and understanding, communication, engagement, education and clinical services.[54] Aboriginal liaison officers (ALO) or similarly focused roles are generally employed by Correctional Services to assist and promote the welfare of Aboriginal and/or Torres Strait Islander prisoners.[54,151] ALOs also have a key role in communication with healthcare staff around health concerns or issues raised by prisoners and can thus support IPC messaging and education in the correctional environment.

Allied health and other health practitioners may be employed within the correctional healthcare team or provide clinical services on a consult basis, including physiotherapy, occupational therapy, audiology, dentists and dental hygienists, podiatrists and speech pathologists.

Some prisons in Australia and overseas also incorporate models of prisoner peer-education and support for specific needs, such as BBV education and support.

Implications for practice

- Prisoner peer education has been shown to be beneficial and effective in supporting knowledge, understanding and disease management initiatives in the prison populations.[152,153] Peer education also supports engagement in health and wellbeing and reduces risk-taking behaviours.

- The IPC risks related to scope of practice will vary between health discipline contexts. Governance and risk management should consider practice context and contemporary professional requirements in all aspects of the spectrum of correctional healthcare.
- Dental services are a high-risk practice for pathogen transmission and require robust practice and risk management in practice and governance.[91,154–157]

39.6 Health information sharing

Health information sharing in the correctional setting may be unintended or mandated to allow for appropriate care, security and safety of the individual and the broader correctional population including staff.

Unintended disclosure of confidential health information can occur through a variety of mechanisms, for example the presence of correctional officers in consultation rooms where security overrides private consultation ability; nearby prisoners waiting to be seen; and overheard or unguarded conversations in healthcare areas. Health staff should be judicious in where, how and when they discuss confidential health information. Information can spread rapidly into the general prison population or workforce, potentially placing the individual, staff and facility security at risk.[158,159] Privacy and confidentiality carries a higher and broader burden in the correctional setting.

Shared responsibilities for the safe care of individuals in custody may require degrees of specific health information sharing with or without consent, in a broad range of circumstances.[16] This can create ethical and professional challenges where policy and governance may override an absolute right to privacy. For example, officers may request to know information about a prisoner's BBV status prior to a transport run, citing information sharing guidelines. However, this knowledge does not change the correctional services management for the prisoner (except for specific high-risk behaviours) and the infectious status is not known for all prisoners. As the same precautions for every prisoner should be taken by correctional officers when responding to situations with potential body-fluid exposure, the health staff member would need to be satisfied that disclosure is in line with 'need to know' and follows jurisdictional policies and guidelines relating to information sharing, handover and inter-agency communication.

Other circumstances where health-related information sharing occurs include prisoner transfers between sites, jurisdictions or other agencies; public guardians/advocates; court or pre-sentencing report preparation; mandatory disease surveillance notifications; correctional supervision of health risk outside health service hours; and complex case management multi-agency meetings and release.

Implications for practice

- Jurisdictional policies and guidelines should clearly define the circumstances in which confidential health information is permitted and be followed by staff in accordance with these, so the process is consistent for circumstances where there are multiple stakeholders and a risk to the safety or wellbeing of the individual to whom the health information pertains.
- Prisoner consent should be obtained for correctional health staff to contact external health providers to continue healthcare, screening and disease prevention,[16,59,160] e.g. general practitioner (GP), homeless health team or other primary health service.
- Health records (electronic or paper) must be protected and only accessed in accordance with health agency and/or correctional agency requirements.[16,59,160] Clear documentation should be entered in the health record of when and what health information has been shared. It should be noted whether this was with or without the knowledge of the individual, as well as the reason for this.

39.7 Common IPC issues in correctional healthcare

In-depth guidance on public health, specific infectious diseases, surveillance and outbreak management is addressed in other chapters. The principles and practice of IPC translate across all settings.

Correctional context considerations for specific infectious diseases are discussed here. A pathogen's ideal environment is one where there is a vulnerable population group with comorbid diseases, held in proximity with inadequate ventilation, shared spaces, environmental and personal hygiene challenges, and no facilities for isolation of infectious respiratory disease.

Mandatory notifiable disease processes within each jurisdiction still apply to prisoners. On the notification, specifically note that screening or diagnosis has occurred by a correctional health provider. This supports location identification in the event of disease prevalence or outbreak and supports targeted health intervention responses in a geographic area.

Where a positive notifiable disease result is returned after release from prison, correctional health providers should endeavour to contact the individual or the nominated health provider for that individual wherever possible. Where the individual is unable to receive their notification of a positive result, service and jurisdictional processes should be followed.

Environmental cleaning may be performed by prisoners in all or part of some facilities. Cleaning methods, education, frequency and available cleaning products may not be to a sufficient standard to control pathogens or infestation. Effective cleaning is proven to reduce environmental pathogen burden and transmission.[109,111,101]

Implications for practice

- Education and audit for cleaning technique, frequency, adequacy, product use, together with risk assessment and response should occur on a regular basis. Clear communication should occur regarding risk ownership of identified issues where more than one agency or service is involved in the facility management process.
- Mandatory disease report notifications should include prison details as the location of screening or diagnosis.

39.8 Contact transmissible diseases

39.8.1 Infestation

Infestation and associated disease or illness occurs through the presence of animals as vectors, including rodents, mosquitoes, cats, bats, birds, amphibians and reptiles. Animals can come into prisons from the natural environment; be introduced with permission under appropriate housing and care conditions; or be kept by prisoners with consent or illicitly as companions or pets.

Personal infestations commonly encountered in the prison population include ectoparasitic infections (head/pubic/body lice, scabies, mites, ticks, impetigo and bedbugs) and endoparasitic infections (worms and flukes).[2,3,16,39,162,163] These may be present on admission into prison or contracted during the period of imprisonment.

Implications for practice

- Correctional and health services policies and protocols should be available for the early identification, control and management of all

causes of pest infestation in individuals and the built environment.

- Proactive scheduled facility maintenance should include regular infestation management.
- Appropriate environmental and personal treatment should be initiated in a timely manner, using appropriate PPE and treatment regimens.
- Laundering practices of clothes, bedding and towels should be compliant with the required temperature controls to eliminate infestation of clothing and bedding.

39.8.2 Multidrug-resistant organisms (MROs)

Routine screening is not undertaken for MROs in prison. Screening may occur in specific circumstances in the same way as in the community or hospital health services. Attention to personal hygiene using soap and water, as well as the importance of not sharing towels or washcloths, should be included in health messaging to prisoners to assist in reducing general bioburden. Routine use of chlorhexidine washes in the correctional community has not been proven significantly more effective than using water and a washcloth, with known risks around chlorhexidine resistance and allergy.[164]

39.8.3 Blood-borne virus (BBV)/sexually transmitted infections (STI)

Prison populations have a far higher prevalence of BBV and STI to the general community, for a complex range of reasons.[58,83,165] BBV and STI infection and associated disease management have a significant global cost impact yet are preventable and largely treatable. Imprisonment provides a significant public health opportunity, as transmission reduction is the cornerstone to manage health and cost-related burdens to society.[37,166-168] Other chapters of this text also address aspects of BBV and STI management.

Body fluid exposure can occur between prisoners, or between workforce and prisoner interaction. Correctional context risks include physical injury; sexual interaction; ingestion (illicit drugs may be ingested, regurgitated and then shared with others); spitting; shared personal care items or injecting equipment; deliberate contamination of shared items or frequently touched surfaces, as well as weaponising and contaminating items to use against workforce members. Such activities may be consensual, forced or bartered.

Tracing an identified source can be problematic in many instances. Essential transmission reduction strategies in prisons for prisoners and workforce alike include education; environmental and personal hygiene; screening; immunisation; access to and use of appropriate PPE; robust adherence to hand hygiene; supervised medication administration for highly desirable/tradeable medications; and effective and timely responses to identified exposure.

Australia has undertaken significant advocacy, research and health promotion over the past decades on BBV and STI prevention and control, through non-government, private and government organisations and clinician groups committed to prevalence and disease burden reduction.[20,21,29,49,58,146] This has led to ongoing improvements across all jurisdictions in all aspects of care including use of newer treatment options, national prevalence data collection and reporting; and care continuation between prison and the community. National strategies, guidelines and surveillance/prevalence audits, including specific Aboriginal and Torres Strait Islander considerations, have been developed with input from key stakeholders across all jurisdictions to support a comprehensive approach[37,48,53,54,169–171] Effective implementation and monitoring is essential to ensure public health gains continue to be made.[172,173]

There are a number of peak bodies working in Australia to improve correctional BBV/STI disease care and prevention, with a wide range of resources, information, research and policy documents available through their respective websites and publications.[174–181]

Implications for practice

* BBV- and STI-related risks or disease assessments must be regularly incorporated into health reviews for prisoners, with targeted management and follow-up for individuals at specific risk.
* Education, vaccination status, medication therapies (whether commenced or supported to continue), treatment response measures and engagement with specialist health providers support transmission reduction strategies.

39.8.4 Injecting drug use, tattooing and safe sex supplies

Prison injecting drug use, tattooing, shared personal care equipment and sexual activity are key disease transmission risk areas.[29,103,159,182,183] Prisoners use 'home-made', illicitly obtained, reused and/or shared supplies for injecting drug use and tattooing.[165,184] Shaving or barbering equipment may be shared between multiple prisoners.

No Australian correctional jurisdiction currently supports access to safe injecting equipment or needle and syringe programs. Injectable equipment cleaning options such as bleach differs across jurisdictions from available to highly limited, despite ongoing public health calls for a comprehensive harm reduction approach to be introduced as a health and cost-effective measure.[182,185–188] Drug use in prison may not be disclosed by prisoners fearful of conviction, additional charges, or fines. Other substance use and harm minimisation treatment programs may be available in prisons to some extent in all jurisdictions, including opioid substitution programs. Reduced illicit injecting drug use in prison may reduce infection risk for some individuals.

Access to safe sex supplies including male condoms or female dental dams, lubricant, or other protections to reduce risk of body-fluid exchange is often limited or may be non-existent in some jurisdictions or prisons. Male condom access may be nominally supported in some correctional policies; however, anecdotal reports indicate that supply may not always be readily available or consistent.[189–192]

Implications for practice

* Consistent and available access to safe sex supplies should occur in all prison environments, regardless of gender.[191,193] Rape does occur in the prison environment globally (prisoner-to-prisoner, staff-to-prisoner or prisoner-to-staff) so clear and contemporary processes should be in place for health responses for individuals disclosing rape that are equivalent to the non-incarcerated community, including assessment and management for disease transmission risks.[3,194,195]
* Correctional health staff are not able to initiate or provide needle and syringe exchange in prison in the current Australian correctional environment. Education and information should be available to prisoners on risks and mitigation strategies for disease transmission reduction. An ongoing correctional and public health focus is required to improve the ability of the correctional setting to meet the priorities of the National Drug Strategy 2017-26.[17,187,196,197]

39.8.5 Other contact pathogens—polio, diphtheria

Polio (faecal-oral transmission) and diphtheria (saliva transmission) are rarely seen due to strong population health vaccination programs in the Australian general community. However, prisoners with incomplete vaccination backgrounds (including prisoners from overseas) come into custody in Australia for a range of reasons and robust health screening may not have occurred. Vaccination status for prisoners should be assessed and catch-up vaccinations offered as required in line with national guidelines for vaccination.[198]

39.8.6 Droplet and/or airborne transmissible diseases

Preparedness and response for droplet and airborne disease in the correctional setting has the same principles and challenges as the wider community—education; preparedness planning; vaccination programs; screening; early identification and reporting; appropriate PPE access and use; and ability to undertake effective isolation.[110,112,114,198,199]

COVID-19, influenza, pertussis, other respiratory virii and mumps are a very real risk for illness and wider contagion in the correctional setting.

Foodborne illnesses can occur more often in prisons than in the community due to communal catering, food hoarding and overcrowding. Prison health services may have no, or extremely limited, capacity to manage unwell prisoners requiring intravenous therapy or clinical monitoring.

Airborne transmissible diseases include, but are not limited to, infective stages of pulmonary tuberculosis (TB), varicella (chicken pox), measles and COVID-19. Prisoners with airborne-transmissible disease, particularly if acutely unwell and requiring frequent monitoring and physical access for care, may not be appropriate to be safely cared for in the correctional setting. Transfer out to hospital for acute care is then required.

Implications for practice

- Prisoners should receive a comprehensive health assessment early in the imprisonment period to assess, identify and screen for transmissible disease.[3,200]
- Clear processes should be in place for health staff,[59,201] correctional staff and prisoners on the early identification, communication, assessment and management of highly transmissible disease.
- Assessment of vaccination status, together with catch-up or ongoing scheduled vaccination is a vital component of health assessment and disease prevention.
- Robust workforce and prisoner education should be in place, including appropriate PPE and hand hygiene for the pathogen involved.
- Incorporation of prisoner-peer educators can be an effective strategy to support public health messaging, reporting and awareness in the wider prison community.[153,202]

- Correctional and correctional health services require clear processes for triage and consideration of transfer out to a higher-level care for individuals who are highly infectious and/or too unwell to be managed within the limitations of available prison facilities and care.

COVID-19 (droplet and airborne transmissible): The COVID-19 novel coronavirus pandemic has without doubt focused a great deal of attention on the need for improved correctional and health system interconnectedness in pandemic preparedness and response. Justice systems globally continue to respond and adapt to the ongoing challenges of managing COVID-19 in the correctional context, for prisoners and staff.[97,100,130,203–207]

The reduction of prisoners and associated crowding through amended sentences of custodial imprisonment or sentence length for the most vulnerable has been one strategy. This may have unintended consequences on other aspects of health post release from prison.[206,208]

Social distancing protective strategies include significant restrictions on visiting prisoners, amending accommodation arrangements and aiming to reduce prisoner 'churn' or flow between sites.[100] Social distancing and isolation measures are known to have consequences on mental and physical health in all populations globally observed to date, including prisons.[100,101]

Temporary facility expansion modules or portable healthcare environments have been incorporated into some correctional facilities.[205] Rapid identification, screening, separation of unwell individuals, quarantining, contact tracing, record keeping, agency and jurisdictional escalation, and all other aspects of effective outbreak management apply.

Already challenging before COVID-19, restrictions on access to specialist external healthcare appointments can continue, especially where telehealth is not in place. Face-to-face visits and access by legal counsel or other community-based services may also be impacted. Workforce and population screening occur in line with jurisdictional guidelines.

Work continues on preparedness, responses and research into the impacts of COVID-19 in Australian correctional systems.[209] The Communicable Diseases Network Australia (CDNA) national guidelines, COVID-19 Outbreaks in Correctional and Detention Facilities, are updated and endorsed by the Australian Health Protection Principal Committee (AHPPC).[130]

39.8.7 Tropical infectious diseases

All prisoners in or from susceptible regions of Australia, and disproportionately affected population groups (not just in tropical climes), may present with or acquire infectious and parasitic diseases with significant health implications, requiring consideration in clinical assessment and diagnostic decision making.[210,211]

Melioidosis, caused by direct contact with bacterium *Burkholderia pseudomallei* (found in contaminated water or soils) can present as mimicking a range of other generalised infective processes.[212,213]

Mycobacterial diseases include lyssavirus and leprosy (Hansen's disease, from *Mycobacterium leprae*). The Australian bat population carries Australian bat lyssavirus (ABLV) which is closely associated to classical rabies.[214] Infected bat bites or scratches can cause paralysis, delirium, convulsions and death, even some years after exposure.[214,215] Leprosy (Hansen's disease), while rare in Australia now, is still seen, and continues to be endemic in some tropical countries. Historically and today, this chronic disease continues to disproportionately affect specific population groups who may be socially disadvantaged, living in crowded households, in remote or endemic areas with limited access to health resources.[216] Aboriginal and Torres Strait Islander peoples are disproportionately represented in Australian case statistics.[217–221] Leprosy is not highly contagious, spreads through nasal droplet secretions and through direct contact with infected skin lesions, with a long incubation period (up to 20 years), affecting the skin, peripheral nerves, upper respiratory tract mucosa and eyes—damage can be progressive and permanent. Treatment includes multidrug antibiotic therapy.[216,221]

Rheumatic fever and associated rheumatic heart disease (RHD) are caused by an immune response to group A streptococcus bacteria—typically *Streptococcus pyogenes*, although *Streptococcal pyoderma* may also be implicated.[222–224] Disease-related prevalence and associated burden of disease (including increased mortality) continues to disproportionately affect specific population groups worldwide, including Aboriginal and Torres Strait Islander, Māori and Pacific Islander peoples.[47,222,223,225–227] Symptom recognition, response and treatment continuity are essential.[223,224,228]

Strongyloidiasis is a helminth-related (intestinal and tissue worm, *Strongyloides stercoralis*) infection which remains endemic in some Australian populations, including Indigenous Australians. Disease can be lifelong, can mimic other disease symptoms and have a high mortality.[229,230]

Trachoma-related eye disease is caused by *Chlamydia trachomatis*. It can progress to blindness and continues to affect populations worldwide living in endemic regions, including some Aboriginal and Torres Strait Islander communities.[231–233] Spread is through personal contact or flies transmitting infected ocular or nasal discharge from one individual to another.[231,233] Trachoma is preventable and Australia is the only high-income country with endemic trachoma. Australian federal and jurisdictional governments continue with essential screening, guidelines and awareness programs.[232–234]

Implications for practice

- Clinical identification, notifiable disease reporting, management and treatment should be in line with contemporary guidelines.

- Prisoners can be transferred intra or interstate for healthcare access or legal reasons. Less common and 'tropical' infectious/parasitic diseases should be considered as a potential contributor or cause in the event of illness during clinical assessment and diagnostic formulation.

- A range of environmental factors including climate change and widespread travel has implications for the increasing range and spread of previously localised or regional disease and illness.

39.8.8 Outbreak identification and management

Outbreak management principles are more specifically addressed elsewhere in this textbook. They remain largely similar in the correctional setting, with due regard given to the increased health and environmental vulnerabilities of this at-risk population. Disease outbreak has the potential to spread extremely rapidly within and across prison sites affecting large numbers of prisoners and potentially staff.

The potential impact of large segments of the prison population becoming unwell from transmissible disease could rapidly overwhelm correctional and health services. Large-scale hospitalisation of unwell prisoners would not be logistically possible nor desirable from both a correctional/security and a health system perspective, for a wide range of reasons.

Jurisdictional preparedness and response plans may be developed by health and correctional agencies in isolation, or have different priorities, resources or logistics; meaning they may not dovetail to effectively provide a cohesive jurisdictional response.

Implications for practice

- Ensure all agency disease preparedness plans interconnect and reflect areas of shared and individual responsibilities and actions in the correctional context.

- Early identification of suspected or confirmed cases; communication, escalation and shared response between correctional and correctional health agencies; case tracking and segregation can assist to reduce spread.

- Practices to restrict disease transmission such as segregation, isolation or lockdown should consider whether other measures to maintain social connection and healthcare access will dovetail into prevention and preparedness planning and response overall.[130,203,235–237] Risk assessment and response plans should be undertaken for highly vulnerable or distressed prisoners.[130]

- A multi-agency and multi-service response is required in a correctional disease outbreak event. Early escalation and notification up the chains of command are essential. Up-line briefings, planning, ministerial and media response preparation and notification may all be required. Health staff should not make public comment to social media or media outlets unless specifically authorised to do so.

39.9 Correctional IPC governance

Principles of sound practice and governance of IPC remain the same, regardless of the contextual setting. Risk management in disease prevention involves the balance and trade-offs between 'the cost of disease transmission and the cost of applying control measures'.[237,238] Personal and societal costs associated with IPC include morbidity and mortality; mental health impact related to stress, anxiety and grief; infrastructure impacts including healthcare services; and financial costs.[238–240]

Every individual coming into the correctional context brings differing knowledge of IPC awareness or practice; has widely variable roles, responsibilities and educational backgrounds; and differing risks for the transmission or contraction of infection. Beyond correctional and correctional health workforces this can include visitors to prisoners; legal or justice staff; inspectors; public guardians; advocates; community advocacy visitors; incoming maintenance services; federal and jurisdictional officers for immigration or police services; co-boarding children or infants; incoming

allied health or health specialists; and, of course, prisoners themselves.

39.9.1 Safety, quality and risk

The correctional healthcare context is a mix of inpatient, clinic, primary care, minor procedural care, dental, aged care, pregnancy and post-delivery care, infancy and paediatric care, mass public health programs and emergency response within the heavily regulated security and facility infrastructure restrictions of the environment.

Effective risk identification and management strategies require navigation across multiple stakeholders, government agencies and the broad variety of personnel who have responsibilities for, and engagement with, prisons and prisoners. Jurisdictional agency or site IPC plans may not communicate or interlink with each other.

Demonstrable leadership and sound governance incorporate robust safety, quality and risk management measures to underpin service delivery and outcomes.[241,242] Clear understanding of risk ownership, risk transference and shared risk management responsibilities is essential, at jurisdictional and agency executive, corporate and operational practice levels.

Implications for practice

- A robust safety, quality and risk management process that includes all elements of IPC practice in a correctional setting is essential.

- Larger correctional health networks may require a distinct role for an IPC practitioner, may require a broader IPC team, and a safety, quality and risk position or equivalent. Effective governance includes audit planning and outcome evaluations, as well as evidence collation and performance monitoring.

- Correctional health representation must be included in relevant broader health service and jurisdictional agency committees, including but not limited to IPC; public health; epidemiology/surveillance; pandemic preparedness; ambulance services; contract development related to infection risks; and relevant input into correctional services site and service practice and governance groups.

- There may also be a jurisdictional representative body or special interest group for non-hospital-based IPC practitioners or service leads, which can be an invaluable source of information sharing, shared education, support, networking and service delivery planning.

39.9.2 Accreditation and service standards

Accreditation and standards help to support robust, high-quality service delivery.[243] In healthcare systems, accrediting bodies assess policy and practice evidenced compliance with a broad range of industry and best practice benchmark standards. Correctional health services may undertake standalone accreditation within the correctional system, or as a part of a broader health network accreditation process where the prison(s) healthcare services are a subset of the wider health agency.

IPC performance standards and measures for healthcare-acquired infection are well established in a hospital and some community setting contexts.[163,244,245] Correctional health services need to apply a broader context for relevance when evidencing health performance review and assessment. Community-based setting guidelines can be a closer 'best-fit' for the general (non-hospital) correctional setting.

There are varying accreditation tools, generally designed for healthcare in a hospital, primary healthcare or GP-led service setting. Individual jurisdictions have differing accreditation requirements, using different standard sets. The main health service accreditation agencies in the Australian healthcare context are the Australian Commission on Safety and Quality in Health Care (ACSQHC) via the National Safety and Quality Health Service Standards (NSQHSS); the Australian Council on Healthcare Standards (ACHS) via the Evaluation and Quality Improvement Program (EQuIP); and the Royal Australian College of General Practitioners (RACGP) via the Standards for General Practice.[244,246,247] Each of these programs has specific foci, contexts and standards, with benefits and limitations to service standard assessment in the correctional context.

The RACGP Standards for General Practice are designed for office-based practices, with accreditation through RACGP accreditation bodies for GP practices. The RACGP Standards for Health Services in Australian Prisons (under review at the time of writing) are predominantly designed to 'support general practitioners working to achieve better health outcomes for people in custody' and are not an accreditation standard of themselves.[16]

NSQHS Standard Three focuses on 'Preventing and Controlling Healthcare Infections' with elements of other NSQHS standards relevant to IPC systems and processes. NSQHS standard guides have been produced for hospital, primary, community health, Aboriginal and Torres Strait Islander health and aged care settings.[52,248–250]

For the correctional health context, the NSQHS Guide for multi-purpose services and small hospitals, and the Guide to the NSQHS Standards for community health services, better reflect a broader setting scope.[248,249] ACHS EQuIP accreditation standard documents are accessible for member bodies only and not made publicly available for viewing. Both NSQHS and EQuIP standards have equivalency mapping of standards requirements to reduce duplication.

All these accreditation standards and guidelines address components of IPC practice relevant to the correctional setting.

Implications for practice

- Correctional healthcare providers should strive to meet accreditation standards, recognising that a 'mix and match' approach may be required.

- Custodial service policy and practice that impacts on the provision of optimal IPC must be reflected in the health service evidence portfolio—for example, this may include risk management and mitigation strategies for prison or area lockdowns limiting access to deliver care; release from prison without prior notice to the health service disrupting planning for continuity of care (including medication access); missed IPC-related specialist appointments due to transfers or transport issues; fixed numbers of healthcare staff providing a service to an increasing prison population; or inability to access required healthcare resources such as internet-based policy, procedure or supporting information in a healthcare delivery site where internet or computer access is not available or is severely limited.

- Critical thinking should be evidenced and demonstrated around the broader application of quality health service standard requirements to best match the correctional setting context. The assessment, practice and scope (including delineation and shared aspects of agency responsibilities) of IPC in the correctional health context must be represented in accreditation preparedness and evidence. Robust processes must exist for risk assessment, management, communication and escalation.

- Where components of resourcing and risk management are shared between or lie solely with other jurisdictional agencies or stakeholders, evidenced systems and processes for inter-agency responsibilities, communication, risk management and escalation processes must be available.

*   Where accreditation is being undertaken as a component of a broader health service process, or by accreditors not familiar with the correctional environment, the service risks and practices specific to the correctional healthcare setting may not be fully reflected. Predominantly hospital-based IPC-related policies and procedures of the broader health service may not be consistent or appropriately represent a prison health service. Where these do not reflect the context of the correctional healthcare setting, processes must be in place to incorporate the correctional context within the wider network policy and procedure management process.

*   Undertaking robust self-assessment at stages in the lead-up to formal accreditation will assist to identify areas for improvement.[251]

39.9.3 Building and supporting correctional IPC governance, expertise and practice

IPC programs that are effective and of high quality are a key component in meeting the duty of care towards those in prison and the correctional custodial and health workforces.[91]

Individual prison sites work within a much larger system where prisoner transfers occur frequently in and out of the community, between sites, with more than one agency involved in care. Staff bring diverse levels of expertise and awareness of the principles and practice of IPC. All staff working in the correctional setting should work cohesively and comprehensively regarding assessment, intervention and communication to support effective IPC.

Implications for practice

Leadership and IPC governance
*   The requirement for robust IPC governance in the correctional setting is not a new concept.[252,253] Strong and clear leadership is required in both health and correctional systems. Robust correctional IPC programs should be modelled on contemporary systems and practices yet be flexible, innovative and agile to meet the specific aims and requirements of the correctional health context.[39,130,254–257]

*   IPC practitioners with expertise in governance, systems development, decision making, oversight,

surveillance, risk management and review should be included at the highest levels of decision making—these may be internal service leads, or jurisdictions working with external specialist expertise as required.

Leads
*   State-wide or multisite services, as well as larger prison facilities, with inpatient, outpatient and community care components may require a dedicated IPC lead position, engaging with governance and operational leads at each site, and developing a network of IPC links to support and drive on-the-ground expertise and activities.[256]

*   Meaningful inclusion of IPC expertise is required in decision making and response processes related to correctional setting risks. This may vary from review and input into cleaning contract renewals, correctional and health equipment purchasing, facility build or renovation design and process, to disease or pandemic preparedness and response across health and correctional agencies.

*   Linking all correctional IPC staff (including portfolio holders) with broader IPC networks (intra-service, inter-service as well as broader regional and state level) is highly beneficial to two-way education; knowledge and network development; and increasing understanding of contextual practice and risks.

Policy
*   All correctional and correctional health services must have policies, procedures and operational processes in place that describe the responsibilities and requirements of all health, correctional and visiting staff in relation to IPC systems, risks, and the meaningful inclusion of individuals in custody to engage in personal and community health through education, peer support and informed decision making. These should be interfaced with other agencies to ensure systems and approaches are effective, timely and seamless wherever possible.

Portfolios
*   Specific IPC nurse-led portfolio positions in each facility (often undertaken with other professional duties) can provide local expertise; support site and service level knowledge; risk management; communication and escalation; audit activities; quality improvement; and early identification of issues of concern. These portfolios may focus broadly on all aspects of IPC, e.g. IPC champions

or IPC link nurses, or be targeted more specifically, e.g. BBV/STI.[258] Portfolio requirements and expectations must be clearly defined to support organisational goals, risk management and performance. The multidisciplinary clinical team has responsibilities and input into IPC practice, audit, surveillance and governance at site and organisational levels.

Expertise

- Correctional and correctional health systems require an 'enquiring mind' approach to the exchange of expertise and information to build knowledge and informed responses relating to IPC. Correctional and correctional health teams should be included in wider conversations that interface with public health, even where those links may seem tenuous e.g. infection control clinical decision-making processes in an acute hospital setting may have considerable implications for prisoners. Correctional liaison/representation in information and knowledge exchange will assist staff and the individual prisoner in other systems to streamline care and communication.

- Expert support may be required to reach into the correctional setting to inform or support IPC governance and/or practice, for example with expertise in infectious diseases, virology, respiratory disease, tropical disease, environmental management, outbreak management, facility design, data and reporting, research and health informatics.

Education/Awareness

- Active IPC education programs and resources should be available for health and correctional workforces and for prisoners, to support knowledge development, clinical practice expertise and preparedness, meet accreditation requirements

and jurisdictional health policies.[259,260] Education and resource development and implementation should address the needs of individuals with different literacy levels and language proficiency. Using health literacy principles, resources and education, communicators will assist in the development of appropriate and effective IPC-related resources.[261,262]

Conclusion

Custodial and correctional settings have a high-risk population in a high-risk environment for infection susceptibility, prevalence and transmission. Prisoners retain rights to healthcare. Custody and imprisonment provide a significant opportunity to have a positive impact on individual and population health, both within the correctional system and the broader population.

The correctional setting poses complex and diverse challenges and risks for IPC, where the navigation and degree of success for systems and intervention is reliant on input from multiple stakeholders.

Prisoner movements and turnover through the correctional system require attention to ensuring continuity of care is supported. This includes ensuring that health information transfer and handover is effective and timely, whilst balancing the principles of confidentiality and information sharing for safety. Effective management of IPC in this setting requires effective working relationships, policies and processes between key agencies and stakeholders at local, jurisdictional and federal levels.

Robust and effective IPC leadership, governance and practice are essential to maintain and improve health, reduce risk to individuals and staff in the correctional system, and support responsible fiscal management.

Useful websites/resources

- Australian Indigenous Health*InfoNet*. https://healthinfonet.ecu.edu.au.
- Australian Government, Australian Institute of Health and Welfare (Reports and Data – Population Groups – Prisoners). www.aihw.gov.au/reports-data/population-groups/prisoners/overview#:,:text=The%20 AIHW%20currently%20collects%20data,diseases%20than%20the%20general%20population.
- Australian Government, Department of Health and Aged Care. National Strategies for bloodborne viruses and sexually transmissible infections. www.health.gov.au/resources/collections/national-strategies-for-bloodborne-viruses-and-sexually-transmissible-infections.
- Public Health Association Australia. www.phaa.net.au.
- Royal Australian College of General Practitioners (RACGP). Standards for health services in Australian prisons. www.racgp.org.au/running-a-practice/practice-standards/standards-for-other-health-care-settings/health-services-in-australian-prisons.

- Worldwide Prison Health Research and Engagement Network (WEPHREN). https://wephren.tghn.org.
- UNSW, Kirby Institute. https://kirby.unsw.edu.au.

References

1. Greig S. Benefits for using a standardised risk management framework to risk assess infection prevention and control. Sydney: ACQHC, 2018. [Accessed 9 July 2022.] Available from: https://www.safetyandquality.gov.au/sites/default/files/migrated/Presentation-1_Benefits-for-Using-a-standardised-risk-management-framework-for-infection-prevention.pdf.

2. Møller L, Stöver H, Jürgens R, et al. Health in prisons – a WHO guide to the essentials in prison health. Geneva: World Health Organization, 2007. [Accessed 9 July 2022.] Available from: https://www.euro.who.int/__data/assets/pdf_file/0009/99018/E90174.pdf.

3. Enggist S, Moller L, Gauden G, Udesen C. Prisons and health. Geneva: World Health Organization, 2014. [Accessed 9 July 2022.] Available from: https://apps.who.int/iris/bitstream/handle/10665/128603/9789289050593-eng.pdf?sequence=3&isAllowed=y.

4. Australian Government, Attorney-General's Department. Right to health. Public sector guidance sheet. Available from: https://www.ag.gov.au/rights-and-protections/human-rights-and-anti-discrimination/human-rights-scrutiny/public-sector-guidance-sheets/right-health.

5. World Health Organization. Human rights and health care. Geneva: WHO, 2017. [Accessed 9 July 2022.] Available from: https://www.who.int/news-room/fact-sheets/detail/human-rights-and-health.

6. General Assembly – United Nations. General Assembly resolution 70/175, United Nations standard minimum rules for the treatment of prisoners (the Nelson Mandela rules). December 17, 2016. [Accessed 9 July 2022.] Available from: https://documents-dds-ny.un.org/doc/UNDOC/GEN/N15/443/41/PDF/N1544341.pdf?OpenElement.

7. Australian Government, Australian Border Force. Detention management. January 24, 2019. [Accessed 9 July 2022.] Available from: https://www.abf.gov.au/about-us/what-we-do/border-protection/immigration-detention/detention-management.

8. Australian Government, Parliamentary Education Office. Three levels of government: governing Australia - Parliamentary Education Office. May 27, 2022. Available from: https://peo.gov.au/understand-our-parliament/how-parliament-works/three-levels-of-government/three-levels-of-government-governing-australia/.

9. Commonwealth of Australia. Commonwealth of Australia Constitution Act - Sect 120 custody of offenders against laws of the Commonwealth, 1900. [Accessed 9 July 2022.] Available from: http://classic.austlii.edu.au/au/legis/cth/consol_act/coacac627/s120.html.

10. Australian Government, Australian Bureau of Statistics. Corrective Services, Australia reference period quarter 2021; 2022. [Accessed 24 July 2022.] Available from: https://www.abs.gov.au/statistics/people/crime-and-justice/corrective-services-australia/dec-quarter-2021.

11. Community Justice Coalition. Prisons in Australia (2015). Prison Insider. 2015. [Accessed 24 July 2022.] Available from: https://www.prison-insider.com/countryprofile/prisonsinaustralia?s=le-systeme-penitentiaire#le-systeme-penitentiaire.

12. Australian Government, Productivity Commission. 8 Corrective services - report on government services 2021.

Productivity Commission, 2021. [Accessed 24 July 2022.] Available from: https://www.pc.gov.au/research/ongoing/report-on-government-services/2021/justice/corrective-services.

13. Australian Institute of Health and Welfare. Health of Prisoners, 2022. [Accessed 24 July 2022.] Available from: https://www.aihw.gov.au/reports/australias-health/health-of-prisoners.

14. Australian Government, Corrective Services Administrators Council. Guiding principles for corrections in Australia (2018). [Accessed 9 July 2022.] Available from: https://www.publications.qld.gov.au/dataset/f18ea162-6af3-4302-b5b4-61dc5286e586/resource/7f4fb1bd-27c5-46a3-8957-249fa227b1ff/download/guiding-principles-for-corrections-in-australia-revised-2018.pdf.

15. Mackay A. Human rights guidance for Australian prisons: complementing implementation of the OPCAT. Alternative Law Journal. 2021;46(1):20-26. doi:10.1177/1037969X20962863

16. Royal Australian College of General Practitioners. Standards for health services in Australian prisons - 1st Edition; 2011. [Accessed 9 July 2022.] Available from: https://www.racgp.org.au/running-a-practice/practice-standards/standards-for-other-health-care-settings/view-all-health-care-standards/health-services-in-australian-prisons.

17. Public Health Association of Australia. Policy position statement: prisoner health. Canberra: PHA, 2017. [Accessed 9 July 2022.] Available from: https://www.phaa.net.au/documents/item/2578.

18. Hendrie D. Expert backs RACGP calls for access to specific MBS items in prison. RACGP, newsGP; 2019. [Accessed 10 July 2022.] Available from: https://www1.racgp.org.au/newsgp/clinical/expert-backs-racgp-calls-for-access-to-specific-me.

19. Australian Government, PBS Drug Utilisation Sub-committee (DUSC). Public Release Document. Direct acting antiviral medicines for the treatment of chronic hepatitis C. 2018. Available from: https://www.pbs.gov.au/pbs/industry/listing/participants/public-release-docs/2018-09/direct-acting-antiviral-medicines-for-hep-c.

20. The Kirby Institute. Annual report 2016. [Accessed 10 July 2022.] Available from: https://kirby.unsw.edu.au/report/annual-report-2016.

21. Clinical Excellence Queensland. Elimination of hepatitis C virus infection from a regional prison - improvement exchange. Queensland Government, 2018. [Accessed 25 July 2022.] Available from: https://clinicalexcellence.qld.gov.au/improvement-exchange/elimination-hepatitis-c-infection-regional-prison.

22. Mitchell G. Coroner calls for Medicare for prisoners after Indigenous man dies of ear infection. The Sydney Morning Herald, June 22, 2022. [Accessed 24 July 2022.] Available from: https://www.smh.com.au/national/nsw/coroner-supports-medicare-becoming-available to-prisoners-after-indigenous-man-dies-of-ear-infection-20220722-p5b3ty.html.

23. Seidel B, O'Mara P, Abbott P. RACGP, Aboriginal and Torres Strait Islander Health. 2017. [Accessed 24 July 2022.] Available from: https://www.racgp.org.au/FSDEDEV/

media/documents/RACGP/Reports%20and%20 submissions/2017/RACGP-Submission-Access-to-Medicare-in-prison.pdf.

24. Plueckhahn TM, Kinner SA, Sutherland G, Butler TG. Are some more equal than others? Challenging the basis for prisoners' exclusion from Medicare. MJA. 2015;203(9): 359-361. doi:10.5694/mja15.00588

25. Mackee N. Call to include prisoners in Medicare and PBS. Insight+. 2017;(27). [Accessed 10 July 2022.] Available from: https://insightplus.mja.com.au/2017/27/call-to-include-prisoners-in-medicare-and-pbs/.

26. Carroll M, Spittal MJ, Kemp-Casey AR, et al. High rates of general practice attendance by former prisoners: a prospective cohort study. MJA. 2017;207(2):75-80. doi:10.5694/mja16.00841

27. Australian Healthcare Associates. Department of Health PBS pharmaceuticals in hospital review - final report. Vol 8006; 2017. Available from: https://www.pbs.gov.au/reviews/pbs-pharmaceuticals-in-hospitals-review-files/PBS-Pharmaceuticals-in-Hospitals-Review.pdf.

28. Meyerowitz-Katz G. Whatever you do, don't get sick. Inside Story. December 20, 2018. [Accessed 10 July 2022.] Available from: https://insidestory.org.au/whatever-you-do-dont-get-sick/.

29. Kinner SA, Streitberg L, Butler T, Levy M. Prisoner and ex-prisoner health - improving access to primary care. Aust Fam Physician. 2012;41(7):535-537. [Accessed 10 July 2022.] Available from: https://www.racgp.org.au/afp/2012/july/prisoner-and-ex-prisoner-health.

30. Young J, Kinner S. Prisoners are excluded from the NDIS – here's why it matters. The Conversation (AU). March 14, 2017. [Accessed 10 July 2022.] Available from: https://theconversation.com/prisoners-are-excluded-from-the-ndis-heres-why-it-matters-73912.

31. Australian Government, Department of Veterans' Affairs. What happens if you are in lawful custody. Department of Veterans' Affairs. June 7, 2022. [Accessed 10 July 2022.] Available from: https://www.dva.gov.au/financial-support/income-support/what-changes-your-payments/what-happens-if-you-are-lawful-custody.

32. Australian Bureau of Statistics. Prisoners in Australia, 2021. December 9, 2021. [Accessed 10 July 2022.] Available from: https://www.abs.gov.au/statistics/people/crime-and-justice/prisoners-australia/2021.

33. Australian Institute of Health and Welfare. Adult prisoners – Australian Institute of Health and Welfare. September 16, 2021. [Accessed 10 July 2022.] Available from: https://www.aihw.gov.au/reports/australias-welfare/adult-prisoners.

34. Ball J. CEDA - Australia pays the price for increasing rates of imprisonment. Committee for economic development of Australia (CEDA). July 2, 2019. [Accessed 10 July 2022.] Available from: https://www.ceda.com.au/Digital-hub/Blogs/CEDA-Blog/July-2019/Australia-pays-the-price-for-increasing-rates-of-imprisonment.

35. Australian Institute of Health and Welfare. Snapshot – profile of Indigenous Australians. Australia's Welfare. September 16, 2021. [Accessed 10 July 2022.] Available from: https://www.aihw.gov.au/reports/australias-welfare/profile-of-indigenous-australians.

36. Lowitja Institute. We nurture our culture for our future, and our culture nurtures us: close the gap report 2020. Lowitja Institute, 2020. Available from: https://www.lowitja.org.au/content/Document/CtG2020_FINAL4_WEB%20(1).pdf.

37. Australian Institute of Health and Welfare 2022. Australian burden of disease study: impact and causes of illness and death in Aboriginal and Torres Strait Islander people 2018. Vol Series 26; 2018. doi:10.25816/xd60-4366

38. Walker JR, Baldry E, Sullivan EA. Residential programmes for mothers and children in prison: key themes and concepts. Criminology and Criminal Justice. 2021;21(1):21-39. doi:10.1177/1748895819848814

39. Bick JA. Infection control in jails and prisons. Clin Infect Dis. 2007;45(8):1047-1055. doi:10.1086/521910

40. Fazel S, Baillargeon J. The health of prisoners. Lancet. 2011; 377(9769):956-965. doi:10.1016/S0140-6736(10)61053-7

41. Herbert K, Plugge E, Foster C, Doll H. Prevalence of risk factors for non-communicable diseases in prison populations worldwide: a systematic review. Lancet. 2012;379(9830): 1975-1982. doi:10.1016/S0140-6736(12)60319-5

42. Winter RJ, Holmes JA, Papaluca TJ, Thompson AJ. The importance of prisons in achieving hepatitis C elimination: insights from the Australian experience. Viruses. 2022;14(3): 497. doi:10.3390/v14030497

43. Australian Institute of Health and Welfare. Australia's health 2018: in brief. 2018. [Accessed 10 July 2022.] Available from: https://www.aihw.gov.au/reports/australias-health/australias-health-2018-in-brief/contents/all-is-not-equal.

44. Australian Law Reform Commission. Pathways to justice – inquiry into the incarceration rate of Aboriginal and Torres Strait Islander Peoples. 2017.

45. Australian Institute of Health and Welfare. Indigenous Australians and the health system. July 7, 2022. [Accessed 10 July 2022.] Available from: https://www.aihw.gov.au/reports/australias-health/indigenous-australians-use-of-health-services.

46. Office of the Aboriginal and Torres Strait Islander Social Justice Commissioner. Indigenous deaths in custody 1989-1996. 1996. [Accessed 2 November 2020.] Available from: https://humanrights.gov.au/our-work/aboriginal-and-torres-strait-islander-social-justice/publications/indigenous-deaths.

47. Colquhoun SM, Condon JR, Steer AC, Li SQ, Guthridge S, Carapetis JR. Disparity in mortality from rheumatic heart disease in Indigenous Australians. J Am Heart Assoc. 2015;4(7). doi:10.1161/JAHA.114.001282

48. Grant E. Approaches to the design and provision of prison accommodation and facilities for Australian Indigenous prisoners after the royal commission into Aboriginal deaths in custody. Australian Indigenous Law Review. 2013;17(1): 47-55. [Accessed 7 November 2020.] Available from: http://www.austlii.edu.au/au/journals/AUIndigLawRw/2013/4.pdf.

49. Gregory V. Infection, prevention and control and Aboriginal and Torres Strait Islander people. IPCCA. [Accessed 7 November 2020.] Available from: https://ipcca.com.au/tag/infection-control/.

50. Kendall S, Lighton S, Sherwood J, Baldry E, Sullivan EA, Sullivan EA. Incarcerated Aboriginal women's experiences of accessing healthcare and the limitations of the "equal treatment" principle. Int J Equity Health. 2020;19(1). doi:10.1186/s12939-020-1155-3

51. Commission HR and EO. Achieving Aboriginal and Torres Strait Islander health equality within a generation – a human rights based approach, 2005. [Accessed 7 November 2020.] Available from: https://humanrights.gov.au/our-work/publications/achieving-aboriginal-and-torres-strait-islander-health-equality-within.

52. Australian Commission on Safety and Quality in Health Care. NSQHS Standards User guide for Aboriginal and Torres Strait Islander health, 2017. [Accessed 8 July 2022.] Available from: https://www.safetyandquality.gov.au/publications-and-resources/resource-library/nsqhs-standards-user-guide-aboriginal-and-torres-strait-islander-health.

53. Halacas C, Adams K. Keeping our mob healthy in and out of prison: exploring prison health in Victoria to improve

quality, culturally appropriate health care for Aboriginal people. 2015. [Accessed 7 November 2020.] Available from: www.vaccho.org.au.

54. Sivak L, Cantley L, Kelly J, Reilly R, Hawke K, Mott K, et al. South Australian Prison Health Service. Model of care for Aboriginal prisoner health and wellbeing for South Australia. Wardliparingga Aboriginal Health Research Unit: SAHMRI, 2017. [Accessed 25 July 2022.] Available from: https://www.sahealth.sa.gov.au/wps/wcm/connect/ d9e831ff-6332-4cc7-95c2-0e3d8e282315/SA+Prison+ Health+Service+MOC+for+Aboriginal+prisoner+ health+and+wellbeing+for+SA.pdf?MOD= AJPERES&CACHEID=ROOTWORKSPACE- d9e831ff-6332-4cc7-95c2-0e3d8e282315-nwLA0VA.

55. Considine J, Currey J. Ensuring a proactive, evidence-based, patient safety approach to patient assessment. J Clin Nurs. 2015;24(1-2):300-307. doi:10.1111/jocn.12641

56. Krogsbøll LT, Jørgensen KJ, Gøtzsche PC. General health checks in adults for reducing morbidity and mortality from disease. (Review). Cochrane Database Syst Rev. 2019; 1(1):CD009009. doi:10.1002/14651858.CD009009.pub3

57. Hinde S, Bojke L, Richardson G, Retat L, Webber L. The cost-effectiveness of population health checks: have the NHS health checks been unfairly maligned? J Public Health (Germany). 2017;25(4):425-431. doi:10.1007/s10389-017-0801-8

58. Kinner SA, Young JT. Understanding and improving the health of people who experience incarceration: an overview and synthesis. Epidemiol Rev. 2018;40(1):4-11. doi:10.1093/ epirev/mxx018

59. Australian Commission on Safety and Quality in Health Care. Communicating for Safety. National Safety and Quality Health Service Standards. 2022. [Accessed 23 July 2022.] Available from: https://www.safetyandquality.gov.au/ standards/nsqhs-standards/communicating-safety-standard.

60. Udoka Nwosu B, Maranda L, Berry R, et al. The vitamin D status of prison inmates. Slominski AT, ed. PLoS ONE. 2014;9(3):e90623. doi:10.1371/journal.pone.0090623

61. Alwarawrah Y, Kiernan K, MacIver NJ. Changes in nutritional status impact immune cell metabolism and function. Front Immunol. 2018;9:1055. doi:10.3389/ fimmu.2018.01055

62. Niki M, Yoshiyama T, Nagai H, et al. Nutritional status positively impacts humoral immunity against its Mycobacterium tuberculosis, disease progression, and vaccine development. Quinn F, ed. PLoS ONE. 2020; 15(8):e0237062. doi:10.1371/journal.pone.0237062

63. Katona P, Katona-Apte J. The interaction between nutrition and infection. Clin Infect Dis.2008;46(10):1582-1588. doi:10.1086/587658

64. Flight H, Marsden J, Creaney S. Crime and nourishment – the link between food and offending behaviour. The Conversation. September 28, 2018. [Accessed 10 July 2022.] Available from: https://theconversation.com/crime-and- nourishment-the-link-between-food-and-offending- behaviour-102791.

65. Calder PC, Carr AC, Gombart AF, Eggersdorfer M. Optimal nutritional status for a well-functioning immune system is an important factor to protect against viral infections. Nutrients. 2020;12(4):1181. doi:10.3390/nu12041181

66. Katona P, Katona-Apte J. The interaction between nutrition and infection. Clin Infect Dis. 2008;46(10):1582-1588. doi:10.1086/587658/2/46-10-1582-FIG004.GIF

67. Crook MA, Hally V, Panteli JV. The importance of the refeeding syndrome. Nutrition. 2001;17(7-8):632-637. doi:10.1016/S0899-9007(01)00542-1

68. Aubry E, Friedli N, Schuetz P, Stanga Z. Refeeding syndrome in the frail elderly population: prevention,

diagnosis and management. Clin Exp Gastroenterol. 2018;11:255-264. doi:10.2147/CEG.S136429

69. Reber E, Friedli N, Vasiloglou MF, Schuetz P, Stanga Z. Management of refeeding syndrome in medical inpatients. J Clin Med. 2019, Vol 8, Page 2202. 2019;8(12):2202. doi:10.3390/JCM8122202

70. Siegelaar SE, Holleman F, Hoekstra JBL, DeVries JH. Glucose variability; does it matter? Endocrine Rev. 2010;31(2):171-182. doi:10.1210/er.2009-0021

71. Calder PC, Dimitriadis G, Newsholme P. Glucose metabolism in lymphoid and inflammatory cells and tissues. Curr Opin Clin Nutr Metab Care. 2007;10(4):531-540. doi:10.1097/MCO.0b013e3281e72ad4

72. Muller LMAJAJ, Gorter KJ, Hak E, et al. Increased risk of common infections in patients with type 1 and type 2 diabetes mellitus. Clin Infect Dis. 2005;41(3):281-288. doi:10.1086/431587

73. Atamna A, Ayada G, Akirov A, Shochat T, Bishara J, Elis A. High blood glucose variability is associated with bacteremia and mortality in patients hospitalized with acute infection. QJM. 2019;112(2):101-106. doi:10.1093/qjmed/hcy235

74. Ismail N, Lazaris A, O'Moore É, Plugge E, Stürup-Toft S. Leaving no one behind in prison: improving the health of people in prison as a key contributor to meeting the sustainable development goals 2030. BMJ Glob Health. 2021;6(3):e004252. doi:10.1136/bmjgh-2020-004252

75. Leach B, Goodwin S. Preventing malnutrition in prison. Nursing Standard. 2014;28(20):50-56. doi:10.7748/ ns2014.01.28.20.50.e7900

76. Hannan-Jones M, Capra S. What do prisoners eat? Nutrient intakes and food practices in a high-secure prison. Br J Nutr. 2016;115(8):1387-1396. doi:10.1017/S000711451600026X

77. Reber E, Gomes F, Vasiloglou MF, Schuetz P, Stanga Z. Nutritional risk screening and assessment. J Clin Med. 2019;8(7). doi:10.3390/JCM8071065

78. Leach B, Goodwin S. Preventing malnutrition in prison. Nurs Stand. 2014;28(20):50-56. doi:10.7748/ns2014.01. 28.20.50.e7900

79. Queensland Health - Nutrition Support Group. Validated malnutrition screening and assessment tools: comparison guide. May 2017. [Accessed 10 July 2022.] Available from: http://www.health.qld.gov.au/masters/copyright.asp.

80. National Institute for Health and Care Excellence (NICE). Physical health of people in prison. NICE Guideline [NG57] (online). November 2, 2016. [Accessed 31 July 2022.] Available from: https://www.nice.org.uk/guidance/ng57/ chapter/Recommendations#managing-deteriorating-health- and-health-emergencies.

81. Australian Government, Australian Institute of Health and Welfare. Medication use by Australia's prisoners 2015: how is it different from the general community? AIHW, 2016.

82. Hassan L, Weston J, Senior J, Shaw J. Prisoners holding their own medications during imprisonment in England and Wales: a survey and qualitative exploration of staff and prisoners' views. Criminal Behaviour and Mental Health. 2012;22(1):29-40. doi:10.1002/cbm.822

83. Australian Government, Australian Institute of Health and Welfare. The health of Australia's prisoners 2018. AIHW; 2019. doi:10.25816/5ec5c381ed17a

84. Ax RK, Fagan TJ, Magaletta PR, Morgan RD, Nussbaum D, White TW. Innovations in correctional assessment and treatment. Criminal Justice and Behavior. 2007;34(7): 893-905. doi:10.1177/0093854807301555

85. Mateo M, Álvarez R, Cobo C, Pallas J, Lopez A, Gaite L. Telemedicine: contributions, difficulties and key factors for implementation in the prison setting. Revista Española de Sanidad Penitenciaria. 2019;21(2):95-105. [Accessed

2 November 2020.] Available from: http://scielo.isciii.es/scielo.php?script=sci_arttext&pid=S1575-06202019000200095&lng=en&nrm=iso.

86. Neuhaus M, Langbecker D, Caffery LJ, et al. Telementoring for hepatitis C treatment in correctional facilities. J Telemed Telecare. 2018;24(10):690-696. doi:10.1177/1357633X18795361

87. Edge C, Black G, King E, George J, Patel S, Hayward A. Improving care quality with prison telemedicine: the effects of context and multiplicity on successful implementation and use. J Telemed Telecare. 2021; 27(6):325-342. doi:10.1177/1357633X19869131

88. Edge C, George J, Black G, et al. Using telemedicine to improve access, cost and quality of secondary care for people in prison in England: a hybrid type 2 implementation effectiveness study. BMJ Open. 2020; 10(2). doi:10.1136/bmjopen-2019-035837

89. Edge C, Hayward A, Whitfield A, Hard J. COVID-19: digital equivalence of health care in English prisons. Lancet Digit Health. 2020;2(9):e450-e452. doi:10.1016/S2589-7500(20)30164-3

90. Aghdam MF, Vodovnik A, Hameed R. Role of telemedicine in multidisciplinary team meetings. J Pathol Inform. 2019; 10(1):35. doi:10.4103/jpi.jpi_20_19

91. National Health and Medical Research Council. Australian guidelines for the prevention and control of infection in healthcare. v11.11. National Health and Medical Research Council, 2022. Available from: https://www.nhmrc.gov.au/about-us/publications/australian-guidelines-prevention-and-control-infection-healthcare-2019#block-views-block-file-attachments-content-block-1.

92. Australasian Health Infrastructure Alliance. Australian health facility guidelines (AusHFG), 2016. [Accessed 10 July 2022.] Available from: https://www.healthfacilityguidelines.com.au/.

93. Grant E. Prison environments and the needs of Australian Aboriginal prisoners: a South Australian case study. Australian Indigenous Law Review. 2008;12(2):66-80. [Accessed 27 October 2020.] Available from: http://www.austlii.edu.au/au/journals/AILRev/2008/34.pdf.

94. Mackay A. Overcrowding in Australian prisons: the human rights implications. precedent (Australian Lawyers Alliance). 2015. [Accessed 5 November 2020.] Available from: http://classic.austlii.edu.au/au/journals/PrecedentAULA/2015/38.html.

95. Victorian Department of Justice. Victorian implementation review of the recommendations from the Royal Commission into Aboriginal deaths in custody. Indigenous Law Bulletin. 2006;6(16):17-20.

96. Semenza DC, Grosholz JM. Mental and physical health in prison: how co-occurring conditions influence inmate misconduct. Health and Justice. 2019;7(1):1. doi:10.1186/s40352-018-0082-5

97. Simpson PL, Butler TG. Covid-19, prison crowding, and release policies. BMJ. 2020;369. doi:10.1136/BMJ.M1551

98. Cloud DH, Drucker E, Browne A, Parsons J. Public health and solitary confinement in the United States. Am J Public Health. 2015;105(1):18-26. doi:10.2105/AJPH.2014.302205

99. Zyvoloski S. Impacts of and alternatives to solitary confinement in adult correctional facilities. Master of Social Work Clinical Research Papers. 2018:1-58. [Accessed 15 February 2021.] Available from: https://sophia.stkate.edu/msw_papers/841.

100. Liotta M. Lockdowns and restricted visits: COVID-19 and the prison population. RACGP / newsGP. May 14, 2020.

[Accessed 10 July 2022.] Available from: https://www1.racgp.org.au/newsgp/clinical/lockdowns-and-restricted-visitation-rights-covid-1.

101. Stewart A, Cossar R, Stoové M. The response to COVID-19 in prisons must consider the broader mental health impacts for people in prison. Aust NZ J Psychiatry. 2020;(0): 000486742093780. doi:10.1177/0004867420937806

102. Turabelidze G, Lin M, Wolkoff B, Dodson D, Gladbach S, Zhu BP. Personal hygiene and methicillin-resistant staphylococcus aureus infection. Emerg Infect Dis. 2006;12(3):422-427. doi:10.3201/eid1203.050625

103. Health Protection Agency and Department of Health – Offender Health. Prevention of infection and communicable disease control in prisons and places of detention: a manual for healthcare workers. 2011:1-138. [Accessed 6 November 2020.] Available from: https://www.gov.uk/government/publications/infection-control-in-prisons-and-places-of-detention.

104. Doyon S, Welsh C. Intoxication of a prison inmate with an ethyl alcohol–based hand sanitizer. N Eng J Med. 2007;356(5):529-530. doi:10.1056/NEJMc063110

105. Hand Hygiene Australia. Alcohol-based handrubs. [Accessed 10 July 2022.] Available from: https://www.hha.org.au/hand-hygiene/alcohol-based-handrubs.

106. Schoenly L. Hand hygiene challenges for correctional nurses. CorrectionalNurse.Net. [Accessed 10 July 2022.] Available from: https://correctionalnurse.net/hand-hygiene-challenges-for-correctional-nurses/.

107. Bloomfield SF, Aiello AE, Cookson B, O'Boyle C, Larson EL. The effectiveness of hand hygiene procedures in reducing the risks of infections in home and community settings including handwashing and alcohol-based hand sanitizers. Am J Infect Control. 2007;35(10):S27-S64. doi:10.1016/j.ajic.2007.07.001

108. Australian Commission on Safety and Quality in Health Care. Environmental cleaning and infection prevention and control. ACSQHC, 2020. [Accessed 3 November 2020.] Available from: https://www.safetyandquality.gov.au/our-work/infection-prevention-and-control/environmental-cleaning-and-infection-prevention-and-control.

109. Mitchell BG, McGhie A, Whiteley G, et al. Evaluating bioburden of frequently touched surfaces using Adenosine Triphosphate bioluminescence (ATP): results from the researching effective approaches to cleaning in hospitals (REACH) trial. Infect Dis Health. 2020;25(3):168-174. doi:10.1016/j.idh.2020.02.001.

110. Sehulster L, Chinn RYW, CDC, HICPAC. Guidelines for environmental infection control in health-care facilities. Recommendations of CDC and the Healthcare Infection Control Practices Advisory Committee (HICPAC) (Updated 2019). MMWR Recomm Rep. 2003;52(RR-10):1-42. [Accessed 7 November 2020.] Available from: https://www.cdc.gov/infectioncontrol/guidelines/environmental/index.html.

111. White NM, Barnett AG, Hall L, et al. Cost-effectiveness of an environmental cleaning bundle for reducing healthcare-associated infections. Clin Infect Dis.2020;70(12). doi:10.1093/cid/ciz717

112. Wei J, Li Y. Airborne spread of infectious agents in the indoor environment. Am J Infect Control. 2016;44(9):S102-S108. doi:10.1016/j.ajic.2016.06.003

113. Li Y, Leung GM, Tang JW, et al. Role of ventilation in airborne transmission of infectious agents in the built environment - a multidisciplinary systematic review. Indoor Air. 2007;17(1):2-18. doi:10.1111/j.1600-0668.2006.00445.x

114. Correia G, Rodrigues L, Gameiro da Silva M, Gonçalves T. Airborne route and bad use of ventilation systems as non-

negligible factors in SARS-CoV-2 transmission. Medical Hypotheses. 2020;141:109781. doi:10.1016/j.mehy.2020.109781

115. Qian H, Zheng X. Ventilation control for airborne transmission of human exhaled bio-aerosols in buildings. J Thorac Dis. 2018; 10(Suppl 19):S2295-S2304. doi:10.21037/jtd.2018.01.24

116. Atkinson J, Chartier Y, Lúcia Pessoa-Silva C, et al. Natural ventilation for infection control in health-care settings. Geneva: World Health Organization. 2016. [Accessed 7 November 2020.] Available from: http://www.who.int/water_sanitation_health/publications/natural_ventilation/en/.

117. Walser SM, Gerstner DG, Brenner B, Höller C, Liebl B, Herr CEW. Assessing the environmental health relevance of cooling towers - a systematic review of legionellosis outbreaks. Int J Hyg Environ Health. 2014;217(2-3): 145-154. doi:10.1016/j.ijheh.2013.08.002

118. Luongo JC, Fennelly KP, Keen JA, Zhai ZJ, Jones BW, Miller SL. Role of mechanical ventilation in the airborne transmission of infectious agents in buildings. Indoor Air. 2016;26(5). doi:10.1111/ina.12267

119. Bouchama A, Aziz MA, Mahri S, et al. A model of exposure to extreme environmental heat uncovers the human transcriptome to heat stress. Scientific Reports. 2017;7(1):9429. doi:10.1038/s41598-017-09819-5

120. Nagai M, Iriki M. Changes in immune activities by heat stress. In: Thermotherapy for neoplasia, inflammation, and pain. Springer Japan, 2001:266-270. doi:10.1007/978-4-431-67035-3_30

121. Grant E, Williamson T, Hansen A, Williamson T. Design issues for prisoner health: thermal conditions in Australian custodial environments. World Health Design. 2012;(July):80-85. [Accessed 18 July 2022.] Available from: https://www.academia.edu/31214904/_Design_issues_for_prisoner_health_Thermal_conditions_in_Australian_custodial_environments.

122. Prisons and Probation Ombudsman. Independent investigation into the death of Mr Rafal Sochacki at Westminster Magistrates Court on 21 June 2017; 2019. [Accessed 18 July 2022.] Available from: https://s3-eu-west-2.amazonaws.com/ppo-prod-storage-1g9rkhjhkjmgw/uploads/2019/07/F3196-17-Death-of-Mr-Rafal-Sochacki-WestminsterMagCourt-21-06-2017-NC-41-50-43.pdf.

123. Watterson R. Inquiry into transportation of detained persons. 2010. Available from: https://www.parliament.wa.gov.au/parliament/commit.nsf/(Evidence+Lookup+by+Com+ID)/D8A1080A011A42E2482578310040D26F/$file/ev.tdp.100514.Ray+Watterson.sub14.d.doc.pdf.

124. Holt D. Heat in US prisons and jails; corrections and the challenge of climate change. Columbia University; 2015. [Accessed 18 July 2022.] Available from: https://web.law.columbia.edu/sites/default/files/microsites/climate-change/holt_-_heat_in_us_prisons_and_jails.pdf.

125. Office of the Inspector of Custodial Services. Thermal conditions of prison cells; 2015. [Accessed 18 July 2022.] Available from: www.oics.wa.gov.au.

126. Epstein Y, Roberts WO, Golan R, Heled Y, Sorkine P, Halpern P. Sepsis, septic shock, and fatal exertional heat stroke. Current Sports Medicine Reports. 2015;14(1):64-69. doi:10.1249/JSR.0000000000000112

127. Uffen JW, Oosterheert JJ, Schweitzer VA, Thursky K, Kaasjager HAH, Ekkelenkamp MB. Interventions for rapid recognition and treatment of sepsis in the emergency department: a narrative review. Clin Microbiol Infect. 2021:27(2) 192-203. doi:10.1016/j.cmi.2020.02.022

128. Chertoff J, Stevenson P, Alnuaimat H. Sepsis outcomes in the correctional system: more potential disparity. Lancet. 2017; 390:25. doi:10.1016/S0140-6736(17)31475-7

129. Chertoff J, Stevenson P, Alnuaimat H. Sepsis mortality in the U.S. correctional system: an underappreciated disparity. J Correct Health Care. 2018;24(4):337-341. doi:10.1177/1078345818792235

130. Australian Government Communicable Diseases Network Australia. CDNA National guidelines for COVID-19 outbreaks in correctional and detention facilities V5; 2022. [Accessed 10 July 2022.] Available from: https://www.health.gov.au/resources/publications/cdna-national-guidelines-for-covid-19-outbreaks-in-correctional-and-detention-facilities.

131. Harvey M. Living conditions of life in prisons. Probation Journal. 2018;65(1):101-102. doi:10.1177/0264550518756527

132. Jewkes Y. Just design: healthy prisons and the architecture of hope. Aust NZ J Criminol. 2018;51(3):319-338. doi:10.1177/0004865818766768

133. López M, Maiello-Reidy L. Prisons and the mentally ill: why design matters. 2017. [Accessed 7 November 2020.] Available from: https://cdn.penalreform.org/wp-content/uploads/2017/06/Prisons-and-the-mentally-ill-why-design-matters-4.pdf.

134. Australian Government, Australian Institute of Health and Welfare. Disease expenditure in Australia, Summary. AIHW, 2019.

135. Reddon JR, Durante SB. Prisoner exposure to nature: benefits for wellbeing and citizenship. Medical Hypotheses. 2019;123:13-18. doi:10.1016/j.mehy.2018.12.003

136. Walsh T, Counter A. Deaths in custody in Australia: a quantitative analysis of coroners' reports. Current Issues in Criminal Justice. 2019;31(2):143-163. doi:10.1080/10345329.2019.1603831

137. Whitehead D. The health promoting prison (HPP) and its imperative for nursing. Int J Nurs Studies. 2006;43(1): 123-131. doi:10.1016/j.ijnurstu.2004.11.008

138. Fries CJ. Healing health care: from sick care towards salutogenic healing systems. Soc Theory Health. 2020;18(1):16-32. doi:10.1057/s41285-019-00103-2

139. Grant E, Hobbs P. West Kimberley regional prison. Architecture Australia. 2013. [Accessed 2 November 2020.] Available from: https://architectureau.com/articles/west-kimberley-regional-prison/.

140. NBRS Architecture. Australia's largest prison: focusing on health and rehabilitation. NBRS Architecture, News. September 4, 2021. Available from: https://nbrs.com.au/ /australias-largest-prison-focusing-on-health-and-rehabilitation.

141. Olmsted RN. Prevention by design: construction and renovation of health care facilities for patient safety and infection prevention. Infect Dis Clin North Am. 2016;30(3): 713-728. doi:10.1016/J.IDC.2016.04.005.

142. Dhaliwal KK, Hirst SP, King-Shier KM, Kent-Wilkinson A. The implementation of correctional nursing practice–caring behind bars: a grounded theory study. J Adv Nurs. 2021; 77(5):2407-2416. doi:10.1111/jan.14772

143. Mathis H, Schoenly L. Healthcare behind bars: what you need to know. Nurse Pract. 2008;33(5):34-41. doi:10.1097/01.NPR.0000317487.35167.C7

144. Gerber L. An inside look at correctional health nursing. Nursing (Brux). 2012;42(4):52-56. doi:10.1097/01.NURSE.0000412925.82265.8d

145. Barbosa ML, Medeiros SG de, Chiavone FBT, Atanásio LL de M, Costa GMC, Santos VEP. Nursing actions for liberty deprived people: a scoping review. Escola Anna Nery. 2019;23(3). doi:10.1590/2177-9465-ean-2019-0098

146. Kelly C, Templeton M, Allen K, Lohan M. Improving sexual healthcare delivery for men in prison: a nurse-led initiative. J Clin Nurs. 2020;29(13-14):2285-2292. doi:10.1111/jocn.15237.

147. Condon L, Gill H, Harris F. A review of prison health and its implications for primary care nursing in England and Wales: the research evidence. J Clin Nurs. 2007;16(7): 1201-1209. doi:10.1111/j.1365-2702.2007.01799.x

148. Schoenly L. Context of correctional nursing. In: Schoenly L, Knox C, eds. Essentials of Correctional Nursing. 1st ed. Springer, 2013:1-18.

149. Wong I, Wright E, Santomauro D, How R, Leary C, Harris M. Implementing two nurse practitioner models of service at an Australian male prison: a quality assurance study. J Clin Nurs. 2018;27(1-2):e287-e300. doi:10.1111/jocn.13935

150. Schoenwald A, Ponting B, How R, Mansfield Y, Meehan T. Consultation with nurse practitioners over the telephone in prison health. J Nurs Practitioner. 2022;18(3):305-309. doi:10.1016/J.NURPRA.2021.12.011

151. Department for Correctional Services. Department for Correctional Services - Aboriginal Liaison Officers. [Accessed 7 November 2020.] Available from: https://www.corrections.sa.gov.au/aboriginal-services/aboriginal-liaison-officers.

152. Bagnall AM, South J, Hulme C, et al. A systematic review of the effectiveness and cost-effectiveness of peer education and peer support in prisons. BMC Public Health. 2015;15(1):290. doi:10.1186/s12889-015-1584-x

153. South J, Bagnall AM, Woodall J. Developing a typology for peer education and peer support delivered by prisoners. J Correctional Health Care. 2017;23(2):214-229. doi:10.1177/1078345817700602

154. Rachael E. Infection prevention and control in dental practice. Int Dent J. 2020;70(1):17-18. doi:10.1111/idj.12557

155. Australian Dental Association. Guidelines for infection control. 4th ed. ADA, 2021. Available from: https://www.ada.org.au/Dental-Professionals/Publications/Infection-Control/Guidelines-for-Infection-Control/Guidelines-for-Infection-Control-V4.aspx.

156. Upendran A, Gupta R, Geiger Z. Dental infection control. StatPearls. August 13, 2020. [Accessed 7 November 2020.] Available from: https://www.ncbi.nlm.nih.gov/books/NBK470356/.

157. Smith AJ, Creanor S, Hurrell DJ. Survey of instrument decontamination in dental surgeries located in Scottish prisons. Am J Infect Control. 2009;37(8):689-690. doi:10.1016/j.ajic.2009.04.282

158. Anno BJ. Correctional healthcare guidelines for the management of an adequate delivery system. (Dubler NN, Faiver K, Harrison B, et al., eds.). US Department of Justice, National Institute of Corrections, 2001. [Accessed 2 November 2020.] Available from: https://nicic.gov/correctional-health-care-guidelines-management-adequate-delivery-system.

159. Hampton S, Abbott P, Turnbull T, Levy M, Lagios K. RACGP Custodial health in Australia tips for providing healthcare to people in prison. Royal Australian College of General Practitioners, 2019. [Accessed 2 November 2020.] Available from: https://www.racgp.org.au/FSDEDEV/media/documents/Faculties/SI/Custodial-health-in-Australia.pdf.

160. Australian Commission on Safety and Quality in Health Care. Partnering with consumers standard. National Safety and Quality (NSQHS) Standards. [Accessed 31 July 2022.] Available from: https://www.safetyandquality.gov.au/standards/nsqhs-standards/partnering-consumers-standard.

161. Australian Commission on Safety and Quality in Health Care. Environmental cleaning and infection prevention and control. ACSQHC, 2020. [Accessed 27 October 2020.] Available from: https://www.safetyandquality.gov.au/our-work/infection-prevention-and-control/environmental-cleaning-and-infection-prevention-and-control.

162. Bartosik K, Tytuła A, Zając Z, et al. Scabies and pediculosis in penitentiary institutions in poland—a study of ectoparasitoses in confinement conditions. Int J Environ Res Public Health. 2020;17(17):6086. doi:10.3390/ijerph17176086

163. National Health and Medical Research Council. Australian guidelines for the prevention and control of infection in healthcare. 2019:1-363. [Accessed 2 November 2020.] Available from: https://www.nhmrc.gov.au/about-us/publications/australian-guidelines-prevention-and-control-infection-healthcare-2019.

164. David MZ, Siegel JD, Henderson J, et al. A randomized, controlled trial of chlorhexidine-soaked cloths to reduce methicillin-resistant and methicillin-susceptible staphylococcus aureus carriage prevalence in an urban jail. Infect Control Hosp Epidemiol. 2014;35(12):1466-1473. doi:10.1086/678606

165. Kinner SA, Jenkinson R, Gouillou M, Milloy MJ. High-risk drug-use practices among a large sample of Australian prisoners. Drug and Alcohol Dependence. 2012;126(1-2): 156-160. doi:10.1016/j.drugalcdep.2012.05.008

166. Spaulding AC, Adee MG, Lawrence RT, Chhatwal J, von Oehsen W. Five questions concerning managing hepatitis C in the justice system: finding practical solutions for hepatitis C virus elimination. Infect Dis Clin North Am. 2018;32(2):323-345. doi:10.1016/j.idc.2018.02.014

167. Kinner SA, Snow K, Wirtz AL, Altice FL, Beyrer C, Dolan K. Age-specific global prevalence of hepatitis B, hepatitis C, HIV, and tuberculosis among incarcerated people: a systematic review. J Adolescent Health. 2018;62(3):S18-S26. doi:10.1016/j.jadohealth.2017.09.030

168. World Health Organization. Fact Sheet: Sexually transmitted infections (STIs). Geneva: WHO, 2021. [Accessed 20 July 2022.] Available from: https://www.who.int/news-room/fact-sheets/detail/sexually-transmitted-infections-(stis).

169. Deloitte Access Economics. Review of the implementation of the recommendations of the Royal Commission into Aboriginal deaths in custody. Department of the Prime Minister and Cabinet, 2018. [Accessed 2 November 2020.] Available from: https://www.niaa.gov.au/sites/default/files/publications/rciadic-review-report.pdf.

170. Australian Government, Australian Institute of Health and Welfare. Profile of Indigenous Australians (Snapshot). AIHW, 2021. [Accessed 3 February 2021.] Available from: https://www.aihw.gov.au/reports/australias-welfare/profile-of-indigenous-australians.

171. Coalition of Aboriginal and Torres Strait Islander Peak Organisations, Australian Governments. National agreement on closing the gap. 2020. [Accessed 25 July 2022.] Available from: https://www.closingthegap.gov.au/.

172. Winter RJ, White B, Kinner SA, Stoové M, Guy R, Hellard ME. A nurse-led intervention improved blood-borne virus testing and vaccination in Victorian prisons. Aust NZ J Public Health. 2016;40(6):592-594. doi:10.1111/1753-6405.12578

173. Tawse A, Tabesh P. Strategy implementation: a review and an introductory framework. European Management Journal. 2021;39(1):22-33. doi:10.1016/j.emj.2020.09.005

174. The Kirby Institute, UNSW Sydney. The Kirby Institute. [Accessed 25 July 2022.] Available from: https://kirby.unsw.edu.au/.

175. Hepatitis Australia. Hepatitis Australia. [Accessed 25 July 2022.] Available from: https://www.hepatitisaustralia.com/.

176. Australasian Society for HIV Medicine. ASHM. [Accessed 25 July 2022.] Available from: https://ashm.org.au/.

177. Australian Federation of AIDS Organisations. [Accessed 25 July 2022.] Available from: https://www.afao.org.au/.

178. National Association of People with HIV Australia. [Accessed 25 July 2022.] Available from: https://napwha.org.au/.

179. Australian Injecting and Illicit Drug Users League (AIVL). [Accessed 25 July 2022.] Available from: https://aivl.org.au/.

180. Aboriginal Health Council of South Australia. Sexual Health and BBV. [Accessed 25 July 2022.] Available from: https://ahcsa.org.au/our-programs/sh-and-bbv.

181. Edith Cowan University, Australian Indigenous HealthInfoNet. Australian Indigenous HealthInfoNet. [Accessed 25 July 2022.] Available from: https://healthinfonet.ecu.edu.au/.

182. Hepatitis Australia. Renewed calls for needle and syringe programs in prisons ahead of International Drug Users Day, Hepatitis Australia. Media releases. 2020. [Accessed 10 November 2020.] Available from: https://www.hepatitisaustralia.com/news/renewed-calls-for-needle-syringe-programs-in-prisons-ahead-of-international-drug-users-day.

183. Moazen B, Saeedi Moghaddam S, Silbernagl MA, et al. Prevalence of drug injection, sexual activity, tattooing, and piercing among prison inmates. Epidemiol Rev. 2018;40(1): 58-69. doi:10.1093/EPIREV/MXY002

184. Hellard ME, Aitken CK, Hocking JS. Tattooing in prisons—not such a pretty picture. Am J Infect Control. 2007;35(7):477-480. doi:10.1016/j.ajic.2006.08.002

185. Kinder S. Ethical justice: needle and syringe programs in Australian prisons. Insight+. April 27, 2020. [Accessed 10 November 2020.] Available from: https://insightplus.mja.com.au/2020/16/ethical-justice-needle-and-syringe-programs-in-australian-prisons/.

186. Lazarus JV, Safreed-Harmon K, Hetherington KL, Bromberg D, Ocampo D, Graf N, et al. Health outcomes for clients of needle and syringe programs in prisons. Epidemiol Rev. 2018;40(1):96-104. doi:10.1093/epirev/mxx019

187. Mogg D, Levy M. Moving beyond non-engagement on regulated needle-syringe exchange programs in Australian prisons. Harm Reduction Journal. 2009;6(1):7. doi:10.1186/1477-7517-6-7

188. Stöver H, Hariga F. Prison-based needle and syringe programmes (PNSP) – still highly controversial after all these years. Drugs: Education, Prevention and Policy. 2016; 23(2):103-112. doi:10.3109/09687637.2016.1148117

189. Dolan K, Lowe D, Shearer J. Evaluation of the condom distribution program in New South Wales prisons, Australia. Journal of Law, Medicine and Ethics. 2004;32(1):124-128. doi:10.1111/j.1748-720X.2004.tb00457.x

190. Moazen B, Owusu PN, Wiessner P, Stöver H. Availability, coverage and barriers towards condom provision in prisons: a review of the evidence, 2019.

191. Moazen B, Mauti J, Meireles P, et al. Principles of condom provision programs in prisons from the standpoint of European prison health experts: a qualitative study. Harm Reduction Journal. 2021;18(1):1-8. doi:10.1186/S12954-021-00462-Y/METRICS

192. Yap L, Butler T, Richters J, et al. Do condoms cause rape and mayhem? The long-term effects of condoms in New South Wales' prisons. Sex Transm Infect. 2007;83(3):219-222. doi:10.1136/sti.2006.022996

193. van den Bergh B, Gatherer A, Atabay T, Hariga F. Women's health in prison action guidance and checklists to review current policies and practices. 2011. [Accessed 23 July 2022.] Available from: https://www.unodc.org/documents/hiv-aids/WHO_UNODC_2011_Checklist_Womens_health_in_prison.pdf.

194. Zweig JM, Naser RL, Blackmore J, Schaffer M. Addressing sexual violence in prisons: a national snapshot of approaches and highlights of innovative strategies, final report, 2007. [Accessed 23 July 2022.] Available from: https://www.ojp.gov/pdffiles1/nij/grants/216856.pdf.

195. National Prison Rape Elimination Commission. Standards for the prevention, detection, response, and monitoring of sexual abuse in adult prisons and jails, (including supplemental standards for facilities with immigration detainees). Walton RB (Chair) ed, 2009. [Accessed 25 July 2022.] Available from: https://www.ojp.gov/pdffiles1/226682.pdf.

196. Ministerial Council on Drug Strategy. National Drug Strategy 2017-2026; 2017. [Accessed 4 December 2020.] Available from: http://www.nationaldrugstrategy.gov.au.

197. Resiak D, Mpofu E, Rothwell R. Harm minimisation drug policy implementation qualities: their efficacy with Australian needle and syringe program providers and people who inject drugs. Healthcare. 2022;10(5):781. doi:10.3390/healthcare10050781

198. Australian Technical Advisory Group on Immunisation (ATAGI). The Australian immunisation handbook. (Online). (ATAGI, ed.). Australian Government Department of Health and Aged Care, 2022. [Accessed 23 July 2022.] Available from: https://immunisationhandbook.health.gov.au/.

199. Infection Prevention Australia, Bibby M. Infection prevention and control review, Port Phillip Prison. COVID-19 risk assessment and compliance report. 2020. [Accessed 10 November 2020.] Available from: https://www.parliament.vic.gov.au/images/stories/committees/paec/COVID-19_Inquiry/Questions_on_Notice/Independent_Final_Port_Phillip_Prison_IC_Review_May_2020.pdf.

200. National Institute for Health and Care Excellence. Physical health of people in prisons (NICE Quality standard). September 7, 2017. [Accessed 23 July 2022.] Available from: www.nice.org.uk/guidance/qs156.

201. Australian Commission on Safety and Quality in Health Care. Partnering with Consumers Standard. (online). ACSQHC, 2022. [Accessed 23 July 2022.] Available from: https://www.safetyandquality.gov.au/standards/nsqhs-standards/partnering-consumers-standard.

202. Ross MW. Pedagogy for prisoners: an approach to peer health education for inmates. J Correctional Health Care. 2011;17(1):6-18. doi:10.1177/1078345810378251

203. ACT Inspector of Correctional Services. Australian responses to COVID-19 in prisons - briefing note. August 25, 2020. [Accessed 2 November 2020.] Available from: https://www.ics.act.gov.au/__data/assets/pdf_file/0004/1618429/Australian-responses_web-version11.pdf.

204. Burki T. Prisons are "in no way equipped" to deal with COVID-19. Lancet. 2020;395(10234):1411-1412. doi:10.1016/S0140-6736(20)30984-3

205. Clun R. Coronavirus Australia: how COVID-19 is being kept out of NSW prisons. The Sydney Morning Herald [online]. Available from: https://www.smh.com.au/national/nsw/the-people-keeping-covid-19-out-of-prison-20200515-p54tg6.html. May 22, 2020. [Accessed 10 November 2020].

206. Shepherd S, Spivak BL. Reconsidering the immediate release of prisoners during COVID-19 community restrictions. MJA.2020;213(2):58-59.e1. doi:10.5694/mja2.50672

207. World Health Organization - Regional Office for Europe. Preparedness, prevention and control of COVID-19 in prisons and other places of detention: interim guidance, 8 February 2021. Copenhagen; WHO, 2021. [Accessed 25 July 2022.] Available from: https://apps.who.int/iris/bitstream/handle/10665/339830/WHO-EURO-2021-1405-41155-57257-eng.pdf?sequence=1&isAllowed=y.

208. Antolak-Saper N. COVID-19 and prisoners: the Australian experience of early release. Oxford Law Faculty. University

of Oxford, Faculty of Law Blogs. June 17, 2020. [Accessed 25 July 2022.] Available from: https://www.law.ox.ac.uk/centres-institutes/centre-criminology/blog/2020/06/covid-19-and-prisoners-australian-experience.

209. Gray R, LLoyd A, Kwon A. Modelling the spread of COVID-19 in NSW prisons, UNSW - The Kirby Institute for infection and immunity in society. UNSW, The Kirby Institute, 2020. [Accessed 25 July 2022.] Available from: https://kirby.unsw.edu.au/project/modelling-spread-covid-19-nsw-prisons.

210. Currie BJ. Infectious diseases of tropical Australia. Medicine Today. 2000;1(3):71-81. [Accessed 10 November 2020.] Available from: https://medicinetoday.com.au/2000/march/feature-article/infectious-diseases-tropical-australia.

211. Kurcheid J, Gordon CA, Clarke NE, et al. Neglected tropical diseases in Australia: a narrative review. MJA. 2022;216(10): 532-538. doi:10.5694/MJA2.51533

212. Cheng A, Hanna J, Norton Robert, et al. Melioidosis in northern Australia, 2001-02. Commun Dis Intell Q Rep. 2003;27(2):272-277. [Accessed 24 July 2022.] Available from: https://www1.health.gov.au/internet/main/publishing.nsf/Content/cda-pubs-cdi-2003-cdi2702-htm-cdi2702n.htm.

213. Chakravorty A, Heath C. Melioidosis: an updated review. Aust J Gen Prac. 2019;48(5). doi:10.31128/AJGP-04-18-4558

214. Queensland Government, Queensland Health. Australian bat lyssavirus. Queensland Government, infections and parasites, viral infections, Australian bat lyssavirus (webpage). 2022. [Accessed 24 July 2022.] Available from: http://conditions.health.qld.gov.au/HealthCondition/condition/14/217/14/Bats-human-health.

215. Merritt T, Taylor K, Cox-Witton K, et al. Australian bat lyssavirus. Aust J Gen Pract. 2018;47(3):93-96. doi:10.31128/AFP-08-17-4314

216. World Health Organization. Leprosy - Fact Sheet. World Health Organization, Fact Sheets, Leprosy, 2022. Geneva: WHO, 2022. [Accessed 24 July 2022.] Available from: https://www.who.int/news-room/fact-sheets/detail/leprosy.

217. Davis J. Stigma, separation, sorrow: leprosy in Australia. Microbiol Aust. 2020;41(4). doi:10.1071/ma20051

218. Riley G. RACGP - Medical history: leprosy is a terror of the past. Right? newsGP; 2018. [Accessed 24 July 2022.] Available from: https://www1.racgp.org.au/newsgp/clinical/medical-history-leprosy-is-a-terror-of-the-past-ri.

219. Hempenstall A, Smith S, Hanson J. Leprosy in Far North Queensland: almost gone, but not to be forgotten. MJA. 2019;211(4):182-183. doi:10.5694/MJA2.50243

220. Leprosy Mission Australia. Do we have leprosy in Australia? The Leprosy Mission Australia, 2017. [Accessed 24 July 2022.] Available from: https://www.leprosymission.org.au/blog/post/do-we-have-leprosy-in-australia.

221. Government of Western Australia. Guidelines for the diagnosis, management and prevention of leprosy; 2019. [Accessed 31 July 2022.] Available from: https://ww2.health.wa.gov.au/,/media/Files/Corporate/general-documents/Leprosy/PDF/WATBCP-WA-Leprosy-Guideline.pdf.

222. Australian Institute of Health and Welfare. Acute rheumatic fever and rheumatic heart disease in Australia 2016–2020. AIHW, 2022. doi:10.25816/tcw7-ws78

223. RHD Australia (ARF / RHD writing group). The 2020 Australian for prevention, diagnosis and management of acute rheumatic and rheumatic disease (3.2 edition); RHD Australia, 2022. [Accessed 10 November 2020.] Available from: https://www.rhdaustralia.org.au/arf-rhd-guideline.

224. Royal Australian College of General Practitioners. Rheumatic fever - identification, management and secondary prevention. Aust Fam Physician. 2012;41(1). [Accessed 24 July 2022.] Available from: https://www.racgp.org.au/afp/2012/january-february/rheumatic-fever.

225. Brown A, McDonald MI, Calma T. Rheumatic fever and social justice. MJA. 2007;186(11):557-558. doi:10.5694/j.1326-5377.2007.tb01052.x

226. Katzenellenbogen JM, Bond-Smith D, Seth RJ, et al. Contemporary incidence and prevalence of rheumatic fever and rheumatic heart disease in Australia using linked data: the case for policy change. J Am Heart Assoc. 2020;9(19):e016851. doi:10.1161/JAHA.120.016851

227. Macleod CK, Bright P, Steer AC, Kim J, Mabey D, Parks T. Neglecting the neglected: the objective evidence of underfunding in rheumatic heart disease. Transactions of The Royal Society of Tropical Medicine and Hygiene. 2019;113(5):287-290. doi:10.1093/TRSTMH/TRZ014

228. RHD Australia, Menzies School of Health Research. RHD Australia (webpage). [Accessed 24 July 2022.] Available from: https://www.rhdaustralia.org.au/.

229. Beknazarova M, Whiley H, Judd J, et al. Argument for inclusion of Strongyloidiasis in the Australian national notifiable disease list. Trop Med Infect Dis. 2018;3(2):61. doi:10.3390/tropicalmed3020061

230. Page WA, Judd JA, MacLaren DJ, Buettner P. Integrating testing for chronic strongyloidiasis within the Indigenous adult preventive health assessment system in endemic communities in the Northern Territory, Australia: an intervention study. Krolewiecki AJ, ed. PLoS Neglected Trop Dis. 2020;14(5): e0008232. doi:10.1371/journal.pntd.0008232

231. Warren JM, Birrell AL. Trachoma in remote Indigenous Australia: a review and public health perspective. Aust NZ J Public Health. 2016. doi:10.1111/1753-6405.12396

232. Australian Government Department of Health and Aged Care. Addressing trachoma. Initiatives and programs. Australian Government. June 30, 2021. [Accessed 24 July 2022.] Available from: https://www.health.gov.au/initiatives-and-programs/addressing-trachoma.

233. Kirby Institute (UNSW Sydney). Australian trachoma surveillance report 2019, Kirby Institute, 2020. [Accessed 24 July 2022.] Available from: https://kirby.unsw.edu.au/report/australian-trachoma-surveillance-report-2019.

234. Australian Government, Department of Health and Aged Care. Trachoma – CDNA national guidelines for public health units. Australian Government, 2014. [Accessed 24 July 2022.] Available from: https://www.health.gov.au/resources/publications/trachoma-cdna-national-guidelines-for-public-health-units.

235. SAHMRI, Health Translation SA, Commission on Excellence and Innovation in Health. COVID-19 Evidence update, optimal methods of reducing spread in long term care facilities. SA Health and Medical Research Institute, 2020. [Accessed 6 November 2020.] Available from: https://www.sahmri.org/m/uploads/2020/05/18/long-term-care-covid-19-evidence-update-22-april-2020_18-may-2020.pdf.

236. Stewart C, Tomossy GF, Lamont S, Brunero S. COVID-19 and Australian prisons: human rights, risks, and responses. J Bioeth Inq. 2020 17:4. 2020;17(4):663-667. doi:10.1007/S11673-020-10054-3

237. United Nations Office on Drugs and Crime. COVID-19 Guidance note: mitigating the disruptive impact of infection prevention and control measures in prisons: core principles and recommendations. UNODC; 2021. [Accessed 24 July 2022.] Available from: https://www.unodc.org/res/justice-and-prison-reform/nelsonmandelarules-GoF_html/COVID_19_Guidance_Note_IPC_ebook.pdf.

238. Fast SM, González MC, Markuzon N. Cost-effective control of infectious disease outbreaks accounting for societal reaction. Bauch CT, ed. PLoS One. 2015;10(8):e0136059. doi:10.1371/journal.pone.0136059

239. Strong P. Epidemic psychology: a model. Sociol Health Illness 1990;12(3):249-259. doi:10.1111/1467-9566.ep11347150

240. Chiu LF, West RM. Health intervention in social context: understanding social networks and neighbourhood. Soc Sci Med. 2007;65(9):1915-1927. doi:10.1016/j.socscimed.2007.05.035

241. Victoria State Government. Delivering high-quality healthcare: Victorian clinical governance framework (Safer Care Victoria), 2017. [Accessed 1 December 2020.] Available from: https://www.safercare.vic.gov.au/sites/default/files/2018-03/SCV%20Clinical%20Governance%20Framework.pdf.

242. Brown A. Understanding corporate governance of healthcare quality: a comparative case study of eight Australian public hospitals. BMC Health Serv Res. 2019;19(1):725. doi:10.1186/s12913-019-4593-0

243. Hussein M, Pavlova M, Ghalwash M, Groot W. The impact of hospital accreditation on the quality of healthcare: a systematic literature review. BMC Health Serv Res. 2021;21(1):1057. doi:10.1186/s12913-021-07097-6

244. Australian Commission on Safety and Quality in Health Care. National Safety and Quality Health Service Standards. 2nd edition. ACSQHC, 2017. [Accessed 10 July 2022.] Available from: https://www.safetyandquality.gov.au/sites/default/files/migrated/National-Safety-and-Quality-Health-Service-Standards-second-edition.pdf.

245. Royal Australian College of General Practitioners. Infection prevention and control standards for general practices and other office-based and community-based practices (5th ed, updated 2016). RACGP, 2014. [Accessed 24 July 2022.] Available from: https://www.racgp.org.au/FSDEDEV/media/documents/Running%20a%20practice/Practice%20standards/Infection-prevention-and-control.pdf.

246. Australian Council on Healthcare Standards. ACHS, EQuIP6. [Accessed 1 November 2020.] Available from: https://www.achs.org.au/programs-services/equip6/.

247. Royal Australian College of General Practitioners. Standards for General Practices, 5th ed. RACGP, 2017. [Accessed 25 July 2022.] Available from: https://www.racgp.org.au/download/Documents/Standards/RACGP-Standards-for-general-practices-5th-edition.pdf.

248. Australian Commission on Safety and Quality in Health Care. NSQHS Standards Guide for multi-purpose services and small hospitals. ACSQHC, 2017. [Accessed 14 November 2020.] Available from: www.safetyandquality.gov.au.

249. Australian Commission on Safety and Quality in Health Care. Guide to the NSQHS standards for community health services. ACSQHC, 2016. [Accessed 15 February 2021.] Available from: http://www.safetyandquality.gov.au/wp-content/uploads/2016/03/Guide-to-the-NSQHS-Standards-for-community-health-services-February-2016.pdf.

250. Australian Commission on Safety and Quality in Health Care. National safety and quality primary and community healthcare standards. ACSQHC, 2021. [Accessed 24 July 2022.] Available from: https://www.safetyandquality.gov.au/publications-and-resources/resource-library/national-safety-and-quality-primary-and-community-healthcare-standards.

251. Australian Commission on Safety and Quality in Health Care. Preparing for an assessment to the NSQHS standards. ACSQHC. [Accessed 24 July 2022.] Available from: https://www.safetyandquality.gov.au/standards/nsqhs-standards/assessment-nsqhs-standards/preparing-assessment-nsqhs-standards.

252. Chisolm SA. Infection control in correctional facilities: a new challenge. Am J Infect Control. 1988;16(3):107-113. doi:10.1016/0196-6553(88)90047-8

253. Levy MH, Mogg D. Infection control standards for Australian prisons: forgotten, but not forgiving. Healthc Infect. 2009;14(1):13-19. doi:10.1071/HI09004

254. Garcia R, Barnes S, Boukidjian R, et al. Recommendations for change in infection prevention programs and practice. Am J Infect Control. 2022. doi:10.1016/J.AJIC.2022.04.007

255. Billings C, Bernard H, Caffery L, et al. Advancing the profession: an updated future-oriented competency model for professional development in infection prevention and control. Am J Infect Control. 2019;47(6):602-614. doi:10.1016/j.ajic.2019.04.003

256. Aziz AM. Infection prevention and control practitioners: improving engagement. Br J Nurs. 2016;25(6):297-302. doi:10.12968/bjon.2016.25.6.297

257. Hall L, Halton K, Macbeth D, Gardner A, Mitchell B. Roles, responsibilities and scope of practice: describing the 'state of play' for infection control professionals in Australia and New Zealand. Healthc Infect. 2015;20(1):29-35. doi:10.1071/HI14037

258. Dekker M, Jongerden IP, van Mansfeld R, et al. Infection control link nurses in acute care hospitals: a scoping review. Antimicrob Resist Infect Control. 2019;8(1):1-13. doi:10.1186/S13756-019-0476-8/TABLES/1

259. Farrington M. Infection control education: how to make an impact - tools for the job. J Hosp Infect. 2007;65(SUPPL. 2):128-132. doi:10.1016/S0195-6701(07)60029-2

260. Flanagan NA, Flanagan TJ. Correctional nurses' perceptions of their role, training requirements, and prisoner health care needs. J Correctional Health Care. 2001;8(1):67-85. doi:10.1177/107834580100800105

261. Castro-Sánchez E, Chang PWS, Vila-Candel R, Escobedo AA, Holmes AH. Health literacy and infectious diseases: why does it matter? Int J Infect Dis. 2016;43:103-110. doi:10.1016/j.ijid.2015.12.019

262. Cox D, Cuddihy M, Hill S, et al. Health literacy: taking action to improve safety and quality, 2014. [Accessed 24 July 2022.] Available from: https://www.safetyandquality.gov.au/sites/default/files/migrated/Health-Literacy-Taking-action-to-improve-safety-and-quality.pdf.

CHAPTER 40

Infection prevention and control in veterinary practice

ASSOCIATE PROFESSOR JANE HELLER[i]
Dr CRISTINA SOTOMAYOR-CASTILLO[ii]
PROFESSOR JACQUELINE NORRIS[iii]

Chapter highlights

- Characteristics and contexts of veterinary practice in Australia
- Explains the healthcare-associated infection (HAI) risks associated with veterinary practice settings in Australia
- Exploration of relevant infection prevention and control (IPC) for HAIs in veterinary practice settings in Australia

i   School of Agricultural, Environmental and Veterinary Sciences, Charles Sturt University, Wagga Wagga, NSW
ii Susan Wakil School of Nursing and Midwifery, Faculty of Medicine and Health, The University of Sydney, Sydney, NSW
iii Sydney School of Veterinary Science, The University of Sydney, Sydney, NSW

Introduction

The overarching goal of IPC in human healthcare settings is to provide an environment in which healthcare staff and patients are protected from any infectious disease hazard, consequently facilitating the expected and required level of care. IPC in animal healthcare settings shares the same goal. However, the very nature of the animal healthcare settings in which IPC is to be implemented dictates that this goal may be realised in vastly differing ways. This chapter presents a holistic view of veterinary practice—along with a justification of the need for, and ideal strategies around, the implementation of IPC measures—to allow protective processes to be realised irrespective of the scenario in which they are applied.

40.1 Setting the scene: characteristics and context of veterinary practice in Australia

There are many different types of veterinary practice in Australia. Broadly speaking, the environments that veterinarians work in fall within three main categories:[1]

1. veterinary clinics/hospitals (static clinical environments)[2]
2. mobile veterinary practices (may be associated with static environments or independent and run from a vehicle);[3] and
3. on-site practice (at animal production sites).

To appropriately appraise a veterinary environment for application of IPC principles we need to consider which animal species are present at each type of practice. As such, practices can be further classified as single or multi-species practices. Examples of single-species practices include a mobile equine practice that consults to private properties or multi-horse establishments, or an on-site poultry veterinarian consulting across multiple establishments owned by the same company. An example of a multi-species practice might be a mixed practice veterinary clinic that consults within the clinic to companion species and through a mobile service to equine and/or food and fibre species (e.g. sheep, cattle and goats) on local properties.

In a clinical/hospital context, individual animals may engage with veterinary services as outpatients or inpatients. Outpatients are presented by their owners for a consultation at a veterinary clinic or may be seen by a veterinarian who visits the home or farm.

A veterinary clinic usually has hospital facilities such as wards (cages, stalls or pens), a treatment room, diagnostic imaging suite (x-ray machine and at some specialists, a CT or MRI), facilities for performing procedures (sample collection, anaesthesia, dentals, endoscopy, etc), and a surgery suite for procedures requiring complete aseptic technique. As a hospital outpatient, the presenting animal will move between the waiting room and consulting rooms with their owner and may spend time in the treatment room of the hospital for minor procedures with the veterinarian but does not spend time out of human contact. Inpatients may be hospitalised (housed within a cage or run) within the clinic environment, or a dedicated area of an intensive farm environment. These patients are more likely to have invasive procedures performed and will potentially move between all areas of the establishment.

40.1.1 Veterinary practice in varied geographical settings

In urban settings, veterinary practice is commonly performed in a small animal hospital environment. Most of these clinics treat (medically and/or surgically) all small companion species (i.e. dogs, cats, pocket pets, pet birds, reptiles and some wildlife). Referral hospitals may be present in some areas, with a high throughput of intensively managed complex medical and surgical cases. These establishments may also have dedicated intensive care facilities. After-hours clinics also exist in some regions, with a similar level of intensive facilities. These may be co-located with referral hospitals. A small number of single species hospital practices (e.g. cat clinics) and mobile small companion clinics exist as well in these regions.

Veterinary clinics in peri-urban regions have a similar profile to those described for urban settings but may also treat larger animals, such as horses or smallholder (backyard) production species (i.e. food and fibre species) with house calls. In some cases, they may attend the clinic in an outpatient capacity. Moving further from the city and in regional areas, the same type of hospital clinics exist but the species that are serviced may include larger numbers. There may be a greater distribution of food and fibre species (e.g. cattle) and a combination of hospital and mobile services is usually provided. There is less likelihood of dedicated referral or after-hours small animal clinics in regional environments, but referral or single species equine or farm animal services may exist.

40.1.2 Intensively raised animals and multi-animal environments

Intensively raised animals (e.g. poultry, pigs, feedlot cattle) will usually require the services of a dedicated veterinarian who will travel to the farm and work on-site for periods of time. In some cases, especially in large companies, a specific in-house veterinarian will be employed to attend to animals across multiple farms. Either way, the veterinarian's workplace is now the farm. This represents a similar scenario to mobile veterinarians, but these visit the farm for prolonged periods and move between cohorts during that time, as opposed to consulting to a particular problem in a particular animal (or group of animals).

Finally, multi-animal environments (e.g. zoos and animal parks) frequently have dedicated on-site veterinarians or engage local veterinarians through a mobile service, depending on location, size of the facilities and resources. Movement of zoo animals to veterinary hospital settings outside of the zoo environment is unusual, with most procedures performed at the facility, including specialist procedures.

40.1.3 Veterinary clinic services

Veterinary hospitals may be purpose-built or converted from existing buildings (houses or commercial premises).[1] Referral and after-hours clinics are almost always purpose-built, whereas general practice environments vary. Mobile veterinary practice may be conducted from a dedicated clinic vehicle or from the veterinarian's personal car.

Personnel that are present in veterinary clinics include veterinarians, veterinary nurses, animal attendants (kennel hands, stable hands) and receptionists. Mobile and on-site veterinary services are usually limited to a single veterinarian. They may also include a veterinary nurse in situations where procedures require additional assistance, for example in the case of specialists in surgery or diagnostic imaging who visit primary care practices to perform specialist procedures. The interaction between species and veterinary service type is displayed in Fig 40.1.

40.2 HAI risks in veterinary practice settings in Australia

IPC in the veterinary space works to prevent transmission of disease from animal to animal (same or different species), from animal to human (veterinarians, other animal health workers and animal owners) and from human to animal. The animal healthcare domain, much like the human healthcare sector, is associated with many potential exposures to biosecurity hazards, which vary depending on the healthcare context (hospital vs farm vs mobile practice), animal species, clinical presentation, and nature of the potential pathogens. It is important to consider that some pathogens pose risks of nosocomial infections in hospitalised patients of the same or different animal species as well as zoonotic infections that can affect veterinary personnel (veterinarians, nurses, animal attendants), and animal owners/carers.[2] Veterinarians are likely to be amongst the first

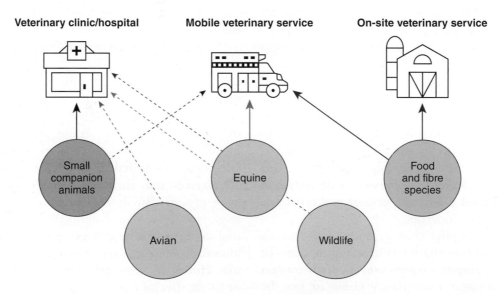

FIGURE 40.1 Representation of interaction between species and veterinary service type

people to engage in high-risk interactions with animals infected with zoonotic pathogens.[3]

40.2.1 Risk-based identification of effective IPC

The hierarchy of hazard control (as explored in Chapter 7), that guides us through the implementation of elimination, substitution, engineering controls, administrative controls and finally the use of PPE, represents a firm basis from which to consider IPC in animal healthcare settings. The hierarchy of control can be combined with targeted analysis of the potential risks to identify effective IPC for each given setting or scenario by asking the following simple questions:

1. What are the likely pathogens involved?

2. What is the likely route(s) of transmission?

3. How can I disrupt the potential route in the most effective way?

Stratification of the first two questions listed here is largely by species, examples of which are listed in Table 40.1. Addressing the third question in light of the likely pathogens and routes of transmission requires additional extensive consideration of the context in which the control or prevention measures are to be applied. Due to the large variation in animal healthcare settings, the appropriateness of measures is highly contextualised, and it is important to appreciate that what might be appropriate for one species/setting combination may not be for another.

40.2.2 Limitations and constraints

In addition to this, it is important to appreciate that almost all settings that call for veterinary IPC have limitations in terms of implementation, with inadequate clinical infrastructure and lack of dedicated IPC staff considered some of the most obvious constraints. While infection control efforts in some veterinary settings such as hospitals or clinics have direct parallels to human healthcare facilities,[4-9] there are specific areas within animal healthcare such as intensive production systems (e.g. piggeries, poultry production, dairy farms) that pose unique challenges for IPC. Disease mitigation in these settings involves assessment of some unique criteria such as stocking density, animal management systems (e.g. is it 'all in–all out', or a 'flow through' system), vaccination programs, infrastructure, airflow, air and water quality and cleaning regimen. Furthermore, conflation between production and clinical environments must also be managed, with some situations requiring control measures that do not provide an immediately obvious benefit to animal

health to be implemented at the level of the production environment, resulting in a cost (and responsibility) for the producer, or owner, rather than the veterinarian.

Despite these issues and limitations, if a holistic view is taken it is possible to identify key opportunities to disrupt the potential route of pathogens, irrespective of the specifics of the situation. Three examples will be used to illustrate how IPC measures can be applied and how they may need to be varied depending on species/setting combination.

CASE STUDY 1

Young dog presented with haemorrhagic diarrhoea

Situation:

A 6-month-old puppy is presented to a veterinary hospital with 24 hours of malaise, vomiting and diarrhoea containing blood. The puppy has been vaccinated against canine parvovirus, canine distemper and canine adenovirus, with this standard primary course finishing at 16 weeks. The puppy is on a mixed diet of fresh beef, chicken and a commercial dry food.

Potential pathogens: canine parvovirus, Campylobacter spp., Salmonella spp., Giardia spp.

Risk assessment: Despite recent completion of vaccination against canine parvovirus, maternal antibody interference can block the development of acquired immune responses to vaccination and leave dogs vulnerable to canine parvoviral disease. This virus is specific to dogs; however, due to the large quantities of virus excretion and environmental resilience, it poses a major nosocomial risk in a hospital setting for all immune-naïve dogs. *Campylobacter spp. and Salmonella spp.* are most frequently acquired from raw meat sources. Transmission from infected dogs to humans and other species is possible; the primary transmission route is in the household. The assemblages of *Giardia duodenalis* seen in dogs and cats are B and C respectively, with most seen in humans being assemblages A and B. While it poses some risk, it is considered low.

IPC measures at the time: Patients presenting to hospitals with these clinical signs need to be isolated from other animals in the hospital. Triage of the patient by veterinary personnel when the appointment is made or when the patient arrives is critical in minimising the patient's time in,

TABLE 40.1 Examples of key healthcare-associated infections (HAIs) in specific animal species in Australia

Animal species	Key HAI	Prominent transmission route	Key species affected
Cats	Bartonella spp.	Scratches	Cats, humans
	Microsporum canis	Cutaneous	Dogs, cats, humans
	Pasteurella and oral anaerobes	Bite wounds	Any animal
	Coxiella burnetii (Q fever)	Respiratory, from birth products	Main species affected are ruminants and humans
Dogs	*Salmonella/Campylobacter*	Faecal-oral	Wide spectrum but transmission to humans is usually foodborne
	Pasteurella and anaerobes	Bite wounds	Any animal
	Coxiella burnetii (Q fever)	Respiratory from birth products	Main species affected are ruminants and humans
	Microsporum canis	Cutaneous	Dogs, cats, humans
Cattle	*Coxiella burnetii* (Q fever)	Respiratory from birth products	Main species affected are ruminants and humans
	Leptospira spp.	Mucous membranes	Serovar dependent
Goats	*Coxiella burnetii* (Q fever)	Respiratory from birth products	Main species affected are ruminants and humans
	Orf (Parapox virus)	Cutaneous	Sheep, goats, humans
Sheep	*Coxiella burnetii* (Q fever)	Respiratory from birth products	Main species affected are ruminants and humans
	Orf (Parapox virus)	Cutaneous	Sheep, goats, humans
Pigs	*Brucella suis* (feral pigs)	Respiratory	Humans, dogs, wildlife
	Leptospira spp.	Mucous membranes	Serovar dependent
	Erysiphelothrix rhusiopathiae	Ingestion or Cutaneous	Humans, pigs, poultry
Horses	Hendra virus	Respiratory	Humans
	Chlamydia psittaci	Respiratory	Humans, most animals
	Leptospira spp.	Mucous membranes	Serovar dependent
	Salmonella spp.	Faeco–oral	Wide spectrum
Poultry	Salmonella spp.	Faeco–oral	Wide spectrum
Bats	Australian Bat Lyssavirus*	Bites and scratches	Humans and all other mammals
Psittacine birds	*Chlamydia psittaci*	Respiratory	Humans, most animals
Australian native reptiles	*Salmonella/Campylobacter*	Faecal–oral	Humans and other mammals

*ABLV is currently the only lyssavirus in Australia. Rabies virus is not present in Australia and if this changed, would elevate the HAI risk across all mammals

and therefore likely contamination of, the waiting room. Use of an isolation ward or an isolated consult room on arrival of the patient is preferable. Immediate closure of the examination space for cleaning following patient assessment is essential. Enhanced cleaning and disinfection procedures are targeted at the most resilient organism, which in this case is canine parvovirus (non-enveloped DNA virus resistant to many standard disinfectants). Most of the other agents of disease are easily contained with standard disinfection procedures.

IPC measures: Acute diarrhoea is a common presentation in small animal practice and standard operating procedures should outline all actions that need to occur from the moment the patient enters the practice. This includes where patients with these signs will be examined, the level of PPE required, cleaning procedures, and isolation of the animal within the hospital setting. If the animal becomes an inpatient, then separate isolation facilities are required.

Different practice setting: If this same patient was seen by a mobile veterinary practice, then the veterinarian's assessment of IPC would depend on whether the dog was to remain at the owner's residence or be admitted to hospital. If the dog was to remain at home, standardised instructions on isolating the dog, cleaning the environment surfaces and appropriate levels of PPE required by the owner are the legal responsibility of the veterinarian.

CASE STUDY 2

Regional equine veterinarian asked to examine a horse with respiratory signs

Situation:

A regional veterinarian in Southeast Queensland receives a phone call about a 7-year-old mare (currently used for pleasure riding) that the owner is concerned about. The owner reports that this morning she was noted to be shifting her weight between legs, was quite wobbly in the paddock when walking, and had twitching muscles that were visible in her shoulder region. She was also off her food. On questioning, the owner revealed that the horse had been vaccinated for tetanus and strangles, but not for Hendra virus.

Potential pathogens: Hendra virus, Australian bat lyssavirus (ABLV), Japanese encephalitis virus (JEV) (or other arboviral diseases such as Kunjin and Murray Valley encephalitis). Other non-infectious causes, such as toxicoses and trauma also need to be considered.

Risk assessment: Given the lack of Hendra virus vaccination and the appropriate clinical signs and geographical location of this case, Hendra virus and ABLV cannot be discounted. Both agents of disease are transmitted to horses from bats, can be transferred to humans from horses (although to date, there has been no demonstrated transfer of ABLV from horse to human) and both have severe outcomes. Given the severity of the outcome of infection in humans, the risk is assessed to be high.

IPC measures: A veterinarian should not travel to see this case without first phoning the Australian National Emergency Animal Disease Watch Hotline (1800 675 888). Similarly, the veterinarian should advise the owners to cease any further direct contact with this horse and direct them to contact their local Public Health unit if they are concerned about prior contact. Any person who approaches this case, given the possibility of these infectious diseases with severe outcomes, will need to be suited in full PPE, until exclusion of Hendra virus (through serological and PCR testing) has occurred.

Different practice setting: If this horse had been presented to a clinic (rather than being an ambulatory case and where the history was known prior to arrival), different IPC implications within that clinical setting would need to be considered. A requirement for immediate isolation of the case is imperative, as is the requirement for full PPE for all contact. As the virus is transmitted via body fluids, extreme caution around any body fluids from an infected horse must be exercised.

CASE STUDY 3

Risk assessment—dystocia in veterinary hospital or farm settings

Situation:

The principal veterinarian at a mixed practice veterinary clinic is discussing the key risks associated with their clinic's response to animals that present with dystocia. The mixed practice has a small animal veterinary hospital in the centre of a regional town and also services the surrounding horse studs, cattle, sheep and goat farms.

Potential pathogens: In this scenario the risks of transmission of infectious agents from an animal to human from birth products is dependent on the animal species and veterinary setting. *Coxiella burnetii* and *Chlamydia psittaci* are the most important agents of disease in the current Australian context, with the relative risk differing between animal species. Other non-zoonotic infectious causes (such as equine herpesvirus 1) or non-infectious causes such as plant toxicosis also need to be considered.

Risk assessment: Veterinarians, and veterinary nurses, should be vaccinated against Q fever (*Coxiella burnetii*) during their training or as part of their workplace vaccinations. Vaccination again Chlamydia spp. is not available. Both agents of disease are transmitted via the respiratory system by aerosolisation of birth products. *Coxiella burnetii* transmission from animals to humans has been reported in cattle, sheep, goats, dogs and cats; however, the risk is much higher in ruminants and is rare in companion animals (dogs and cats). *Chlamydia psittaci* has been transmitted from horses to humans through exposure to fetal membranes and critically unwell equine neonates. Given the severity of outcomes of infection with both agents of disease, precautions for all personnel attending animals with dystocia are required.

Infection prevention and disease control measures: Q fever vaccination is critical for all veterinary hospital personnel. This, however, does not protect transient staff (e.g. work experience) or members of the public (animal owners) attending the clinic or being present during farm visits. Isolation and containment of the patient and rapid disinfection or cautious disposal of all bedding, equipment and surfaces is essential, as some agents such as *Coxiella burnetii* can be transmissible in their dried form and have been spread throughout a hospital setting through the process of washing gowns, drapes and bedding.[10-12]

Different practice setting: In a farm setting, the veterinarian must be conscious of birth fluid contamination of the paddock, farm sheds, nearby animals and humans. PPE— such as masks, eye protection and face shields that prevent inhalation and splashes of fluid—is required during procedures on the animal and during decontamination procedures. Contamination of the clothing must be considered with use of disposable PPE. Disinfection of the environment and equipment is critical. These same measures are required in the hospital setting.

40.3 IPC in veterinary practice

The prevention of infections in the veterinary setting is an essential daily activity. It is acknowledged that all Australian veterinary hospitals face challenges in preventing the spread of infectious diseases, and that these settings have the potential to harbour or amplify their spread.[13] An increase in awareness around implementing effective IPC practices in veterinary hospitals has been shown to occur within professionals as well as patient owners after the emergence of specific cases of disease, for example methicillin-resistant and multidrug-resistant *Staphylococcus* infections in dogs and cats.[14,15] Although there are available guidelines developed by groups of experts from various countries, veterinary IPC practices often escalate when a zoonotic infection is present, for example around infections with Leptospira spp. ABLV, *Coxiella burnetii*, *Brucella suis* or Hendra virus. In these circumstances, highly contagious animal diseases tend to generate increased awareness and rapid implementation of effective infection control practices.[13] This approach is not at all uncommon for the healthcare setting in general. When managing situations where there is no perceived risk, human behaviour can drift towards reduced adherence to various IPC practices. This may lead to poor attention to specific IPC measures which will eventually result in a need for immediate and/or long-term pharmaceutical intervention at a much higher cost, contributing to a potential risk of extending well-known issues such as antimicrobial resistance, or resulting in the death of a patient.

The currently available veterinary IPC guidelines have been developed by expert groups and committees specific to each of the countries and/or regions developing them, focusing on certain animal species as well as types of practice. This section will describe Australia's approach to IPC measures in terms of existing guidelines and briefly explore some of those available internationally, classifying them based on the country of origin.

The Australian Veterinary Association (AVA) and the Australian Infectious Diseases Advisory Panel (AIDAP) have developed guidelines aiming to firstly support clinical and other practices ensuring the safety and welfare of all animals under veterinary care, and secondly to provide a safe and healthy environment for veterinary personnel as well as owners.[16,17] The Guidelines for Veterinary Personal Biosecurity developed by the AVA is a practical IPC resource that covers veterinary practices of all types. It includes overall principles and a framework for developing and implementing a series of IPC procedures to prevent the spread of diseases between animals, from animals to staff, and from staff to animals.[16] Similarly, the AIDAP guidelines provide a resource for IPC within the small animal clinical setting.[17]

In appreciating the variety of settings where veterinary healthcare takes place, the guidelines emphasise that the appropriateness and applicability of the procedures will vary according to the size and nature of the practice as well as the facilities into which these will be applied. These factors will frame the scope of actions to be taken based on the particular and multiple settings where veterinary practice occurs, keeping in mind four general guiding principles:

1. identifying potential source(s) of organisms
2. decreasing transmission
3. decreasing exposure risks; and
4. maximising patient resilience and immunity.[17]

Having these four principles in mind, every clinic 'should develop an infection control program and every practice should have a designated infection control champion/officer'.[17] It will be their role to develop a written set of guidelines, specific to the requirements of the practice in which they are to be implemented and which should be conceptually framed, taking into consideration the IPC guidelines. This document should, alongside the broader guidelines, assist the training of new and existing staff as well as serving as a quality control program in the field of IPC. Further actions including, but not limited to, surveillance of surgical infection rates, antimicrobial resistance detection in samples cultured from hospitalised patients, and investigation of disease outbreaks, are also suggested as these may identify potential breaches in the performance of procedures.

The AIDAP guidelines contain five different sections which will be used to highlight the key messages around IPC that are imparted through both currently available guidelines:

1. Hand hygiene
2. Personal protective equipment (PPE)
3. Environmental hygiene
4. General procedures
5. Biosecurity, infection control and prevention of common zoonotic infections.

40.3.1 Hand hygiene

Both sets of guidelines emphasise the importance of hand hygiene for all individuals who play a role during veterinary care, namely veterinarians, veterinary nurses and technicians, receptionists, animal attendants, cleaners and animal owners. Routine hand hygiene is key for reducing the number of microorganisms on the hands, particularly those that are potential opportunistic pathogens. The use of alcohol-based hand hygiene as well as handwashing with soap and running water are well recognised as hand hygiene measures, with the use of alcohol-based hand sanitisers identified as the preferred method for decontaminating hands that are not visibly soiled. The use of gloves is not a substitute for hand hygiene. The Australian Commission on Safety and Quality in Health Care's (ACSQHC) National Hand Hygiene Initiative (NHHI) website and manual is the key resource for data, research and methods of hand hygiene.[18] Practical tips and schematics on particulars to consider when performing a correct hand hygiene technique can be found in both sets of guidelines. Hand hygiene considerations in veterinary practice are in line with those in human medicine and have been further heightened following the COVID-19 global pandemic.

40.3.2 Personal protective equipment

The use of PPE sits at the bottom or the lowest level of the hierarchy of infection control measures, and should be seen as an adjunct to other means of infection control (elimination, substitution, engineering controls and administrative controls). Both sets of Australian-based veterinary guidelines offer practical guidance on which PPE should be used when, including sub-sections on the use of laboratory coats/scrubs, non-sterile gowns, gloves, face protection, respiratory protection such as the use of N95 masks/respirators and footwear. The guidelines also describe the specific context required for situations with varied levels of risk, ranging from routine examinations of healthy animals (low risk) to high-risk procedures such as performing a necropsy on animals suspected to have died from ABLV Hendra virus or herpes virus B (from primates).

Advice includes the use of the National Emergency Animal Disease Watch Hotline (1800 675 888) as well as important information about donning and doffing PPE presented in an easily accessible format (see the AVA guidelines).[16] Additional resources have been developed by the AVA and are available through the AVA website (see Useful websites/resources at the end of this chapter). Among the AVA's resources are two videos for equine clinical staff that cover PPE use in equine practice.

40.3.3 Environmental hygiene

Environmental hygiene relates to the array of measures used to reduce the overall burden of infectious disease agents in the veterinary clinic and hospital, with a focus on specific cleaning and disinfection practices. Both sets of guidelines emphasise the importance of combining cleaning (removal of visible organic matter using soap or detergent) and disinfection (the use of a chemical or other procedure to kill or inactivate remaining microbes), noting that methods will vary depending on the surface or equipment to be used and the setting in which it is to be applied (e.g. the difference between consulting room and isolation ward). Specific information is included in both sets of guidelines around the selection of appropriate PPE and disinfection processes to take into consideration relative to the exposure risks.[19] Both guidelines contain two user-friendly tables that detail disinfectant properties and their antimicrobial spectrum, to allow for appropriate selection. Additional tables are included to further assist selection of specific disinfectants.

40.3.4 General procedures

Practical applications of IPC are covered in a dedicated section within the AIDAP guidelines and are also discussed throughout the AVA document. The importance of overall routine disinfection of the examination room cannot be understated, along with an understanding of how to properly clean and disinfect all equipment and environments. Every animal patient that enters an examination room or undergoes a procedure carries the risk of harbouring a transmissible infectious disease, with some animal/procedure combinations assessed as a greater risk than others in terms of transmission of pathogen (e.g. otoscopic examination, dental procedures, resuscitation, obstetrics and post-mortem examinations). For this reason, it is essential that dedicated procedural documentation is maintained within any clinic IPC program. Procedures for cleaning stethoscopes and smart devices, otoscopes—which in the veterinary setting come with reusable specula video-otoscopy units—diagnostic equipment (ultrasound and x-ray machines), anaesthetic equipment and endoscopes are discussed in the AIDAP guidelines and the information in the guidelines is generalisable to any setting.

40.3.5 Biosecurity and IPC for common zoonotic infections

Processes to ensure that biosecurity is maintained when visiting properties where there is a high risk of infectious disease (zoonotic or otherwise) are essential to prevent serious personal illness. AVA guidelines clearly document the required risk assessment, process and flow for any visit. A risk assessment must cover both the risk of:

- zoonoses; and
- the disease spreading from the affected property.

Veterinarians should have good knowledge of the potential major personal risks—inclusive of zoonotic pathogens (animal bites, brucellosis, leptospirosis, psittacosis and Q fever, amongst others)—which are covered in depth in the AIDAP guidelines. Potential routes of exposure should be known so that pre-emptive strategies can be put in place and risk can be assessed appropriately for all activities and procedures. Pre-emptive strategies include employee vaccinations for diseases, such as rabies, to cover ABLV, tetanus and Q fever. Similarly, the level of baseline risk for employees (i.e. level of immunocompetence) should be assessed and activities adjusted accordingly to manage risk.

40.3.6 Other international guidelines

IPC guidelines for the veterinary healthcare setting have also been developed and made available in various countries including Canada, the United States of America and the United Kingdom. These documents encompass various topics integral to the field of IPC and related areas, such as the surveillance methods for effective detection of pathogen entries to veterinary practices, and detailed biosafety-related risks and recommendations to manage certain infectious agents. Table 40.2 summarises some of the most relevant international guidelines on veterinary IPC.

Conclusion

A bespoke, updateable, written IPC plan that is specific to the facility it covers and based on the recommendations in the currently available national guidelines should be developed for each clinical veterinary environment.

The plan should be clearly based on the hierarchy of hazard control, and its implementation should result in the disruption of all potential pathogen pathways that exist within the setting in which it is to be applied. An effective IPC plan identifies and addresses all of the pathways by answering the following questions for each animal, setting or procedural combination:

1. What is the likely pathogen(s) involved?
2. What is the likely route(s) of transmission?
3. How can I disrupt the potential route in the most effective way?

The characteristics and contexts of veterinary practice in Australia are highly variable. However, with an understanding of the HAI risks likely to be associated with different species or setting combinations, and by application of IPC guidelines both holistically and through a targeted IPC plan, protection across all veterinary settings can be achieved.

TABLE 40.2 Examples of available international veterinary IPC guidelines

Country	Year of publication	Leading committee/ association	Field	Themes	Source
USA	2009	American Veterinary Association sponsored by the Canadian Committee on Antibiotic Resistance	Small animal practice	Pathogen transmission risk reduction Best practices for surgical site management Use of appropriate PPE Disinfectant use Cleaning and disinfection practices	https://www.avma.org/javma-news/2009-04-15/infection-control-guide-available-canadian-committee
United States of America	2018	American Animal Hospital Association (AAHA) (experts from Canada and the US)	Small and large animal hospitals	Minimise and reduce breaches in IPC as well as biosecurity (ICPB). Surveillance methods to detect pathogen entries into the practice	https://www.aaha.org/aaha-guidelines/infection-control-configuration/aaha-infection-control-prevention-and-biosecurity-guidelines/
Canada	2008 (1st edition) 2019 (2nd edition)	Ontario Animal Health Network (OAHN) and the Center for Public Health and Zoonoses (CPHAZ)	Small animal veterinary clinics	Infection Prevention and Control Best Practices for Small Animal Veterinary. To support and guide small animal clinical practice, providing assistance for decision making specifically in IPC Issues	https://www.oahn.ca/resource-type/infection-prevention-and-control/
Canada	2011	Ontario Veterinary College Teaching Hospital (OVCTH)	Small and large animal veterinary teaching hospital (OVCTH)	Infection Control Manual containing all approved infection control protocols which frame the way clinical activities take care in the referred healthcare facility. This resource is available in the OVCTH website and is regularly updated.	https://ovc.uoguelph.ca/doc/InfectionControlManual_Aug_2011_V2.pdf
Canada	2017	Public Health Agency of Canada (PHAC) Biosafety and Biosecurity (Government of Canada) in collaboration with the Canadian Food Inspection Agency (CFIA)	Veterinary practices performing diagnostic activities	Risk-based biosafety precautions and recommendations for veterinary facilities performing laboratory analyses and diagnostic testing with Risk Group 2 (RG2) human pathogens. To provide guidance on how to mitigate risks when handling pathogens, toxins, or other infectious material within veterinary practices. To delineate physical design features and operational practices for veterinary facilities handling pathogens	https://www.canada.ca/content/dam/phac-aspc/documents/services/canadian-biosafety-standards-guidelines/guidance/veterinary-practices-physical-design-operational-practices-diagnostic-activities/pub-eng.pdf

Continued

TABLE 40.2 Examples of available international veterinary IPC guidelines—cont'd

Country	Year of publication	Leading committee/ association	Field	Themes	Source
United Kingdom	2020	The Royal College of Veterinary Surgeons (RCVS)	Veterinary practices across the UK	The RCVS Practice Standards Scheme (PSS) to guide and encourage the effective implementation of IPC practices in any establishment providing veterinary services. Since 2020, the RCVS has established the creation of an Infection Control Group, the development of biosecurity policy as well as framing the role of the infection control veterinary nurses and the specific considerations for infection control in practice	https://knowledge. rcvs.org.uk/quality-improvement/tools-and-resources/qi-cpd/

Useful websites/resources

*   The Australian Veterinary Association. www.ava.com.au.
*   Australian Infectious Diseases Advisory Panel (AIDAP).
*   National Emergency Animal Disease Watch Hotline (1800 675 888).

References

1. Australian Small Animal Veterinarians (ASAV). Manual of hospital standards and accreditation 2019. St Leonards NSW: ASAV, 2019. Available from: https://www.ava.com.au/siteassets/about-us/programs-and-awards/2019-asav-manual-of-hospital-standards-and-accreditation.pdf.
2. Benedict KM, Morley PS, Van Metre DC. Characteristics of biosecurity and infection control programs at veterinary teaching hospitals. J Am Vet Med Assoc. 2008;233(5):767-773. https://doi.org/10.2460/javma.233.5.767
3. Dowd K, Taylor M, Toribio JA, Hooker C, Dhand NK. Zoonotic disease risk perceptions and infection control practices of Australian veterinarians: call for change in work culture. Prev Vet Med. 2013;111(1-2):17-24. https://doi.org/10.1016/j.prevetmed.2013.04.002
4. Morley PS. Evidence-based infection control in clinical practice: if you buy clothes for the emperor, will he wear them? J Vet Intern Med. 2013;27(3):430-438. https://doi.org/10.1111/jvim.12060
5. Ekiri AB, House AM, Krueger TM, Hernandez JA. Awareness, perceived relevance, and acceptance of large animal hospital surveillance and infection control practices by referring veterinarians and clients. J Am Vet Med Assoc. 2014;244(7): 835-843. https://doi.org/10.2460/javma.244.7.835
6. Ekiri AB, MacKay RJ, Gaskin JM, Freeman DE, House AM, Giguère S, et al. Epidemiologic analysis of nosocomial Salmonella infections in hospitalized horses. J Am Vet Med Assoc. 2009;234(1):108-119. https://doi.org/10.2460/javma.234.1.108
7. Morley PS. Surveillance for nosocomial infections in veterinary hospitals. Vet Clin North Am Equine Pract. 2004;20(3): 561-576. https://doi.org/10.1016/j.cveq.2004.08.002
8. Smith BP. Evolution of equine infection control programs. Vet Clin North Am Equine Pract. 2004;20(3):521-530. v. https://doi.org/10.1016/j.cveq.2004.07.002
9. Traub-Dargatz JL, Dargatz DA, Morley PS, Dunowska M. An overview of infection control strategies for equine facilities, with an emphasis on veterinary hospitals. Vet Clin North Am Equine Pract. 2004;20(3):507-520. https://doi.org/10.1016/j.cveq.2004.07.004
10. Maywood P, Boyd R. (2011) Q fever in a small animal hospital. In: Australian College of Veterinary Scientists College Science Week Scientific Meeting: Epidemiology Chapter and Aquatic Animal Health Chapter Proceedings, 30 June–2 July 2011, Gold Coast, Australia, p 4. Eight Mile Plains, Queensland: Australian College of Veterinary Scientists, 2011.
11. Kopecny L, Boswate KL, Shapiro AJ, Norris JM. (2013) Using serological assays and fluorescent in situ hybridisation to investigate Coxiella burnetii infection in a breeding cattery. J Feline Med Surg. 2013;15(12):1037-1045.
12. Eastwood K, Graves SR, Massey PD, Boswate K, van den Berg D, Hutchinson P. Q fever: a rural disease with potential urban consequences. Aust J Gen Pract. 2018;47(3):5555. https://doi.org/10.31128/AFP-08-17-4299

13. Willemsen A, Cobbold R, Gibson J, Wilks K, Lwaler S, Reid S. Infection control practices employed within small animal veterinary practices – a systematic review. Zoonoses Public Health. 2019;66(5):439-457. https://doi.org/10.1111/zph.12589

14. Chai MH, Sukiman MZ, Liew YW, Shapawi MS, Roslan FS, Hashim SN, et al. Detection, molecular characterization, and antibiogram of multi-drug resistant and methicillin resistant Staphylococcus aureus (MRSA) isolated from pets and pet owners in Malaysia. Iran J Vet Res. 2021;22(4):277-287. https://doi.org/10.22099/ijvr.2021.39586.5752

15. Dazio V, Nigg A, Schmidt JS, Brilhante M, Campos-Madueno EI, Mauri N, et al. Duration of carriage of multidrug-resistant bacteria in dogs and cats in veterinary care and co-carriage with their owners. One Health. 2021; 13:100322. https://doi.org/10.1016/j.onehlt.2021.100322

16. Australian Veterinary Association. Guidelines for veterinary personal biosecurity, 2017. AVA, 2017. Available from: www.ava.com.au.

17. Australian Veterinary Association, Australian Infectious Diseases Advisory panel practical infection control guideline. AVA, 2018. Available from: www.ava.com.au.

18. Australian Commission on Safety and Quality in Health Care. Infection prevention and control: national hand hygiene initiative. ACSQHC, 2019. Available from: https://www.safetyandquality.gov.au/our-work/infection-prevention-and-control/national-hand-hygiene-initiative.

19. New South Wales Government, Department of Primary Industries. Animal biosecurity: zoonoses – animal diseases that can infect people. State Government of NSW, 2022. Available from https://www.dpi.nsw.gov.au/biosecurity/animal/humans.

CHAPTER 41

Infection prevention and control in pharmacy practice and antimicrobial stewardship

ASSOCIATE PROFESSOR GARY DEAN GRANT[i,ii]

TEJASWINI KALKUNDRI[i]

Chapter highlights

- Pharmacists' knowledge, skills and capabilities make them essential members of the fight against antimicrobial resistance
- The expanding scope of pharmacy practice bolsters infection prevention and control (IPC) efforts
- Pharmacist involvement in antimicrobial stewardship efforts enhances the effectiveness of programs
- There is scope to further utilise the skills and capabilities of pharmacists in IPC to reduce the risk of antimicrobial resistance

i   School of Pharmacy and Medical Sciences, Griffith University, Gold Coast, QLD
ii School of Pharmacy and Medical Sciences, Griffith University, Gold Coast, QLD

Introduction

The availability of safe, cost–effective and readily available effective antimicrobials has significantly contributed to our modern way of life. Antimicrobials provide a means to cure life-threatening infections, control infectious diseases, prevent surgical complications and increase life expectancy.[1,2] Antimicrobial resistance (AMR) is a predictable and inevitable outcome of increasing antimicrobial use (AU).[3] Levy (1998) highlighted five important considerations about AMR that should influence our actions, namely:

1. resistance affects all antibiotics;

2. resistance is progressive, and increasing minimum inhibitor concentrations (MICs) are a marker for future resistance;

3. organisms resistant to one antimicrobial are likely to become resistant to others;

4. once resistance appears it is likely to decline slowly (*if at all*); and

5. the use of antimicrobials in one person affects others in the immediate and extended environment.[4]

These considerations highlight the critical importance of IPC efforts. As the pressure on AMR mounts, there is a need to maximise these mitigating efforts.

Surveillance systems now demonstrate how variable the incidence and pattern of AMR are between different settings. Researchers have provided compelling evidence on how the pattern of AU has contributed to this. The pace and extent of AMR are governed by human behaviour, and essential drivers include antibiotic consumption, hygiene, sanitation and infection control.[5] The consumption of antimicrobials is not limited to the clinical setting (i.e. human use). However, the inappropriate and excessive use of antimicrobials to treat human infections has significantly contributed to selective pressure, accelerating the development of clinically relevant AMR across all settings.[6] The overuse, misuse, underuse and abuse of antimicrobials represent important modifiable drivers of AMR, as outlined by Hand (2013) (Fig 41.1).

AMR impacts every location where antimicrobials are used. Research has demonstrated the link between AU and AMR at the institutional and patient levels in the hospital setting.[7–9] But research has also highlighted

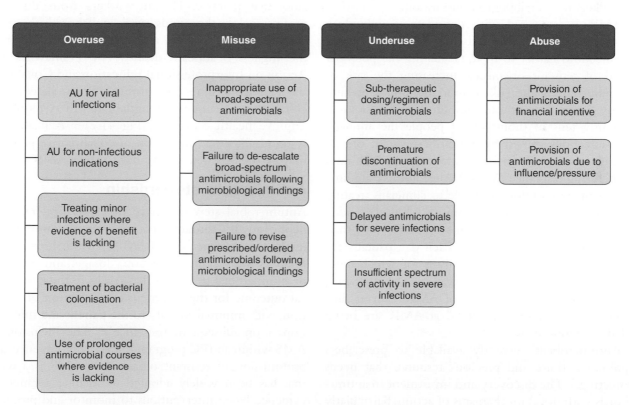

FIGURE 41.1 Examples of antimicrobial overuse, misuse, underuse and abuse

Source: From Doron S, Davidson LE. Antimicrobial stewardship. Mayo Clin Proc 2011;86:1113–23. 10.4065/mcp.2011.0358 and Dryden M, Johnson AP, Ashiru-Oredope D, Sharland M. Using antibiotics responsibly: right drug, right time, right dose, right duration. J Antimicrob Chemother 2011;66:2441–3. 10.1093/jac/dkr370

that AMR is an increasing problem outside hospitals, which is not surprising given the extent of antimicrobial consumption in the community compared to the hospital setting.[10] The relationship between AU and AMR in the community has been evidenced.[11] In 1999, a geographically localised association between AMR and AU in the community setting was demonstrated. The local pattern of AU was shown to directly affect the regional patterns of AMR.[12] AMR is further complicated because the effects of AU may have a prolonged or sustained impact on AMR patterns of organisms. AU is associated with an increased risk of antibiotic-resistant respiratory and urinary tract bacteria up to 12 months after exposure.[13] At an individual level, patients exposed to antibiotics can be at higher risk of being infected by resistant organisms.[14,15] The prescribing of ineffective antimicrobials to patients infected with resistant organisms can, in some cases, increase the risk of mortality from infection when compared to patients not infected with resistant organisms.[16] Patients who receive inappropriate antimicrobial treatment are also at risk of a longer course of the disease or fatal outcomes, increased risk of morbidity, and are more likely to contribute to transmission.[17]

AMR is associated with considerable individual, healthcare system and societal costs.[18,19] AMR is making infections harder to treat, facilitating the potential spread of resistant organisms, increasing the risk of morbidity, raising the risk of mortality and stretching already strained healthcare resources and systems.[20] Currently, tens of thousands of people die annually from infections caused by antibiotic-resistant organisms. The situation is further complicated by high rates of multidrug resistance (MDR). Already there are limited therapeutic options available to clinicians treating infections caused by MDR organisms. Clinical care duration is extended and treatments are more costly than traditional therapeutic options. Each day, patients die from infections caused by organisms for which there are no effective antimicrobials available.[14] Future predictions on the broader cost of AMR remain dire. Maximising interventions aimed at AMR are being called for almost daily.

Antimicrobials currently available to prescribers represent a finite and precious resource that needs protecting.[14] The discovery and investment in antimicrobials with novel mechanisms of action, particularly against Gram-negative bacteria, is challenging, risky and costly.[5,21–23] Indeed, novel treatments for resistant bacterial infections are limited.[24–27] The use of any new antibiotic is compromised by the potential development of rapid resistance from the time it is first used. This hinders the incentive to invest significant amounts of money and time into antibiotic drug discovery.[6] Antibiotics currently in development belong to existing pharmacological classes, targeting existing mechanisms of action, and are often broad spectrum in nature, which has the potential to promote the development of further resistance. Broader spectrum antibiotic consumption has been shown to cause extensive destruction of normal flora, compromise host immune function and render patients vulnerable to opportunistic pathogens.[5]

Without a sustainable pipeline of novel antimicrobials, several strategies have been devised and implemented to mitigate the growing risk of AMR, including more robust infection control practices, a focus on better infection prevention, and plans to improve the use of existing antimicrobials.[9,28] Early attempts to reduce the emergence of AMR were principally aimed at altering prescriber behaviour. However, AMR is everyone's responsibility, including the clients. The most effective strategy to manage this global threat is to enhance interprofessional and collaborative practice. Health workers from different professional backgrounds work collaboratively with patients, families, carers and communities to deliver the highest healthcare quality. The Framework for Action on Interprofessional Education and Collaborative Practice outlines mechanisms to shape successfully collaborative teams to strengthen health systems and improve health outcomes (Fig 41.2).[29] A healthcare system built on a foundation of collaborative practice may be the best defence we have against AMR.

Antimicrobial stewardship

Antimicrobial stewardship (AMS), a critical component of any IPC program, is a vital critical control point in the risk management of AMR. AMS is broadly defined as 'the optimal selection, dosage, and duration of antimicrobial treatment that results in the best clinical outcome for the treatment or prevention of infection, with minimal toxicity to the patient and minimal impact on subsequent resistance'.[30] The inclusion of AMS within an IPC program limits the emergence and transmission of resistant organisms.[31] AMS is a term that has been widely adopted to include a range of evidence-based interventions to monitor and promote the judicious and appropriate use of antimicrobials.[5,18,32] AMS interventions are diverse, and the strategies adopted vary between healthcare settings depending on the best fit (Fig 41.3).

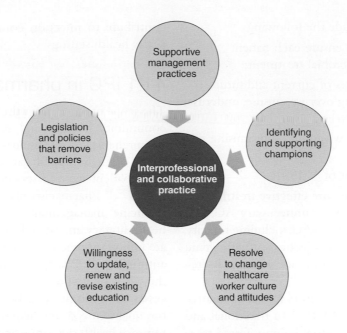

FIGURE 41.2 Mechanisms suggested for shaping effective interprofessional education and collaborative practice
Source: Gilbert JHV, Yan J, Hoffman SJ. A WHO report: Framework for action on interprofessional education and collaborative practice. J Allied Health. 2010;39(SUPPL. 1):196–197

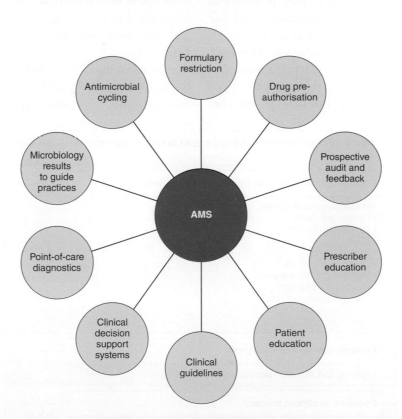

FIGURE 41.3 Examples of AMS interventions
Source: Based on Hand K. Antibiotic stewardship. Vol. 13, Clin Med. 2013;13(5):499-503; Tamma PD, Cosgrove SE. Antimicrobial Stewardship. Infect Dis Clin North Am. 2011;25(1); 245-260; Davey P, Marwick CA, Scott CL, Charani E, Mcneil K, Brown E, et al. Interventions to improve antibiotic prescribing practices for hospital inpatients. Cochrane Database Syst Rev. 2017;2(2):CD003543.

The goals of AMS include the following:

1. work collaboratively to ensure each patient receives optimal antimicrobial treatment;
2. preserve the effectiveness of current and future antibiotics by preventing overuse, misuse, underuse, or abuse;
3. reduce healthcare costs without compromising the quality of care; and
4. reduce the development of AMR.

AMS programs aim to ensure effective treatment of patients with infection, reduce unnecessary AU, and minimise collateral damage from AU, including toxicity, increased risk of colonisation, selection of pathogenic organisms, or infection with antibiotic-resistant bacteria following antibiotic treatment.[5,14,18,31,33,34]

Pharmacists are vital contributors to a collaborative that is tasked with tackling AMR.[35] In traditional and expanded scopes of practice (now being referred to as a full scope of practice), pharmacists play a critical role in contributing to IPC. Pharmacist involvement has traditionally been related to the proper preparation, handling, storage and dispensing of medications, education, development and implementation of guidelines, point-of-care testing and patient counselling. However, the expanded scope of pharmacy practice means that pharmacists are equipped to play a more prominent role in AMS.[36] This chapter explores how pharmacists contribute to infection control, prevention and AMS across health settings.

41.1 IPC in pharmacy practice

The scope of practice for the modern pharmacist in the community, hospital and other healthcare settings, is comprehensive and extends well beyond the mere provision of medicines. Pharmacist roles now encompass a more patient-centred service to optimise patient outcomes.[37,38] Pharmacists play a more significant role in medicine management to improve medicine safety, health literacy and the effective use of medicines. These are important practices to ensure the appropriate use of antimicrobials. Pharmacists have long been involved in the safe supply of drugs through robust dispensing processes. Community and hospital pharmacists promote the quality use of medicines (QUM), which strives to improve health outcomes and reduce preventable harm (Fig 41.4).[39] Pharmacists apply these QUM principles during the provision of any prescription medicine and in all client interactions. When the principles of QUM are applied to reviewing or recommending antimicrobials and managing minor ailments, it contributes to IPC efforts.

Overall reduction of AMR impact can only be effectively achieved by addressing the outpatient use of antimicrobials. Most antimicrobials for human use are

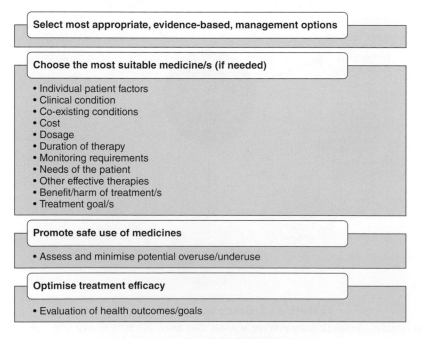

FIGURE 41.4 Elements of QUM practices

Source: Australian Government Department of Health and Ageing. Quality use of medicines (QUM). Canberra: Australian Government, 2022.

in the outpatient setting, and a considerable proportion of these may be inappropriate.[40–44] Around 75% of all antibiotic prescribing is estimated to occur in the community setting.[45] However, not all AU can be attributed to this in the community setting. Over-the-counter supply and access to antibiotics without prescription must be accounted for and critically reviewed. Although the scope of practice and service delivery model of pharmacy varies across the globe, pharmacy practice and pharmacists play an essential collaborative role in managing the risk of AMR.[46,47]

Pharmacists play an essential role in infection control by reducing infection transmission through the proper preparation, handling, storage and dispensing of medicines. Contamination of products may occur during manufacture, compounding, improper preparation, handling, storage, or when the product is expired. The administration of drugs contaminated by microbes may result in infection and harm patients.[48,49]

Aseptic practices, proper compounding, handling, and storing sterile products are critically important in IPC. Contamination of intravenous fluids at any stage of the process is significant due to the substantial risk of harm.[50–52] To reduce the risk of microbial contamination, pharmacists must have the required training and aseptic skills, work within appropriate facilities, and abide by rigorous policies, procedures and quality control programs to prevent contamination, irrespective of the healthcare setting.[48,49,53] Despite attempts at best practice, microbial contamination of these parenteral products still occurs.[54,55] Suvikas-Peltonen et al. (2017) provided a systematic review of incorrect aseptic techniques in medicine preparation. Their work highlighted significant safety risks and offered several recommendations to avoid contamination of these critical medicines. Their findings suggest that improvements are still required for both theoretical knowledge and practical skills to ensure safer preparation and administration of these high-risk medicines. Microbial contamination is more likely to occur when these products are prepared on the ward when compared to pharmacy environments.[56] Evidence shows that greater involvement of pharmacists in the process reduces overall risk due to their aseptic skills and access to purpose-built pharmacy facilities.[55–58] Risk management procedure is proposed to transfer identified high-risk parenteral medicines to pharmacy services for preparation.[59] Improvements in this area will go a long way to improve IPC outcomes.

41.1.1 Expanding the scope of pharmacy practice

Community pharmacies are among the most accessible, frequently accessed health destinations. Pharmacists are well placed with knowledge, skills and capabilities to improve health outcomes across all healthcare settings. Evidence already demonstrates how pharmacists reduce unnecessary prescribing and increase the appropriateness of prescribing antibiotics.[60–62] Pharmacists' traditional roles continue to contribute to IPC strategies in the hospital and community setting through activities that form part of the preventative aspects of pharmaceutical care. Clients present to community pharmacies to help manage a range of minor ailments. Pharmacists play an essential role in triaging these patients. In the context of infections, pharmacists have the knowledge, skills and capabilities to identify when to treat or refer. Hence, pharmacists play an essential role in reducing AU to treat viral infections. Pharmacy practice ensures appropriate and timely access to up-to-date, evidence-based treatment. The education and advice provided by pharmacists in this setting promote self-care, which can reduce AMR through simple, cost-effective interventions.

Embedded, enabled and fully equipped pharmacists will promote antibiotic management (e.g. general practice, hospitals, residential aged care facilities). However, a team approach is needed to improve AU, and every effort should be made to enhance the collaborative practice between prescribers and pharmacists.[47] Collaborative practice agreements (CPAs) centred around physician–pharmacist collaboration have been promoted as a powerful strategy to improve the effectiveness of antibiotic stewardship, particularly in the community setting. These agreements can give community pharmacists autonomy in the care they provide to patients and optimise the effectiveness and efficiency of the collaboration.[60]

41.1.2 The availability of antimicrobials directly from pharmacies

The availability of antimicrobials without prescription from pharmacies directly is cause for concern.[63] Although this type of antibiotic provision can provide timely access to effective treatment, there is concern that it contributes to excessive use of antimicrobials.[64] The lack of access to tools or services required to assist in the accurate diagnosis of infection is misaligned with the ideal objectives of AMS. Technological advances in rapid diagnostics will likely change this perspective soon. For now, however, there is concern from a range of stakeholders that this type of antibiotic availability could lead to inappropriate use, resulting in increasing rates of antibiotic-resistant bacteria. Evidence, however, is lending support to the role of community pharmacists in antimicrobial prescribing. The role of pharmacists in antimicrobial prescribing and the integration of AMS practices in the community setting is associated with patient benefits, healthcare benefits and high patient satisfaction. Importantly, pharmacists involved in these studies were also shown to adhere strictly to the provided guidelines.[36] The provision of antibiotics without prescription or pharmacist prescribing must be accounted for by rigorous evaluation, including surveillance of both AU and antimicrobial appropriateness. In addition, long-term evaluation is needed to ensure that it is fit for purpose and not negatively contributing to AMR. In the absence of this data, more emphasis should be placed on maximising the physician-pharmacist-patient collaboration rather than moving down a pathway of pharmacists prescribing antimicrobials.

41.1.3 The importance of pharmacy education

Delivering a pharmacy workforce with enhanced skills in AMR and AMR-related activities could be an efficient and cost-effective strategy to influence the behaviours of prescribers and the public.[60,65,66] The education of pharmacy students and pharmacists must ensure that they have the appropriate knowledge, skills and capabilities to address contemporary AMR and AMR-related issues. Research shows a disparity between pharmacy students' understanding of AU and knowledge of AMR in various parts of the world. There is a need to standardise the required educational outcomes for all pharmacists. Appropriate education and training, which delivers contemporary AMS skills to pharmacy students, has the potential to have a positive impact on patterns of AU in all healthcare settings. There is also a need to make AMR a core component of professional education, training, continuing education and development to ensure that the latest evidence-based information informs AMS interventions.

This doesn't seem to be the current status. Analysis of prescribing patterns highlights frequent inappropriate prescribing of antibiotics.[67] Blame must not be pointed at any specific profession. Prescribers face daily pressure from patients to provide antibiotics for infections when they are not warranted. There is a need to improve public education to alter antimicrobial prescribing and use expectations.[21] There is a need to

support prescribers when dealing with patient expectations regarding when antibiotics should be prescribed. Prescribers need assistance to strengthen skills in discussing antibiotic resistance with patients. Prescribers should not be pressured to prescribe antibiotics because of patient expectations.[68]

Pharmacists are well placed to support prescribers by providing timely, evidence-based patient education to the public on antimicrobials, AMR and AMR-related issues. Education delivered through pharmacy can reduce the unnecessary use of antibiotics for infections caused by viruses (e.g. common sore throats and colds), which would help reduce expectations and pressures placed on prescribers. Patient education interventions delivered before illness can significantly reduce inappropriate AU and may slow or reverse resistance trends.[67]

Self-medication with antimicrobials (use of antimicrobials without prescription, use of delayed repeats, left-over, or someone else's antimicrobials) is a concerning practice. It is estimated that self-medication accounts for two-thirds of antibiotic use within the pharmaceutical sector and has become a significant factor driving AMR.[69,70] Self-medication with antimicrobials contributes to AMR, increasing the risk of adverse drug reactions (ADRs). Pharmacist education is critically important to prevent self-medication with antimicrobials by clients. Pharmacies should be better used in campaigns to promote and conduct awareness on infection prevention, AMR and appropriate antimicrobials.

Pharmacists prevent the spread of disease by participating in vaccination efforts, providing evidence-based advice regarding exclusion periods for infectious diseases and promoting adequate hygiene precautions and practices.[71] Due to their accessibility, community pharmacists are often the first point of contact for advice about infectious diseases. Pharmacists routinely provide disease information, proper hygiene measures, appropriate minimum exclusion periods if required, treatment advice and critical points for referral. The evidence-based information provided by pharmacists is an essential element of IPC. It is no surprise that this has led to the delivery of expanding pharmacy vaccination services.

41.1.4 The role of pharmacy practice in vaccination

Pharmacists remain among the most trusted, accessible healthcare professionals. Hence, they play a vital role in educating the public on the actual value of vaccination, managing vaccine hesitancy and dispelling false and misleading information about vaccines.[72,73] This evidence-based information is provided free of charge. Pharmacists play an essential role in promoting immunisations across all healthcare settings.[71] More recently, pharmacist-led vaccination services have grown as a critical service to prevent infectious diseases and support improved herd immunity. Pharmacist involvement in vaccination (i.e., as educators, facilitators or administrators) has increased the uptake of immunisations.[74-78] People choosing to be vaccinated by pharmacist-led vaccination services report that convenience was the primary factor in selecting a pharmacy as the site for their vaccination. Other factors influencing their choice included: the positive environment in the pharmacy, the professionalism and knowledge of the pharmacist, and the wait-time post-vaccination.[74]

Pharmacists have become important vaccinators during the pandemic. The accessibility of pharmacies has proven beneficial in boosting vaccination numbers. Pharmacists played an important role in educating people about the benefits of COVID-19 vaccination whilst addressing their concerns. The unique expertise of the pharmacist has also played an important role in the proper storage and handling of the vaccines.[79,80] Czech et al. (2020) presented a review of pharmacists' involvement in providing vaccinations. Shown benefits extend beyond the patient, reducing pressures across the healthcare system.[80] Importantly, pharmacist involvement in vaccination has increased vaccination rates and improved herd immunity.[80]

While novel antibiotic drug discovery is limited, vaccine technologies are increasing.[81-85] The ability to vaccinate more people against more infections may have a vital role in reducing AMR. Vaccinations prevent diseases, but they also prevent secondary diseases by reducing the need for antimicrobial treatment. Enhanced vaccination rates may reduce AMR indirectly by decreasing the need for antimicrobial therapy.[86]

41.1.5 Role of pharmacy practice in antimicrobial disposal

The role of pharmacists is critical to ensure the safe, appropriate disposal of medicines. Pharmacies provide services to collect and dispose of unused and expired antimicrobials through the proper waste management processes. These services reducing the amount of microbials that eventually end up in the environment. Although there is a need for more evidence to determine the extent to which inappropriate antimicrobial disposal contributes to AMR, it seems logical that appropriate disposal has a more negligible effect on the environment and human health. Proper disposal further helps prevent left-over medicines and the sharing

of antimicrobials. Research suggests a need for more uniform guidelines and monitoring in pharmacy practice worldwide and better public education to ensure that unused and expired antimicrobials are safely disposed of.[87-91]

41.1.6 Role of pharmacist in therapeutic drug monitoring

Pharmacists, particularly those in the hospital setting, are routinely involved in the therapeutic drug monitoring (TDM) of antimicrobials to ensure optimal therapeutic outcomes. The optimisation of antimicrobial dosing improves clinical outcomes from infections and reduces the development of AMR.[92] Preventing sub-therapeutic doses of antimicrobials is an essential control to prevent AMR. Pharmacists routinely recommend dosing adjustments to reach the desired PK and PD targets. The dose optimisation of vancomycin by pharmacist recommendation is an excellent example of this significant role.[93-95] Pharmacist involvement improves the optimisation of the initiating dose, enhances the accuracy and timeliness of TDM, achieves the target therapeutic range more frequently and lowers the incidence of harm.[93,96] Ensuring that therapeutic drug concentrations are reached and maintained during antibiotic therapy will reduce the potential risk of AMR.

41.2 AMS and the role of the pharmacist

AMS programs across the healthcare sector prove invaluable in the fight against AMR, with evidence demonstrating pharmacists' vital role.[97,98] The pharmacist's role in hospital AMS is well established and clearly defined (Fig 41.5).[63]

However, community pharmacists appear to be a critical control point in reducing AMR-associated risks.[63] There is still a lot that can be done in a community pharmacy setting to contribute to AMS efforts. Irrespective of the setting, pharmacists' knowledge, skills and capabilities in AMS programs will most likely improve successful outcomes.

AMS activities are unlikely to be effective if they are not built on a collaborative practice framework. AMS strategies adopted need to be consultative to be contextual and relative to a specific clinical setting. Stakeholder consultation is critical when developing and deploying AMS initiatives. Early engagement with leaders, prescribing groups and other key stakeholders will improve acceptance and implementation of AMS.[14]

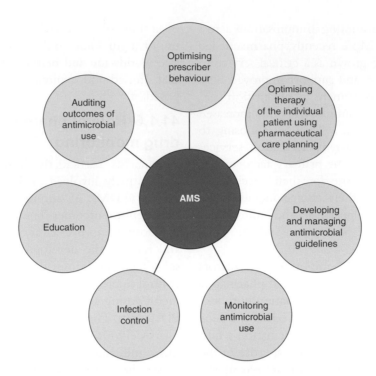

FIGURE 41.5 Essential roles of pharmacists in AMS programs

Source: Garau J, Bassetti M. Role of pharmacists in antimicrobial stewardship programmes.
Int J Clin Pharm. 2018;40(5):948-952.

There is a risk that prescribers may consider AMS interventions condescending or insulting and a threat to clinical autonomy.

The most effective AMS efforts reported in the literature include multiple strategies after collaborating with various stakeholders in a particular clinical setting.[18] AMS programs are not standalone efforts to curb AMR—they aim to supplement IPC strategies. The cooperation of AMS, infection control and healthcare policymakers is essential to tackling AMR.[100]

AMS teams are varied, often influenced by setting, staff availability and budget. Multidisciplinary teams typically run AMS programs. Groups usually include infectious disease physicians, pharmacists (with or without specialised training in infectious disease), nurses, clinical microbiologists and administrative staff. Pharmacists are essential to any AMS effort, given their expertise in medication management.[101] Pharmacists are best positioned to influence the appropriate use of antibiotics. However, there are still numerous barriers to overcome to ensure full participation.[102]

AMS programs or interventions reported in the literature are diverse and their applicability in different settings varies considerably.[100] AMS programs should be multifaceted and comprise policies, guidelines, surveillance, prevalence reports, education and audit practice to optimise prescribing.[103] A one-size-fits-all approach to AMS is unlikely to suit all healthcare settings. What is clear from the literature is that AMS programs and interventions need to target specific factors that influence antimicrobial prescribing and focus efforts to better assist in decision-making.

Additionally, interventions need to be evidence-based in the context of the clinical setting. There is a range of strategies reported in the literature which optimise AU. Despite most of these AMS strategies emerging in hospital practice, the principles and procedures apply to all healthcare settings, including outpatient clinics, long-term care facilities (e.g. residential aged care facilities) and community or primary practice.

41.2.1 Categories of AMS interventions

AMS practices or interventions to influence prescribing behaviour are broadly categorised into restrictive, persuasive, enablement and structural interventions (Fig 41.6).[32]

Despite being more labour intensive and potentially more costly, persuasive interventions, such as prospective audit and feedback, are the most widely practised and more readily accepted by clinicians when compared to restrictive interventions (formulary restriction and pre-authorisation strategies). This is because prescribers

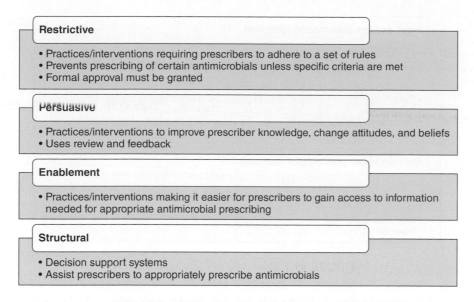

Restrictive

- Practices/interventions requiring prescribers to adhere to a set of rules
- Prevents prescribing of certain antimicrobials unless specific criteria are met
- Formal approval must be granted

Persuasive

- Practices/interventions to improve prescriber knowledge, change attitudes, and beliefs
- Uses review and feedback

Enablement

- Practices/interventions making it easier for prescribers to gain access to information needed for appropriate antimicrobial prescribing

Structural

- Decision support systems
- Assist prescribers to appropriately prescribe antimicrobials

FIGURE 41.6 Categories of AMS interventions

Source: Davey P, Marwick CA, Scott CL, Charani E, Mcneil K, Brown E, et al. Interventions to improve antibiotic prescribing practices for hospital inpatients. Cochrane Database Syst Rev. 2017;2(2):CD003543.

still feel like they have autonomy as the acceptance of recommendations is only voluntary. The feedback mechanisms of the persuasive approach can be tailored to fit the needs of a particular setting, but the effective collaborative practice is still critical for maximised success. Importantly, through feedback mechanisms, persuasive interventions provide opportunities to educate prescribers.[100] Given that AMS outcomes are reliant on changes in the behaviour of individual prescribers, the inclusion of behavioural change strategies is needed to supplement persuasive approaches.[100,104]

The adoption of AI to assist AMS programs to deliver effective persuasive interventions is an important development in the fight against AMR. Prospective audit and feedback are more labour intensive, requiring tailored processes for case selection to maximise outcomes. The availability of electronic medical records and opportunities offered by advances in artificial intelligence will enhance the effectiveness of this approach. Predictive AI models can be developed to identify and triage cases that need review and provide automated workflow alerts to the AMS team. The AI models can be sensitive to patient factors, types of infections and local antibiotic sensitivity patterns.

Both enablement and restriction of AMS interventions increased compliance with antibiotic policies. Enablement interventions enhance the effect of restrictive interventions. When feedback was included with enabling interventions, they were more likely to be effective than those that did not. There are concerns that

restrictive interventions may delay treatment resulting in adverse outcomes. This approach could lead to a negative professional cultural breakdown in communication and trust between infection specialists and clinical teams.[32] There is also the potential that restricting specific antibiotics may increase prescribing of other, not delayed, antibiotics.[14]

41.2.2 Front-end and back-end AMS approaches

AMS approaches can also be categorised as either front-end or pre-prescription authorisation or back-end or post-prescription (Fig 41.7).

Formulary restrictions coupled with continued comprehensive education and guidelines have been shown to reduce AU, improve appropriate antibiotic prescribing, and lower related costs over an extended period.[105] An important activity associated with the back-end approach is de-escalation. De-escalation practices include modifying the initial antibiotic regimen (based on culture data, laboratory tests and patient clinical status); changing from a broad-spectrum antibiotic to one with a narrower spectrum of activity; switching from combination therapy to monotherapy; and stopping antibiotic therapy altogether when justified. The availability of more rapid, accurate tools to support diagnosis will further enhance the efficacy of this back-end approach. A literature survey in this field of study shows an array of impressive technologies that fit the brief. Furthermore, real-time antibiogram data

---

Front-end/pre-prescription approach

- Restrict specific antimicrobials
- Controls needed to specify indication/s, duration of use, when review is required, stop dates
- Targeted reduction of specific antimicrobial use
- Select prescribers have authority to prescribe specific antimicrobials without need for approval
- Prescribers without authority must obtain approval from designated antimicrobial stewards

Back-end/post-prescription approach

- Review of antimicrobial orders
- Recommendations given to continue, adjust, change or discontinue therapy
- Review guided by microbiological and clinical findings
- Evidence-based approach used to guide antimicrobial therapy for each infection type

FIGURE 41.7 Overview of AMS approaches

Source: From Doron S, Davidson LE. Antimicrobial stewardship. Mayo Clin Proc 2011;86:1113–1123. 10.4065/mcp.2011.0358; and Dryden M, Johnson AP, Ashiru-Oredope D, Sharland M. Using antibiotics responsibly: right drug, right time, right dose, right duration. J Antimicrob Chemother 2011;66:2441–2443. 10.1093/jac/dkr370

specific to the setting and local community has the potential to strengthen clinical outcomes.[14]

41.2.3 Antibiotic appropriateness

Appropriate antibiotic use involves selecting a 'targeted spectrum' antibiotic and proper dose and duration.[28] Maximising antibiotic effectiveness depends on pharmacokinetic (PK) and pharmacodynamic (PD) considerations. Therapeutic failure can be avoided by considering PK/PD factors when choosing an appropriate antimicrobial regimen. A sufficient dose and a reasonable administration interval are necessary to ensure that the antimicrobial concentration at the site of infection is high enough to kill or inhibit the growth of the pathogen.[35] Low doses of antimicrobials reduce effectiveness, potentially prolong therapy, and encourage resistance through various mechanisms.[67]

Hand (2013) provided practical guidelines to support effective antibiotic prescribing, including:[5]

1. starting antibiotics immediately in patients with life-threatening infections;

2. prescribing following local policies and guidelines

3. avoiding broad-spectrum agents;

4. documenting indications for prescribing antibiotic in clinical notes;

5. optimising therapy based on microbiology results;

6. using antimicrobial susceptibility data to de-escalate, substitute and add agents, and switch from intravenous to oral antibiotics;

7. prescribing the shortest antibiotic course likely to be effective;

8. always selecting agents to minimise collateral damage;

9. monitoring antibiotic drug levels, where relevant;

10. using single-dose antibiotic prophylaxis where possible; and

11. consulting local infection experts where there is a need.

Schiff et al. (2001) provided a series of practical approaches and suggestions to improve the appropriateness of antimicrobial prescribing (Table 41.1).[106]

The enhanced integration of these guidelines and practical suggestions into pharmacists' education and standard practices will further assist AMS efforts irrespective of setting.

41.2.4 Outcomes associated with AMS

The outcomes of any AMS program need to be carefully assessed to ensure that it delivers the intended goals. Several studies have demonstrated the outcomes AMS interventions and programs have on reducing AU.[32,107,108] Well-designed AMS programs can improve the appropriateness of antimicrobial prescribing, increase antimicrobial effectiveness and improve patient outcomes.[32,109] They can reduce parenteral broad-spectrum AU even when patient care increases and reduce the risk of nosocomial infections.[110] Importantly, several studies have shown that a reduction of AU by AMS interventions does not adversely affect clinical outcomes.[32,111] Comprehensive management programs directed by multidisciplinary teams, computer-assisted decision making and antibiotic cycling have been beneficial in controlling

TABLE 41.1 A practical approach to improving antimicrobial prescribing

Adopt a general approach to improving antibiotic prescribing • Gather credible evidence, address prescriber concerns and scepticism, remove barriers to make it easier for prescribers to change practices
Rethink guidelines • Provide syndrome-based guidance, revise national guidelines for local use, define scenarios in which antibiotics can be safely withheld, offer alternatives, prospectively resolve conflicts over drug choice and empiric regimens, define situations in which immediate treatment is indicated
Get the message out and ensure the change is implemented • Use antibiotic order forms, computer order entry, and infectious diseases specialist consultation
Build viable linkages to leverage change • Bridge disciplines
Improve measurement
Promote non-drug strategies
Increase the patient's roles in treating and preventing infection

Source: Schiff GD, Wisniewski M, Bult J, Parada JP, Aggarwal H, Schwartz DN. Improving inpatient antibiotic prescribing: insights from participation in a national collaborative. Jt Comm J Qual Improv. 2001;27(8):387-402.

antibiotic use, decreasing cost without impacting patient outcomes and potentially decreasing AMR.[112] To date, only a few studies report short-term reductions in AMR associated with AMS programs. Research is still needed to demonstrate the long-term benefits of AMS interventions on AMR.[18]

Pharmacists' contribution to reducing the development and spread of AMR is continuously evolving. AMR interventions led by clinical pharmacists have promoted the rational use of antimicrobials and decreased AU.[113] The benefits shown include both clinical and economic outcomes.[114] Adequately trained pharmacists can considerably minimise inappropriate AU, adding to efforts to contain global AMR.[114] Education appears to be a vital component of programs to combat AMR. Pharmacist-led education-based interventions effectively increase guideline compliance and reduce the duration of antimicrobial therapy.[115] Pharmacists have been shown to facilitate the intravenous-to-oral switch, reduce the use of broad-spectrum antibiotics, reduce costs associated with antimicrobial agent use, reduce associated adverse effects, identify patients

suitable for outpatient antimicrobial therapy (OPAT), and identify patients suitable for outpatient antimicrobial therapy (patients suitable for discharge on oral therapies).[116,117]

What is clear from the published literature on AMS outcomes is these positive outcomes are due to the complementary knowledge, skills and capabilities of the multidisciplinary team driving the interventions and practices. In most cases, the pharmacist is an essential player in these AMS teams. If we are to truly make a difference in AMR, then the pharmacist needs to be fully utilised in AMS programs across the globe.

Conclusion

AMS should be informed by effective, evidence-based programs or interventions, supported by systems to monitor AMR and AU and assess the appropriateness of direct antibiotic prescribing.[5] The success of any AMS program depends on rapid, reliable surveillance systems which monitor AMR and AU. Routine antimicrobial susceptibility surveillance can detect the emergence of resistant pathogens and allow for prompt, targeted interventions.[35] Prescribers may be aware of current guidelines, but local sensitivity data may not always be available.[68] Individual patient-level and community-level antibiotic use changes susceptibility patterns.[14]

Improving the availability of local sensitivity data across all healthcare sectors will better inform prescribing and AMS efforts. Monitoring of antibiotic usage should accompany surveillance programs for antibiotic resistance.[3] Local antimicrobial resistance patterns are essential to update local protocols and prescribe antibiotics appropriately. Population-level surveillance can be effectively achieved by public health personnel working with hospitals and laboratories in their jurisdiction to develop aggregated antibiograms.[10] Clinicians should report any identified trends in antibiotic treatment failure suggestive of resistance.[10]

The timely reporting of microbial culture and susceptibility data is essential for the appropriate management of infected patients. However, there is little value unless patients directly benefit from this rapidly reported data.[108] Currently, available data sources are not readily available in real-time, reducing their value to prescribers rationalising their empiric antibiotic choice. The real-time computer link between a pharmacy (antibiotic orders) and a microbiology laboratory (culture results) provides rapid and clinically useful information. Automated software processes can automatically screen all patients for mismatches between pathogens and drugs and screen for doses inappropriate to MIC or renal function.[108]

Strategies to minimise the risk of AMR are multi-faceted, and the involvement of pharmacists is encouraged. There remains a critical need for investment in novel antibiotic drug discovery to ensure a sustainable pipeline of antibiotics available to clinicians. Evidence-based AMS programs, supported by real-time informatics, in all settings are needed to preserve current and future antimicrobials. Embracing innovative technologies will further bolster the fight against AMR. Digital technologies such as AI, ML, big data and real-time interactive digital dashboards will provide invaluable support tools to all those involved in the battle against AMR. The real-time flow of AMR, AU data and associated factors that are geographically located can provide incredible insights to modify drivers of AU. AI and ML interrogation of the data will facilitate the development of clinician decision support applications with more significant value to prescribers.

The effectiveness of these strategies will no doubt still be dependent on the foundations of better inter-professional and collaborative practice. There remains a need for research to assess AMS program interventions' long-term outcomes objectively, and pharmacists will be essential players in this ongoing challenge.[100] Pharmacists will undoubtedly play an ever-increasing role in these programs across all healthcare settings. Standardising pharmacy practice and associated education and training is essential to ensure that pharmacists can provide a consistent service to support AMR programs to reduce the risk of AMR across the globe.

Useful websites/resources

- National Centre for Antimicrobial Stewardship. https://www.ncas-australia.org/
- Australian Government: Antimicrobial Resistance and Antimicrobial Stewardship. https://www.amr.gov.au/what-you-can-do/hospitals/antimicrobial-stewardship
- Aged Care Quality and Safety Commission: Antimicrobial Stewardship. https://www.agedcarequality.gov.au/antimicrobial-stewardship
- Australian Commission on Safety and Quality in Health Care: Antimicrobial stewardship. https://www.safetyandquality.gov.au/our-work/antimicrobial-stewardship

References

1. Ozkaya-Parlakay A, Polat M. Antibiotic stewardship in urinary tract infection in paediatrics. Pediatr Infect Dis. 2020;39(8):e218-219.
2. Aminov RI. A brief history of the antibiotic era: lessons learned and challenges for the future. Front Microbiol. 2010;8;1:134
3. Goossens H. Antibiotic consumption and link to resistance. Clin Microbiol Infect. 2009;15 Suppl 3:12-15.
4. Levy SB. Multidrug resistance — a sign of the times. N Eng J Med. 1998;338(19):1376-1378.
5. Hand K. Antibiotic stewardship. Vol. 13, Clin Med. 2013;13(5):499-503.
6. Davies J, Davies D. Origins and evolution of antibiotic resistance. Microbiol Mol Biol Rev. 2010;74(3):417-433.
7. Tacconelli E, De Angelis G, Cataldo MA, Mantengoli E, Spanu T, Pan A, et al. Antibiotic usage and risk of colonization and infection with antibiotic-resistant bacteria: a hospital population-based study. Antimicrob Agents Chemother.2009;53(10):4264-4269.
8. Skjøt-Rasmussen L, Olsen SS, Jensen US, Hammerum AM. Increasing consumption of antimicrobial agents in Denmark parallels increasing resistance in Escherichia coli bloodstream isolates. Int J Antimicrob Agents. 2012;40(1):86-88.
9. McGowan J, Tenover FC. Control of antimicrobial resistance in the health care system. Infectious Disease Clinics North America. 1997;11(2):297-311.
10. Bancroft EA. Antimicrobial resistance: it's not just for hospitals. JAMA: 2007:298(15):1803–1804.
11. Bronzwaer SLAM, Cars O, Buchholz U, Mölstad S, Goettsch W, Veldhuijzen IK, et al. The relationship between antimicrobial use and antimicrobial resistance in Europe. Emerg Infect Dis. 2002;8(3):278-82.
12. Magee JT, Pritchard EL, Fitzgerald KA, Dunstan FDJ, Howard AJ. Antibiotic prescribing and antibiotic resistance in community practice: retrospective study, 1996-8. BMJ. 1999;319(7219):1239-40.
13. Costelloe C, Metcalfe C, Lovering A, Mant D, Hay AD. Effect of antibiotic prescribing in primary care on antimicrobial resistance in individual patients: systematic review and meta-analysis. BMJ. 2010;340(may18_2):c2096.
14. Doron S, Davidson LE. Antimicrobial stewardship. In: Mayo Clinic Proceedings. Elsevier Ltd, 2011.
15. Tacconelli E, De Angelis G, Cataldo MA, Pozzi E, Cauda R. Does antibiotic exposure increase the risk of methicillin-resistant Staphylococcus aureus (MRSA) isolation? A systematic review and meta-analysis. J Antimicrob Chemother. 2008;61(1):26-38.
16. Paul M, Shani V, Muchtar E, Kariv G, Robenshtok E, Leibovici L. Systematic review and meta-analysis of the efficacy of appropriate empiric antibiotic therapy for sepsis. Antimicrob Agents Chemother. 2010;54(11)4851-4863.

17. Acar JF. Consequences of bacterial resistance to antibiotics in medical practice. Clin Infect Dis. 1997;24 Suppl 1:S17-18.

18. Tamma PD, Cosgrove SE. Antimicrobial stewardship. Infect Dis Clin North Am. 2011;25(1); 245-260.

19. Roberts RR, Hota B, Ahmad I, Scott RD, Foster SD, Abbasi F et al, Hospital and societal costs of antimicrobial-resistant infections in a Chicago teaching hospital: implications for antibiotic stewardship. Clin Infect Dis. 2009;49(8):1175-1184.

20. World Health Organization. WHO policy guidance on integrated antimicrobial stewardship activities. Geneva: WHO, 2021.

21. Höjgård S. Antibiotic resistance – why is the problem so difficult to solve? Infect Ecol Epidemiol. 2012; 2;10.3402/iee.v2i0.18165. Published online 2012 Aug 20.

22. Wright H, Bonomo RA, Paterson DL. New agents for the treatment of infections with Gram-negative bacteria: restoring the miracle or false dawn? Clin Microbiol Infect. 2017;23(10):704-712.

23. Mo Y, Lorenzo M, Farghaly S, Kaur K, Housman ST. What's new in the treatment of multidrug-resistant gram-negative infections? Diagn Microbiol Infect Dis. 2019;93(2):171-181.

24. Butler MS, Paterson DL. Antibiotics in the clinical pipeline in October 2019. J Antibiot (Tokyo). 2020;73(6):329-364

25. Theuretzbacher U, Gottwalt S, Beyer P, Butler M, Czaplewski L, Lienhardt C, et al. Analysis of the clinical antibacterial and antituberculosis pipeline. Lancet Infect Dis. 2019;19(2):e40-e50

26. da Cunha BR, Fonseca LP, Calado CRC. Antibiotic discovery: where have we come from, where do we go? Antibiotics (Basel). 2019;8(2):45.

27. Theuretzbacher U, Outterson K, Engel A, Karlén A. The global preclinical antibacterial pipeline. Nat Rev Microbiol. 2020;18(5):275-285.

28. Lieberman JM. Appropriate antibiotic use and why it is important: the challenges of bacterial resistance. In: Pediatr Infect Dis. 2003;22(12):1143-1151.

29. Gilbert JHV, Yan J, Hoffman SJ. A WHO report: framework for action on interprofessional education and collaborative practice. J Allied Health. 2010;39(SUPPL. 1):196-197.

30. Gerding DN. The search for good antimicrobial stewardship. Jt Comm J Qual Improv. 2001;27(8):403-404.

31. Dellit TH, Owens RC, McGowan JE, Gerding DN, Weinstein RA, Burke JP, et al. Infectious Diseases Society of America and the Society for Healthcare Epidemiology of America guidelines for developing an institutional program to enhance antimicrobial stewardship. Clin Infect Dis. 2007; 44(2):159-177.

32. Davey P, Marwick CA, Scott CL, Charani E, Mcneil K, Brown E, et al. Interventions to improve antibiotic prescribing practices for hospital inpatients. Cochrane Database Syst Rev. 2017;2(2):CD003543.

33. Davey P, Sneddon J, Nathwani D. Overview of strategies for overcoming the challenge of antimicrobial resistance. Expert Rev Clin Pharmacol. 2010;3(5):667-86.

34. Cunha CB, Opal SM. Antibiotic stewardship. Med Clin North Am. 2018;102(5):831-843.

35. Pflomm JM. Strategies for minimizing antimicrobial resistance. In: Am J Health Syst Pharm. 2002;59(8 Suppl 3):S12-15.

36. Wu JH-C, Khalid F, Langford BJ, Beahm NP, McIntyre M, Schwartz KL, et al. Community pharmacist prescribing of antimicrobials: a systematic review from an antimicrobial stewardship perspective. Can Pharm J (Ott). 2021 May 1;154(3):179-92.

37. Holland RW, Nimmo CM. Transitions, part 1: beyond pharmaceutical care. Am J Health Syst Pharm. 1999;56(17): 1758-64.

38. Tsuyuki RT, Schindel TJ. Changing pharmacy practice: the leadership challenge. Los Angeles, CA: Sage Publications, 2008. http://dx.doi.org/10.3821/1913701X2008141174CP PTLC20CO2

39. Australian Government Department of Health and Ageing. Quality use of medicines (QUM). [cited 3 April 2022]. Canberra, Australian Government. Available from: https://www1.health.gov.au/Internet/main/publishing.nsf/Content/nmp-quality.htm.

40. Fleming-Dutra KE, Hersh AL, Shapiro DJ, Bartoces M, Enns EA, File TM, et al. Prevalence of inappropriate antibiotic prescriptions among us ambulatory care visits, 2010-2011. JAMA. 2016;315(17):1864-1873.

41. Chua KP, Fischer MA, Linder JA. Appropriateness of outpatient antibiotic prescribing among privately insured US patients: ICD-10-CM based cross sectional study. BMJ (Online). 2019;364.

42. Kitano T, Langford BJ, Brown KA, Pang A, Chen B, Garber G, et al. The association between high and unnecessary antibiotic prescribing: a cohort study using family physician electronic medical records. Clin Infect Dis. 2021;72(9): e345-351.

43. Schwartz KL, Langford BJ, Daneman N, Chen B, Brown KA, McIsaac W, et al. Unnecessary antibiotic prescribing in a Canadian primary care setting: a descriptive analysis using routinely collected electronic medical record data. CMAJ Open. 2020;8(2):E360-369.

44. Dolk FCK, Pouwels KB, Smith DRM, Robotham J V., Smieszek T. Antibiotics in primary care in England: which antibiotics are prescribed and for which conditions? J Antimicrob Chemother. 2018;73(Suppl 2):ii2-10.

45. Zuckerman IH, Perencevich EN, Harris AD. Concurrent acute illness and comorbid conditions poorly predict antibiotic use in upper respiratory tract infections: a cross-sectional analysis. BMC Infect Dis. 2007;7;47.

46. Ahmed Abousheishaa A, Hatim Sulaiman A, Zaman Huri H, Zaini S, Adha Othman N, bin Aladdin Z, et al. Global scope of hospital pharmacy practice: a scoping review. Healthcare. 2020;8(2):143.

47. World Health Organization. The role of pharmacist in encouraging prudent use of antibiotics and averting antimicrobial resistance: a review of policy and experience. Geneva: WHO, 2014.

48. Gudeman J, Jozwiakowski M, Chollet J, Randell M. Potential risks of pharmacy compounding. Drugs R D. 2013;13(1):1-8.

49. Rich DS, Fricker MP, Cohen MR, Levine SR. Guidelines for the safe preparation of sterile compounds: results of the ISMP Sterile Preparation Compounding Safety Summit of October 2011. Hosp Pharm. 2013;48(4):282-294.

50. Gershman MD, Kennedy DJ, Noble-Wang J, Kim C, Gullion J, Kacica M, et al. Multistate outbreak of Pseudomonas fluorescens bloodstream infection after exposure to contaminated heparinized saline flush prepared by a compounding pharmacy. Clin Infect Dis. 2008;47(11): 1372-1379.

51. Civen R, Vugia DJ, Alexander R, Brunner W, Taylor S, Partis N, et al. Outbreak of Serratia marcescens infections following injection of betamethasone compounded at a community pharmacy. Clin Infect Dis. 2006;43(7): 831-837.

52. Held MR, Begier EM, Beardsley DS, Browne FA, Martinello RA, Baltimore RS, et al. Life-threatening sepsis caused by Burkholderia cepacia from contaminated intravenous flush solutions prepared by a compounding pharmacy in another state. Pediatrics. 2006;118(1): e212-215.

53. Cairns KA, Avent M, Buono E, Cheah R, Devchand M, Khumra S, et al. Standard of practice in infectious diseases for pharmacy services. JPPR. 2021;51(3):247-264.

54. Austin P, Elia M. A systematic review and meta-analysis of the risk of microbial contamination of aseptically prepared doses in different environments. J Pharm Pharm Sci. 2009; 12(2):233-242.

55. Austin PD, Hand KS, Elia M. Systematic review and meta-analysis of the risk of microbial contamination of parenteral doses prepared under aseptic techniques in clinical and pharmaceutical environments: an update. J Hosp Infect. 2015;91(4):306-18.

56. Suvikas-Peltonen E, Hakoinen S, Celikkayalar E, Laaksonen R, Airaksinen M. Incorrect aseptic techniques in medicine preparation and recommendations for safer practices: a systematic review. Eur J Hosp Pharm. 2017;24(3):175-181.

57. Larmené-Beld KHM, Frijlink HW, Taxis K. A systematic review and meta-analysis of microbial contamination of parenteral medication prepared in a clinical versus pharmacy environment. Eur J Clin Pharmacol. 2019;75(5):609-617.

58. Austin PD, Hand KS, Elia M. Systematic review and meta-analysis of the risk of microbial contamination of parenteral doses prepared under aseptic techniques in clinical and pharmaceutical environments: an update. J Hosp Infect. 2015;91(4):306-318.

59. Beaney AM. Preparation of parenteral medicines in clinical areas: how can the risks be managed – a UK perspective? J Clin Nurs. 2010;19(11-12):1569-1577.

60. Bishop C, Yacoob Z, Knobloch MJ, Safdar N. Community pharmacy interventions to improve antibiotic stewardship and implications for pharmacy education: a narrative overview. Res Social Adm Pharm. 2019;15(6):627-631.

61. Saha SK, Hawes L, Mazza D. Improving antibiotic prescribing by general practitioners: a protocol for a systematic review of interventions involving pharmacists. BMJ Open. 2018;8(4): e020583.

62. Saha SK, Hawes L, Mazza D. Effectiveness of interventions involving pharmacists on antibiotic prescribing by general practitioners: a systematic review and meta-analysis. J Antimicrob Chemother. 2019;74(5):1173-1181.

63. Bishop BM. Antimicrobial stewardship in the emergency department: challenges, opportunities, and a call to action for pharmacists. J Pharm Pract. 2016;29(6):556-563.

64. Frost I, Laxminarayan R, McKenna N, Chai S, Joshi J. Antimicrobial resistance and primary health care. World Health Organization. 2018;3-6.

65. Sakeena MHF, Bennett AA, Carter SJ, McLachlan AJ. A comparative study regarding antibiotic consumption and knowledge of antimicrobial resistance among pharmacy students in Australia and Sri Lanka. PLoS ONE. 2019;14(3):e0213520.

66. Sakeena MHF, Bennett AA, Jamshed S, Mohamed F, Herath DR, Gawarammana I, et al. Investigating knowledge regarding antibiotics and antimicrobial resistance among pharmacy students in Sri Lankan universities. BMC Infect Dis. 2018;18(1):1-11.

67. Steinberg I. Clinical choices of antibiotics: judging judicious use. Am J Manag Care. 2000;6(23 Suppl):S1178-88.

68. Hardy-Holbrook R, Aristidi S, Chandnani V, DeWindt D, Dinh K. Antibiotic resistance and prescribing in Australia: current attitudes and practice of GPs. Healthcare Infect. 2013;18(4):147-151.

69. World Health Organization. Antimicrobial resistance global report on surveillance. Geneva: WHO, 2014.

70. Torres NF, Chibi B, Middleton LE, Solomon VP, Mashamba-Thompson T. Evidence of factors influencing self-medication with antibiotics in LMICs: a systematic scoping review protocol. Systematic Reviews. 2018;7(1):1-5.

71. Rich DS, Kwan JW, Pelham LD, Smaglia RA. ASHP guidelines on the pharmacist's role in home care. Am J Hosp Pharm. 1993;50(9)1940-1944.

72. Hogue MD, Grabenstein JD, Foster SL, Rothholz MC. Pharmacist involvement with immunizations: a decade of professional advancement. J Am Pharm Assoc (2003). 2006; 46(2):168-82.

73. Gatewood S, Goode JVR, Stanley D. Keeping up-to-date on immunizations: a framework and review for pharmacists. J Am Pharm Assoc. 2006;46(2):183-92.

74. Isenor JE, Wagg AC, Bowles SK. Patient experiences with influenza immunizations administered by pharmacists. Hum Vaccin Immunother. 2018;14(3):706-711.

75. Isenor JE, Alia TA, Killen JL, Billard BA, Halperin BA, Slayter KL, et al. Impact of pharmacists as immunizers on influenza vaccination coverage in Nova Scotia, Canada. Hum Vaccin Immunother. 2016;12(5)1225-1228.

76. Baroy J, Chung D, Frisch R, Apgar D, Slack MK. The impact of pharmacist immunization programs on adult immunization rates: a systematic review and meta-analysis. J Am Pharm Assoc. 2016;56(4):418-426.

77. Isenor JE, O'Reilly BA, Bowles SK. Evaluation of the impact of immunization policies, including the addition of pharmacists as immunizers, on influenza vaccination coverage in Nova Scotia, Canada: 2006 to 2016. BMC Public Health. 2018 Jun 26;18(1):787.

78. Isenor JE, Edwards NT, Alia TA, Slayter KL, MacDougall DM, McNeil SA, et al. Impact of pharmacists as immunizers on vaccination rates: a systematic review and meta-analysis. Vaccine. 2016;;34(47):5708-5723

79. Mukattash TL, Jarab AS, Farha RKA, Nusair MB, Muqatash S al. Pharmacists' perspectives on providing the COVID-19 vaccine in community pharmacies. J Pharm Health Serv Res. 2021;12(2):313-316.

80. Czech M, Balcerzak M, Antczak A, Byliniak M, Piotrowska-Rutkowska E, Drozd M, et al. Flu vaccinations in pharmacies—a review of pharmacists fighting pandemics and infectious diseases. Int J Environ Res Public Health. 2020;17(21):1-12.

81. Buchy P, Ascioglu S, Buisson Y, Datta S, Nissen M, Tambyah PA, et al. Impact of vaccines on antimicrobial resistance. Int J Infect Dis. 2020 Jan;90:188-196.

82. Lipsitch M, Siber GR. How can vaccines contribute to solving the antimicrobial resistance problem? mBio. 2016 Jun 7;7(3):e00428-16.

83. Jansen KU, Knirsch C, Anderson AS. The role of vaccines in preventing bacterial antimicrobial resistance. Nature Medicine. 2018;24:10-20.

84. Spika J, Rud E. Immunization as a tool to combat antimicrobial resistance. Canada Communicable Disease Report. 2015;41(S5):7-10.

85. Jansen KU, Anderson AS. The role of vaccines in fighting antimicrobial resistance (AMR). Vol. 14, Hum Vaccin Immunother. 2018. p. 2142-9.

86. Spika J, Rud E. Immunization as a tool to combat antimicrobial resistance. Can Commun Dis Rep. 2015; 41(S5):7-10.

87. Abahussain E, Waheedi M, Koshy S. Practice, awareness and opinion of pharmacists toward disposal of unwanted medications in Kuwait. Saudi Pharm J. 2012 Jul;20(3):195-201.

88. Caban M, Stepnowski P. How to decrease pharmaceuticals in the environment? A review. Environmental Chemistry Letters. Springer; 2021;1:3.

89. Kuspis DA, Krenzelok EP. What happens to expired medications? A survey of community medication disposal. Vet Hum Toxicol. 1996;38(1):48-49.

90. Jones OAH, Voulvoulis N, Lester JN. Potential impact of pharmaceuticals on environmental health. Bull World Health Organ; 2003;81(10):768-769.

91. Michael I, Ogbonna B, Sunday N, Anetoh M, Matthew O. Assessment of disposal practices of expired and unused medications among community pharmacies in Anambra State southeast Nigeria: a mixed study design. J Pharm Policy Pract. 2019;12(1):1-10.

92. Roberts JA, Norris R, Paterson DL, Martin JH. Therapeutic drug monitoring of antimicrobials. Vol. 73, Br J Clin Pharmacol. 2012;73(1):27-36.

93. Xu G, Chen E, Mao E, Che Z, He J. [Research of optimal dosing regimens and therapeutic drug monitoring for vancomycin by clinical pharmacists: Analysis of 7-year data]. Zhonghua Wei Zhong Bing Ji Jiu Yi Xue. 2018;30(7):640-645.

94. Alhameed AF, Khansa S al, Hasan H, Ismail S, Aseeri M. Bridging the gap between theory and practice; the active role of inpatient pharmacists in therapeutic drug monitoring. Pharmacy (Basel). 2019;7(1):20.

95. Hussain K, Ikram R, Ambreen G, Salat MS. Pharmacist-directed vancomycin therapeutic drug monitoring in pediatric patients: a collaborative-practice model. J Pharm Policy Pract. 2021;14(1):100.

96. Imai S, Momo K, Kashiwagi H, Miyai T, Sugawara M, Takekuma Y. Association of the ward pharmacy service with active implementation of therapeutic drug monitoring for vancomycin and teicoplanin-an epidemiological surveillance study using Japanese large health insurance claims database. J Pharm Health Care Sci. 2020;6(1):18.

97. Garau J, Bassetti M. Role of pharmacists in antimicrobial stewardship programmes. Int J Clin Pharm. 2018;40(5):948-952.

98. Gilchrist M, Wade P, Ashiru-Oredope D, Howard P, Sneddon J, Whitney L, et al. Antimicrobial stewardship from policy to practice: experiences from UK antimicrobial pharmacists. Infect Dis Ther. 2015;4(Supp 1):51-64.

99. Garau J, Bassetti M. Role of pharmacists in antimicrobial stewardship programmes. Int J Clin Pharm. 2018;40(5):948-952.

100. Chung GW, Wu JE, Yeo CL, Chan D, Hsu LY. Antimicrobial stewardship: a review of prospective audit and feedback systems and an objective evaluation of outcomes. Virulence. 2013;4(2):151-157.

101. Blanchette L, Gauthier T, Heil E, Klepser M, Kelly KM, Nailor M, et al. The essential role of pharmacists in antibiotic stewardship in outpatient care: an official position statement of the Society of Infectious Diseases Pharmacists. Vol. 58, J Am Pharm Assoc (2003). 2018;58(5):481-484.

102. Weier N, Tebano G, Thilly N, Demoré B, Pulcini C, Zaidi STR. Pharmacist participation in antimicrobial stewardship in Australian and French hospitals: a cross-sectional nationwide survey. J Antimicrob Chemother. 2018;73(3):804-13.

103. Al-Hamad A. The need for antimicrobial stewardship: a public health concern. J Infect Public Health. 2014;7(2):174-175.

104. Charani E, Edwards R, Sevdalis N, Alexandrou B, Sibley E, Mullett D, et al. Behavior change strategies to influence antimicrobial prescribing in acute care: a systematic review. Clin Infect Dis. 2011;53(7):651-62.

105. Rüttimann S, Keck B, Hartmeier C, Maetzel A, Bucher HC. Long-term antibiotic cost savings from a comprehensive intervention program in a medical department of a university-affiliated teaching hospital. Clin Infect Dis. 2004;38(3):348-356.

106. Schiff GD, Wisniewski M, Bult J, Parada JP, Aggarwal H, Schwartz DN. Improving inpatient antibiotic prescribing: insights from participation in a national collaborative. Jt Comm J Qual Improv. 2001;27(8):387-402.

107. Finkelstein JA, Huang SS, Kleinman K, Rifas-Shiman SL, Stille CJ, Daniel J, et al. Impact of a 16-community trial to promote judicious antibiotic use in Massachusetts. Pediatrics. 2008;121(1):e15-23.

108. Schentag JJ, Ballow CH, Fritz AL, Paladino JA, Williams JD, Cumbo TJ, et al. Changes in antimicrobial agent usage resulting from interactions among clinical pharmacy, the infectious disease division, and the microbiology laboratory. Diagn Microbiol Infect Dis. 1993;16(3):255-264.

109. Nguyen-Thi H-Y, Nguyen D-A, Huynh P-T, Le NDT. Impact of antimicrobial stewardship program on vancomycin usage: costs and outcomes at hospital for tropical diseases in Ho Chi Minh City, Vietnam. Risk Manag Healthc Policy. 2021;14:2637-2646.

110. Carling P, Fung T, Killion A, Terrin N, Barza M. Favorable impact of a multidisciplinary antibiotic management program conducted during 7 years. Infect Control Hosp Epidemiol. 2003;24(9):699-706.

111. Lutters M, Harbarth S, Janssens JP, Freudiger H, Herrmann F, Michel JP, et al. Effect of a comprehensive, multidisciplinary, educational program on the use of antibiotics in a geriatric university hospital. J Am Geriatr Soc. 2004;52(1):112-116.

112. Monroe S, Polk R. Antimicrobial use and bacterial resistance. Curr Opin Microbiol. 2000;3(5):496-501.

113. Xu J, Huang J, Yu Y, Zhou D, Wang Y, Xue S, et al. The impact of a multifaceted pharmacist-led antimicrobial stewardship program on antibiotic use: evidence from a quasi-experimental study in the department of vascular and interventional radiology in a Chinese tertiary hospital. Front Pharmacol. 2022;13:832078. Published online 2022 Feb 28. doi: 10.3389/fphar.2022.832078.

114. Sakeena MHF, Bennett AA, Mclachlan AJ. Enhancing pharmacists' role in developing countries to overcome the challenge of antimicrobial resistance: a narrative review. Antimicrob Resist Infect Control. 2018;7:63.

115. Monmaturapoj T, Scott J, Smith P, Abutheraa N, Watson MC. Pharmacist-led education-based antimicrobial stewardship interventions and their effect on antimicrobial use in hospital inpatients: a systematic review and narrative synthesis. J Hosp Infect. 2021;115:93-116.

116. Morrill HJ, Caffrey AR, Gaitanis MM, LaPlante KL. Impact of a prospective audit and feedback antimicrobial stewardship program at a veterans affairs medical center: a six-point assessment. PLoS One. 2016;11(3):e0150795.

117. Taggart LR, Leung E, Muller MP, Matukas LM, Daneman N. Differential outcome of an antimicrobial stewardship audit and feedback program in two intensive care units: a controlled interrupted time series study. BMC Infect Dis. 2015;15:480.

CHAPTER 42

Infection prevention and control in maternity settings

Dr LYNDALL J. MOLLART[i]

RACHEL NEWELL[i]

Chapter highlights

- In the context of the maternity setting, comorbidities such as obesity, diabetes and other chronic diseases impact on women's health and immune systems, with increased risk of infections and sepsis
- Blood-borne pathogen (hepatitis B, C and HIV) transmission within healthcare settings (such as maternity care) continues to occur
- Caesarean section (CS) can increase women's risk of infection
- The safe disposal of clinical waste, such as the placenta, is important to discuss with women to reduce risk of infection
- The chance of women becoming infected with group A streptococcus (GAS) in the postpartum period is 20 times greater than the risk for women in general. Identification of GAS by healthcare professionals is vital

i   School of Nursing and Midwifery, University of Newcastle, Gosford, NSW

Introduction

Midwives, nurse–midwives and obstetric medical officers must use standard precautions as the basic level of infection prevention and control (IPC) when delivering care to all patients (women and babies), regardless of the patient's presumed infection status.[1] Midwives need to have sound knowledge and compliance with standard infection control precautions which are covered in other chapters. Chapter 14 discusses standard precautions in more detail.

Pregnancy (also known as the antenatal or prenatal period: 'natal' meaning birth) is measured in trimesters from the first day of the last menstrual period, totalling 42 weeks or 294 days. The first trimester of pregnancy is weeks 1–12, or about 3 months; the second trimester is weeks 13–27; and the third trimester spans from week 28 to the birth. What happens in the antenatal environment can directly impact on maternal risk factors for infection, and this influences birth and neonatal outcomes. The nature of the woman's pregnancy and fetal environment during pregnancy and labour are important factors influencing the health status of the neonate at birth.

This chapter will focus on:

1. *the risk, prevention and control of healthcare-acquired infections (HAIs)*—also called nosocomial infections—in maternity settings, i.e. pregnancy, childbirth and the postnatal (perinatal period), and newborns

2. *maternity-setting-specific infections*, such as those following waterbirths, caesarean sections and regional anaesthetics, as well as perineal infections and mastitis. Data on HAI data in the maternity setting is currently not publicly available for all jurisdictions in Australia. Victoria is the only state to publicly report the incidence of CS infection.[2]

42.1 Characteristics and contexts of maternity care (midwifery/obstetric practice)

The rate of women giving birth in Australia has decreased from 65 per 1000 women in 2008 to 58 per 1000 women in 2018.[3] The average age of mothers has been rising over time, for both first-time mothers and those who have given birth previously. Pregnant women have increasing rates of comorbidities, such as obesity, diabetes and other chronic diseases, and these conditions impact on women's health and immune systems, with increased risk of sepsis.[4,5]

In developed countries, most women birth in a hospital or birth centre, with few birthing at home. For example, in Australia, 96.3% of women birthed in a hospital, and 2.7% in a birth centre.[3] The rates of women birthing at home varies between 0.3% in Australia,[3] 0.1% in Sweden, 2.3% in the UK, 2.5% in New Zealand, and up to 20% in the Netherlands.[6] Although possibly very small, still concerning is the number of women 'free birthing', meaning that they are *intentionally* unattended by a registered, qualified midwife or obstetrically trained registered professional. However, data are not collected on freebirths.[7]

Caesarean section operations have been steadily increasing worldwide over the past 8 years. In developing countries this increase is needed to reduce maternal and neonatal morbidity and mortality; however, in many developed and high-income countries the CS operation rate has reached alarming levels for non-medical reasons, resulting in no change or improvement in outcomes. For example, in Australia CS operations have increased from 31.6% in 2010 to 35.3% in 2018, which is higher than the CS average of 28 per 100 live births in most Organisation for Economic Co-operation and Development (OECD) countries.[8] As with any operation, women having a CS have increased risk of infection, especially in low-income countries which may lack sterile equipment, educated staff, and infection control policies and guidelines.[9]

42.1.1 Workforce

In many countries, including Australia, the main healthcare providers in the hospital maternity setting are registered midwives (who may also be registered nurses), obstetricians, and in some countries registered nurses that usually work in the postnatal wards. Homebirths in Western countries like the UK, Europe, New Zealand and Australia are attended by registered midwives either in private practice or as part of a publicly funded homebirth program conducted by the public health system.[7,10]

All registered midwives are required to comply with their professional code of conduct and practice standards in relation to IPC. Refer to your country's relevant professional documents and the International Council of Midwives (ICM) Code of Ethics.[11]

42.1.2 Standard IPC practices in maternity setting (midwifery/obstetric practice)

Midwives, medical officers and nurses are involved in all aspects of patient (women/newborns) care and apply a person-centred and holistic approach to their practice. Midwives are a constant in the women's journey, with their valuable contribution to patient safety and quality of care.[1]

The need for personal protective equipment (PPE), safe management of care equipment, and safe management of blood and body fluid spillages in the birth suite is slightly different than in other hospital settings and will be covered in more depth later in this chapter, in the sections on blood-borne pathogens and waterbirths. Disposal of clinical waste, such as consuming or burying the placenta at the woman's home, will be briefly discussed. Human tissue and organs such as the placenta, amniotic sac and umbilical cord are classified as medical or clinical waste.[12] However, some see the placenta as the 'tree of life' and many cultures have rituals and ceremonies with the placenta.[13,14] It is important to remember that the placenta has the potential to harbour microorganisms or subsequently become contaminated. Inappropriate handling or management of the placenta can result in the transmission of infection.[12,14] More information on placental tissue is in section 4.2.3 Horizontal transmission.

42.2 Mode of infection transmission in the perinatal period

42.2.1 Vertical transmission

Vertical transmission of infection means that a pathogen is transmitted from one host/source to its descendants.[15] The time of infection is often critical to the consequences of infection and the extent of childhood harm. Prenatal infection occurs during the pregnancy, labour and postnatal period. Perinatal infection occurs via the transmission of a pathogen during labour/childbirth through blood or vaginal secretions, such as blood-borne viruses (hepatitis C, HIV) and group B streptococcus (GBS).[15] Postnatal infection occurs when the transmission of a pathogen occurs after birth, such as via breast milk.

42.2.2 Transplacental

The placenta serves as the portal of entry for the intrauterine transmission from the mother to the fetus during pregnancy and/or labour (Fig 42.1). Prerequisites are maternal viremia and the ability of the virus to infect the placenta, such as rubella, mumps, smallpox, syphilis, malaria, toxoplasmosis, cytomegalovirus (CMV), Zika virus (ZIKV) and herpes simplex virus, to name a few.[15,16]

An infection of the embryo during organogenesis when the fetus's important organs are developing

(5–10 weeks from conception; heart starts beating by day 22–23) can lead to a developmental disorder of the affected organs called embryopathy. Embryopathogenic viruses cause congenital disease and include rubella virus, parvovirus B19, cytomegalovirus (CMV) and Zika virus (ZIKV).[15,16]

Some microbes can cross the placental barrier, and placental infections are major causes of maternal and fetal disease. Transmission of pathogens from mother to fetus can occur at two sites of direct contact between maternal cells and specialised fetal cells (trophoblasts) in the human placenta:[17]

1. maternal immune and endothelial cells juxtaposed to extra-villous trophoblasts in the uterine implantation site and supportive immune cell types (such as macrophages, T-lymphocytes, T-regulatory cells, natural killer cells, and dendritic cells) that regulate immune defence mechanisms at the maternal-fetal interface[18]

2. maternal blood surrounding the syncytiotrophoblast. As syncytiotrophoblasts are in direct contact with maternal blood, they form the initial line of defence against the hematogenous spread of viruses and other pathogens.[19]

PRACTICE TIP 1

- Infectious agents can reach the placenta either via maternal blood or by ascending the genital tract.
- The membrane around the fetus at conception is a metabolically active tissue.

42.2.3 Horizontal transmission

Horizontal transmission of infection means that a pathogen is transmitted between host/source and susceptible individuals via direct contact such as the faecal–oral route, ingestion of contaminated water or food, or infected blood or blood products (e.g. hepatitis B, HIV).[15,20]

Safe management of the placenta at home: consumption and burying: A placenta provides a perfect environment for bacteria growth, which can be a threat to the health of women if ingested. There are no laws or guidelines regarding the consumption of the placenta but there are precautions that parents can take for health and safety. There are laws regarding the burial of the placenta in the backyard in some countries. Parents are responsible for contacting their local council for any particular guidelines in their municipality on burying human tissue/clinical

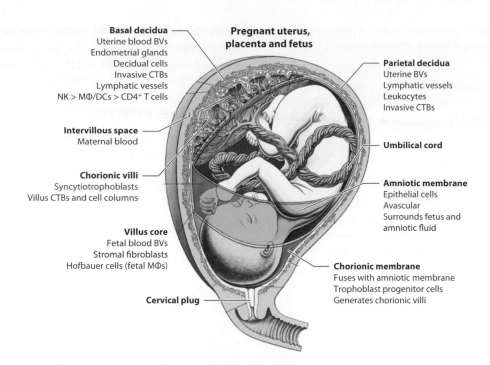

Basal decidua
Uterine blood BVs
Endometrial glands
Decidual cells
Invasive CTBs
Lymphatic vessels
NK > MΦ/DCs > CD4⁺ T cells

Pregnant uterus, placenta and fetus

Parietal decidua
Uterine BVs
Lymphatic vessels
Leukocytes
Invasive CTBs

Intervillous space
Maternal blood

Umbilical cord

Chorionic villi
Syncytiotrophoblasts
Villus CTBs and cell columns

Amniotic membrane
Epithelial cells
Avascular
Surrounds fetus and
amniotic fluid

Villus core
Fetal blood BVs
Stromal fibroblasts
Hofbauer cells (fetal MΦs)

Chorionic membrane
Fuses with amniotic membrane
Trophoblast progenitor cells
Generates chorionic villi

Cervical plug

FIGURE 42.1 Anatomy of third-trimester pregnant uterus depicting the interfaces between the fetus and placenta. The pregnant uterus is composed of the decidualised endometrium: basal decidua, underlying the placenta and parietal decidua in contact with the amniochorionic membrane. Basal decidua contains uterine BVs, endometrial glands, decidual cells, invasive CTBs (placental), lymphatic vessels, and maternal leukocytes: NK cells, macrophage/dendritic cells, and CD4 T-cells. Intervillous blood space, bounded by the placenta and basal decidua, contains maternal blood. Villus cores contain fetal BVs (which receive substances crossing syncytiotrophoblasts and transport them to the fetus via the umbilical cord) and Hofbauer cells (fetal macrophages). The avascular amniotic membrane is lined by epithelial cells, contains the amniotic fluid, and is fused with the chorionic membrane creating a secondary interface with parietal decidua. The cervical plug functions as a barrier to ascending infection.

BV: blood vessel; CTB: cytotrophoblast; DC: dendritic cell; MΦ: macrophage; NK: natural killer.

Source: Figure modified from Standring S, ed. Gray's Anatomy: The Anatomical Basis of Clinical Practice. 39th edn. London: Churchill Livingstone, 2005.

waste.[13,21] While the risk of getting an infection from a healthy placenta is not high, standard hygiene precautions should always be followed.

Placenta consumption: Women consume their placentas to achieve claimed health benefits, including improved mood, energy and lactation.[14] Women have eaten the placenta raw, cooked, roasted, dehydrated, or encapsulated or through smoothies and tinctures.[14,22] The most frequently used preparation appears to be placenta encapsulation after steaming and dehydration.[22]

Placentas for consumption should be treated similar to fresh, raw meat and should be placed in a cooler as soon as possible after birthing. It is recommended that the raw placenta should not be stored in a fridge where food is kept.[21]

PRACTICE TIP 2

Steps for packaging the placenta for transport home are as below:

1. The placenta should be double-bagged and sealed in a plastic 'clinical waste' bag
2. It should then be placed in a rigid-walled, leakproof plastic container for storage and transport
3. The container should be labelled with a date and 'Human tissue for collection by (mother's name)'; and
4. The container must be handed to the mother for removal from the hospital premises.[12]

It is recommended that the placenta is not released from the hospital if the woman has been diagnosed with an infectious condition, or in the interim period when the infectious status of the woman is being determined.[12]

It is recommended that midwives instruct the parents on how to handle the placenta.[12] When handling the placenta:

- cover any cuts or abrasions
- wear protective gloves
- wash hands thoroughly afterwards
- avoid eating or smoking around the placenta; and
- if to be buried, the placenta is to remain in a leakproof plastic container and be buried within 8 hours of its removal from cold storage.

42.3 Blood-borne pathogens (BBPs)

Although routine pregnancy screening for hepatitis B, C and human immunodeficiency virus (HIV) has dramatically decreased the incidence of healthcare-associated BBP infections, transmission of these pathogens within healthcare settings, including maternity care, continues to occur.[23]

42.3.1 Human immunodeficiency virus (HIV)

HIV risk in pregnancy and labour: Perinatal transmission from an HIV-infected woman to her fetus, also known as mother-to-child transmission (MTCT), can occur during pregnancy, labour, delivery or with breastfeeding, and in the absence of any intervention, transmission rates range from 15–45% globally.[24] This wide range is due to access to antiretroviral medications during and after pregnancy by low-income to high-income countries.[25]

Over the last 30 years, 804 cases of perinatal HIV exposure among children born in Australia have been reported.[26] Among 246 children born to HIV-positive mothers in the period 2013–17, the HIV transmission rate from mothers was 1%, compared to 44% in the period 1988–92, and 27% in 1993–97 (prior to the routine antenatal screening and antiretroviral medications during and after pregnancy). In the past 10 years, the transmission rate in Australia was highest in 2015 (4.1%) but has been 0.0% in 6 of the last 10 years, including 2017.[26]

Prevention and control of mother–newborn transmission: Since 1995, the Centers for Disease Control and Prevention (CDC) has recommended all pregnant women be tested for HIV, and if found to be infected, offered treatment to improve their health and to prevent passing the virus to their baby.[27]

Since 2016, the World Health Organization (WHO) has recommended that all people living with HIV, including pregnant and breastfeeding women, be provided with lifelong antiretroviral therapy (ART), regardless of clinical status or CD4 cell count.[28] HIV disease can be managed by treatment regimens composed of a combination of three or more antiretroviral (ARV) drugs. Current antiretroviral therapy (ART), commenced in early pregnancy and continuing throughout pregnancy, does not cure HIV infection but highly suppresses viral replication within the woman's body. It allows the immune system to recover sufficiently to regain the capacity to fight off opportunistic infections, thus reducing the viral load at time of birthing and transfer to the baby.[28]

For current advice on antiviral medications during pregnancy, refer to your local or national guidelines.

Mode of birth: The recommended mode of delivery internationally for HIV-infected women has been CS operation; however, the numbers of planned vaginal deliveries (VD) are increasing.[25] USA Department of Health Guidelines released in December 2019 state that elective scheduled CS is *not routinely recommended* solely for prevention of perinatal transmission in women receiving ART with HIV RNA ≤1000 copies/mL, given the low rate of perinatal transmission in this group.[29] The best mode of delivery should be discussed with the woman.

However, it is recommended that CS occurs before labour and before ruptured membranes among women with HIV not taking antiretrovirals or taking only zidovudine, and the CS be performed if HIV viral load is >1000 copies/ml in the last few weeks of pregnancy (38 weeks gestation).[24]

Breastfeeding: Breastfeeding is recognised as a risk factor for vertical transmission of HIV to the infant and current recommendations vary between high- and low-resource countries.[30,31] The 2016 guideline on HIV and infant feeding developed by the WHO and United Nations Children's Fund[32] states:

'In settings where health services provide and support lifelong ART, including adherence counselling, and promote and support breastfeeding among women living with HIV, the duration of breastfeeding should not be restricted.

Mothers known to be HIV-infected (and whose infants are HIV-uninfected or of unknown HIV status) should exclusively breastfeed their infants for the first six months of life, introducing appropriate complementary foods thereafter and continue breastfeeding.

Breastfeeding should then only stop once a nutritionally adequate and safe diet without breast milk can be provided.'

42.3.2 Hepatitis C virus (HCV)

Risk: It appears that risk of HCV vertical transmission is proportional to the degree of viraemia at the time of delivery; however, the overall (mean) risk of vertical transmission is estimated to be 5.8% (95% CI 4.2–7.8%) among antibody-positive and RNA-positive women.[33] However, this data needs to be interpreted with caution due to the asymptomatic nature of HCV infection, lack of universal antenatal HCV screening for all pregnant women, and the fact that in some countries HCV screening may only be undertaken in pregnant women with risk factors for HCV infection.[34] A well-described risk factor for mother-to-child transmission (MTCT) of HCV is HIV coinfection.[34]

Prevention and control: The CDC and American College of Obstetricians and Gynaecologists (ACOG) have recently revised their HCV screening recommendations to screen all women during pregnancy.[35] This comes into line with the Australian recommendations, with RANZCOG and the Australian Pregnancy Care Guidelines recommending that all pregnant women be tested for HCV early in pregnancy.[36,37]

During the childbearing period, transmission risk of HCV is increased with intrapartum invasive procedures. Fetal scalp electrode insertion is invasive; therefore, *fetal scalp monitoring and blood sampling is contraindicated for HCV RNA-positive women due to the increased risk of vertical transmission.*[34,38] Prolonged rupture of membranes may increase the risk of transmission; however, this could be related to maternal viral load and length of membrane rupture.[39]

Scheduled elective CS are not recommended for HCV RNA-positive women. Several large meta-analyses have demonstrated that vertical transmission of HCV is not influenced by the mode of delivery in women without HIV coinfection.[34]

Newborn: The baby should be bathed or the skin at the injection site should be cleaned with soap and water (if visible blood) OR with an alcohol swab before administering injections of hepatitis B vaccine, immunoglobulin, vitamin K to prevent risk of transmission.[40]

Breastfeeding: Breastfeeding should not be discouraged as there is no evidence of association with an increased risk of transmission of HCV to the newborn unless the mother's nipples are cracked or bleeding.[34] Women should be advised, if they have cracked or bleeding nipples, to express and discard the breast milk until healed.

PRACTICE TIP 3

- Midwives and medical officers need to take care when performing an artificial rupture of membranes (ARM) to not scratch the baby's head with the amihook, i.e. not break the fetus' skin integrity and thereby increase the risk of vertical transmission with HCV RNA-positive women.
- If fetal distress, as assessed by non-invasive means, is sufficiently severe and would normally require invasive fetal monitoring, then consultation between senior obstetric medical staff and the woman and partner is to be undertaken to discuss the need for emergency CS.

CASE STUDY 1

Caring for women that are HCV RNA positive

Situation:

You are working in the postnatal ward and receive handover of a woman with HCV RNA-positive who has just birthed.

Questions:

1. What do you need to consider regarding your clinical care of her in relation to her HCV status?
2. What education or information do you need to provide?

Answer: Careful disposal of peri pad with blood, shared postnatal ward rooms and bathrooms re blood, breastfeeding and cracked nipples.

42.3.3 Hepatitis B virus (HBV)

Risk: Preventing mother-to-child transmission (MTCT) is crucial in reducing the HBV infection rate which is still a major global health issue—257 million people have chronic HBV infection.[41] HBV infection in infancy or early childhood often leads to chronic infection, so appropriate prophylaxis and management of HBV in pregnancy is crucial to prevent MTCT.[42] This is important, because more than 90% of infants with the infection will develop chronic infection, with the potential for significant adverse health outcomes.[43] Perinatal transmission in China has been reported as being as low as 0.9%.[44] Perinatal transmission in Australia has not been reported and is not routinely monitored.[45]

When a mother has high levels of circulating virus HBV DNA, approximately 10% of babies are still at risk of infection despite the current strategy of giving HBIG and HBV vaccination at birth.[43] A theory to explain these infants' failure to resolve HBV infection is that the maternal hepatitis Be antigen (HBeAg) crosses the placenta, resulting in a tolerising effect on the developing fetal immune system.[43,46]

Prevention and control—screening: It is recommended that all pregnant women are screened for hepatitis B surface antigen (HBsAg) at the first antenatal visit, and should be provided with verbal and written information.[47,48]

A woman identified as HBsAg positive should be tested for hepatitis Be antigen (HBeAg) and hepatitis B virus (HBV) DNA, to determine risk of transmission to the neonate and the degree of infectivity.[46,47] It is recommended that HBsAg-positive women with high viral loads (>200,000 IU/mL) be referred to a specialist for consideration of antiviral therapy (between 28–32 weeks gestation) to further reduce the MTCT risk.[43,47]

Labour/birth: Based on available evidence, MTCT HBV transmission usually occurs during the birth (as opposed to pregnancy) but evidence supporting elective CS delivery being a protective factor is conflicting and not high quality. Consequently, there are no international guidelines recommending elective CS to prevent MTCT.[46] However, transmission risk of HBV is increased with intrapartum invasive procedures (fetal scalp electrode insertion); therefore, fetal scalp monitoring and blood sampling is contraindicated for women with positive HBeAg and HBsAg.[49]

Neonates of HBeAg positive and HBsAg-carrier mothers: As perinatal transmission of HBV occurs through exposure to blood and blood-contaminated fluids at or around birth, it is recommended that the newborn be bathed or the skin at the injection site should be cleaned with soap and water OR with an alcohol swab before administering any injections to reduce any risk of transmission.[50]

The neonate should be given hepatitis B immunoglobulin (HBIG) 100 international units (0.5 ml) intramuscularly into one thigh, preferably within 4–12 hours after birth (and certainly within 24 hours), irrespective of gestational age; AND monovalent hepatitis B vaccine is given at the same time but in the other thigh.[46,51,52]

Breastfeeding: HBsAg-positive mothers are encouraged to breastfeed as long as the newborn receives doses of HBIG and hepatitis B vaccine at birth.[46,48] Women should be advised if they have cracked or bleeding nipples to express and discard the breast milk until healed as a precaution, as HBV is spread via blood.[48]

Follow-up: It is recommended that all babies of HBsAg-positive mothers should have three or four subsequent doses of HBV vaccine depending on the country (different schedule guidelines for preterm babies); and be tested for HBsAg and anti-HBs after 9–12 months of age (at least three months after final dose of HBV vaccine).[46,48,52,53]

PRACTICE TIP 4

- For a schedule of HBIG, check your country's requirements. For example, in Australia refer to the Australian Immunisation Handbook, which is online and regularly updated.

  Note: HBIG is a blood product made from human plasma (CSL Behring.com.au) and in accordance with country's legislative health policies requires written consent prior to administration.

42.4 Common pathogens in the perinatal period and HAIs

Perinatal infections occur during, shortly before or shortly after birth. Common infections and their respective pathogens are:

- sepsis or meningitis due to *Listeria monocytogenes*, beta-haemolytic streptococci group B (*Streptococcus agalactiae*), or *Escherichia coli*
- eye infection or sepsis due to *Neisseria gonorrhoeae*
- eye infection due to *Chlamydia trachomatis*

- hepatitis B
- primary genital herpes simplex; and
- primary varicella.[15]

The major pathogens causing fatal perinatal infections are *E. coli* and coliforms, *Streptococcus pneumoniae*, and *Streptococcus pyogenes*, also known as group A streptococcus or GAS (Phillips and Walsh 2019).

42.4.1 Group A beta-haemolytic streptococci (GAS)

Background and risk: GAS is a Gram-positive, b-haemolytic organism that is adaptable and can cause a variety of wound infections, such as pharyngitis, impetigo, pneumonia, meningitis and endometritis.[54]

In the maternity setting, postnatal or puerperal infection is usually caused by GAS, and it has been reported that 120 different strains of GAS have emerged in recent times. The chance of women becoming infected with GAS in the postpartum period is 20 times greater than the risk in general women.[54]

Modern hospital-associated epidemics of postpartum GAS infection, though rare, still occur. Only 15–25% of GAS postpartum infections are from nosocomial acquisition, largely due to improved infection control practices and shorter hospital stays after delivery.[55]

Risk factors include invasive procedures such as CS, regional anaesthesia, intravenous (IV) lines and indwelling catheters.[56] Even after an uncomplicated vaginal birth, mucosal barriers can be compromised due to vaginal tears, an open cervix, and altered vaginal pH due to the postpartum uterus being a conducive environment for organisms to invade. Bacteria thrive in necrotic decidual tissue and blood.[54] The spectrum of GAS postpartum infections can develop rapidly—ranging from mild endomyometritis (absence of tachycardia and leukocytosis) to fulminant endomyonecrosis and death.[57]

Prevention and control: The CDC recommends in-depth epidemiologic investigations for two or more cases of invasive GAS infection occurring at an institution in a 6-month period, including screening of healthcare personnel.[58]

Mother: There are no recommendations for screening pregnant women for GAS infection before delivery, because of the relatively low (0.03–0.37%) reported prevalence of vaginorectal colonisation of GAS during pregnancy.[59]

In the early postpartum period, diagnosis of GAS infections is often difficult due to a low prevalence of these infections and to initial non-specific symptoms.[59] Because postpartum GAS infections remain relatively uncommon, midwives and obstetricians often misconstrue the pain of developing infection as typical postpartum discomfort.[54] The occurrence of fever, chills and abdominal pain in an early postpartum woman warrants an aggressive attempt to provide a definitive diagnosis[59] and staff to be alert for increased respiration rate and SaO2 which are the first signs for sepsis.[54]

Neonate: In neonatal sepsis, *Streptococcus pyogenes* can be detected in blood culture, cerebrospinal fluid and urine of newborns.[15] A GAS infection is rare in neonates, presenting in late onset sepsis—and nosocomial transmission is the likely cause. The presence of soft tissue infection or toxic shock-like syndrome should prompt clinical consideration (Table 42.1).

42.4.2 Group B beta-haemolytic streptococci (GBS)

Background and risk: GBS is part of the normal bacteria that lives in the body (e.g. the vaginal canal). However, maternal colonisation of the lower genital tract with GBS during pregnancy increases the risk of neonatal infection by vertical transmission.[60] Maternal colonisation rates vary, with estimated prevalence of 10–30%, as colonisation may be transient, intermittent or persistent.[61]

Streptococcus agalactiae or group B streptococcus (GBS) is the most frequent cause of early onset neonatal streptococcus disease (EOGBSD), with 50% of babies with EODBS showing signs at birth.[61] Neonatal EODBSD occurs in approximately 3–6 per 1000 births[62] and mortality from EOSBSD is estimated at 6%.[63] Late onset neonatal GBS disease (LOD) occurs at 5–8 days of age (estimated incidence 2 per 1000 births), and is associated with meningitis and pneumonia.[15]

Prevention and control: *Pregnancy: risk reduction— universal screening versus risk factor treatment:* Most countries recommend offering all women screening for GBS at 35–37 weeks gestation (low vaginal/rectum swab/s). This includes women with planned CS because of their risk of labour or ruptured membranes earlier than the scheduled CS.[60]

Both routine antenatal screening (35–37 weeks) and risk-based treatment approaches are currently used in various states and territories of Australia as there is limited high-quality scientific evidence (no randomised controlled trials) and a lack of expert consensus.[64] The risk factor approach involves no universal antenatal

TABLE 42.1 Group A versus group B Streptococcus

Characteristic	Streptococcus pyogenes (Group A)	Streptococcus agalactiae (Group B)
Common sites of colonisation	Throat and skin	Intestinal and genital tracts
Manifestations	Impetigo	Asymptomatic bacteriuria
	Strep throat	Urinary tract infection
	Scarlet fever	Pyelonephritis
	Cellulitis	Postpartum endometritis
	Invasive disease	Amnionitis
	Necrotising fasciitis	Neonatal infection (e.g. meningitis, pneumonia)
Source	Community-acquired nosocomial	Ascending
	Descending (originating in respiratory tract)	Passage through birth canal
Screening	No routine screening pharyngeal culture in pregnant women with upper respiratory infection symptoms	Vaginal and rectal culture at 35–37 weeks gestation (plus urine culture considered with heavy colonisation)
Treatment	Penicillin	Amoxicillin or cephalexin for urinary tract infection
	Clindamycin	Prophylactic intrapartum antibiotics
	Source control (e.g. debridement, hysterectomy)	
Sequelae	Toxic shock syndrome, rheumatic fever, glomerulonephritis	Neonatal infection and/or death, intrauterine fetal demise
Risk factors	Postpartum period, comorbidities, history of upper respiratory symptoms or risks (e.g. exposure to children)	Vaginal colonisation, urinary tract infection (group B Streptococcus), previous pregnancy with neonatal infection, premature rupture of membranes, preterm birth
Onset of symptoms	Rapid Postpartum (usually 1–2 days)	Neonatal Early onset (within 24 hours of birth) Late onset (up to 30 days after birth)

Lees E, Carrol E. Treating invasive Group A Streptococcal infections. Paediatrics & Child Health, 2014;24(6);242–247, 10.1016/j.paed.2014.01.001

screening; treat all women with risk factors for EOGBS with intrapartum antibiotics.[61]

Risk factors for EOGBS and for routine intrapartum antibiotics prophylaxis (IAP) include:[61]

- GBS colonisation in current pregnancy
- GBS bacteriuria in current pregnancy
- preterm labour (<37+0 weeks)
- previous baby with EOGBSD
- rupture of membranes (ROM) >18 hours. If labour established: at 14 hours after ROM and birth is unlikely by 18 hours, then commence IAP
- maternal temperature ≥38°C intrapartum or within 24 hours of giving birth

Newer and quicker PCR testing: A major limitation with universal antenatal screening at 35–37 weeks gestation is its low positive predictive value for GBS colonisation at term (at time of birthing) due to considerable fluctuations in GBS colonisation over time. It has been reported that 41% of women who are positive for GBS at 35–37 weeks are negative at the time of birth, which leads to unnecessary use of antibiotics for the mother and transmission to the newborn.[65]

The alternative is a rapid test based on qPCR technology whereby rectal and vaginal swabs are collected when a woman presents in labour and a result is obtained in approximately 50 minutes. An Australian study found GBS PCR sensitivity and specificity were 89.0% (95% CI–82.8–93.6%) and 97.9% (95% CI–96.0–99.0%) respectively, higher than compared with swab culture.[66] Compared with the historical cohort, PCR reduced the requirement for intrapartum antibiotics by 25.6% (P < 0.001) and there were no significant differences in maternal outcomes or combined rates of admissions to neonatal intensive care or special care nursery.[66] It is unclear why this newer, more specific test has not been introduced more widely as the qPCR has demonstrated high sensitivity for GBS detection in Australian and international studies.[66-69]

Pregnancy: Women with a GBS positive swab at 35–37 weeks gestation *are not treated in pregnancy* and it does not reduce the likelihood of GBS colonisation at the time of birth.[70] However, women with GBS urinary tract infection (growth of greater than 105 cfu/ml) during pregnancy should receive appropriate treatment at the time of diagnosis as well as IAP.[70]

Labour: management and treatment
- Membrane sweeping (to stimulate contractions) *is not contraindicated* in women who are carriers of GBS.[70] Birth in a pool *is not contraindicated* if the woman is a known GBS carrier provided she receives appropriate IAP.[70]
- Women with GBS positive culture or unknown status with ruptured membranes: induction of labour is recommended and commence IAP.[60]
- Women with GBS positive culture at 35–37 weeks, or confirmed preterm labour/birth *where GBS carriage status is unknown*, maternal GBS bacteriuria during pregnancy or previous infant with EOGBS: treat with IAP.[60]
- Women with risk factors: administration of IAP to all women at risk of transmitting GBS to their baby.[61]
- Women with positive GBS culture or risk factors are advised to remain in hospital for 24–48 hours after the birth so that the baby can be observed for signs of group B streptococcus infection.[64]

Neonatal: *Early onset (EOGBSD):* The Royal College of Obstetricians and Gynaecology released an updated Green-top guideline with new recommendations;[70] these include:
- term babies who are clinically well at birth and whose mothers have received IAP for prevention of EOGBS disease more than 4 hours before delivery do not require special observation

- women with known GBS colonisation who decline IAP should be advised that the baby should be very closely monitored for 12 hours after birth, and discouraged from seeking very early discharge from the maternity hospital.

Late onset GBS: The symptoms most often occur from the second week of life.[15] It is important to remember that intrapartum antibiotic prophylaxis (IAP) does not prevent late onset GBS disease (LOD).[61]

At discharge offer parents of babies, at increased risk of late onset (LOD), advice about: signs of sepsis in the newborn; and importance of seeking medical assistance if baby unwell.[61]

PRACTICE TIP 5

- Routinely provide written information (in appropriate languages) about GBS and EOGBSD to women during the antenatal period to ensure they can provide informed consent.[61]
- Request antibiotic susceptibility testing on GBS vaginal/rectal swab cultures (and MSU) in women who are thought to have a significant risk of anaphylaxis from penicillin.[60]

CASE STUDY 2

GBS screening during pregnancy

You are providing antenatal care with a primigravida with no GBS risk factors and she is undecided about having the GBS swab screening at 35–37 weeks gestation (your hospital policy). What evidence-based information could you provide her that could assist her in her decision?

Answer:
- *Maternal colonisation rates vary with estimated prevalence of 10–30% as colonisation may be transient, intermittent or persistent*
- *Neonatal EODBSD occurs in approximately 3–6 per 1000 births, with 50% at birth and mortality from EOSBSD is estimated at 6%*
- *If chooses not to swab screen at 35–37 weeks, and experiences ruptured membranes, she needs to present to hospital as soon as possible. When presenting or in labour, staff will assess for any GBS risk factors*

- *Provide written information about GBS and EOGBSD for her to read and consider. She needs to be aware that many websites do not provide evidence-based information*
- *Document the discussion in her medical records*

42.4.3 Escherichia coli

Background and risk: In pregnancy, renal physiology changes, with marked volume expansion and vasodilation (ureters dilate, particularly on the right). The dilated collecting system promotes urinary stasis, increasing the risk of pyelonephritis with asymptomatic bacteriuria (ASB).[71]

Escherichia coli is part of the normal physiological intestinal flora but the most frequent cause of HAIs and the common pathogen of urinary tract infections (UTIs) and sepsis[15] in pregnancy.[72]

Asymptomatic bacteriuria (ASB) incidence during pregnancy has been reported to be 2–10%[71] and if untreated, up to 30% of women will develop acute pyelonephritis.[72] How a UTI may cause premature labour is not fully understood, but the theory is that proinflammatory cytokines secreted in response to bacterial endotoxins likely initiate labour in these women.[71]

Pyelonephritis most often presents between 20–28 weeks gestation. Bacteraemia is a common and usually transient complication of pyelonephritis. Without treatment, the complications of acute pyelonephritis during pregnancy can be severe, more so than in non-pregnant women.[71] Occasionally, women may become septicemic and develop endotoxemia with shock, with sequelae including respiratory failure, disseminated intravascular coagulation (DIC) and acute kidney injury.[71] In pregnancy, if untreated there is an increased risk of fetal morbidity such as preterm birth, low birth weight and stillbirth.[73]

Catheter-associated UTI (CAUTI): Due to the hormonal changes in the urinary system during pregnancy, there is an increased risk for women to develop a CAUTI during pregnancy and the postnatal period. Until recently, indwelling urethral catheters were inserted routinely prior to or immediately after a CS operation. There is emerging evidence that suggests that immediate postoperative removal of catheters after CS may decrease rates of CAUTI and facilitate early ambulation; however, urinary catheters are still used widely and remain in longer than necessary.[74] It is routine practice that women receive antibiotic prophylaxis 60 minutes prior to skin incision, dosed on a weight-based schedule to reduce risk of infection, not necessarily to address possible CAUTI. Other prevention measures related to the prevention of CAUTI are detailed in Chapter 17.

Prevention and control: The current recommendation is that all women have a midstream urine sample collected on the first antenatal visit to identify asymptomatic urinary tract infection.[64] Discuss with the woman at the first antenatal visit, the importance of identifying UTI early in pregnancy.

Treating ASB during pregnancy may reduce the incidence of pyelonephritis, low birthweight and preterm delivery.[72]

The challenge with identifying pyelonephritis in pregnant women is they may only have lower urinary tract symptoms, or present with acute abdominal pain or premature labour.[71]

Diagnosis of pyelonephritis is usually made on clinical symptoms such as fever with chills, nausea/vomiting, dysuria, increased frequency, urgency and CVA tenderness (usually unilateral).[73] Treatment with a 3–7 day antibiotics regimen should not be delayed while waiting for a definitive diagnosis by positive urine culture.[71]

PRACTICE TIP 6

- When possible, urethral catheters should be avoided or removed as early as possible, even in women having CS section, because the incidence of UTI in these women is twice that of those not catheterised.[71]

42.4.4 Herpes simplex virus

Background and risk: Women with genital herpes can be infected with either herpes simplex virus (HSV) type 1 (herpes labialis) or HSV type 2 (herpes genitalis) or both, although HSV-2 is more common.[75] The primary concern of HSV in pregnancy is maternal-fetal transmission at the time of birthing as a result of direct contact with the virus shed from lesions around the cervix and vaginal canal; shedding can occur without symptoms.[24,76] The incidence of neonatal HSV rate has been reported to be 1 per 17,000 live births in Canada,[76] 1 in 3500 in the USA,[75] and 3.27 per 100,000 in Australia.[77]

Distinguishing a primary from a non-primary infection of HSV in pregnancy cannot be based on clinical findings. Diagnosis is based on a combination of positive viral findings and negative serological tests or evidence of seroconversion.[78]

Pregnant women who have preexisting genital HSV have a very low risk of transmitting the virus to the baby during labour/birth as the maternal acquired antibodies help to protect the newborn.[15] If a genital lesion is present at the time of birthing with preexisting HSV, the risk of neonatal infection is reported to be 2–5%.[75]

It is especially problematic when a woman's first contact with herpes simplex virus type 2 occurs during the third trimester of pregnancy, since it increases the risk of a perinatal infection of the newborn with *herpes neonatorum*. As the woman is unable to complete seroconversion to IgG prior to labour and the baby is birthed in the absence of protective passive maternal (IgG), the virus can spread to the newborn, with local infections of the skin and mucous membranes to generalised infection involving the internal organs and the central nervous system (CNS).[15,75]

Neonatal HSV may be classified into three main categories for therapeutic and prognostic considerations: localised skin, eye and mouth (SEM) lesions; CNS (encephalitis); and disseminated disease. There is a high risk of progression from SEM lesions to CNS or disseminated disease if untreated; eye involvement can lead to permanent vision impairment.[75] Mortality of disseminated disease exceeds by 80% if untreated.[24] *Kerato-conjunctivitis herpetica* is inflammation of the cornea and possibly also the conjunctiva, dominantly by herpes simplex type 1.[15]

Prevention and control: This is the most challenging issue, as many infants with neonatal HSV (NHSV) are born to mothers with no history of genital HSV infection.[76] However, routine HSV screening of pregnant women is not recommended.[78] It has been recommended that a pregnant woman who does not have a HSV history but who has a partner with genital HSV should have type-specific serology testing to determine her risk of acquiring genital HSV in pregnancy or as early in pregnancy as possible; and testing repeated at 32–34 weeks gestation.[75]

It is best practice that women are asked at the first antenatal visit if there is a history of or current genital herpes. For women with preexisting HSV infection it is important to document confirmed diagnosis, occurrence and last episode of outbreak.

If a pregnant woman (with no prior history of genital herpes) presents with clinical features suggestive of genital herpes, it is recommended to obtain HSV serology (type specific) and swab the genital lesion for HSV PCR (preferably within 36 hours of lesion appearance).

A primary infection will be HSV Ab negative to type from a genital HSV PCR test.[78]

For women with recurrent outbreaks during pregnancy, antiviral therapy can be commenced regardless of gestation if manifestations are very severe or unacceptable to the woman.[24,77] Suppressive antiviral therapy is recommended from 36 weeks gestation through to birthing for women with a history of genital HSV to reduce the risk of viral shedding at the time of birthing and the need for a CS operation.[24,75]

Although the risk of transmission is low (2–5%), the mode of delivery (i.e. vaginal birth or CS) needs to be discussed with the woman. However, if there are prodromal symptoms or in the presence of a lesion suggestive of HSV at the time of labour, the woman should be offered a CS operation.[75]

For women who develop a primary HSV infection in late pregnancy, a scheduled elective CS operation at term is recommended because of more prolonged viral shedding, lack of maternal protective antibodies and higher risk (30–50%) of neonatal transmission.[15,24,75]

PRACTICE TIP 7

- Provide education to women on the risks related to genital herpes outbreak. Remind women that they need to inform staff if they experience an outbreak during pregnancy or when presenting in labour.

42.4.5 Influenza and pertussis (whooping cough) vaccinations

Influenza—risk: Influenza is more likely to cause severe illness in pregnant and postpartum women than in women who are not pregnant/postpartum. Changes in the immune system, heart and lungs during pregnancy make pregnant women more prone to severe illness from influenza.[79] Pregnant women and their babies are at increased risk of influenza-related complications and infection during seasonal and pandemic influenza outbreaks.[79,80]

Pertussis (whooping cough)—risk: Pertussis can be a life-threatening infection in babies, with mortality up to 2% in the first year of life.[15] Pertussis in babies can lead to apnoea, pneumonia, feeding problems and weight loss, seizures and brain damage. Older children and adults can get whooping cough too, and pass it on to babies.[81]

Prevention and control: Immunisation of pregnant women against influenza and pertussis has now been shown to be effective in not only protecting the mother but also the fetus/newborn via transfer of transplacental antibodies and through breastfeeding.[80] Pertussis and influenza immunisation is recommended during pregnancy and in every pregnancy.[82]

Influenza immunisation for pregnant women is recommended at any time during pregnancy and in every pregnancy.[79,83] Maternal vaccination in the second and third trimester will elevate newborn antibody levels.[82]

Pertussis immunisation for pregnant women is a single dose adult vaccine in combination with tetanus and diphtheria toxoids for women in the third trimester of pregnancy (27–36 weeks) and in every pregnancy.[81] Earlier in this trimester is preferred as it takes about 2 weeks for maternal antibodies to peak and for active transfer of transplacental antibodies.[81,82]

Postpartum pertussis vaccination is not optimal as it does not provide immunity to the newborn who remains at risk of contracting pertussis from others, including siblings, grandparents and other care providers.[81] 'Cocooning' means vaccinating anyone who comes in close contact with the newborn; however, cocooning alone is not effective and difficult to implement to ensure everyone who is around the baby is vaccinated, for example, shopping centres.[81,82]

PRACTICE TIP 8

- It is recommended to discuss vaccination with pregnant women at their first visit, and at the 24-week visit check-up in advance of the 28-week visit so there has been time to consider, thus ensuring informed consent for the vaccination.

- Women have the right to decline care or advice if they choose, or to withdraw consent at any time and have these choices respected. It is important that the level of care provided does not alter because of this choice.[64]

- Midwives and nurses are entitled to hold personal beliefs on vaccinations/immunisations, but they must ensure that they do not contradict or counter public health campaigns, including about the efficacy or safety of public health initiatives. In response to practitioners who have advocated against evidence-based vaccination programs, National Registration Boards have released position statements.[84] For Australian health professionals, refer to the NMBA position statement on nurses, midwives and vaccination. (See Useful websites/ resources at the end of this chapter.)

Special considerations for First Nations peoples: Influenza and pertussis infections are disproportionately higher among Aboriginal and Torres Strait Islander women and their infants compared to other Australians.[85] The limited data available suggest there is a lower uptake of maternal vaccination among Australian First Nations women compared to other women, possibly due to lack of equitable access to quality culturally appropriate antenatal care; perceived lack of evidence on the safety of vaccines early in pregnancy; and possible pregnancy loss <20 weeks gestation.[85] To address this gap, and facilitate access to, and use of, appropriate and acceptable antenatal care and vaccination program, McHugh et al recommend to:[85]

- strengthen an Indigenous health workforce that will provide culturally competent and responsive healthcare that is holistic, culturally inclusive, and involves respectful and meaningful collaborative partnerships; and

- involve Indigenous peoples in the development, implementation and dissemination of health programs such as vaccination programs.

42.4.6 Varicella zoster virus (chicken pox) prevention and control

Background and risk: Congenital varicella syndrome, maternal varicella zoster virus (VZV) pneumonia and neonatal varicella infection are linked to serious maternal–fetal morbidity.[86]

If maternal varicella occurs in the first and second trimesters of pregnancy, congenital varicella syndrome (FVS) may occur.[87] FVS is characterised by segmental skin lesions (ulcers, scars), neurological disorders and malformations (atrophy of the brain, paresis, seizures), eye damage and skeletal abnormalities.[15] The reported mortality rate of varicella in newborns exposed around birth is 14–31%.[87]

Newborn infants whose mothers had onset of varicella within 5 days before delivery or within 48 hours after delivery are at especially high risk because they do not receive protective transplacental VZV antibodies before birth.[15,87]

Prevention and control: Vaccination against varicella zoster virus (VZV) *prior to pregnancy* can prevent the disease and limits the exposure of pregnant women to the infectious agent and severe impact on the fetus.[88] Because the effects of the varicella virus on the fetus are unknown, *pregnant women should not be vaccinated*.[89]

Varicella zoster immune globulin (human) (VARIZIG) is recommended for postexposure prophylaxis to prevent or attenuate varicella zoster virus infection in pregnant women.[87]

Varicella zoster immune globulin (VARIZIG) administration up to 10 days after varicella exposure in pregnant women has been well tolerated and is safe.[87]

42.4.7 Staphylococcus aureus

Background and risk: *Staphylococcus aureus* (*S. aureus*) is carried by up to one-third of the general population; about 2% are carriers for methicillin-resistant *S. aureus* (MRSA).[90] *S. aureus* can produce many other antigens and toxins eliciting significant immune response in the human host and is the pathogen most frequently isolated from infection sites in the skin, soft tissue, mucous membranes and internal organs.[15] Horizontal transmission from the mother is probably the major source for *S. aureus* carriage in newborns.[91] *S. aureus* is a major pathogen in hospitalised infants and is the second most common cause of late onset neonatal sepsis which is associated with morbidity and prolonged hospital admissions.[91]

Prevention and control: *S. aureus* is a common pathogen of gestational mastitis. For more information on mastitis, refer to Section 42.5.6.

42.5 Maternity-specific site infections

This section will focus on maternity-specific site infections such as waterbirth and potential infections; postnatal wound care (CS operation and perineal laceration); regional anaesthesia; and mastitis and breast abscess.

42.5.1 Waterbirth

Background and risk: This section focuses on potential infections for birthing a baby underwater. Concerns have been raised that neonatal infection can occur through contact with contaminated water because of faecal matter, and unclean pipes and hoses when being birthed in water.[92] A Vanderlaan et al. systematic review and meta-analysis reported no difference in odds of neonatal pneumonia between waterbirth and land birth (OR 1.88 95% CI 0.36), and surprisingly a lower odds of non-pneumonia infections with waterbirth compared to land births

(OR 0.60 95% CI 0.37–0.97).[93] A Sidebottom et al. study found admissions to the neonatal intensive care unit (NICU) or special care nursery (SCN) were lower for second-stage water immersion births than those in the control group (odds ratio [OR] 0.3, 95% CI 0.2–0.7) and no difference in chorioamnionitis.[94] The Cochrane review on water immersion during labour and birth concluded that there is *no evidence of increased adverse effects to the fetus/neonate or woman from labouring or giving birth in water.*[95] There have been single cases reported in the literature of neonates infected with infections such as legionellosis[96] and herpes simplex.[76]

Prevention and control: Cleaning and maintaining all equipment used for a waterbirth (hospital and homebirths) will prevent the spread of infection.[97] For staff safety, PPE can include additional requirements: non-sterile single use shoulder-length gloves, waterproof gowns and shoe covers.

GBS: Birth in a pool is *not contraindicated* if the woman is a known GBS carrier provided she receives appropriate intrapartum antibiotic prophylaxis (IAP).[70]

Clean bath: The literature indicates that there is no increase in neonatal or maternal infection if baths are adequately cleaned with detergent/soap and water, then an antibacterial solution that is effective against HIV and both hepatitis B and hepatitis C (according to the hospital infection control policy), rinsed with hot water and then allowed to air dry.[92,98,99]

Using disposable liners has become the norm for use with portable birth pools (hospitals and home) but attention must also be paid to proper cleaning of drain pumps, hoses, filter nets, taps and any other items that are reused from one birth to the next (e.g. waterproof thermometers, mirrors).[97-99]

Homebirth baths/pools: The CDC and/or manufacturer's recommendations for disinfecting pools is using a 1:10 mix of chlorine bleach:water. The dwell time is 5 minutes to disinfect the pool. Large spills of blood require that the surface be cleaned before an EPA-registered disinfectant or a 1:10 bleach:water solution is applied.[99]

Spas and cleaning of jets: The issue of cleaning the jets of permanently installed baths in hospitals has generated some concern and discussion over the past years. The protocol for cleaning jetted tubs is simply to completely clean the tub with an ammonium solution, refill with water and add a brominating agent to circulate through the jet system for a minimum of 10 minutes. A number of hospitals report that they use a half cup of powdered dishwashing crystals.[97]

PRACTICE TIP 9

Reflect on these questions:

1. What are your own perceptions of infection risk related to waterbirths?

2. How would you communicate the 'risks' to well women without risk factors?

42.5.2 Caesarean section (CS) operation

Background and risk: While CS is the most appropriate delivery method for many conditions and complications that can affect the mother and/or baby, the benefits need to be weighed against the risks.[1] Risks of having a CS operation to the mother include postoperative infection, haemorrhage and complications during future births.[100] Risks of being delivered by CS to the baby include increased rates of asthma and obesity, and breathing difficulties and developmental issues in babies born by CS at less than 39 weeks gestation.

Surgical site infection (SSI) is one of the most common complications following CS and has an incidence varying worldwide from 3–15%.[101] Most wound infections do not become clinically apparent until postoperative days 4–7, when most women have already been discharged from the hospital.[102] *Since early treatment has an important role in preventing severe consequences, it is essential to instruct the women on signs and symptoms that require further evaluation by a healthcare professional.*[15]

Risk factors can be divided into three categories:

1. host-related factors (age, morbidity, pregestational diabetes mellitus and previous caesarean delivery)

2. pregnancy and intrapartum-related factors (hypertensive disorder, gestational diabetes mellitus, twin pregnancy, preterm rupture of membranes, greater number of vaginal examinations)

3. procedure-related factors (emergency delivery, caesarean hysterectomy, surgery duration of more than 60 minutes).[103]

The infections after CS are usually caused by Gram-positive cocci, although a polymicrobial infection consisting of both aerobic and anaerobic organisms is not rare.

Besides daily inspection of the caesarean incision, the following evidence-based interventions may significantly reduce post-caesarean delivery wound complications:[15]

• appropriate timing of perioperative prophylaxis (before the skin slit)

• alcohol-based antiseptic solutions based on chlorhexidine for surgical site skin preparation.

CS surgical site infection (SSI): Bacterial spectrum depending on the site of surgery performed: *S. aureus* (in surgery of soft tissues, bone and joint, cardiothoracic), *E. coli* and other Gram-negative bacteria after intraabdominal surgery.[15] For microbiological sampling, the wound should be cleansed with sterile saline before sample collection. A local wound cleansing with an antiseptic is necessary. For severe symptoms, systemic antibiotic treatment is necessary.[15]

Prevention and control: It has been shown to reduce the risk of lower postoperative CS SSI, strategies include: use of sterile technique, antiseptic skin preparation, administration of antimicrobial prophylaxis within 60 minutes before an incision is made, maintaining normothermia, and controlling glucose levels during surgery.[104]

42.5.3 Perineal wound

Background and risk: Perineal status refers to the state of the perineum after vaginal birth, and is categorised as intact, first-degree laceration, second-degree laceration, third- or fourth-degree laceration (includes anal/rectal damage), episiotomy, and episiotomy with tear.[105] Second-degree lacerations (30%) have been reported as the most common perineal trauma. Potential morbidities after repair of perineal tear/episiotomy include pain, dyspareunia, incontinence and infection.[106]

Episiotomy is one of the most common surgical procedures in women after childbirth and prolongs postnatal recovery and can result in complications such as wound infection and dehiscence.[107] Perineal wound dehiscence occurs in the first 7–14 days following delivery and is often associated with infection. The true prevalence of perineal wound infection and dehiscence is unknown; a recent systematic review has reported the incidence as 0.1–23.6% and 0.2–24.6% respectively.[107]

Prevention and control: The UK National Institute of Health and Clinical Excellence (NICE) guideline on intrapartum care for healthy women has highlighted best practice measures. These include restrictive use of episiotomies, prompt suturing of all tears (with the exception of non-bleeding first-degree tears), synthetic suture materials, standardised suturing techniques, aseptic suturing procedures, and the use of prophylactic antibiotics for anal sphincter injuries (OASIS).[108]

- Routine review of perineal trauma by the healthcare professional to identify any signs of infection, and maternal education on perineal hygiene, diet and pelvic floor exercises.[108]
- Healthcare professionals (midwives, nurses and medical officers) need to monitor postnatal perineal wounds for infection. However, midwifery care usually ceases (hospital or home) at around 7–10 days postnatal. Therefore, education of women on symptoms of infection is important.

REFLECTION

It is standard practice to wash/prep the skin prior to incision to reduce the risk of infection. As the perineal area is usually contaminated with faecal matter/fluid during labour, any incision or disruption of skin integrity to this area has a potential risk of infection.

When preparing perineum skin prior to an episiotomy, what do you or your organisation recommend using to wash/prep the area prior to cutting (episiotomy) to reduce risk of infection?

42.5.4 Chorioamnionitis

Background and risk: The term chorioamnionitis refers to an acute inflammation of the membranes and umbilical cord, and chorion of the placenta, usually caused by ascending polymicrobial bacteria during pregnancy or birth. Most commonly, the infection originates in the lower genital tract (cervix and vagina), with hematogenous/transplacental passage, or through iatrogenic contamination during amniocentesis.[109] Chorioamnionitis can occur as an infection that can be acute, subacute or chronic. Bacteria in chorioamnionitis include colonisations of group B streptococcus, bacterial vaginosis, sexually transmissible genital infections and vaginal colonisation with urea plasma.

The most common factors associated with chorioamnionitis are preterm labour, prolonged rupture of membranes, prolonged labour, tobacco use, nulliparous pregnancy, meconium-stained fluid, and repeated vaginal exams following rupture of membranes.[110] HAI

risks include the use of fetal scalp electrodes and repeated vaginal exams during labour.[111]

Chorioamnionitis is linked to chronic pulmonary disease in infants. In premature infants, chronic chorioamnionitis is associated with retinopathy of prematurity, very low birthweight, and impaired brain development.[112] If left untreated, chorioamnionitis can result in increased maternal and neonatal mortality.[111]

Prevention and control: Treat GBS bacteriuria during pregnancy. It may be the high concentration of GBS in the genital tract that drives the link between untreated GBS bacteriuria and chorioamnionitis.[113]

Reduce vaginal examinations (VEs) in labour, as repeated VEs increase the risk of HAI and chorioamnionitis.[111]

Antibiotic therapy reduces the incidence and severity of infection in both the mother and the newborn.[114]

- Sloane et al. highlighted that although infants with early onset sepsis require antibiotics, there is little evidence to support routinely administering antibiotics to asymptomatic infants who have been exposed to chorioamnionitis and more research is needed. The risk of early onset sepsis in asymptomatic term infants of mothers with chorioamnionitis is low.[115]

REFLECTION

1. What is the practice at your organisation?
2. Does your organisation recommence routine antibiotics to asymptomatic infants who have been exposed to chorioamnionitis?

Neonatal cord infection: Infection-related neonatal mortality due to omphalitis in developing country homebirths is an important public health problem.[116] Upon birth, the devitalised umbilical cord is an ideal site for bacterial growth from the uterine environment, as well as providing direct access to the neonate's bloodstream. Omphalitis, thrombophlebitis, cellulitis and necrotising fasciitis are commonly caused by bacterial colonisation of the cord. In various countries, topical substances are still used to mitigate the risk of infection.[117]

CASE STUDY 3

Caring for women with GBS positive with preterm ruptured membranes

A 38-year-old woman, G1P0+1 (1st trimester miscarriages), presents to birth unit at 31+4 weeks gestation with a history of 2 hours of clear vaginal fluid draining and GBS-positive screening swab. A vaginal examination with Amnicator testing is positive confirming preterm premature rupture of membranes (PPROM). She is afebrile and haemodynamically stable, has no abdominal pain so she was admitted to the postnatal ward for monitoring. Is she at risk of chorioamnionitis?

Answer:

YES. There are three risk factors:

1. *Vaginal examination is a risk factor; it could introduce ascending bacteria into the uterus.*
2. *This fetus is compromised due to PPROM; once the amniotic sac breaks, you have an increased risk for infection.*
3. *GBS infection may cause chorioamnionitis infecting the chorion and amnion, and placenta.*

42.5.5 Regional anaesthesia

Risk: The most common pathogens for catheter-associated infections are *S. aureus*, coagulase-negative staphylococci, enterococci, *E. coli*, *Klebsiella* spp., other enterobacteria, *Pseudomonas* spp. and Candida (yeast).[15] Although epidural anaesthesia is generally considered safe, serious complications including spinal abscess can occur, potentially leading to irreversible neurological deficit.[118] Infections may occur more frequently in birthing suites where the environment is less aseptic than the operating theatre room.[119]

Rosero and Joshi, in a 2016 study, found incidence of 0.6 per 100,000 for spinal abscess and no epidural abscesses for obstetric patients in the 13-year period (1998–2010) of 2.32 million USA obstetric cases.[118] A Yin and Hu study found that having epidural anaesthesia for 6 hours or more significantly increased the risk of

maternal intrapartum fever (independent risk factor–odds ratio 3.28), and more likely to receive antibiotics but the underlying mechanism is thought to be non-infectious inflammation.[120] A recent systematic review and meta-analysis supported this increased risk of intrapartum fever but was unable to determine a proven maternal and/or neonatal bacteraemia due to the low quality of data.[121]

Prevention and control: As per general patients, to prevent HAI, infection control is pivotal as well as other clinical measures:

- absolute skin disinfection, aseptic injection technique, careful implantation care[119]
- patients should be mobilised as soon as possible and catheters removed as soon as possible[15]
- unnecessary antibiotic therapy or therapy with broad-spectrum antibiotics should be avoided.[15]

42.5.6 Mastitis

Background and risk: Mastitis occurs predominantly in women who are breastfeeding and is usually caused by a staphylococcal infection of the breast tissue and milk ducts. The bacteria enter the breast through a crack in the nipple or break in skin integrity.[122] Infection is often associated with poor hand hygiene, stress, reduced immunity, or missed or increased intervals between feedings of a breastfed baby. Milk stasis or inefficient removal of milk from the breast is a common cause of non-infectious mastitis and may be due to ineffective infant suckling, poor latching of the infant at the breast, or blockage of the milk ducts.[123]

The incidence of mastitis is approximately 20% of lactating women and 3% developed a breast abscess as cited by the CASTLE (Candida and Staphylococcus Transmission: Longitudinal Evaluation) prospective cohort study conducted in Melbourne, Australia.[124]

Breast abscess: Approximately 11% of the time, mastitis is complicated by a breast abscess. Up to 100% of culture-confirmed cases of postpartum breast abscesses are caused by *S. aureus*.[125] Some studies have identified risk factors such as increasing maternal age, being a first-time mother, breastfeeding difficulties and MRSA.[126]

Prevention and control: Regular breastfeeding and milk removal are necessary since breast milk is not sterile and is high in lactose, which promotes bacterial growth. Emptying the affected breast prevents more bacteria from collecting and shortens the length of the infection.[123]

Early management includes:[126]

- breastfeeding should be continued during the treatment of mastitis. Increased milk expression from the affected breast can help ease discomfort
- alternate hot and cold packs applied to the symptomatic breast help reduce the inflammation and pain and provide comfort
- gently massaging the tender area/s increases circulation and helps loosen any blocked ducts; and
- fever can be treated with paracetamol or ibuprofen without any harm to a breastfeeding baby.

Once a diagnosis of mastitis is made, antibiotics will be required, and symptoms should resolve in 2–5 days. The WHO suggests that breast milk culture and sensitivity testing should be undertaken if there is no response to antibiotics within 2 days, the mastitis recurs, or if it is hospital-acquired mastitis.[127] If not treated in a timely manner, mastitis can lead to a breast abscess that requires surgical draining.[123]

Probiotics: Antibiotic resistance is the reason for the development of new approaches in mastitis treatment, such as using probiotics. Some strains of lactobacilli isolated from milk have already demonstrated high efficacy in the prevention and treatment of mastitis in lactating women.[128] Treatment with lactobacilli probiotics is associated with lower recurrence rates and decreased pain compared to antibiotic therapy in women with infectious mastitis.[128,129]

PRACTICE TIP 12

Healthcare professionals must be aware of the early signs of mastitis (and breast abscess) such as swelling, redness, heat, tenderness, hardness of a reddened area, and pain; and flu-like symptoms, such as tiredness, aches, fever and fatigue, often prior to onset of pain.[123]

CASE STUDY 4

Caring for a woman with a history of mastitis

You are caring for a pregnant multipara woman who has a history of mastitis. She asks you what she can do to reduce her chance of getting mastitis this time.

Answer:

- *Regular breastfeeding and ensure breasts are emptied regularly; every 3–5 hours, try and empty each breast*
- *Regularly check breasts for any redness, heat, tenderness or hardened areas*
- *Gently massage any lumps towards nipple area*
- *Consider taking prophylactic probiotics*

42.6 Homebirth—use of reusable equipment/cleaning practices

Background and risk: Some of the reasons women choose a homebirth over a hospital experience are that they believe having a homebirth will:

- optimise choice
- allow for increased comfort and control in decision making
- reduce intervention; and
- allow them to have family and friends involved in the birth.[130]

In 2012, Murray-Davis et al. reported that some women voiced concern about acquiring infections during hospital stays compared to birthing in a safe home environment; however, more recent articles have focused on women's choice to birth at home due to concerns about their risk of contracting coronavirus (COVD-19) specifically and restrictions in hospitals such as support people and waterbirths.[10,131-133]

Prevention and control: Privately practising registered midwives (PPM) or nurse-midwives providing homebirths are required to adhere to the *national practice standards relating to infection control* similarly to midwives practising in the hospital setting. Independent homebirth midwives and nurse-midwives are required to personally purchase PPE, hand sanitiser, disinfectant and other relevant equipment such as a sharps disposal container and sterile equipment.[10] Maintaining infection control in the home environment, such as cleaning baby-weighing scales and equipment bags that will be taken from house to house, is important.[10]

Some Australian publicly funded homebirth programs specifically require the woman's house to have running water, electricity and line or mobile phone coverage to be eligible for the homebirth option.[134-136]

Many women choosing homebirth also *choose water-birth* and there is a potential risk of infection due to poor cleaning practices. Refer to Section 42.1.1.

Conclusion

This chapter focused on the risk, prevention and control of healthcare-acquired infections in maternity settings for women and newborns. Although women are inpatients for very short periods of time, there are risks for maternity-setting-specific infections associated with caesarean section operations and regional anaesthetics, as well as potential perineal infections.

Useful websites/resources

- International Confederation of Midwives (2017). Midwives and prevention of antimicrobial resistance. The Hague, The Netherlands: https://www.internationalmidwives.org/assets/files/statement-files/2018/04/eng-midwives_preventio_amr.pdf.

- Australian Commission on Safety and Quality in Health Care (2018). Role of nurses, midwives and infection control practitioners in antimicrobial stewardship: https://www.safetyandquality.gov.au/sites/default/files/migrated/Chapter12-Role-of-nurses-midwives-and-infection-control-practitioners-in-antimicrobial-stewardship.pdf.

- Nursing and Midwifery Board of Australia (NMBA): www.nursingmidwiferyboard.gov.au.

- Australian Government (2020). Pregnancy Care Guidelines, Part F: Routine maternal screening tests including hepatitis B, C, and HIV: https://www.health.gov.au/resources/pregnancy-care-guidelines/part-f-routine-maternal-health-tests.

- Australian Government Department of Health: Immunisation for pregnancy (influenza and pertussis): https://www.health.gov.au/topics/immunisation/when-to-get-vaccinated/immunisation-for-pregnancy?language=und.

- Australian Government (2022). Top 3 questions – flu vaccination & pregnancy with Professor Alison McMillan (Chief Nursing and Midwifery Officer): https://www.health.gov.au/news/top-3-questions-flu-vaccination-pregnancy-with-professor-alison-mcmillan.

References

1. Australian Commission on Safety and Quality in Health Care. Role of nurses, midwives and infection control practitioners in antimicrobial stewardship. Sydney: ACSQHC, 2018.
2. Shaban RZ, Mitchell BG, Russo PL, Macbeth D. Epidemiology of healthcare-associated infections in Australia. 1st ed. Elsevier, 2021.
3. Australian Institute of Health and Welfare. Australia's mothers and babies data 2019. Canberra: AIHW, 2021. [Updated 24 June 2021. Mothers and babies report 2019]. Available from: https://www.aihw.gov.au/reports/mothers-babies/australias-mothers-babies.
4. Orr K, Chien P. Sepsis in obese pregnant women. Best Pract Res Clin Obstet Gynaecol. 2015;29(3):377-393.
5. Krieger Y, Walfisch A, Sheiner E. Surgical site infection following cesarean deliveries: trends and risk factors. J Matern Fetal Neonatal Med. 2017;30(1):8-12.
6. Zielinski R, Ackerson K, Kane Low L. Planned home birth: benefits, risks, and opportunities. Int J Womens Health. 2015; 7:361-377.
7. Jackson M, Dahlen H, Schmied V. Birthing outside the system: perceptions of risk amongst Australian women who have freebirths and high risk homebirths. Midwifery. 2020;28(5): 561-567.
8. Organisation for Economic Cooperation and Development. Caesarean sections: OECD Library, 2019. [cited 2021.] Available from: https://www.oecd-ilibrary.org/sites/fa1f7281-en/index.html?itemId=/content/component/fa1f7281-en.
9. Miller S, Abalos E, Chamillard M, Ciapponi A, Colaci D, Comande D, et al. Beyond too little, too late and too much, too soon: a pathway towards evidence-based, respectful maternity care worldwide. Lancet. 2016;388(10056): 2176-2192.
10. Homer CSE, Davies-Tuck M, Dahlen HG, Scarf VL. The impact of planning for COVID-19 on private practising midwives in Australia. Women Birth. 2021;34(1):e32-e37.
11. International Confederation of Midwives. International code of ethics for midwives [code of ethics]. The Hague, The Netherlands: ICM, 2014 [3]. Available from: https://www.internationalmidwives.org/assets/files/general-files/2019/10/eng-international-code-of-ethics-for-midwives.pdf.
12. South Australia Health. Policy for the management of the release of a placenta for private use in South Australian Public Health Services. 1st ed. Adelaide: SA Department of Health, 2016.

13. Burns E. More than clinical waste? Placenta rituals among Australian home-birthing women. J Perinat Educ. 2014;23(1): 41-49.

14. Hayes EH. Consumption of the placenta in the postpartum period. J Obstet Gynecol Neonatal Nurs. 2016;45(1):78-89.

15. Presterl E, Diab-El Schahawi M, Reilly JS. Basic microbiology and infection control for midwives. Springer International Publishing, 2019.

16. Pereira L. Congenital viral infection: traversing the uterine-placental interface. Annu Rev Virol. 2018;5(1):273-299.

17. Heerema-McKenney A. Defense and infection of the human placenta. APMIS. 2018;126(7):570-588.

18. Pollheimer J, Vondra S, Baltayeva J, Beristain AG, Knofler M. Regulation of placental extravillous trophoblasts by the maternal uterine environment. Front Immunol. 2018;9:2597.

19. Zaga-Clavellina V, Diaz L, Olmos-Ortiz A, Godinez-Rubi M, Rojas-Mayorquin AE, Ortuno-Sahagun D. Central role of the placenta during viral infection: Immuno-competences and miRNA defensive responses. Biochim Biophys Acta Mol Basis Dis. 2021;1867(10):166182.

20. Li Z, Hou X, Cao G. Is mother-to-infant transmission the most important factor for persistent HBV infection? Emerg Microbes Infect. 2015;4(5):e30.

21. Royal Women's Hospital. Taking our placenta home. RWH D16-229 ed. Victoria: RWH, 2018.

22. Farr A, Chervenak FA, McCullough LB, Baergen RN, Grunebaum A. Human placentophagy: a review. Am J Obstet Gynecol. 2018;218(4):401.e1-401.e11.

23. Calfee D. Prevention and control of health care-associated infections. Goldman L, Schafer A, eds. Goldman-Cecil Medicine. 26th ed. Elsevier Health Series, 2019.

24. Desale M, Thinkhamrop J, Lumbiganon P, Qazi S, Anderson J. Ending preventable maternal and newborn deaths due to infection. Best Pract Res Clin Obstet Gynaecol. 2016;36: 116-130.

25. O'Donovan K, Emeto TI. Mother-to-child transmission of HIV in Australia and other high-income countries: trends in perinatal exposure, demography and uptake of prevention strategies. Aust N Z J Obstet Gynaecol. 2018;58(5): 499-505.

26. Kirby Institute. HIV in Australia: annual surveillance short report 2018. Sydney: UNSW, 2018.

27. Centers for Disease Control and Prevention. An opt-out approach to HIV screening. https://www.cdc.gov/hiv/ default.html. US Dept of Health and Human Services, 2019 [Updated 2019.] Available from: https://www.cdc.gov/hiv/ group/gender/pregnantwomen/opt-out.html.

28. World Health Organization. HIV/AIDS [Fact sheet]. WHO, 2021 [Updated 14 July 2021.] Available from: https://www. who.int/news-room/fact-sheets/detail/hiv-aids.

29. Panel on treatment of pregnant women with HIV infection and prevention of perinatal transmission. Recommendations for the use of antiretroviral drugs in pregnant women with HIV infection and interventions to reduce perinatal HIV transmission in the United States. Dept Health and Human Services USA, 2021.

30. Li KMC, Li KYC, Bick D, Chang YS. Human immunodeficiency virus-positive women's perspectives on breastfeeding with antiretrovirals: a qualitative evidence synthesis. Matern Child Nutr. 2021:e13244.

31. Ruppe LB, Spencer LA, Kriebs JM. Pre-exposure prophylaxis for HIV infection and the role of the women's health care provider in HIV prevention. J Midwifery Womens Health. 2021;66(3):322-333.

32. WHO/UNICEF. Guideline updates on HIV and infant feeding. The duration of breastfeeding and support from health services to improve feeding practices among mothers living with HIV. Geneva: WHO, 2016. Report ISBN 978 92 4 154970 7.

33. Benova L, Mohamoud YA, Calvert C, Abu-Raddad LJ. Vertical transmission of hepatitis C virus: systematic review and meta-analysis. Clin Infect Dis. 2014;59(6):765-773.

34. Altinbas S, Holmes JA, Altinbas A. Hepatitis C virus infection in pregnancy: an update. Gastroenterol Nurs. 2020;43(1):12-21.

35. American College of Obstetricians and Gynecologists. Practice advisory. Routine hepatitis C virus screening in pregnant individuals. Washington DC: ACOG, 2021 [Updated May 2021.] Available from: https://www.acog. org/clinical/clinical-guidance/practice-advisory/articles/ 2021/05/routine-hepatitis-c-virus-screening-in-pregnant-individuals.

36. RANZCOG. Management of hepatitis C in pregnancy. Melbourne: RANZCOG, 2020. [Updated March 2020.] Available from: https://ranzcog.edu.au/RANZCOG_SITE/ media/RANZCOG-MEDIA/Women%27s%20Health/ Statement%20and%20guidelines/Clinical-Obstetrics/ Management-of-Hepatitis-C-in-Pregnancy-(C-Obs-51). pdf?ext=.pdf.

37. Australian Department of Health. Pregnancy care guidelines: 35. Hepatitis C. Part F: Routine maternal health tests. Canberra: Australian Government Department of Health, 2020. Available from: https://www.health.gov.au/resources/ pregnancy-care-guidelines/part-f-routine-maternal-health-tests/hepatitis-c.

38. Garcia-Tejedor A, Maiques-Montesinos V, Diago-Almela VJ, Pereda-Perez A, Alberola-Cunat V, Lopez-Hontangas JL, et al. Risk factors for vertical transmission of hepatitis C virus: a single center experience with 710 HCV-infected mothers. Eur J Obstet Gynecol Reprod Biol. 2015;194:173-177.

39. Rac MW, Sheffield JS. Prevention and management of viral hepatitis in pregnancy. Obstet Gynecol Clin North Am. 2014;41(4):573-592.

40. South Australia Health. Hepatitis C in pregnancy clinical guideline. In: SA maternal and neonatal clinical network. 5th ed. Adelaide: SA Health, 2015.

41. Boucheron P, Lu Y, Yoshida K, Zhao T, Funk AL, Lunel-Fabiani F, et al. Accuracy of HBeAg to identify pregnant women at risk of transmitting hepatitis B virus to their neonates: a systematic review and meta-analysis. Lancet Infect Dis. 2021;21(1):85-96.

42. Visvanathan K, Dusheiko G, Giles M, Wong ML, Phung N, Walker S, et al. Managing HBV in pregnancy. Prevention, prophylaxis, treatment and follow-up: position paper produced by Australian, UK and New Zealand key opinion leaders. Gut. 2016;65(2):340-350.

43. Thilakanathan C, Wark G, Maley M, Davison S, Lawler J, Lee A, et al. Mother-to-child transmission of hepatitis B: examining viral cut-offs, maternal HBsAg serology and infant testing. Liver Int. 2018;38(7):1212-1219.

44. Peng S, Wan Z, Liu T, Zhu H, Du Y. Incidence and risk factors of intrauterine transmission among pregnant women with chronic hepatitis B virus infection. J Clin Gastroenterol. 2019;53(1):51-57.

45. Wiseman E, Fraser MA, Holden S, Glass A, Kidson BL, Heron LG, et al. Perinatal transmission of hepatitis B virus: an Australian experience. Med J Aust. 2009;190(9): 489-492.

46. Levy MT, Giles M, Hardikar W. Managing hepatitis B virus in pregnancy and children. In: Australasian Society for HIV Medicine, ed; 2018. Available from: www.hepatitisb.org.au/ managing-hepatitis-b-virus-in-pregnancy-and-children/.

47. National Hepatitis B Virus (HBV) Testing Policy Expert Reference Committee. National hepatitis B testing policy

2020. In: Australasian Society for HIV Medicine, ed. Vol 1.2. Canberra: Australian Department of Health, 2020.

48. Centers for Disease Control and Prevention. Breastfeeding – hepatitic B or C infections. CDC; 2020 [Updated 10 Aug 2021.] Available from: https://www.cdc.gov/breastfeeding/breastfeeding-special-circumstances/maternal-or-infant-illnesses/hepatitis.html.

49. RANZCOG. Management of hepatitis B in pregnancy [Statement]. www.ranzcog.edu.au: RANZCOG; 2019. [Updated Nov 2019.] Available from: https://ranzcog.edu.au/RANZCOG_SITE/media/RANZCOG-MEDIA/Women%27s%20Health/Statement%20and%20guidelines/Clinical-Obstetrics/Management-of-Hepatitis-B-in-pregnancy-(C-Obs-50).pdf?ext=.pdf.

50. KEMH Western Australia Government. Hepatitis B virus (HBV): care of the infant born to HBV positive women - clinical practice guideline. 2nd ed. Perth WA: KEMH, 2017. Available from: https://www.kemh.health.wa.gov.au/~/media/Files/Hospitals/WNHS/For%20health%20professionals/Clinical%20guidelines/NEOPN/WNHS.NEOPN.MaternalHepatitisBVirusHBV.pdf.

51. ATAGI. Australian immunisation handbook. Canberra: Australian Department of Health, 2018.

52. World Health Organization. Prevention of mother-to-child transmission of hepatitis B virus: guidelines on antiviral prophylaxis in pregnancy. Geneva: WHO, 2020. Contract No. ISBN 978-92-4-000270-8 (electronic version) ISBN 978-92-4-000271-5 (print version).

53. Centers for Disease Control and Prevention. Hepatitis B vaccination: protect your baby for life [pamphlet]. CDC, 2019 [Updated 12 Nov 2019.] Available from: https://www.cdc.gov/hepatitis/HBV/PDFs/HepBPerinatal-ProtectHepBYourBaby.pdf.

54. Phillips C, Walsh E. Group A Streptococcal infection during pregnancy and the postpartum period. Nurs Womens Health. 2020;24(1):13-23.

55. Nguyen M, Bendi VS, Guduru M, Olson E, Vivekanandan R, Foral PA, et al. Postpartum invasive Group A Streptococcus infection: case report and mini-review. Cureus. 2018;10(8): e3184.

56. Cooper JD, Cooper SR, Wolk DM, Tice AM, Persing TF, Esolen LM. Postpartum Streptococcus pyogenes outbreak in the labor and delivery unit of a quaternary referral center: a case series and review of the literature. Clinical Microbiology Newsletter. 2017;39(2):11-15.

57. Hayata E, Nakata M, Hasegawa J, Tanaka H, Murakoshi T, Mitsuda N, et al. Nationwide study of mortality and survival in pregnancy-related streptococcal toxic shock syndrome. J Obstet Gynaecol Res. 2021;47(3):928-934.

58. Mahida N, Prescott K, Yates C, Spencer F, Weston V, Boswell T. Outbreak of invasive group A streptococcus: investigations using agar settle plates detect perineal shedding from a healthcare worker. J Hosp Infect. 2018; 100(4):e209-e215.

59. Rottenstreich A, Benenson S, Levin G, Kleinstern G, Moses AE, Amit S. Risk factors, clinical course and outcomes of pregnancy-related group A streptococcal infections: retrospective 13-year cohort study. Clin Microbiol Infect. 2019;25(2):251.e1-e4.

60. Money D, Allen VM. No. 298 -The prevention of early-onset neonatal group B Streptococcal disease. J Obstet Gynaecol Can. 2018;40(8):e665-e674.

61. Queensland Health. Queensland clinical guidelines: early onset group B Streptococcal disease (EOGBSD). Brisbane: Queensland Government, 2020. Available from: Guideline: Early onset Group B Streptococcal Disease (health.qld.gov.au).

62. Steer PJ, Russell AB, Kochhar S, Cox P, Plumb J, Gopal Rao G. Group B Streptococcal disease in the mother and newborn-a review. Eur J Obstet Gynecol Reprod Biol. 2020;252:526-533.

63. Ko DW, Zurynski Y, Gilbert GL, Group GBSS. Group B Streptococcal disease and genotypes in Australian infants. J Paediatr Child Health. 2015;51(8):808-814.

64. Australian Department of Health. Clinical practice guidelines: pregnancy care. Canberra: Australian Government, 2019.

65. Wang M, Keighley C, Watts M, Plymoth M, McGee TM. Preventing early-onset group B Streptococcus neonatal infection and reducing antibiotic exposure using a rapid PCR test in term prelabour rupture of membranes. Aust N Z J Obstet Gynaecol. 2020;60(5):753-759.

66. Chan WS, Chua SC, Gidding HF, Ramjan D, Wong MY, Olma T, et al. Rapid identification of group B streptococcus carriage by PCR to assist in the management of women with prelabour rupture of membranes in term pregnancy. Aust N Z J Obstet Gynaecol. 2014;54(2):138-145.

67. Buchan BW, Faron ML, Fuller D, Davis TE, Mayne D, Ledeboer NA. Multicenter clinical evaluation of the Xpert GBS LB assay for detection of group B Streptococcus in prenatal screening specimens. J Clin Microbiol. 2015;53(2):443-448.

68. Vieira LL, Perez AV, Machado MM, Kayser ML, Vettori DV, Alegretti AP, et al. Group B Streptococcus detection in pregnant women: comparison of qPCR assay, culture, and the Xpert GBS rapid test. BMC Pregnancy Childbirth. 2019;19(1):532.

69. Plainvert C, El Alaoui F, Tazi A, Joubrel C, Anselem O, Ballon M, et al. Intrapartum group B Streptococcus screening in the labor ward by Xpert(R) GBS real-time PCR. Eur J Clin Microbiol Infect Dis. 2018;37(2):265-270.

70. Hughes RG, Brocklehurst P, Steer PJ, Heath P, Stenson BM. Prevention of early-onset neonatal group B Streptococcal disease. Green-top guideline No. 36. BJOG. 2017;124(12): e280-e305.

71. Aggarwal S, Brown MA. Renal physiology and complications in normal pregnancy. In: Feehally J, Floege J, Tonelli M, Johnson RJ, editors. Comprehensive clinical nephrology. Edinburgh: Elsevier Inc, 2019.

72. Smaill FM, Vazquez JC. Antibiotics for asymptomatic bacteriuria in pregnancy. Cochrane Database Syst Rev. 2019;2019(11).

73. Zanatta DAL, Rossini MM, Trapani Junior A. Pyelonephritis in pregnancy: clinical and laboratorial aspects and perinatal results. Rev Bras Ginecol Obstet. 2017;39(12):653-658.

74. Moulton L, Lachiewicz M, Liu X, Goje O. Catheter-associated urinary tract infection (CAUTI) after term cesarean delivery: incidence and risk factors at a multi-center academic institution. J Matern Fetal Neonatal Med. 2018;31(3):395-400.

75. Money DM, Steben M. No. 208-Guidelines for the management of herpes simplex virus in pregnancy. J Obstet Gynaecol Can. 2017;39(8):e199-e205.

76. Al-Assaf N, Moore H, Leifso K, Ben Fadel N, Ferretti E. Disseminated neonatal herpes simplex virus type 1 after a water birth. J Pediatric Infect Dis Soc. 2017;6(3):e169-e172.

77. Jones CA, Raynes-Greenow C, Isaacs D. Neonatal HSVSI, contributors to the Australian Paediatric Surveillance U. Population-based surveillance of neonatal herpes simplex virus infection in Australia, 1997-2011. Clin Infect Dis. 2014;59(4):525-531.

78. ACOG. Management of genital herpes in pregnancy: ACOG Practice Bulletin No. 220. Obstet Gynecol. 2020;135(5): e193-e202.

79. Centers for Disease Control and Prevention. Influenza (flu) vaccine and pregnancy. US Department of Health and Human Services, 2019 [Updated December 2019.] Available from: https://www.cdc.gov/vaccines/pregnancy/hcp-toolkit/flu-vaccine-pregnancy.html.

80. Mohammed H, Clarke M, Koehler A, Watson M, Marshall H. Factors associated with uptake of influenza and pertussis vaccines among pregnant women in South Australia. PLoS One. 2018;13(6):e0197867.

81. Centers for Disease Control and Prevention. Tdap (pertussis) vaccine and pregnancy. CDC, 2017.] Available from: https://www.cdc.gov/vaccines/pregnancy/hcp-toolkit/tdap-vaccine-pregnancy.html.

82. Royal Australian New Zealand College of Obstetricians and Gynaecologists. Pre-pregnancy and pregnancy related vaccinations. RANZCOG, 2019.

83. Australian Government Department of Health. Immunisation for pregnancy. Canberra: Australian Government, 2021 [Updated 23 July 2021.] Available from: https://www.health.gov.au/health-topics/immunisation/immunisation-throughout-life/immunisation-for-pregnancy.

84. NMBA. Nurses, midwives and vaccination: position statement, (2016). NMBA, 2016. Available from: Nursing and Midwifery Board of Australia - position statement on nurses, midwives and vaccination (nursingmidwiferyboard.gov.au).

85. McHugh L, Crooks K, Creighton A, Binks M, Andrews RM. Safety, equity and monitoring: a review of the gaps in maternal vaccination strategies for Aboriginal and Torres Strait Islander women. Hum Vaccin Immunother. 2020;16(2):371-376.

86. Benoit G, Etchemendigaray C, Nguyen-Xuan HT, Vauloup-Fellous C, Ayoubi JM, Picone O. Management of varicella-zoster virus primary infection during pregnancy: a national survey of practice. J Clin Virol. 2015;72:4-10.

87. Levin MJ, Duchon JM, Swamy GK, Gershon AA. Varicella zoster immune globulin (VARIZIG) administration up to 10 days after varicella exposure in pregnant women, immunocompromised participants, and infants: varicella outcomes and safety results from a large, open-label, expanded-access program. PLoS One. 2019;14(7):e0217749.

88. Blumental S, Lepage P. Management of varicella in neonates and infants. BMJ Paediatr Open. 2019;3(1):e000433.

89. Centers for Disease Control and Prevention. Guidelines for vaccinating pregnant women. USA: CDC, 2016. [Updated 31 August.] Available from: https://www.cdc.gov/vaccines/pregnancy/hcp-toolkit/guidelines.html#varicella.

90. Kriebs JM. Staphylococcus infections in pregnancy: maternal and neonatal risks. J Perinat Neonatal Nurs. 2016;30(2):115-123.

91. Cho HK, Yang JN, Cunningham SA, Greenwood-Quaintance KE, Dalton ML, Collura CA, et al. Molecular epidemiology of methicillin-susceptible Staphylococcus aureus in infants in a neonatal intensive care unit. Infect Control Hosp Epidemiol. 2020;41(12):1402-1408.

92. Maude R, Caplice S. Using water for labour and birth. In: Pairman S, Tracy S, Dahlen H, Dixon L, eds. Midwifery preparation for practice 2. 4th ed. Chatswood: Elsevier, 2019.

93. Vanderlaan J, Hall PJ, Lewitt M. Neonatal outcomes with water birth: a systematic review and meta-analysis. Midwifery. 2018;59:27-38.

94. Sidebottom AC, Vacquier M, Simon K, Wunderlich W, Fontaine P, Dahlgren-Roemmich D, et al. Maternal and neonatal outcomes in hospital-based deliveries with water immersion. Obstet Gynecol. 2020;136(4):707-715.

95. Cluett ER, Burns E, Cuthbert A. Immersion in water during labour and birth. Cochrane Database Syst Rev. 2018;5(5):CD000111.

96. Barton M, McKelvie B, Campigotto A, Mullowney T. Legionellosis following water birth in a hot tub in a Canadian neonate. CMAJ. 2017;189(42):E1311-E1313.

97. Harper B. Waterbirth basics: from newborn breathing to hospital protocols. Midwifery Today Int Midwife. 2016(117):32-35.

98. Nutter E, Shaw-Battista J, Marowitz A. Waterbirth fundamentals for clinicians. J Midwifery Womens Health. 2014;59(3):350-354.

99. American College of Nurse-Midwives. A model practice template for hydrotherapy in labor and birth. J Midwifery Womens Health. 2017;62(1):120-126.

100. Ketcheson F, Woolcott C, Allen V, Langley JM. Risk factors for surgical site infection following cesarean delivery: a retrospective cohort study. CMAJ Open. 2017;5(3):E546-E56.

101. Bolte M, Knapman B, Leibenson L, Ball J, Giles M. Reducing surgical site infections post-caesarean section in an Australian hospital, using a bundled care approach. Infect Dis Health. 2020;25(3):158-167.

102. Martin EK, Beckmann MM, Barnsbee LN, Halton KA, Merollini K, Graves N. Best practice perioperative strategies and surgical techniques for preventing caesarean section surgical site infections: a systematic review of reviews and meta-analyses. BJOG. 2018;125(8):956-964.

103. Scheck SM, Blackmore T, Maharaj D, Langdana F, Elder RE. Caesarean section wound infection surveillance: information for action. Aust N Z J Obstet Gynaecol. 2018;58(5):518-524.

104. Shea SK, Soper DE. Prevention of cesarean delivery surgical site infections. Obstet Gynecol Surv. 2019;74(2):99-110.

105. O'Kelly SM, Moore ZE. Antenatal maternal education for improving postnatal perineal healing for women who have birthed in a hospital setting. Cochrane Database Syst Rev. 2017;12(12):CD012258.

106. Diaz MP, Steen M. Perineal wound care: education and training in Australia. Aust Nurs Midwifery J. 2017;24(8):41.

107. Jones K, Webb S, Manresa M, Hodgetts-Morton V, Morris RK. The incidence of wound infection and dehiscence following childbirth-related perineal trauma: a systematic review of the evidence. Eur J Obstet Gynecol Reprod Biol. 2019;240:1-8.

108. National Institute for Health and Care Excellence. Intrapartum care for healthy women and babies. [Clinical Guideline 190, updated 21 Feb 2017.] United Kingdom: NICE, 2017.

109. Cappelletti M, Presicce P, Kallapur SG. Immunobiology of acute chorioamnionitis. Front Immunol. 2020;11:649.

110. Kim CY, Jung E, Kim EN, Kim CJ, Lee JY, Hwang JH, et al. Chronic placental inflammation as a risk factor of severe retinopathy of prematurity. J Pathol Transl Med. 2018;52(5):290-297.

111. Venkatesh KK, Glover AV, Vladutiu CJ, Stamilio DM. Association of chorioamnionitis and its duration with adverse maternal outcomes by mode of delivery: a cohort study. BJOG. 2019;126(6):719-727.

112. Fowler JR, Simon LV. Chorioamnionitis: Treasure Island. 2020. [Updated Jan, 2021.] Available from: https://www.ncbi.nlm.nih.gov/books/NBK532251/.

113. Doyle RM, Harris K, Kamiza S, Harjunmaa U, Ashorn U, Nkhoma M, et al. Bacterial communities found in placental tissues are associated with severe chorioamnionitis and adverse birth outcomes. PLoS One. 2017;12(7):e0180167.

114. Johnson CT, Adami RR, Farzin A. Antibiotic therapy for chorioamnionitis to reduce the global burden of associated disease. Front Pharmacol. 2017;8:97.

115. Sloane AJ, Coleman C, Carola DL, Lafferty MA, Edwards C, Greenspan J, et al. Use of a modified early-onset sepsis risk calculator for neonates exposed to chorioamnionitis. J Pediatr. 2019;213:52-57.

116. Oh JW, Park CW, Moon KC, Park JS, Jun JK. The relationship among the progression of inflammation in umbilical cord, fetal inflammatory response, early-onset neonatal sepsis, and chorioamnionitis. PLoS One. 2019;14(11):e0225328.

117. Stewart D, Benitz W, Committee on Fetus and Newborn. Umbilical cord care in the newborn infant. Pediatrics. 2016;138(3):e20162149.

118. Rosero EB, Joshi GP. Nationwide incidence of serious complications of epidural analgesia in the United States. Acta Anaesthesiol Scand. 2016;60(6):810-820.

119. Xue X, Song J, Liang Q, Qin J. Bacterial infection in deep paraspinal muscles in a parturient following epidural analgesia: a case report and literature review: A CARE-Compliant Article. Medicine (Baltimore). 2015;94(50): e2149.

120. Yin H, Hu R. A cohort study of the impact of epidural analgesia on maternal and neonatal outcomes. J Obstet Gynaecol Res. 2019;45(8):1435-1441.

121. Jansen S, Lopriore E, Naaktgeboren C, Sueters M, Limpens J, van Leeuwen E, et al. Epidural-related fever and maternal and neonatal morbidity: a systematic review and meta-analysis. Neonatology. 2020;117(3):259-270.

122. Angelopoulou A, Field D, Ryan CA, Stanton C, Hill C, Ross RP. The microbiology and treatment of human mastitis. Med Microbiol Immunol. 2018;207(2):83-94.

123. Pevzner M, Dahan A. Mastitis while breastfeeding: prevention, the importance of proper treatment, and potential complications. J Clin Med. 2020;9(8):2328.

124. Cullinane M, Amir LH, Donath SM, Garland SM, Tabrizi SN, Payne MS, et al. Determinants of mastitis in women in the CASTLE study: a cohort study. BMC Fam Pract. 2015; 16(1):181.

125. Jena P, Duggal S, Gur R, Kumar A, Bharara T, Dewan R. Staphylococcus aureus in breast abscess-major culprit besides others. Indian Journal of Medical Sciences. 2019; 71(1):40-44.

126. Boakes E, Woods A, Johnson N, Kadoglou N. Breast infection: a review of diagnosis and management practices. Eur J Breast Health. 2018;14(3):136-143.

127. World Health Organization. Mastitis: causes and management. Geneva: WHO; 2000 [WHO/FCH/CAH/00.13.] Available from: https://apps.who.int/iris/bitstream/handle/10665/66230/WHO_FCH_CAH_00.13_eng.pdf?sequence=1&isAllowed=y.

128. Barker M, Adelson P, Peters MDJ, Steen M. Probiotics and human lactational mastitis: a scoping review. Women Birth. 2020;33(6):e483-e91.

129. Bond DM, Morris JM, Nassar N. Study protocol: evaluation of the probiotic Lactobacillus Fermentum CECT5716 for the prevention of mastitis in breastfeeding women: a randomised controlled trial. BMC Pregnancy Childbirth. 2017;17(1):148.

130. Tedesco-Schneck M. Planned home births: the role of the primary care NP. Nurse Pract. 2020;45(4):18-24.

131. Murray-Davis B, McNiven P, McDonald H, Malott A, Elarar L, Hutton E. Why home birth? A qualitative study exploring women's decision making about place of birth in two Canadian provinces. Midwifery. 2012;28(5):576-581.

132. Davis-Floyd R, Gutschow K, Schwartz DA. Pregnancy, birth and the COVID-19 pandemic in the United States. Med Anthropol. 2020;39(5):413-427.

133. Blums T, Donnellan-Fernandez R, Sweet L. Women's perceptions of inclusion and exclusion criteria for publicly-funded homebirth — a survey. Women and Birth. 2022;35(4): 413-422.

134. South Australia Health. Planned birth at home in SA: Clinical Directive. In: SA Health Safety and Quality Strategic Governance Committee. 3rd ed. Adelaide: South Australia Government, 2018.

135. Western Australia Department of Health. Public home birth program standard. Perth: Women and Newborn Health Network, WA Dept of Health, 2021. Available from: https://ww2.health.wa.gov.au/~/media/Corp/Policy-Frameworks/Clinical-Services-Planning-and-Programs/Public-Home-Birth-Program-Policy/Supporting/Public-Home-Birth-Program-Standard.pdf.

136. Northern NSW LHD. Planned home birth. NSW Health, 2014. Available from: https://nnswlhd.health.nsw.gov.au/about/hospitals/byron-central-hospital/birthing-suite/the-home-birth-program/.

CHAPTER 43

Infection prevention and control in neonatal and paediatric health

PROFESSOR RAMON Z. SHABAN[i-iv]

Dr DEBOROUGH MACBETH[v]

PROFESSOR DONNA WATERS[vi]

Dr CATHERINE VIENGKHAM[i]

Chapter highlights

- Outlines the current characteristics of infants, children and young people living in Australia
- Identifies the context and unique features of neonatal and paediatric care, why it is important, and how it is different from adult healthcare services
- Describes the epidemiology of healthcare-associated infections (HAIs) in paediatric settings, including how the characteristics and frequency of infections change as children become older
- Examines the intrinsic and extrinsic factors that increase the risk of acquiring HAIs, such as the impact of preterm births, low birthweight, and the care environment
- Summarises evidence-based infection prevention and control (IPC) practices that best reduce the risk of acquiring HAIs and protect the health of infants, children and young people

i Susan Wakil School of Nursing and Midwifery, Faculty of Medicine and Health, University of Sydney, Sydney, NSW
ii Sydney Infectious Diseases Institute, Faculty of Medicine and Health, University of Sydney, Sydney, NSW
iii Public Health Unit, Centre for Population Health, Western Sydney Local Health District, North Parramatta, NSW
iv New South Wales Biocontainment Centre, Western Sydney Local Health District, Westmead, NSW
v Gold Coast Hospital and Health Service, Southport, QLD
vi Faculty of Medicine and Health, University of Sydney, Sydney, NSW

Introduction

Little over a century ago, infectious diseases caused disproportionate morbidity and mortality in newborn babies and children. From birth, infants with immature immune systems and underdeveloped protective mechanisms are abruptly transitioned from the safe environment of the womb to one that is abundant with new microorganisms. First encounters with novel disease-causing bacteria and viruses will occur throughout infancy, childhood and adolescence. In addition to being highly dependent on parents and caregivers, many infants and children also rely on healthcare workers (HCWs) to provide safe environments to ensure their health needs are met and that they are protected from disease. While modern medicine, pharmacotherapies and improved hygiene practices have significantly reduced the burden of pathogenic threats, they have also presented new problems for healthcare, such as the increased risk of healthcare-associated infections (HAIs) resulting from the reliance on invasive devices and antibiotics to facilitate the survival of preterm infants. This chapter will summarise the unique infectious disease and IPC challenges that emerge across different stages of childhood. Infection control plays a crucial role in paediatric healthcare, and it is important to recognise that we cannot simply apply recommendations from adult care. Interventions must carefully account for the physiological and developmental characteristics of the paediatric patient, as well as realise the importance of shared decision making with children, parents and caregivers, and the provision of family-centred care.

43.1 Characteristics of infants, children and young people in Australia

43.1.1 Definitions

This chapter will examine IPC issues and practices that affect neonates, infants, children, young people and the HCWs that care for them.

The neonatal period encompasses the first 4 weeks of life. Following on from Chapter 42, this chapter examines the key risk factors, microorganisms, infectious diseases and IPC practices that are pertinent during a newborn baby's first weeks of life. Care of the neonate is encompassed within the broader speciality of paediatrics, which engages a wider focus in the provision of healthcare to infants, children, adolescents and, occasionally, young adults.

Infancy is usually defined as the first 12 months of life; however, definitions of what constitutes each age group vary across different systems of data reporting and legislation in Australia. For example, the Australian Bureau of Statistics (ABS) defines children as those under 15 years of age and young adults as those between 15–24 years of age.[1] Alternatively, 18 is the age of legal adulthood in Australia and thereby children can also be defined as anyone under the age of 18.

In this chapter, we will use the definitions established by the Australian Institute of Health and Welfare (AIHW) (Fig 43.1), as well as those used in existing paediatric healthcare texts.[2,3] Infancy will cover the age range of 0–1 year, early childhood 1–4 years, childhood 5–12 years, and adolescence 13–18 years. More specifically, we will be examining the unique IPC issues relevant to the neonates, infants and children, covering the age range of 0–12 years. For clarity, we will use the term 'neonatal' and 'neonate' when referring to care for babies under 1 month of age, and 'paediatric' for all ages up to 12 years after that period. Statistics reported in the chapter that are drawn from sources using different age ranges will be specified where relevant.

43.1.2 Australia's children and young people

As of 2021, there were approximately 4.6 million children aged between 0–14 living in Australia, accounting for 18.2% of the country's total population.[4] Although the total number of children has been increasing, children make up a smaller and smaller

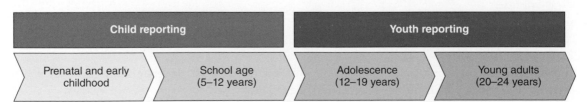

FIGURE 43.1 Age groups of children and youth defined by the Australian Institute of Health and Welfare
Source: AIHW. Reports and data, Population groups, Children & youth. Canberra: Australian Government, 2022.
https://www.aihw.gov.au/reports-data/population-groups/children-youth/data

proportion of the total population as a result of falling fertility rates and greater life expectancy.[2] In 2020, there were 295,976 babies born to 291,712 mothers, equating to a birth rate of 56 per 1000 women—a notable decline from the rate of 66 per 1000 women reported over a decade earlier.[3] In contrast, children between the ages of 0–14 comprised almost one-third of the Aboriginal and Torres Strait Islander population, reflecting the higher fertility rate and shorter life expectancy in this population.

The first 28 days of life is the most vulnerable time for a child's survival. Australia is one of the safest countries for babies to be born in; however, infant deaths do still occur and rates of infant mortality have remained relatively unchanged over the last 20 years.[6] In 2019, there were 2897 perinatal deaths—75% of which were stillbirths and the remaining 25% were neonatal deaths. This is equivalent to a rate of 7.2 stillbirths per 1000 births and 2.4 neonatal deaths per 1000 live births. This is lower than the average global rate of 17 deaths per 1000 live births, and is consistent with other high-income countries with similar access to healthcare.[7] However, infant mortality is not the same across the Australian population, with higher rates observed in Aboriginal and Torres Strait Islander peoples and those who live in very remote areas of Australia. In 2019, infection accounted for approximately 6.7% of neonatal deaths.[6] Following the first few weeks of life, rates of mortality decrease considerably, with a mortality rate of approximately 15 deaths per 100,000 children aged between 1–4 years of age, and 8.7 per 100,000 children for those between 5–14 years.[2]

43.2 Features and settings of neonatal and paediatric healthcare

43.2.1 Neonatal and paediatric healthcare services

Paediatricians and paediatric nurses: Paediatricians are medical practitioners who specialise in the diagnosis and treatment of infants, children and adolescents. In Australia, this typically requires 6 additional years of full-time training after becoming a doctor. All public and private children's hospitals, neonatal and paediatric intensive care units, and general hospitals with neonatal and paediatric wards employ paediatricians. They may also work in surgeries, clinics and community health centres, as well as being part of larger multidisciplinary teams that include

general practitioners (GPs), nurses, social workers, and other allied health professionals. Paediatricians can also sub-specialise in areas like paediatric emergency care, neonatal and perinatal care, and mental healthcare and behavioural development. A neonatologist is an example of a paediatrician who specialises in caring for fetuses and newborns, particularly those who are severely ill or born prematurely. Neonatologists usually work in neonatal intensive care units in maternity and/or children's hospitals. Most paediatric healthcare services will also employ neonatal and paediatric nurses that have similarly completed specialty training in the care of newborns and/or children.

Specialisation in paediatric care equips HCWs with an important set of knowledge and skills in the assessment and treatment of children. The health of children differs from that of adults on many levels, including physiologically, psychosocially, immunologically and developmentally. Childhood also presents a period of substantial development and growth. HCWs require a comprehensive understanding of infant, child and adolescent development to respond and adapt appropriately to the rapidly changing physiology of their patients. For example, paediatric HCWs must be cognisant of factors such as:

* how a child's normal biophysical parameters differ from that of an adult (e.g. blood pressure, heart rate)
* age-appropriate methods of assessing subjective measures like pain
* how hospitalisation and treatments affect the wellbeing of a child and their family
* how to safely calculate and administer medication and perform procedures; and
* how to communicate and partner with the child and their family in their care.

Partnering in care: Caregivers, such as parents, family members and designated guardians, play an integral role in caring for children. As in adult healthcare settings, the paediatric 'patient' of any age is considered first and foremost a 'person', and care is delivered in partnership with both the child and their family. Depending on personal capability and maturity, children often do not have the ability to seek medical attention for themselves when they are feeling unwell. They may not always display or have the ability to coherently communicate symptoms or distress, or to understand the strategies and treatments implemented for their care. Caregivers are therefore responsible for ensuring that the health and medical needs of their child are met. Parents and caregivers will typically accompany, communicate, and make decisions with, and sometimes on behalf of, their child during their encounters with the healthcare system. Many children and young people, particularly those with protracted or chronic illnesses, become highly experienced in managing their own care. Caregivers also take responsibility for ensuring that treatment, medication and other prophylactic activities prescribed to the child by a health professional are being adhered to, both within and outside of the healthcare setting. In the context of IPC, caregivers are instrumental in supporting children's health literacy, hygiene practices, healthy food choices, and the scheduled administration of age-appropriate vaccinations.

43.2.2 Settings for neonatal and paediatric healthcare services

Children's hospitals, paediatric wards and ambulatory services: The vastly different physiological, developmental and medical needs of neonatal and paediatric patients necessitate the establishment of dedicated healthcare services and facilities. These include emergency, inpatient and outpatient services, all of which must be constructed and fitted with age-appropriate equipment and staffed with a specialist paediatric workforce. Most encounters between the paediatric population and the healthcare system occur in ambulatory and outpatient settings, where general health checks, scheduled immunisations and medical assessment and treatment for non-urgent health issues occur. These settings may be attached to a larger healthcare facility, such as a hospital or healthcare centre, or be an independent office-based practice. Virtual hospital care is also appropriate in some contexts. Children with more severe illness or chronic conditions may require inpatient care at dedicated healthcare services provided at children's hospitals or paediatric and adolescent wards within larger general hospitals (Table 43.1). Neonatal wards and intensive care services are typically located adjacent to maternity wards to ensure that urgent care is available to unwell newborns and mothers with high-risk pregnancies, or who experience complications during delivery.[8]

Healthcare facilities specialising in neonatal and paediatric care generally have some notable features that distinguish them from adult-oriented facilities. These include differences in the hospital or ward's

TABLE 43.1 List of dedicated children's hospitals in Australia

State/ Territory	Hospital/s
ACT	1. Centenary Hospital for Women and Children
NSW	2. John Hunter Children's Hospital, Newcastle 3. Sydney Children's Hospital Randwick, Sydney 4. The Children's Hospital at Westmead, Sydney
NT	1. Alice Springs Hospital, Alice Springs (Paediatric Ward) 2. Royal Darwin Hospital, Darwin (Paediatric Ward)
QLD	3. Queensland Children's Hospital, Brisbane
SA	4. Women's and Children's Hospital, Adelaide
Vic	5. The Royal Children's Hospital, Melbourne 6. Monash Children's Hospital, Melbourne
Tas	7. The Royal Hobart Hospital, Hobart (Paediatric Ward)
WA	8. Princess Margaret Hospital for Children, Perth

physical layout, staffing levels and skills, supervision requirements, family accommodation, education initiatives, and treatment and recreational facilities. Importantly, any dedicated paediatric healthcare service, whether inpatient or outpatient, will be staffed by HCWs specialising in the care of children. As described above, these staff have additional skills and knowledge to assess, communicate with, and treat children and young people across various developmental stages, as well as the interpersonal skills to facilitate person- and family-centred partnerships in care. Paediatric facilities also employ specially trained nutrition, speech, movement and play therapists, for example, to support normal physical and psychosocial development. Pharmacists and nurses formulate medications for children based on their age and weight, and ensure that the concentration, dose, route and rate of medication delivery is appropriate for their needs. This may involve making medications easier to administer, such as providing liquid alternatives for oral medications for children who cannot swallow pills.

Additionally, the physical environment and facilities are designed to accommodate patients across a range of ages. For example, the age and size of the patient will determine whether they are placed in an incubator, cot or bed. Similarly, the size and characteristics of monitoring, diagnostic and treatment equipment, such as catheters and chest tubes, are selected based on the physiology of the child. Careful thought is given to the physical design of the auxiliary healthcare environment, which includes the use of age appropriate décor, furniture and artwork, to provide a comfortable and reassuring environment for both the child and their family. Furnishings are usually selected to be made of smooth, durable and easy-to-clean materials that are free of sharp corners, are pram and wheelchair friendly, and come in a variety of sizes that are height-appropriate for both children and adolescents. Paediatric settings also feature additional facilities for the family/carer, such as foldable bed/recliners, kitchenettes, showers and toilets, and baby-changing facilities. Depending on the size of the facility, many paediatric healthcare services incorporate areas for play, recreation, learning and socialisation. Smaller office-based settings typically offer a range of toys or games in the waiting room. Larger facilities like children's hospitals offer dedicated play, quiet spaces or games rooms, hospital 'school', as well as outdoor areas like gardens, playgrounds and art installations.

Neonatal intensive care unit (NICU) and paediatric intensive care unit (PICU): Mothers who are identified as being at additional risk during labour, or are more likely to experience a high-risk birth may be transferred to birthing facilities with co-located neonatal care services. The neonatal intensive care unit (NICU) specialises in the care and ongoing support of premature and ill neonates. The NICU is fitted with highly trained staff and advanced life support equipment designed to meet the unique physiological needs of newborn infants.[9] Babies may be transferred directly to a NICU if they are preterm, experienced complications during labour, have a low birthweight (<2.5 kg), experience complications such as breathing problems, infections or birth defects, multiple birth (e.g. twins, triplets) or require surgery.

In the NICU, each baby is placed in an incubator to maintain their body temperature and monitor their vital signs. Depending on the baby's condition, they may also be connected to a ventilator to assist with breathing and other machines to administer fluids and medication intravenously.

While staff aim to handle small or unwell babies as little as possible, NICUs are also designed to facilitate and support attachment, bonding and family involvement in care. Parents are encouraged to be in the NICU at any time. Support for greater involvement in their baby's health and recovery has catalysed the more recent move away from open-bay wards to private, single-family rooms in NICUs.

The environment within NICUs is carefully maintained to ensure babies are not disturbed by excessive noise or light. Single-family rooms have been shown to provide better privacy, enable easier parental access, control noise and reduce the length of hospital stay.[9] This model has also had implications for infection control. One US study found the use of single-family rooms reduced the rate of catheter-associated bloodstream infections in NICUs from 10.1 to 3.3 per 1000 device-days over a 9-month period. The introduction of hand-basins and hand-sanitiser dispensers within each room also saw an increase in hand hygiene practices.[10,11]

Similarly, paediatric intensive care units (PICU) provide specialised medical care and support to severely ill children. Children are admitted to the PICU when they are critically ill and have medical needs that extend beyond the expertise or facilities of the general hospital or paediatric ward. This may include children experiencing severe breathing problems, serious infections, injuries, near-drownings, or complications related to existing conditions and comorbidities. Additionally, children who have undergone major surgeries may also be cared for in the PICU in the days following the procedure. High-dependency patients, who are otherwise unsuitable for care in regular wards due to physiological instability or dependence on specialist technology, may also require periods of specialist, intensive care. Like the NICU, the PICU includes specialist facilities and life support equipment designed for paediatric populations.

43.3 Epidemiology of HAIs in neonatal and paediatric populations

Data on the incidence of HAIs in adult care settings is already patchy, and is even more difficult to obtain for the calculation of HAI incidence in neonatal and paediatric populations. A repeated prevalence survey, conducted over a 5-year period starting in 1989, reported the incidence of several HAIs in an Australian children's hospital at 6-month intervals.[12] Averaging over different HAI types and patient age, the study reported a mean HAI prevalence rate of 7.7%. This value falls within the prevalence range established in more recent international studies, which reports an average prevalence of 4.2% and a range between 1.2 to 10.4% across different countries.[13] Data obtained from surveillance systems in the US and Europe offer comparable, recent estimates for the epidemiology of different types of HAIs and allow further clarity for their health impacts and risk (Fig 43.2). Variations in infection rates, mortality, sites and distribution of causal pathogens depend on patient susceptibility, immune status, age, and healthcare setting. For example, while the Australian study did not observe a significant effect of age on HAI incidence, modern studies have consistently established a greater prevalence of HAIs in infants <1 year of age compared to children >1 years of age, in those who receive invasive devices and with longer length of hospital stay.[13-16]

The prevalence of HAIs also varies considerably between different types of healthcare units. Infection rates are unsurprisingly greater in intensive care settings, such as NICU and PICU, with patients who are experiencing more severe illness, and who are more likely to require the use of invasive treatments and devices. In intensive care settings, reported rates of HAIs have been as high as 23.6%,[14] whereas rates observed

in paediatric hospitals, paediatric wards in general hospitals and in neonatology wards typically range between <1 to 3.5%.[13,14,17] The frequency of different infection types also varies across age. Bloodstream infections (BSIs) are the most commonly reported HAI in neonates. While BSIs continue to encompass a substantial proportion of HAIs in paediatric populations, the rates of respiratory, gastrointestinal, urinary tract and surgical site infections also increase as children grow older.[13] Respiratory tract and gastrointestinal infections are the most commonly reported HAIs in general paediatric settings.[14,15,18]

Mortality rates vary widely depending on the type of HAI, the pathogen and the health and age of the infant.[19] A 3% mortality rate has been reported for BSIs in paediatric settings. Much steeper BSI mortality rates have been observed in neonatal settings, reaching as high as 11% and even higher still for patients with additional risk factors, such as low birthweight.[19,20] More specific examinations of mortality and morbidity for

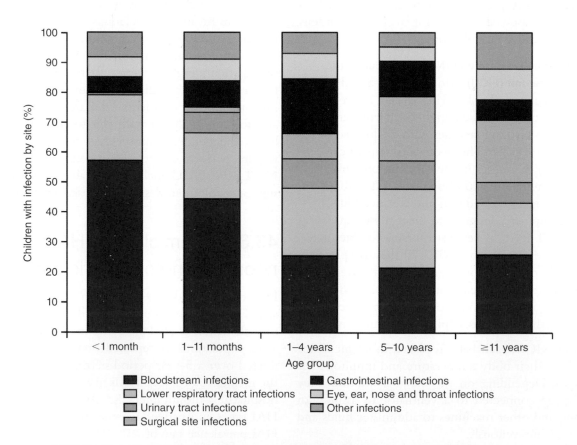

FIGURE 43.2 Proportion of HAIs from a multinational European point prevalence survey

Source: Zingg W. et al. Health-care-associated infections in neonates, children, and adolescents: an analysis of paediatric data from the European Centre for Disease Prevention and Control point-prevalence survey. Lancet Infect Dis. 2017;17(4):381-389.

the different types of HAIs are provided later in this chapter.

In neonatal settings, bacteria are the most common cause of HAIs, followed by fungi and viruses. With respect to bacteria, Coagulase-negative staphylococci (CoNS) is the most frequently isolated pathogen, due to the higher incidence of BSIs in the neonatal population, resulting from the treatment of low birthweight neonates and the subsequent increased use of invasive devices and prolonged hospital stay.[21] As respiratory, gastrointestinal, urinary tract and surgical site infections become more prevalent in older children, the types of causal pathogens isolated change accordingly. Similar to the adult population, bacteria like *Staphylococcus aureus*, *Escherichia coli*, *Pseudomonas aeruginosa* and Enterobacter spp. are also commonly associated with HAIs in paediatric patients. Other common infections, including fungi, like Candida spp., and viruses, like rotavirus and respiratory syncytial virus (RSV), also become more frequent.

In general, viral infections are more prevalent in non-intensive paediatric care settings.[14,17] In contrast to NICUs and PICUs, HAIs within general paediatric wards more closely reflect the occurrence of circulating pathogens and disease epidemics in the community. Many pathogens cause more severe disease in children compared to adults, which naturally result in increased hospital admission rates. These include viruses that lead to respiratory and gastrointestinal infections, many of which circulate in the community, are highly contagious

and cause seasonal epidemics. Once admitted to hospital care, the infected child becomes a source of the infection themselves and poses a risk for spreading the disease to family, healthcare staff and other patients. While viruses remain a concern in neonatal units, they contribute to a much greater HAI burden in general paediatric settings where infection is further exacerbated by their ease of spread through both direct and indirect contact.[14] Table 43.2 provides a broad overview of the distribution of the most commonly isolated microorganisms in HAIs across neonatal and paediatric populations in Europe, the United States (US) and Australia.

43.4 HAI risks in neonatal and paediatric health

Given the developmental and physiological characteristics of neonatal and paediatric patients, the role and often constant presence of the parent/caregiver, and the unique environment in which care is delivered, a number of critical risk factors must be considered when managing HAIs in these settings. Some risk factors are shared across neonatal, paediatric and adult populations, such as the use of intravascular devices, mechanical ventilation, comorbid disease and immunosuppression.[20] However, there are certain factors unique to children that put them at a higher risk of

TABLE 43.2 Common causal microorganisms (bacteria and fungi) of HAIs in neonatal and paediatric populations

Organisms	Europe[13]*	US[22]**	Australia[23]***
Gram-positive bacteria			
Coagulase-negative staphylococcus	21	16.6	24.2
Staphylococcus aureus	11	17.3	16.1
Streptococcus spp.	5	2.6	1.1
Gram-negative bacteria			
Escherichia coli	9	10.5	11.1
Klebsiella spp.	9	8.7	11.6
Enterobacter spp.	7	6.1	8.8
Pseudomonas aeruginosa	7	5.8	2.8
Fungi			
Candida albicans	6	3.4	5.6

*All HAIs. ** CLABSI, CAUTI, SSI, VAP. *** CLABSI, PLABSI.

acquiring HAIs and experiencing more severe disease compared to their adult counterparts. The following sections will distinguish these into:

- 'intrinsic' risk factors—those that are inherent to the child and which cannot be changed; and
- 'extrinsic' risk factors—those involving external forces such as the environment, family and HCWs that can be minimised.

43.4.1 Intrinsic risk factors

Immature immune system: Infant mortality and the burden of HAIs is greatest during the first year of the child's life. This vulnerability is likely caused by several factors, such as an immature and underdeveloped immune system and gastrointestinal tract, and fragile, easily damaged skin.[20] Neonates are exposed before birth and during labour to microorganisms from the mother. This normal flora is established within a few days of birth and has the protective effect of preventing the growth of pathogenic microorganisms. However, abnormal flora may be acquired rapidly in hospital settings, especially for infants in NICUs that might have limited maternal contact, delayed feeding, and multiple invasive treatments. This immunological naivety increases the neonates' susceptibility, usually resulting in a higher rate of infection, greater severity of disease and longer duration of microorganism shedding.[24,25] Furthermore, both the innate and adaptive immune functions of an infant are inexperienced and limited with, for example, lower levels of immune cells like neutrophils and immunoglobulins compared to adults. An infant's immune system exhibits overall reduced antigen-presenting functions, with lower levels of dendritic cell function upon pathogen encounter, reduced phagocytic and chemotactic function of monocytes during sepsis and impaired T-cell function and ability to produce antibodies.[26,27] Neonates can also exhibit overactive innate immune responses, which may incur severe organ damage. Systemic inflammation during neonatal infections is closely linked to brain injury and neurological impairments.[24]

Preterm births: The effects of an immature immune system are further exacerbated in preterm (or premature) infants compared to term infants.[28] Preterm births are defined as those occurring before 37 weeks' gestation. In 2020, 8.3% of babies were born preterm in Australia and this proportion has remained stable over the past decade.[29] Factors that increase the likelihood of preterm births include mothers who smoke and those giving birth to multiple babies. Preterm infants are more likely to have immature defence mechanisms or be born with severe medical conditions that put them at higher risk of acquiring HAIs and experiencing worse health outcomes.[30] Organs such as the lungs and the gastrointestinal tract are at greater risk of complications following infection, such as necrotising enterocolitis (NEC), which is seen almost exclusively, and has a higher case fatality rate, in preterm infants.[31] More severe immune defects and a dependence on lifesaving procedures such as mechanical ventilation, intravascular access devices and parenteral nutrition are also more common in the preterm infant.[17] The development of treatments, devices and intensive care practices has substantially improved the health outcomes and survival of preterm infants in recent decades. However, many of these treatments also carry their own inherent risk for infection, particularly the use of invasive interventions, ventilators, catheters, and central and peripheral lines.

Low birthweight (LBW): Infants of low birthweight are those who weigh less than 2500 grams at birth. Low birthweight infants may be further categorised into 'very low birthweight' for babies weighing less than 1500 grams, and 'extremely low birthweight' for those weighing less than 1000 grams. Low birthweight is frequently associated with lower gestational age and preterm birth, but is also an independent risk factor for infection. These infants are also more likely to require longer care in neonatology units, be exposed to more invasive devices, have underdeveloped mechanical barriers, an immature immune system, as well as low levels of trans-placentally acquired antibodies.[32]

Low birthweight has been observed to increase the risk of BSIs and ventilator-associated pneumonia, even after adjusting for exposure to central-line and ventilator use.[33] This has also led to considerably greater mortality rates. Whereas BSIs have an estimated mortality rate of 3% in paediatric patients, it is approximately 11% among neonates of very low birthweight.[20,34,35] Surveillance studies have revealed similar patterns in healthcare-associated respiratory, skin and urinary tract infections where infection rates in low to extremely low birthweight infants were up to 4 times greater, and mortality rates up to 2 times greater, compared to normal birthweight infants.[36] Furthermore, low birthweight is also a predictor of long-term disease and morbidity following infections. For example, extremely low birthweight infants with systemic Candida spp. infections have been observed to have higher rates of chronic lung disease, periventricular leukomalacia, severe retinopathy of prematurity, and adverse neurological outcomes.[37] Ostensibly, the smaller the infant, the higher the risk of acquiring

an HAI and experiencing more severe illness, morbidity and mortality (Fig 43.3).[20]

Age and developmental stages: Normal child development, in terms of physical, behavioural and psychosocial growth, also affects the risk of infection in important ways.[20] As infants develop, they pass through several stages which determine how they interact with the world around them.

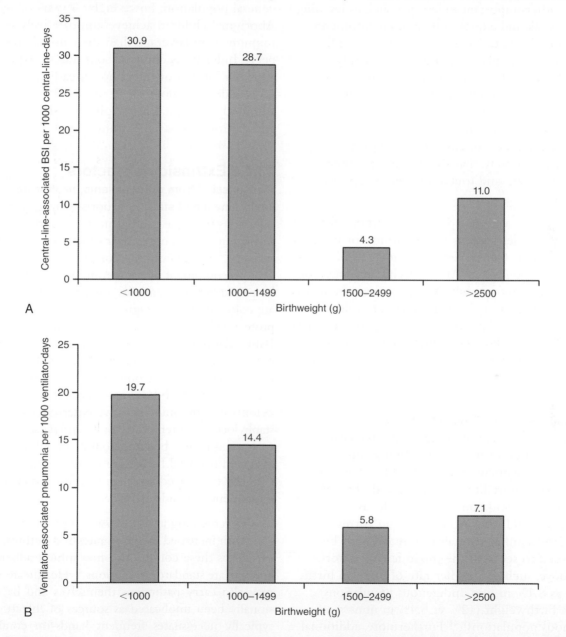

FIGURE 43.3 Rates of central-line associated bloodstream infection (A) and ventilator-associated pneumonia (B) in normal, low, very low and extremely low birthweight infants

Source: Adapted from van der Zwet WC, Kaiser AM, van Elburg RM, Berkhof J, Fetter WPF, Parlevliet GA, et al. Nosocomial infections in a Dutch neonatal intensive care unit: surveillance study with definitions for infection specifically adapted for neonates. J Hosp Infect. 2005;61(4):300-11.

Parents and carers take full responsibility for the hygiene safety of babies and young children until they become physically and developmentally capable of undertaking simple personal hygiene practices themselves.[39] For example, infants and young children will use their mouths to explore objects throughout the first 3 years of life (and often beyond), during what many child developmentalists call an 'oral' stage.[39] Infancy and toddlerhood also includes other important milestones such as learning to crawl, walk and explore different environments, eating solid foods, toilet training, and moving from individual to peer play. The toddler frequently mouths hands and environmental objects, and is yet to master the timing of hand washing and respiratory etiquette in response to normal sneezing, coughing and wiping the nose. This similarly extends to awareness of environmental grime on their hands and body, sharing objects with other children and pets, and touching open wounds or skin lesions.[40]

Children are also susceptible to infections that are prevented in older patients by vaccination or previous natural exposure. Consequently, the nosocomial pathogens and most common HAI sites in children differ from those observed among adults. Many vaccine-preventable diseases like respiratory virus infections, rotavirus, varicella zoster virus and pertussis represent persistent challenges in children's hospitals. Child immunisation schedules are therefore timed to ensure that children receive protection at age- and stage-appropriate periods throughout childhood.

Aboriginal and Torres Strait Islander peoples:
Indigenous Australians experience poorer health and wellbeing compared to non-Indigenous Australians. This includes a shorter life expectancy, greater infant mortality, and significantly higher rates of chronic and communicable diseases throughout childhood. Aboriginal and Torres Strait Islander infants are also more likely to be predisposed to some of the intrinsic risk factors listed above, such as a higher rate of preterm births (13.9% vs 8.1% in non-Indigenous populations) and low birthweight (12% vs 6.4% in non-Indigenous populations).[41] Furthermore, additional socio-economic, environmental and cultural factors contribute to ill health in Indigenous Australians, including inadequate housing, overcrowding and less consistent access to health services.[42] This is exacerbated by a greater proportion of Aboriginal

people living in remote to very remote areas of Australia compared to the general population (21.4% vs 1.7%). Higher rates of maternal risk factors are also observed, such as lack of access to maternity services and higher smoking rates among Indigenous mothers (43% vs 9.2%). Finally, immunisation coverage is also lower in 1- and 2-year-old Aboriginal infants, averaging a rate of 91.5% compared to 93.6% in the general population; however, by 5 years of age, Aboriginal children achieve comparatively greater immunisation coverage than their non-Indigenous peers. Indigenous children continue to experience a greater burden of infectious disease and as they grow older, are more likely to be affected and admitted to hospital for respiratory, skin infections and gastrointestinal infections.[42-45]

43.4.2 Extrinsic risk factors

Transmission from other patients, healthcare environment and staff: Newborns may acquire infections from the mother in utero, during birth or from maternal, hospital or other sources post-delivery.[46] In these settings, organisms that can survive on care equipment and environmental surfaces may be passed between patients. Infants delivered vaginally are colonised with a vaginal microbiota, which offer a protective boost to the newborn immune system. Babies delivered via caesarean section develop early colonisation similar to maternal skin and through contact with their surroundings and caregivers. Newborns in the NICU are more likely to be colonised with Gram-negative enteric rods, staphylococci, enterococci and Candida spp.[28] Colonised infants become potentially infectious agents in neonatal healthcare settings, with infection typically transferred between infants on contaminated equipment or hands of HCWs.[28]

Overcrowding and understaffing have been associated with increased infection rates and outbreaks in the NICU, as these conditions often inhibit adherence to appropriate standard precautions.[47] Healthcare workers may also carry pathogens themselves and have occasionally been implicated as sources of infection. Care typically necessitates frequent hands-on contact and use of medical equipment by healthcare personnel and parents, both of which have been implicated as sources of pathogenic microorganisms.[47-49] Methicillin-resistant *Staphylococcus aureus* (MRSA), *Clostridium difficile*, vancomycin-resistant enterococcus (VRE) and respiratory syncytial virus have previously been isolated on stethoscope diaphragms and other equipment.[50-52] A wide host of bacteria and fungi have been cultured from HCWs' hands resulting from poor hand hygiene compliance and the use of artificial fingernails.[49,53]

While physiological systems are still maturing, children's responses to infection are highly variable and deterioration can occur quickly. Outside of intensive care settings, it is common for children to be admitted to general hospital care with community-acquired respiratory and gastrointestinal infections. As a result, the hospitalised child serves as a potential source for transmission of the community-acquired pathogen in the healthcare setting.[20] Transmission in general paediatric settings is facilitated by close physical contact between children in waiting rooms, shared multi-bed rooms, and other communal rooms and play areas. Additionally, interactions between children, family and visitors provide abundant opportunities for infection spread.[20] Young children frequently harbour infectious organisms and may shed pathogens, like respiratory and gastrointestinal viruses, even if they are asymptomatic. Heavy environmental contamination enhances transmission potential, as does a low infective dose. Respiratory viruses and rotavirus have low infective doses and persist for prolonged periods on inanimate objects. The normal behavioural characteristics of young children amplify transmission opportunity through such activities as mouthing and drooling, direct contact between children during play, and dependence on others for hygienic feeding and toileting practices.

Breastfeeding and the handling of milk and formula: Exclusive infant breastfeeding is recommended for the first 6 months of life.[54] Breast milk is not sterile and while not common, breastfeeding and breast milk can be a source of HAIs. The main infection risks include exposure to maternal viral pathogens such as HIV, human T-cell lymphotropic viruses and cytomegalovirus.[55] Bacteria, like *S. aureus*, Group B Streptococci, *E. coli*, Pseudomonas spp., Klebsiella spp., Serratia spp. and Salmonella spp. have also been identified in breast milk but rarely cause infection in the infant.[56] In most cases these infections have occurred when mothers had mastitis or skin lesions on the breast, or have been linked to the improper handling and storage of expressed breast milk.[57] For example, previous outbreaks of breast-milk-associated *P. aeruginosa* have been linked to contaminated milk bank pasteurisers, and an outbreak of *Klebsiella pneumoniae* has been linked to contaminated

breast-pump tubing.[58,59] Powdered infant formula (PIF) is frequently used as an alternative to breast milk. Its use has been previously linked to neonatal infections with *Cronobacter sakazakii* and Salmonella.[60-63] Pathogens in PIF can be introduced either during the manufacturing process or during reconstitution through the use of contaminated water, bottles or utensils.

Toys and shared equipment: Toys are a common feature of many paediatric settings and serve to provide entertainment, distraction and enrichment to infants and children who are unwell. Toys are an indispensable, therapeutic component of the hospital environment, which can be an intimidating and distressing place for children. However, the sharing of communal toys and other equipment for play, seating support and transport (e.g. highchairs, bouncinettes and prams), presents a broad opportunity for fomite transmission of HAIs. For example, toys frequently become contaminated with pathogens including, but not limited to, *S. aureus*, CoNS, Bacillus spp., Streptococcus spp. and Pseudomonas spp.[64-66] Bath toys have been previously linked to an outbreak of *P. aeruginosa* infection in a paediatric oncology ward after a multi-resistant strain of the bacteria was isolated from a toy-box that contained water-retaining bath toys.[67] Improperly cleaned toys have also been responsible for the transmission of viral infections, most notably rotaviruses and other enteric pathogens.[68,69]

A study examining the level of contamination on hard and soft toys in the waiting rooms of general practitioners found the presence of coliforms on 13.5% of hard toys and 90% of soft toys.[70] Only one-third of practices reported cleaning the toys regularly (weekly to fortnightly basis). Hard toys were effectively decontaminated by soaking them in a dilute sodium hypochlorite solution for at least one hour, or cleaned by wiping them with disinfectant spray. However, there was no significant difference in levels of bacterial or coliform growth when soft toys were cleaned in a washing machine, compared to soft toys that were not cleaned at all. Hard toys were found to not recontaminate as rapidly as soft toys, although both types of toys generally returned to the same level of contamination prior to cleaning approximately one week after decontamination.[41]

To remain a constant feature in paediatric healthcare settings, strategies must be implemented to ensure that toys and other communally used equipment are not a vector for disease spread. This will necessarily include the use of non-soft toys or the provision of dedicated toys where possible if they cannot be cleaned easily (e.g. asking parents to bring the child's personal toys and not sharing these with other children). However, even recent studies of healthcare settings that have transitioned to predominantly hard toys made out of plastic, wood, metal, cardboard and rubber, continue to report high levels of contamination.[71] Like any shared equipment, healthcare facilities must include toys and other equipment as part of a strict cleaning protocol that is documented, monitored and regularly audited.[39] Due to the frequency of exposure, all equipment should optimally be cleaned between each patient. Though if this is not feasible, then at least daily or immediately after the toy or object has been visibly soiled.[40]

43.5 Types of HAIs

43.5.1 Sepsis

Sepsis is the body's systemic response to infection. Sepsis represents a major cause of morbidity and mortality in neonates, particularly in those who are preterm and/ or have very low birthweight.[24] In neonates, sepsis is typically categorised into two stages: early onset and late onset sepsis, and while there is some overlap, the predominant microorganisms responsible for sepsis differs between these stages.[72-75] Early onset sepsis (EOS) is defined by sepsis that occurs during the first 72 hours of life. Infection in utero is a significant risk factor for the development of EOS,[62,63] with vertical transmission of infection from the mother occurring during the perinatal period or as the baby is delivered. Group B Streptococcus and *E. coli* are more commonly isolated during EOS. Additionally, viral infections, including herpes simplex virus (HSV), enteroviruses and parechoviruses, are also implicated in EOS.[24] Late onset sepsis (LOS) is characterised by sepsis that occurs between the first 4–30 days after birth and is usually caused by pathogenic bacteria in the environment after delivery, such as from contact with HCWs, caregivers, equipment and the use of invasive devices. However, a small proportion of LOS may be the result of the late manifestation of vertically transmitted infection. CoNS and *S. aureus* are more commonly implicated in LOS.[76] Some literature has also proposed the inclusion of a third stage of sepsis—very late-onset sepsis, which encompasses all cases of sepsis in newborns occurring after the first 30 days of birth until discharge.[72]

The incidence of sepsis decreases past the neonatal period and as children get older.[77] Microorganisms like *S. aureus*, CoNS and Enterococcus spp., which are associated with LOS, persist as the most commonly identified microorganisms in sepsis for the paediatric population.[78] Sepsis resulting from respiratory infection is more common in infants and children compared to neonates, and typically originates from bacteria like *Pneumococcus* and *H. influenzae* and viruses like influenza and RSV.[77,79] Infections caused by meningococcus bacteria causing meningitis and other forms of meningococcal disease also become more prevalent in older children. The signs and symptoms of neonatal sepsis will differ depending on the age of the child. In neonates and younger children, the symptoms tend to be vague and non-specific and may include apnoea, bradycardia/tachycardia, hypotension, respiratory distress, lethargy, poor feeding, fever/ hypothermia, jaundice, vomiting/diarrhoea, abdominal distension, abscesses, petechiae and more. Paediatric sepsis is a serious medical emergency often accompanied by rapid deterioration, and is characterised by a triad of fever, tachycardia and vasodilation, as well as a change in mental status or prolonged capillary refill greater than 2 seconds.[80]

43.5.2 Bloodstream infections

Healthcare-associated BSIs carry a high rate of morbidity and mortality across both neonatal and paediatric populations. In neonates, BSIs are the most commonly reported HAIs and are particularly problematic for neonates in the NICU who are more likely to require invasive life support measures, such as the insertion of intravascular devices.[20] Some studies report that BSIs represent more than 75% of all nosocomial infections among neonates; however, this proportion generally decreases as children get older.[32] The use of intravascular devices substantially increases the risk of central (CLABSI) and peripheral line-associated bloodstream infection (PLABSI) and has previously been reported as responsible for approximately 50% of healthcare-associated BSIs.[34] Due to differences in the criteria used to define line-related BSIs, the reported incidence of these HAIs exhibit a wide range. For example, the reported incidence of CLABSIs in neonates ranges from 3.2 to 21.8 CLABSIs per 1000 central line days.[13,76] BSIs have also been associated with umbilical artery catheters and umbilical vein catheters, which have reported approximate CLABSI incidence rates of 5% and 3–8% respectively. If left untreated, BSIs will progress to sepsis, which as indicated above, is clinically characterised by severe illness with vital sign instability, central nervous system manifestations such as irritability, lethargy or seizures and, ultimately, multi-organ system dysfunction and failure.[76] In longitudinal studies across both neonatal and paediatric populations, mortality rates following BSIs are reported to range from 2.4–6.1%.[34,81] Mortality rates are highest for neonates and those with low birthweights, with risk decreasing steadily with age. CLABSIs that occur within the first 30 days of life are most commonly caused by CoNS, followed by *S. aureus*, Enterococcus species and Gram-negative rods. Beyond 30 days of life, fungi become an important consideration, but CoNS remain the most common causative organism.

43.5.3 Respiratory tract infections and pneumonia

Respiratory infections are the second most common HAI affecting neonatal and paediatric populations, with rates remaining stable across age groups. Both bacterial and viral respiratory infections contribute to significant morbidity and mortality in children. Bacterial infections typically occur following the use of ventilators and are a common source of ventilator-associated pneumonia (VAP)—the second most common HAI in neonatal and paediatric ICUs.[32,82] The incidence of VAP is dependent on gestational age, intubation status, case definition, the level and standard of neonatal care, geography and socio-economic status. In developed countries, the incidence of VAP ranges from between 0.9-2.7 episodes per 1000 ventilator days for neonates, and between 1.4–7 episodes per 1000 ventilator days for paediatric patients.[82,83] Group B Streptococcus accounts for most cases of early-onset pneumonia, while the most common bacteria causing late-onset pneumonia are *S. aureus* and Gram-negative bacilli such as *E coli*, *P. aeruginosa* and Klebsiella spp.[84] Additionally, bacteria such as *Bordetella pertussis*, the cause of pertussis (whooping cough), remain a serious concern. Pertussis is highly contagious and can cause severe disease and mortality in infants, particularly in neonates who are too young to be vaccinated. In Australia, infants under one year of age comprised over one-third of the 445 pertussis hospitalisations in 2016.[85] While deaths caused by pertussis are now exceptionally rare, infants remain at greatest risk of complications (apnoea, severe pneumonia, encephalopathy). The high infectivity and long infectious period of the disease significantly magnify the risk of outbreaks in the healthcare setting.

Newborns and young children are also highly susceptible to viral respiratory infections. These infections may be acquired from family members, carers, HCWs or other infants in nursery, childcare or healthcare settings. A prevalence rate of up to 30% is reported for outbreaks of respiratory viruses in NICUs.[86] Most respiratory viruses are transmitted directly or indirectly via respiratory droplets and exhibit a prolonged shedding period in newborns. RSV is a common viral cause of respiratory tract infection in children under 2 years of age and is responsible for approximately 45% of all hospital admissions for acute respiratory disease in that population.[87] In most cases, RSV manifests as a mild respiratory illness with general symptoms of coughing, sneezing, runny nose and fever. However, in severe cases, RSV infectious can spread to the lower respiratory tract and cause bronchiolitis and pneumonia. Epidemics of RSV occur seasonally and peak during the winter months. The virus is highly infectious and nosocomial transmission of RSV occurs readily via respiratory droplets and contaminated fomites. The general prevalence of RSV is estimated to range between 1–4%;[86] however, a review of RSV outbreaks in NICUs observed substantially greater infection rates of approximately 23.8%.[87] Other commonly reported causes of viral respiratory infection include human metapneumovirus, influenza, parainfluenza 3 and rhinoviruses.[88,89] Many of these viruses circulate widely within the community and as a result occur more frequently in paediatric patients compared to neonates, with incidence decreasing as children become older.[39]

43.5.4 Gastrointestinal infections

Healthcare-associated gastrointestinal infections have been reported in both neonatal and paediatric populations, however, comprise a greater proportion of HAIs for those in the paediatric age group. Rotavirus is the leading cause of nosocomial gastroenteritis in children, followed by norovirus, adenovirus and astrovirus. Additionally, microorganisms such as Salmonella spp., Campylobacter spp., Shigella spp., *E coli* and *C difficile* are also common bacterial causes of gastrointestinal infection, though are less frequently reported compared to viral pathogens.[90] Clinical symptoms of gastroenteritis in children include vomiting, severe watery diarrhoea, mild-to-moderate fever, abdominal pain and dehydration. Severe complications in infants may include necrotising enterocolitis, which occurs following inflammation of an immature gastrointestinal tract. Premature babies, as well as those with a low birthweight or those fed enterally, are most at risk of NEC.

Healthcare-associated transmission of viral gastroenteritis and outbreaks are well documented. These are often associated with faecal–oral spread due to poor hygiene measures among children and/or caregivers.[39] Prospective studies of hospitalised children have shown HAI rates for rotavirus to be as high as 27%.[91] Such high rates are likely sustained by patients with rotavirus gastroenteritis excreting high amounts of the virus in stools, and because the virus is capable of surviving on hands and surfaces for long periods of time. Thus, both the environment and the hands of children themselves, parents/carers and HCWs have the potential to become contaminated and serve as reservoirs for the virus. Although rotavirus may manifest as an asymptomatic infection, in particular amongst older children, it can also cause severe infection and even mortality in young children, especially those with comorbidities. A study describing the impact of nosocomial rotavirus infection on paediatric patients estimated the excess length of hospital stay to be 4.9 days.[20]

43.5.5 Skin and other infections

Varicella zoster virus (VZV) commonly causes chicken pox (varicella) in paediatric populations. Chicken pox manifests as a blistering and itchy skin rash that can form all over the body and head, typically resolving within 1 to 2 weeks. While the disease is usually mild, VZV infections can lead to complications such as pneumonia and meningitis. It is also more likely to cause severe disease and mortality in immunocompromised populations and in preterm newborns. VZV is also highly contagious, making healthcare-associated outbreaks in neonatal and paediatric settings particularly hazardous. However, in general, healthcare-associated transmission of VZV is considerably less frequent compared to household transmission.[92] Secondary transmission rates in a paediatric hospital with both inpatient and ambulatory services has been observed to be approximately 4.5% compared to 96% in households. Fortunately, the uptake of the varicella vaccine has substantially reduced the burden of disease in both children and adults.

Healthcare-associated urinary tract infections (UTIs) are more infrequent in neonatal and paediatric populations compared to adults. Neonatal UTI occurs in approximately 0.5–1% of full-term infants and in 4–25% of premature infants.[93] In paediatric settings, the incidence of UTI ranges between 0.36–5.2%.[94,95] UTIs are more common in infants that have other infectious diseases, and/or are undergoing treatment with broad-spectrum antibiotics, mechanical ventilation, parenteral nutrition and those requiring intravascular and urinary catheters.[96] In general, approximately 80% of UTIs are catheter-related.[97] *E coli* is the most common cause of UTI, followed by Candida spp., Enterococcus spp., Pseudomonas spp., Enterobacter spp. and Klebsiella spp.[94] UTIs pose a smaller burden of disease compared to other HAIs in children.[94]

43.6 Specific IPC practices for neonatal and paediatric health

43.6.1 Breastfeeding and the handling of milk

Breastfeeding provides the neonate with many health benefits, including protection against some infectious diseases caused by bacteria, viruses and parasites.[55] Breastfeeding reduces infant mortality and facilitates the development of the baby's microbiome. Breastfed neonates have higher concentrations of protective bifidobacteria and lactobacillus in their gastrointestinal tract, which increase resistance of the tract to pathogenic organisms.[57,98,99] Compared to infant formula feeding, breastfeeding is associated with significantly lower rates of gastrointestinal and respiratory infection in infants under 6 months of age. Australian and international guidelines recommend that mother's exclusively breastfeed newborns for up to 6 months, after which solid food can be introduced in addition to breastfeeding.[100] Maternal infections that require breast milk to be withheld from neonates include:

1. The presence of a breast abscess

2. HSV lesions on the breast

3. Infection with HIV, West Nile virus or human T-cell lymphotropic virus type I or II

4. Active pulmonary tuberculosis, to active tuberculous breast lesion or tuberculous mastitis.

If mastitis is present, breastfeeding can continue (see Chapter 42). If a breast abscess is present, the mother should pump the breast milk and discard it until 24 to 48 hours after surgical drainage and antimicrobial therapy.[55] If no such infections are present, breastfeeding may proceed with standard precautions such as hand hygiene.

Expressed breast milk (EBM) is milk that is pumped and collected from the breast, and which is typically stored and fed to the baby at a later time. As breast milk is not sterile, the pumping, collection and storage of breast milk can create opportunities for bacterial contamination and cross-infection if equipment is not adequately cleaned and/or is shared between mothers. To ensure the safety of expressed milk, mothers and caregivers should be instructed on hygienic methods for collecting milk as well as for the cleaning and disinfection of breast-pumps. In the healthcare setting, breast milk must be collected into sterile and aseptic containers, appropriately labelled, dated and refrigerated. Refrigerated milk should be maintained at a temperature below 5°C and be used within 72 hours of collection. Alternatively, EBM can be stored in freezer compartments for longer periods—up to 2–3 weeks at -15°C and up to several months under deep freeze at -20°C. Refrigerators and freezers used within healthcare facilities must be monitored for constant temperature and trigger an alarm if the temperature is outside the accepted range. EBM should be stored at the back of the fridge as opposed to by the door, where the temperature may fluctuate. Milk that needs to be transported must be under refrigeration, which can be achieved with the use of freezer pads.

Milk must be prepared for the infant using aseptic technique and, therefore, not at the bedside. Frozen breast milk should be thawed in the refrigerator and used within 24 hours of thawing.[101] EBM is warmed by placing the container in a ziplocked bag that is then placed under warm running water, or by placing the bag into another large container of warm water. The capped tip of the feeding syringe (if the infant is tube-fed), the bottle top or teat is not immersed in the water.

EBM must never be refrozen or reheated or thawed at room temperature or in a microwave as this will result in the loss of nutrients. Small amounts of unused EBM should be discarded via the sewage system and large amounts should be discarded as clinical waste when in a healthcare facility.

43.6.2 Childhood immunisation and vaccine-preventable disease (VPD)

Childhood immunisation is a powerful and effective means for preventing infectious disease spread and HAIs in children. The development of vaccines and increased adherence to the childhood immunisation schedule over the past century has greatly reduced child mortality and the burden of severely debilitating diseases like measles and polio. Immunisation also further protects people who are not immunised through a process called 'herd immunity', where enough people are immunised against a disease to stop the infection from spreading. Children who do not receive their vaccinations on time are at risk of acquiring VPDs, spreading the disease to others (including within a healthcare setting) and experiencing the short- and long-term health consequences associated with the disease.

The National Immunisation Program (NIP) is an Australian initiative that provides free vaccines against 17 diseases (Table 43.3). Eligibility for specific vaccines

TABLE 43.3 The National Immunisation Program schedule for non-Indigenous and Indigenous Australian children from birth to 16 years old

Age	Vaccine
Birth	Hepatitis B
2 months	Diphtheria, tetanus, pertussis, hepatitis B, polio, *Haemophilus influenzae* type b (Hib)
	Rotavirus
	Pneumococcal
	Meningococcal B (Indigenous children)
4 months	Diphtheria, tetanus, pertussis, hepatitis, polio, *Haemophilus influenzae* type b (Hib)
	Rotavirus
	Pneumococcal
	Meningococcal B (Indigenous children)
6 months	Diphtheria, tetanus, pertussis, hepatitis, polio, *Haemophilus influenzae* type b (Hib)
	Pneumococcal (additional dose for children with specified medical risk conditions)
	Pneumococcal (Indigenous children living in WA, NT, SA, QLD)
	Meningococcal B (Indigenous children with specified medical risk conditions)

Continued

TABLE 43.3 The National Immunisation Program schedule for non-Indigenous and Indigenous Australian children from birth to 16 years old—cont'd

Age	Vaccine
12 months	Meningococcal ACWY
	Measles, mumps, rubella
	Pneumococcal
	Meningococcal B (Indigenous children)
18 months	*Haemophilus influenzae* type b (Hib)
	Measles, mumps, rubella, varicella (chickenpox)
	Pneumococcal
	Diphtheria, tetanus, pertussis
	Hepatitis A (Indigenous children in WA, NT, SA and QLD)
4 years	Diphtheria, tetanus, pertussis, polio
	Pneumococcal (additional dose for children with specified medical risk conditions)
	Pneumococcal (Indigenous children living in WA, NT, SA, QLD)
	Hepatitis A (Indigenous children in WA, NT, SA, QLD)
12–13 years	Diphtheria, tetanus, pertussis
	Human papillomavirus (HPV)
14–16 years	Meningococcal ACWY

is determined by age and considers the different needs of at-risk groups and Indigenous populations for earlier immunisation or additional doses. Vaccination plays a strong role in preventing respiratory and other serious infections in the paediatric population. Pertussis, influenza, Haemophilus influenza type B, hepatitis A and B and rotavirus can all be prevented by immunisation, especially among at-risk patients such as candidates for transplantation or immunosuppressed children. Preterm and low birthweight infants can be vaccinated during a hospital stay with few side effects and the possibility of considerable benefit. Fig 43.4 shows vaccination coverage across 1-, 2- and 5-year-olds in Australia for a range of VPD, including diphtheria, meningococcal, hepatitis B, pertussis, polio and measles.

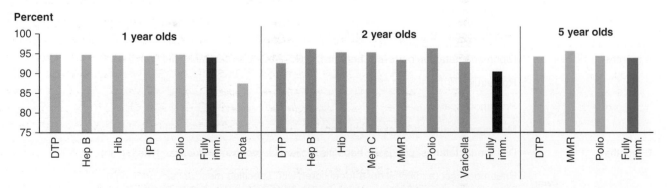

FIGURE 43.4 Vaccination coverage across 1-, 2- and 5-year-olds in Australia

Source: AIHW. Immunisation:vaccine-preventable diseases. Canberra: Australian Government, 2019.

https://www.aihw.gov.au/reports/immunisation/vaccine-preventable-diseases/contents/about

43.6.3 Caregiver involvement

Close caregiver involvement provides an important protective function against infections and begins at the very start of a child's life. In neonates, 'kangaroo care', or skin to skin contact between a parent/carer and the baby, has many positive functions including regulating the baby's body temperature, heart and breathing rate. Kangaroo care has also been shown to increase neonatal weight gain and improve the mother's breast milk production. The practice of kangaroo care is observed to be particularly critical in ensuring better health outcomes in preterm, low weight and/or very ill babies.[102,103] A Cochrane review that explored the effect of kangaroo care on low birthweight infants found the practice reduced mortality, severe illness and length of hospital stay.[103] Notably, the practice also decreased the incidence of HAIs and sepsis and increased infant colonisation with protective maternal flora.

As children develop they will continue to rely on adult caregivers to protect them from disease.[39] Starting from a position of full dependence at birth, children's developmental capacity gradually extends to learning the importance of basic hygiene and engaging in appropriate IPC practices such as hand hygiene, respiratory etiquette, toilet use and bathing. Healthcare staff can support caregivers with strategies, role modelling behaviours and physical resources for the development of age-appropriate health literacy. In addition to hygiene, this may also include healthy nutrition and recommending the administration of vaccines according to the national schedule and their child's unique needs. This is particularly critical in the healthcare setting, where children are likely to be closely interacting with healthcare staff and other young children who are unwell or compromised.

43.6.4 Hand hygiene

Hand hygiene by all direct and indirect caregivers is one of the most important interventions in interrupting the transmission of microorganisms and preventing HAIs across all stages of neonatal and paediatric healthcare (Table 43.4).[47,104] Healthcare workers' hands may include microorganisms such as *S. aureus*, *Klebsiella pneumoniae*, Enterobacter spp., Acinetobacter spp. and Candida spp.[49] Healthcare facilities must ensure the establishment and enforcement of appropriate hand hygiene protocols. This includes regulations around the use of artificial fingernails and jewellery that interfere with hand sanitising. Outbreaks caused by bacteria like *P. aeruginosa* and *Klebsiella pneumoniae*, as well as fungi, in neonatal intensive care settings have previously been linked to carriage under long and/or artificial fingernails.[53,105-107] Viable organisms on the HCWs' hands can contaminate patient clothing, bed linen, furniture and medical equipment if they are not cleaned before and after patient contact.[21] In addition to HCWs, parents, siblings and other visitors are responsible for reducing the risk of infection transmission. Hand hygiene must be emphasised to all visitors and caregivers in neonatal and paediatric healthcare settings. While this intervention may appear simple, implementation can often prove challenging, with low compliance rates even in intensive care areas. A considered effort is required to improve compliance through the education of HCWs, audit programs, performance feedback, the introduction of automated taps over handbasins and system-wide incorporation of alcohol-based hand rubs.

TABLE 43.4 WHO recommendations for the prevention of early and late neonatal infections

Early neonatal infections	Late neonatal infections

• Avoid unnecessary separation of the newborn from the mother
• Handwashing before delivering and handling the infant
• Good basic hygiene and cleanliness during delivery
• Appropriate umbilical cord care
• Appropriate eye care
• Give prophylactic antibiotic only to neonates with documented risk factors for infection, such as:
  ◦ Membranes ruptured >18 hrs before delivery
  ◦ Mother had fever >38C before delivery or during labour
  ◦ Amniotic fluid was foul-smelling or purulent
• Give IM or IV ampicillin and gentamicin for at least 2 days and reassess; continue treatment only if there are signs of sepsis (or a positive blood culture).
	• Exclusive breastfeeding
	• Strict procedures for handwashing or alcohol-based hand rubs for all staff and for families before and after handling infants
	• Using kangaroo mother care and avoiding use of incubators for preterm infants. If an incubator is used, do not use water for humidification (where Pseudomonas will easily colonise) and ensure that it was thoroughly cleaned with an antiseptic
	• Strict sterility for all procedures. Clean injection practices. Removing intravenous drips when they are no longer necessary

43.6.5 Equipment reprocessing

Reusable equipment must be appropriately cleaned, disinfected or sterilised between patient use (see Chapter 16). In neonatal settings, any equipment that makes contact with the neonate's skin or mucous membrane should be sterilised or disinfected. Equipment and utensils used for collecting, preparing and delivering breast milk or infant formula pose a frequent risk for contamination and must be handled with care. This includes sanitising hands and workspaces prior to preparation, and separating all of the component parts of breast pumps and bottles for thorough cleaning between each use. These items should be washed with hot soapy water, dried and stored in a clean, dry place after each use. For very young infants (<2 months), those who are born preterm or are immunocompromised, pacifiers and feeding items should be sanitised at least daily by either boiling, steaming or soaking in a bleach solution.[108] Items must also be sterilised if they are to be used between different mothers. As noted earlier, toys present a common source of microorganisms and HAIs in paediatric settings. Ideally, toys should be reserved for the use of a single patient, or caregivers should be instructed to bring toys for the sole use of their child. Toys that are shared in communal play areas must be easy to clean and sterilised on a regular basis. It is the responsibility of healthcare facilities to ensure a routine protocol is in place to enforce and monitor the cleaning of toys, play equipment, bouncinettes and prams. Extra attention should be placed on cleaning surfaces like the wall and floors of areas where children may traverse or play.

43.6.6 Visitor and staff screening

The child's family is a core part of the care team in person-centred approaches to healthcare. However, the promotion of family care and access to visitors must be balanced with the risk of the introduction of infectious diseases and the wellbeing of the paediatric patient. Visitor screening policies differ between hospitals and may change in response to external conditions. Special considerations include the role of parents or other visitors as primary caregivers, the child's condition and respect of cultural norms. Visitors are made aware of expectations to ensure they do not transmit pathogens to their child or to other children. This includes adherence to hand hygiene policies, respiratory and cough etiquette, reducing socialisation with other parents and patients, limiting visitor numbers, and limiting contact with ill or symptomatic persons.[39] Caregivers and staff should be appropriately immunised against vaccine-preventable diseases prior to contact with neonatal and paediatric patients. Those who are not immune to common childhood diseases, like varicella, measles, rubella and mumps, should not provide direct care to an infectious patient as they themselves are at risk of acquiring the disease and spreading it to others. This is particularly critical in HCWs, who may spread the disease to other patients.

Conclusion

Healthcare-associated infections pose a significant challenge in neonatal and paediatric settings. Young children are particularly at risk of acquiring HAIs and experiencing poor outcomes due to underdeveloped defences, vulnerability to novel pathogens and developmental inability to adhere to basic hygiene and infection control practices. Healthcare workers must be aware of how the nature and burden of HAIs also varies considerably across age groups and is heavily impacted by the presence of certain risk factors like birthweight, gestational age and immunocompetence. Bacterial BSIs associated with the use of intravascular devices are more prevalent in neonates and children in intensive care units. On the other hand, children who are older and who present at general paediatric units are more likely to have acquired viral pathogens that cause respiratory and gastrointestinal infections.

The widespread adoption of vaccines and implementation of a national immunisation schedule have greatly reduced the prevalence of infectious diseases, such as whooping cough, which have previously caused significant illness in infants. Similarly, the development of new treatments and medical devices has substantially improved our ability to care for critically ill neonates, such as those born too early and at extremely low weights. However, new infection risks have emerged as a result, including catheter-related bloodstream infections, ventilator-associated pneumonia and increasing antimicrobial resistance. Balancing the benefits and costs of prevention, preventing infections associated with invasive procedures and devices, and protecting immunocompromised patients will continue to be major challenges in paediatric care. Effective infection control programs require qualified infection control professionals, the involvement of physicians, nurses, allied health practitioners and administrators, and strategies to ensure that all hospital personnel are aware of their responsibility for the safe care of children and young people. Programs must be visible and proactive, and must evolve with the changing epidemiology of paediatric nosocomial infections.

Useful websites/resources

- Australian Paediatric Society. https://auspaediatrics.org.au/
- Royal Australian College of Physicians. Paediatrics and Child Health. https://www.racp.edu.au/about/college-structure/paediatrics-child-health-division
- Australian Society for Infectious Diseases Paediatric Infectious Diseases Group. https://www.asid.net.au/groups/overview-2
- Maternal, Child and Family Health Nurses Australia. https://www.mcafhna.org.au/
- World Society for Pediatric Infectious Diseases. https://wspid.org/

References

1. Australian Bureau of Statistics. Child Canberra: ABS, 2016 [cited 26 August 2022]. Available from: https://www.abs.gov.au/ausstats/abs@.nsf/Lookup/2901.0Chapter25702016#:~:text=%3E%20Glossary%20%3E%3E%20Child-,Child,another%20member%20of%20the%20household.
2. Australian Institute of Health and Welfare. Australia's children: the health of Australia's children. Canberra: Australian Government, 2022. Available from: https://www.aihw.gov.au/reports/children-youth/australias-children/contents/health/the-health-of-australias-children.
3. Fraser J, Waters D, Forster E, Brown N. Paediatric nursing in Australia. Sydney: Cambridge University Press, 2017.
4. Australian Bureau of Statistics. Census of population and housing: snapshot of Australia data summary, 2021. Canberra: Australian Government, 2021.
5. Australian Institute of Health and Welfare. Australia's mothers and babies: overview. Canberra: Australian Government, 2022. Available from: https://www.aihw.gov.au/reports-data/population-groups/mothers-babies/overview.
6. Australian Institute of Health and Welfare. Australia's mothers and babies: stillbirths and neonatal deaths. Canberra: Australian Government, 2021. Available from: https://www.aihw.gov.au/reports/mothers-babies/stillbirths-and-neonatal-deaths.
7. UNICEF. Neonatal mortality 2021 [cited 26 August 2022]. Available from: https://data.unicef.org/topic/child-survival/neonatal-mortality/.
8. Casimir G. Why children's hospitals are unique and so essential. Front Pediatr. 2019;7:305.
9. Shahheidari M, Homer C. Impact of the design of neonatal intensive care units on neonates, staff, and families: a systematic literature review. J Perinatal Neonatal Nurs. 2012;26(3):260-266.
10. Walsh WF, McCullough KL, White RD. Room for improvement: nurses' perceptions of providing care in a single room newborn intensive care setting. Adv Neonatal Care. 2006;6(5):261-270.
11. Cone SK, Short S, Gutcher G. From "baby barn" to the "single family room designed NICU": a report of staff perceptions one year post occupancy. Newborn Infant Nurs Rev. 2010;10(2):97-103.
12. Burgner D, Dalton D, Hanlon M, Wong M, Kakakios A, Isaacs D. Repeated prevalence surveys of paediatric hospital-acquired infection. J Hosp Infect. 1996;34(3):163-170.
13. Zingg W, Hopkins S, Gayet-Ageron A, Holmes A, Sharland M, Suetens C, et al. Health-care-associated infections in neonates, children, and adolescents: an analysis of paediatric data from the European Centre for Disease Prevention and Control point-prevalence survey. Lancet Infect Dis. 2017;17(4):381-389.
14. Raymond J, Aujard Y, Group ES. Nosocomial infections in pediatric patients: a European, multicenter prospective study. Infect Control Hosp Epidemiol. 2000;21(4):260-263.
15. Raymond J. Epidemiology of nosocomial infections in pediatrics. Pathologie-biologie. 2000;48(10):879-884.
16. Cavalcante SS, Mota E, Silva LR, Teixeira LF, Cavalcante LB. Risk factors for developing nosocomial infections among pediatric patients. Pediatr Infect Dis J. 2006;25(5):438-445.
17. Moore DL. Essentials of paediatric infection control. Paediatr Child Health. 2001;6(8):571-579.
18. Welliver RC, McLaughlin S. Unique epidemiology of nosocomial infection in a children's hospital. Am J Dis Child. 1984;138(2):131-135.
19. Dramowski A, Madide A, Bekker A. Neonatal nosocomial bloodstream infections at a referral hospital in a middle-income country: burden, pathogens, antimicrobial resistance and mortality. Paediatr Int Child Health. 2015;35(3):265-272.
20. Posfay-Barbe KM, Zerr DM, Pittet D. Infection control in paediatrics. Lancet Infect Dis. 2008;8(1):19-31.
21. Ramasethu J. Prevention and treatment of neonatal nosocomial infections. Matern Health Neonatol Perinatol. 2017;3(1):1-11.
22. Lake JG, Weiner LM, Milstone AM, Saiman L, Magill SS, See I. Pathogen distribution and antimicrobial resistance among pediatric healthcare-associated infections reported to the National Healthcare Safety Network, 2011–2014. Infect Control Hosp Epidemiol. 2018;39(1):1-11.
23. Worth L, Daley A, Spelman T, Bull A, Brett J, Richards M. Central and peripheral line-associated bloodstream infections in Australian neonatal and paediatric intensive care units: findings from a comprehensive Victorian surveillance network, 2008–2016. J Hosp Infect. 2018;99(1):55-61.
24. Tsafaras GP, Ntontsi P, Xanthou G. Advantages and limitations of the neonatal immune system. Front Pediatr. 2020;8:5.
25. Kemp AS, Campbell DE, editors. The neonatal immune system. Seminars in Neonatology. Elsevier; 1996:
26. Rangelova V, Kevorkyan A, Krasteva M. Nosocomial infections in the neonatal intensive care unit. Arch Balk Med Union. 2020;55(1):121-127.
27. Futata EA, Fusaro AE, De Brito CA, Sato MN. The neonatal immune system: immunomodulation of infections in early life. Expert Review of Anti-infective Therapy. 2012;10(3):289-298.
28. Hooven TA, Polin RA. Healthcare-associated infections in the hospitalized neonate: a review. Early Human Development. 2014;90:S4-S6.
29. Australian Institute of Health and Welfare. Gestational age. Canberra: Australian Government, 2022. Available from: https://www.aihw.gov.au/reports/mothers-babies/australias-mothers-babies/contents/baby-outcomes/gestational-age.
30. Platt M. Outcomes in preterm infants. Public Health. 2014;128(5):399-403.
31. Lin PW, Stoll BJ. Necrotising enterocolitis. Lancet. 2006;368(9543):1271-1283.

32. Zingg W, Posfay-Barbe KM, Pittet D. Healthcare-associated infections in neonates. Curr Opin Infect Dis. 2008;21(3): 228-234.

33. Gaynes RP, Edwards JR, Jarvis WR, Culver DH, Tolson JS, Martone WJ, et al. Nosocomial infections among neonates in high-risk nurseries in the United States. Pediatrics. 1996; 98(3):357-361.

34. Gray JW. A 7-year study of bloodstream infections in an English children's hospital. European Journal of Pediatrics. 2004;163(9):530-535.

35. Stoll BJ, Hansen N, Fanaroff AA, Wright LL, Carlo WA, Ehrenkranz RA, et al. Late-onset sepsis in very low birth weight neonates: the experience of the NICHD Neonatal Research Network. Pediatrics. 2002;110(2):285-291.

36. Drews M, Ludwig A, Leititis J, Daschner F. Low birth weight and nosocomial infection of neonates in a neonatal intensive care unit. J Hosp Infect. 1995;30(1):65-72.

37. Friedman S, Richardson SE, Jacobs SE, O'Brien K. Systemic Candida infection in extremely low birth weight infants: short term morbidity and long term neurodevelopmental outcome. Pediatr Infect Dis J. 2000;19(6):499-504.

38. van der Zwet WC, Kaiser AM, van Elburg RM, Berkhof J, Fetter WPF, Parlevliet GA, et al. Nosocomial infections in a Dutch neonatal intensive care unit: surveillance study with definitions for infection specifically adapted for neonates. J Hosp Infect. 2005;61(4):300-311.

39. Koutlakis-Barron I, Hayden TA. Essentials of infection prevention in the pediatric population. Int J Pediatr Adolesc Med. 2016;3(4):143-152.

40. Moore DL, Society CP, Diseases I, Committee I. Infection control in paediatric office settings. Paediatr Child Health. 2008;13(5):408-419.

41. Australian Institute of Health and Welfare. Australia's mothers and babies: Aboriginal and Torres Strait Islander mothers and babies. Canberra: Australian Government, 2022. Available from: https://www.aihw.gov.au/reports/mothers-babies/australias-mothers-babies/contents/focus-population-groups/aboriginal-and-torres-strait-islander-mothers-and-babies.

42. Hendrickx D, Bowen AC, Marsh JA, Carapetis JR, Walker R. Ascertaining infectious disease burden through primary care clinic attendance among young Aboriginal children living in four remote communities in Western Australia. PLoS One. 2018;13(9):e0203684.

43. Carville KS, Lehmann D, Hall G, Moore H, Richmond P, De Klerk N, et al. Infection is the major component of the disease burden in Aboriginal and non-Aboriginal Australian children: a population-based study. Pediatr Infect Dis J. 2007;26(3):210-216.

44. Davidson L, Knight J, Bowen AC. Skin infections in Australian Aboriginal children: a narrative review. MJA. 2020;212(5): 231-237.

44. Cuningham W, McVernon J, Lydeamore MJ, Andrews RM, Carapetis J, Kearns T, et al. High burden of infectious disease and antibiotic use in early life in Australian Aboriginal communities. Aust N Z J Public Health. 2019;43(2):149-155.

45. Moore D, Morrell G, Biel M. Neonates. In: Carrico R, editor. APIC text of infection control and epidemiology, 3rd ed, vol 2. Scientific and practice elements. Washington DC: APIC, 2009.

46. Goldmann DA, Durbin Jr WA, Freeman J. Nosocomial infections in a neonatal intensive care unit. J Infect Dis. 1981;144(5):449-459.

47. Won SP CH, Hsieh WS, Chen CY, Huang SM, Tsou KI, Tsao PN. Handwashing program for the prevention of nosocomial infections in a neonatal intensive care unit. Infect Control Hosp Epidemiol. 2004;25(9):742.

49. Waters V LE, Wu F, San Gabriel P, Haas J, Cimiotti J, Della-Latta P, Saiman L. Molecular epidemiology of gram-negative bacilli from infected neonates and health care workers' hands in neonatal intensive care units. Clin Infect Dis. 2004;38(12):1682-1687.

50. McFee RB. Nosocomial or hospital-acquired infections: an overview. Disease-a-Month. 2009;55(7):422-438.

51. Marinella MA PC, Chenoweth C. The stethoscope: a potential source of nosocomial infection?. Arch Intern Med. 1997;157(7): 786-790.

52. Youngster I BM, Heyman E, Lazarovitch Z, Goldman M. The stethoscope as a vector of infectious diseases in the paediatric division. Acta Paediatr. 2008;97(9):1253-1255.

53. Foca M, Jakob K, Whittier S, Latta PD, Factor S, Rubenstein D, et al. Endemic Pseudomonas aeruginosa infection in a neonatal intensive care unit. N Eng J Med. 2000;343(10):695-700.

54. Blackshaw K, Valtchev P, Koolaji N, Berry N, Schindeler A, Dehghani F, et al. The risk of infectious pathogens in breast-feeding, donated human milk and breast milk substitutes. Public Health Nutr. 2021;24(7):1725-1740.

55. Thomas E, Hunter R. Perinatal care. In: Carrico R, editor. APIC text of infection control and epidemiology, 3rd ed, vol 2. Scientific and practice elements. Washington DC: APIC, 2009.

56. Cossey V, Jeurissen A, Thelissen M-J, Vanhole C, Schuermans A. Expressed breast milk on a neonatal unit: a hazard analysis and critical control points approach. Am J Infect Control. 2011;39(10):832-838.

57. Lawrence RM, Lawrence RA. Breast milk and infection. Clin Perinatol. 2004;31(3):501-528.

58. Gras-Le Guen C, Lepelletier D, Debillon T, Gournay V, Espaze E, Roze J-C. Contamination of a milk bank pasteuriser causing a Pseudomonas aeruginosa outbreak in a neonatal intensive care unit. Arch Dis Child-Fetal Neonatal Ed. 2003; 88(5):F434-F435.

59. Donowitz LG, Marsik FJ, Fisher KA, Wenzel RP. Contaminated breast milk: a source of Klebsiella bacteremia in a newborn intensive care unit. Rev Infect Dis. 1981;3(4):716-720.

60. McMullan R, Menon V, Beukers AG, Jensen SO, van Hal SJ, Davis R. Cronobacter sakazakii infection from expressed breast milk, Australia. Emerg Infect Dis. 2018;24(2):393-394.

61. Control CfD, Prevention. Enterobacter sakazakii infections associated with the use of powdered infant formula—Tennessee, 2001. MMWR. 2002;51(14):297-300.

62. Angulo FJ, Cahill SM, Wachsmuth IK, Costarrica MdL, Embarek PKB. Powdered infant formula as a source of Salmonella infection in infants. Clin Infect Dis. 2008;46(2): 268-273.

63. Drudy D, Mullane N, Quinn T, Wall P, Fanning S. Enterobacter sakazakii: an emerging pathogen in powdered infant formula. Clin Infect Dis. 2006;42(7):996-1002.

64. Avila-Aguero MaL, German G, Paris MaM, Herrera JF, Group STS. Toys in a pediatric hospital: are they a bacterial source? Am J Infect Control. 2004;32(5):287-290.

65. Morley C, Davies M, Mehr S. Bacterial on toys in neonatal intensive care cots. Pediatr Res. 1999;45(6):900.

66. Davies MW, Mehr S, Garland ST, Morley F, J C. Bacterial colonization of toys in neonatal intensive care cots. Pediatrics. 2000;106(2):e18.

67. Buttery JP, Alabaster SJ, Heine RG, Scott SM, Crutchfield RA, Garland SM. Multiresistant Pseudomonas aeruginosa outbreak in a pediatric oncology ward related to bath toys. Pediatr Infect Dis J. 1998;17(6):509-513.

68. Rogers M, Weinstock DM, Eagan J, Kiehn T, Armstrong D, Sepkowitz KA. Rotavirus outbreak on a pediatric oncology floor: possible association with toys. Am J Infect Control. 2000;28(5):378-380.

69. Soule H, Genoulaz O, Gratacap-Cavallier B, Mallaret MR, Morand P, François P, et al. Monitoring rotavirus environmental contamination in a pediatric unit using polymerase chain reaction. Infect Control Hosp Epidemiol. 1999;20(6):432-434.

70. Merriman E, Corwin P, Ikram R. Toys are a potential source of cross-infection in general practitioners' waiting rooms. Br J Gen Pract. 2002;52(475):138-140.

71. Aleksejeva V, Dovbenko A, KroiČa J, Skadiņš I. Toys in the playrooms of children's hospitals: a potential source of nosocomial bacterial infections? Children (Basel). 2021; 8(10):914.

72. Odabasi IO, Bulbul A. Neonatal sepsis. Sisli Etfal Hastan Tip Bull. 2020;54(2):142-158.

73. Kim F, Polin RA, Hooven TA. Neonatal sepsis. BMJ. 2020;371.

74. Ershad M, Mostafa A, Dela Cruz M, Vearrier D. Neonatal sepsis. Curr Emerg Hosp Med Rep. 2019;7(3):83-90.

75. Fleischmann C, Reichert F, Cassini A, Horner R, Harder T, Markwart R, et al. Global incidence and mortality of neonatal sepsis: a systematic review and meta-analysis. Arch Dis Childhood. 2021;106(8):745-52.

76. Payne V, Hall M, Prieto J, Johnson M. Care bundles to reduce central line-associated bloodstream infections in the neonatal unit: a systematic review and meta-analysis. Arch Dis Child-Fetal Neonatal Ed. 2018;103(5):F422-F429.

77. Watson RS, Carcillo JA, Linde-Zwirble WT, Clermont G, Lidicker J, Angus DC. The epidemiology of severe sepsis in children in the United States. Am J Resp Crit Care Med. 2003;167(5):695-701.

78. Niedner MF, Huskins WC, Colantuoni E, Muschelli J, Harris JM, Rice TB, et al. Epidemiology of central line-associated bloodstream infections in the pediatric intensive care unit. Infect Control Hosp Epidemiol. 2011;32(12):1200-1208.

79. Gupta N, Richter R, Robert S, Kong M. Viral sepsis in children. Front Pediatr. 2018;6:252.

80. Emr BM, Alcamo AM, Carcillo JA, Aneja RK, Mollen KP. Pediatric sepsis update: how are children different? Surg Infect. 2018;19(2):176-183.

81. Verstraete E, Boelens J, De Coen K, Claeys G, Vogelaers D, Vanhaesebrouck P, et al. Healthcare-associated bloodstream infections in a neonatal intensive care unit over a 20-year period (1992–2011): trends in incidence, pathogens, and mortality. Infect Control Hosp Epidemiol. 2014;35(5):511-518.

82. Foglia E, Meier MD, Elward A. Ventilator-associated pneumonia in neonatal and pediatric intensive care unit patients. Clinical Microbiol Rev. 2007;20(3):409-425.

83. Cernada M, Brugada M, Golombek S, Vento M. Ventilator-associated pneumonia in neonatal patients: an update. Neonatology. 2014;105(2):98-107.

84. Reiterer F. Neonatal Pneumonia. In: Resch B, editor. Neonatal bacterial infection. London: IntechOpen, 2013.

85. Australian Institute of Health and Welfare. Whooping cough in Australia. Canberra: Australian Government, 2018. Available from: https://www.aihw.gov.au/getmedia/ 303c1ab7-9b04-4544-9c5d-852c533ac87a/aihw-phe-236_ WhoopingCough.pdf.aspx.

86. Pichler K, Assadian O, Berger A. Viral respiratory infections in the neonatal intensive care unit—a review. Front Microbiol. 2018;9:2484.

87. Mosalli R, Alqarni SA, Khayyat WW, Alsaidi ST, Almatrafi AS, Bawakid AS, et al. Respiratory syncytial virus nosocomial outbreak in neonatal intensive care: a review of the incidence, management, and outcomes. Am J Infect Control. 2022; 50(7):801-808.

88. Manchal N, Mohamed MRS, Ting M, Luetchford H, Francis F, Carrucan J, et al. Hospital acquired viral respiratory tract infections: an underrecognized nosocomial infection. Infect Dis Health. 2020;25(3):175-180.

89. Chow EJ, Mermel LA, editors. Hospital-acquired respiratory viral infections: incidence, morbidity, and mortality in pediatric and adult patients. Open Forum Infect Dis. 2017:4(1):ofx006.

90. Lam B, Tam J, Ng M, Yeung C. Nosocomial gastroenteritis in paediatric patients. J Hosp Infect. 1989;14(4):351-355.

91. Gianino P, Mastretta E, Longo P, Laccisaglia A, Sartore M, Russo R, et al. Incidence of nosocomial rotavirus infections, symptomatic and asymptomatic, in breast-fed and non-breast-fed infants. J Hosp Infect. 2002;50(1):13-17.

92. Langley J, Hanakowski M. Variation in risk for nosocomial chickenpox after inadvertent exposure. J Hosp Infect. 2000; 44(3):224-226.

93. Mohamed W, Algameel A, Bassyouni R, Mahmoud AeT. Prevalence and predictors of urinary tract infection in full-term and preterm neonates. Egyptian Pediatric Association Gazette. 2020;68(1):1-7.

94. Langley J, Hanakowski M, LeBlanc JC. Unique epidemiology of nosocomial urinary tract infection in children. Am J Infect Control. 2001;29(2):94-98.

95. Matlow AG, Wray RD, Cox PN. Nosocomial urinary tract infections in children in a pediatric intensive care unit: a follow-up after 10 years. Pediatr Crit Care Med. 2003; 4(1):74-77.

96. Jones C, Kausman J. Newborn urinary tract infections. Rickham's Neonatal Surgery. Springer, 2018. p.1153-1160.

97. Wagenlehner F, Naber K. Hospital-acquired urinary tract infections. J Hosp Infect. 2000;46(3):171-181.

98. Palmeira P, Carneiro-Sampaio M. Immunology of breast milk. Revista da Associação Médica Brasileira. 2016;62: 584-593.

99. Walker A. Breast milk as the gold standard for protective nutrients. J Pediatr. 2010;156(2):S3-S7.

100. World Health Organization. Breastfeeding. Geneva, WHO. [cited 28 August 2022]. Available from: https://www.who. int/health-topics/breastfeeding.

101. Clinical Excellence Queensland. Establishing breastfeeding. In: Health Q, editor. Brisbane: Queensland Health, 2021.

102. Jefferies AL, Society CP, Fetus, Committee N. Kangaroo care for the preterm infant and family. Paediatr Child Health. 2012;17(3):141-143.

103. Conde-Agudelo A, Belizán JM, Diaz-Rossello J. Cochrane Review: Kangaroo mother care to reduce morbidity and mortality in low birthweight infants. Cochrane Database Syst Rev. 2012;7(2):760-876.

104. Brady MT. Health care–associated infections in the neonatal intensive care unit. Am J Infect Control. 2005;33(5): 268-275.

105. Moolenaar RL, Crutcher JM, San Joaquin VH, Sewell LV, Hutwagner LC, Carson LA, et al. A prolonged outbreak of Pseudomonas aeruginosa in a neonatal intensive care unit: did staff fingernails play a role in disease transmission? Infect Control Hosp Epidemiol. 2000;21(2):80-85.

106. Jefferies J, Cooper T, Yam T, Clarke S. Pseudomonas aeruginosa outbreaks in the neonatal intensive care unit—a systematic review of risk factors and environmental sources. J Med Microbiol. 2012;61(8):1052-1061.

107. Gupta A, Della-Latta P, Todd B, San Gabriel P, Haas J, Wu F, et al. Outbreak of extended-spectrum beta-lactamase–producing Klebsiella pneumoniae in a neonatal intensive care unit linked to artificial nails. Infect Control Hosp Epidemiol. 2004;25(3):210-215.

108. Centers for Disease Control and Prevention. How to clean, sanitize, and store infant feeding items. Atlanta, GA: CDC, 2022. [cited 28 August 2022.] Available from: https://www.cdc.gov/hygiene/childcare/clean-sanitize.html.

CHAPTER 44

Infection prevention and control in primary healthcare settings

KAREN BOOTH[i]

Chapter highlights

- High volumes of people pass through community-based primary healthcare settings every year. The chances of crossing paths with someone with a communicable disease is quite high. Good triage practices are essential
- Mitigating risk plays a key role in preventing transmission and keeping your patient base and staff safe and healthy and your business in operation
- Good clinical governance structures and strong policies and procedures are essential
- Educating staff about the Hierarchy of Controls and appointing an infection control coordinator for your clinic are the major tools in infection prevention and control (IPC)

i Australian Primary Health Care Nurses Association (APNA), Melbourne, VIC

Introduction

According to the Australian Institute for Health and Welfare, in 2018–19, 88% of Australians saw a general practitioner (GP).[1] This equates to 154 million Medicare-rebated services to 21.9 million people entering and being cared for in a primary healthcare setting such as general practice. In private allied health services during the same period, the AIHW notes there were 24 million Medicare-subsidised health services and another 52 million visits reportedly claimed via private health insurers.[1] With high volumes of patients transiting in and out of community-based healthcare settings there exists a high possibility of transmission of various communicable diseases as people pass by or sit in waiting rooms, shared treatment rooms and consulting rooms.

Primary healthcare settings are much less formal than hospital settings and staff have a wide range of skills sets in awareness, understanding and managing any potential for infection transmission and risk management control. A formal hospital setting is more likely to have an appointed infection control team and a commercial cleaning service trained to higher levels of IPC and risk management. Smaller primary healthcare settings often do not have access to, or cannot afford, the type of infrastructure used in acute settings to support IPC regimes. In smaller services these roles are often shared between different healthcare team members.

Cleaning services are often provided by community-based private cleaning contractors that visit twice weekly, and cleaning is maintained by the administration team on the days between formal cleanings. There is a rapidly emerging role for healthcare assistants who move between clerical and simple patient care roles to support clinician care and IPC. In some primary healthcare settings, healthcare assistants also perform instrument reprocessing as part of their role. The vocational education and training (VET) sector offers certificate-level training, and some VET courses, such as medical practice assistants, cover basic infection control and reprocessing of instruments as a course subject.[2] While small office-based health services must adhere to national safety guidelines for reprocessing instruments, there is no mandated training for staff.

Staff turnover is also more likely to have an impact on smaller services. There is a need to continually review staff training and orientation to their role, including personal and organisational occupational health and safety, especially for IPC.

Patient seating is often closely placed in waiting rooms. While most practices try to be efficient with their time keeping, waiting times can vary depending on demand and the complexity of patients. There exists the potential for an infectious person to sit in the waiting room for some time, in close contact with multiple other patients and staff unless good triage processes are in place. The 2020 SARS-CoV-2 virus and subsequent COVID-19 pandemic heightened the awareness of the need for social distancing and respiratory hygiene etiquette in primary healthcare settings.

The Royal Australian College of General Practitioners (RACGP) Standards for General Practices has a mandatory indicator that states, 'Our practice has an emergency response plan for unexpected events such as natural disasters, pandemic diseases, or unplanned absences of clinical team member'.[3] Despite the RACGP having developed a practical Pandemic Influenza Toolkit and the Emergency Response Planning Toolkit (ERPT) in 2014, as well as running successful workshops nationally in response to the H1N1 pandemic, it became apparent that few general practices and small primary healthcare settings had either used the resources or had plans in place when the COVID-19 pandemic erupted.

Primary healthcare is predominantly made up of small to medium-sized private medical and allied health businesses, Aboriginal-controlled community health organisations (ACCHOs), nurse practitioner services and community health clinics. Services such as general practices are required to undergo accreditation on a continuous three-yearly cycle to comply with both the RACGP Accreditation Standards for General Practice[3] and the RACGP Infection Prevention and Control Guidelines for general practices and other office-based and community-based practices (IPC Guidelines).[4] Many primary healthcare settings such as general practices, dentists and other small office-based practices, such as podiatrists and dermatologists, do minor surgical procedures and reprocess instruments on-site. There needs to be strong infection and quality control systems in place for both reprocessing and tracking of instruments, whether using reprocessed or disposable kits, ensuring appropriate and ongoing training for all staff involved.

While infection control standards apply to all primary healthcare settings, there is often a lack of surveillance data monitoring infection control breaches and no formal reporting pathway for these in private primary healthcare settings. Unless services are regularly monitoring IPC systems, breaches can be missed and patients put at risk. There can also be significant medico-legal risk for the service if injury occurs to a patient. Too often, high-profile media stories are the first we hear of IPC breaches and the subsequent public health efforts to follow up patients that have been potentially exposed. Infection prevention and control requires a whole-of-team approach.

44.1 Clinical governance

The National Safety and Quality Health Service Standards (2021) describe clinical governance as the safety and quality systems that are required to maintain and improve the reliability, safety and quality of healthcare, and improve health outcomes for patients. Clinical governance is the approach through which organisations are responsible for continuously safeguarding high standards of care which ensures patient safety, while improving the quality of their services.[5]

The RACGP guide, the General Practice Management Toolkit: Clinical Governance, recommends a systematic approach to quality and safety where general practice owners and teams share responsibility and accountability for agreed outcomes and create a supportive culture. It also recommends there be a clear assignment of roles, responsibilities and accountabilities for achieving agreed outcomes, and that individual and collective performance is proactively managed.[6]

All team members should be educated about the Hierarchy of Controls and its role in categorising, prioritising and managing IPC risk (Fig 44.1). Primary

healthcare services can be at an increased exposure risk to COVID-19 due to the setting and activities they undertake.[7]

It is the healthcare business owner's responsibility to ensure that all treatments and care given on their premises are safe and fit for purpose. It is crucial that services have in place systems and controls to ensure the safety of patients and workers. Clear measures must be implemented to guide staff on acceptable practices by implementing policies and protocols, especially for IPC, to measure risk for each service and care procedure, measuring deviation from protocol and breaches, as well as clear lines of responsibility and a reporting pathway in the event of a breach or incident.

Healthcare business owners also need to ensure that employees have the training, skills and supervision to provide safe, high-quality care to patients.[5]

44.2 The role of the IPC coordinator

The guidelines recommend that general practice and other office-based health services appoint an IPC coordinator.[4] Infection control professionals should have the skills, experience and qualifications relevant to their specific clinical setting.[8] In many primary healthcare settings, responsibility for oversight of IPC risk assessment, auditing and monitoring is delegated to a nurse. Nurses play a key role in developing

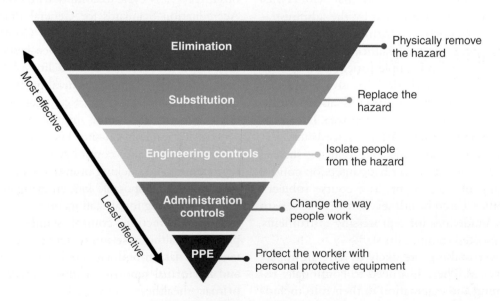

FIGURE 44.1 The Hierarchy of Controls

policies, procedures and training, and in the competency checking of staff. This was highlighted during the COVID-19 pandemic, when nurses in primary healthcare settings played key roles in developing and organising COVID-safe IPC facilities and work and patient flow plans for their services as well as staff training and ongoing IPC surveillance.

The IPC coordinator's role includes assessing the risks of infection transmission throughout the service, reviewing policies and procedures for IPC, and monitoring compliance. The nurse IPC coordinator has a key role in organising education and training for team members relevant to their roles as well as assessing and regularly checking ongoing skill competencies. They also have oversight of activities, such as ensuring adequate PPE supplies are maintained in the service and monitoring that essential equipment is in good working order.

During times of disease outbreaks, primary healthcare settings will be inundated by messages coming from state and federal government health sources, health professional peak bodies and local primary health networks. The IPC coordinator can play a role in ensuring that health messages filter through to all team members and are appropriate for the role they perform within the service. It is recommended that IPC be a regular agenda item at team meetings.

Both the RACGP and the NSQHS (2021) recommend a team-based approach to foster ownership of IPC activities. It is also good risk management for practices to have more than one team member monitoring IPC risk. Staff members are likely to need additional training and perhaps ongoing external support in managing IPC issues.[5,8]

44.3 Staff induction and training

While most workplaces have a core of long-term employees, casual and temporary workforce in small private practice is commonplace, particularly in reception and administration roles. There is also the rotation of registrars and healthcare students that add to the mix of workers passing through primary healthcare settings.

Health service employees have a major influence on the quality and safety of care provided to patients. All team members, especially in small business, have key roles to perform to ensure high-quality, efficient service delivery. A consistent high-quality orientation program is essential for staff training and setting the ground rules for IPC standards early in their employment.

Training, particularly for new team members, both clinical and non-clinical, is key to not only quality IPC activity but also occupational health and safety. Owners and administrators of primary healthcare settings need to ensure all team members have a good understanding of standard and transmission-based precautions and when to use them. All employees should understand their roles and responsibilities and have appropriate training to maintain a safe work environment.[8]

The Australian Guidelines for the Prevention and Control of Infection in Healthcare (2019) note that infection control is everybody's business. 'Understanding the modes of transmission of infectious organisms and knowing how and when to apply the basic principles of IPC is critical to the success of an infection control program. This responsibility applies to everybody working in and visiting a healthcare facility.'[8]

Policies must reinforce that all members of the team are responsible for implementing IPC activities. Team members should be able to demonstrate how any potential risks of cross-infection are managed and the reporting pathway should a breach occur.

Protection of all team members and patients begins with using correct hand hygiene techniques. While not mandatory in office-based primary healthcare settings, it is recommended that all team members complete the ACSQHC National Hand Hygiene Initiative (NHHI) modules applicable to their role. Education should include the best type of product to use depending on the situation requiring hand hygiene. A list of suitable products can be found on the Hand Hygiene Australia (HHA),[9] Therapeutic Goods Administration (TGA)[10] and the National Hand Hygiene Initiative (NHHI)[11] websites.

Competency checking should occur for use of both handwash and alcohol-based hand rub (ABHR) products. Completed NHHI certificates can be added to the team member training profiles and used as a whole-of-practice, quality improvement and continuing professional development exercise. It is recommended that the certificates be updated annually.[9]

The Australian Government Department of Health developed specific COVID-19 infection control online training. The modules are available for healthcare workers (HCWs) in all settings and cover the fundamentals of IPC for COVID-19.[12] Both the Hand Hygiene Australia certification and the COVID-19 IPC training should be built into the practice orientation program to ensure that all new staff members are systematically and safely inducted into the workplace.

Services also need to be flexible and have staff health policies that support team members to stay home when they are unwell. Having multiple team members on sick leave can have a severe impact on the operations and business continuity of small-to-medium primary healthcare settings. As part of good risk management and occupational health and safety practice all health employers should know the vaccination status of all team members. The Australian Immunisation Handbook sets out the recommended schedule for those working in health and people with increased risk of occupational exposure to vaccine-preventable diseases. Employers should have a clear vaccination policy identifying required vaccines and maintain evidence of staff vaccinations in employee records. Employers should also have a clear policy for managing unvaccinated HCWs and are advised to have a policy for documenting and managing vaccine refusal amongst staff.[13]

For general practices, the RACGP accreditation standards criterion covering occupational health and safety states that the practice team is encouraged to obtain the immunisations recommended by the current edition of the Australian Immunisation Handbook, based on their duties and immunisation status. In times of disease outbreak, the criterion notes the need to consider the wellbeing of practice team members who are not immunised, balanced against the need to help prevent transmission of disease to patients who cannot be immunised for medical reasons.[3]

Public health orders, such as those put in place during the COVID-19 pandemic covering vaccination status and permission to work in healthcare services, must be followed. This may lead to the exclusion of face-to-face care given by unvaccinated HCWs.

Staff training also includes the application and removal of personal protective equipment (PPE) for standard precautions and transmission-based precautions. Self-contamination is a frequent problem associated with incorrect doffing procedures of PPE and likely contributes to the spread of viral infections.[14] A 2019 study of 125 HCWs found that 39% made errors in removing PPE, including gowns and gloves, increasing the incidence of contamination.[15]

Both clinical and non-clinical team members require training in the appropriate PPE required for activities such as patient contact, handling of specimens, cleaning of the environment, instrument cleaning and spillages. Correct mask fitting should be included in the team induction. All team members should be competency checked regularly, at least annually, for correct donning, doffing and disposal of PPE to avoid contamination of self and others. The use of a PPE spotter, where possible, is recommended to provide support and guidance in observing and correcting the technique for staff when donning and doffing. The use of a PPE spotter adds a level of IPC risk management for staff providing care and support to patients, and when staff are in common areas interacting with other staff members.[16]

44.3.1 Sharps

All team members need to know what to do in the case of a needlestick injury. Health services and clinics must have an easily accessible instruction poster displaying needlestick hotlines and first aid management, as well as an accessible policy and procedure for managing needlestick injury, body fluid contact with mucous membranes, and incident reporting.

Staff need to be taught how to manage sharps and this must be covered in the practice protocols. All clinical team members are accountable for the safe use and disposal of sharps they use in procedures, and this must be reflected in practice policy documents. Sharps should be disposed of at point of use.

It is important to have a clear procedure for staff who discover an accidentally discarded sharp. The procedure must include a non-touch technique for isolating the sharp and instructions on how to pick the sharp up without using the hands. This may be, for example, with forceps or similar grasping device. The procedure should also indicate to staff to bring a portable sharps container to the point of discovery, or if needed, transport the sharp in a puncture-proof container to the point of disposal into a sharps container. Such incidents must be reported, and a risk assessment and review of the sharps disposal procedure conducted. Systems should then be improved accordingly.

44.3.2 Body fluids and spills

Staff training is required in managing body fluids and blood spills, including where to find and how to use the service's biohazard spills kit. Cleaning training includes knowing where to access the procedure for cleaning spills, and learning the correct techniques for isolating the area, the proper application and removal of personal protective equipment, and no-flick methods for removing soil and debris.

The RACGP Infection Prevention and Control Standards for general practices and other office-based and community-based practices has sample templates for practice staff task competency checking and staff records.[4]

44.4 Triage and waiting room management

People make appointments to visit a GP, nurse, specialist or allied health practitioner for a wide range of conditions. Some of these are planned appointments and some are unexpected, urgent treatment requests. New, smart technologies now allow patients to book appointments to see their health professionals several ways, including via online bookings through either the service's website or an online third-party booking provider, phone apps or the traditional phone call. The phone call method can be a more predictable mode as it allows for a degree of triage activity and scaling of urgency of an appointment during a conversation with a patient. Online booking systems are popular and convenient for patients, and save staff time, but can make triage at the time of making an appointment problematic for services.

Clinical risk management is the process of improving the quality and safety of healthcare services by identifying the circumstances and opportunities that put patients and/or staff at risk of harm, and then acting to prevent or control those risks. Triage is part of a good risk management system.

It is essential that staff respond rapidly when confronted by a patient with a suspected or confirmed infectious illness. All team members should be aware and mindful of the application of the Hierarchy of Control in the context of COVID-19, and the triage and management of other infectious diseases. This includes:

- when and how to appropriately use PPE
- policies and procedures
- engineering controls in small offices such as ventilation, distancing shields or barriers to promote patient distancing
- the use of isolation areas or rooms
- the substitution of services and elimination of risk by keeping infected persons away from the health practice; and
- the use of care by telehealth where appropriate.[17]

The aim of any triage system is to provide efficient delivery of care based on the level of urgency for treatment, the options available, and determining priorities to meet the patient's health needs. There is much written about triage scales, stratifying levels of clinical urgency and providing access to the most appropriate health professionals or health service to meet patient needs.[18] Primary healthcare services are often the first point of contact for most people, especially when they are unwell. Early recognition of symptoms, especially for potentially infectious patients, facilitates appropriate patient management.[19]

Patients must be educated to advise reception staff of a possible infectious illness prior to arrival at the service. This may be as simple as having messaging on the service website, in newsletters, signage at entry to the service, and on-hold phone call messaging.

Screening either prior to, or on arrival at a service, especially during times of known communicable disease outbreaks such as influenza, gastroenteritis and COVID-19, is essential for reducing risk of harm to both staff and patients. Administration staff are very aware of the need for patient privacy, yet they play a key role in triage and screening patients when making bookings and when patients arrive at a service for care.

The administration team are often the first point of contact, the first to ask questions and to gauge the sense of urgency or need for immediate access to care. The administration team need to be supported to triage patients for symptoms of respiratory transmitted infectious illness and to report upwards to on-site health professionals. This requires appropriate training, triage guidelines and ongoing support from the clinical team.[18] Primary healthcare settings should have a hygiene station with alcohol-based hand rub (ABHR) and face masks for patient use, at the entry point into the service.

A sample triage script might include:

1. Do you have a fever or flu-like symptoms?
2. Do you have a rash?
3. Do you have a cough?
4. Do you have vomiting or diarrhoea?
5. Have you lost your taste or sense of smell?
6. Have you been overseas recently, and if so, where?
7. Have you recently had contact with an infectious disease?

Keeping infectious people out of the primary healthcare setting is the ideal. A person with a highly transmissible infectious illness has the potential to infect staff and other patients. Such an event not only puts people at risk but can lead to closure of a practice or clinic for a quarantine period, staff shortage and reduced ability to provide health services to the local community. Risk reduction strategies include offering telehealth appointments where possible. Other options include consults where patients remain in their cars if appropriate. Screening before entry into the clinic is essential. If clinically indicated for potentially infectious patients who must be seen in person, schedule appointments at the end of the day or session to avoid crossover with other people in waiting rooms.

44.4.1 Cleaning

Routine cleaning of a health service is not only an imperative risk management strategy for IPC but is also important for managing occupational health and safety. Environmental cleaning and disinfection is an important strategy to reduce environmental contamination with pathogens such as COVID-19 and reduce the risk of transmission. The importance of environmental cleaning applies to any and all settings.[20]

Frequently touched surfaces include door handles, beds, desks, telephones, light switches and shared computers. Clean these surfaces frequently (at least twice daily) and when visibly dirty. Use detergent solution or combined detergent and disinfectant solution or wipes. Follow the instructions on the cleaning product label (Table 44.1).

The RACGP Standards for General Practices[3] recommends that health services engage formal cleaning contractors and have a formal signed contract outlining the cleaning schedule. Contract cleaners need to clearly understand their role in the service's IPC policy and procedure, including when, how and why they clean specific surfaces and equipment.[4] Services should

consider keeping their own cleaning products and equipment on-site, so as not to expose the service's environment to cleaning equipment that may have been used in multiple other premises.

Non-clinical staff in office-based primary healthcare settings are often tasked with cleaning duties in between formal contractor cleaning. Training should include environmental management such as cleaning procedures, cleaning schedules and the correct use of chemicals and detergents. Services should use a cleaning schedule and cleaning log to ensure all duties are performed on a regular basis and demonstrate accountability for safe IPC environmental management.[3]

The use of aerosol cleaning sprays should be avoided to reduce the risk of inhalation of products that may cause airway irritation and potential inhalation of infectious materials that can be dislodged from surfaces into the air from the force of the sprays. Data safety sheets for all chemicals and cleaning agents used in the setting need to be kept in an easily accessible area.

Toys are not recommended in waiting areas due to risk of fomite transmission. If primary healthcare settings choose to have toys, they must be non-porous, easily cleaned and not have small parts that can fit inside children's mouths. Toys need to be cleaned at least twice daily and be included in the routine cleaning schedule.

The RACGP Infection Prevention and Control Standards: For general practices and other office-based and community-based practices, has sample cleaning schedules with products and cleaning methods listed

TABLE 44.1   Routine environmental cleaning

	Minimally Touched Surfaces	Frequently Touched Surfaces
Examples	Floors, ceilings, walls, blinds/curtains, interior décor	Door handles, stair railings, bed rails, tabletops, light switches, remote controls, elevator panels, IV poles, touch screens, toys, kitchen equipment and appliances, bathroom facilities
Recommendations	• Use detergent solution and/or wipes for cleaning general surfaces and non-patient areas. • Damp mopping preferred to dry mopping. • Walls and blinds should be cleaned when visible dusty or soiled. • Window curtains should be changed regularly or cleaned when soiled. • Sinks and basins should be regularly cleaned.	• These surfaces require frequent cleaning. • Use a detergent solution that is suitable based on the type of surface and the degree of contamination. • Detergent-impregnated wipes can also be used; however, they should not replace mechanical cleaning processes.

that can help guide the development of staff training and practice procedure development.[4]

Links to template examples of health clinic cleaning schedules can be found in the resource section of this chapter.

44.4.2 Handling of linen

While the widespread use of fabric bedcovers has reduced during the COVID-19 pandemic, some small office-based services still use linen bed sheets and pillow slips (although not recommended). All members of the team should receive education regarding the management of soiled linen, including when to change linen, washing and drying, storage, and the use of appropriate precautions during the handling of linen. Linen will be managed using the AS/NZS 4146: 2000 standards.[8] Bed linen and other fabrics such as bed privacy and treatment room curtains should be handled using standard precautions, and with minimal agitation to avoid contamination of air, surfaces and persons. Linen should be bagged ready for transfer to laundering facilities. Blood-soaked, contaminated linen should be put into plastic biohazard bags and labelled for easy recognition by the laundry contractors. Bagging should preferably be done at the point of generation then safely transported to the storage bay. Staff should use PPE suitable for the task at hand and perform hand hygiene as part of their personal protection after handling used linen.[17]

The use of fabric handtowels should be actively discouraged in favour of single use paper towels. Fabric towels are slow to dry, and the same towel should not be used by multiple people. They remain moist for long periods, which can encourage the growth and spread of organisms.

44.4.3 Waste management

Staff need to know the correct procedures for emptying waste bins (clinical and non-clinical waste), using correct PPE, and avoiding touching the base or sides of waste bags due to potential injury from inadvertent discarding of sharps into waste bins. Hand hygiene should be performed after the task. All staff should understand how to categorise waste to ensure disposal into the correct waste stream (i.e. clinical/non-clinical, infectious/hazardous waste for destruction vs household waste).[4,17]

Services must have an up-to-date waste handling and management policy, included in the staff orientation program, and must demonstrate that the handling and destruction of sharps and other clinical waste conforms to state and territory waste disposal regulations and the AS/NZ 3186. Services also need to demonstrate evidence, such as a contract with an authorised clinical waste disposal company, and destruction certificates to prove that waste has been correctly managed and destroyed. Apart from being good practice, this is a mandatory criterion for meeting the RACGP general practice accreditation standards.[3]

Clinical waste is stored and disposed of in yellow biohazard bags or bins. Examples of biohazardous, clinical waste in primary healthcare settings include materials with expressible blood, body tissue and fluids. Clinical waste also includes contact materials from people with known wound infection, such as MRSA, or known to have a significant communicable disease (e.g. influenza or measles). Rarely, cytotoxic waste may be encountered in primary healthcare settings and specialist advice should be sought regarding risk and the correct handling and disposal of such materials.

Waste considered non-hazardous includes urine, faeces, teeth, nappies, pads, tongue depressors and speculums. These can be disposed of in the general waste bins.[4] Clinical waste storage bins and used linen carriers must be stored securely away from patient care and access areas.

44.5 Immunisation and vaccine potency

In Australia, the majority of vaccines for both children and adults are given through general practices, ACCHOs and similar office-based primary healthcare settings. It is important to note that in small office-based settings a nurse will not always be on duty, so it takes a whole-of-team approach to ensure that vaccines are safely stored and managed.

Administration staff will receive vaccine deliveries and need to know how to quickly and safely handle them to ensure vaccine potency and maintenance of the cold chain. All team members should be aware of the National Vaccine Storage Guidelines—Strive for 5. Primary healthcare settings that store and handle vaccines should have a purpose-built vaccine fridge that is serviced at least annually to ensure optimal function. Staff need to know how to monitor the vaccine fridge temperatures and how to respond in accordance with the practice's vaccine management protocol in the event of a power failure or temperature excursion from the recommended temperature range of +2°C to +8°C.[21]

Staff training must include temperature chart recording systems, data loggers, thermometers, disposable cold chain monitors, automated temperature-monitoring systems and back-to-base systems. The Strive for 5 guideline recommends that at a minimum, all vaccine refrigerators must have a basic data logger and thermometer to continuously monitor refrigerator temperature.[21]

All documentation and records of refrigerator maintenance, for example electrical checks and servicing by a refrigeration technician, need to be kept in the clinic equipment register. For general practices, both are compulsory 'flagged' indicators for practice accreditation. Records of cold chain management include twice daily temperature recording, data logging and refrigerator maintenance.[3,21]

When ordering new vaccine fridges, consideration should be given to the population size and demographics of the community serviced by the primary healthcare setting. Most general practice-based clinical software will give an age breakdown of currently registered patients. This can help with planning and ordering of vaccine stock to meet those needs and avoid over- or under-ordering (e.g. adult and paediatric vaccines for flu seasons, the number of childhood vaccines expected to be given between ordering cycles, coverage and expected need for special vaccines such as the COVID-19 vaccines during the pandemic).

All staff must be competent in vaccine storage management in the event of an emergency or power failure. Practices need clear policy and procedures that are readily accessible to staff, with clear reporting pathways should a breach occur. These documents are to include how to isolate vaccines and how to manage vaccines in case of power outage. The phone contact details for the local public health unit should be readily accessible to the team. Some states and primary health networks have online cold chain training modules that are easily accessible and suitable for a range of team members.

44.6 Reprocessing of reusable instruments in small office-based settings

Many small office-based health settings perform clinical procedures that require the use of surgical instruments. Single use equipment has advantages for minimising cross-infection and reducing the workload associated with reprocessing instruments. While there has been a move towards the use of disposable instruments in many primary healthcare settings, many services continue to use reusable instruments due to the higher cost of disposable surgical instruments, and the need to either absorb or pass on those costs to patients. Others will choose reusable instruments for environmental considerations and not wanting to add to waste. General practices, dentist, dermatology and podiatry practices are all clinical settings where small operative or cutting type procedures are performed.

While instrument cleaning and reprocessing is covered in Chapter 16, there are some special contexts that need to be considered in small office-based settings. General practices may have the services of a nurse to monitor instrument cleaning, reprocessing/sterilising, storage and tracking of instruments, but some general practices and many other primary healthcare services do not have a nurse to manage instrument reprocessing.

Primary healthcare settings that do not have a nurse may use care assistants, such as dental assistants, medical practice assistants or administration staff to reprocess instruments. Training and risk management oversight is critical. It is essential that any staff reprocessing instruments have adequate IPC training to protect both themselves and the person on whom any instruments will be used from the risk of infection.

Regardless of the setting, procedures for the reprocessing of reusable instruments must consider the manufacturer's instructions for use. Disposable instruments must not be reprocessed as the safety of the disposable item cannot be guaranteed after reprocessing. Reprocessing must be consistent with relevant national guidelines—such as 3.14 set out in the National Safety and Quality Health Service (NSQHS) Standards—and align with AS/NZ Standard ASNZ 4185:2006 for the Reprocessing of reusable medical devices in health service organisations.[5,22]

ASNZ 4185:2006 states that 'management should ensure that personnel involved in the cleaning, disinfecting, sterilisation, storage and distribution of items are trained and educated to enable them to correctly undertake any task that they will be required to perform'.[22]

Any staff involved in the reprocessing of instruments also need training to ensure they know how to keep instruments in good working order, check that packaging meets expected guidelines, and they can safely load, program and unload the steriliser. Whether using reprocessed or single use items, staff should know how to log and track instruments. Regular competency checking by a person trained in instrument reprocessing is also advised for ongoing quality control.

There are multiple training options for upskilling staff in infection control and for managing instrument reprocessing. The VET sector offers certificates in instrument reprocessing[7] and primary health networks offer CPD events in infection control and instrument processing. A record of training and competency checking should be kept in the staff file.

44.7 Antimicrobial resistance and primary care

Antimicrobial resistance (AMR) continues to be one of the greatest threats to human and animal health, and to food safety. Overuse and inappropriate use of antimicrobials is a key factor contributing to multiresistance and reduces the effectiveness of treatments for infections that were previously readily treatable with antimicrobials.[23] Primary healthcare clinicians play a key role in antimicrobial stewardship as gatekeepers for managing access to, and the use of, antimicrobial therapies in the community.

Despite a downward trend, Australia still has relatively high rates of antibiotic prescribing in the community, compared with other OECD nations.[24,25]

The Australian Government reported that in 2015:
- 44.7% of the Australian population (about 10.7 million people) received a prescription for at least one antibiotic
- more than 30 million antibiotic prescriptions were dispensed under the Pharmaceutical Benefits Scheme (PBS) and Repatriation PBS
- 60% of people with an acute respiratory condition such as sore throat, bronchitis, otitis media and sinusitis were prescribed antibiotics.[26]

The findings from the 2017 General Practice National Antimicrobial Prescribing Survey (GPNAPS) notes the majority of antibiotic prescribing in humans occurs in general practice. Primary care clinicians play a key role in antimicrobial stewardship (AMS) and in the prevention of antimicrobial resistance (AMR). Antibiotics are only indicated in populations at increased risk of complications or when symptoms are severe.[24]

There is also widespread antibiotic prescribing in aged care. Topical antibiotics for skin conditions, high levels of prescribing of antibiotics used for long-term prophylaxis to suppress potential respiratory and urinary infections, and antibiotics prescribed by telephone without a clinical examination have all been observed in the annual Aged Care National Antimicrobial Prescribing Survey (ACNAPS). The 2020 ACNAPS found that 50–75% of aged care residents received at least one course of antimicrobials annually and more than 1 in 10 residents are given an antimicrobial at any given time. Between 40% and 75% of antibiotic use in residential aged care facilities is considered inappropriate and not consistent with clinical practice guidelines.[27]

It is well accepted that wide use of broad-spectrum antibiotics is more likely to lead to antimicrobial resistance in the population. Despite healthcare authorities discouraging the use of broad-spectrum antibiotics in favour of narrow-spectrum antibiotics, GPs often choose to prescribe broad-spectrum antibiotics to avoid time-consuming microbiological tests and discussions with patients who may prefer quick treatment.[28]

Often patients have the expectation that they will be prescribed antibiotics for an acute infection. Many prescribers complain of feeling pressured to prescribe antibiotics. A 2020 survey of 386 Australian GPs found that major barriers to improving antimicrobial prescribing include:
- patient expectations and desire for quick recovery
- lack of awareness regarding the risk of antibiotic use
- late presentation of patients despite severe symptoms
- desire for a quick recovery; and
- poor health literacy.[29]

The same study found barriers to reducing antimicrobial prescribing by GPs include willingness to follow AMS guidance, AMS training, and confidence to not prescribe antibiotics. The study also observed that 'although GPs were familiar with AMS, it is concerning that approximately half of the respondents still did not firmly believe that their individual efforts have the potential to reduce AMR'.[29]

Having access to therapeutic guidelines, prescribing tools in clinical software, and education for all team members on appropriate and judicious antimicrobial use helps to support prescriber behaviour and decision making.

Ensuring there are readily available resources for clinicians to use, such as information handouts, and decision-making tools for managing specific issues, such as acute respiratory illnesses, will assist health professionals to reinforce key messages and educate consumers about appropriate antibiotic use and actions that can be taken to reduce AMR.[30]

Encouraging shared decision making about antibiotic use, using evidence-based resources, and providing patients with information on simple measures to self-manage their symptoms may help clarify misconceptions about the need for antibiotics.

- Have your infection, prevention and control policy ready and reachable by ALL team members
- Symptom check all patients booking appointments by phone or online AND when they arrive
- No-one gets through the door without hand hygiene
- Enforce cough etiquette rules—adults and children
- Anyone coughing wears a mask and waits outside
- Check that vaccines are up to date for all staff and offer a booster as needed
- Check that vaccines are up to date for all patients and offer a booster as needed
- Staff: If you are sick stay home—you could force the closure of the practice
- Keep hands away from your face
- Practise hand hygiene, putting gloves on and off with your team
- Regular hand hygiene
- Do not have food at reception
- Do not have a shared water dispenser in the waiting room
- Avoid handling cash and use EFTPOS for billing transactions where possible

- Stop wearing hand jewellery and keep nails short to make hand hygiene more effective
- Consider separate clinic session times for over 65s and other vulnerable people during disease outbreaks
- Have a script ready and ensure triage training for the staff taking calls and greeting patients
- Debriefing for staff—dealing with sick patients can be stressful, especially during high-load disease outbreaks such as influenza and COVID-19.

Conclusion

Primary healthcare settings strive to ensure safe and high-quality care. High-quality IPC in both clinical activities and environmental safety are of critical importance. For those primary healthcare settings where nurses are employed, they will be leaders and key drivers of IPC processes, policy and procedure development, monitoring, auditing risk and training staff.

In some small office-based primary healthcare settings, responsibility may be handed to an allied health professional or a non-clinical team member. All healthcare professionals and practice team members need to have a full understanding of the risk of acquiring and transmitting infection. Education and communication are important components of risk management including IPC. Employers need to have strong policies and procedures in place to guarantee adequate staff training is in line with their role in the workplace and to ensure the safety of staff and the community they service. IPC is everybody's business.

Useful websites/resources

- Royal Australian College of General Practitioners. Infection-prevention-and-control.pdf (racgp.org.au)
- Practice Assist. https://www.practiceassist.com.au/PracticeAssist/media/ResourceLibrary/General%20Practice%20Accreditation/General-Practice-Cleaning-Schedule-Template-Editable.pdf

References

1. Australian Institute of Health and Welfare. Medicare-subsidised GP, allied health and specialist health care across local areas: 2013–14 to 2017–18. AIHW, 2019. [cited 26 September 2019.] Available from: https://www.aihw.gov.au/reports/primary-health-care/medicare-subsidised-gp-allied-health-and-specialis/contents/introduction.
2. National Register on Vocational Education and Training (VET) in Australia Training.gov.au. HLT47715 - Certificate IV in Medical Practice Assisting (Release 2) 2022. Canberra: Australian Government, 2022. Available from: Training.gov.au: https://training.gov.au/Training/Details/HLT47715.
3. Royal Australian College of General Practitioners. Standards for general practice, 5th ed. Melbourne: RACGP, 2017. [Updated Feb 2022.] Available from: https://www.racgp.org.au/getmedia/b4047a62-9477-46b1-a5ce-22b1f5abcd51/Standards-for-general-practices-5th-edition_1.pdf.aspx.
4. Royal Australian College of General Practitioners. Infection prevention and control standards for general practices and other office-based and community based practices 5th ed. [Updated June 2022.] Available from: https://www.racgp.org.au/running-a-practice/practice-standards/standards-5th-edition/infection-prevention-and-control.

5. Australian Commission for Quality and Safety in Health Care. National safety and quality health service standards, 2nd ed. Sydney: ACQSHC, 2021. Available from: https://www.safetyandquality.gov.au/sites/default/files/2021-05/national_safety_and_quality_health_service_nsqhs_standards_second_edition_-_updated_may_2021.pdf.

6. Royal Australian College of General Practitioners. General practice management toolkit: clinical governance, module 12. Melbourne: RACGP, 2014. Available from: Clinical-governance.pdf (racgp.org.au).

7. Australian Government Department of Health. Minimising the risk of COVID-19 transmission in a primary health care setting. Canberra: Australian Government Department of Health, 2022. Available from: www.health.gov.au/resources/publications: https://www.health.gov.au/sites/default/files/documents/2022/01/minimising-the-risk-of-covid-19-transmission-in-a-primary-health-care-setting.pdf.

8. National Health and Medical Research Council (NHMRC). Australian Guidelines for the prevention and control of infection in healthcare. NHMRC: Building a healthy Australia; 2019. Canberra: Australian Government, 2019. Available from: https://www.nhmrc.gov.au/about-us/publications/australian-guidelines-prevention-and-control-infection-healthcare-2019.

9. Hand Hygiene Australia. What is hand hygiene? Melbourne: Hand Hygiene Australia, 2021. Available from: https://www.hha.org.au/hand-hygiene/what-is-hand-hygiene.

10. Therapeutic Goods Administration. Hand sanitisers: information for consumers. Canberra: Australian Government, 2020. [cited 31 August 2020.] Available from: https://www.tga.gov.au/hand-sanitisers-information-consumers.

11. Australian Commission for Quality and Safety in Health Care. The National Hand Hygiene Initiative (NHHI) Learning Management System (LMS). Sydney: ACSQHC, 2022. Available from https://www.safetyandquality.gov.au: Hand hygiene online learning modules.

12. Australian Government Department of Health. COVID-19 infection control training. Canberra: Australian Government, 2020, May. Available from: https://www.health.gov.au/resources/apps-and-tools/covid-19-infection-control-training.

13. Australian Government Department of Health. Vaccination for people at occupational risk. In: Australian immunisation handbook. Canberra: Australian Government, 2021. Available from: https://immunisationhandbook.health.gov.au/vaccination-for-special-risk-groups/vaccination-for-people-at-occupational-risk.

14. Barycka K, Torlinski T, Filipiak K, Jaguszewski M, Nadolny K, Szarpak L. Risk of self-contamination among healthcare workers in the COVID-19 pandemic. Am J Emerg Med. 2021;46:751–752.

15. Society for Healthcare Epidemiology of America. Improper removal of personal protective equipment contaminates health care workers. Science Daily; 2019, March 20. Available from: https://www.sciencedaily.com/releases/2019/03/190320110630.htm.

16. Victoria State Government Department of Health. Position description - personal protective equipment spotter - coronavirus (COVID-19). Melbourne: State Government of Victoria, 2020. [Updated October 17 2021.] Available from: https://www.health.vic.gov.au/personal-protective-equipment-spotter-position-description-covid-19-doc.

17. Clinical Excellence Commission. COVID-19 infection prevention and control manual: for acute and non-acute healthcare settings (internet). Sydney: CEC, 2022. Available from: https://www.cec.health.nsw.gov.au/__data/assets/pdf_file/0018/644004/COVID-19-IPAC-manual.pdf.

18. Evans J, Gerddtz M. Triage in general practice. In: Walker L, Patterson E, Wong W, Young D. General practice nursing. Sydney: McGraw-Hill Australia Pty Ltd, 2010.

19. Royal Australian College of General Practitioners Pandemic Taskforce. Preparedness: organizational and environmental measures. In: Managing pandemic influenza in general practice: a guide for preparation, response and recovery. Melbourne: RACGP, 2014.

20. Australian Government Department of Health. Environmental cleaning and disinfection principles for COVID-19. Canberra: Australian Government, 2020. Available from: https://www.health.gov.au/sites/default/files/documents/2020/03/environmental-cleaning-and-disinfection-principles-for-covid-19.pdf.

21. Australian Government Department of Health. National vaccine storage guidelines - Strive for 5. 3rd ed. Canberra: Australian Government, 2020. Available from: https://www.health.gov.au/resources/publications/national-vaccine-storage-guidelines-strive-for-5.

22. Standards Australia/Standards New Zealand. AS/NZS 4815:2006 Office-based health care facilities - reprocessing of reusable medical and surgical instruments and equipment, and maintenance of the associated envirinment. SAI Global Assurance, 2006. Available from: AS/NZS 4815:2006 Office-based health care facilities - reprocessing of reusable medical and surgical instruments and equipment, and maintenance of the associated environment (saiglobal.com).

23. Australian Commission for Quality and Safety in Health Care. AURA 2021 highlights - fourth Australian report on antimicrobial use. Sydney: ACSQHC, 2021. Available from: https://www.safetyandquality.gov.au/sites/default/files/2021-08/aura_2021_-_highlights_resource_-_august_17.pdf.

24. Monaghan T, Biezen R, Buising K, Hallinan C, Cheah R, Manski-Nankervis J. (2022). Clinical insights into appropriate choice of antimicrobials for acute respiratory tract infections. Aust J Gen Pract. 2022;51(1–2):33-37.

25. Buising K, Mansi-Nankervis J, Ingram R, James R, Biezen R. Evaluating antimicrobial prescribing in general practice in Australia. Melbourne: National Centre for Antimicrobial Stewardship, 2019. Available from: https://www.youtube.com/watch?v=6Keq38nSic0.

26. Australian Government Antimicrobial Resistance. For general practice: what you can do. Canberra: Australian Government, 2017. Available from: https://www.amr.gov.au/what-you-can-do/general-practice.

27. Australian Commission for Quality and Safety in Health Care. Role of general practice in antimicrobial stewardship Chapter 13. In: Antimicrobial stewardship in Australian healthcare. Sydney: ACSQHC, 2018. [Updated November 2021.] Available from: chapter_13_ams_book_-_final_-_general_practice_gp_-_nov_2021.pdf (safetyandquality.gov.au).

28. Allen T, Gyrd-Hansen D, Kristensen S, Oxholm A, Pedersen L, Pezzino, M. Physicians under pressure: evidence from antibiotics prescribing in England. Med Decis Making. 2022;42(3):303-312.

29. Sajal K, Konf D, Thursky K, Mazza D. A nationwide survey of Australian general practitioners on antimicrobial stewardship: awareness, uptake, collaboration with pharmacists and improvement strategies. Antibiotics (Basel) 2020;9(6):310.

30. Australian Government Antimicrobial Resistance. Objective one: increase awareness and understanding of AMR, its implications, and actions to combat it through effective communication, education and training. In: Implementation plan: Australia's first national antimicrobial resistence strategy 2015-2019. Canberra: Australian Government, 2017. Available from: file: https://www.amr.gov.au/resources/national-amr-implementation-plan.

CHAPTER 45

Infection prevention and control in cosmetic, tattooing, piercing and personal appearance practice and settings

Dr CATHERINE VIENGKHAM[i]

Dr DEBOROUGH MACBETH[ii]

PROFESSOR RAMON Z. SHABAN[i,iii,iv,v]

Chapter highlights

- The current state of the cosmetic, tattooing, piercing and personal services industry in Australia, describing what each service involves, the most common procedures and current regulations and licensing requirements for industry professionals
- A review of the healthcare-associated infection (HAI) and communicable diseases risks observed across these cosmetic, tattooing, piercing and personal services
- An overview of context-specific infection prevention and control (IPC) measures for cosmetic, tattooing, piercing and personal service settings

i   Susan Wakil School of Nursing and Midwifery, Faculty of Medicine and Health, University of Sydney, Sydney, NSW
ii Gold Coast Hospital and Health Service, Southport, QLD
iii Sydney Infectious Diseases Institute, Faculty of Medicine and Health, University of Sydney, Sydney, NSW
iv Public Health Unit, Centre for Population Health, Western Sydney Local Health District, Westmead, NSW
v   New South Wales Biocontainment Centre, Western Sydney Local Health District, Westmead, NSW

Introduction

Personal appearance services encompass a wide array of aesthetic procedures ranging from those that are completely non-invasive such as hairdressing, to those requiring deep skin incision and surgical reconstructions. Services like tattooing, piercing and cosmetic surgery have become increasingly popular in recent decades, due in no small part to reduced stigma and social media advocacy. This in turn has facilitated greater accessibility to such services within the community, many of which exist as completely distinct entities from healthcare settings. Nevertheless, the spread of infections in these contexts still represents a major risk due to the frequent use of shared equipment and surfaces, close interactions with service providers and most importantly, the high prevalence of skin penetration procedures.

45.1 Infection prevention and control in cosmetic, tattooing, piercing and personal appearance practice and settings

45.1.1 Cosmetic services

The Medical Board of Australia defines cosmetic medical and surgical procedures as 'operations and other procedures that revise or change the appearance, colour, texture, structure or position of normal bodily features with the dominant purpose of achieving what the patient perceives to be a more desirable appearance or boosting the patient's self-esteem'.[1] Furthermore, it specifically distinguishes 'major' and 'minor' cosmetic medical and surgical procedures. Major procedures encompass those that cut 'beneath the skin' and include breast augmentation, breast reduction, rhinoplasty, surgical face lifts and liposuction. Minor procedures do not cut beneath the skin but may still include piercing the skin to some degree, and include procedures like non-surgical varicose vein treatment, laser skin treatments, mole removal, laser hair removal, dermabrasion, chemical peels, injections and hair replacement therapy. Cosmetic surgery falls within the broader specialty of 'plastic surgery' and is also commonly referred to as 'aesthetic surgery'. It differentiates itself from reconstructive surgery, in that its primary purpose is the improvement of appearance in otherwise healthy patients, whereas reconstructive surgery necessarily serves to restore function to where there is impairment.

Both globally and in Australia, cosmetic procedures are becoming increasingly diverse and more widely accessed. The prevalence of cosmetic surgery in Australia is difficult to accurately quantify, as it is not covered by Medicare or private health insurance and there is no central framework for the reporting of procedures.[2] A broader snapshot is provided by the *International Survey on Aesthetic/Cosmetic Procedures*, a global survey of over 1000 cosmetic surgeons that is published annually by the International Society of Aesthetic Plastic Surgery (ISAPS).[3] In 2020, the most common surgical procedures performed in women included breast augmentation, liposuction, eyelid surgery, abdominoplasty (tummy tuck) and rhinoplasty. For men, the most common procedures also included eyelid surgery, liposuction and rhinoplasty, in addition to gynecomastia and ear surgery. The most common types of non-surgical cosmetic procedures requested were the same across both men and women, including botulinum toxin injections, hyaluronic acid, hair removal, photo rejuvenation and non-surgical fat reduction. Women accounted for over 85% of clients receiving both surgical and non-surgical cosmetic procedures.[3]

Regulation of cosmetic services and 'cosmetic surgeons': The Australian Health Practitioner Regulation Agency (AHPRA) and the Medical Board of Australia (MBA) form part of the multi-jurisdictional system that regulates cosmetic surgery in Australia.[2] Specifically, AHPRA and the MBA regulate individual medical practitioners registered under the National Registration and Accreditation Scheme, which includes 'cosmetic surgeons'. They are responsible for handling complaints and concerns, as well as issuing codes of conduct, guidelines and standards that inform good practice.

They also oversee the appropriate and protected use of specialist titles by medical practitioners, which are gained by seeking specialist registration following completion of accredited specialist training. There are 11 specialist surgical titles accredited by the Australian Medical Council (AMC); however, 'cosmetic surgery' is currently not recognised as a medical specialty and there exist no restrictions on use of the title 'cosmetic surgeon' or 'surgeon'. Under Australian law, cosmetic procedures may be performed by a range of registered medical practitioners with significant differences in training, qualifications and experience. These include, and are not limited to, plastic surgeons, general surgeons, otolaryngologists, dermatologists, ophthalmologists, general practitioners and practitioners with no specialty qualifications.[4] Similar to the surgeon title, the speciality of 'cosmetic surgery' is not recognised in Australia and does not have a protected title under Australian legislation.[5] The *Health Practitioner Regulation National Law Act 2009* asserts that medical practitioners must not make claims about their qualifications, experience or expertise, or use their title, to mislead patients with respect to their skill and ability to perform requested procedures.[6] The MBA Guidelines[1] further state that procedures should only be provided given the practitioner has the appropriate training and they may only broaden the scope of their practice after undertaking the necessary training. Additional national laws include the *Competition and Consumer Act 2010* and the *Therapeutic Goods Act 1989*, which encompass both the regulation of therapeutic goods advertising in Australia and the Therapeutic Goods Advertising Code.

Regulatory responsibilities are also shared by Australian states and territories and vary across jurisdictions (Table 45.1). Most state and territory laws have placed specific restrictions on where specific types of cosmetic procedures can be performed. For example, in New South Wales, the Private Health Facilities Regulation 2017 (NSW) requires that all cosmetic surgeries involving the use of general anaesthetic be performed in a licensed private health facility. Similarly, both Queensland and Victoria require surgical procedures such as breast augmentation, liposuction, implants, or those which require high doses of local anaesthesia, to be performed in facilities like a day hospital or day procedure centre.[2] In general, facilities such as public and private hospitals and day procedure services must be accredited to the National Safety and Quality Health Service Standards (NSQHS), which include standards for infection control.

Cosmetic surgery also has several representative groups in Australia that provide either educational support for members or have minimum entry requirements for membership:[5]

- The Australasian Society of Aesthetic Plastic Surgery
- The Australian Society of Plastic Surgeons
- The Australasian College of Dermatologists
- The Australasian College of Cosmetic Surgery and Medicine
- The Cosmetic Physicians College of Australasia
- The Australasian College of Aesthetic Medicine.

However, membership is not required to perform cosmetic surgery in Australia and there remain no specific qualification requirements to classify a medical practitioner as a 'cosmetic surgeon'. As of 2016, there were 424 plastic surgeons in Australia. Approximately 76.9%

TABLE 45.1 Summary of state and territory legislation for personal appearance services and skin penetration procedures

State	Cosmetic surgical procedures	Tattooing, piercing and other personal appearance services
NSW	Private Health Facilities Regulation 2017, Private Health Facilities Act 2007, Medical Practice Regulation 2008	Public Health Act 2010, Public Health Regulation 2012, Tattoo Parlour Act 2012
QLD	Private Health Facilities Act 1999, Private Health Facilities Regulation 2016	Public Health (Infection Control for Personal Appearance Services) Act 2003, Tattoo Industry Act 2013
VIC	Health Services (Health Service Establishments) Regulations 2013, Health Services Act 1988	Public Health and Wellbeing Act 2008, Public Health and Wellbeing Regulations 2019
ACT	Health Professionals (ACT Medical Board Standards Statements) Approval 2006	Public Health Act 1997, Public Health Regulation 2000
SA	Health Care Act 2008, Health Care Regulations 2008	South Australian Public Health Act 2011, Tattoo Industry Control Act 2015
NT	Health Practitioners Act 2004	Public and Environmental Health Regulations 2014
WA	Health Practitioner Regulation National Law (WA) Act 2010	Health (Skin Penetration Procedures) Regulations 1998
TAS	Health Practitioner Regulation National Law (Tasmania) Act 2010	Public Health Act 1997

worked in the private sector and 97% indicated they were clinicians.[7] NSW and VIC have the highest proportion of cosmetic surgeons, though the distribution across jurisdictions was roughly proportional to population size.

45.1.2 Tattooing services

Tattooing is a form of body decoration and its practice can be dated as far back as 3000 BCE.[8] Tattooing involves the insertion of ink or pigment into the upper and middle dermis with the intention of creating a permanent (sometimes semi-permanent) design on the skin. While tattooing tools have evolved substantially over time, the basic application principle remains the same. Traditionally, tattoos were created using sharp instruments to make incisions on the surface of the skin, into which a pigment would be pressed. Pigment could be made from any number of substances, including ash, oil and synthetic dyes. Modern day tattooing typically involves commercial ink and an electric tattoo machine, which is a hand-held device fitted with single to multiple needles that oscillate rapidly to push ink into the skin. Modern tattoo needles are produced in many configurations that are suitable for different functions, ranging from fine detail work to the shading and filling of large areas.

'Decorative' tattoos are usually received at tattoo parlours or studios from professional tattoo artists. Other forms of tattoo include cosmetic tattoos, sometimes referred to as 'permanent makeup', which usually serve to alter or add pigmentation and form to certain facial features such as on the lips and eyebrows. These services are typically provided by beauticians within beauty clinics. Tattoos have also been introduced in the medical field, sometimes as a means of providing medical information or to act as fiducial markers in some forms of therapy. Most commonly, they may be applied to disguise a medical condition or the result of certain treatments. For example, they have been used to replace the removed areola on the breast following mastectomies or breast reduction surgeries.

Scarification and branding are similar, though considerably less common, procedures for creating permanent body art. They differ from tattoos as they do not involve the insertion of ink to create designs. Branding is a method of scarification that uses the precise application of extreme heat or cold to permanently scar the skin. This can be achieved via 'strike branding' where strips of metal are repeatedly heated and pressed onto the skin. Alternatively, 'cautery branding' uses surgical-grade electrocautery equipment to deliver extreme heat through a small wire tip. Other methods of scarification involve the deliberate scratching, etching and cutting of the skin to create patterns and designs.[9]

The number of Australians receiving tattoos has been increasing since the turn of the century. A survey conducted in 2004–05 revealed that approximately 14.5% of Australians have been the recipient of a tattoo.[10] Subsequent surveys in more recent years have found this has increased to around 1 in 5 Australians in 2016–18 and to 1 in 4 in 2019.[11] The rising prevalence of tattooing parallels shifts in consumer attitudes and perceptions. As tattoos become more commonplace in the general population, they have also become less associated with delinquency and crime, and more as a means of self-expression. Nevertheless, stigma and negative attitudes towards individuals with tattoos remain widespread and a large proportion of tattooed people still indicate the need to cover their tattoos when attending formal occasions or job interviews.[11,12] For the purpose of this chapter, we will examine the regulation and IPC practices of tattoo services provided in the community, such as those by tattoo artists in tattoo parlours and beauticians in beauty clinics.

Regulation of tattooing and tattoo parlours: Regulation of tattooists, tattooing services and operating venues is the responsibility of state and territory governments, and local jurisdictions. As a result, requirements for individuals intending to provide professional tattoo services differ from state to state. Some jurisdictions like QLD, NSW and Western Australia require licences for both individual tattooists and business operators. Applications for licences typically involve identification documents, a criminal history check, employment/training history, mandatory fingerprinting and associated fees. Evidence of additional training and qualifications is required in some jurisdictions. For example, tattooists in QLD are required by the *Tattoo Industry Act 2013* to hold a certificate for Maintain Infection Prevention for Skin Penetration Treatments (HLTINF005). They are also required to maintain a record of any procedure performed at a parlour for a fee or reward, which includes the tattooist's name and licence number. Western Australia similarly requires applicants to obtain certification for blood-borne pathogens, and licence applications for some cities, such as Hobart in Tasmania, uniquely involve the completion of a set of questions in relation to infection control. Victoria and South Australia do not require individual tattooists to be licensed but do require registration of businesses that perform tattoos, and conduct monitoring and compliance of mandatory record-keeping activities accordingly.

Outside of state-mandated licensing requirements, there are generally no other additional certification or qualifications legally needed to become a professional tattoo artist. Courses and training programs from both educational colleges and professional organisations are available to provide both theoretical and practical experience. Most professionals are trained through apprenticeships under experienced artists in existing establishments. There is no formal or regulated structure for apprenticeships, they can last on average from two to three years and are often completed without pay.

45.1.3 Piercing services

Body piercing is a body modification procedure that involves the puncturing or cutting of a part of the body to create an opening for jewellery or decorative implants to be inserted.

The techniques used for body piercing vary depending on the site of the piercing but will typically be administered using a sharp, hollow needle. The piercing site is held in place by a surgical clamp or by hand, during which the needle is pushed through. Piercings using a hollow needle will have the jewellery to be inserted attached to the blunt end, so that it can be pulled through and into the opening created by the needle. An open end of the jewellery is introduced into the rear blunt end of the piercing needle and pulled through the opening made by the needle. Piercing guns with spring-loaded or hand clasp mechanisms are also available and have been commonly used for earlobe piercings. However, these have generally fallen out of favour by professional body piercers due to their reliance on blunt force to create openings. Notably, some states, including QLD, only allow the use of piercing guns for the earlobe and no other part of the body.

Some piercing procedures such as dermal piercings (also known as microdermal piercings) and transdermal implants do not create two-ended openings. Instead, the jewellery that is visible on the surface of the skin is held in place using an anchor that is inserted underneath the skin.[13] Dermal punching is a related procedure that involves removing a small amount of tissue or cartilage to create a hole that can accommodate larger piercings. Subdermal transplants describe a type of body modification procedure that involves the insertion of objects fully beneath the skin to create raised surfaces and textures.

The jewellery inserted during the initial piercing is most commonly made from hypoallergenic materials such as stainless steel, titanium, niobium or acrylic. Jewellery usually comes in pre-sterilised packaging that is only opened immediately prior to the piercing procedure. There are many styles of jewellery and implants, which vary widely in shape, size and placement. Additionally, traditional jewellery used in cultural practices may include items made of bone, wood, metal, shells or feather quills.

Similar to tattooing, the prevalence of body piercing in Australia has been increasing, due in no small part to increasing availability, trends in fashion and reduced social stigmatisation.[14] The practice was noted as a 'worldwide fashion craze' at the beginning of the 21st century and was primarily driven by its increasing popularity among the younger generation at the time. Ear piercing remains the most prevalent form of the procedure, with almost half of women and around 1 in 5 men having received at least one ear piercing in Australia.[14,15] Individuals with piercings on other parts of the body remain less frequent compared to both ear piercings and tattoos. The most common locations to receive piercings outside the ear include the nose, tongue, navel, eyebrow, nipples and genitalia.[15]

Regulation of body piercing services: Like tattoo services, body piercing services are regulated by state and territory governments, and by local councils. In NSW and WA, body piercing is classified as a 'skin penetration procedure' and premises seeking to undertake such procedures in a non-medical context must notify and be registered with their local council and are required to undergo routine inspections. In NSW, regulation of body piercing services and skin penetration procedures is enforced via the *Public Health Act 2010* and *Public Health Regulation 2012*. These regulations set out specific requirements for body piercing services, including those relating to infrastructure (e.g. installation of surfaces to prioritise efficient cleaning, separate sinks for cleaning hands and equipment, single use towels, gloves and gowns and a waste disposal bin), equipment reuse and sterilisation, appropriate disposal of sharps, hygiene procedures and personal hygiene. Some councils will require proof of completion of additional training, such as the Maintain Infection Prevention for Skin Penetration Treatments (HLTINF005) in QLD and the submission of how the premises will be laid out to best promote flow of service and good hygiene practice. Broadly speaking, there are no additional certifications that individuals who perform body piercings are legally required to obtain. As with tattooing, training in body piercing can be accessed via a wide range of avenues, ranging from formal courses to apprenticeships.

45.1.4 Other beauty and cosmetic services

There are a diverse range of everyday beauty and cosmetic services that do not inherently involve any degree of skin penetration and where the risk of infection transmission is low. Hairdressing and barbering services offer a variety of procedures that are performed to the hair on a person's head or face, such as cutting, shaving, cleaning, colouring, bleaching, heat-styling and the application of extensions and chemical treatments. While these procedures are localised to the hair and hold a low risk of infection, the use of shears and razors does carry the risk of cutting the client (or the hairdresser) and creating an opening for microorganisms.

Hair removal services are also popular and widely used. They encompass a wide range of techniques used to remove hair from different areas of the body. The technique used differs based on the area where hair is to be removed, the size of the area and the desire to inhibit further hair growth in those areas. For example, waxing is suitable for small to large areas of skin across the face and body, whereas threading and tweezing are appropriate for achieving precise hair removal on smaller areas such as the eyebrows and face. Electrolysis and laser hair removal are examples of services that involve the precise application of current or heat to individual hair follicles. The application destroys each follicle to achieve long-term to permanent reduction of hair growth in the targeted area. While none of these procedures involve skin penetration, excessive application or inappropriate technique may cause skin damage and small amounts of bleeding. It is vital for providers to ensure the correct practice of single-use, disposable materials and that all reusable equipment is reprocessed appropriately between clients.

Manicure and pedicure services offer a variety of treatments for an individual's hand and feet, respectively. Treatments typically include the filing and shaping of the nails, pushing and clipping the cuticles, removing dead skin, buffing, soaking, massaging and the application of nail polish, acrylic nails and/or other forms of nail decor. These services employ a variety of single-use and reusable equipment including nail files, buffers, clippers, scissors, cuticle pushers and brushes. Pedicures commonly include the use of footbaths and a pumice block or similarly abrasive device to remove calluses. Similar to the cosmetic services described above, infection risks may arise from the accidental cutting of skin and the inappropriate reprocessing of equipment and hygiene across clients.

45.2 HAI risks in cosmetic, tattooing, piercing and personal service settings

45.2.1 Factors increasing the risk of infection

The skin is a natural barrier and the first line of defence against infection. However, the process of skin penetration is inherent to many cosmetic procedures and personal appearance services. In some cases, the risk may be unintentional, such as accidental cuts caused by sharp instruments in hair salons and nail services. On the other hand, wounds are unavoidable in the case of surgical cosmetic procedures and those involving injections, piercings and tattooing. These may range from small, localised punctures or deep incisions, to shallow wounds that cover a large surface of the body. Any site of skin penetration presents an opportunity for disease-causing microorganisms to enter and trigger serious complications.

There are several factors that greatly increase the risk of infection in the cosmetic industry and personal appearance services. As highlighted in the previous section, there is a large degree of heterogeneity in which these services are regulated within Australia, both in regard to the qualification of the service providers, and the premises in which the services are performed. While some jurisdictions have limited the performance of certain cosmetic procedures to private hospitals, which are accredited against national infection control standards, many others remain unaccredited and unregulated. Common sources of infection, such as through contaminated products, also remain an issue, particularly in the tattooing industry. For example, most tattoo inks used in commercial studios are imported internationally but are currently exempt from national or jurisdictional regulation. However, contaminated ink is often implicated in tattoo-associated infections, and bacterial cultures have previously been observed in unopened, 'sterile' labelled ink containers.[16]

45.2.2 Bacterial infections

Bacterial infections are a common complication following skin penetration procedures. The risk of such infections occurring may be compounded throughout multiple stages of many services, including inadequate sterilisation (antisepsis instead of sterilisation—especially as it relates to persons) of persons and equipment during the procedure, to improper aftercare and healing of fresh wounds post-procedure. Infectious complications range from local skin infections—such as the appearance of abscesses, pustules or papules, erythema, necrotising fasciitis, tissue necrosis and cellulitis—to more serious systemic infections, such as septicaemia, septic shock, endocarditis and multiple organ failure.[17] The most common bacterial infections reported across cosmetic, tattooing, piercing and personal services are summarised in Table 45.2, and further described in the sections below.

Pseudomonas aeruginosa: Local and systemic infection with *Pseudomonas aeruginosa* has been reported following both tattooing and skin piercing procedures. In tattooing, *P. aeruginosa* has been the pathogen responsible for several reported life-threatening cases following traditional tattooing procedures.[36-39] For example, traditional Samoan tattooing (ta tatau) is an important cultural practice and is still commonly sought by young Samoan men as a rite of passage over conventional tattoo services. Historically, traditional tattooing methods utilised a range of handmade tools created from natural materials, such as combs derived from boars' husks, turtle shell and coconut fibres, and custom pigments mixed from candlenut soot and sometimes kerosene. The tattoos created are large, often starting at the waist and ending at the knee (known as pe'a). More modern tools have since been adopted, in particular, the use of commercial tattoo ink; however, minimal infection control measures and sanitation precautions are in place. The tattoo is typically completed across multiple several hour-long sessions and may be spread over several days to several weeks.

P. aeruginosa is also implicated in bacterial infections following certain piercing procedures, particularly transcartilaginous ear piercings, which have become increasing popular in recent decades as an alternative to more conventional lobe piercings. Transcartilaginous ear piercings commonly include the piercing of the upper cartilage of the ear, the scapha and the helix. A review of transcartilaginous ear piercing complications found *P. aeruginosa* accounted for 87.2% of infections and 92.3% of required hospitalisations.[40] The symptoms of infection may present as ear chondritis, perichondritis, abscesses and cellulitis, and treatment involves drainage and antibiotics. Severe complications may result from delayed intervention, including the complete collapse of the ear cartilage and subsequent deformation requiring reconstructive surgery.[41] Multiple sources of *P. aeruginosa* bacteria have been implicated across multiple case reports, including contaminated disinfectants and the use of inappropriate piercing equipment.[18] Infection via bacteria already present on the patient or

TABLE 45.2 Common bacterial infections across cosmetic, tattooing, piercing and personal appearance services

Bacteria	Service	Commons sources
Pseudomonas aeruginosa	Tattoo, piercing	• Contaminated tattoo ink[16] and non-professional or traditional tattooing services • Improper use of piercing equipment, disinfection and aftercare practices, exposure to water post-procedure[18,19]
Mycobacteria (non-tuberculous; chelonae, fortuitum, abscessus)	Tattoo, piercing, cosmetic surgery, nail salons	• Contaminated water used to dilute tattoo ink[20] • Contaminated piercing equipment and jewellery[21] • Inadequate sterilisation of surgical equipment or implants[22] • Contaminated footbaths in nail salons[23-27]
Staphylococcus aureus	Tattoo, piercing	• Contaminated ink, unsanitary conditions[16,28-30] • Non-professional piercing procedures, pre-existing cardiac conditions[31-33]
Streptococcus pyogenes	Tattoo, piercing, cosmetic surgery	• Inadequate IPC and hand hygiene during procedures, droplet transmission[34] • Contaminated equipment and jewellery[35]

practitioner skin is also likely, and further exacerbated by hot weather, sweat and the specific, inherent risk of transcartilaginous piercing procedures.[42,43]

Mycobacteria infections: Mycobacteria is a large family of bacteria best known for the species of bacteria that cause tuberculosis (*Mycobacterium tuberculosis* complex) and leprosy (*M. leprae*) in humans. However, it is predominantly the non-tuberculous species of mycobacteria (NTM) that are responsible for infectious complications, such as skin and soft tissue infections, following skin penetration procedures. NTMs are widespread in the environment and can be isolated in water (most relevantly, tap water), soil, dust, animals and food sources.[20] While there are many species of mycobacteria, the following species of rapidly growing mycobacteria (RGM) are the most commonly reported sources of skin and soft tissue infection: *M. chelonae*, *M. abscessus* and *M. fortuitum*. RGMs are particularly problematic in the context of HAIs due to their environmental ubiquity, resistance to common methods of disinfection and sterilisation and difficulty to diagnose and treat.[44]

The majority of NTM infections following tattooing are caused by *M. chelonae*, which typically manifest in the form of red papules, pustules and rashes on the tattooed area within several weeks after the procedure.[20] Notably, many cases reported localisation of the infection to grey coloured areas of the tattoo, which are usually created using diluted black ink. As such, it is highly likely that contaminated water used to dilute the tattoo ink is the source of many tattoo-related NTM infections. *M. fortuitum* infections have been increasingly reported following piercings, specifically nipple piercings, which typically present as an abscess at the site of piercing that requires antibiotic treatment and surgical removal.[45-49] Outbreaks of mycobacteria infections following cosmetic surgeries are also well documented in the contexts of cosmetic or medical 'tourism' where patients travel abroad for surgical procedures.[50] In 2003, the CDC reported a large-scale outbreak of *M. abscessus* across 12 North American patients who underwent cosmetic surgery procedures in the Dominican Republic.[51] The infections, typically presenting as subcutaneous or deep-tissue abscesses, arose out of a wide range of cosmetic procedures, including abdominoplasty, liposuction, breast lift, breast reduction and breast implant. Treatment included incision, drainage and antibiotic therapy and 9 of the 12 patients required hospitalisation as a result of the infection.

Systemic NTM infection complications include bacteraemia and infection of the central nervous, ocular and pulmonary systems, and disseminated infection in the immunocompromised.[22] Pulmonary infections are a concern in high-risk populations such as individuals with underlying lung diseases like cystic fibrosis, bronchiectasis and prior tuberculosis.[52] Patients with cancer and/or chronic kidney disease are also susceptible to disseminated and invasive disease due to *M. chelonae*.[53]

Staphylococcus aureus: *S. aureus* remains a primary source of bacterial skin and soft tissue infection following skin penetration procedures.[32,54] Both methicillin-sensitive (MSSA) and methicillin-resistant (MRSA) strains are commonly reported as the causative agents of complications in cosmetic surgeries, tattooing and piercing procedures. Local skin infections are the most frequently observed complication and typically include the development of benign boils, folliculitis, impetigo and cellulitis, or the more severe staphylococcal scalded skin syndrome (SSSS) in paediatric patients.[55] Receiving tattoos has been identified as a risk factor for community-acquired and Panton-Valentine leucocidin-producing *S. aureus* and has been linked with multiple outbreaks since the beginning of the 21st century.[28,30,56,57] The majority of reported outbreaks were identified in inmates held in correctional facilities or prisons, where the sharing of makeshift tattooing instruments and suboptimal sanitary conditions were implicated in the outbreak. An investigation of 6 unlinked CA-MRSA outbreaks across 44 tattoo recipients across 3 states in the USA led to the identification of 13 unlicensed tattooists.[28] They determined inadequate adherence to IPC precautions, such as changing gloves, sterilising equipment and hand hygiene, and the use of home-made tattoo equipment and performance of services in private residences (i.e. homes of the client) were the likely causes of both primary and secondary *S. aureus* infection.

S. aureus infections may also lead to systemic complications, including septicaemia, toxic shock syndrome (TSS), septic arthritis and endocarditis.[31,58,59] Infective endocarditis (IE) is a particularly serious and widely reported complication resulting from body piercing, caused by the introduction of bacteria like *S. aureus* into the bloodstream and subsequent infection of the lining of the heart.[33] Approximately half of reported cases require surgical intervention and valve replacement operations. The disease is more common in those with underlying cardiac issues but has also been reported following body piercing procedures in individuals without underlying conditions.[60] *S. aureus* associated IE has been reported following both tattooing and piercing of the ear, eyebrow, nose, tongue and navel.[44] Toxic shock syndrome resulting from independent ear and nipple piercing procedures has also been reported, with the latter case resulting in death.[31,61] While the fatal case was determined to likely have been the result of a home-administered piercing, the majority of reported piercing complications, like infectious endocarditis, involved professional services. These complications highlight the need to clarify the risk of infection with respect to their interactions with preexisting conditions, and to educate both clients and service providers accordingly.

Streptococcus pyogenes: Similar to Staphylococcus spp., Streptococcus spp. and specifically *S. pyogenes* is a well-documented cause of bacterial skin infections following skin penetration procedures. The bacteria is commonly found in the throat and on the skin and is primarily spread through direct contact and respiratory droplets. It is most known for causing illnesses such as strep throat, cellulitis, scarlet fever and impetigo, but infection resulting from surgical complications can also lead to greater systemic illnesses. *S. pyogenes* has also been observed as a causative agent of bacteraemia and infective endocarditis following piercing procedures, particularly those in the oral cavity.[62] In the context of cosmetic surgery, it is the most commonly documented cause of necrotising fasciitis (NF), a severe and sometimes fatal condition characterised by an infection of the superficial soft tissues with rapid spread to the fascia.[63] In the US, NF complications resulting from *S. pyogenes* have been reported following procedures such as liposuction, blepharoplasty and breast implants, with the former two operations commonly performed in outpatient settings.[34,63,64] The infection was found to be lethal in 20% of cases. Other complications include toxic shock syndrome, pneumonia and bacteraemia.

45.2.3 Viral infections

Infections due to exogenous agents are caused by inoculation of a microbe not present on the host initially and should typically be preventable if hygienic techniques are followed. Reuse of tattoo ink or needles, contamination of equipment between tattoo recipients, and use of contaminated body fluids during the

tattoo process (e.g. saliva used to wet the needle) have all been implicated in transmission of pathogenic microbes. Viral hepatitis, tuberculosis, syphilis and human immunodeficiency virus (HIV) disease are examples of infections following inoculation from an exogenous source. Both endogenously and exogenously acquired infections have the potential to widely disseminate in the body via the bloodstream (Table 45.3).

Hepatitis virus: Hepatitis viruses are comprised of several distinct viral species that all cause infection and inflammation of the liver. Currently, there are five main types of hepatitis virus: A, B, C, D and E. Two of these—hepatitis B virus (HBV) and hepatitis C virus (HCV)—are transmitted through blood and sexual contact, making them a considerable risk in any service involving skin penetration procedures and the sharing of equipment, such as tattooing and skin piercing. Infection with hepatitis D virus (HDV) is also a notable risk as the virus can only infect hosts in which HBV is already present. Viral hepatitis remains one of the most commonly reported viral infections following tattooing procedures and is strongly associated with the reusing of tattoo needles, contaminated equipment and receiving any skin penetrating procedure in non–professional settings.[65,68,69,72,93]

Human papillomavirus (HPV): Both common (verruca vulgaris) and flat warts (verruca plana) are benign growths caused by human papillomavirus (HPV), of which more than 200 different types have so far been identified. HPV infections are most commonly reported following tattoo procedures, with warts typically occurring at the site of the tattoo within a month or up to several years post-procedure. A review found that for 70% of reported cases, warts appeared within 3 years after receiving a tattoo, with the remaining minority seeing the warts 5–21 years later.[75,94] The number of warts may range from one to 'many', with a median reported quantity of approximately 17.[75,95]

Contaminated tattoo ink is heavily implicated for HPV infection as the appearance of most warts is observed to be localised to areas of skin treated with one specific pigment (e.g. growing only along a black outline or within a uniformly coloured-in section). Dark coloured inks, in particular black pigments, have been found to be the most common sites for wart growth.[74,96] Other possible infection sources include contact with contaminated needles during the tattooing procedure,

TABLE 45.3 Possible viral infections resulting from cosmetic, tattooing, piercing and personal services

Virus	Service	Common sources
HBV	Tattoo, piercing	• Sharing contaminated needles,[65-67] equipment and contamination of jewellery[68]
HCV	Tattoo, piercing	• Sharing contaminated needles,[69-73] equipment and contamination of jewellery[68]
HPV	Tattoo, hair removal	• Contaminated needles or tattoo ink, infected tattooist, reactivation of virus at site of damaged skin[74-76] • Contaminated equipment or reactivation of virus at site of damaged skin following hair removal procedures, such as threading[77-79] and waxing[79,80]
Molluscum contagiosum	Tattoo, hair removal	• Contaminated needles or tattoo ink, infected tattooist, reactivation of virus at site of damaged skin[29,76] • Weakening of the skin barrier facilitating viral infection, particularly in the pubic region[81-83]
HSV	Tattoo, hair removal	• Primary infection through superinfection of damaged skin[84,85] or reactivation of virus[86] • Reactivation of virus at site of damaged skin following hair removal procedures, such as waxing[81,87] and laser-assisted hair removal[88-90]
HIV	Tattoo, piercing	• Unsterilised needles[91,92]

contact with contaminated surfaces in the environment during or after the procedure, or contact with bodily fluids (e.g. saliva) on the hands of an infected tattoo artist.[95,97] Koebnerisation (also known as the Koebner phenomenon) has also been asserted as an alternative hypothesis, suggesting that skin trauma and localised immunosuppression caused by the tattooing process creates an area that is more susceptible to wart growth in individuals who are already infected, or have previously been infected, with HPV.[76] The high latency between receiving the tattoo and the appearance of warts may also be influenced by environmental stressors and other external factors modulating skin integrity and immunocompetency, such as excessive ultraviolet exposure and sunburn.[98]

Molluscum contagiosum and pox-related viral infections: Several pox-related viral infections have also been reported, primarily following tattooing procedures. These include both rubella and *vaccinia*, the virus that causes smallpox; however, both instances of disease are exceedingly rare and either limited to singular case reports or specific circumstances.[99] For example, tattoo-associated smallpox infections have only been reported in patients who received tattoos immediately prior to, or following, smallpox inoculation in the same area.[100] The subsequent smallpox autoinoculation leads to a considerably greater presentation of disease over the tattooed area, longer recovery and larger areas of scarring post-recovery.

Molluscum contagiosum virus (MCV) is a double-stranded DNA virus that also belongs in the Poxviridae family, and is the most commonly reported pox-related infection following tattooing procedures.[29,101-103] The virus causes *Molluscum contagiosum* (MC), which is a self-limited cutaneous viral infection that affects the epidermis and replicates in the cytoplasm of cells but which does not exceed the basement membrane. It is characterised by firm, pearly white or pink, dome-shaped, centrally umbilicated papules that range in size from 1–5 mm in diameter.[74] Similar to HPV, case reports of MC infection observe lesions which are localised to areas of tattooed skin and most frequently occurred in black ink. Additionally, there is also a latency between patients receiving the tattoo and the onset of visible lesions, though the period is considerably shorter, ranging from between 2 weeks to 5 months.

Other viral infections: The frequent use of skin penetration procedures will also increase the risk of viral infections such as those caused by herpes simplex virus (HSV) and human immunodeficiency virus (HIV).[104] Despite being commonly cited as cause for concern, the actual case incidence HSV and HIV infection occurring following personal appearance procedures is exceedingly rare. Moreover, most reported cases involve the use of unregulated, non-professional avenues. For example, to date there have been three patients with tattoo-associated HIV infection, two of which received these tattoos in prison using unsterilised needles.[91,92] Similarly, HSV infection is possible but also rarely reported. Furthermore, cases of HSV have predominantly implicated superinfection of tattoo-associated wounds that occurs post-procedure, or in one case the reactivation of HSV, as opposed to transmission of the viral infection during the procedure itself.[84-86]

45.3 IPC in cosmetic, tattooing, piercing and personal service settings

Standard and transmission-based precautions apply to cosmetic, tattooing, piercing and personal service settings in the same way they do in any other health or health-related settings. Similar to the healthcare industry, standard precautions remain an integral foundation of IPC practices across all cosmetic and personal appearance services. These include practices of good personal hygiene, particularly handwashing before and after contact with clients, appropriate reprocessing of reusable equipment and instruments, management of contaminated linen and waste, and the use of personal protective equipment (Chapter 13). There are nonetheless some contextual considerations that are important in these settings. A range of jurisdictional IPC guidelines for services outside of hospital settings are available and can be broadly applied to most personal appearance services.[105-111] The following sections will provide an overview of key infection control precautions with context-specific examples.

45.3.1 Skin preparation

Many infections following the use of personal appearance services and skin penetration procedures are caused by bacteria that are commonly found on the surface of skin, including *S. aureus* and *S. pyogenes*. Aseptic non-touch technique remains an important standard precaution to be practised throughout this process. Prior to performing any skin penetration procedures, it is integral to ensure that the skin of both clients and service providers are appropriately cleaned and disinfected. Service providers must ensure appropriate hand hygiene both prior to and immediately after the procedure, the removal of hand and wrist jewellery, intact and non-damaged skin, and the use of gloves and personal protective equipment where appropriate. For clients, this includes removing any

visible signs of dirt with water and liquid soap, and ensuring the site is free of any existing wounds, sores or infection. In some instances, hair will need to be removed from the area prior to the procedure. This should be achieved using a single use, disposable safety razor that is disposed of immediately after use. Washed skin should be dried before an alcohol, chlorhexidine or iodine-based antiseptic solution is applied with a clean, single use swab. The type of antiseptic used will vary depending on the service to be performed, the location of the body it is applied and the allergies of the client. For example, iodine solutions are ill-suited to procedures like tattooing, as the solution may alter and obstruct the colour of the skin and the ink of the applied tattoo.

Single use swab packets or sachets of skin antiseptic products are recommended over large containers of solution designed for multiple uses. If containers are used, then a portion of the solution should be dispensed into a smaller, clean, dry container for use on an individual client. After use, any leftover antiseptic must be discarded and the container cleaned before being used again (or simply disposed of if it is a single use container). Both single use antiseptic packets and multi-use containers must be discarded if they have passed the manufacturer's use-by date. The antiseptic must also be dry prior to beginning the procedure and the swabbed area must not be touched with the hand after swabbing.

45.3.2 Cleaning and reprocessing of reusable instruments

Reprocessing involves the cleaning, disinfecting or sterilising of instruments and equipment for reuse on another client (Chapter 16). While single use items are recommended, many personal appearance services use specialised equipment that must be appropriately cleaned and reprocessed prior to use across different clients. Equipment that penetrates the skin is intrinsic to tattooing and piercing instruments, which generally do not have single use alternatives but will come with specific manufacturer instructions for reprocessing. Services may also involve the use of shared equipment that does not necessarily penetrate the skin, such as scissors, razors, heating appliances and small utensils used in hair and nail salons. Nevertheless, all equipment shared across multiple people presents a non-zero risk for the spread of infection, or similar issues like head lice. The minimum reprocessing requirement for shared equipment is dependent on the level of risk of infection transmission. As examined in detail in Chapter 16, reprocessing of reusable instruments and equipment can include:

- *cleaning:* removal of general contamination and foreign material from equipment, typically using warm water and detergent
- *disinfection:* a process that involves the inactivation of microorganisms on equipment, typically involving the application of a disinfectant solution; and
- *sterilisation:* a process that removes any viable microorganisms, including bacterial spores, using either heat (e.g. autoclave), chemical or radiation treatment.

The Spaulding Classification distinguishes items based on the degree of risk of infection from how the equipment is used. Table 45.4 provides a general overview of the Spaulding Classification of items that are commonly used in personal appearance service settings.

The reprocessing of instruments and equipment must be completed in an area dedicated to this task. As a result, services that utilise reusable equipment must design their facilities to include a separate, dedicated room or a section within the larger treatment area for the purpose of reprocessing. The placement of these areas is also important and should facilitate a one-way movement of dirtied items from cleaning, disinfection and/or sterilisation, storage and then return to use. This aims to prevent the cross-contamination of clean and dirty equipment (Fig 45.1).

Cleaning is a fundamental tenet of standard precautions. Reusable equipment may undergo manual or automated cleaning depending on suitability. Manual cleaning is typically utilised when the equipment requires careful handling and is not suited to automated cleaning methods. In most cases, these items can and should be disassembled and immersed in warm water following use, thoroughly cleansed using a low-foaming, non-abrasive and non-corrosive detergent, scrubbed using a nylon brush and then rinsed with clean water from a second sink. This should be done as soon as practically possible for items that come into contact with blood or body fluids. Depending on the instrument, it may also be appropriate to don PPE prior to cleaning (see Chapters 13 and 14). This may include the use of heavy utility gloves when handling needles and sharps, or an apron and face protection to prevent splashes. Items that cannot be immersed in water (e.g. electric powered tools) should be carefully cleaned with a moistened disposable paper towel and detergent and then disinfected immediately after use. After cleaning, all items should be dried within a drying cabinet or with a clean lint-free cloth. It is important that all items are dry prior to storage and that no items are left on the counter to air dry as this may lead to airborne contamination.

Thermal or chemical disinfection offers an additional layer of protection and may be utilised for reusable equipment after they have already been cleaned. For items that can be fully immersed in water, thermal disinfection in boiling water offers an effective and efficient means of destroying microorganisms. Chemical disinfection with alcohol solutions should only be used when the equipment cannot be fully immersed. The disinfectant should be wiped onto the dry surface of the item and left to dry again prior to storage. For all equipment classified as 'critical', sterilisation is the only recommended method to ensure adequate and safe reprocessing. Sterilisation destroys all microorganisms on the item and is most commonly achieved using heat and pressure. The use of autoclaves and steam

TABLE 45.4 Spaulding Classification of examples encountered in cosmetic, tattooing and piercing services

Spaulding Classification	Level of risk	Application	Examples	Level of reprocessing required
Non-critical	Low	Contact with intact skin only	Hairbrush, scissors, makeup brushes	Cleaning, and low-level disinfection
Semi-critical	Medium	Contact with mucous membranes or non-intact skin	Eyelash extension tweezers, lip brush, eyeliner brushes	Sterilisation where possible, otherwise high-level disinfection
Critical	High	Penetration into sterile tissue, cavity or bloodstream	Tattoo needles, piercing needles, surgical equipment	Sterilisation

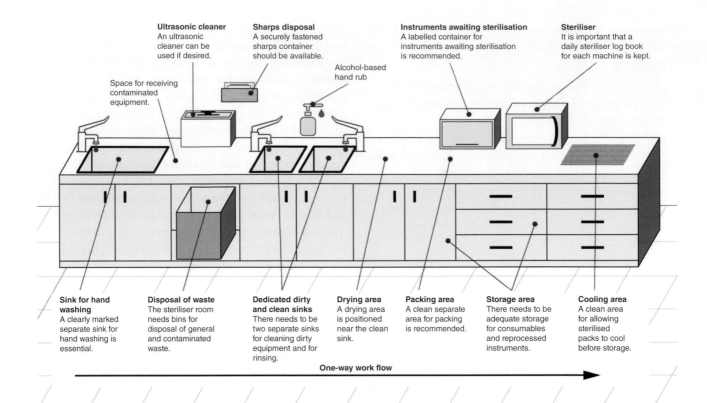

Ultrasonic cleaner
An ultrasonic cleaner can be used if desired.

Sharps disposal
A securely fastened sharps container should be available.

Alcohol-based hand rub

Instruments awaiting sterilisation
A labelled container for instruments awaiting sterilisation is recommended.

Steriliser
It is important that a daily steriliser log book for each machine is kept.

Space for receiving contaminated equipment.

Sink for hand washing
A clearly marked separate sink for hand washing is essential.

Disposal of waste
The steriliser room needs bins for disposal of general and contaminated waste.

Dedicated dirty and clean sinks
There needs to be two separate sinks for cleaning dirty equipment and for rinsing.

Drying area
A drying area is positioned near the clean sink.

Packing area
A clean separate area for packing is recommended.

Storage area
There needs to be adequate storage for consumables and reprocessed instruments.

Cooling area
A clean area for allowing sterilised packs to cool before storage.

One-way work flow →

FIGURE 45.1 Suggested layout for reprocessing area

Source: Adapted from Royal Australian College of General Practitioners (RACGP) 2014, Infection prevention and control standards for general practices and other office-based and community-based practices, 5th edn, and from the College of Physicians and Surgeons of Alberta IPAC Physician Toolkit, Suggested reprocessing area design and layout, p. 27. http://cpsa.ca/wpcontent/uploads/2015/04/IPAC_Reprocessing__A_Physician_Toolkit.pdf?pdf=Reprocessing-Toolkit

sterilisation under pressure is the most reliable means of sterilising reusable items within the personal appearance service industry.

Once reprocessed, all items must be stored in a way that prevents further contamination. This may be achieved using closed cupboards or in washable plastic containers with sealable lids. These storage devices should be maintained in a clean, dry condition to ensure that sterile items are not contaminated. Many manufacturer-sterilised items, like jewellery and other implants/inserts, are pre-packaged. However, if the packaging of these items is torn, broken or affected by moisture, the items within will no longer be sterile. Furthermore, common sources of infection reported in the literature include tattoo inks and refillable bottles of disinfectant solutions that become contaminated from environmental sources over time. It is important that procedures are in place to ensure that the stock of sterile items is regularly rotated based either on the date of sterilisation or the steriliser load number.

45.3.3 Environmental cleaning and waste disposal

The physical environment in which personal appearance services are provided also presents many opportunities for contamination and infection spread. This may occur when clients have direct contact with contaminated surfaces or when the service provider transfers the contamination indirectly to the client. Many personal appearance services are provided within an open and relatively communal area, where individual benches, beds and surfaces may be shared across multiple clients in a single day. Specific cleaning requirements will vary from service to service. As such, all facilities should develop and enforce a written cleaning policy that includes specific protocols for the routine and scheduled cleaning of different surfaces within the environment, as well as the unscheduled cleaning procedure for blood, body fluids and other spills. These protocols should be informed by a thorough risk assessment to determine what needs to be cleaned, how frequently, the types of cleaning materials and tools to be used, and how the effectiveness of the cleaning should be monitored. For example, surfaces like client beds, which encounter heavy traffic and that may become exposed to infectious agents or body fluids during use, will need to be cleaned after each client. More general environmental surfaces like floors, washbasins and desks should be cleaned at least once daily. Service providers must also carefully consider the types of equipment, furnishings, flooring and interior decor in their facility. These objects should be durable, have surfaces that prioritise easy cleaning and which prevent the accumulation of grime and bacterial growth.

Furthermore, most personal appearance services result in the generation of clinical waste, including human blood, body fluids and tissue, sharps and disposable equipment that are contaminated with blood or body fluids. The definition of what constitutes clinical waste varies between jurisdictions. Nevertheless, safe waste handling and management at the point of generation is essential to protect clients, workers and the wider community from infection and blood-borne viruses. Separate bins, identified using a label or by colour, should be used to distinguish clinical and general waste and staff must be trained in correct procedures for handling waste. Similar to the reprocessing of dirtied equipment, waste should follow a one-way flow within the facility. All waste should eventually collect within a designated storage area that is inaccessible to the public and be held securely until disposal. Bins for both clinical and general waste should be cleaned regularly and be lined appropriately with a plastic bag to facilitate handling, sealing and disposal.

45.3.4 Occupational safety and record keeping

Services involving the use of sharps and skin penetration procedures present significant risks of needlestick injuries and infection with blood-borne viruses, like hepatitis B. In addition to the practice of standard precautions, vaccination against hepatitis B and other vaccine-preventable diseases, such as influenza and varicella, provides the most efficient means of prophylaxis. Furthermore, service providers must ensure that staff are trained in the event of needlestick injury and exposure to blood or other body fluids. Additionally, while not strictly required across all jurisdictions, all services that involve skin penetrating procedures should maintain a

comprehensive record of both staff and clients. For staff, this includes records of immunisation, training compliance and qualifications. For clients, this may include the name and address of the client, the date the personal appearance service procedure was performed, the site and type of high-risk personal appearance service procedure, the staff member who provided the service/administered the procedure, and the instruments used (including sterilising batch number).

Conclusion

Most cosmetic and personal appearance services are not performed within healthcare settings, and yet many will involve the frequent, and usually inherent, administration of high-risk and skin penetrating procedures. This chapter provided an overview of the most common types of infections reported following the use of personal appearance services, including cosmetic surgery, tattooing and body piercing. Bacterial infections remain the greatest risk and are most commonly caused by contact with contaminated equipment and surfaces in the environment. Blood-borne viral infections, such as HBV and HCV, as well as viral skin infections, such as HPV and MCV, have also been reported following the sharing of equipment, such as tattoo needles.

In Australia, licensing requirements and the regulation of personal appearance services are enforced differently across different services and also vary between jurisdictions. Most notably, 'cosmetic surgery' is currently not recognised as a medical specialty and there exists no restrictions on use of the title 'cosmetic surgeon'. Any registered medical practitioner, regardless of their qualifications or designated specialty, may use the title of 'cosmetic surgeon' and perform cosmetic procedures. However, in many states, high-risk cosmetic procedures that involve the use of anaesthesia must be performed within a hospital setting and therefore meet the national standards for IPC. On the other hand, infection control standards and qualifications for non-hospital-based services and service providers remain highly heterogenous. Some jurisdictions have formal licensing obligations, which require the completion of infection control training prior to practice, while others require no licence to practice at all. As cosmetic, tattooing and piercing services become increasingly accessible and used by the broader Australian community, the need to ensure that adequate levels of IPC are met grows ever more critical.

Useful websites/resources

- Hair, beauty, tattooing and skin penetration industries, Department of Health, Victorian Government. https://www.health.vic.gov.au/infectious-diseases/hair-beauty-tattooing-and-skin-penetration-industries
- Body art and tattoo businesses—infection prevention and control. Department of Health, Victorian Government. https://www.health.vic.gov.au/infectious-diseases/body-art-and-tattoo-businesses-infection-prevention-and-control
- Skin penetration procedures and the law. Department of Health, Western Australian Government. https://ww2.health.wa.gov.au/Articles/S_T/Skin-penetration-procedures-and-the-law
- Guidelines for registered medical practitioners who perform cosmetic medical and surgical procedures. Medical Board of Australia. https://www.medicalboard.gov.au/Codes-Guidelines-Policies/Cosmetic-medical-and-surgical-procedures-guidelines.aspx

References

1. Medical Board of Australia. Guidelines for registered medical practitioners who perform cosmetic medical and surgical procedures. Medical Board of Australia, 2016.
2. Australian Health Practitioner Regulation Agency and Medical Board of Australia. Independent review of the regulation of health practitioners in cosmetic surgery. Melbourne: APHRA, 2022.
3. International Society of Aesthetic Plastic Surgery. ISAPS International Survey on Aesthetic/Cosmetic Procedures performed in 2020. ISAPS, 2020. Available from: https://www.isaps.org/media/hprkl132/isaps-global-survey_2020.pdf.
4. NSW Department of Health. Cosmetic surgical procedures by registered medical practitioners. [cited 11 July 2022] Sydney: State Government of New South Wales, 2018.
5. Jobson D, Freckelton I. The changing face of cosmetic surgery regulation: a review of controversies and potential reforms. ANZ J Surg. 2022;92(5):964-969.
6. Health Practitioner Regulation National Law Act 2009 (Qld).
7. Australian Government Department of Health. Plastic surgery. Canberra: Australian Government, 2016.
8. Pesapane F, Nazzaro G, Gianotti R, Coggi A. A short history of tattoo. JAMA Dermatol. 2014;150(2):145.
9. Braverman PK. Body art: piercing, tattooing, and scarification. Adolescent Medicine Clinics. 2006;17(3):505-19; abstract ix.
10. Heywood W, Patrick K, Smith AM, Simpson JM, Pitts MK, Richters J, et al. Who gets tattoos? Demographic and behavioral correlates of ever being tattooed in a representative sample of men and women. Ann Epidemiol. 2012;22(1):51-56.
11. Fell A. Tattoos in Australia; perceptions, trends and regrets. Norwest: McCrindle Research, 2019.
12. Broussard KA, Harton HC. Tattoo or taboo? Tattoo stigma and negative attitudes toward tattooed individuals. J Social Psychol. 2018;158(5):521-540.
13. Breuner CC, Levine DA, Alderman EM, Garofalo R, Grubb LK, Powers ME, et al. Adolescent and young adult tattooing, piercing, and scarification. Pediatrics. 2017;140(4).
14. Makkai T, McAllister I. Prevalence of tattooing and body piercing in the Australian community. Commun Dis Intell Q R. 2001;25(2):67-72.
15. Gold MA, Schorzman CM, Murray PJ, Downs J, Tolentino G. Body piercing practices and attitudes among urban adolescents. J Adolesc Health. 2005;36(4):352.e15-.e21.
16. Høgsberg T, Saunte D, Frimodt-Møller N, Serup J. Microbial status and product labelling of 58 original tattoo inks. J Eur Acad Dermatol Venereol. 2013;27(1):73-80.
17. Dieckmann R, Boone I, Brockmann SO, Hammerl JA, Kolb-Mäurer A, Goebeler M, et al. The risk of bacterial infection after tattooing: a systematic review of the literature. Deutsches Ärzteblatt International. 2016;113(40):665.
18. Fisher CG, Kacica MA, Bennett NM. Risk factors for cartilage infections of the ear. Am J Prev Med. 2005; 29(3):204-209.
19. Keene WE, Markum AC, Samadpour M. Outbreak of Pseudomonas aeruginosa infections caused by commercial piercing of upper ear cartilage. Jama. 2004;291(8):981-985.
20. Mudedla S, Avendano EE, Raman G. Non-tuberculous mycobacterium skin infections after tattooing in healthy individuals: a systematic review of case reports. Dermatol Online J. 2015;21(6):13030/qt8mr3r4f0.
21. Patel T, Scroggins-Markle L, Kelly B. A dermal piercing complicated by Mycobacterium fortuitum. Case Rep Dermatol Med. 2013;2013:149829.
22. Green DA, Whittier S, Greendyke W, Win C, Chen X, Hamele-Bena D. Outbreak of rapidly growing nontuberculous mycobacteria among patients undergoing cosmetic surgery in the Dominican Republic. Ann Plast Surg. 2017;78(1):17-21.
23. Winthrop KL, Albridge K, South D, Albrecht P, Abrams M, Samuel MC, et al. The clinical management and outcome of nail salon—acquired Mycobacterium fortuitum skin infection. Clin Infect Dis. 2004;38(1):38-44.
24. Cooksey RC, de Waard JH, Yakrus MA, Rivera I, Chopite M, Toney SR, et al. Mycobacterium cosmeticum sp. nov., a novel rapidly growing species isolated from a cosmetic infection and from a nail salon. Int J Systematic Evolutionary Microbiol. 2004;54(6):2385-2391.
25. Vugia DJ, Jang Y, Zizek C, Ely J, Winthrop KL, Desmond E. Mycobacteria in nail salon whirlpool footbaths, California. Emerg Infect Dis. 2005;11(4):616.
26. Stout JE, Gadkowski LB, Rath S, Alspaugh JA, Miller MB, Cox GM. Pedicure-associated rapidly growing mycobacterial infection: an endemic disease. Clin Infect Dis. 2011;53(8): 787-792.
27. Schmidt AN, Zic JA, Boyd AS. Pedicure-associated Mycobacterium chelonae infection in a hospitalized patient. J Am Acad Dermatol. 2014;71(6):e248-e250.
28. Control CfD, Prevention. Methicillin-resistant Staphylococcus aureus skin infections among tattoo recipients—Ohio, Kentucky, and Vermont, 2004-2005. MMWR. 2006;55(24): 677-679.

29. Blasco-Morente G, Naranjo-Díaz MJ, Pérez-López I, Martínez-López A, Garrido-Colmenero C. Molluscum contagiosum over tattooed skin. Sultan Qaboos Univ Med J [SQUMJ]. 2016;16(2):257-258.

30. Stemper ME, Brady JM, Qutaishat SS, Borlaug G, Reed J, Reed KD, et al. Shift in Staphylococcus aureus clone linked to an infected tattoo. Emerging Infect Dis. 2006;12(9):1444.

31. Bader MS, Hamodat M, Hutchinson J. A fatal case of Staphylococcus aureus: associated toxic shock syndrome following nipple piercing. Scand J Infect Dis. 2007;39(8): 741-743.

32. Holbrook J, Minocha J, Laumann A. Body piercing. Am J Clin Dermatol. 2012;13(1):1-17.

33. Dähnert I, Schneider P, Handrick W. Piercing and tattoos in patients with congenital heart disease–is it a problem? Zeitschrift für Kardiologie. 2004;93(8):618-623.

34. Beaudoin AL, Torso L, Richards K, Said M, Van Beneden C, Longenberger A, et al. Invasive group A Streptococcus infections associated with liposuction surgery at outpatient facilities not subject to state or federal regulation. JAMA Int Med. 2014;174(7):1136-1142.

35. Garcia-Pola MJ, Garcia-Martin JM, Varela-Centelles P, Bilbao-Alonso A, Cerero-Lapiedra R, Seoane J. Oral and facial piercing: associated complications and clinical repercussion. Quintessence Int. 2008;39(1):51-59.

36. McLean M, D'Souza A. Life-threatening cellulitis after traditional Samoan tattooing. Aust N Z J Public Health. 2011;35(1):27-29.

37. Mathur D, Sahoo A. Pseudomonas septicaemia following tribal tatoo marks. Trop Geogr Med. 1984;36(3):301-302.

38. Korman T, Grayson M, Turnidge J. Polymicrobial septicaemia with Pseudomonas aeruginosa and Streptococcus pyogenes following traditional tattooing [4]. J Infection. 1997;35(2):203.

39. Porter CJ, Simcock JW, MacKinnon CA. Necrotising fasciitis and cellulitis after traditional Samoan tattooing. J Infection. 2005;50(2):149-152.

40. Sosin M, Weissler JM, Pulcrano M, Rodriguez ED. Transcartilaginous ear piercing and infectious complications: a systematic review and critical analysis of outcomes. Laryngoscope. 2015;125(8):1827-1834.

41. Cicchetti S, Skillman J, Gault DT. Piercing the upper ear: a simple infection, a difficult reconstruction. Br J Plast Surg. 2002;55(3):194-197.

42. Lee TC, Gold WL. Necrotizing Pseudomonas chondritis after piercing of the upper ear. CMAJ. 2011;183(7):819-821.

43. Rowshan HH, Keith K, Baur D, Skidmore P. Pseudomonas aeruginosa infection of the auricular cartilage caused by "high ear piercing": a case report and review of the literature. J Oral Maxillofac Surg. 2008;66(3):543-546.

44. Patel M, Cobbs CG. Infections from body piercing and tattoos. Infections of Leisure. 2016;307-323.

45. Acuña-Chávez LM, Alva-Alayo CA, Aguilar-Villanueva GA, Zavala-Alvarado KA, Alverca-Meza CA, Aguirre-Sánchez MM, et al. Bacterial infections in patients with nipple piercings: a qualitative systematic review of case reports and case series. GMS Infect Dis. 2022;10.

46. Abbass K, Adnan MK, Markert RJ, Emig M, Khan NA. Mycobacterium fortuitum breast abscess after nipple piercing. Can Fam Physician. 2014;60(1):51-52.

47. Bengualid V, Singh V, Singh H, Berger J. Mycobacterium fortuitum and anaerobic breast abscess following nipple piercing: case presentation and review of the literature. J Adolesc Health. 2008;42(5):530-532.

48. Ferringer T, Pride H, Tyler W. Body piercing complicated by atypical mycobacterial infections. Pediatric Dermatol. 2008; 25(2):219-222.

49. Lewis CG, Wells MK, Jennings WC. Mycobacterium fortuitum breast infection following nipple-piercing, mimicking carcinoma. Breast J. 2004;10(4):363-365.

50. Cusumano LR, Tran V, Tlamsa A, Chung P, Grossberg R, Weston G, et al. Rapidly growing Mycobacterium infections after cosmetic surgery in medical tourists: the Bronx experience and a review of the literature. Int J Infect Dis. 2017;63:1-6.

51. Control CfD, Prevention. Nontuberculous mycobacterial infections after cosmetic surgery—Santo Domingo, Dominican Republic, 2003-2004. MMWR. 2004;53(23):509.

52. Lee M-R, Sheng W-H, Hung C-C, Yu C-J, Lee L-N, Hsueh P-R. Mycobacterium abscessus complex infections in humans. Emerg Infect Dis. 2015;21(9):1638-1646.

53. Akram SM, Rathish B, Saleh D. Mycobacterium chelonae. StatPearls [Internet] 2017.

54. Tweeten SSM, Rickman LS. Infectious complications of body piercing. Clin Infect Dis. 1998;26(3):735-740.

55. Iyer S, Jones DH. Community-acquired methicillin-resistant Staphylococcus aureus skin infection: a retrospective analysis of clinical presentation and treatment of a local outbreak. J Am Acad Dermatol. 2004;50(6):854-858.

56. Cohen PR. Community-acquired methicillin-resistant Staphylococcus aureus skin infections. Am J Clin Dermatol. 2007;8(5):259-270.

57. Bourigault C, Corvec S, Brulet V, Robert P-Y, Mounoury O, Goubin C, et al. Outbreak of skin infections due to Panton-valentine Leukocidin-positive methicillin-susceptible Staphylococcus aureus in a French prison in 2010-2011. PLoS Curr. 2014;6.

58. Weinberg JB, Blackwood RA. Case report of Staphylococcus aureus endocarditis after navel piercing. Pediatr Infect Dis J. 2003;22(1):94-96.

59. Battin M, Fong L, Monro J. Gerbode ventricular septal defect following endocarditis. Eur J Cardiothorac Surg. 1991;5(11): 613-614.

60. Lee S-H, Chung M-H, Lee J-S, Sil Kim E, Suh J-G. A case of Staphylococcus aureus endocarditis after ear piercing in a patient with normal cardiac valve and a questionnaire survey on adverse events of body piercing in college students of Korea. Scand J Infect Dis. 2006;38(2):130-132.

61. McCarthy VP, Peoples WM. Toxic shock syndrome after ear piercing. Pediatr Infect Dis J. 1988;7(10):741-742.

62. Kloppenburg G, Maessen JG. Streptococcus endocarditis after tongue piercing. J Heart Valve Dis. 2007;16(3):328-230.

63. Marchesi A, Marcelli S, Parodi PC, Perrotta RE, Riccio M, Vaienti L. Necrotizing fasciitis in aesthetic surgery: a review of the literature. Aesthetic Plast Surg. 2017;41(2):352-358.

64. Klapper SR, Patrinely JR, editors. Management of cosmetic eyelid surgery complications. Seminars in plastic surgery. New York: Thieme Medical Publishers, Inc, 2007.

65. Jafari S, Buxton JA, Afshar K, Copes R, Baharlou S. Tattooing and risk of hepatitis B: a systematic review and meta-analysis. Can J Public Health. 2012;103(3):207-212.

66. Limentani A, Elliott L, Noah N, Lamborn J. An outbreak of hepatitis B from tattooing. Lancet. 1979;314(8133):86-88.

67. Sebastian V, Ray S, Bhattacharya S, Maung OT, Saini HM, Jalani HD. Tattooing and hepatitis B infection. J Gastroenterol Hepatol. 1992;7(4):385-387.

68. Yang S, Wang D, Zhang Y, Yu C, Ren J, Xu K, et al. Transmission of hepatitis B and C virus infection through body piercing: a systematic review and meta-analysis. Medicine. 2015;94(47).

69. Jafari S, Copes R, Baharlou S, Etminan M, Buxton J. Tattooing and the risk of transmission of hepatitis C: a systematic review and meta-analysis. Int J Infect Dis. 2010;14(11):e928-e40.

70. Khodadost M, Maajani K, Arabsalmani M, Mahdavi N, Tabrizi R, Alavian SM. Is tattooing a risk factor for hepatitis c transmission?: an updated systematic review and meta-analysis. Hepatitis Monthly. 2017;17(9).

71. Haley RW, Fischer RP. Commercial tattooing as a potentially important source of hepatitis C infection: clinical epidemiology of 626 consecutive patients unaware of their hepatitis C serologic status. Medicine. 2001;80(2):134-151.

72. Carney K, Dhalla S, Aytaman A, Tenner CT, Francois F. Association of tattooing and hepatitis C virus infection: a multicenter case-control study. Hepatology. 2013;57(6): 2117-2123.

73. Ko YC, Ho MS, Chiang TA, Chang SJ, Chang PY. Tattooing as a risk of hepatitis C virus infection. J Med Virol. 1992; 38(4):288-291.

74. Tampa M, Mitran MI, Mitran CI, Matei C, Amuzescu A, Buzatu AA, et al. Viral infections confined to tattoos—a narrative review. Medicina. 2022;58(3):342.

75. Cohen PR. Verruca vulgaris occurring on a tattoo: case report and review of tattoo-associated human papillomavirus infections. Cureus. 2021;13(8).

76. Huynh TN, Jackson JD, Brodell RT. Tattoo and vaccination sites: possible nest for opportunistic infections, tumors, and dysimmune reactions. Clin Dermatol. 2014;32(5):678-684.

77. Litak J, Krunic AL, Antonijevic S, Pouryazdanparast P, Gerami P. Eyebrow epilation by threading: an increasingly popular procedure with some less-popular outcomes—a comprehensive review. Dermatol Surg. 2011;37(7):1051-1054.

78. Kumar R, Zawar V. Threading warts: a beauty parlor dermatosis. J Cosmet Dermatol. 2007;6(4):279-282.

79. Sidharth S, Rahul A, Rashmi S. Cosmetic warts: pseudo-koebnerization of warts after cosmetic procedures for hair removal. J Clin Aesthet Dermatol. 2015;8(7):52-56.

80. Kirchhof MG, Au S. Brazilian waxing and human papillomavirus: a case of acquired epidermodysplasia verruciformis. CMAJ. 2015;187(2):126-128.

81. Schmidtberger L, Ladizinski B, Ramirez-Fort MK. Wax on, wax off: pubic hair grooming and potential complications. JAMA Dermatol. 2014;150(2):122.

82. Desruelles F, Cunningham SA, Dubois D. Pubic hair removal: a risk factor for 'minor' STI such as molluscum contagiosum? Sexually Transmitted Infections. 2013;89(3):216.

83. Veraldi S, Nazzaro G, Ramoni S. Pubic hair removal and molluscum contagiosum. London: Sage Publications UK, 2016.

84. Kluger N, Armingaud P. Herpes simplex infection on a recent tattoo. A new case of "herpes compuctorum". Int J Dermatol. 2016;56(1):e9-e10.

85. Marshall CS, Murphy F, McCarthy SE, Cheng AC. Herpes compunctorum: cutaneous herpes simplex virus infection complicating tattooing. MJA. 2007;187(10):598.

86. Begolli Gerqari A, Ferizi M, Kotori M, Halimi S, Daka A, Hapciu S, et al. Activation of herpes simplex infection after tattoo. Acta Dermatovenerol Croat. 2018;26(1):75-76.

87. Dendle C, Mulvey S, Pyrlis F, Grayson ML, Johnson PD. Severe complications of a "Brazilian" bikini wax. Clin Infect Dis. 2007;45(3):e29-e31.

88. Reis J, Santos FV. Perianal reactivation of herpes simplex virus type 2 after laser-assisted hair removal. Sex Transm Dis. 2021;48(2):e30-e31.

89. Rasheed AI. Uncommonly reported side effects of hair removal by long pulsed-alexandrite laser. J Cosmet Dermatol. 2009;8(4):267-274.

90. Dierickx CC. Hair removal by lasers and intense pulsed light sources. Dermatologic Clin. 2002;20(1):135-146.

91. Doll D. Tattooing in prison and HIV infection. Lancet. 1988;331(8575):66-67.

92. Garland SM, Ung L, Vujovic OV, Said JM. Cosmetic tattooing: a potential transmission route for HIV? Aust N Z J Obstet Gynaecol. 2006;46(5):458-459.

93. Tohme RA, Holmberg SD. Transmission of hepatitis C virus infection through tattooing and piercing: a critical review. Clin Infect Dis. 2012;54(8):1167-1178.

94. Kirchhof MG, Wong SM. Tattoos and human papilloma virus: a case report of tattoo-associated flat warts (verrucae planae). SAGE Open Med Case Rep. 2019; 7:2050313X19857416.

95. Wanat KA, Tyring S, Rady P, Kovarik CL. Human papillomavirus type 27 associated with multiple verruca within a tattoo: report of a case and review of the literature. Int J Dermatol. 2014;53(7):882-884.

96. Miller DM, Brodell RT. Verruca restricted to the areas of black dye within a tattoo. Arch Dermatol. 1994;130(11): 1453-1454.

97. Nemer KM, Hurst EA. Confluent verruca vulgaris arising within bilateral eyebrow tattoos: successful treatment with ablative laser and topical 5% imiquimod cream. Dermatol Surg. 2019;45(3):473-475.

98. Brajac I, LonČarek K, Stojnić-Soša L, Gruber F. Delayed onset of warts over tattoo mark provoked by sunburn. J Eur Acad Dermatol Venereol. 2005;19(2):247-248.

99. Goldstein N IV. Complications from tattoos. J Dermatol Surg Oncol. 1979;5(11):869-878.

100. Carius BM, Dodge PM, Randles JD. Smallpox autoinoculation via tattoo in a soldier. Mil Med. 2019;184(1-2):e275-e279.

101. Foulds I. Molluscum contagiosum: an unusual complication of tattooing. BMJ (Clinical research ed). 1982;285(6342):607.

102. De Giorgi V, Grazzini M, Lotti T. A three-dimensional tattoo: Molluscum contagiosum. CMAJ. 2010;182(9):E382.

103. Molina L, Romiti R. Molluscum contagiosum on tattoo. Anais Brasileiros de Dermatologia. 2011;86:352-354.

104. Cohen PR. Tattoo-associated viral infections: a review. Clin Cosmet Investig Dermatol. 2021;14:1529-1540.

105. ACT Government. Infection control guidelines for office pratices and other community based services. Canberra: ACT Government, 2006.

106. State Government of Tasmania Department of Health and Community Services. Guidelines for ear and body piercing. Hobart: State Government of Tasmania, 1998.

107. State Government of Victoria Department of Human Services. Health guidelines for personal care and body art industries. Melbourne: State Government of Victoria, 2004.

108. Government of Western. Australia Department of Health. Code of practice for skin penetration procedures. Perth: Government of Western Australia, 1998.

109. Northern Territory Government. Public and environment health guidelines for hairdressing, beauty therapy and body art. Darwin: Northern Territory Government of Health Environmental Health Branch, 2014.

110. Queensland Government. Infection control guidelines for personal appearance services. Brisbane: Queensland Government, 2012.

111. South Australian Department of Health. Guideline on the safe and hygienic practice of skin penetration. Adelaide: South Australian Government, 1995.

Index